REPORTING CHANGES IN ASSESSMENT — cont'd

Fluid/renal (compare to past status)
Urine Output_____ ml/hr ☐ Edema _____ (location/amount) ☐ Increased ☐ Decreased
Fluid Balance _____ ml ☐ Weight Gained _____ lbs ☐ CAPD (Status) _____
Last Hemodialysis (date/time)_____ Tolerated? _____ UF (last hemodialysis) _____ liters

Medications (that may have contributed to the change)
Medications given during the past 12 hours: _____
Medications held during the past 12 hours: _____

Most recent lab values (compare to past values)
WBC _____ Hgb _____ Hct _____ Platelets _____
Any blood products given during the past 12 hrs?
☐ Packed RBC ☐ Platelets ☐ FFP ☐ Cryo ☐ Other _____
PT _____ INR _____ PTT _____ ☐ On Heparin ☐ On Coumadin ☐ On Plavix ☐ On Aspirin
Glucose _____ Na _____ K+ _____ Cl− _____ CO_2 _____ BUN _____ Creatinine _____
Magnesium _____ Calcium _____ CPK _____ CKMB _____ Troponins _____ BNP _____

Today's activity:
Did the patient have a procedure today? Surgery/Radiology/GIDU _____ Cardiac Intervention _____
Rehab/HBO _____
Explain _____
Diagnostic testing _____ Falls _____ Other_____

RN signature _____   **RN signature** _____
RRT signature _____

D1025944

Manual of CRITICAL CARE NURSING

NURSING INTERVENTIONS AND COLLABORATIVE MANAGEMENT

Manual of CRITICAL CARE NURSING

NURSING INTERVENTIONS AND COLLABORATIVE MANAGEMENT

SIXTH EDITION

MARIANNE SAUNORUS BAIRD, MN, RN
Clinical Nurse Specialist
Acute Care
Magnet Program Coordinator
Center for Nursing Excellence
Saint Joseph's Hospital
Atlanta, Georgia

SUSAN BETHEL, MS, RN
Director of Clinical Programs & Research
Greenville Hospital System
University Medical Center
Greenville, South Carolina

ELSEVIER
MOSBY

3251 Riverport Lane
St. Louis, Missouri 63043

MANUAL OF CRITICAL CARE NURSING: NURSING INTERVENTIONS
AND COLLABORATIVE MANAGEMENT, SIXTH EDITION ISBN 978-0-323-06376-0
Copyright © 2011, 2005, 2001, 1998, 1995, 1991 by Mosby, Inc., Elsevier Inc.

Notice

Knowledge and best practice in this field are constantly changing. As new research and experience broaden
our understanding, changes in research methods, professional practices, or medical treatment may become
necessary. Practitioners and researchers must always rely on their own experience and knowledge in evaluating and using any information, methods, compounds, or experiments described herein. In using such
information or methods they should be mindful of their own safety and the safety of others, including
parties for whom they have a professional responsibility.

With respect to any drug or pharmaceutical products identified, readers are advised to check the most
current information provided (i) on procedures featured or (ii) by the manufacturer of each product to be
administered, to verify the recommended dose or formula, the method and duration of administration,
and contraindications. It is the responsibility of practitioners, relying on their own experience and knowledge of their patients, to make diagnoses, to determine dosages and the best treatment for each individual
patient, and to take all appropriate safety precautions.

To the fullest extent of the law, neither the Publisher nor the authors, contributors, or editors, assume
any liability for any injury and/or damage to persons or property as a matter of products liability, negligence or otherwise, or from any use or operation of any methods, products, instructions, or ideas contained
in the material herein.

Library of Congress Cataloging-in-Publication Data
Baird, Marianne Saunorus.
    Manual of critical care nursing : nursing interventions and collaborative management/Marianne Saunorus
Baird, Susan Bethel.—6th ed.
        p. ; cm.
    Rev. ed. of: Manual of critical care nursing. 5th ed. c2005.
    Includes bibliographical references and index.
    ISBN 978-0-323-06376-0 (hardcover : alk. paper)
    1. Intensive care nursing. 2. Nursing diagnosis. I. Bethel, Susan. II. Manual of critical care nursing. III. Title.
    [DNLM: 1. Critical Care. 2. Nursing Assessment. 3. Nursing Care.
WY 154]
    RT120.I5M3644 2011
    616.02'8–dc22

                                                                                        2010031645

Managing Editor: Maureen Iannuzzi   *Publishing Services Manager:* Pat Joiner-Myers
Senior Developmental Editor: Robin Richman   *Senior Project Manager:* Joy Moore
Developmental Editor: Laurie Sparks   *Senior Book Designer:* Amy Buxton

Printed in The United States of America

Last digit is the print number: 9   8   7   6   5   4   3   2   1

Contributors

Jenni Jordan Abel, RN, CME
Staff Nurse
Surgical Intensive Care Unit
University of Colorado Hospital
Denver, Colorado

Patrice C. Al-Saden, RN, CCRC
Senior Clinical Research Coordinator
Comprehensive Transplant Center
Feinberg School of Medicine
Northwestern University
Northwestern Memorial Hospital
Chicago, Illinois

Marianne Saunorus Baird, MN, RN
Clinical Nurse Specialist
Acute Care
Magnet Program Coordinator
Center for Nursing Excellence
Saint Joseph's Hospital
Atlanta, Georgia

Laura Barrett, BSN, MN, RNC
Curriculum Consultant
Greenville HealthCare Simulation Center
Greenville Hospital System
University Medical Center
Greenville, South Carolina

Risa Benoit, MSN, RN, CCRN-CSC, CNS-BC
Clinical Nurse Specialist
Critical Care
Center for Nursing Excellence
Saint Joseph's Hospital
Atlanta, Georgia

Susan Bethel, MS, RN
Director of Clinical Programs & Research
Greenville Hospital System
University Medical Center
Greenville, South Carolina

Cheryl Bittel, MSN, RN, CCRN
Cardiac Transplant Coordinator
Transplant Services
Piedmont Heart Institute
Atlanta, Georgia

Carolyn Blayney, BSN, RN
Nurse Manager
Burn Intensive Care Unit
University of Washington Burn Center
Harborview Medical Center
Seattle, Washington

Mimi Callanan, MSN, RN
Clinical Nurse Specialist
Department of Neurology
Epilepsy Center
Stanford University Medical Center
Stanford, California

Gretchen J. Carrougher, MN, RN
Clinical Instructor
University of Washington School of Nursing
NIDRR Research Nurse Supervisor
Department of Surgery
University of Washington Burn Center
Harborview Medical Center
Seattle, Washington

Cynthia Rebik Christensen, MSN, FNP, ARNP-BC
Nurse Practitioner
Mobile Medical Professionals
Des Moines, Iowa

A. Suzanne Cosby, MSN, RN, CCRN
Clinical Nurse Specialist
St. Joseph's/Candler Health System
Savannah, Georgia

Alice Davis, PhD, APRN, FNP
Assistant Professor, Nursing
University of Hawaii at Hilo
Hilo, Hawaii

Joni Dirks, MSN, RN, CCRN
Critical Care Educator
Providence Sacred Heart Medical Center
   and Children's Hospital
Spokane, Washington

Carey Freeland, MSN, RN, CCRN
Clinical Manager and Clinical Nurse Specialist
Coronary Care Unit and Intensive Care Unit
St. Joseph's/Candler
Savannah, Georgia

Beverly George-Gay, MSN, RN, CCRN
Assistant Professor
Department of Nurse Anesthesia
Virginia Commonwealth University
Richmond, Virginia

Vicki Good, MSN, RN, CCRN, CENP
Director of Nursing
Cox Health System
Springfield, Missouri

Phyllis Gordon, MSN, RN, CS, APRN-BC
Clinical Assistant Professor
School of Nursing
Clinical Nurse Specialist
Department of Surgery, Vascular Division
University of Texas Health Science Center at
    San Antonio
San Antonio, Texas

Kathleen Halvey, MN, RN, NP-BC
Nurse Practitioner
Heart Failure Center
Saint Joseph's Hospital
Atlanta, Georgia

Adina Chaya Hirsch, PharmD
Nutrition Support Pharmacist
Pharmaceutical Care Pharmacist
Saint Joseph's Hospital of Atlanta
Atlanta, Georgia

Shari Honari, BSN, RN
Burn Research Supervisor
Department of Surgery
University of Washington Burn Center
Harborview Medical Center
Seattle, Washington

Alice Kerber, MSN, RN, AOCN, APNG
Clinical Nurse Specialist
Cancer Screening and Genetics
Saint Joseph's Hospital
Atlanta, Georgia

Cathie Osika Landreth, BSN, MS, CCRN, CEN
Trauma Program Coordinator
Clinical Nurse Specialist
Greenville Hospital System
University Medical Center
Greenville, South Carolina

Laura Leigh Leary, MS, RN-BC, OCN
Nursing Instructor
Mary Black School of Nursing
University of South Carolina Upstate
Spartanburg, South Carolina

Lynda Liles, RN, MBA, CCRN
Performance Improvement Specialist
Department of Patient Safety and Quality
Saint Joseph's Hospital
Atlanta, Georgia

Barbara McLean, MN, RN, CCRN, CCNS-NP, FCCM
Consultant in Critical Care
Atlanta, Georgia

Mary Ann Mullaney, MS, RN, CWCN, CGNP
Wound/Ostomy Care Nurse
Greenville Hospital System
University Medical Center
Greenville, South Carolina

Barbara Nickles, MN, BSN, RN
Associate Dean, Nursing Specialties and
    Simulation Project
Greenville Technical College
Greenville, South Carolina

Paul E. Schmidt, RPh, BCPS
Adjunct Faculty, Pharmacy
University of Georgia
Athens, Georgia;
Mercer University
Atlanta, Georgia;
Clinical Pharmacist
Saint Joseph's Hospital
Atlanta, Georgia

Elizabeth Scruth, MN, RN, MPH, CCRN, CCNS, PhD(c)
Assistant Clinical Professor
School of Nursing
University of California
San Francisco, California;
Critical Care Clinical Nurse Specialist
Nursing Education
Kaiser Permanente
San Jose, California

Connie Steed, MSN, RN, CIC
Director, Infection Prevention and Control
Greenville Hospital System
University Medical Center
Greenville, South Carolina

Joyce C. Warner, MN, RN, CCRN
Nurse Clinician
Surgical Intensive Care Unit
Emory Healthcare
Atlanta, Georgia

Patricia Weiskittel, MSN, RN, CNN, ACNP-BC
Renal/Hypertension Nurse Practitioner
Department of Internal Medicine
Cincinnati Veteran's Administration Medical
  Center
Cincinnati, Ohio

Karen Zorn, MSN, RN, ONC
Wellstar School of Nursing
Kennesaw State University
Kennesaw, Georgia;
Clinical Nurse Specialist
Acute Care and Informatics
Center for Nursing Excellence
Saint Joseph's Hospital
Atlanta, Georgia

REVIEWERS

Michael D. Aldridge, MSN, RN, CCRN
Assistant Professor of Nursing
Concordia University Texas
Austin, Texas

Earnest Alexander, PharmD, FCCM
Manager, Clinical Pharmacy Services
Program Director
PGY2 Critical Care Residency
Department of Pharmacy Services
Tampa General Hospital
Tampa, Florida

Olga Amusina, MSN, RN, ACNP-BC
Pulmonary/Critical Care Nurse Practitioner
NorthShore University HealthSystem
Highland Park, Illinois;
Doctoral Student
University of Illinois at Chicago
Chicago, Illinois

Patricia N. Bradshaw, MSN, MS, RN, CEN, CCRN, CCNS
Critical Care Clinical Nurse Specialist
Lieutenant Colonel, United States Air Force
San Antonio, Texas

Marylee Rollins Bressie, MSN, RN, BCCVN, CEN, CCRN, CCNS
Division of Nursing
Spring Hill College
Providence Hospital
Mobile, Alabama

Beth Broering, MSN, RN, CCRN, CEN, CPEN, FAEN
Director of Nursing
Bokamoso Private Hospital
Gaborone, Botswana

Mary Brune, MS, RN, CNE
Instructor
Division of Nursing
Northwestern Oklahoma State University
Alva, Oklahoma

Denise Buonocore, MSN, RN, CCRN, ACNP-BC
Nurse Practitioner, Heart Failure Service
St. Vincent's Medical Center
Bridgeport, Connecticut

Diane Byrum, MSN, RN, CCRN, CCNS, FCCM
Clinical Nurse Specialist
Presbyterian Hospital Huntersville
Huntersville, North Carolina

Susan Marie Chioffi, MSN, RN, CCRN, ACNP-BC
Acute Care Nurse Practitioner
Adult Neurosciences ICU
Duke University Medical Center
Durham, North Carolina

Damon Cottrell, MS, RN, CEN, CCRN, CCNS, ACNS-BC
Assistant Professor
Department of Nursing
Westbrook College of Health Professions
University of New England
Portland, Maine

Heide Rose Cygan, BSN, RN, DNP(c)
Public Health Nurse
NorthShore University HealthSystem
Evanston, Illinois;
Graduate Student
College of Nursing
University of Illinois at Chicago
Chicago, Illinois

Laura Dechant, MSN, RN, CCRN, CCNS
Clinical Nurse Specialist
Christiana Care Health System
Newark, Delaware

Joni L. Dirks, MS, RN, CCRN
Critical Care Educator
Providence Sacred Heart Medical Center
Spokane, Washington

Sonya Flanders, MSN, RN, ACNS-BC
Clinical Nurse Specialist for Internal
   Medicine
Baylor University Medical Center
Dallas, Texas

**Joyce Foresman-Capuzzi, BSN, RN, CEN,
CCRN, CTRN, CPN, CPEN, SANE-A, EMT-P**
Clinical Nurse Educator
Emergency Department
Lankenau Hospital
Wynnewood, Pennsylvania

James Graves, RPh
Licensed Pharmacist
Walgreens
Moberly, Missouri

**Joellen W. Hawkins, Phd, RN, WHNP-BC,
FAAN, FAANP**
Professor Emeritus
William F. Connell School of Nursing
Boston College
Chestnut Hill, Massachusetts;
Writer-in-Residence
Nursing Department
Simmons College
Boston, Massachusetts

Adina Chaya Hirsch, PharmD, RPH
Nutrition Support Pharmacist
Pharmaceutical Care Pharmacist
St. Joseph's Hospital of Atlanta
Atlanta, Georgia

**Reneé S. Holleran, PhD, RN, CEN, CCRN,
CFRN, CTRN, FAEN**
Staff Nurse
Emergency Department
Intermountain Medical Center
Salt Lake City, Utah

Barbara Konopka, MSN, RN, CNE, CCRN, CEN
Instructor, Nursing
Pennsylvania State University, Worthington
   Scranton
Dunmore, Pennsylvania

Adisa Tokacha Kudomovic, MSN, RN
Assistant Professor
Allen College
Waterloo, Iowa

Robert E. Lamb, PharmD
Independent Clinical Consultant
REL & Associates, LLC
Downingtown, Pennsylvania

Sheryl E. Leary, MS, RN, PCCN, CCRN, CCNS
Clinical Nurse Specialist–Progressive Care
VA San Diego Healthcare System
San Diego, California

**Rosemary Koehl Lee, MSN, RN-CS,
CCRN, CCNS, ACNP-BC**
Homestead Hospital
Homestead, Florida

Elizabeth A. Mann, RN, PhD(c), CCRN, CCNS
Major (P), United States Army
US Army Institute of Surgical Research
Fort Sam Houston, Texas

Elizabeth M. Mendeloff, MS, RN, FNP-BC
Adjunct Faculty
College of Nursing
University of Illinois at Chicago
Chicago, Illinois;
Faculty Member
College of Medicine
UIC at Rockford
Rockford, Illinois

**Joshua J. Neumiller, PharmD, CDE, CGP,
FASCP**
Assistant Professor
Department of Pharmacotherapy
College of Pharmacy
Washington State University
Spokane, Washington

Christopher T. Owens, PharmD, BCPS
Associate Professor and Chair
Department of Pharmacy Practice
College of Pharmacy
Idaho State University
Pocatello, Idaho

Michaelynn Paul, MS, RN, CCRN
Assistant Professor
School of Nursing
Walla Walla University
College Place, Washington

Beth Anne Phelps, MS, RN, ACNP-BC, DNP(c)
Assistant Professor
College of Nursing
Illinois State University
Normal, Illinois;
Graduate Student
University of Illinois at Chicago
Chicago, Illinois;
Nurse Practitioner, Otolaryngology
Springfield Clinic
Springfield, Illinois

Jan Powers, PhD, RN, CCRN, CCNS, CNRN, FCCM
Director of Clinical Nurse Specialists and
    Nursing Research
Critical Care Clinical Nurse Specialist
St. Vincent Hospital
Indianapolis, Indiana

Candace L. Rouse, MSN, RNC, CNS-BC
Advanced Practice Nurse, Obstetrics
Sinai Hospital of Baltimore
Baltimore, Maryland

Stephen M. Setter, PharmD, DVM, CDE, CGP, FASCP
Associate Professor of Pharmacotherapy
College of Pharmacy
Washington State University
Elder Services/Visiting Nurse Association
Spokane, Washington

Eva Sheets, BSN, RNC, CCRN, MBA
Critical Care Nurse–Special Staffing Team
Tampa General Hospital
Adjunct Professor
Hillsborough Community College
Tampa, Florida

Suzanne Sutherland, PhD, RN, CCRN
Staff Nurse, Burn Unit
University of California Davis Medical Center
Professor of Nursing
Sacramento State University Sacramento
Sacramento, California

Paul Thurman, MS, RN, CNRN, CCRN, CCNS, ACNPC-BC
Clinical Nurse Specialist
University of Maryland Medical Center
Baltimore, Maryland

Jeanne Malcom Widener, PhD, RN, CCRN
Critical Care Float Nurse
King's Daughters Medical Center
Ashland, Kentucky

Lindy D. Wood, PharmD
Fellow in Geriatrics
Department of Pharmacotherapy
College of Pharmacy
Washington State University
Spokane, Washington

Tresa E. Zielinski, MS, RN, PCCN, PNP-BC
APN Manager Outpatient Cardiology
Children's Memorial Hospital
Chicago, Illinois

Preface

Manual of Critical Care Nursing is a clinical reference for both practicing and student critical care nurses. It is the most comprehensive of the critical care handbooks available, yet is concise and easy to use because of its abbreviated outline format and its portable trim size. This handbook provides quick information for more than 75 clinical phenomena seen in critical care and can be used in the clinical setting to plan nursing care.

WHO WILL BENEFIT FROM THIS BOOK?

Nurses from novice to expert will derive help with assessing, managing, and evaluating their acutely ill patients. The textual information and numerous tables will serve as a quick review for the practicing nurse. Academicians can use the book in teaching students to apply theoretical concepts to clinical practice. Students will find the book to be an excellent tool for assessing the patient systematically, as well as for learning how to set priorities for nursing interventions.

WHY IS THIS BOOK IMPORTANT?

Given the increasing acuity of hospitalized patients, information previously considered exclusive to critical care such as managing acid-base balance and arterial blood gas interpretation is becoming common knowledge in progressive care, telemetry, stepdown units, and high-acuity medical-surgical units. Accordingly, the care outlined here is applicable across the spectrum of high-acuity care, from high-acuity medical-surgical to critical care.

BENEFITS OF USING THIS BOOK

Our primary goal is to present the information necessary to provide patient-centered care in a technologically advanced environment in a quick and easy-to-use format. Throughout the text, we strive to consider the whole patient with care recommendations that address the physical, emotional, mental, and spiritual distress involved in illness. The prevention of potentially life-threatening complications is of primary importance and therefore addressed through assessment, planning, implementation, and evaluation of interdisciplinary collaborative care, and nursing plans of care.

To best assess changes in status, knowledge of the patient's condition before acute, critical illness is essential. This book offers many interventions for each disorder, but not all interventions are appropriate for every patient. Our intent is to offer a thorough selection of prioritized actions that can be chosen as needed in planning individualized care.

HOW TO USE THIS BOOK

Manual of Critical Care Nursing has been reorganized for easy access and logical presentation. Information regarding general concepts of patient care, including those unique to the critical care environment, is presented in the first two chapters, General Concepts in Caring for the Critically Ill and Managing the Critical Care Environment. Following is a chapter on Trauma and related disorders. Chapters 4 through 10 cover disorders classified by body system, and Chapter 11 addresses Complex Special Situations, such as high-risk obstetrics and organ transplantation.

Each body system–specific chapter includes a general physical assessment, and several chapters include generic plans of care applicable to patients with all disease processes affecting that body system. Each disorder includes a brief review of pathophysiology, physical assessment, diagnostic testing, collaborative management, NANDA-approved nursing diagnoses and nursing interventions, patient/significant other teaching, desired outcomes, and disease-specific discharge planning considerations. Gerontologic icons highlight material relevant to the care of older adults. Desired nursing care outcomes and interventions are based on the University of

Iowa's Nursing Intervention Classification (NIC) and Nursing Outcomes Classification (NOC) systems and are highlighted throughout the text. Nursing interventions are linked to nursing diagnoses, and suggested outcomes include specific measurement criteria for physical parameters and time frames for attainment of expected outcomes. The time frames are guidelines, because each patient's response time to both illness and intervention is unique.

For clarity and consistency throughout the book, normal values are given for hemodynamic monitoring and other measurements. All values should be individualized to each patient's baseline health status.

NEW TO THIS EDITION

The sixth edition has been extensively revised and reorganized to mirror a practicing nurse's approach to patient care and allow even easier access to information. Changes include:

- New information on patient safety, organ transplantation, emotional and spiritual support of the patient and significant others, peripheral vascular disease, continuous renal replacement therapy, brain death, neuromuscular diseases, hyperglycemia, and oncologic emergencies.
- Updated guidelines and recommendations for mechanical ventilation, hemodynamic monitoring, and the management of heart and respiratory failure including evolving mechanical devices.
- A composite chapter reflecting the evolution of management of hyperglycemia and associated emergency conditions.
- Enhanced information on acid-base balance, acute asthma, burns, sepsis, cardiogenic shock, aortic dissection, and the management of delirium.
- Physical assessment and generic plans of care for disorders of each body system.
- Collaborative care and nursing care plans with prioritized interventions and outcomes based on the Nursing Outcomes Classification (NOC).
- Organization of information by alphabetical order, with color tabs for easy access.
- Appropriate resuscitation interventions within the section on Dysrhythmias and Conduction Disturbances.

We hope that critical care practitioners, students, and academicians will find that the new edition of *Manual of Critical Care Nursing* provides them with a wealth of easy-to-access knowledge to apply in practice and in the classroom.

ACKNOWLEDGMENTS

We want to thank many individuals who supported the development of this manuscript. In particular, we are grateful for the time and efforts of Laurie Sparks, Developmental Editor, and Jeff Somers. We appreciate the guidance of Maureen Iannuzzi, Editor, and Robin Levin Richman, Senior Developmental Editor. We thank all the contributors for their hard work and attention to detail, as well as all the reviewers whose comments helped guide our revisions. All are recognized as shining stars in their own right. Both perseverance and patience are the fundamental characteristics inherent in all participants.

We extend special recognition to Barbara McLean, for "going the extra mile" to enhance her content; to Phyllis Gordon and Cynthia Rebik Christensen for their excellent job in creating the new Peripheral Vascular Disease section; Patricia Weiskittel for taking on several additional sections; Elizabeth Scruth for her extensive enhancement to the Cardiogenic Shock section; Gretchen J. Carrougher, Shari Honari, and Carolyn Blayney for extensive work on the Burn section; and Vicki Good for creating the new Patient Safety section.

Marianne Saunorus Baird and Susan Bethel

I acknowledge the support of my daughter Rachel, my husband Thom, and my mother, Irene Saunorus. I could not have done it without all of you.

MSB

I acknowledge the support of my husband Terry, and the team effort of my team of authors within the Greenville Health System. You are the best!

SB

Contents

Appendixes

General Concepts in Caring for the Critically Ill

ACID-BASE IMBALANCES

Cells must transport ions, metabolites and gases in order to respond appropriately. For this to occur, the bloodstream's chemical environment must be electrically stable. *The stability of the environment is measured by the arterial pH and must be chemically neutral (pH 7.40) for all systems to function properly. The arterial blood gas (ABG) is the most commonly used analysis to measure acid-base balance and to assess the efficacy of oxygenation.* Respiratory (CO_2) and metabolic acids (H^+) are generated as cells work and must be buffered or eliminated to maintain a neutral chemical environment. When the chemical environment is no longer neutral, the patient has an acid-base imbalance. Ineffective metabolism (tissue level), renal dysfunction, and/or problems with ventilation (breathing gasses effectively) are often the cause of acid-base imbalance.

There are two main types of acid-base imbalance: *acidosis* and *alkalosis*. The kidneys and lungs work in tandem to maintain chemical neutrality, but it is actually cellular function which produces acid. When either the kidneys or lungs are over or under functioning, the other system is designed to have the opposite response in order to compensate and bring the pH back to a normal range. When the kidneys fail to regulate metabolic acids (H^+), the lungs must compensate. When the lungs fail to regulate respiratory acid (CO_2), the kidneys must compensate. Additional buffering mechanisms are also available to help regulate the accumulation of acids. Control of alkaline states, resulting from accumulation of bases or loss of acids, is maintained in a similar fashion between the lungs and kidneys.

PATHOPHYSIOLOGY OF ACID-BASE REGULATION

Arterial pH is an indirect measurement of CO_2 and H^+ concentration, which reflects the overall level of acid and effectiveness of maintaining the balance. The normal acid-base ratio is 1:20—1 part acid (the H^+ and CO_2 component of H_2CO_3) to 20 parts base (HCO_3^-). If the ratio is altered through an increase or a decrease in either acid H^+ or CO_2 or the base, HCO_3^-, the pH changes. Chemically, the CO_2 does not contain H^+, but when dissolved in water (plasma), $CO_2 + H_2O$ yields H_2CO_3 (carbonic acid). CO_2, when combined with H_2O, becomes the largest contributor of H^+ (acids), which must be eliminated or buffered to maintain normal pH. Too many H^+ ions in the plasma creates *acidemia* (pH less than 7.35), while too few H^+ ions creates *alkalemia* (pH greater than 7.45).

Maintaining the 1:20 ratio ("the balance") depends on the ability of the lungs and kidneys to help normalize concentrations of carbonic acid (H_2CO_3) a product of hydrogen ion (H^+) plus bicarbonate buffer (HCO_3). Both the kidney and lung are designed to eliminate carbonic acid effectively and therefore the pH should always be in the range of normal. A pH change is a symptom that there is a significant problem with one or both of the systems.

- *Acidosis:* Extra acids are present or base is lost, with a pH less than 7.35.
  1. *Cellular acidosis:* When cells are hypoxic or processing proteins to yield glucose, there is an increase in lactic acid or ketoacid.
  2. *Respiratory acidosis:* If the function of the lungs is inadequate, such as in COPD disease, the failure to effectively ventilate results in the inability to excrete CO_2, and that failure causes carbonic acid to go up (more acid) and pH to go down.

   3. *Renal acidosis:* If the kidney function is inadequate, the ability to break carbonic acid
      from H_2CO_3 into hydrogen ions (H^+) and HCO_3^-. When this failure occurs, car-
      bonic acid goes up (more acid) and pH goes down.
- Buffering of acid or compensation for an acid state, occurs in three primary ways:
   1. *Plasma and cellular buffering:* Using bicarbonate, proteins, intracellular electrolytes,
      and chloride to buffer H^+. Most common is the marriage of H^+ to HCO_3^- which
      yields carbonic acid H_2CO_3.
   2. *Hyperventilation (lungs):* The presence of increased carbonic acid stimulates a hyper-
      ventilation response. This allows for exhaling ("blow off") more of the CO_2
      component of carbonic acid. This compensatory response for metabolic acidosis
      occurs within minutes and should bring pH to a normal range.
   3. *Acid excretion (kidneys):* A functional kidney will utilize increased carbonic acid by
      breaking the H_2CO_3 into bicarbonate and H^+, excreting the H^+ and retaining the
      bicarbonate. This should compensate for the increased respiratory acidosis but is very
      slow, taking 4 to 48 hours for compensation to occur.
- *Alkalosis:* Extra base is present or there is loss of acid, with a pH greater than 7.45.
   1. *Respiratory alkalosis:* When hyperventilation is the primary problem, there is a very
      rapid removal of CO_2, causing carbonic acid to go down (less acid) and pH to go up.
   2. *Renal alkalosis:* If the kidney function is overstimulated (for example with aggressive
      diuresis), there may be excessive loss of hydrogen ions (H^+), causing carbonic acid to
      go down (less acid) and pH to go up.
   3. *Other contributors:* Gastric and intestinal removal of acids may occur when patients
      have diarrhea, vomiting, or when excessive gastric drainage influences the acid-base
      balance.
- *Alkalosis:* Compensating for an alkaline state occurs in two ways:
   1. *Hypoventilation:* The respiratory system responds by slowing ventilation and retain-
      ing CO_2 (acid), to help compensate for metabolic alkalosis from any cause. This re-
      sponse occurs within minutes.
   2. *Renal response:* The kidneys respond by retaining more acid (H^+) and excreting more
      bicarbonate to help correct respiratory alkalosis. This response occurs within 4 to
      48 hours.

Example of Compensation (pH Regulation):

When metabolic acids accumulate, they are attracted to bicarbonate. The marriage of H^+ and
HCO_3^- buffers the acid. This yields an increase in carbonic acid and causes the pH to go down.
Chemoreceptors are stimulated by this acid presence and the hypothalamus, if not damaged,
triggers a hyperventilation response. Since H^+ is not measured directly, the indirect calculation of bicarbonate or the base is used to evaluate the presence or absence of metabolic acid. As
H^+ goes up, the bicarbonate or base goes down. When evaluating the acid base balance, it is
simplest to look at bicarbonate but to think in terms of H^+. They travel in completely opposite
directions (when bicarbonate is down, H^+ is up and vice versa).

The lungs increase buffering *to compensate* for a failure of the kidneys or a cellular excess
acid production to keep the pH balanced. The lungs do this by effectively exhaling more
CO_2 than usual, breaking down the carbonic acid and therefore bringing pH back towards
normal.

When CO_2 is retained or increased because of respiratory failure, the kidneys should, in
turn, respond by processing the increased H_2CO_3. The kidneys separate the carbonic acid into
H^+ and HCO_3^- and excrete the H^+ while retaining HCO_3^- bicarbonate. If either the kidneys
or lungs do not respond to a pH change (*no compensation*) or they provide an ineffective response (*partial compensation*), the patient will remain in acid-base imbalance. If the pH is outside of the range of normal, then there is a primary problem and *compensation* is inadequate or
has failed. Patients may have a pure acidosis or alkalosis and the overall problem may be
masked by compensation or two problems presenting at the same time.

It is essential to understand that unless the patient has ingested acid (aspirin, ethanol,
etc.), all acid in the bloodstream was produced at the cellular level (Table 1-1). When evaluating patients, care providers must have a basic understanding of the acid-base balancing system.
The main formula for maintenance of acid-base balance is the following:

$$CO_2 + H_2O \leftrightarrow H_2CO_3 \leftrightarrow HCO_3^- \text{ and } H^+$$

Table 1-1	PRODUCERS AND REGULATORS OF ACID	
Acid Pathways	**Cause**	**Measure**
Cells produce acid (acid production increases).	Hypermetabolic states, such as pain, hyperthermia, or inflammation. The respiratory and heart rates increase, and bicarbonate is initially consumed by buffering.	HCO_3 ↓
	Tissues are hypoxic; anaerobic metabolism ensues resulting in lactic acidosis.	Lactate level ↑
	Absolute insulin deficiency results in failure of glucose to be transported into cells.	Blood glucose level ↑ Ketoacids ↑
Cells regulate acids.	When acid production (H^+) increases, pH decreases, bicarbonate is initially consumed by buffering, and CO_2 is exhaled in larger amounts, and H^+ exchanges for K^+ as cells buffer acid.	pH ↓ HCO_3 ↓ K^+ ↑ Total serum CO_2 ↓
Lungs regulate acid.	When acid increases due to hypermetabolic states such as pain, hyperthermia, or inflammation, carbonic acid (H_2CO_3) increases and rapidly converts to CO_2 and H_2O. The respiratory rate increases to blow off CO_2.	$Paco_2$ ↓
Kidneys regulate acid.	When acid increases, tubules are affected by low blood pH, and work to neutralize increased carbonic acid (H_2CO_3) by separating it into H^+ and bicarbonate HCO_3. Kidneys excrete what is necessary to sustain normal pH if renal function is normal. If abnormal, kidneys may not perform this task.	HCO_3 ↑ Kidney function is assessed by serum BUN and creatinine; elevated BUN and creatinine indicate abnormal kidney function.

The most important component identified is the H_2CO_3, or *carbonic acid*. As carbonic acid increases ("goes up"), the pH decreases ("goes down"), reflecting the presence of acid. If the carbonic acid decreases ("goes down"), the pH increases ("goes up"), reflecting the absence of acid. The equation is constantly shifting from left to right and right to left to maintain a normal H_2CO_3 and therefore a normal pH. Whatever causes the change of carbonic acid concentration (may be related to a regulation failure by either the lungs or kidneys or a metabolic acid production state) is the "primary culprit." Identifying the origin or cause of the change in pH direction identifies the problem. Therefore, if the problem is too much acid (either increased CO_2 or H^+), the carbonic acid goes up and the pH goes down. The primary problem is acidosis. Further evaluation is needed to determine whether failure to regulate the acid was ineffective regulation by the lungs, the kidneys or an increase in cellular acid production (ketoacidosis or lactic acidosis).

Safety Alert *Changes in pH are associated with changes in the potassium level. As the plasma level of nonvolatile or metabolic acid (H^+) increases, H^+ moves into the cells in order to buffer the acid effect. In this case H^+ "exchanges places" with the intracellular potassium (K^+), resulting in a measured serum hyperkalemia but is actually an intracellular hypokalemia. The positively charged intracellular potassium ions are replaced by positively charged hydrogen ions. During an alkalotic state, K^+ may shift into cells as H^+ is released into the serum, creating a transient hypokalemia. As pH changes, it is imperative for the care providers to observe the corresponding changes in the K^+ level, and manage K^+ carefully. When the pH normalizes, the K^+ will shift back to its original location. If a transient K^+ change is managed too aggressively, the patient may experience dangerous hypokalemia or hyperkalemia when pH normalizes.*

UNDERSTANDING THE ARTERIAL BLOOD GAS

The ABG is the most commonly used measurement to help assess the origins of problems with acid-base imbalance and to guide treatment designed to restore pH balance and effective oxygenation. *"Perfect" values* for each reflects *chemical neutrality*. There are normal variations or a range for each value.

ABG Values

Blood gas analysis is usually based on sampling of arterial blood. Mixed venous blood sampling from a pulmonary artery (PA) catheter (Svo_2) and central venous sampling from a central intravenous (IV) line ($Scvo_2$) may also be performed for very critically ill patients. Venous values are given for reference only.

Normal Arterial Values	Normal Venous Values
pH: 7.35–7.45	pH: 7.32–7.38
$Paco_2$: 35–45 mm Hg	$Pvco_2$: 42–50 mm Hg
Pao_2: 80–100 mm Hg	Pvo_2: 40 mm Hg
Sao_2: 95%–100%	Svo_2: 60%–80%
Base excess (BE): −2 to +2	BE: −2 to +2 (only calculated on ABG analyzer)
HCO_3^-: 22–26 mEq/L	total Serum CO_2^-: 23–27 mEq/L

pH (perfect 7.40, range of normal 7.35 to 7.45): This reflects the level of respiratory and metabolic acids found in the blood during the continuous "balancing act" that regulates the acid environment. If this balance is altered, derangements in pH occur. Any alteration in pH should be evaluated. If the pH has changed from perfect, it can only be one of two reasons: normal variation, or abnormality with compensation. When pH is less than 7.35 or greater than 7.45, it is considered an acute change that is uncompensated. When *full compensation* is attained for an acid-base imbalance, *the pH normalizes.* Failure to bring pH to range of normal means that there is failure to compensate, even if there is an attempt. Traditionally this was known as partial compensation. That term is no longer advocated.

Paco₂ (perfect 40, range of normal 35 to 45 mm Hg): This is a measure of pressure (partial pressure which is designated by the P) that the dissolved CO_2 exerts in the arterial blood. The dissolved gas exerts the pressure of CO_2, enabling it to diffuse across the capillary and alveolar cell wall.

CO_2 is released during aerobic metabolism and is the main contributor to serum acid. CO_2 is controlled through ventilation. In the normal lung, CO_2 is regulated by changes in the rate and depth of alveolar ventilation. CO_2 is carried both bound to hemoglobin and dissolved in the blood. The measured CO_2 is termed $Paco_2$. $Paco_2$ is directly measured (not calculated) and is a reliable indicator of respiratory acid-base regulation. The correlation between $Paco_2$ and respiratory-based pH changes is direct, consistent, and linear. In other words if $Paco_2$ is up and pH is down, the cause is respiratory deregulation. If the issue is metabolic, and respiratory compensation has occurred, the $Paco_2$ will decrease in order to bring pH back to normal levels. Respiratory compensation typically occurs rapidly in metabolic acid-base disturbances as long as respiratory function is not impaired. When a patient hyperventilates, $Paco_2$ decreases as it is "blown off" by rapid exhalations. During hypoventilation (slow and/or shallow breathing), $Paco_2$ increases. Although the only way to evaluate true lung function is by the gas exchange, the *capacity of the lungs (CO_2 regulation response) is measured via the minute ventilation* (V_E or MV). This measures the amount of volume exhaled per minute (V_E) calculated as respiratory rate (RR) × V_T. Normal MV is about 8 to 10 L/min. B

Pao₂ (perfect 95 to 100 mm Hg, normal range 80 to 100 mm Hg): The partial pressure of oxygen (O_2), or Pao_2, is a measure of the dissolved (usable) gas in the arteries. The dissolved gas exerts the pressure of O_2, enabling it to diffuse across the capillary and cell wall to oxygenate cells. Pao_2 normally declines in the older adult.

- *Hypoxemia (Pao₂ less than 80 mm Hg):* Low partial pressure of O_2 affects the cellular levels of oxygen available and may result in cellular metabolic dysfunction reflected by lactic acid production and metabolic acidosis.

- FIO_2: Fraction of inspired O_2 or the percentage of the atmospheric pressure which is oxygenated. Room air is 21% or 0.21 O_2. O_2 delivery devices can increase the FIO_2 to 100% or 1.00.

  P/F ratio (greater than 300): PaO_2 is evaluated in relationship to FIO_2; that is, the higher the percent O_2 pressure that is delivered to the lungs, the higher the O_2 in the blood should be.

$$PaO_2/FIO_2 \text{ (in the decimal)} = \text{the P/F ratio}$$
$$100/0.21 = 476$$
$$\text{Normal P/F} > 300$$
$$\text{Hypoxemia P/F} < 300 \text{ on} > 0.40 \text{ FIO}_2$$

  SaO_2 (perfect 100% or 1.0, normal range 95% to 100% or 0.95 to 1.0): O_2 saturation (SaO_2) reflects the loading of O_2 onto hemoglobin (Hgb) in the lungs. When Hgb is loaded with O_2, it is termed oxyhemoglobin. Hgb is the primary transporter of O_2 and supplies a reservoir (reserve) of O_2 for cellular use. Each Hgb molecule carries 1.34 to 1.36 ml of O_2. O_2 must be released from the Hgb, dissolve in blood (PaO_2), and exert pressure to diffuse across the cell wall. The uptake/use of O_2 by the tissues is measured by SvO_2 and/or $ScvO_2$ (mixed venous and/or central venous saturation of Hgb, respectively). Cellular metabolism and O_2 utilization are affected by changes in stress level, temperature, pH, blood flow, and $PaCO_2$. When the PaO_2 falls to less than 60 mm Hg, there is a large drop in saturation, reflected in the oxyhemoglobin dissociation curve.

- Pulse oximetry (SpO_2): This can be used to noninvasively trend the arterial O_2 saturation and determine ventilation status using a probe fastened to the patient's finger, earlobe, or forehead. This monitoring technique is frequently used in critical care areas for patients at high risk of ventilation problems, in operating rooms, and in emergency departments. SpO_2 should be correlated with SaO_2 (or oxyhemoglobin) via blood gas analysis when pulse oximetry is initiated, to assess accuracy of SpO_2 readings. Pulse oximetry is a close correlate to SaO_2 under normal physiologic conditions, but if perfusion decreases, the pulse needed for accurate measurement by the SpO_2 probe is decreased, prompting inaccurate readings. Anemic patients should have consistently high readings, so what is usually considered a normal SpO_2 reading may be too low in an anemic patient. The measure of true oxyhemoglobin (Hgb saturated with O_2) requires an ABG analysis. Many centers do not perform a correlation analysis when oximetry is initiated.

  BE (perfect 0, normal range -2 to $+2$): Base excess or base deficit uses a calculation to reflect the presence (excess) or absence (deficit) of buffers. The calculation reflects the tissue and renal tubular presence (or absence) of acid. As the proportion of acid rises, the relative amount of base decreases (and vice versa). Abnormally high values (greater than $+2$) reflect alkalosis, or an excess of base; low values (less than -2) reflect acidosis, or a deficit of base (base deficit).

- All buffers: Absorb acids (H^+), but do so with a varying affinity. Buffers are present in all body fluids and cells and act within 1 second after acid accumulation begins. They combine with excess acid to form substances that may not greatly affect pH. Some buffers have a strong affinity to acid; others are weak. The three primary plasma buffers are bicarbonate (HCO_3^-), intracellular proteins, and chloride (Cl^-). All are negatively charged to facilitate attraction to positively charged hydrogen ions (H^+). Combining positively charged with negatively charged hydrogen ions yields a neutral substance.

- Proteins: Serum and intracellular proteins offer a significant contribution to buffering acids. Hgb not only transports O_2 but also provides a very strong buffer for hydrogen ions (H^+). Albumin is also a significant buffer, and hypoalbuminemia must be considered when performing anion gap calculations.

- HCO_3^- (perfect 24, normal range 22 to 26 mEq/L): Serum bicarbonate (HCO_3^-) is one of the major components of acid-base regulation by the kidney. Bicarbonate is generated and/or excreted by normally functioning kidneys in direct proportion to the amount of circulating acid to maintain acid-base balance. Because bicarbonate is affected by both the respiratory and metabolic components of the acid-base system, the relationship between metabolic acidosis and bicarbonate is not particularly linear or predictable. When the bicarbonate level changes, the acid level changes in the opposite direction. To determine the cause of bicarbonate changes (as the source of a pH problem versus compensation), the relationship to pH must be evaluated. The pH changes in the presence or absence of acid, and the directional relationship reflects what caused the pH alteration. The kidney is responsible for the regeneration of bicarbonate ions, as well as excretion of the hydrogen ions. Although serum bicarbonate is a buffer, it is usually reported in the standard electrolyte panel from a venous blood sample as "CO_2 content" or "total CO_2" rather than as bicarbonate (HCO_3^-). The serum HCO_3^- concentration is usually calculated and reported separately with ABG analysis. Either value may be used as part of the assessment of acid-base balance (Table 1-2).

- *Chloride (Cl$^-$):* The number of positive and negative ions in the plasma must balance at all times. Aside from the plasma proteins, bicarbonate and chloride are the two most abundant negative ions (anions) in the plasma. *To maintain electrical neutrality, any change in chloride must be accompanied by the opposite change in bicarbonate concentration.* If chloride increases, bicarbonate decreases (hyperchloremic acidosis) and vice versa. However the combination of H$^+$ and chloride actually exerts an acid effect (HCl). Chloride concentration may influence acid-base balance (see anion gap). Chloride concentration should be observed closely when large amounts of normal saline are administered to patients.

- *Other buffers:* Other buffers, including phosphate and ammonium, are present in very limited quantities and have a lesser impact on the regulation of acid.

Table 1-2	DIAGNOSTIC TESTS FOR ACID-BASE BALANCE	
Role of the ABG	**Measures**	**Normals**
Evaluation of arterial oxygen (dissolved oxygen and oxygen bound to hemoglobin)	Arterial oxygen saturation (oxygen bound to hemoglobin)	Sao_2: 0.95–1.0 or 95%–100%
	Partial pressure of arterial oxygen (dissolved oxygen)	Pao_2: 80–100 mm Hg (decreased over the age of 70)
Calculation of alveolar-arterial (A-a) oxygen gradient	Alveolar-arterial gradient	A-a Do_2: <20 mm Hg
	Pao_2/Fio_2 ratio	PF ratio: .300
Evaluation of cellular environment	pH (reflects H_2CO_3) i.e., ↑↑ H_2CO_3 then pH ↓↓	pH Perfect: 7.40 Normal range: 7.35–7.45
Evaluation of ventilation	$Paco_2$	$Paco_2$ Normal range: 35–45 mm Hg
Evaluation of tissue metabolism	H$^+$ inversely (indirectly) reflected by buffers: Bicarbonate (HCO_3^-) Base measures (+ or −) Total CO_2 i.e., ↑↑ H$^+$ then buffers ↓↓	pH Perfect: 7.40 Normal range: 7.35–7.45 HCO_3^-: 22–26 mEq/L Total CO_2: 20–26 Base Normal range: −2 to +2 Anion gap: 12 + or −2
Additional measures of tissue metabolism	Both contribute H$^+$ to blood lactic acid Ketoacids	Lactic acid: 1–2 mmol/L Ketoacids Blood: 0.27–0.5 mmol/L Urine levels Small: <20 mg/dl Moderate: 30–40 mg/dl Large: >80 mg/dl
Evaluation of renal clearance	Appropriate clearance of excessive components: H$^+$ or HCO_3^- Appropriate clearance of excessive components: BUN and creatinine	pH Perfect: 7.40 Range: 7.35–7.45 BUN: 0–20 mg/dl Creatinine: <2.0 mEq/L

- *Cellular electrolytes:* The cells also offer protection in the metabolic acid environment. H^+ may exchange across the cell wall, attracted by negatively charged intracellular proteins in a cellular buffering process. When this happens, K^+ is released from the proteins and shifts out of the cell, causing an excess of K^+ in the blood.
- *Anion gap:* Anion gap is an estimate of the differences between measured and unmeasured cations (positively charged particles, such as Na and H^+ respectively) and measured and unmeasured anions (negatively charged particles such as HCO_3^- and Cl^-. Normally, cations and anions are equally balanced in live humans (in vivo), but when measured in the laboratory (in vitro), the difference may be between 10 to 12 mmol/L. This difference is termed a normal gap (between + and – ions). Particles that possess charges tend to have high affinity to bind to other particles that possess charges that are opposite their own (hence the term, "opposites attract"). *Anion gap is used to determine if a metabolic acidosis is due to an accumulation of nonvolatile acids such as lactic acid or ketoacids.* Both contribute a positive charge due to excess H^+ or from net loss of bicarbonate (e.g., diarrhea). The *gap is not affected when a patient has metabolic acidosis purely from kidney failure.* The formula for calculation of anion gap is

$$AG = [Na^+] + [K^+] - [Cl^-] - [HCO_3^-]$$
$$(\text{Normal range: } 10\text{--}14)$$

Unmeasured cations: Calcium, magnesium, gamma globulins, potassium (bind negative charged particles)

Unmeasured anions: Albumin, phosphate, sulfate, lactate, hydrogen ion (bind positive charge particles)

Step-by-Step Guide to ABG Analysis

A systematic analysis is critical to the accurate interpretation of ABG values to determine the origin of acid-base imbalance, and level of compensation (see Table 1-2).

Step 1: Check the pH: Determine if pH is perfect (7.40)   When there is a perfect balance of acid and buffer (base), the pH is termed *neutral* or *perfect*. If it is not perfect, determine if the direction of the difference is above or below 7.40. Next, determine if it is in the range of normal (7.35 to 7.45). If it is abnormal, identify whether it is on the *acidotic (less than 7.35)* or *alkalotic (greater than 7.45)* side of normal. *"Perfect pH" occurs when the system preserves neutrality (pH 6.8) inside the cells, where most chemistry occurs, and maintains the serum pH at 7.40.* For the purposes of learning, the perfect pH is where all measurement begins. When the system contains too many acid ions (in the form of ↑CO_2 or ↑H^+), this causes acidemia. When the system contains too few acid ions (in the form of ↓CO_2 or ↓H^+), this causes alkalemia, and the pH will reflect the change. Any variation in the pH in relationship to perfect (7.40) must be noted by the provider. If the pH is in the range of 7.35 to 7.45, there are only two possibilities: First, the deviation is a normal variation, wherein no abnormalities exist on either the respiratory side ($Paco_2$) or the metabolic side (HCO_3^-) of the pH equation. The second possibility is there is a problem with ventilation (respiratory), cellular acid production (metabolic), or the ability of the kidneys (metabolic) to balance the pH. Diagnosis of a problem with metabolic acid-base balance is more complex, as many conditions generate metabolic acids and renal failure creates an acid clearance deficit.

pH less than 7.35, Acidosis: Extra acids are present or base is lost. If pH is 7.35 to 7.39, the pH is normal but not perfect (7.40); the pH is considered "on the acidotic side."

- *Acidosis: Extra acids are present or base is lost, with a pH less than 7.35*
  1. *Cellular acidosis:* When cells are hypoxic or processing proteins to yield glucose, there is an increase in lactic acid or ketoacid.
  2. *Respiratory acidosis:* If the function of the lungs is inadequate, such as in COPD disease, the failure to effectively ventilate results in the inability to exhale CO_2, and that failure causes carbonic acid to go up (more acid) and pH to go down.
  3. *Renal acidosis:* If the kidney function is inadequate, the ability to break carbonic acid from H_2CO_3 into hydrogen ions (H^+) and HCO_3^- is reduced or lost. When this failure occurs, carbonic acid goes up (more acid) and pH goes down.

pH greater than 7.45, Alkalosis: Extra base is present or there is loss of acid. If pH is 7.41 to 7.45, the pH is normal but not perfect (7.40); the pH is considered "on the alkalotic side."

- *Alkalosis: Extra base is present or there is loss of acid, with a pH greater than 7.45.*
  1. *Respiratory alkalosis:* When hyperventilation is the primary problem, there is a very rapid removal of CO_2, causing carbonic acid to go down (less acid) and pH to go up.

2. *Renal alkalosis:* If the kidney function is overstimulated (for example, with aggressive diuresis), there may be excessive loss of hydrogen ions (H^+), causing carbonic acid to go down (less acid) and pH to go up.

3. *Other contributors:* Gastric and intestinal removal of acids may occur when patients have diarrhea, vomiting, or when excessive gastric drainage removes acidic secretions and influences the acid-base balance.

Step 2: Check the $Paco_2$ Check $Paco_2$ for perfect levels (40 mm Hg). If not perfect, determine if the direction of change is above or below 40 mm Hg. Next, determine if CO_2 is in the range of normal (35 to 45 mm Hg). If abnormal, identify whether it is on the acidotic (greater than 45 mm Hg) or alkalotic (less than 35 mm Hg) side of normal. If $Paco_2$ has been retained as a result of hypoventilation or overly removed through hyperventilation, the change in pH will be in the opposite direction of the $Paco_2$. Elevated CO_2 lowers pH, while decreased CO_2 increases pH. *If the change in pH is in normal range but not perfect, or is out of range, with a $Paco_2$ value that has traveled in the opposite direction, respiratory acid retentions caused the imbalance.* Using this technique helps determine whether the primary problem is respiratory (involving $Paco_2$) or metabolic (reflected by HCO_3^-). *The $Paco_2$ has to be outside of the normal range for there to be a problem.*

Step 3: Check for base (deficit or excess)   Check bicarbonate (HCO_3^-) (24 mEq/L) and base (0) for perfect levels. If not perfect, determine if the direction of change is above or below perfect. Next, determine if HCO_3^- (22 to 26 mEq/L) and/or base (+2 to −2) is in the normal range. If the values are abnormal, relate the two values to metabolic acid (H^+). If bicarbonate and base are decreased (a deficit), metabolic acid is increased. If bicarbonate and base are increased (in excess), metabolic acid is decreased. *If the change in pH is in normal range but not perfect, or out of range and the assumed H^+ is in the opposite direction (meaning that the HCO_3^- (and/or base are in the same direction as the pH) metabolic issues caused the imbalance.* Using this technique helps determine whether the primary problem is respiratory (involving $Paco_2$) or metabolic (reflected by HCO_3^-) or both.

Step 4: (Evaluate both $Paco_2$ and HCO_3^-)   Correlating the direction of the pH change with the direction of change in $Paco_2$ and H^+ (HCO_3^-) is essential. The value that deviates in the opposite direction from the pH suggests the primary disturbance responsible for the altered pH. Assess pH for acidosis or alkalosis, and then evaluate whether the change in CO_2 or H^+ (HCO_3^-) is most reflective of the "direction" of the pH change.

A mixed metabolic-respiratory acid-base imbalance or compensation may be responsible for the values reflected by the ABG.

Step 5: Check Pao_2 and Sao_2   Check Pao_2 and O_2 saturation to determine whether they are decreased, normal, or increased. Decreased Pao_2 and O_2 saturation may signal the need for increased concentrations of O_2 or alveolar recruitment strategies. Conversely, high Pao_2 may indicate the need to decrease delivered concentrations of O_2. Oxygen evaluation is the same for all arterial blood gases, although in the presence of metabolic acidosis, a more in-depth investigation will require evaluation of tissue metabolic functions.

RESPIRATORY ACIDOSIS

PATHOPHYSIOLOGY

Evaluation of an Abnormal Arterial Blood Gas Resulting in a Decreased pH due to Hypoventilation

Example: pH 7.28, $Paco_2$ 55, HCO_3^- 24, Pao_2 92 mm Hg, Sao_2 91%

Step 1: pH is 7.28, not perfect or neutral (7.40) and outside the normal range of 7.35 to 7.45.

Ideally the pH should always be perfect (7.40), but a small variation is acceptable (range of 7.35 to 7.45). One must remember that pH changes are a symptom of a problem. So the first issue is to identify the problem.

pH: The primary problem with pH regulation is identified by the direction of the pH change in respect to *perfect*: Is it on the *acid side (less than 7.40)* or the *alkaline side (greater than 7.40)*?

1. pH 7.28: *Acid side*, outside of range of normal
2. Question: Is there a problem? YES, acidosis (identified by the pH)
3. Where is the acid being generated? Are the acids respiratory or metabolic?

4. $Paco_2$: 55 (elevated outside the normal range) → respiratory acid is accumulating
5. HCO_3^-: 24 (perfect) → metabolic acid is not present, perfect HCO_3

Step 2: $Paco_2$ is 55 mm Hg, not perfect (40 mm Hg) and above the normal range of 35 to 45 mm Hg indicating an excess of respiratory acid.

Investigation begins:

1. *Hypercapnia/elevated Paco2 (Paco2 greater than 45 mm Hg): Signals alveolar hypoventilation. This problem occurs when alveoli are not recruited, there is poor blood flow, the respiratory rate or tidal volume is inadequate, or there is fluid or an increase in the space between alveoli and blood vessel. These conditions may be chronic or acute.*
2. If this is the causative problem, the pH has to be below 7.40, reflecting excess acid (CO2) or an increase in carbonic acid (H2CO3), which is a primary acidosis. So now one must investigate what caused the increase in carbonic acid (H2CO3). For every 10 mm Hg increase in CO2, the pH will acutely decrease 0.08 (on the acid side).
3. Problem: Respiratory acidosis
    Respiratory acidosis (hypercapnia, hypoventilation) is always related to a ventilation problem caused by inadequate therapeutic interventions or lung pathophysiology, resulting in retention of $Paco_2$. $Paco_2$ derangements are direct reflections of the degree of ventilatory function or dysfunction. The degree to which the increased $Paco_2$ alters the pH depends on the rapidity of onset and the blood and kidney's ability to compensate via the blood buffer and renal regulation systems. The pH may be profoundly affected initially because of the time required (hours to days) for kidney compensation to occur. The most common cause of inadequate CO_2 excretion (CO_2 retention) is inadequate alveolar ventilation, or alveolar hypoventilation. Alveolar hypoventilation can occur when there is airway obstruction, loss of alveolar recoil, or inadequate time for exhalation affecting the ability to express carbon gas into the environment. For CO_2 to be removed from the blood, the partial pressure of CO_2 in the alveoli must be less than that in the blood. In air-trapping syndrome (loss of alveolar recoil or elasticity or airway obstructive disease) or profound hypoventilation states, the alveolar concentration of CO_2 increases, which then limits the removal of CO_2 from the blood. If the problem is not properly managed, the patient may deteriorate into acute respiratory failure.

Step 3: The HCO_3^- in the example is perfect at 24 mEq/L. The normal range of bicarbonate is 22 to 26 mEq/L.

Investigation begins:

1. Normal HCO_3^- indicates that there is not a metabolic problem, although compensation should begin within 4 to 48 hours, as opposed to respiratory compensation for metabolic pH imbalances, which happens in minutes.
2. Problem: *No apparent kidney or metabolic problems*

Is there compensation for the respiratory acidosis?

In order for compensation to occur, the carbonic acid must be presented to the kidney and separated into H^+ and HCO_3^-. In other words, the excess CO_2 will be processed into carbonic acid and ultimately into H^+ (which will be excreted in a functional kidney state) and HCO_3^-. Kidney or renal compensation for accumulation of respiratory acids is a slow process, After 48 hours if there continues to be an acidotic pH, one must assume that the kidneys have lost the ability to eliminate H^+ or retain HCO_3^-.

Step 4: Diagnosis begins:

1. Only the CO_2 is elevated, without a change in the HCO_3^-.
2. pH is down and outside range reflecting the presence of acid in the blood.
3. Problem: The patient has acute respiratory failure, causing an accumulation of respiratory acid (CO_2). There is no compensation, but no evidence is available at this time.
    Diagnosis: Acute Respiratory Acidosis

Step 5: Pao_2 92 mm Hg (not perfect 98 to 100 mm Hg but within normal range 80 to 100 mm Hg), Sao_2 91% (not perfect 100% and below normal range of 95% to 100%).

Investigation begins: Slight decrease is apparent in Pao_2 and Sao_2

1. *Use of O_2:* If O_2 is not in use on a patient with reduced Pao_2 and Sao_2, applying O_2 often corrects the readings. If O_2 is in use, changing to a device that delivers a higher concentration of O_2, such as changing from a nasal cannula to a face mask, may be sufficient to correct the

alveolar levels of O_2. If the Pao_2 and Sao_2 do not respond to the first device change or values further deteriorate, a 100% nonrebreather mask may be applied to provide close to 100% O_2. Note: *All ABG readings must be recorded with consideration of the mode of O_2 delivery recorded, as well as the Fio_2 or concentration of O_2. Otherwise, evaluation of the Pao_2 and $Sao2$ values is meaningless. If the values are NOT recorded, the assumption is made the readings are done on room air, without O_2 in place.*

2. *Evaluating risk for poor tissue oxygenation:* Thus far, ventilation has been evaluated using the ABG, but both ventilation AND perfusion must be evaluated as part of O_2 delivery to the cell level. To objectively and proactively identify the patient at risk for tissue hypoxia, early signs of the perfusion changes that precede increases in serum lactate and the widening anion gap associated with lactic acidosis may be noted. Changes in heart rate (HR), blood pressure (BP), respiratory rate, urine output, saturation of continuous central or mixed venous Hgb, and serum creatinine are common. In the shock setting, normal or near normal Pao_2 and Sao_2 readings are possible on an ABG while capillary bed dysfunction ensues. Normal readings indicate O_2 is being provided in adequate amounts to saturate Hgb effectively; but the ABG is unable to assess whether all tissue beds are receiving O_2 or whether the cells are able to use the O_2. Until metabolic acidosis ensues due to accumulation of lactic acid byproducts of anaerobic metabolism due to hypoperfusion, the ABG and Spo_2 readings may be misleading.

COLLABORATIVE MANAGEMENT: ACUTE RESPIRATORY ACIDOSIS
Care Priorities
1. **Restore effective alveolar ventilation.**
   - *Symmetrical lung expansion:* Always check for symmetrical lung expansion, particularly if the patient was recently admitted for trauma, has recently had central line placement, or been recently intubated or extubated. A pneumothorax may be present, which may cause ineffective ventilation.
   - *Support ventilation:* If $Paco_2$ is greater than 50 to 60 mm Hg, there may be a need to intubate and place the patient on mechanical ventilation, or if already ventilated, there may be a need to reevaluate the ventilation settings. The primary mechanism to treat respiratory acidosis is to increase the tidal volume (V_T) and/or the respiratory rate (F), to increase minute ventilation ($V_T \times F$). Care must be taken to ensure the adequate minute ventilation; therefore, if low tidal volumes are applied, the respiratory rate may need to be increased. If the lung compliance allows, the flow rate (how rapidly the volume is delivered) may also be increased. This will prolong exhalation time and allow adequate time for CO_2 excretion.
- *Bronchodilation:* Consider the use of inhaled beta-agonists to maintain open airways.
2. **Normalize the pH.**
   - Although a life-threatening pH must be corrected to an acceptable level promptly, a normal pH is not the immediate goal. Generally, the use of bicarbonate is avoided because of the risk of alkalosis when the respiratory disturbance has been corrected and the secondary effect of blocking the signal to the hemoglobin to release the oxygen (shift to the left). Note: If lactic acidosis is present, the patient has *metabolic* acidosis, which has resulted from ineffective tissue oxygenation. Supporting ventilation will not resolve lactic acidosis. And bicarbonate may temporarily neutralize the pH, but may actually worsen tissue hypoxia.
3. **Evaluate compensation (occurs in the presence of normal renal function).**
   - Although the kidneys' response to an abnormal pH level is slow (4 to 48 hours), they are able to facilitate a nearly normal pH level by excreting or retaining large quantities of HCO_3^- or H^+ from the body. Remember that the level of available HCO_3^- is always opposite the level of H^+ present in the plasma. HCO_3 is partnered as it buffers H^+, which yields carbonic acid.

Compensatory Response for Acute Respiratory Acidosis   When the respiratory acid level (CO_2) increases, carbonic acid increases and the pH decreases. The increased H_2CO_3 (carbonic acid) is presented to the kidney, where the H^+ is separated from the bond, yielding HCO_3^-. The "free" bicarbonate (HCO_3^-) provides additional buffer. In addition, the kidneys excrete the "free" H^+ (hydrogen ions) in the urine to reduce the acid level. When the kidneys are functional, the pH decrease seen from increased respiratory acid is less dramatic. The decrease in pH is modified to a small degree by intracellular buffering. To compensate for the acidosis created by increased CO_2, K^+ ions are released from cellular proteins and H^+

ions take their place, bound to the proteins. The result is frequently serum hyperkalemia (reflective of intracellular hypokalemia). This is much more common and dangerous in the presence of metabolic acidosis (particularly diabetic ketoacidosis [DKA]).

Renal or kidney compensation via synthesis and retention of HCO_3 regulates much of the acid; however, the pH will not be returned to perfect. When the carbonic acid is converted into HCO_3^- (bicarbonate buffer), the pH will only be decreased by about 0.03 for every 10 mm Hg increase in CO_2.

1. Original problem: pH 7.28, $Paco_2$ 55, HCO_3^- 24 [Pao_2 92 mm Hg, Sao_2 91%]
2. With kidney compensation: pH 7.35, $Paco_2$ 55, HCO_3^- 32 [Pao_2 100mm Hg, Sao_2 100%]

With compensation: Over time, if ventilation is not effectively managed, the HCO_3^- will increase to 32, which will correct the pH to 7.35. The CO_2 remains 55. O_2 provided at 4 L/ min by nasal cannula increases the Pao_2 to 100% and the Sao_2 to 100%.

$$\text{Problem: } \uparrow\uparrow CO_2 + H_2O \rightarrow \uparrow\uparrow H_2CO_3 \leftrightarrow HCO_3^- + H^+$$

With the same $Paco_2$, the pH is corrected to 7.35, on the acid side but in the normal range. Whenever the pH is less than 7.40, it reflects either a normal variation OR abnormality with compensation.

With compensation:

pH 7.35: Acid side but in range of normal
$Paco_2$ 55 mm Hg: Acid and outside of range of normal
Problem: Respiratory acidosis, but pH is in range of normal
HCO_3^- 32 mEq/L: The kidneys took the H_2CO_3, separated it into HCO_3^- and H^+; then, excreted the H^+ and retained the end product, the bicarbonate (made from the CO_2).

Renal compensation: $\uparrow\uparrow CO_2 + H_2O \rightarrow \uparrow H_2CO_3 \rightarrow \uparrow\uparrow HCO_3^- + \downarrow\downarrow H^+$

Ultimately, the increase in $Paco_2$, which created an increase in carbonic acid, made the pH decrease. When the increased carbonic acid was presented to the kidney, it was separated into $\uparrow\uparrow$ bicarbonate ($H^+ \downarrow\downarrow$) and yielded the end diagnosis: compensated respiratory acidosis! The kidneys must be functional for compensation to occur in the presence of respiratory acidosis.

CHRONIC RESPIRATORY ACIDOSIS

The compensated scenario just described is what is often seen with chronic hypercapnia, which occurs with chronic obstructive pulmonary disorders (e.g., chronic emphysema and bronchitis, cystic fibrosis), restrictive disorders (e.g., pneumothorax, hemothorax, Pickwickian syndrome), neuromuscular abnormalities (e.g., myasthenia gravis, Guillain-Barré syndrome, amyotrophic lateral sclerosis), respiratory center depression (e.g., brain tumor, stroke, bleed, head injury), and poor ventilation management. In patients with a chronic lung disease, a near-normal pH is the result of kidney compensatory mechanisms as discussed earlier.

Patients with chronic lung disease can experience acute rises in $Paco_2$ or lose their metabolic compensation (increased production of metabolic acid or loss of renal function) secondary to superimposed disease states such as pneumonia, hypermetabolic cellular hypoxia, or renal dysfunction. If the chronic compensatory mechanisms in place (e.g., elevated) are inadequate to meet the sudden increase in $Paco_2$ or if the circulation of metabolic acids increases, pH may change rapidly. In fact, these patients frequently have normal HCO_3^- measures upward of 30. As an acute (on top of chronic) process begins, the pH drops, but the bicarbonate may be slower to reflect the real problem. Care must be taken when evaluating patients with chronic respiratory acidosis who have secondary issues.

Clinical Presentation

Patients have possible increased work of breathing, anxiety, pallor, sweating; reflective of respiratory distress. In advanced respiratory acidosis, somnolence and inability to awaken patient are common. CO_2-based acidosis has a sedative-like effect on patients. Sleep may ensue following distress, giving the false impression the problem has resolved, when in reality, the problem has resulted in sufficient CO_2 accumulation for the patient to lose consciousness. Patients with obstructive sleep apnea (OSA) are at risk for developing respiratory acidosis.

Physical Assessment

Patients have decreased depth of respirations with an initially increased rate or decreased rate and depth of respirations in severe respiratory acidosis. With obstructive lung disease or acute asthma exacerbation, audible wheezing may be present. With severe asthma, the chest can become silent, indicative gas exchange is extremely impaired, and the patient is close to respiratory arrest.

Monitoring Parameters

Use pulse oximetry to assess if hypoxemia ensues due to ineffective ventilation. The patient needs close observation for deterioration, so appropriate steps can be taken to provide noninvasive positive pressure ventilation (NPPV) such as bilevel positive airway pressure (BiPAP) or endotracheal (ET) intubation with mechanical ventilation.

CARE PLAN: RESPIRATORY ACIDOSIS

Impaired gas exchange *related to alveolar-capillary membrane changes secondary to pulmonary tissue destruction*

- -

GOALS/OUTCOMES Within 24 hours of initiation of treatment, patient improves and is reevaluated. The ultimate goal of adequate gas exchange is evidenced by $Paco_2$, pH, and Sao_2 that are normal or within 10% of patient's baseline.
NOC Respiratory Status Ventilation, Vital Signs Status, Respiratory Status: Gas Exchange, Symptom Control Behavior, Comfort Level, Endurance, Acid-Base Management: Respiratory Acidosis

Respiratory Monitoring
1. Monitor serial ABG results to assess patient's response to therapy. Consult physician for significant findings: increasing $Paco_2$ with decreasing pH, Pao_2, and Sao_2 values.
2. Monitor O_2 saturation via pulse oximetry (Spo_2). Compare Spo_2 with Sao_2 values to assess reliability. Watch Spo_2 closely, especially when changing Fio_2 or to evaluate patient's response to treatment (e.g., repositioning, chest physiotherapy).
3. Assess and document patient's respiratory status: respiratory rate and rhythm, exertional effort, and breath sounds. Compare pretreatment findings with posttreatment findings (e.g., O_2 therapy, physiotherapy, medications) for evidence of improvement.
4. Assess and document patient's level of consciousness (LOC). If $Paco_2$ increases, be alert to subtle, progressive changes in mental status. A common progression is agitation $\longrightarrow$ insomnia $\longrightarrow$ somnolence $\longrightarrow$ coma. To avoid a comatose state caused by rising CO_2 levels, always evaluate the arousability of a patient with elevated $Paco_2$ who appears to be sleeping. Consult physician if the patient is difficult to arouse.

Oxygen Therapy
1. Ensure appropriate delivery of prescribed O_2 therapy. Assess the patient's respiratory status after every change in Fio_2. Patients with chronic CO_2 retention may be very sensitive to increases in Fio_2, resulting in depressed ventilatory drive. If the patient requires mechanical ventilation, be aware of the importance of maintaining the compensated acid-base status. If the $Paco_2$ is rapidly decreased by excessive mechanical ventilation (dropping $Paco_2$, but a remaining excess of bicarbonate), a severe metabolic alkalosis (posthypercapnic metabolic alkalosis) could develop. The sudden onset of metabolic alkalosis may lead to hypocalcemia or hypokalemia, which can result in tetany (see *Hypocalcemia*, 57). Severe alkalosis also can precipitate cardiac dysrhythmias.

Ventilation Assistance
1. Assess for presence of bowel sounds, and monitor for gastrointestinal (GI) distention, which can impede movement of the diaphragm and further restrict ventilatory effort.
2. Assess for presence of symmetric lung expansion and normal resonance of lung fields. Hyperresonance and asymmetry indicate pneumothorax; dullness and asymmetry indicate solid tissue or fluid occupation of lung or pleural space (e.g., hemothorax, pleural effusion, hyperplasia).
3. In patients who have obstructive lung disease and are not intubated, encourage use of pursed-lip breathing (inhalation through nose, with slow exhalation through pursed lips), which helps airways to remain open and allows for better air excursion. Optimally, this technique will diminish air entrapment in the lungs and make respiratory effort more efficient.

NIC Cough Enhancement, Acid-Base Management, Respiratory Acidosis, Mechanical Ventilation, Artificial Airway Management, Oral Health Maintenance

ADDITIONAL NURSING DIAGNOSES AND INTERVENTIONS:

Nursing diagnoses and interventions are specific to the pathophysiologic process. See *Acute Pneumonia*, (p. 373), *Acute Lung Injury and Acute Respiratory Distress Syndrome*, (p. 365) and *Acute Respiratory Failure*, (p. 383), along with *Mechanical Ventilation*, (p. 99).

RESPIRATORY ALKALOSIS

PATHOPHYSIOLOGY

The problem is alveolar hyperventilation, which results in an increased pH
Example: pH 7.48, $Paco_2$ 30, HCO_3 23

Step 1: The pH is not perfect.

The problem is named by the direction of the pH in respect to perfect: Is the pH on the alkaline side greater than 7.40 or the acid side less than 7.40? The pH of 7.48 is on *the alkaline side.*

Step 2: The $Paco_2$ has decreased to 30 mm Hg, reflecting *hypocapnia ($Paco_2$ less than 35 mm Hg).*

This signals alveolar hyperventilation (decreased respiratory acid causing an alkaline pH). When minute ventilation is increased, CO_2 decreases, which causes H_2CO_3 to also decrease (production of carbonic acid decreases) and the pH becomes alkalotic. Question: Is there a problem? The CO_2 has decreased and the pH has gone up. The problem is respiratory alkalosis.

Step 3: The HCO_3^- is 23, which is less than perfect but still in the normal range.

It must be determined if there is a metabolic contribution to the alkalosis or if there is compensation provided by the kidney retaining acid and excreting bicarbonate. The BE is +1, within the normal range.

Step 4: The Pco_2 is low, the pH is high and the HCO_3 is normal.

The patient is exhibiting a rapid respiratory rate, with deep breaths.

Step 5: The Spo_2 may be normal, as the patient is breathing very rapidly, but effectively. However, when the respiratory rate is very rapid, there is less time for oxygen diffusion, so it is possible that the patient's oxygen levels may decrease.

$$Problem: \downarrow\downarrow CO_2 + H_2O \leftrightarrow \downarrow\downarrow H_2CO_3 \leftrightarrow HCO_3^- + H^+$$

ACUTE RESPIRATORY ALKALOSIS

Respiratory alkalosis occurs as a result of an increase in the minute ventilation (alveolar hyperventilation). Defined as $Paco_2$ less than 35 mm Hg, acute alveolar hyperventilation results most frequently from anxiety and is commonly referred to as hyperventilation syndrome. *Caution must be applied to evaluate whether hyperventilation is actually a compensatory mechanism for primary metabolic acidosis.* Although it may become necessary to control the patient's minute ventilation, in the presence of metabolic acidosis, loss of the hyperventilation compensation may create a life-threatening acidotic pH and profound refractory hypotension and asystole.

In the alkalotic environment, cells release H^+ and take up K^+. The result is frequently serum hypokalemia (with intracellular hyperkalemia). Kidney compensation for the respiratory alkalosis is not clinically apparent for 4 to 48 hours. Acute respiratory alkalosis progresses to chronic respiratory alkalosis if it persists for longer than 6 hours and/or renal compensation occurs.

Compensatory Response to Respiratory Alkalosis:

The kidneys, within 4 to 48 hours, should excrete bicarbonate and retain additional H^+ in an attempt to compensate for the lack of respiratory acid.
- *Acute respiratory alkalosis:* First 4 to 48 hours HCO_3^- (and therefore the increase in H^+) will decrease 2 mEq/L for every 10 mm Hg decrease in PCO_2.

- *Chronic respiratory alkalosis:* After about 48 hours, the amount of bicarbonate should decrease 4 mEq/L of HCO_3 for every 10 mm Hg decrease in PCO_2.
1. Original problem: pH 7.48, $Paco_2$ 30, HCO_3^- 23
2. With compensation: pH 7.44, $Paco_2$ 30, HCO_3^- 19

If there is only one problem contributing to the pH abnormalities, the pH should behave as expected. In other words, a removal of acid by the problem system should be compensated by acid retention by the opposing system.
1. Original problem: $\downarrow\downarrow CO_2 + H_2O \leftarrow \downarrow\downarrow H_2CO_3 \leftrightarrow HCO_3^- + H^+$
2. With compensation: $\downarrow\downarrow CO_2 + H_2O \leftarrow \downarrow H_2CO_3 \leftarrow \downarrow\downarrow HCO_3^- + \uparrow\uparrow H^+$

CHRONIC RESPIRATORY ALKALOSIS

Chronic respiratory alkalosis is a state of chronic hypocapnia caused by stimulation of the respiratory center. The decreased $Paco_2$ stimulates the renal compensatory response and results in a proportionate decrease in plasma bicarbonate (and retention of H^+) until a new, steady state is reached. Maximal renal compensatory response requires several days to occur and can result in a normal or near-normal pH. Chronic respiratory alkalosis is not commonly seen in acutely ill patients but, when present, it can signal a poor prognosis.

Safety Alert *In alkalotic environments*

- *Sodium and potassium:* May be decreased slightly to profoundly (potassium will shift from the extra cellular space to the intracellular space in exchange for H^+).
- *Serum calcium:* May be decreased because of increased calcium and bicarbonate binding. Signs of hypocalcemia include muscle cramps, hyperactive reflexes, carpal spasm, tetany, and convulsions.
- *Serum phosphorus:* May decrease (less than 2.5 mg/dl), especially with salicylate intoxication and sepsis, because the alkalosis causes increased uptake of phosphorus by the cells. No symptoms occur, and treatment usually is not required unless a preexisting phosphorus deficit is present.

Clinical Presentation
Presentation includes lightheadedness, anxiety, paresthesias (especially of the fingers), and circumoral numbness. In extreme alkalosis, confusion, tetany, syncope, and seizures may occur.

Physical Assessment
Increased rate and depth of respirations (hyperventilation) are present.

Monitoring Parameters
Cardiac dysrhythmias are present.

CARE PLAN: RESPIRATORY ALKALOSIS
Ineffective breathing pattern Related to anxiety, tissue hypoxia, or work of breathing

GOALS/OUTCOMES If the respiratory alkalosis is primary, within 4 hours of initiating treatment, the patient has improved. Final outcome is that the patient's breathing pattern is effective as evidenced by a state of eupnea: $Paco_2 \geq$ 35 mm Hg and pH 7.45.

NOC Respiratory Status: Ventilation, Vital Signs Status, Respiratory Status: Gas Exchange, Symptom Control Behavior, Comfort Level, Endurance; Electrolyte and Acid-Base Balance.

Ventilation Assistance
1. To help alleviate anxiety, reassure the patient that a staff member will remain with him or her.
2. Encourage patient to breathe slowly. Pace the patient's breathing pattern by having him or her mimic your own breathing pattern.
3. Monitor patient's cardiac rhythm. Consult physician for new or increased dysrhythmias. With acute respiratory alkalosis, even a modest alkalosis can precipitate dysrhythmias in a patient with a preexisting heart disease who is also taking inotropic drugs (see Appendix 6). In part, this is caused by the hypokalemia that occurs with alkalosis.
4. Administer sedatives or tranquilizers as prescribed. Assess and document effectiveness.

5. Have the patient rebreathe into a paper bag as indicated (if practice is supported by institution).
6. Ensure that the patient rests undisturbed after his or her breathing pattern has stabilized. Hyperventilation can result in fatigue.

> **Safety Alert**   *Hyperventilation may lead to hypocalcemic tetany despite a normal or near-normal calcium level because of increased binding of calcium. For chronic respiratory alkalosis, nursing diagnoses and interventions are specific to the pathophysiologic process.*

ADDITIONAL NURSING DIAGNOSES AND INTERVENTIONS
Nursing diagnoses and interventions are specific to the pathophysiologic process.

METABOLIC ACIDOSIS

PATHOPHYSIOLOGY
Accumulation of metabolic acids, reflected by decreased HCO_3^- (less than 22 mEq/L) with a pH decreased below 7.40. Metabolic acids are circulating acids that cannot be exhaled. These acids should be neutralized by buffers, excreted by the kidneys, or metabolized.
Example: pH 7.28, $Paco_2$ 39, HCO_3^- 16, Pao_2 98 mm Hg, Sao_2 99%

Step 1: The pH is not perfect.
The problem is named by the direction of the pH in respect to perfect: Is the pH on the alkaline side greater than 7.40 or the acid side less than 7.40? The pH of 7.28 is on the acid side.
- *Increased acid production:* Excessive lactate and ketones cause acidosis and contribute more unmeasured positives (H^+) into circulation. When an increase in H^+ occurs, HCO_3^- goes down as the role of bicarbonate is to buffer H^+. The conjugation of H^+ and HCO_3^- yields an increase in carbonic acid. As carbonic acid (H_2CO_3) goes up, the pH goes down.
- *Decreased renal tubular function (acute tubular necrosis [ATN] or chronic failure):* If the kidney is unable to excrete H^+, or if the load is beyond tubular transport capabilities, an increase in H^+ occurs. HCO_3^- decreases as the role of bicarbonate is to buffer H^+ and the kidney has lost the capability to regulate and create appropriate bicarbonate. The conjugation of H^+ and available HCO_3^- yields an increase in carbonic acid. As carbonic acid (H_2CO_3) increases (goes up), the pH decreases (goes down).
- *Ingestion of exogenous acids:* Certain medications can cause an increase in circulating acids. Alcohols and other ingested acids can facilitate a wide anion gap.

Step 2: The Paco₂ is slightly decreased to 39 but within the normal range.
The patient does not have respiratory alkalosis or acidosis. The lungs are not retaining CO_2 and are not exhaling excessive amounts of CO_2.

Step 3: The HCO₃⁻ is 16, which is less than perfect and below the normal range.
This means the metabolic acid (H^+) is increased. The BE is −6, below the normal range. It must be determined if the acidosis is the problem or a compensatory mechanism for metabolic alkalosis.
Problem: Metabolic acidosis caused by *any/or any combination thereof:*
- Kidney failure to regulate and excrete acid appropriately (acute or chronic kidney failure)
- Cellular production of acid increases beyond normal regulatory capacity due to metabolic alterations (lactic acidosis or ketosis)
- Ingestion of acids (aspirin, methanol)

> **Safety Alert**   *Metabolic acidosis is much more difficult to diagnose than the simple presence or absence of acid. One must first diagnose the cause of the acid-base imbalance.*

Step 4: The PCO_2 is normal, while the HCO_3^- is decreased.

The patient is exhibiting a normal respiratory rate, with normal depth. With a decreased HCO_3^- and normal $Paco_2$, the patient is not compensating for a respiratory alkalosis. The $Paco_2$ would be decreased with respiratory alkalosis if the decreased HCO_3^- was a compensatory response. The decreased HCO_3^- is the primary problem; an acute metabolic acidosis. Question: What is the problem? The HCO_3^- has decreased, and no compensation is apparent by the lungs. The respiratory rate and depth have not increased.

Step 5: The Pao_2 and Sao_2 are normal, as the patient is breathing normally.

The patient has normal oxygenation.

Step 6 : Performed only in metabolic acidosis: Evaluate glucose, ketones, lactate and tissue oxygenation (if necessary).

Example: pH 7.28, $Paco_2$ 39, HCO_3^- 16, Pao_2 98 mm Hg, Sao_2 99%
One must investigate why H+ is increased and bicarbonate is down.

- Is it a compensatory response? If so the $H_2CO_3\downarrow$ (H$^+\uparrow$) and the patient would have a pH on the alkaline side, indicating compensatory response for respiratory alkalosis.
- Is it a kidney problem? In this case, BUN and/or Creatinine would be elevated.
- Is it a high chloride (inadequate buffer) problem? If so, the chloride would have to be high.
- Did the patient ingest acids?
- Is it a tissue metabolism issue? In this case, the patient will have high ketones and/or lactic acidosis.

If the answer to the first four questions is no, or those problems do not seem significant enough for the pH change, a further investigation must be performed.

Evaluation of glucose and ketones may be reviewed (*Diabetic Ketoacidosis* [DKA], p. 713). Evaluation of tissue perfusion and oxygenation requires more testing.

1. Lactic acidosis may be caused by an *oxygenation-related, metabolic acidosis,* which results from a significant increase in lactate production during anaerobic metabolism. This excess lactate production also yields H$^+$.
2. *Lactic acidosis IS NOT respiratory acidosis!* Respiratory acidosis is primarily a ventilation problem, while lactic acidosis is primarily a perfusion-, metabolic stress-, or cellular O_2 consumption or extraction–related problem. Lactic acidosis will be discussed further as part of the section on metabolic acidosis.
3. Additional measures are sometimes used in critically ill patients for evaluation of tissue hypoxia. Mixed venous and/or central venous saturation of Hgb evaluates the tissue use of O_2. The comparison of arterial (precellular) saturation to central or mixed venous (postcellular) is most commonly used to evaluate the tissue O_2 consumption compared to O_2 delivery.
4. *Mixed venous (Svo_2) or central venous oxygen saturation ($Scvo_2$):* This value is measured by an indwelling O_2 probe/sensor on the tip of a catheter placed in the central vein (CVP catheter) or PA (PA catheter). Measurement may provide an early indication of perfusion failure or increased tissue demands for O_2, reflected by a decreased mixed venous saturation of Hgb. If this saturation is normal or high but the patient has an increased lactate level, the cells may be unable to extract or use the O_2, which frequently occurs in the later stages of severe sepsis.
5. *Mixed venous saturation values (Svo_2):* This value should always be correlated with other tissue indicators of hypoxia, base deficit, widening anion gap, serum bicarbonate, and lactate levels. The difference between arterial and venous blood gases is reflective of global O_2 consumption. The following standard parameters are based on mixed venous blood gas and have not yet been standardized for central venous gases; however, the basic principles are the same.
6. Sao_2 reflects reservoir bound O_2 and very indirectly reflects delivery.
   a . Normal Sao_2 is 0.95 to 1.00.
7. Svo_2 or $Scvo_2$ reflects unused O_2 or remaining reservoir after release of needed O_2 has occurred.
   b. Normal Svo_2 is 0.60 to 0.80 OR $Scvo_2$ of 0.65 to 0.85.
8. Sao_2 minus $Scvo_2$ reflects O_2 consumption.
   c. $1.00 - 0.70 = 0.30$, about 30% consumption

9. Sao_2 minus Svo_2 divided by Sao_2 reflects O_2 extraction ratio, valued at around 20% to 30%.

   d. $1.00 - 0.70 \div 1.00 = 30\%$

10. *Normal oxygen extraction ratio is 20% to 30%:* In other words, the patient should use normally between 20% and 30% of their total available O_2. O_2 extraction is a mathematical formula that assists in evaluating the compensatory mechanisms: First line of compensation is to *increase the delivery* of O_2 (increase the cardiac output [CO], amount of Hgb, and O_2 saturation), and the second line is to *release O_2 from Hgb* to provide more dissolved O_2 at the cell level, resulting in a shift to the right in the dissociation curve (Figure 1-1).

11. *Patients presenting with a normal Svo_2 and persistent lactic acidosis are NOT normal.* They are not using O_2 appropriately. Patients who are using more than 20% to 30% are signaling inadequate O_2 delivery, dipping into second-line compensation, which is very risky, because the cells may undergo acute hypoxia.

LACTIC ACIDOSIS (LACTATE LEVEL GREATER THAN 4 mmol/L)
Assessing Perfusion and Oxygen Consumption at the Cellular Level

Since the early work of Dr. William Shoemaker, it has been well identified that global tissue hypoxia accompanies all categories of shock, including both O_2 delivery and O_2 utilization shock. The work of the Surviving Sepsis Campaign to establish early goal-directed therapy validated the role of lactate measurement as a guide to therapy. When cells are in a shock state, *O_2 delivery shock* is present. Shock effects the mechanics of delivery, while *systemic inflammatory response* or *severe sepsis*, with the secondary effects of endothelial dysfunction, vasodilation, inflammatory mediation, and unopposed procoagulation, interfere with the utilization of O_2 at a microcirculatory and cellular level. Large areas of the capillary beds may be hypoperfused, resulting in cells resorting to anaerobic metabolism to survive. Anaerobic metabolism results in the production of lactic acid, a metabolic acid that can create acidosis if compensation fails. The ABG reflects a decreased pH but does NOT always reflect a markedly decreased Pao_2 and Sao_2. Persistent tissue-level hypoxia further exacerbates the systemic inflammatory response and may lead to multiple organ dysfunction (MODS) and eventually death.

Arterial lactate concentration is dependent on the balance between its production and consumption. In the critically ill septic population, increased glucose metabolism, increased energy expenditures, and profound catabolism are the norm. The corresponding lactic acidosis signals physiologic stress but may not necessarily be evidence of tissue hypoxia. The concomitant energy expenditures—along with metabolic dysfunction—will increase lactate production, but high levels of clearance may mask this disturbing trend.

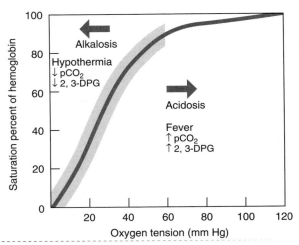

Figure 1-1 The oxyhemoglobin dissociation curve. (From Stillwell SB: *Mosby's critical care nursing reference,* ed. 4. St. Louis, 2006, Mosby.)

These conditions, coupled with an out-of-control inflammatory response and increasing oxygenation dysfunction at the tissue level, combine to produce a profound tissue acidosis. The lactate production is further increased via other abnormal pathways that are specifically related to metabolic dysfunction, even in the absence of tissue hypoxia (type B lactic acidosis). The main cause of the significantly increased lactate is still a puzzle. One factor is the failure of ATP production, which clearly occurs in the presence of a profound O_2 supply/demand imbalance (type A lactic acidosis). This in turn affects the mitochondrial ability to utilize pyruvate, and the increased pyruvate is indicative of a profound metabolic hyperlactatemia, an elevated lactate/pyruvate ratio, increased glucose, and low energy production. Ultimately, as severe sepsis progresses, it evolves into a mediator-induced cardiac failure state, with profound intra-arterial hypovolemia.

Special Considerations for Patients with Lactic Acidosis

Nguyen et al. (2004), in their work related to early goal-directed therapy when treating sepsis, validated that the higher the clearance of lactate in the first 6 hours after resuscitation, the lower is the mortality. In those first hours of evaluation and resuscitation, achieving a normal Scvo$_2$ along with an increasing lactate clearance is the desired therapeutic endpoint, reducing the potential for MODS.

Measuring Lactic Acids

In any patient whose condition arouses suspicion (e.g., with tachycardia, tachypnea, hyperventilation, and/or hypotension), it is essential to directly measure acid.

1. Lactate level: All patients who run the risk of cellular hypoxia must have a sample drawn for a lactate level to evaluate for lactic acidosis. An arterial lactate sample should be placed on ice and taken as soon as possible to the lab. Any lactate greater than 4 mmol/dL needs to be investigated for severe tissue hypoxia and hypoperfusion. Lactates > 2 mmol/dL should be observed along with the clinical conditions of the patient. Serial lactates should be performed to evaluate therapy effectiveness and follow the clearance level. A lactate clearance greater than 10%/24 hr is considered a successful measure of therapeutic intervention for severe sepsis.

   a. Limitations to lactate level: The value of lactate is obviously limited due to lactate concentrations that are affected by both production as well as elimination. Liver dysfunction, ketosis, and many medications administered in the critical care unit may affect the measured lactate levels. Therefore, lactate levels by themselves will not give as much beneficial information as those in the presence of wide anion gap and low or normal Scvo2.

Serum ketone level: If the glucose is elevated, a serum ketone level should also be drawn to evaluate for ketoacidosis.

ACUTE METABOLIC ACIDOSIS

Example: pH 7.28, Paco$_2$ 39, HCO$_3^-$ 16, Pao$_2$ 98 mm Hg, Sao$_2$ 99%

Bicarbonate is decreased, which always means that H$^+$ is elevated. If H$^+$ is elevated, resulting in increased carbonic acid, and the pH is down even slightly, the problem is acid accumulation. In this case, it is acute metabolic acidosis, without compensation!

 Safety Alert *As the nonvolatile acid H$^+$ increases, it will displace the intracellular potassium, resulting in a serum hyperkalemia but an intracellular hypokalemia. The lungs should increase the rate and depth of respirations to exhale CO_2, to compensate for the excess metabolic acid, so the pH can return to normal range.*

Consideration must be allowed for glucose and ketones. If lactic acid is elevated, it may become necessary to find the culprit utilizing tissue oxygenation measures.

Glucose 120, Ketones -, Lactate 6.8

This then points to acute metabolic (lactic) acidosis!

COMPENSATORY RESPONSE TO ACUTE METABOLIC ACIDOSIS

When H$^+$ (acid) increases, pH decreases in the plasma. The central respiratory center in the brain responds by *increasing the rate and depth of ventilation* to 4 to 5 times the normal level to exhale significant amounts of CO_2 and returning the carbonic acid; therefore, the pH is back to normal (but never perfect if there is a problem). The decrease in pH (high presence of H^+) stimulates respirations. Attempts to compensate occur rapidly, as manifested by lowering of the $Paco_2$, which may be reduced to as little as 10 to 15 mm Hg. The most important mechanism for ridding the body of excess H^+ is the increase in acid excretion through ventilation. In addition, if the kidney is functional, acid will be excreted and bicarbonate reabsorbed. Nonvolatile acids, however, may accumulate more rapidly than the body's buffers can neutralize them, compensated for by the respiratory system, or excreted by the kidneys.

1. Original problem: Acute metabolic acidosis: pH 7.28, $Paco_2$ 39, HCO_3^- 16
2. With compensation: pH 7.36, $Paco_2$ 30, HCO_3^- 16, Sao_2 99%, Pao_2 100%

   Original problem: $CO_2 + H_2O \leftrightarrow \uparrow\uparrow H_2CO_3 \leftarrow \downarrow\downarrow HCO_3^- + H^+\uparrow\uparrow$

   With compensation: $\downarrow\downarrow CO_2 + H_2O \leftarrow H_2CO_3 \leftarrow \downarrow\downarrow HCO_3^- + H^+\uparrow\uparrow$

Step 1: pH 7.36: Acid side but in range of normal.

- Question: Is there a problem? Normal variation in pH from perfect, OR a compensated acid-base imbalance?
- Answer: Yes, there is a problem. The pH decrease is not a normal variation because the $Paco_2$ and HCO_3 are out of range.

Step 2: $Paco_2$ 30 mm Hg.

On the alkaline side, which does not coincide with the direction of the pH change.

Step 3: HCO_3^- 16 mEq/L.

Decreased and out of range, which means the metabolic acid (H^+) is increased! HERE is the CAUSE of the problem that decreased the HCO_3^-.

Step 4: The $Paco_2$ is increased in the presence of a decreased HCO_3^-.

Acid reduced the pH, and the lungs compensated by separating the H_2CO_3 into CO_2 and H_2O and, with the help of the respiratory center, exhaled the CO_2. The problem is *COMPENSATED metabolic acidosis.*

Step 5: The Pao_2 and Sao_2 are normal, as the patient is breathing normally.

The patient has normal oxygenation.

COLLABORATIVE MANAGEMENT: ACUTE METABOLIC ACIDOSIS
Care Priorities

1. **It is most important to treat the underlying disorder if possible.**
- *Diabetic ketoacidosis:* Insulin and fluids. If acidosis is severe (with a pH of less than 7.15 or HCO_3^- 6 to 8 mEq/L), judicious administration of $NaHCO_3$ may be necessary.
- *Alcoholism-related ketoacidosis:* Glucose and saline.
- *Diarrhea:* Usually occurs in association with other fluid and electrolyte disturbances; correction addresses concurrent imbalances.
- *Acute renal failure:* Hemodialysis or peritoneal dialysis to maintain an adequate level of plasma HCO_3^-.
- *Renal tubular acidosis:* May require modest amounts (less than 100 mEq/day) of bicarbonate.
- *Poisoning and drug toxicity:* Treatment depends on drug ingested or infused. Hemodialysis or peritoneal dialysis may be necessary.
- *Lactic acidosis:* Correction of underlying disorder related to hypoxia and/or hypoperfusion. Mortality associated with lactic acidosis is high. Unless pH is life-threatening, treatment with $NaHCO_3$ is generally not indicated and may actually be harmful.
2. **Measure Anion gap:** Anion gap is an estimate of the differences between measured and unmeasured cations (positively charged particles, such as Na and H^+ respectively) and measured and unmeasured anions (negatively charged particles such as HCO_3^- and Cl^-). Normally, cations and anions are equally balanced in live humans (in vivo), but when measured in the laboratory (in vitro), the difference may be between 10 to 12 mmol/L. This difference is termed a normal gap (between + and – ions). Particles that possess charges tend to have high affinity to bind to other particles that possess charges that are opposite their own (hence the term, "opposites attract"). *Anion gap is used to determine if a metabolic acidosis is due to an accumulation of nonvolatile acids such as lactic acid or ketoacids.* Both contribute a positive charge due to excess H^+ or from net loss of bicarbonate

(e.g., diarrhea). The *gap is not affected* when a patient has *metabolic acidosis purely from kidney failure*. The formula for calculation of anion gap is:

$$Na - (Cl^- + HCO_3)$$
$$\text{Normal Value: } 12 \pm 2 \text{ (10 to 14)}$$

Unmeasured cations: Calcium, magnesium, gamma globulins, potassium (bind negative charged particles)

Unmeasured anions: Albumin, phosphate, sulfate, lactate, hydrogen ion (bind positive charge particles)

3. **Treat the pH:** Only if the patient's life is threatened by the pH. Sodium bicarbonate ($NaHCO_3$) may be indicated when arterial pH is ≤ 7.15. The usual mode of delivery is IV drip: 2 or 3 ampules (44.5 mEq/ampule) in 1000 ml D_5W, although $NaHCO_3$ may be given by IV push in emergencies. Deficit should be calculated and replaced accordingly. Concentration depends on severity of the acidosis and presence of any serum sodium disorders. $NaHCO_3$ must be given very cautiously to avoid metabolic alkalosis and pulmonary edema as a result of the sodium load. Total body weight $\times$ Base deficit/4 = Amount of sodium bicarbonate that must be replaced.

4. **Manage hyperkalemia:** Usually, serum hyperkalemia is present, but an intracellular potassium deficit may be present. If a potassium deficit exists (K^+ less than 3.5), it must be corrected before $NaHCO_3$ is administered, because when the acidosis is corrected, the potassium shifts back to intracellular spaces. This shift in K^+ could result in a profound serum hypokalemia with serious consequences, such as cardiac irritability with fatal dysrhythmias and generalized muscle weakness. See *Hypokalemia,* p. 52, for more information.

5. **Support ventilation:** If mechanical ventilation is required on the basis of ABG results and clinical signs, it is important that the patient's compensatory hyperventilation be allowed to continue to prevent acidosis from becoming more severe. Therefore the respiratory rate on the ventilator should not be set lower than the rate at which patient has been breathing spontaneously, and the tidal volume should be large enough to maintain compensatory hyperventilation until the underlying disorder can be resolved.

NURSING DIAGNOSES AND INTERVENTIONS

Nursing diagnoses and interventions are specific to the pathophysiologic process. See nursing diagnoses and interventions in *Mechanical Ventilation* (p. 99), *Acute Respiratory Failure* (p. 383), *Emotional and Spiritual Support of the Patient and Significant Others* (p. 200), *Acute Renal Failure/ Acute Kidney Injury* (p. 584), and *Diabetic Ketoacidosis* (p. 713).

CHRONIC METABOLIC ACIDOSIS

ASSESSMENT
History and Risk Factors
Affected patients generally include those with chronic renal failure, renal tubular acidosis, loss of alkaline fluid (e.g., with diarrhea or pancreatic or biliary drainage) for greater than 3 to 5 days.

Clinical Presentation
Usually the process leading to chronic metabolic acidosis is gradual and the patient is symptom free until serum HCO_3^- is ≤ 15 mEq/L. Fatigue, malaise, and anorexia may be present in relation to the underlying disease.

Clinical Presentation
Findings vary, depending on underlying disease states and the severity of the acid-base disturbance and the speed with which it developed. There may be changes in LOC that range from fatigue and confusion to stupor and coma.

Physical Assessment
Tachycardia (until pH less than 7, then bradycardia), decreased BP, tachypnea leading to alveolar hyperventilation (may be Kussmaul respirations), dysrhythmias, and shock state. Depending on the type of shock and the vascular response, skin temperature and color will be

affected. Mild metabolic acidosis (HCO_3^- 15 to 18 mEq/L) may result in no symptoms, whereas symptoms will develop with a pH less than 7.2.

Monitoring Parameters

A waveform suggestive of hyperkalemia (prolonged PR interval, widened QRS, and peaked T waves) may occur. Persistent tachycardia may indicate tissue hypoperfusion.

ECG: Detects dysrhythmias, which may be caused by metabolic acidosis or hyperkalemia. Changes seen with hyperkalemia include peaked T waves, depressed ST segment, decreased size of R waves, decreased or absent P waves, and widened QRS complex. Ventricular fibrillation may occur.

COLLABORATIVE MANAGEMENT: CHRONIC METABOLIC ACIDOSIS

Care Priorities

1. **Normalize the pH with alkalizing agents:**
   - For serum HCO_3^- levels less than 15 mEq/L, oral alkalis may be administered ($NaHCO_3$ tablets or sodium citrate and citric acid oral solution [Shohl solution]). They are used cautiously to prevent fluid overload and tetany caused by hypocalcemia.
   - *Caution:* Be alert to the possibility of pulmonary edema, if bicarbonate is administered parenterally to patients with renal insufficiency or cardiovascular disorders.
2. **Manage hypophosphatemia with oral phosphates:**
   - These are given if hypophosphatemia is present; it is not common with chronic renal failure but may result from overuse of phosphate binders given to treat hyperphosphatemia (very common with chronic renal failure).
3. **Provide renal replacement therapies:**
   - Hemodialysis, citrated blood and renal replacement therapy (CRRT), or peritoneal dialysis may be indicated for chronic renal failure or other disease processes (see *Acute Renal Failure/Acute Kidney Injury*, p. 584).

NURSING DIAGNOSES AND INTERVENTIONS FOR CHRONIC METABOLIC ACIDOSIS

Nursing diagnoses and interventions are specific to the underlying pathophysiologic process.

METABOLIC ALKALOSIS

PATHOPHYSIOLOGY

Elevated HCO_3^- levels (greater than 26 mEq/L) reflect decreasing circulating metabolic acids (H^+). Caution must be applied to differentiate compensatory alterations in response to respiratory acidosis versus primary disorder. The diagnosis is made by the presence of elevated serum HCO_3^- (up to 45 to 50 mEq/L). Acute metabolic alkalosis most commonly reflects:

- *Excessive loss of hydrogen ions:* Loss of gastric acid from vomiting or gastric suction, diuretic therapy
- *Excessive resorption of bicarbonate:* Post hypercapnic alkalosis (which occurs when chronic CO_2 retention is corrected rapidly)
- *Ingestion or administration of alkaline:* Excessive $NaHCO_3$ administration (i.e., overcorrection of a metabolic acidosis) or ingestion of over-the-counter antacids

Even when the causative factors have been removed, the alkalosis will be sustained until volume and electrolyte disturbances that are contributing to the alkalosis have been corrected. Severe alkalosis (pH greater than 7.6) is associated with high morbidity and mortality. Acidosis is better tolerated than alkalosis. Spo_2 *will be used for Step 5*, because a discussion of Pao_2 and Sao_2 does not add to knowledge of metabolic alkalosis.

Example: pH 7.58, $Paco_2$ 40 mm Hg, HCO_3^- 35, Sao_2 99%, Pao_2 99 mm Hg

Problem: $CO_2 + H_2O \leftrightarrow H_2CO_3 \downarrow\downarrow \leftrightarrow \uparrow\uparrow HCO_3^- + H^+ \downarrow\downarrow$

Step 1: The pH is not perfect.

The problem is named by the direction of the pH in respect to *perfect*: on the acid side less than 7.40 or the alkaline side greater than 7.40.

Example: pH 7.58 on alkaline side, outside of range of normal

Question: Is there a problem? YES

Step 2: The Paco$_2$ is 40 mm Hg, which is perfect.
This indicates Paco$_2$ is not driving the increase in pH.

Step 3: HCO$_3^-$ has increased to 35 mEq/L, indicating the kidneys are retaining bicarbonate (H$^+$ is decreased).
HERE is the cause of the problem: ACUTE metabolic alkalosis.

HCO$_3^-$ is 35 (up and out of range), which means the metabolic acid, and H$^+$ is decreased.

Step 4: The Paco$_2$ has not increased in an attempt to help correct or compensate for the increased HCO$_3^-$.
The patient is exhibiting a normal respiratory rate, with normal depth. With an increased HCO$_3^-$, and normal Paco$_2$, the patient is not compensating for a metabolic alkalosis.

Step 5: The Pao$_2$ and Sao$_2$ are normal, as the patient is breathing normally. The patient has a normal oxygenation.
Compensatory Response to Metabolic Alkalosis When H$^+$ (acid) decreases, pH increases. The central respiratory center in the brain responds by *decreasing the rate and depth of ventilation* (in the normal lung) to 50% to 75% of the normal level. This method of compensation is very poorly tolerated, as patients will almost stop breathing.
   Original problem: pH 7.58, Paco$_2$ 40 mm Hg, HCO$_3^-$ 35
   With compensation: pH 7.45, Paco$_2$ 59 mm Hg, HCO$_3^-$ 35

$$\text{Compensation:} \uparrow\uparrow CO_2 + H_2O \longrightarrow H_2CO_3\downarrow\downarrow \leftrightarrow \uparrow\uparrow HCO_3^- + H^+\downarrow\downarrow$$

   In this example: pH 7.45, Paco$_2$ 59 mm Hg, HCO$_3^-$ 35, Sao$_2$ 99%, Pao$_2$ 99 mm Hg

Step 1: pH 7.45.
Alkaline side, inside the normal range
   • Question: Is there a problem, despite the normal pH? *YES!* Other values are *abnormal.*

Step 2: Paco$_2$ 59 mm Hg.
On the acid side, opposite the pH, which is toward the alkaline side. The Paco$_2$ is not the problem but rather a COMPENSATION. The increased Paco$_2$ would not increase the pH to alkaline. This measure is in the wrong direction to be the cause.

Step 3: HCO$_3^-$ 35 mEq/L.
Increased and out of range. HERE is the cause of the problem. *Metabolic alkalosis* is present because the metabolic acid (H$^+$) is decreased.

Step 4: The Paco$_2$ is elevated at 59 mm Hg.
The Paco$_2$ has increased response to an increased HCO$_3^-$ level. When HCO$_3^-$ increases, the pH goes up, indicating less H$^+$ is present in the body. The pH normalized on the alkaline side, so the patient has *fully compensated metabolic alkalosis.*

Step 5: The Sao$_2$ is normal.
The patient has a normal rate and depth of respirations.

COLLABORATIVE MANAGEMENT: ACUTE METABOLIC ALKALOSIS
Management will depend on the underlying disorder. Mild or moderate metabolic alkalosis usually does not require specific therapeutic interventions. Correction of chloride deficits is a priority for treatment with many underlying disorders.

Care Priorities
1. **Manage chloride deficit:** Normal saline infusion may correct volume (chloride) deficit in patients with gastric alkalosis because of gastric losses. Metabolic alkalosis is difficult to correct if hypovolemia and chloride deficit are not corrected.

2. **Correct hypokalemia:** Potassium chloride (KCl) is indicated for patients with low potassium levels. KCl is preferred over other potassium salts because chloride losses can be replaced simultaneously.
3. **Sodium and potassium chloride:** Effective for post hypercapnic alkalosis, which occurs when chronic CO_2 retention is corrected rapidly (e.g., via mechanical ventilation). If adequate amounts of chloride and potassium are not available, renal excretion of excess HCO_3^2 is impaired and metabolic alkalosis continues.
4. **Cautious IV administration of isotonic hydrochloride solution, ammonium chloride, or arginine hydrochloride:** May be warranted if severe metabolic alkalosis (pH greater than 7.6 and HCO_3^2 greater than 40 to 45 mEq/L) exists, especially if chloride or potassium salts are contraindicated. The medication is delivered via continuous IV infusion at a slow rate, with frequent monitoring of IV insertion site for signs of infiltration. Ammonium chloride and arginine hydrochloride may be dangerous to patients with renal or hepatic failure.

NURSING DIAGNOSES AND INTERVENTIONS FOR ACUTE METABOLIC ALKALOSIS

Nursing diagnoses and interventions are specific to the underlying pathophysiologic process.

CHRONIC METABOLIC ALKALOSIS

PATHOPHYSIOLOGY

Chronic metabolic alkalosis results in a pH greater than 7.45 and HCO_3^- greater than 26 mEq/L. $Paco_2$ will be elevated (greater than 45 mm Hg) to compensate for the loss of H^+ or excess serum HCO_3^-. The three clinical situations in which this can occur are the following:

1. Abnormalities in the kidneys' excretion of HCO_3^- related to a mineralocorticoid effect
2. Loss of H^+ through the GI tract
3. Long-term diuretic therapy, especially with the thiazides and furosemide. A compensatory increase in $Paco_2$ (up to 50 to 60 mm Hg) may be seen. Respiratory compensation is very limited because of the hypoxemia, which develops as a result of decreased alveolar ventilation.

Compensatory Response to Chronic Alkalosis When extracellular fluid is alkalotic, the kidneys conserve H^+ and eliminate HCO_3^-, resulting in excretion of alkalotic urine. Renal excretion of acid load and increase in circulating buffer represent the major compensation for respiratory deficits and require a normally functioning kidney. Although the kidneys' response to an abnormal pH level is slow (4 to 48 hours), they are able to facilitate a nearly normal pH level by excreting or retaining large quantities of HCO_3^- or H^+ from the body. Acid-base balance is regulated by increasing or decreasing H^+ and bicarbonate (HCO_3^-) concentration in body fluids. A series of complex reactions with H^+ secretion, sodium ion (Na^+) resorption, HCO_3^- retention, and ammonia synthesis (excretes H^+ in the urine) occurs.

Clinical Presentation

Muscular weakness, neuromuscular instability, and hyporeflexia because of accompanying hypokalemia are present. Decrease in GI tract motility may result in an ileus. Severe alkalosis can result in apathy, confusion, and stupor. Seizures may occur.

PHYSICAL ASSESSMENT

Decreased respiratory rate and depth, periods of apnea, tachycardia (atrial or ventricular) are present.

Monitoring Parameters

Atrioventricular dysrhythmias as a result of cardiac irritability secondary to hypokalemia; prolonged QT intervals are present. See *Hypokalemia*, p. 52.

- *Urinalysis:* Urine chloride levels can help identify the cause of the metabolic alkalosis. Urine chloride level will be less than 15 mEq/L if hypovolemia and hypochloremia are present, and greater than 20 mEq/L with excess retained HCO_3^-. This test is not reliable if diuretics have been used within the previous 12 hours.
- *ECG findings:* To assess for dysrhythmias, especially if profound hypokalemia or alkalosis is present.

COLLABORATIVE MANAGEMENT: CHRONIC METABOLIC ALKALOSIS

The goal is to correct the underlying acid-base disorder via the following interventions.

Care Priorities

1. **Fluid management:** If volume depletion exists, normal saline infusions are given.
2. **Potassium replacement:** If a chloride deficit also is present, KCl is the drug of choice. If a chloride deficit does not exist, other potassium salts are acceptable.
   - *IV potassium:* If the patient is undergoing cardiac monitoring, up to 20 mEq/hr of KCl is given for serious hypokalemia. Concentrated doses of KCl (greater than 40 mEq/L) require administration through a central venous line because of blood vessel irritation.
   - *Oral potassium:* This tastes very unpleasant; 15 mEq/glass is all most patients can tolerate, with a maximum daily dose of 60 to 80 mEq. Slow-release potassium tablets are an acceptable form of KCl. All forms of KCl may be irritating to gastric mucosa.
3. **Dietary:** The normal diet contains 3 g or 75 mEq of potassium but not in the form of KCl. Dietary supplementation of potassium is not effective if a concurrent chloride deficit also is present.
4. **Potassium-sparing diuretics:** These may be added to treatment if thiazide diuretics are the cause of hypokalemia and metabolic alkalosis.

Clinical Presentation

Patient may be free of symptoms. With severe potassium depletion and profound alkalosis, patient may experience weakness, neuromuscular instability, and a decrease in GI tract motility, which can result in ileus.

Physical Assessment

Decreased respiratory rate and depth, and tachycardia (atrial or ventricular) are present.

Monitoring Parameters

Frequent PVCs or U waves with hypokalemia and alkalosis are present.

NURSING DIAGNOSES AND INTERVENTIONS FOR CHRONIC METABOLIC ALKALOSIS

Nursing diagnoses and interventions are specific to the underlying pathophysiologic process. For NIC and NOC, see Acute Metabolic Alkalosis.

ALTERATIONS IN CONSCIOUSNESS

PATHOPHYSIOLOGY

Consciousness is a state of awareness of the self and environment composed of three aspects: arousal (ability to awaken), ability to perceive internal and external stimuli, and ability to perform goal-directed behavior. Alterations in these aspects of consciousness result in a broad spectrum of syndromes including coma, delirium, and cognitive dysfunction. Factors precipitating various alterations in consciousness are listed in Table 1-3. These precipitating factors arise from intrinsic causes (medical condition and associated problems) and extrinsic causes (environmentally produced). Impaired consciousness, regardless of etiology, results in higher complication rates, puts the patient's safety at risk, causes longer hospital stays, and is linked to higher morbidity and mortality. Three states of impaired consciousness can be recognized in hospitalized patients—coma, delirium, and cognitive dysfunction. While each of these conditions may arise from distinct medical problems, the clinical features often are similar and may be superimposed on each other, making diagnosis and treatment more complex. *Change in mental status is often the early warning sign of a medical emergency.* The differential diagnosis is critical to the proper treatment of these mental status changes. The following are descriptions of normal mental status variants that require further evaluation.

Delirium

This is a state of disordered attention that reflects an underlying acute or subacute process. It is usually a transient condition (may be prolonged) that develops along a continuum including a clouding of consciousness, confusion, attention deficit, global cognitive impairment, and psychosis. Symptoms include disorientation to time, place, and person; disorganized thinking; fear;

Table 1-3	**FACTORS PRECIPITATING ALTERATIONS IN CONSCIOUSNESS**		
Delirium	**Coma**	**Cognitive Dysfunction**	**Others**
Age	Cerebral structural	Chronic Alcohol (ETOH)	Coma related to cerebral
Aggressive/dominant	changes (brain injury)	abuse	or metabolic disorders
personality	Cerebrovascular impair-	Dementia	Diffuse organic cerebral
Anesthesia time	ment (hemorrhage,	Huntington disease	dysfunction (confused
Arrhythmias	ischemia, or edema)	Hydrocephalus	with the catatonic
Body temperature	CNS dysfunction	Hypoxic/anoxic injury	behavior of schizophrenia
Cardiac dysrhythmia	Metabolic conditions	Parkinson disease	or severe depressive
Cerebral disorders	(liver/renal failure, dia-	Stroke	reaction)
Dehydration	betic coma, ketoacidosis)	Thiamine, vitamin B	Drug overdose
Disease severity in ICU		deficiencies	Alcohol (ETOH)
Drug interactions		Traumatic brain injury	intoxication
Electrolyte imbalances			Locked-in syndrome
End-stage disease (renal,			Stupor
liver)			Supranuclear motor
Impaired communication			deafferentation related to
Infection			brainstem injury
Metabolic disturbances			Vegetative state
Neuropsychiatric disorders			(coma vigil)
Pulmonary disorders			
Sleep deprivation			
Surgery (hip, cardiac,			
neurologic)			
Toxins			
Use of physical restraints			
Withdrawal syndromes			

irritability; misinterpretation of sensory stimuli (e.g., pulling at tubes and dressings); appearance of being distracted; altered psychomotor activity; altered sleep-wake cycles; memory impairment; hallucinations; inappropriate communication (e.g., yelling, swearing, nonsensical speech); and dreamlike delusions. Lucid intervals alternate with episodes of delirium. Patients may have difficulty following commands. Daytime drowsiness is contrasted with nighttime agitation. Clinical variants of delirium include the hyperactive-hyperalert form, the quiet form, and a combination form that combines the hyperactive-hyperalert and quiet forms to produce both lethargy and agitation (Figure 1-2).

Coma
Coma is an alteration in arousal and diminished awareness of self and environment. No understandable response to external stimuli or inner need is elicited. No language is spoken. There are no covert or overt attempts at communication or eye opening. Spontaneous purposeful movement and/or localizing movements are absent. Motor responses to noxious stimuli are reflexive and do not result in recognizable defensive movements. Sleep-wake cycles are absent on the electroencephalogram (EEG). The extent of coma is difficult to quantify because limits of consciousness are difficult to define. Self-awareness can only be inferred from appearance and actions. Coma occurs when normal central nervous system (CNS) function is disrupted by alteration in the cerebral structure (brain injury), cerebrovascular impairment (hemorrhage, ischemia, or edema), or metabolic conditions (hepatic encephalopathy). If coma persists for longer than 4 weeks, it is defined as transitioning to a vegetative state.

Differential Diagnosis of Coma   The characteristics of syndromes or mental states described next are useful in determining the differential diagnosis because many have similar presentations.

- *Stupor*—Deep sleep with responsiveness only to vigorous and repeated stimuli with return to unresponsiveness when the stimulus is removed. Stupor usually is related to

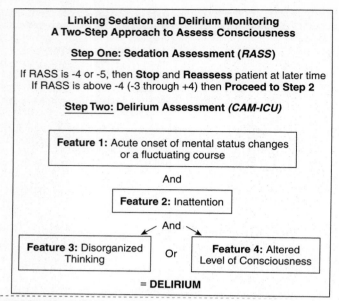

Figure 1-2 Linking sedation and delirium monitoring; a two-step approach to assess consciousness.
(Copyright E. Wesley Ely, MD, MPH, and Vanderbilt University, 2002.)

diffuse organic cerebral dysfunction but may be confused with the catatonic behavior of schizophrenia or the behavior associated with a severe depressive reaction.

- *Minimally conscious state (MCS)*–Describes patients who demonstrate inconsistent but reproducible behavior indicating awareness of self and environment. Generally they cannot reliably follow commands or communicate but show visual fixation and tracking and have emotional and/or behavioral responses to external stimuli. Once the patient consistently follows commands, can reliably communicate, and uses objects in a functional way, the minimal conscious state ends. Although the etiology is uncertain, MCS seems to be related to diffuse, bilateral, subcortical, and hemispheric damage.

- *Akinetic mutism (AM)*–Subcategory of MCS in which a decrease in spontaneity and initiation of actions, thoughts, speech, or emotion is present. Sensory motor function is normal. Visual tracking and eye movements are intact, and there is occasional speech and movement to commands. However, internally guided behavior is absent because cortical activation is inadequate. AM is associated with orbitomesial frontal cortex, limbic system, and reticular formation lesions.

- *Vegetative state (VS)*–Vegetative state is a subacute or chronic condition that may follow the coma of brain injury or occur independently of coma (e.g., dementia). Transition from coma to VS occurs if coma without detectable awareness of environment persists for longer than 4 weeks. Onset of VS is signaled by a return of wakefulness (eyes are open and sleep patterns may be observed) with return of spontaneous control of autonomic function but without observable signs of cognitive function. The patient cannot follow commands, offers no comprehensible sounds, and displays no localization to stimuli. There is complete loss of meaningful interaction with the environment. When the VS continues for weeks or months, it is considered persistent vegetative state (PVS). PVS may exist for many years because the autonomic and vegetative functions necessary for life have been preserved. PVS generally resolves more quickly in traumatic brain–injured patients than in nontrauma patients.

- *Locked-in syndrome (LIS)* –Characterized by paralysis of all four extremities and the lower cranial nerves but with preservation of cognition. Associated with deafferentation (disruption of the pathways of the brainstem motor neurons), this condition prevents the patient from communicating with a full range of language and body movement. Generally, consciousness, vertical eye movement, and eyelid blinking are intact and provide a mechanism for communication. LIS is classified by the degree of voluntary speech and motor function preservation. In complete LIS, there is total immobility and anarthria (inability to speak). In incomplete LIS, there is vertical eye movement and blinking function. LIS can be distinguished from a vegetative state because patients give appropriate signs of being aware of themselves and their environment. Often, sleep patterns are disrupted (see Spinal cord injury)

Cognitive Dysfunction

This is an alteration in thought process involving many of the following brain functions: memory, learning, language, attention, judgment, reasoning, reading, and writing. Aphasia, or difficulty understanding language or with responding with the proper words, may also be present. Dysphagia, or difficulty swallowing, occurs because of attention deficits or muscle weakness. These cognitive impairments, whether permanent or transitory, are overlooked and therefore underdiagnosed or incorrectly diagnosed. See Table 1-3 for factors contributing to cognitive dysfunction during critical illness.

ASSESSMENT: ALTERATIONS IN CONSCIOUSNESS
Goal of Assessment

- Evaluate for changes in behavior, including ability to both understand and comply with directions.
- Determine if altered behaviors have occurred in the past or occur regularly; new-onset changes in mental status should be very closely evaluated. Considerations of cause may include withdrawal from abused substances, a reaction to a new medication, hypoxia, and hypoglycemia.
- Determine the severity of the change in behavior from baseline; acute changes require prompt action.
- *An acute or unexpected change in mental status that occurs should be investigated immediately and requires an extensive medical evaluation with labs, physical examination, and neuroimaging.* These patients may need immediate transfer to a higher level of care. **Change in mental status is often the earliest warning sign of a medical emergency!**
- Resist the temptation to sedate an agitated patient prior to completing a full assessment, to ensure the patient is not hypoxic or hypoglycemic. Assessment for hypoxia should include both a ventilation and a perfusion assessment. The ABG includes an estimated Hgb level, which can prove to be invaluable to determine if patient may have internal bleeding.

History and Risk Factors

- *Age*—Older adults (age 60 years and older) more prone to alterations in consciousness, especially with changes in the environment
- *Brain injury*—Lesions of the cortex, subcortex, and brainstem caused by global or focal ischemia, stroke, or traumatic brain injury (see *Traumatic Brain Injury*, p. 331)
- *Cerebral disorders*—Deteriorating brain conditions, such as expanding lesions, hydrocephalus, Parkinson disease, dementia, or mental health disorders (bipolar, depression, schizophrenia)
- *Cardiovascular status*—Disorders that lower CO (heart failure, myocardial infarction, shock states), procedures that cause post cardiotomy delirium, intra-aortic balloon pump sequelae, hypoperfusion states (altered cerebral perfusion pressure [CPP] and dysrhythmias)
- *Pulmonary disorders*—Those causing hypoxia and hypoxemia such as pneumonia, ARDS, pulmonary emboli
- *Drug therapy*—Sedation, analgesia, drug toxicity, drug interactions, drug withdrawal, or drug sensitivity
- *Surgical factors*—Nature (hip, cardiac, neurosurgery patients at increased risk) and extent of surgery and anesthesia time
- *Infection*—Bacteremia, urinary tract infections, pneumonia, or sepsis
- *Perceptual/sensory factors*—Sleep deprivation, sensory overload, sensory deprivation, impaired sensation (hypesthesia, decreased hearing or vision), impaired perception (inability to identify environmental stimuli), and impaired integration (inability to integrate environmental stimuli)

- *Metabolic factors*–Changes in glucose level, hypermetabolism, hypometabolism, and endocrine crises (diabetic coma, ketoacidosis, pituitary dysfunction or injury)
- *Fluid and electrolyte disturbances*–Sodium and potassium imbalances, hypovolemia, or dehydration

Vital Signs

All of the following vital sign changes may be associated with an alteration in consciousness:
- Fever may indicate possible sepsis and/or bacteremia.
- Tachycardia may indicate hypovolemia, resulting from dehydration or bleeding. If patient has undergone a recent invasive procedure, evaluation for internal bleeding is warranted. Tachycardia is also present with fever and hypoglycemia.
- Tachypnea, if coinciding with tachycardia, may reflect the same findings but is also a compensatory mechanism to help control acidosis. Tachypnea is also present during a panic attack, as well as hypoxia.
- Bradypnea may be associated with high doses of narcotics used for pain control.
- Head-injured patients may exhibit signs of increased intracranial pressure (ICP), which vary depending on the degree of pressure elevation (see *Traumatic Brain Injury*, p. 331)
- Hypotension may indicate a later sign of shock or may be associated with higher doses of antihypertensive medications, narcotics, or other medications that can slow the HR or reduce the BP.

Observation and Neurologic Evaluation

- The patient's normal baseline neurologic status must be documented and used for comparison.
- Baseline neurologic findings elicited from each component of the examination must be documented.
- Requires a thorough evaluation of mental/emotional status, cranial nerve function, motor function, sensory function, and reflex activity. When alterations in consciousness are manifested, the mental/emotional component of the examination is of particular importance.
- In patients who are unconscious or demonstrate low-level function, assessment techniques are used that do not require patient participation, such as coma and cognitive functioning scales. The purpose of assessment is to determine the extent of wakefulness and cognition through observed responses, such as eye opening, movement of the head and body, verbalization, and ability to follow commands. These observations alone will not fully discriminate the subtle differences in altered states of arousal.
- Assessment should be accompanied by an in-depth history focusing on the possible etiology of the change in mental status. Extensive cognitive testing including attention, concentration, memory, and learning assessments is performed when the patient is arousable and aware.

Screening Labwork

- ABGs evaluate ventilation, perfusion, estimated Hgb and acid-base status.
- Point-of-care blood glucose readings evaluate for hypoglycemia or extreme hyperglycemia.
- Biochemical panel evaluates for electrolyte imbalances, such as hyponatremia, which are associated with alterations in behavior.

Neurologic Evaluation

- *Mental status testing*–Subjective assessment requiring patient cooperation for best results (Box 1-1).
- *Mini-Mental Status Examination*–Objective neuropsychologic tool used to measure orientation, recall, attention, calculation, and language. Scores less than 23 (total 25) indicate cognitive dysfunction. Patient participation is necessary for this examination (Box 1-2).
- *Glasgow Coma Scale*–Quantitative, three-part scale that assesses the patient's ability to open his or her eyes, to move, and to speak/communicate. Scores range from 3 to 15, with 3 being unresponsive to all stimuli and 15 being awake, alert, and oriented. Patients who are unable to cooperate can be evaluated using this scale. See Appendix 1.

| Box 1-1 | **MENTAL STATUS COMPONENT OF THE NEUROLOGIC EXAMINATION** |

1. General appearance
2. Behavior (with and without stimulation)
3. Language and speech characteristics (organization, coherence, and relevance)
4. Mood and affect
5. Judgment
6. Abstract thinking
7. Orientation (time, place, person)
8. Attention and concentration
9. Memory (recent, remote)
10. Cognition (following commands, fund of knowledge, interpretation of information, problem solving)

| Box 1-2 | **MINI-MENTAL STATUS EXAMINATION** |

1. What is the year, season, date, day, month? (5 points)
2. Where are we: state, county, town, hospital, room? (5 points)
3. Name three objects. (3 points)
4. Count backward by sevens (e.g., 100, 93, 86, 79, 72). (5 points)
5. Repeat same three objects from item number 3 above. (3 points)
6. Name a pencil and watch. (2 points)
7. Follow a three-step command. (3 points)
8. Write a sentence. (1 point)
9. Follow the command "close your eyes." (1 point)
10. Copy a design (e.g., two hexagons). (1 point)

- *Coma Recovery Scale*–Quantitative 35-item scale used to assess brain function at four levels (generalized, localized, emergent, cognitively mediated). Seven responses are evaluated: arousal and attention, auditory perception, visual perception, motor function, oromotor ability, communication, and initiative. Patients who are unable to cooperate can be evaluated using this scale.
- *Confusion Assessment Method (CAM, CAM-intensive care unit)*–Four-part scale used to evaluate confusion. Onset and course, inattention, disorganized thinking, and level of consciousness are assessed (Box 1-3).
- *Intensive Care Delirium Screening Checklist (ICDSC)*–Eight-item scale that rates behavioral responses exhibited by patients in intensive care; delirium is indicated with scores *greater than* 4 to 8 (Table 1-4).
- *Richmond Agitation-Sedation Scale (RASS)*–Scores sedation and agitation with a 10-point scale using verbal and physical stimulation to determine patient's response; used to titrate medications (Table 1-5).
- *Rancho Los Amigos (RLA) Cognitive Functioning Scale*–Seven-level scale that describes levels of cognitive functioning. Levels range from unresponsive to sensory stimuli to purposeful/appropriate actions. Patients who cannot cooperate can be evaluated using this scale (Table 1-6).

DIAGNOSTIC TESTS
Neurodiagnostic Testing
See *Traumatic Brain Injury*, p. 331.

Neuropsychological Testing
Although not a routine part of critical care, neuropsychological testing should be planned and implemented for patients with brain injury or altered consciousness when they enter the recovery phase. This testing provides a comprehensive baseline for rehabilitation by evaluating higher cortical functions, such as memory, learning, and language.

Box 1-3	CAM-ICU WORKSHEET

Feature 1: acute onset or fluctuating course
Positive if you answer 'yes' to either 1A or 1B.
> Positive or Negative
> 1A: Is the patient different than his/her baseline mental status?
> Or
> 1B: Has the patient had any fluctuation in mental status in the past 24 hours as evidenced by fluctuation on a sedation scale (e.g., RASS), GCS, or previous delirium assessment?
> Yes or No

Feature 2: inattention
Positive if either score for 2A or 2B is less than 8.
> Attempt the ASE letters first. If patient is able to perform this test and the score is clear, record this score and move to Feature 3. If patient is unable to perform this test or the score is unclear, then perform the ASE Pictures. If you perform both tests, use the ASE Pictures' results to score the feature.
> Positive or Negative
> 2A: ASE Letters: record score (enter NT for not tested)
> Directions: Say to the patient, "*I am going to read you a series of 10 letters. Whenever you hear the letter 'A,' indicate by squeezing my hand.*" Read letters from the following letter list in a normal tone.
> S A V E A H A A R T
> Scoring: Errors are counted when patient fails to squeeze on the letter "A" and when the patient squeezes on any letter other than "A."
> Score (out of 10): _____
> 2B: ASE Pictures: record score (enter NT for not tested)
> Directions are included on the picture packets.
> Score (out of 10): _____

Feature 3: disorganized thinking
Positive if the combined score is less than 4
> Positive or Negative
> 3A: Yes/No Questions
> (Use either Set A or Set B, alternate on consecutive days if necessary):

Set A	Set B
1. Will a stone float on water?	1. Will a leaf float on water?
2. Are there fish in the sea?	2. Are there elephants in the sea?
3. Does one pound weigh more than two pounds?	3. Do two pounds weigh more than one pound?
4. Can you use a hammer to pound a nail?	4. Can you use a hammer to cut wood?

> Score ____ (Patient earns 1 point for each correct answer out of 4)
> 3B: Command
> Say to patient: "Hold up this many fingers" (Examiner holds two fingers in front of patient). "Now do the same thing with the other hand" (Not repeating the number of fingers). (If patient is unable to move both arms, for the second part of the command ask patient "Add one more finger"). Score____ (Patient earns 1 point if able to successfully complete the entire command)
> Combined Score (3A+3B):_____ (out of 5)

Feature 4: altered level of consciousness
Positive if the Actual RASS score is anything other than "0" (zero)
> Positive Negative
> Overall CAM-ICU (Features 1 and 2 and either Feature 3 or 4): Positive Negative

Table 1-4 — INTENSIVE CARE DELIRIUM SCREENING CHECKLIST

Symptom Checklist (total 0–8)	Level of Consciousness Scoring
Level of Consciousness	*Level of Consciousness*
Inattentiveness	
Disorientation	A = no response: none
Hallucination, delusion, psychosis	B = response to intense, repeated stimuli (loud voice or pain): none
Agitation	C = response to mild or moderate stimulation: 1
Inappropriate speech or mood	D = normal wakefulness: 0
Sleep/wake cycle disturbance	E = exaggerated response to normal stimulation: 1
Symptom fluctuation	(if A or B above do not complete evaluation for the day)

Adapted from Bergeron N, Dubois M-J, Dumont M, Dial S, Skrobik Y: Intensive care delirium screening checklist: evaluation of a new screening tool. *Intens Care Med* 27(5):859–864, 2001.

Table 1-5 — RICHMOND AGITATION-SEDATION SCALE (RASS)*

+4 Combative	Overtly combative or violent, immediate danger to staff
+3 Very agitated	Pulls on or removes tubes or catheters, aggressive behavior toward staff
+2 Agitated	Frequent nonpurposeful movement or patient-ventilator dyssynchrony
+1 Restless	Anxious or apprehensive but movements not aggressive or vigorous
0 Alert and calm	
−1 Drowsy	Not fully alert, sustained (>10 seconds) awakening, eye contact to voice
−2 Light sedation	Briefly (<10 seconds) awakens with eye contact to voice
−3 Moderate sedation	Any movement (but no eye contact) to voice
−4 Deep sedation	No response to voice, any movement to physical stimulation
−5 Unarousable	No response to voice or physical stimulation

Procedure

1. Observe patient. Is patient alert and calm (score 0)?
   Does patient have behavior that is consistent with restlessness or agitation?
   Assign score +1 to +4 using the criteria listed above.

2. If patient is not alert, in a loud speaking voice state patient's name and direct patient to open eyes and look at speaker. Repeat once if necessary. Can prompt patient to continue looking at speaker.
   Patient has eye opening and eye contact, which is sustained for more than 10 seconds (score −1).
   Patient has eye opening and eye contact, but this is not sustained for 10 seconds (score −2).
   Patient has any movement in response to voice, excluding eye contact (score −3).

3. If patient does not respond to voice, physically stimulate patient by shaking shoulder and then rubbing sternum if there is no response.
   Patient has any movement to physical stimulation (score −4).
   Patient has no response to voice or physical stimulation (score −5).

Reproduced with permission from Sessler CN, Gosnell M, Grap MJ, et al: The Richmond Agitation-Sedation scale: Validity and reliability in adult intensive care unit patients. *Am J Respir Crit Care Med* 166:1338, 2002. Copyright © 2002 American Thoracic Society.

Continued

Table 1-5	RICHMOND AGITATION-SEDATION SCALE (RASS)—cont'd

Score Term Description

+4 Combative	Overtly combative, violent, immediate danger to staff
+3 Very agitated	Pulls or removes tube(s) or catheter(s); aggressive
+2 Agitated	Frequent non purposeful movement, fights ventilator
+1 Restless	Anxious but movements not aggressive or vigorous
0 Alert and calm	
−1 Drowsy	Not fully alert, but has sustained awakening (eye-opening/eye contact) to voice (>10 seconds)
−2 Light sedation	Briefly awakens with eye contact to voice (<10 seconds)
−3 Moderate sedation	Movement or eye opening to voice (but no eye contact)
−4 Deep sedation	No response to voice, but movement or eye opening to physical stimulation
−5 Unarousable	No response to voice or physical stimulation

Procedure for RASS Assessment

1. Observe patient
   a. Patient is alert, restless, or agitated. (score 0 to +4)

2. If not alert, state patient's name and say to open eyes and look at speaker.
   b. Patient awakens with sustained eye opening and eye contact. (score −1)
   c. Patient awakens with eye opening and eye contact, but not sustained. (score −2)
   d. Patient has any movement in response to voice but no eye contact. (score −3)

3. When no response to verbal stimulation, physically stimulate patient by shaking shoulder and/or rubbing sternum.
   e. Patient has any movement to physical stimulation. (score −4)
   f. Patient has no response to any stimulation. (score −5)

*From Sessler CN, Gosnell M, Grap MJ, et al: The Richmond Agitation-Sedation Scale: validity and reliability in adult intensive care patients. *Am J Respir Crit Care Med* 2002; 166:1338–1344, 2002; and Ely EW, Truman B, Shintani A, et al: Monitoring sedation status over time in ICU patients: the reliability and validity of the Richmond Agitation-Sedation Scale (RASS). *JAMA* 2003; 289:2983–2991, 2003.

Laboratory Studies
If there is an acute or unexpected mental status change, lab studies include CBC, electrolytes, cardiac profile, blood and sputum cultures, urinalysis and culture, chest radiograph, and other tests as determined by signs and symptoms.

COLLABORATIVE MANAGEMENT
Care Priorities
When evaluating an alteration in consciousness or a change in mental status, acute and/or life-threatening problems must be ruled out before proceeding. Although severe agitation is difficult to manage, it is imperative that physiologic causes of agitation are ruled out before sedating the patient. Once acute causes of the problem are ruled out, the following measures may be implemented for other causes of behavioral changes:
1. For Delirium
   - Determine and correct physiologic imbalances and drug interactions.
   - Correct sensory/perceptual deficits (e.g., provide hearing aid, eyeglasses).
   - Reorient patient to the self and environment.
   - Perform neuropsychologic testing.
   - Implement appropriate medications to help control behavior.
   - Consider geriatric consult.
   - Manage pain and assess effectiveness.

Table 1-6 COGNITIVE REHABILITATION GOALS

Level	Response	Goal/intervention
I	None	*Goal:* Provide sensory input to elicit responses of increased quality, frequency, duration, and variety.
II	Generalized	
III	Localized	*Intervention:* Give brief but frequent stimulation sessions, and present stimuli in an organized manner, focusing on one sensory channel at a time; for example: *Visual:* Intermittent television, family pictures, bright objects *Auditory:* Tape recordings of family or favorite song, talking to patient, intermittent TV or radio *Olfactory:* Favorite perfume, shaving lotion, coffee, lemon, orange *Cutaneous:* Touch or rub skin with different textures such as velvet, ice bag, warm cloth *Movement:* Turn, ROM exercises, up in chair *Oral:* Oral care, lemon swabs, ice, sugar on tongue, peppermint, chocolate
IV	Confused, agitated	*Goal:* Decrease agitation, and increase awareness of environment. This stage usually lasts 2–4 weeks. *Intervention:* Remove offending devices (e.g., NG tube, restraints), if possible. Do not demand patient follow through with task. Provide human contact unless this increases agitation. Provide a quiet, controlled environment. Use a calm, soft voice and manner around patient.
V	Confused, inappropriate	*Goal:* Decrease confusion and incorporate improved cognitive abilities into functional activity.
VI	Confused, appropriate	*Intervention:* Begin each interaction with introduction, orientation, and interaction purpose. List and number daily activity in the sequence in which it will be done throughout the day. Maintain a consistent environment. Provide memory aids (e.g., calendar, clock). Use gentle repetition, which aids learning. Provide supervision and structure. Reorient as needed.
VII	Automatic, appropriate	*Goal:* Integrate increased cognitive function into functional community activities with minimal structuring. *Intervention:* Enable practicing of activities. Reduce supervision and environmental structure. Help patient plan adaptation of ADLs and home living skills to home environment.

Modified from Rancho Los Amigos Hospital, Inc. Levels of Cognitive Functioning (scale based on behavioral descriptions or responses to stimuli). From Swift CM: Neurologic disorders. In Swearingen PL, editor: *Manual of medical-surgical nursing care*, ed 4, St. Louis, 1999, Mosby.
ADLs, activities of daily living; *NG,* nasogastric; *ROM,* range of motion.

- Minimize sedative medications; benzodiazepines are not recommended.
- Check bowel and bladder function.
- Establish sleep/wake cycle.
- Treat agitation.
- See Sedation and neuromuscular blockade, p. 158).

Safety Alert *For mild confusion, good outcomes have been reported with the use of reorientation techniques and observation (use of "sitters"), especially by family members. Prophylactic low-dose haloperidol did not prevent delirium but was noted to reduce the severity of delirium in one study. Newer atypical antipsychotic medications, those with fewer extrapyramidal side effects such as quetiapine, olanzapine, and risperidone, have been shown to have an efficacy similar to haloperidol.*

2. **For Coma**
   - Assess cognitive function using the RLA score or Coma Recovery Scale.
   - Initiate a sensory stimulation program for patients with low-level cognition.
   - Minimize stimulation for confused or agitated patients.
   - Consult with rehabilitation services including physical, occupational, and speech therapy.
   - Plan care to prevent or minimize problems related to the injury (e.g., spasticity, swallowing disorders) and complications of immobility (e.g., disuse syndrome, contractures, pressure ulcers).

3. **For Locked-In Syndrome**
   - Establish a communication system/pattern.
   - Consult a mental health professional to assess the psychological impact of this syndrome.
   - Consult with rehabilitation (see preceding section on Coma).
   - Provide a normal day/night routine to help minimize sleep-wake cycle disturbances.

4. **For Vegetative State**
   - Perform neurodiagnostic and neuropsychological testing to confirm the diagnosis.
   - Provide essential supportive care to minimize complications such as pressure ulcers and aspiration.
   - Initiate a sensory stimulation program for low-level cognitive function, including visual, auditory, tactile, gustatory, and vestibular stimuli (Figure 1-3).

Safety Alert *Research has demonstrated positive outcomes from two interventions designed to reduce delirium in the intensive care unit—one was to reduce delirium in postoperative patients by controlling disturbances in the sleep-wake cycle. The second involved the daily visit of a geriatric consult service, which provided targeted recommendations using a 10-item protocol. The protocol included (1) maintenance of CNS O_2 delivery, (2) fluid and electrolyte corrections, (3) pain management, (4) removal of unnecessary medications, (5) bowel/bladder regulation, (6) establishing adequate nutrition, (7) mobilization and rehabilitation, (8) detection/prevention and treatment of surgical complications, (9) sensory stimulation, and (10) treatment of agitational variant of delirium.*

CARE PLANS: ALTERATION IN CONSCIOUSNESS

 Disturbed sensory perception *related to physiologic changes; psychological changes; environmental changes; sensory deprivation; sensory overload; drug interactions*

GOALS/OUTCOMES If cause of alteration in consciousness is an extracerebral event, within 72 hours of this diagnosis, the patient's level of arousal and cognition improve and the patient responds consistently and appropriately to stimuli. If the cause is cerebral, increased arousal and improvements in cognition may take days to weeks.

NOC Cognitive Orientation, Distorted Thought Self-Control, Information Processing, Neurological Status: Consciousness

COGNITIVE ABILITY: Ability to execute complex mental processes; Ability to identify person, place, and time; Information Processing: Ability to acquire, organize, and use information

1. Eliminate environmental causes of sensory/perceptual deficit.
   - Assess patient for potential causes of sensory/perceptual deficits. For the hearing- or vision-impaired patient, wearing eyeglasses or hearing aids will decrease misinterpretation of visual and auditory stimuli.
   - Assess environment for potential causes of disorientation and confusion. Maintain day/night environment as much as possible. Keep clocks and calendars within patient's field of vision.

SENSORY STIMULATION (SS) PROGRAMS AS AN INTERVENTION TECHNIQUE IN THE CRITICALLY ILL

STRONG EVIDENCE	INSUFFICIENT EVIDENCE	RECOMMENDATIONS
SS programs appear to be safe to administer.	There is still no clear evidence that increased arousal is brain injury recovery or SS program enhanced recovery.	SS programs can be initiated as an adjustment therapy.
SS programs do not increase ICP or CPP and do not affect HR or BP. A positive trajectory of recovery has been documented in all studies.	It is unclear how the time when SS was started (early or late) influences outcome. It is unclear how the type of program (multimodal or unimodal) influences outcome.	SS program can be incorporated into daily nursing routine. Use rest periods between sessions to diminish fatigue.
	It is unclear what type of stimulation is most useful for increasing arousal (e.g., novel, familiar music, voices). It is unclear how long daily stimulation should last (concentrated or multiple short sessions).	Stop intervention if an unstable medical status develops, and resume when patient is stable. Include family in intervention program.

BP, blood pressure; CPP, cerebral perfusion pressure; HR, heart rate; ICP, intracranial pressure

Figure 1-3 Sensory stimulation (SS) programs as an intervention technique in the critically ill. (From Kater K: Response of head-injured patients to sensory stimulation. *West J Nurs Res* 11[1]:20–33, 1989; Lewinn E, Dimancescu M: Environmental deprivation and enrichment in coma. *Lancet* 2:156–157, 1978; Mackay L, et al: Early intervention in severe head injury: long-term benefits of a formalized program. *Arch Phys Med Rehabil* 73:635–641, 1992; Mitchell S, et al: Coma arousal procedure: a therapeutic intervention in the treatment of head injury. *Brain Inj* 4:273–279, 1990; Schinner K, et al: Effects of auditory stimuli on intracranial pressure and cerebral perfusion pressure in traumatic brain injury. *J Neurosci Nurs* 27[6]:336–341, 1994; and Wilson S, et al: Vegetative state and response to sensory stimulation: an analysis of 24 cases. *Brain Inj* 10(11):807–818, 1996.)

2. Develop a plan of care consistent with sensory/perceptual deficit.
3. Assess patient for sensory deprivation and sensory overload. Decrease or increase stimulation based on RLA assessment (see Figure 1-3, above) and patient's needs. For example, agitated and confused individuals require structure and reorientation interventions, whereas those who are comatose or stuporous require stimulation techniques.
   - Orient patient to time, place, and person during all interactions. Explain procedures in terms patient can understand.
   - Teach significant others reorientation and sensory stimulation strategies, and provide liberal visitation to facilitate their assistance.
   - Assess underlying cause of confusion or delirium before using sedation, anxiolytic, analgesic, or antipsychotic drug therapy (see Sedation and neuromuscular blockade, p. 158).

NIC Cognitive Restructuring; Cognitive Stimulation; Environmental Management; Reality Orientation; Dementia Management; Electrolyte Management; Delirium Management

Impaired verbal communication *related to neurologic deficits*

GOALS/OUTCOMES If cause of alteration in consciousness is an extracerebral event, within 72 hours of this diagnosis, patient communicates needs and feelings and exhibits decreased frustration and fear related to communication barriers. If cause is cerebral, improvement in communication may take days to weeks.
NOC Communication: Expressive; Communication; Communication: Receptive

Communication Enhancement
1. Determine underlying cause of impaired communication, including physiologic (cortical, brainstem, or cranial nerve injury) or psychological (depression, fear, or anger).
2. When communicating with these patients, use their name, face them, use eye contact if they are awake, speak clearly, and use a normal tone of voice.
3. Be alert to nonverbal messages, especially eye movement, blinking, facial expressions, and head and hand movements. Attempt to validate these signals with the patient.
4. Assure patient that you are attempting to find methods that promote communication if the patient's needs cannot always be understood.
5. For the patient who does not respond to or acknowledge verbal stimulation, continue communication attempts.
6. Teach significant others methods of communication, and encourage them to continue attempts at communication.
7. Brainstem-evoked potentials and audiometry (hearing test) can provide useful information related to a patient's ability to receive and process auditory stimuli. Detection and treatment of otitis media in patients who have ET tubes will improve hearing.
8. Obtain a speech therapy consultation to assess nature and severity of communication impairment and assist in developing a communication plan. Special attention is required for individuals with locked-in syndrome.
9. Obtain a mental health consultation to assist with a patient who is angry, frustrated, and fearful because of the communication impairment.

NIC Communication Enhancement: Speech Deficit; Support System Enhancement

Impaired physical mobility *related to perceptual or cognitive impairment; imposed restrictions of movement*

GOALS/OUTCOMES By the time of discharge from the critical care unit, patient demonstrates range of motion (ROM) and muscle strength within 10% of baseline parameters.
NOC Mobility, Ambulation

Exercise Therapy: Joint Mobility
1. Assess muscle strength and tone to determine type of interventions required. Consult physical therapy and occupational therapy for evaluation and treatment plan.
2. Manage decreased muscle tone (flaccidity):
   - Maintain body alignment and positioning.
   - Perform passive ROM and stretching exercises.
   - Avoid prolonged periods of limb flexion.
   - Apply splints and other adaptive devices to maintain functional position of the extremities.
   - Turn patient every 2 hours.
   - Consider chair sitting as the patient stabilizes.
3. Manage increased muscle tone (spasticity):
   - Avoid supine position; use side-lying, semiprone, prone, and high Fowler's positions.
   - Position limbs opposite flexion posture.
   - Use skeletal muscle relaxant, such as baclofen (Lioresal), as prescribed for decreasing tone.
4. Monitor calcium and alkaline phosphatase levels. Increased levels can lead to the development of heterogeneous ossification, which often is seen with states of impaired mobility, such as spinal cord injury. See Fluid and Electrolyte Disturbances, p. 37.
5. Maintain patient's skin integrity. See Wound and Skin Care, p. 167.
6. Prevent pulmonary complications in the following ways:
   - Encourage deep breathing if patient is able, or suction as needed. Coughing is warranted only if sputum is present.
   - Assess swallowing ability before initiating oral feedings. Obtain dysphagia consultation (usually from a speech therapist) if swallowing reflexes are impaired.

- Initiate enteral feeding protocol for patients with feeding tubes to prevent aspiration. See Nutritional Support, p. 117.

NIC Bed Rest Care; Positioning; Exercise Promotion; Self-Care Assistance

ADDITIONAL NURSING DIAGNOSES

Also see nursing diagnoses and interventions under *Nutritional Support* (p. 117), *Sedation and neuro-muscular blockade* (p. 158), *Prolonged Immobility* (p. 149), and *Risk for Disuse Syndrome*, in *Traumatic Brain Injury* (p. 331), *Acute Spinal Cord Injury* (p. 264), and *SIRS, Sepsis, and MODS* (p. 924).

FLUID AND ELECTROLYTE DISTURBANCES

The volume and composition of body fluids and electrolytes are affected by hormonal, renal, vascular, and exogenous factors. An understanding of the complexity of chemical currents, cellular function, and distribution of water between the cells and vessels provides the information used to facilitate the best patient outcome.

Water is the major constituent of the human body, comprising 55% to 72% of body mass. Body water decreases with both age and increasing body fat. The average male adult is approximately 60% water by weight, while the average female adult is 55% water by weight. *Two-thirds* of body fluid is within the *intracellular fluid compartment* (ICF). ICF contains a high concentration of potassium (K^+), magnesium (Mg^+), phosphates (PO_4^-), proteins, and sulfates. The *extracellular fluid* (ECF) compartment is composed of *interstitial fluid*, which surrounds the cells, and *intravascular fluid*, contained within blood vessels. ECF contains the remaining *third* of body fluid and has a high concentration of the plasma ions sodium (Na^+), chloride (Cl^-), and bicarbonate (HCO_3^-).

The composition and concentration of ECF are primarily regulated by the concentration of Na^+, which defines the relative relationship of sodium and water. Although ECF is altered and then modified as the body reacts with its surrounding environment, ICF remains relatively stable. Intracellular stability is important for maintaining normal cellular function.

In addition to water, body fluids contain two types of dissolved substances: electrolytes and nonelectrolytes. *Electrolytes* are substances that carry an electrical current and can dissociate into ions, which have either a positive or a negative charge. They are measured by their capacity to combine (milliequivalents/liter [mEq/L]) or by the molecular weight in milligrams (millimoles/liter [mmol/L]). *Nonelectrolytes* are substances such as glucose and urea that do not dissociate in solution and are measured by weight (milligrams per 100 milliliters, or mg/dl). The body fluid compartments are separated by a semipermeable membrane, which allows movement of dissolved substances/particles between compartments, while maintaining the unique composition of each compartment (Table 1-7).

OSMOLALITY

Osmolality is the number of particles in solution. This concentration of particles determines the relationship of fluid between the ICF and ECF. Normal osmolality is regulated by a wide variety of mechanisms, which include arterial BP, sympathetic stimulation, renal regulation, and hormonal outflow.

$$\text{Osmolality} = 2(Na^+) + \text{Glucose}/18 + \text{Blood urea nitrogen (BUN)}/2.8$$
$$\text{normal 265 to 285 mOsm/L}$$

HORMONAL INFLUENCE

Antidiuretic hormone (ADH), or vasopressin, is a hormone released by the posterior pituitary in response to a reduction in intravascular volume (hypovolemia) or an increase in extracellular osmolality. It acts on the kidney at both the glomerulus and the tubules to conserve water by increasing urine concentration. The hormone regulates the electrolyte and fluid balance to keep serum in "perfect" concentration (osmolality). Thirst is stimulated by hypovolemia and increased osmolality.

Table 1-7	PRIMARY CONSTITUENTS OF BODY WATER COMPARTMENTS*		
Element	**Intravascular**	**Interstitial**	**Intracellular (skeletal muscle cell)**
Na^+	142 mEq/L	145 mEq/L	12 mEq/L
Cl^-	104 mEq/L	117 mEq/L	4 mEq/L
HCO_3^-	24 mEq/L	27 mEq/L	12 mEq/L
K^+	4.5 mEq/L	4.5 mEq/L	150 mEq/L
HPO_4^-	2 mEq/L	2 mEq/L	40 mEq/L

*This is a partial list. Other constituents include calcium (Ca^{2+}), magnesium (Mg^{2+}), and proteins. Cl^-, chloride; HCO_3^-, bicarbonate; HPO_4^-, phosphate; K^+, potassium; Na^+, sodium.

Aldosterone is another regulator of fluid volume. It is released by the adrenal cortex in response to an increased plasma renin level, acts on the kidney to conserve sodium (along with water), and increases potassium and hydrogen excretion.

Atrial natriuretic peptide (ANP) is a hormone released by the cardiac atria in response to increased atrial pressure (e.g., acute volume expansion). ANP reduces BP and vascular volume by increasing excretion of sodium and water by the kidneys, decreasing release of aldosterone and ADH, and by direct vasodilation.

FLUID DISTURBANCES
Fluid changes affect the volume status, regulation, and the composition of body fluids. Fluid loss or gain changes the concentration of particles in fluid compartments.

HYPOVOLEMIA

PATHOPHYSIOLOGY
ECF volume depletion or *hypovolemia* may be caused by abnormal skin losses, GI losses, polyuria/diuresis, bleeding, decreased intake, and movement of fluid into a third space (e.g., pleura, peritoneum, interstitium). Depending on the type of fluid lost or "third-spaced," hypovolemia may be accompanied by acid-base, osmolar, or electrolyte imbalances. Severe ECF volume depletion can lead to *hypovolemic shock* and cellular dehydration, which causes alterations in electric potentials (the ability to conduct impulse) throughout the body.

Compensatory mechanisms in hypovolemia include increased sympathetic nervous system stimulation: increased HR, increased force of cardiac contraction (positive inotropic effect), vasoconstriction to maintain perfusion to O_2–dependent organs (i.e., heart, lungs, brain), increased thirst, and increased release of aldosterone and ADH (vasopressin). Reduced perfusion to high-flow, low O_2-consuming organs (i.e., kidney, mesenteric bed, skeletal muscles) may lead to acute renal failure, ischemic bowel, and skeletal muscle cell rupture.

Hypovolemic shock develops when the intravascular volume decreases to the point where compensatory mechanisms can no longer maintain the perfusion needed for normal, aerobic cellular function. Without normal levels of O_2, cellular metabolism becomes anaerobic, resulting in acidosis, cardiac depression, intravascular coagulation, increased capillary permeability, and release of toxins. If shock is not adequately treated, it may become irreversible, leading to death.

HYPOVOLEMIA ASSESSMENT
Goal of Assessment
Identify the signs and symptoms of hypovolemia

History and Risk Factors
The following list of factors may be associated with loss of intravascular fluids or overall blood volume:
- *Abnormal GI losses*: Vomiting, nasogastric suctioning, diarrhea, intestinal drainage
- *Abnormal skin losses*: Excessive diaphoresis secondary to fever or exercise, burns

- *Abnormal renal losses:* Diuretic therapy, polyuria/osmotic diuresis seen with DKA, hyperglycemic hyperosmolar nonketotic syndrome (HHNS), nephrotoxicity, rhabdomyolysis, diabetes insipidus, diuretic phase of acute renal failure/acute kidney injury, adrenal insufficiency
- *Third-spacing or plasma to interstitial fluid shift:* Peritonitis, intestinal obstruction, burns, ascites, severe sepsis
- *Hemorrhage:* Major trauma, GI bleeding, obstetric complications, postoperative bleeding, high dosage of anticoagulants or antiplatelet medications
- *Altered intake:* Coma, fluid deprivation

Vital Signs
Evaluate BP, HR, temperature, weight, CVP, PAWP, and urine output to determine the extent of volume depletion.
- Check BP lying, sitting, and standing to determine presence of orthostasis.
- HR will be increased (tachycardia).
- Narrowed pulse pressure
- Low CVP (less than 2 mm Hg)
- Low PAWP (less than 3 mm Hg)
- Urine output decreased and may be less than 0.5 ml/kg/hour
- Increased temperature
- Acute weight loss unless third spacing is occurring (Table 1-8)

Observation
Evaluate the skin, mucous membranes, and clinical presentation for signs of dehydration including furrowed tongue, dry mucous membranes, sunken eyeballs, flat neck veins, clinical pallor, dizziness, weakness, fatigue, syncope, anorexia, nausea, vomiting, thirst, confusion, and constipation.

Palpation
Chest and abdominal palpation are performed to elicit pain in the abdomen or chest.

Screening Labwork
Blood studies can reveal the extent of hypovolemia, as the blood becomes more concentrated as fluid is lost. If bleeding is present, studies will reveal blood loss.
- Hematocrit levels are elevated with dehydration and decreased with bleeding.
- BUN values may be elevated, with a BUN/creatinine ratio of greater than 20:1 suggesting hypovolemia.
- Electrolyte levels will vary depending on the type of fluid lost.
- ABG values depend on the type of fluid lost.
- Serum and urine osmolality depend on the type of fluid lost, and comparison assists in the diagnosis of renal insufficiency.

Safety Alert *Early hypovolemic shock is often missed. As the HR increases and arteries constrict, BP may be compensated and remain normal or slightly elevated. Widening of pulse pressure (systolic BP + diastolic BP = pulse pressure) is a more accurate tool in early shock. A pulse pressure of 40 mm Hg may indicate shock. CO and mean arterial pressure (MAP) may be compensated by HR and vasoconstriction consecutively.*

Table 1-8	WEIGHT LOSS AS AN INDICATOR OF EXTRACELLULAR FLUID DEFICIT IN THE ADULT
Acute Weight Loss	**Severity of Deficit**
2%–5%	Mild
5%–10%	Moderate
10%–15%	Severe
15%–20%	Fatal

Safety Alert   *As shock progresses, HR decreases, and ventricular compliance and filling time decrease, resulting in decreased CVP and PA pressure (PAP). Volume status may be underestimated.*

Diagnostic Tests for Hypovolemia

Test	Purpose	Abnormal Findings
Blood urea nitrogen (BUN)	Evaluates the renal response to decreased perfusion. Renal clearance of urea is reduced when renal blood supply is compromised.	Elevated with dehydration, decreased renal perfusion or decreased renal function. *BUN/creatinine ratio* greater than 20:1 suggests hypovolemia.
Hematocrit	Evaluates for hemoconcentration resulting from loss of fluid in the blood, or blood itself.	*Elevated:* with dehydration *Decreased:* with bleeding If both blood and fluid are lost, blood loss may be underestimated due to hemoconcentration.
Serum electrolytes	Assesses abnormalities that may increase morbidity. Changes are dependent on the type of fluid lost.	*Hypokalemia:* May occur with abnormal GI or renal loss. *Hyperkalemia:* Associated with adrenal insufficiency. *Hypernatremia:* Seen with increased insensible loss, and diabetes insipidus. *Hyponatremia:* Associated with increased thirst and ADH release; may lead to increased water intake, retention and dilution of serum sodium.
Serum total CO_2 (CO_2 content)	Evaluates for metabolic acidosis or alkalosis	Decreased with metabolic acidosis and increased with metabolic alkalosis.
ABG values	Assesses the body's chemical environment. Acidosis and alkalosis can have a profound effect on electrolyte balance.	Metabolic acidosis may occur with lower GI loses, shock, or diabetic ketoacidosis. Metabolic alkalosis may occur with upper GI losses and diuretic therapy.
Urine specific gravity	Assesses the ability of the kidneys to concentrate urine. With hypovolemia, urine should be more concentrated.	Increased with kidneys' attempt to conserve water. May be fixed at approximately 1.010 in the presence of renal disease.
Urine sodium	Assesses the ability of the kidneys to conserve sodium in response to increased aldosterone levels	In the absence of renal disease, osmotic diuresis or diuretic therapy, the value should be less than 20 mEq/L.
Serum osmolality	Assess compensation	Variable, depending on the type of fluid lost and the body's ability to compensate with thirst and ADH
Urine osmolality	Assess concentrating ability of the kidneys. The role of urine production and concentration is to keep serum osmolality perfect.	Level should be increased greater than 450 mOsm/kg as the kidneys attempt to conserve water. If serum is concentrated, urine should be more concentrated. Comparing urine osmolality to serum osmolality assists in the diagnosis of renal insufficiency.

COLLABORATIVE MANAGEMENT
Care Priorities
Identification of patients at risk for volume loss and prevention of continued losses and fluid replacement guide the care plan for these patients.
1. Restore tissue perfusion with fluid volume replacement and correct electrolyte disturbances: Administer and monitor fluid replacement with crystalloids, colloids, or blood.
2. Document response to fluid administration.
3. Maintain a safe environment for patients with neurologic symptoms.
4. Monitor for the signs and symptoms of dehydration.
   - Monitor urine output.
   - Moisten mucous membranes.
5. Protect skin with lotions and egg crate or alternating pressure mattress.

Management of Hypovolemia

1. Restore Normal Fluid Volume and Correct Acid-Base and Electrolyte Disturbances

The type of fluid replacement depends on the type of fluid lost and the severity of the deficit and on serum electrolytes, serum osmolality, and acid-base status. IV fluids are provided to expand intravascular volume or to correct an underlying imbalance in fluids or electrolytes. Fluids should be infused at a rate resulting in a positive fluid balance (e.g., 50–100 ml in excess of all hourly losses).

Replacement fluids

- Isotonic solutions (Normal Saline 0.9%): Expand ECF only; do not enter ICF. Appropriate for rapid volume replacement.
- Hypotonic saline solutions (0.45% saline): Expand the ECF and provide some free water to the cells. Used in the management of the patient who is both volume-depleted and hyperosmolar (e.g., in cases of hypernatremia or hyperglycemia).
- Dextrose and water (5% dextrose in water): Provides free water only and will be distributed evenly through both the ICF and ECF; used to treat water deficit.
- Mixed isotonic saline/electrolyte solutions: Provide additional electrolytes (e.g., potassium and calcium) and a buffer (e.g., lactate or acetate). Example: lactated Ringer's solution (Ringer's lactate): isotonic solution containing a small amount of K^+ and lactate, which metabolizes to bicarbonate in the liver to assist blood buffering.
- Blood and albumin: Expand only the intravascular portion of the ECF. Both packed red blood cells and fresh-frozen plasma expand the intravascular volume.
- Dextran or hetastarch, hypertonic saline, hextend: Synthetic colloidal solutions used to expand the intravascular volume.

2. Restore Tissue Perfusion (Hypovolemic Shock)

- *Rapid volume replacement with crystalloids:* Fluids may be given rapidly as long as cardiac filling pressures and BP remain low. Overaggressive fluid resuscitation in uncontrolled hemorrhage can increase the risk of secondary hemorrhage as the intravascular hydrostatic pressure increases.
- *Volume replacement with colloids:* Use of volume replacement with colloids to prevent the development of pulmonary edema secondary to rapid volume replacement remains controversial. Solutions include albumin and synthetics such as hetastarch.
- *Blood:* Administered only if necessary to maintain oxygen-carrying capacity. Hct should not be raised >35%.
- *Vasopressors:* Used to reduce the size of blood vessels while volume infusions continue to increase blood pressure. Effective for false hypovolemia induced by vasogenic (septic, anaphylactic, neurogenic) shock to control severe vasodilation.

CARE PLANS FOR HYPOVOLEMIA
Deficient fluid volume *related to loss of body fluid or blood*

GOALS/OUTCOMES Within 24 hours of starting fluid therapy, patient becomes normovolemic as evidenced by urine output ≥0.5 ml/kg/hr, specific gravity 1.010 to 1.030, stable weight, no clinical evidence of hypovolemia (e.g., furrowed tongue), BP within patient's normal range, HR and pulse pressure normalized, CVP 2 to 6 mm Hg, PAP 20 to 30/8 to 15 mm Hg, CO 4 to 7 L/min, MAP 70 to 105 mm Hg, HR 60 to 100 beats per minute (bpm), and systemic vascular resistance (SVR) 900 to 1200 dynes•sec•cm^{-5}.

NOC Fluid Balance, Hydration, Kidney Function

Fluid Monitoring

1. *Monitor input and output (I&O) hourly.* During initial therapy, intake should exceed output. Consult physician for urine output less than 0.5 ml/kg/hr for 2 consecutive hours. Measure urine specific gravity every 4 hours as available. Normal range is 1.010 to 1.030. Expect it to decrease with therapy.
2. *Monitor vital signs (VS) and hemodynamic pressures for continued hypovolemia.* Be alert to decreased BP, CVP, PAP, CO, and MAP and to increased HR and SVR.
3. *Weigh patient daily.* Daily weight measurements are the single most important indicator of fluid status, because acute weight changes usually indicate fluid changes. A decrease in daily weight of 1 kg is equal to the loss of 1 L of fluid. The adult who is not eating or receiving enteral or parenteral nutrition (PN) may lose 0.25 kg of nonfluid weight daily as body tissues are used for glucose production. Weigh patient at the same time of day (preferably before breakfast) on a balanced scale, with patient wearing approximately the same clothing. Document type of scale used (i.e., standing, bed, chair).
4. *Monitor for signs of fluid overload or too-rapid fluid administration:* Crackles (rales), decreased O_2 saturation (pulse oximetry/SpO$_2$), shortness of breath (SOB), tachypnea, tachycardia, increased CVP, increased PA pressures, neck vein distention, and edema.
5. *Monitor patient for hidden fluid losses.* Measure/record abdominal girth or limb size if indicated.
6. *Monitor for signs of abdominal compartment syndrome:* Acute increase in ventilator pressures and a decrease in SpO$_2$.
7. *Monitor for signs of bleeding:* Decreased hematocrit (Hct), Hgb, tachycardia. Remember that Hct, serum Na$^+$, and BUN may decrease in dehydrated patients as rehydration progresses.
8. *Monitor for hypocalcemia:* May develop in rapidly transfused patients due to the citrate used in banked blood (citrate binds calcium, making it unavailable for cellular uptake). Sudden symptoms may include refractory hypotension (see hypocalcemia p. 57). Calcium chloride or gluconate may be prescribed.

Fluid Management

1. Place hypotensive patients in supine position with the legs elevated to 45 degrees to increase venous return. Avoid Trendelenburg position, which causes abdominal organs to lean on the diaphragm, thereby impairing ventilation.
2. Administer oral (PO) and IV fluids as prescribed. Ensure adequate intake, especially in older adults, a population at higher risk for volume depletion. Give water with enteral feedings and supplements.
3. Ensure a patent IV access and availability of blood products if needed.

NIC Fluid Monitoring; Hypovolemia Management; Fluid Resuscitation; Intravenous (IV) Therapy; Invasive Hemodynamic Monitoring; Shock Management; Volume

---

Ineffective peripheral tissue perfusion *related to lack of blood volume*

GOALS/OUTCOMES Within 12 hours after initiation of volume resuscitation, patient has adequate perfusion as evidenced by alertness; warm and dry skin; BP within patient's normal range; HR ≤100 bpm; urinary output ≥0.5 ml/kg/hr; and capillary refill less than 2 seconds.

NOC Circulation Status, Tissue Integrity: Skin and Mucous Membranes

Circulatory Care: Arterial Insufficiency

1. Monitor for signs of decreased cerebral perfusion: vertigo, syncope, confusion, restlessness, anxiety, agitation, excitability, weakness, nausea, and cool and clammy skin. Consult physician or midlevel practitioner for worsening symptoms.
2. To avoid unnecessary vasodilation, treat fevers promptly.
3. Cover patient with a light blanket to maintain body temperature.
4. Palpate peripheral pulses bilaterally in arms and legs (radial, brachial, dorsalis pedis, posterior tibial). Use a Doppler ultrasonic device if unable to palpate pulses. Rate pulses (0 to 4+ scale). Consult physician for weak/absent pulses.

Safety Alert *Abnormal pulses also may be caused by a local vascular disorder.*

5. Consult physician or midlevel practitioner for urinary output less than 0.5 ml/kg/hr for 2 consecutive hours.

Positioning
1. Protect patients who are at high risk for falling: those who are confused, dizzy, or weak. Keep side rails up and bed in lowest position with wheels locked. Assist with ambulation. Raise patient to sitting or standing positions slowly.
2. Monitor for orthostatic hypotension: decreased BP, increased HR, dizziness, and diaphoresis. If symptoms occur, return patient to supine position.

NIC Neurologic Monitoring

ADDITIONAL NURSING DIAGNOSES
For additional nursing diagnoses, see specific medical disorder, electrolyte imbalance, or acid-base disturbance.

HYPERVOLEMIA

PATHOPHYSIOLOGY
Hypervolemia is a state of higher-than-normal intravascular volume that occurs in four situations: (1) excessive retention of sodium and water caused by a chronic renal stimulus to conserve sodium and water, (2) abnormal renal functioning causing reduced excretion of sodium and water, (3) excessive administration of IV fluids, and (4) interstitial-to-plasma fluid shifting. Hypervolemia may lead to heart failure and pulmonary edema, especially in the patient with cardiovascular dysfunction.

HYPERVOLEMIA ASSESSMENT
Goal of Assessment
- Evaluate the potential causes and sequelae of hypervolemia

History and Risk Factors
- *Retention of sodium and/or water:* Heart failure, hepatic failure, nephrotic syndrome, excessive administration of glucocorticosteroids, syndrome of inappropriate antidiuretic hormone (SIADH)
- *Abnormal renal function:* Acute or chronic renal failure, oliguria, anuria, excessive administration of IV fluids
- *Interstitial-to-plasma fluid shifting:* Remobilization of fluid after burn treatment, excessive administration of hypertonic solutions (i.e., mannitol, hypertonic saline), excessive administration of colloid oncotic solutions (i.e., albumin)

Observation
- *Evaluate for the clinical signs of volume overload:* SOB, orthopnea, peripheral edema, distended neck veins, moist skin

Vital Signs
- HR, BP, and hemodynamic measurements to evaluate volume status
  - Increased BP
  - BP: will decrease as the heart fails
  - HR: tachycardia
  - Respirations: tachypnea
  - O_2 saturation decreased
  - Increased CVP, PAP, PAWP
  - MAP: increased unless heart failure is present

Palpation
- *Pulse assessment to evaluate tissue perfusion:* Bounding pulses, ascites, peripheral and sacral edema

Auscultation
- *Heart and lung assessment to evaluate signs of volume overload:* Tachycardia, gallop rhythm, crackles, rhonchi, and wheezes

Screening Labwork
- *Blood studies are variable and nonspecific:* Hematocrit, BUN and creatinine, arterial blood gases, serum sodium and osmolality, urinary sodium, urine specific gravity

Radiology
- Chest radiograph may reveal signs of pulmonary vascular congestion.

Diagnostic Tests for Hypervolemia		
Test	**Purpose**	**Abnormal Findings**
Hematocrit	Assesses for anemia	*Decreased:* Due to hemodilution by excess fluids in the vasculature
Blood urea nitrogen	Evaluates for presence of renal dysfunction	*Decreased:* In pure hypervolemia. *Increased:* With renal failure
Arterial blood gases	Assesses for hypoxemia and acid-base imbalance (acidosis or alkalosis)	*Hypoxemia with alkalosis:* May be present due to tachypnea associated with early pulmonary edema. *Respiratory acidosis:* May be present in severe pulmonary edema. Diffusion of oxygen is difficult across the edematous alveolar-capillary membrane.
Serum sodium and serum osmolality	Assesses for water retention	*Decreased:* If hypervolemia is from water retention (i.e., chronic renal failure)
Urinary sodium	Evaluates efficacy of renal handling of sodium	*Elevated:* Results from kidneys excreting excess sodium. Sodium excretion prompts fluid excretion. NOTE: Urinary sodium *is not elevated* with secondary hyperaldosteronism (e.g., heart failure, cirrhosis, nephrotic syndrome) because hypervolemia occurs secondary to a chronic renal stimulus; the aldosterone increases resorption of Na^+
Urine specific gravity	Evaluates the solute concentrating ability of the kidney	*Decreased:* If the kidney is excreting excess volume. May be fixed at 1.010 in acute renal failure
Chest radiograph	Assesses for pulmonary edema	May reveal signs of pulmonary vascular congestion ("whiter" appearance)

COLLABORATIVE MANAGEMENT
Care Priorities
The priorities include prevention of further volume overload and returning the patient to a euvolemic state.
1. **Restrict intake of sodium and water** Monitor intake of oral, enteral and parenteral fluids. Prevent the intake of high sodium foods. Box 1-4 lists foods high in sodium.
2. **Administer diuretics** May be given IV or PO. Loop diuretics (i.e., furosemide) are indicated for severe hypervolemia or heart failure. Diuresis may prompt profound electrolyte loss.
3. **Monitor weight and output** To assess the response to diuretics. Monitor for electrolyte loss.
4. **Renal replacement therapy** Used in renal failure or life-threatening fluid overload (see *Acute Renal Failure/Acute Kidney Injury,* p. 584)
5. **Patient education** Signs and symptoms of volume overload. Information provided regarding high sodium-containing foods
6. **VS** Monitor for changes in BP and CO with diuresis.

Box 1-4	FOODS HIGH IN SODIUM

Bouillon	Pickles
Celery	Preserved meat
Cheeses	Salad dressings and prepared sauces
Dried fruits	Sauerkraut
Frozen, canned, or packaged foods	Snack foods (e.g., crackers, chips,
Monosodium glutamate (MSG)	pretzels)
Mustard	Soy sauce
Olives	

Safety Alert *Also see specific discussions under Burns (p. 279), Acute Lung Injury and Acute Respiratory Distress Syndrome (p. 365), and Acute Renal Failure/Acute Kidney Injury (p. 584).*

CARE PLANS FOR HYPERVOLEMIA

Excess fluid volume *related to patient's disease state(s), medications, and/or other therapies*

GOALS/OUTCOMES Within 24 hours of starting treatment, patient is improved as evidenced by reduced edema, BP approaching patient's normal range, HR 60 to 100 bpm, CVP 2 to 6 mm Hg, PAP 20 to 30/8 to 15 mm Hg, MAP 70 to 105 mm Hg, and CO 4 to 7 L/min.

NOC Electrolyte and Acid-Base Balance, Fluid Balance, Fluid Overload Severity

Fluid/Electrolyte Management

1. *Monitor intake and output hourly.* Urine output should be greater than/equal to 0.5 ml/kg/hr unless the patient is in oliguric renal failure.
2. *Measure urine specific gravity or urine osmolality every 4 hours.* If the patient is receiving diuretic therapy, specific gravity should be 1.010 to 1.020 with osmolality less than 500 mOsm/L.
3. *Monitor and manage edema* (pretibial, sacral, periorbital), using a 0 to 4+ rating scale.
4. *Weigh patient daily.* Daily weight measurements are the single most important indicator of fluid status.
5. *Limit oral, enteral, and parenteral sodium intake* as prescribed. Be aware that medications may contain sodium (e.g., penicillins, bicarbonate). See Box 1-4 for some foods high in sodium.
6. *Limit fluids as prescribed.* Offer a portion of allotted fluids as ice chips to minimize patient's thirst. Teach patient and significant others the importance of fluid restriction and how to measure fluid volume.
7. *Provide oral hygiene* at frequent intervals to keep oral mucous membrane moist and intact.
8. *Document response to diuretic therapy* (e.g., increased urine output, decreased CVP/PAP, decreased adventitious breath sounds, decreased edema). Many diuretics (e.g., furosemide, thiazides) cause hypokalemia. Observe for indicators of hypokalemia: muscle weakness, dysrhythmias (especially PVCs and ECG changes such as flattened T wave, presence of U waves). (See *Hypokalemia* [p. 52].) Potassium-sparing diuretics (e.g., spironolactone, triamterene) may cause hyperkalemia: signs include weakness, ECG changes (e.g., peaked T wave, prolonged PR interval, widened QRS complex). (See *Hyperkalemia* [p. 55]) Consult physician or midlevel practitioner for significant findings.
9. *Observe for indicators of overcorrection and dangerous volume depletion:* Vertigo, weakness, syncope, thirst, confusion, poor skin turgor, flat neck veins, and acute weight loss.
10. *Monitor VS and hemodynamic parameters for volume depletion occurring with therapy:* Decreased BP, CVP, PAP, MAP, and CO; increased HR. Consult physician or midlevel practitioner for significant changes or findings.
11. *Monitor appropriate laboratory tests* (e.g., BUN and creatinine in renal failure). Consult with physician or midlevel practitioner for abnormal trends.

NIC Fluid Monitoring; Hypervolemia Management; Fluid/Electrolyte Management; Invasive Hemodynamic Monitoring; Hemodialysis Therapy

Impaired gas exchange *related to fluid volume overload*

GOALS/OUTCOMES Within 12 hours of initiating treatment, patient has improved gas exchange as evidenced by RR ≤20 breaths/min with normal depth and pattern (eupnea); HR ≤100 bpm; Pao$_2$ ≥80 mm Hg; pH 7.35 to 7.45; Paco$_2$ 35 to 45 mm Hg; and Spo$_2$ ≥92%. Patient exhibits reduction in or absence of crackles, gallops, or other clinical indicators of pulmonary edema. PAP is ≤30/15 mm Hg and PAWP is 6–12 mm Hg.
NOC Respiratory Status: Gas Exchange; Respiratory Status: Ventilation

Respiratory Monitoring
1. *Monitor patient for signs of acute pulmonary edema,* a potentially life-threatening complication of hypervolemia: air hunger, decreased pulse oximetry, anxiety, cough with production of frothy sputum, crackles, rhonchi, tachypnea, increasing ventilator pressures, tachycardia, gallop rhythm, and elevation of PAP and PAWP. Administer diuretics and other medications to reduce venous return to the heart as prescribed.
2. *Monitor ABG values for hypoxemia and respiratory alkalosis.* Monitor O$_2$ saturation. Administer O$_2$ to maintain Spo$_2$ ≥92%. Increased O$_2$ requirements may signal increased pulmonary vascular congestion.
3. *Keep patient in semi-Fowler's position* or position of comfort to minimize dyspnea.

NIC Ventilation Assistance, Positioning

Impaired skin integrity *related to edematous, possibly friable tissue*

GOALS/OUTCOMES Patient's skin and tissue remain intact.
NOC Tissue Integrity: Skin and Mucous Membranes

Pressure Management
1. Assess and document circulation to extremities at least each shift. Note color, temperature, capillary refill, and peripheral pulses. Consult physician or midlevel practitioner if capillary refill is delayed or if pulses are diminished or absent.
2. Turn and reposition patient at least every 2 hours to minimize tissue pressure.
3. Check tissue areas at risk with each position change (e.g., heels, sacrum, areas over bony prominences).
4. Use pressure-relief mattress as indicated.
5. Support arms and hands on pillows and elevate legs to decrease dependent edema. Do not elevate legs in the presence of pulmonary congestion.
6. Treat pressure ulcers per unit protocol. Consult physician or midlevel practitioner if sores, ulcers, or areas of tissue breakdown are present; especially with patients who are at high risk for infection (i.e., those with diabetes mellitus or renal failure or who are immunosuppressed).
7. Consult a skin/wound care nurse specialist for advanced tissue breakdown or any alteration in tissue integrity in high-risk patients.

NIC Circulatory Care; Skin Surveillance

HYPONATREMIA (serum sodium less than 135 mEq/L)

PATHOPHYSIOLOGY
Hyponatremia occurs from a net gain of water or a loss of sodium-rich fluids that have been replaced by water (net gain fluid > net gain Na$^+$). The most common cause of hyponatremia is water gain from renal dysfunction. The kidneys should increase output if intake increases. As serum osmolality decreases, fluid shifts into cells, causing swelling and sometimes compartment syndromes.

There are three types of hyponatremia: *hypovolemic, hypervolemic,* and *euvolemic.* Dilutional states are the most frequent cause of hyponatremia in the critically ill. Clinical indicators and treatments depend on the cause of hyponatremia and whether it is associated with normal, decreased, or increased ECF volume. For more information, see *Burns* (p. 279), *Heart Failure* (p. 421), *Acute Renal Failure/Acute Kidney Injury* (p. 584), and *Syndrome of Inappropriate Antidiuretic Hormone* (p. 734).

 Safety Alert *Hyperlipidemia, hyperproteinemia, and hyperglycemia may cause a pseudohyponatremia. Pseudohyponatremia reduces the Na^+ content but also causes a reduction in volume. Actual osmolality may be normal or high. If blood glucose, lipids, or proteins are elevated, an osmolality calculation or laboratory determination should be performed. Hyperlipidemia and hyperproteinemia reduce the percentage of plasma water. With hyperglycemia, the osmotic action of elevated glucose causes water to shift out of the cells into the ECF, thus diluting the serum sodium. For every 100 mg/dl that glucose is elevated, sodium is diluted by 1.6 mEq/L. The sodium-to-water ratio of plasma is unchanged, but the amount of sodium in the plasma is reduced.*

HYPONATREMIA ASSESSMENT
Goal of Assessment
- Evaluate for the signs and symptoms of hyponatremia.

History and Risk Factors
- *Decreased ECF volume*: GI losses: diarrhea, vomiting, fistulas, nasogastric suction, renal losses: diuretics, salt-wasting kidney disease and adrenal insufficiency, skin losses: burns, wound drainage, excessive diaphoresis
- *Normal/increased ECF volume*: Hypothyroidism, SIADH, edematous states: heart failure, cirrhosis and nephrotic syndrome; vigorous administration of hypotonic IV fluids; very dilute enteral feedings; oliguric renal failure; primary polydipsia; any patient with impaired ability to excrete free water (e.g., those being treated with thiazide diuretics) is at risk if given hypotonic fluids.

Vital Sign Assessment
- Blood pressure and HR will vary based on the state of ECF volume.
    - Postural hypotension with decreased ECF volume
    - Elevated BP with normal or increased ECF volume
    - Weight gain with normal or increased ECF volume
- Hemodynamic measurements
    - Decreased ECF volume: decreased CVP, PAP, CO, MAP; increased SVR
    - Increased ECF volume: increased CVP, PAP, MAP

Observation
- *Hyponatremia with decreased ECF volume*: Irritability, apprehension, dizziness, personality changes, poor skin turgor, dry mucous membranes, tremors, seizures, coma
- *Hyponatremia with normal or increased ECF volume*: Headache, lassitude, apathy, confusion, weakness, edema, convulsions, coma

Palpation
- Cold clammy skin with decreased ECF volume
- Hyperreflexia and muscle spasms with normal on increased ECF volume

Screening Labwork
- Serum sodium
- Serum osmolality
- Urine specific osmolality
- Urine sodium

Diagnostic Tests for Hyponatremia

Test	Purpose	Abnormal Findings
Serum sodium	Evaluate sodium level	*Decreased*: Less than 135 mEq/L
Serum osmolality	Assess hydration status	*Decreased*: Except in cases of pseudohyponatremia
Urine specific osmolality	Assess renal concentrating ability	*Elevated*: Usually more than 100 mOsm/kg, but less than the plasma level. *SIADH*: The urine will be inappropriately concentrated.
Urine sodium	Assess renal ability to conserve sodium	*Decreased*: Usually less than 20 mEq/L EXCEPT with SIADH, salt-wasting kidney disease, adrenal insufficiency, or excessive diuretic therapy

COLLABORATIVE MANAGEMENT

Care Priorities

1. **Replace sodium and fluid losses with reduced ECF volume.**   Adequate replacement of fluid volume is essential to turn off the physiologic stimulus to ADH release and enable the kidneys to restore sodium and water balance. Administer IV fluids while monitoring for further signs and symptoms of hyponatremia and I&O.
2. **Replace other electrolyte losses,** such as potassium and bicarbonate.
3. **Administer IV hypertonic saline (3% NaCl).** AUse if serum sodium is dangerously low or the patient has extreme symptoms. Therapeutic goal is to slowly shrink the cerebral cells. The dose is based on the patient's response. Therapy is sufficient when symptoms resolve and may be discontinued. Therapy MUST BE administered carefully, as too rapid correction can result in a life-threatening demyelination syndrome.
4. **Monitor rate of sodium replacement to prevent too rapid correction of hyponatremia.** Mild symptoms/no symptoms of hyponatremia: Strive to increase in serum sodium 0.5 to 1 mEq/L/hr. Severe symptoms, including seizures: Increase serum sodium no more than 1 to 2 mEq/L/hr for 3–4 hours. Sodium should not increase more than 10 mEq/L in any 24 hour period, and no more than 6 mEq/L during the first 3–4 hours.
5. **For hyponatremia with expanded ECF volume:**
   - Remove or treat the underlying cause.
   - Administer diuretics.
   - Restrict fluid intake to 1000 ml/daily to establish a negative water balance and increase sodium levels.
6. **Assess for resolution of the signs and symptoms of neurologic changes.**
7. **For dilutional hyponatremia:** Administer diuretics and restrict water intake.

 Safety Alert   *See Syndrome of Inappropriate Antidiuretic Hormone, Chapter 8, for specific treatment of hyponatremia.*

HIGH ALERT!   **Osmotic Demyelination Syndrome**

Overly aggressive or inappropriate treatment of hyponatremia can also cause permanent neurologic damage secondary to osmotic demyelination syndrome. Osmotic demyelination is poorly understood but should always be suspected after hypertonic resuscitation when patients display bilateral neurologic deficits, flaccidity, and quadriparesis. Initially, sodium levels should not increase at a level greater than 0.5 to 1.0 mEq/L/hr in patients being treated for symptomatic hyponatremia with hypertonic NaCl. For those symptomatic with severe hyponatremia (less than 120 mEq/L), the rate of correct should be 1–2mEq/hr for 3–4 hr. After an initial 6 to 8 mEq/L increase in the serum sodium level, the rate of increase should not be greater than 0.5 mEq/L/hr. Levels should not increase at an average rate of greater than 0.5 mEq/L/hr in patients without symptoms. The total increase in the first 24 hours of treatment should not exceed 12 mEq/L.

CARE PLANS FOR HYPONATREMIA

Readiness for enhanced fluid balance *related to the dynamic fluid and electrolyte changes that prompt sodium imbalance*

GOALS/OUTCOMES Within 24 hours of initiating treatment, patient's volume status is improving as evidenced by normalization of the heart and respiratory rates (HR 60 to 100 bpm, RR 12 to 20 breaths/min), BP within patient's normal range, CVP 2 to 6 mm Hg, and PAP 20 to 30/8 to 15 mm Hg or within patient's normal range.

NOC Fluid Balance, Kidney Function, Hydration

Fluid Monitoring
If patient is receiving hypertonic saline, assess carefully for signs of intravascular fluid overload: tachypnea, tachycardia, acute SOB, crackles (rales), rhonchi, increased CVP and PAP, gallop rhythm, and increased BP. For other interventions, see *Hypovolemia* (p. 38) or *Hypervolemia* (p. 43).

NIC Electrolyte Management: Hyponatremia; Fluid/Electrolyte Management; Intravenous (IV) Therapy; Invasive Hemodynamic Monitoring

Acute confusion *related to hyponatremia*

GOALS/OUTCOMES Within 48 hours of treatment, the patient more consistently verbalizes orientation to time, place, and person and has not sustained physical injury related to altered sensorium. Serum sodium level should ideally increase to greater than 125 mEq/L in the first 48 hours after treatment.

NOC Cognitive Orientation, Distorted Thought Self-Control, Information Processing, Neurological Status: Consciousness

Neurologic Monitoring
1. Assess and document LOC, orientation, and neurologic status with each vital sign check. Reorient patient as necessary. Consult physician or midlevel practitioner for significant changes.
2. If seizures are expected, pad side rails and keep an appropriate-size airway at the bedside.
3. Inform patient and significant others that altered sensorium is temporary and will improve with treatment.
4. Keep side rails up and bed in lowest position with wheels locked.
5. Use reality therapy such as clocks, calendars, and familiar objects; keep these items at the bedside within patient's visual field.
6. Monitor serum sodium levels closely. Permanent neurologic damage may occur with untreated, severely symptomatic hyponatremia secondary to cerebral edema.

HIGH ALERT! Overly rapid correction of chronic hyponatremia may result in permanent neurologic damage.

NIC Electrolyte Management: Hyponatremia; Seizure Precautions, Reality Orientation, Fall Prevention

HYPERNATREMIA (serum sodium greater than 145 mEq/L)

PATHOPHYSIOLOGY

Hypernatremia may occur with either free water loss or sodium gain. Hypernatremia always causes hypertonicity because sodium is the major determinant of ECF osmolality. Hypertonicity causes a shift of water out of the cells, which leads to intracellular dehydration. Hypernatremia usually results from volume depletion (hypovolemia) and is rarely caused by increased sodium intake.

HYPERNATREMIA ASSESSMENT
Goal of Assessment
Evaluate the risk factors and clinical symptoms of hypernatremia.

History and Risk Factors
- *Water (volume) loss:* Increased diaphoresis, respiratory infection, mechanical ventilation, diabetes insipidus, osmotic diuresis (e.g., hyperglycemia), osmotic diarrhea
- *Sodium gains:* IV administration of hypertonic saline or sodium bicarbonate, increased oral intake, primary aldosteronism, drugs such as sodium polystyrene sulfonate (Kayexalate)

Observation
- *Symptoms related to hypertonicity, intracellular dehydration, and electrolyte imbalance:* Intense thirst, fatigue, restlessness, agitation, coma, flushed skin, peripheral edema

Vital Signs
- Low-grade fever
- Postural hypotension
- Increased CVP and PAP: With sodium excess
- Decreased CVP and PAP with water loss: May be minimized by the extracellular shift of fluid that occurs with hypernatremia
- Tachycardia may be present.

 Safety Alert *Symptoms of hypernatremia occur only in individuals who do not have access to water or who have an altered thirst mechanism (e.g., infants, older adults, those who are comatose).*

Safety Alert *Symptoms are most likely to develop with a sudden increase in plasma sodium. After 24 hours, brain cells adjust to ECF hypertonicity by increasing intracellular osmolality. The mechanism of action is unclear, but the increased osmolality helps to rehydrate the cells. Individuals with chronic hypernatremia exhibit few symptoms. This adaptive mechanism plays a key role in treatment of hypernatremia.*

 HIGH ALERT!   Overly aggressive water administration may cause rapid movement of water into the cells, which can result in dangerous cerebral edema due to a too-rapid reduction of sodium.

Diagnostic Tests for Hypernatremia		
Test	**Purpose**	**Abnormal Findings**
Serum sodium	Assesses level of sodium	*Increased:* More than 145 mEq/L
Serum osmolality	Determines concentration of solutes	*Increased:* Due to elevated serum sodium; more than 300 mOsm/kg.
Urine specific gravity	Assesses kidneys' ability to retain water	*Increased:* More than 1.030. Lower than expected in diabetes insipidus and too dilute in early osmotic diuresis (e.g., hyperglycemia).

COLLABORATIVE MANAGEMENT
Care Priorities
1. Assess the patient for fluid losses or gains
2. Administer IV or PO water replacement: Used for water loss. If sodium is greater than 160 mEq/L, IV 5% dextrose or hypotonic (0.45%) saline is given to replace pure water deficit (see *Diabetes Insipidus*, p. 703).
3. Monitor intake to prevent too rapid correction of water loss.

4. Administer diuretics with water replacement: Use for sodium gain.
5. Provide information to the patient to help decrease sodium intake.

Safety Alert   *Hypernatremia is corrected slowly, over approximately 2 days, to avoid too great a shift of water into brain cells.*

CARE PLANS FOR HYPERNATREMIA
Acute confusion   *related to hypernatremia*

- -

GOALS/OUTCOMES Within 48 hours after treatment, patient more consistently verbalizes orientation to time, place, and person and has not sustained an injury caused by altered sensorium or seizures. Serum sodium level has decreased and is approaching high normal (145 mEq/L).

NOC Cognitive Orientation, Distorted Thought Self-Control, Information Processing, Neurological Status: Consciousness

Fluid/Electrolyte Management
1. Monitor serial serum sodium levels (sodium should not decrease at a rate greater than 0.5 to 1.0 mEq/L/hr); consult physician for rapid decreases. *Cerebral edema may occur if hypernatremia is corrected too rapidly.*
2. Assess patient for signs of cerebral edema: lethargy, headache, nausea, vomiting, increased BP, widening pulse pressure, decreased HR, altered sensorium, and seizures.
3. Assess and document LOC, orientation, and neurologic status with each vital sign check. Reorient patient as necessary. Consult physician or midlevel practitioner for deterioration.
4. Inform patient and significant others that altered sensorium is temporary and will improve with treatment.
5. Keep side rails up and bed in lowest position with wheels locked.
6. Use reality therapy such as clocks, calendars, and familiar objects; keep these items at the bedside within patient's visual field.
7. *If seizures are anticipated, pad side rails and keep an appropriate-size airway at the bedside.*
8. Provide comfort measures to decrease thirst.

NIC Neurologic Monitoring; Electrolyte Management: Hypernatremia; Seizure Precautions; Surveillance: Safety

---

ADDITIONAL NURSING DIAGNOSES
See *Hypovolemia for Fluid Volume Deficit* (p. 41) and *Hypervolemia for Fluid Volume Excess* (p. 45)

POTASSIUM IMBALANCE
(Normal serum K⁺ level 3.5 to 5 mEq/dl)

Potassium is the primary intracellular cation ($^+$ or positive ion), with normal levels inside cells of 150 mEq/dl. Of total potassium, 98% is inside the cell and markedly affects cell metabolism. Abnormal serum K^+ levels may adversely affect neuromuscular and cardiac function, because they affect resting membrane potential and conduction velocity of nerve and cardiac cells. A relatively small amount of potassium is present in ECF, and concentrations are maintained within a narrow range. Potassium is constantly moving into and out of the cell. Distribution of potassium between ECF and ICF is maintained by the sodium-potassium pump located in the membrane of all body cells and is affected by ECF pH, glucose and protein metabolism, insulin levels, and stimulation of beta₂-adrenergic receptors. Acute changes in serum pH are accompanied by reciprocal changes in serum potassium concentration as the exchange of K^+ and H^+ takes place.

The body gains potassium through foods (primarily meats, fruits, and vegetables) and medications. ECF also gains potassium from breakdown or death of cells, when a large amount of intracellular K^+ is released from the cell contents. Potassium is eliminated from the body through the kidneys, the GI tract, and the skin. The potassium level may decrease in the serum (ECF) when K^+ shifts inside the cells. The serum potassium level increases when renal function decreases, when circulation is reduced to a large amount of cells causing cell death, with cellular lysis, and with rhabdomyolysis. Changes in insulin production, insulin and other receptor activity, and catecholamine level affect the movement of K^+ across the cell wall. The kidneys are the primary regulators of potassium balance.

 Safety Alert *Disorders of potassium balance are potentially life-threatening because of the effects of altered potassium levels on neuromuscular and cardiac function. Suspected alterations in potassium balance require prompt consultation with the physician.*

HYPOKALEMIA (serum potassium level less than 3.5 mEq/L)

PATHOPHYSIOLOGY

Hypokalemia occurs because of a loss of potassium from the body or a movement of potassium into the cells. Acid-base imbalances are associated with changes in serum potassium level. Management of shifts in the K^+ level must be done judiciously if an acid-base imbalance is present. Hypokalemia is sometimes associated with alkalosis (see *Acid-Base Imbalances*, p. 1). Serum K^+ levels are an inadequate measure of intracellular K^+, but intracellular measurement is not clinically available.

 Safety Alert *Changes in serum potassium levels reflect changes in ECF potassium—not necessarily changes in total body levels.*

HYPOKALEMIA ASSESSMENT
Goal of Assessment
Evaluate for the risk factors and signs and symptoms of hypokalemia and use the information to manage the symptoms. Patient is at risk for torsades de pointes and ventricular tachycardia.

History and Risk Factors
- *Reduction in total body potassium*: Hyperaldosteronism, diuretic therapy or abnormal urinary losses, increased GI losses, increased loss through diaphoresis, decreased intake, dialysis
- *Intracellular shift*: Increased insulin (e.g., from TPN or aggressive IV insulin), acute alkalosis: K^+ moves into the cells in exchange for H^+ to electrically and pH balance the serum, stress causing a loss of potassium in the urine secondary to increased release of aldosterone, intracellular shift of potassium secondary to increased stimulation of $beta_2$-adrenergic receptors

Vital Signs
- Postural hypotension
- Irregular respiratory pattern due to respiratory muscle weakness

Auscultation
- Decreased bowel sounds

Palpation
- Weak and irregular pulse
- Decreased reflexes
- Decreased muscle tone
- Paresthesias

Screening
12-Lead ECG: Evaluate changes typically seen with hypokalemia, including ST-segment depression, flattened T waves, presence of U waves; with *severe hypokalemia*, P-wave amplitude is increased, PR interval is prolonged, QRS and QT complexes widen, and *patient is at risk for torsades de pointes.*

Safety Alert *An inadequate diet may contribute to but will rarely cause hypokalemia. Large amounts of potassium are contained in many common foods. Hypokalemia sometimes develops when patients are maintained on parenteral fluid therapy with inadequate replacement of potassium or when increased losses occur when oral intake is poor.*

Diagnostic Tests for Hypokalemia		
Test	**Purpose**	**Abnormal Findings**
Serum potassium	Determine if hypokalemia is present	*Decreased:* Less than 3.5 mEq/L
Arterial blood gases	Evaluate for the presence of alkalosis	*Increased pH and bicarbonate.* Hypokalemia is associated with metabolic alkalosis.

Safety Alert *Hypokalemia potentiates the effect of digitalis. ECG may reveal signs of digitalis toxicity despite a normal serum digitalis level.*

COLLABORATIVE MANAGEMENT
Care Priorities
1. **Replace potassium (K^+).** Administer IV potassium as an infusion if less than 3.0 mEq/L. IV infusion is 40 to 80 mEq/L given in divided doses. Generally, 10 mEq of K^1 is diluted in 50 mL IV solution and given over 30 minutes. The process is repeated until the K^1 is normalized. NEVER ADMINISTER potassium IV PUSH! If K^1 level is 3.0 to 3.5 mEq/L, increase dietary intake and use oral supplements (see Box 1-5 for high-K^1 foods).
2. **Document dietary intake of potassium.**
3. **Administer potassium-sparing diuretics** in place of thiazide or loop diuretics, which promote potassium loss. Diuretics are often associated with hypokalemia.
4. **Monitor for signs of hyperkalemia** when replacing K^+.

HIGH ALERT! Patients receiving 10 to 20 mEq/hr should be on a continuous cardiac monitor. If potassium is administered via a peripheral line, the rate of administration may require reduction to prevent irritation of vessels. The development of tall, peaked T waves suggests the presence of hyperkalemia and should be reported to a physician. IV potassium may be administered as potassium chloride or potassium phosphate.

Box 1-5	Foods High in Potassium
Apricots	Nuts
Artichokes	Oranges, orange juice
Avocados	Peanuts
Bananas	Potatoes
Cantaloupes	Prune juice
Carrots	Pumpkins
Cauliflower	Spinach
Chocolate	Swiss chard
Dried beans, peas	Sweet potatoes
Dried fruit	Tomatoes, tomato juice, tomato sauce
Mushrooms	

CARE PLANS FOR HYPOKALEMIA
Decreased cardiac output *related to dysrhythmias caused by hypokalemia*

GOALS/OUTCOMES Within 2 hours of treatment, patient is normalizing cardiac conduction as evidenced by normal T-wave configuration and normal sinus rhythm without ectopy on ECG.
NOC Cardiac Pump Effectiveness, Circulation Status

Electrolyte Management
1. *Administer potassium supplement as prescribed.* Avoid giving IV potassium chloride at a rate faster than recommended, because this can lead to life-threatening hyperkalemia. K^+ supplements for symptomatic hypokalemia may be given in isotonic saline, as sometimes D_5W increases insulin-induced intracellular shift of potassium. Concentrated solutions of potassium may be administered in limited volumes (i.e., 20 mEq in 100 ml of isotonic NaCl), administered at less than 20 mEq/hr. Concentrated solutions are used only with severe hypokalemia.

 Safety Alert *Potassium chloride should not be added to IV bags while they are hanging on a pole, to avoid accumulation of K^+ at the bottom of the IV bag. The solution container should be inverted before adding the medication and mixed well.*

2. *Be aware that IV potassium chloride (KCl) can cause local irritation of veins and chemical phlebitis.* Assess IV insertion site for erythema, heat, or pain. Irritation may be relieved by applying an ice bag, giving mild sedation, or numbing insertion site with a small amount of local anesthetic. Phlebitis may necessitate changing of IV site.
3. *Oral supplements may cause GI irritation.* Administer with a full glass of water or fruit juice; encourage patient to sip slowly. Consult physician or midlevel practitioner for symptoms of abdominal pain, distention, nausea, or vomiting. Do not switch potassium supplements without physician prescription.
4. *Monitor I&O hourly.* Consult physician or midlevel practitioner for urine output less than 0.5 ml/kg/hr. Unless severe symptoms of hypokalemia are present, potassium supplements should not be given to patients with low urine output; hyperkalemia may develop in patients with oliguria (output less than 15 to 20 ml/hr). High urine output (diuresis or polyuria) increases the risk of hypokalemia.
5. *Monitor ECG for signs of continuing hypokalemia* (i.e., ST-segment depression, flattened T wave, presence of U wave, ventricular dysrhythmias) or hyperkalemia during potassium replacement (i.e., tall, thin T waves; prolonged PR interval; ST depression; widened QRS complex; loss of P wave).
6. *Monitor serum potassium levels in patients at risk for hypokalemia,* such as patients taking diuretics or undergoing gastric suction.
7. *Administer potassium cautiously in patients at risk to develop hyperkalemia:* those receiving potassium-sparing diuretics (e.g., spironolactone or triamterene) or angiotensin-converting enzyme (ACE) inhibitors (e.g., captopril).
8. *Monitor patients on digitalis, because hypokalemia potentiates the effects.* Signs of increased digitalis effect include multifocal or bigeminal PVCs, paroxysmal atrial tachycardia with atrioventricular block, and other heart blocks.

NIC Electrolyte Management: Hypokalemia; Medication Administration; Dysrhythmia Management

Ineffective breathing pattern *related to respiratory muscle weakness associated with severe hypokalemia*

GOALS/OUTCOMES Within 2 hours of treatment, patient has effective breathing pattern as evidenced by normal respiratory depth and pattern and rate of 12 to 20 breaths/min.
NOC Respiratory Status: Ventilation; Vital Signs

Respiratory Monitoring
1. If patient has worsening hypokalemia, if respirations become rapid and shallow, notify physician or midlevel practitioner. Severe hypokalemia causes respiratory muscle weakness. Shallow respirations, apnea, and respiratory arrest may occur.

2. Keep manual resuscitator (Ambu bag) at patient's bedside when severe hypokalemia is present. Reposition patient every 2 hours to prevent stasis of secretions; suction airway as needed.
3. Encourage deep breathing (and coughing if indicated) every 2 hours.

NIC Ventilation Assistance

HYPERKALEMIA (serum potassium level greater than 5 mEq/L)

PATHOPHYSIOLOGY

Hyperkalemia results from increased intake of potassium, decreased urinary excretion of K^+, or sudden movement of K^+ out of cells. The rate of change in serum K^+ is as important as the level. Rapid increases do not allow time to compensate. Hyperkalemia is often associated with acidosis.

> **Safety Alert**   *Changes in serum potassium levels reflect changes in ECF potassium—not necessarily changes in total body levels of potassium.*

HYPERKALEMIA ASSESSMENT
Goal of Assessment

Evaluate for the risk factors and signs and symptoms of hyperkalemia. Information should be used immediately to manage potentially life threatening dysrhythmias. Hyperkalemia is often associated with acidosis.

History and Risk Factors

- *Inappropriately high intake of potassium:* IV potassium delivery, aggressive red blood cell administration, symptomatic hyperkalemia may develop when doses of IV potassium are administered too rapidly
- *Decreased excretion of potassium:* Renal disease both acute and chronic, potassium sparing diuretics and ACE inhibitors, Addison disease (hypoaldosteronism)
- *Movement of potassium out of the cells:* Acidosis, insulin deficiency particulary in dialysis patients, tissue catabolism (e.g., fever, sepsis, trauma, surgery)

Observation

- Irritability
- Abdominal distention
- Diarrhea
- Ascending weakness
- Parathesias

Vital Signs

- Irregular pulse
- Cardiac arrest at levels greater than 8.5 mEq/L
- Hypotension

Screening

- *12-Lead ECG:* Tall, thin T waves, prolonged PR interval, ST depression, widened QRS complex with progression to cardiac arrest, loss of P wave; eventually, QRS widens further and cardiac arrest occurs.

Diagnostic Tests for Hyperkalemia		
Test	**Purpose**	**Abnormal Findings**
Serum potassium	Evaluate potassium level	*Elevated:* greater than 5 mEq/L
Arterial blood gases	Evaluate acid base status	*Decreased pH and bicarbonate.* Hyperkalemia associated with acidosis

Pseudohyperkalemia may occur with mechanical trauma during venipuncture or incorrect handling of the laboratory specimen. If red blood cells (RBCs) hemolyze (are injured), potassium is released from damaged cells while or after specimen has been drawn.

COLLABORATIVE MANAGEMENT
Care Priorities
1. **Administer calcium gluconate to decrease myocardial irritability for severe hyperkalemia.** IV calcium gluconate is given to counteract the neuromuscular and cardiac effects of hyperkalemia. Serum K^+ may remain elevated.
2. **Administer insulin and IV glucose and bicarbonate to move potassium into the cell for severe hyperkalemia.** AThis strategy provides a temporary reduction in serum potassium. Sodium bicarbonate shifts K^+ into the cells.
3. **Administer beta$_2$-adrenergic agonists (albuterol) to shift K^+ back into the cells** to provide a temporary reduction in K^+ level.
4. **Take precautions when drawing blood to prevent hemolysis,** because damaged cells release intracellular contents into the blood sample, which elevates the sample's K^+ level. Most laboratories can provide information about whether the sample was hemolyzed.
5. **Administer cation exchange resins orally or rectally.** Cation exchange resins (e.g., Kayexelate) is given orally, or as a retention enema to exchange sodium for potassium in the gut. The oral form is combined with sorbitol to promote rapid transit through the gut and to induce diarrhea. Recommended rectal dose is 30 to 60 g every 6 hours.
6. **Provide hemodialysis to lower K^+ level if rapid removal for K^+ is needed.**
7. **Monitor for signs of hypokalemia,** which may result from aggressive management of hyperkalemia.

The effects of calcium, glucose and insulin, sodium bicarbonate, and beta$_2$-adrenergic agonists are temporary, lasting only a few hours. These medications should be followed by therapy to remove potassium from the body (i.e., hemodialysis or administration of cation exchange resins).

CARE PLANS FOR HYPERKALEMIA
Decreased cardiac output *related to dysrhythmias induced by hyperkalemia*

GOALS/OUTCOMES Within 6 hours after initiation of treatment, patient's CO is adequate as evidenced by PAP 20 to 30/8 to 15 mm Hg, CVP ≤6 mm Hg, CO 4 to 7 L/min, HR ≤100 bpm, BP within patient's normal range, and absence of the clinical signs of heart failure or pulmonary edema (e.g., crackles, SOB). ECG shows normal sinus rhythm without ectopy or other electrical disturbances. Serum K^+ levels normalize.

 Cardiac Pump Effectiveness, Circulation Status

Fluid/Electrolyte Management
1. *Monitor I&O.* Consult physician for urine output less than 0.5 ml/kg/hr. Oliguria increases the risk for development of hyperkalemia.
2. *Monitor for signs of hyperkalemia:* Irritability, anxiety, abdominal cramping, diarrhea, ascending weakness, paresthesias, irregular pulse. Assess for hidden sources of potassium: medications (e.g., potassium penicillin G), banked blood, salt substitute, GI bleeding, or catabolic conditions (i.e., infection or trauma).
3. *Monitor for signs of hypokalemia after treatment:* Muscle weakness, cramps, nausea, vomiting, decreased bowel sounds, paresthesias, weak and irregular pulse.
4. *Monitor serum potassium levels, especially in high-risk patients* (i.e., those with renal failure). Monitor other lab values associated with conditions that alter potassium levels (e.g., BUN, creatinine, ABGs, glucose). Consult physician or midlevel practitioner for abnormal values.
5. *Monitor ECG for signs of hypokalemia* (i.e., ST-segment depression, flattened T waves, presence of U wave, ventricular dysrhythmias), or continuing hyperkalemia (i.e., tall, thin T waves, prolonged PR interval, ST depression, widened QRS complex, loss of P wave). Report changes to physician or midlevel practitioner as soon as possible.
6. *Administer insulin and glucose in the order prescribed.*

7. *Administer calcium gluconate as prescribed.* Use caution in patients receiving digitalis. Monitor for digitalis toxicity. Do not add calcium gluconate to solutions containing sodium bicarbonate, because precipitates may form. For more information about calcium administration, see *Hypocalcemia,* p. 57.

8. *If administering cation exchange resins by enema, encourage patient to retain the solution for at least 30 to 60 minutes to ensure therapeutic effects.* Administer Kayexalate (without sorbitol) via a Foley catheter inserted into the rectum. The balloon is filled with sterile water to keep the catheter in place, and the catheter is clamped. Cleansing enemas may be done prior to administering Kayexelate to enhance absorption, and afterward to reduce the risk of bowel complications.

NIC Electrolyte Management: Hyperkalemia; Dysrhythmia Management; Hemodialysis Therapy

CALCIUM IMBALANCE (normal serum Ca²⁺ level: 8.5 to 10.5 mg/dl, ionized 4.5–5.5 mEq/L)

Calcium, one of the body's most abundant ions, combines with phosphorus to form the mineral salts of the bones and teeth. Calcium exerts a sedative effect on nerve cells and has important intracellular functions, including development of the cardiac action potential and contraction of muscles. Only 1% of the body's calcium is contained within ECF, yet this concentration is regulated carefully by the *hormones parathyroid hormone (PTH) and calcitonin.*

Slightly less than half of the calcium in the plasma is *free or ionized calcium.* The percentage of ionized calcium is affected by plasma pH and the albumin level. About 40% of calcium is bound to protein, primarily albumin. Calcium bound to albumin is not ionized and cannot be used. Albumin releases calcium to the ionized state when needed. Only the ionized calcium exerts physiologic effects and combines with nonprotein anions such as phosphate, citrate, and carbonate. Patients with alkalosis may show signs of hypocalcemia because of increased calcium binding. Changes in the plasma albumin level will affect the total serum calcium level without changing the level of ionized calcium.

> **Safety Alert**   *To determine the "true calcium level" or calcium correction factor: for every gram of albumin less than 4, add 0.8 to the serum calcium value.*

PTH is released by the parathyroid gland in response to low serum Ca²⁺ levels to increase movement of Ca²⁺ and phosphorus out of the bone (resorption of bone); to activate vitamin D (increases the absorption of calcium from the GI tract); and to stimulate the kidneys to conserve calcium and excrete phosphorus. *Calcitonin* is produced by the thyroid gland when serum Ca²⁺ increases to inhibit bone resorption.

Calcium regulates skeletal and cardiac muscle contractions, is part of the clotting cascade, and has other essential functions. It is imperative to maintain the Ca²⁺ balance.

HYPOCALCEMIA (serum calcium less than 8.5 mg/dl, ionized less than 4.5 mEq/L)

PATHOPHYSIOLOGY

Symptoms of hypocalcemia result from decreased total body calcium or a decreased percentage of ionized calcium. Low total calcium levels may be caused by increased calcium loss, reduced intake secondary to altered intestinal absorption, altered regulation (i.e., hypoparathyroidism); aggressive infusion of citrated blood or CRRT if citrate is used for anticoagulation. *Elevated phosphorus levels and decreased magnesium levels may precipitate hypocalcemia.*

HYPOCALCEMIA ASSESSMENT
Goal of the Assessment

Evaluate the signs and symptoms of hypocalcemia.

History and Risk Factors

- Decreased ionized calcium
  - Alkalosis

- Rapid administration of citrated blood. Citrate added to the blood to prevent clotting may bind with calcium, causing hypocalcemia.
  - Hemodilution (e.g., occurring with volume replacement with normal saline after massive hemorrhage)
- Increased calcium loss in body fluids
  - Large volume diuresis from loop diuretics
- *Decreased intestinal absorption:* Decreased intake, impaired vitamin D metabolism, chronic diarrhea, postoperatively following a gastrectomy
- *Other causes:* Acute and chronic renal failure, hypoparathyroidism, hyperphosphatemia, hypomagnesemia, acute pancreatitis, chemotherapy, treatment with bisphosphonates

Observation
- Numbness with tingling of fingers and circumoral region
- Tetany
- Convulsions
- Alteration in mental status (anxiety, depression, frank psychosis)

Vital Signs
- Hypotension secondary to vasodilation
- Heart failure secondary to decreased myocardial contractility

Percussion
- Positive Trousseau sign: Ischemia-induced carpopedal spasms. Elicited by applying a BP cuff to the upper arm and inflating it past systolic BP for 2 minutes.
- Positive Chvostek sign: Unilateral contraction of facial and eyelid muscles. Elicited by stimulating the facial nerve during percussion of the face just in front of the ear.

Screening
- *12-Lead ECG:* Prolonged QT interval caused by elongation and elevation of ST segment

Diagnostic Tests for Hypocalcemia		
Test	**Purpose**	**Abnormal Findings**
Total serum calcium level	Evaluate total calcium level	*Decreased:* Less than 8.5 mg/dl. Evaluate with serum albumin. For every 1 g/dl drop in the serum albumin level there is a 0.8–1 mg/dl drop in the total calcium.
Ionized calcium level	Evaluate the free calcium level	*Decreased:* less than 4.5 mg/dl
Parathyroid (PTH) level	Evaluate for hyperparathyroidism or hypoparathyroidism	*Hypoparathyroidism:* Less than 150 pg/ml. *Hyperparathyroidism:* More than 350 pg/ml. Varies among labs
Magnesium level	Evaluate for hypomagnesemia	*Decreased:* Less than 1.5 mEq/L
Phosphorus level	Evaluate for hyperphosphatemia	*Increased:* More than 4.5 mEq/L

COLLABORATIVE MANAGEMENT
Care Priorities
1. **Administer IV calcium by continuous infusion over 4 to 6 hours** May give PO or IV calcium. Tetany is treated with 10 to 20 ml of 10% calcium gluconate administered IV or by continuous infusion of 100 ml of 10% calcium gluconate diluted in 1000 ml D$_5$W over at least 4 to 6 hours.
2. **Administer vitamin D therapy** Provide additional vitamin D (e.g., dihydrotachysterol, calcitriol) to increase vitamin D absorption from the GI tract. Use of oral vitamin D$_3$ (activated vitamin D, available over the counter) is helpful to maintain calcium levels over time.

3. **Administer magnesium replacement** Used for magnesium depletion; hypomagnesemia-induced hypocalcemia is often refractory to calcium therapy alone.
4. **Administer phosphate binders if needed** Used to reduce elevated phosphorous before treating hypocalcemia. Used primarily in renal failure.
5. **Monitor for signs of hypercalcemia during calcium replacement therapy** Lethargy, weakness, anorexia, nausea, vomiting, constipation, itching, polyuria, confusion, personality changes, stupor, coma

CARE PLANS FOR HYPOCALCEMIA
Ineffective protection *related to the potential complications of hypocalcemia*

GOALS/OUTCOMES Patient is not permanently harmed by severe hypocalcemia.
NOC Electrolyte and Acid-Base Balance, Nutritional Status: Food and Fluid Intake, Kidney Function, Fluid Balance

Electrolyte Management: Hypocalcemia
1. Monitor patient for worsening hypocalcemia and consult physician or midlevel practitioner promptly for symptoms that occur before overt tetany: Numbness and tingling of fingers and circumoral region, hyperactive reflexes, and muscle cramps. Positive Trousseau or Chvostek sign also signals latent tetany. Monitor total and ionized calcium levels as available.

HIGH ALERT! *Administer IV calcium slowly.* Undiluted IV 10% calcium should not be given faster than 0.5 to 1 ml/min. Diluted calcium given in an infusion is preferred. *Rapid administration can cause hypotension.* Observe IV insertion site for infiltration; calcium will slough tissue. *Concentrated calcium solutions (calcium chloride) should be administered through a central line.* Do not add calcium to solutions containing sodium bicarbonate or sodium phosphate to avoid dangerous precipitates. Digitalis toxicity may develop, because calcium potentiates digitalis. Monitor for hypercalcemia: lethargy, confusion, irritability, nausea, and vomiting.

Safety Alert *Always clarify the type of IV calcium to be given. Both calcium chloride and calcium gluconate come in 10-ml ampules. One ampule of calcium chloride contains 13.6 mEq of calcium, whereas one ampule of calcium gluconate contains 4.5 mEq of calcium.*

2. For patients with chronic hypocalcemia, administer oral calcium supplements and vitamin D preparations as prescribed. Administer oral calcium 30 minutes before meals or at bedtime for maximal absorption. Administer phosphorus-binding antacids with meals. If calcium carbonate is being administered primarily to bind phosphorus, administer with food.
3. Consult physician or midlevel practitioner if response to calcium therapy is ineffective. Tetany that does not respond to IV calcium may be caused by hypomagnesemia.
4. Maintain seizure precautions for affected patients.
5. Avoid hyperventilation if hypocalcemia is suspected. Respiratory alkalosis may cause tetany if pH increases when ionized calcium is low.
6. Monitor for calcium loss (e.g., with loop diuretics, renal tubular dysfunction) or conditions that place the patient at risk for it (e.g., acute pancreatitis).
7. Inform patient and significant others that the neuropsychiatric symptoms of hypocalcemia will improve with treatment.

NIC Neurologic Monitoring; Seizure Precautions; Medication Administration

Decreased cardiac output *related to abnormal action of calcium in myocardial contractile tissues*

GOALS/OUTCOMES Within 12 hours of initiation of treatment, patient's CO is improving as evidenced by readings approaching normal baseline or PAP 20 to 30/8 to 15 mm Hg, CVP less than 6 mm Hg, CO 4 to 7 L/min, HR 100 bpm, BP within patient's normal range, and diminishing clinical signs of heart failure or pulmonary edema (e.g., crackles, SOB). ECG shows a sinus rhythm without ectopy or other electrical disturbances.
NOC Cardiac Pump Effectiveness

Cardiac Care: Acute Hemodynamic Regulation
1. Monitor ECG for signs of worsening hypocalcemia (e.g., prolonged QT interval) or of digitalis toxicity with calcium replacement: multifocal or bigeminal PVCs, paroxysmal atrial tachycardia with AV block, and other heart blocks.
2. Hypocalcemia may decrease cardiac contractility. Monitor patient for signs of heart failure or pulmonary edema: crackles, rhonchi, SOB, decreased BP, increased HR, increased PAP, or increased CVP.

NIC Dysrhythmia Management; Cardiac Care

Ineffective breathing pattern *related to abnormal rigidity of upper airway and respiratory muscles*

GOALS/OUTCOMES Within 1 hour of initiation of treatment, the patient is regaining an effective breathing pattern as evidenced by more comfortable work of breathing with RR 12 to 20 breaths/min and absence of the indicators of laryngeal spasm: laryngeal stridor, dyspnea, or crowing.
NOC Respiratory Status: Ventilation, Respiratory Status: Airway Patency

Respiratory Monitoring
1. Assess patient's respiratory rate, character, and rhythm. Be alert to laryngeal stridor, dyspnea, and crowing, which occur with laryngeal spasm, a life-threatening complication of hypocalcemia.
2. Keep an emergency tracheostomy tray at the bedside of all patients with symptoms of hypocalcemia.

NIC Airway Management; Ventilation Assistance

HYPERCALCEMIA (serum calcium level greater than 10.5 mEq/L, ionized greater than 5.5)

PATHOPHYSIOLOGY

Hypercalcemia is caused by increased total serum calcium or increased percentage of free, ionized calcium. If hypercalcemia is accompanied by a normal or elevated serum phosphorus level, calcium phosphate crystals may precipitate in the serum and deposit throughout the body. Soft tissue calcifications usually occur when the product of the serum calcium and serum phosphorus (i.e., calcium level $\times$ phosphorus level) exceeds 70 mg/dl.

HYPERCALCEMIA ASSESSMENT
Goal of the Assessment

Evaluate the signs, symptoms, and risk factors for hypercalcemia.

History and Risk Factors

- *Hyperparathyroidism:* May be stress-related in critical illness
- *Lymphoproliferative disorders:* Which prompt parathyroid protein production
- *Increased intake of calcium:* Excessive administration during cardiopulmonary arrest; milk-alkali syndrome
- *Increased intestinal absorption:* Vitamin D overdose or hyperparathyroidsm. Increased release of calcium from bone: hyperparathyroidism, malignancies, prolonged immobilization; Paget disease
- *Decreased urinary excretion:* Renal failure, thiazide diuretics, hyperparathyroidism
- *Increased ionized calcium:* Acidosis

Observation

- Symptoms absent unless serum calcium is more than 11 mg/dl
- Behavioral changes: Personality changes, depression
- Neurological changes: Lethargy, weakness, confusion, paresthesias, stupor, coma
- GI/digestive changes: Anorexia, nausea, vomiting, constipation
- Other: Polyuria, itching, bone pain

Vital Signs
- Hypertension
- Heart block
- Cardiac arrest

12-Lead ECG
- Shortening ST segment and QT interval
- PR interval is sometimes prolonged.
- Ventricular dysrhythmias

Diagnostic Tests for Hypercalcemia		
Test	**Purpose**	**Abnormal Findings**
Total serum calcium	Evaluate total calcium level; calcium is bound to albumin; if albumin is low, calcium is low.	*Elevated:* More than 10.5 mg/dl. Evaluate with serum albumin level to avoid false lows.
Ionized calcium	Evaluate free calcium level.	*Elevated:* More than 5.5 mg/dl
PTH (parathyroid hormone)	Assess for hyperparathyroidism or hypoparathyroidism.	*Elevated:* More than 350 pg/ml
Radiographs (bone scan, DEXA scan, KUB)	Evaluate for bone changes or urinary calculi.	Osteoporosis, bone cavitations, or urinary calculi

COLLABORATIVE MANAGEMENT
Care Priorities
1. **Administer loop diuretics and isotonic saline** Administered rapidly to increase urinary calcium excretion. Concomitant administration of furosemide prevents the development of fluid volume excess and further increases urinary calcium excretion.
2. **Discontinue vitamin supplements and thiazide diuretics** *if* patient has been taking them.
3. **Treat the underlying cause** May include antitumor chemotherapy for malignancy, partial parathyroidectomy for hyperparathyroidism; discontinuation of calcium supplements, vitamins A and D, and thiazide diuretics
4. **Facilitate rebuilding of bone.**
   - *Increase activity level.* Weight-bearing stimulates bone deposition; increased activity decreases bone resorption.
   - *Administer bisphosphonates (etidronate and pamidronate):* Act directly on bone to reduce decalcification; used primarily to treat hypercalcemia associated with neoplastic disease. May take several days to work but the effects last for days to weeks.
   - *Mithramycin* is a cytotoxic antibiotic that decreases bone resorption.
   - *Calcitonin:* Reduces bone resorption and increases bone deposition of calcium and phosphorus; increases urinary calcium and phosphate excretion.
   - *Gallium nitrate:* Inhibits osteoclasts and increased bone calcium. Used in the treatment of malignancy-induced hypercalcemia.
5. **Reduce calcium intake and intestinal absorption** Administer steroids to compete with Vitamin D, thereby reducing intestinal absorption of calcium.
6. **Monitor for signs of hypocalcemia** May result from hypercalcemia therapies.

CARE PLANS FOR HYPERCALCEMIA
Ineffective protection *related to inability to guard self from internal and external threats due to impaired decision making resulting from changes in mental status*

GOALS/OUTCOMES Within 24 to 48 hours of initiating treatment, patient more consistently verbalizes orientation to time, place, and person. Patient does not exhibit evidence of injury caused by neurosensory changes.
NOC Cognitive Orientation, Distorted Thought Self-Control, Neurologic Status

⚕ Neurologic Monitoring
1. Monitor patient for worsening hypercalcemia: disorientation to time, place, and person; and deterioration in neurologic status.
2. Note personality changes, hallucinations, paranoia, and memory loss. Inform patient and significant others that altered sensorium is temporary and will improve with treatment. Use reality therapy: clocks, calendars, and familiar objects; keep them at the bedside within patient's visual field.

Electrolyte Monitoring: Hypercalcemia
1. Administer fluids and diuretics as prescribed. Evaluate response to therapy. Monitor serum calcium levels and albumin levels. Observe for signs of fluid volume excess that develop with treatment.
2. Hypercalcemia causes neuromuscular depression with poor coordination, weakness, and altered gait. Provide a safe environment. Keep side rails up and bed in lowest position with wheels locked. Assist with ambulation.
3. Monitor for signs of digitalis toxicity (hypercalcemia potentiates digitalis): multifocal or bigeminal PVCs, paroxysmal atrial tachycardia with AV block, other heart blocks.
4. Monitor serum electrolytes: calcium, potassium, and phosphorus (normal range is 2.5 to 4.5 mg/dl). Note changes that result from therapy. Consult physician or midlevel practitioner for abnormal values.
5. Encourage increased mobility to reduce bone resorption. Ideally patient should be out of bed and up in a chair at least 6 hours a day.

NIC Fluid Monitoring; Dysrhythmia Management; Fluid Management

⚕ Impaired urinary elimination *related to hypercalcemia decreasing the ability of the kidneys to concentrate urine, which can lead to polyuria and possible fluid volume deficit. Hypercalcemia can impair renal function.*

GOALS/OUTCOMES Within 24 hours of initiation of treatment, the patient exhibits voiding pattern and urine characteristics that are moving toward normal for the patient.
NOC Urinary Elimination

Fluid Management
1. Monitor I&O hourly. Consult physician or midlevel practitioner for unusual changes in urine volume (e.g., oliguria alternating with polyuria, which may signal urinary tract obstruction, or continuous polyuria). This is a type of nephrogenic diabetes insipidus (see *Diabetes Insipidus*, p. 703). Monitor for signs of volume depletion when giving diuretics: decreased BP, CVP, and PAP and increased HR.
2. Monitor patient's renal function carefully: Urine output, BUN, creatinine values (see *Acute Renal Failure/Acute Kidney Injury*, p. 584).
3. Provide patient with a low-calcium diet and avoid use of calcium-containing medications (e.g., antacids such as Tums). Encourage intake of fruits (e.g., cranberries, prunes, plums) that leave an acid ash in the urine. Acidic urine reduces the risk of calcium stone formation. Also increase fluid intake (at least 3 L in nonrestricted patients) to reduce the risk of renal stone formation.
4. Assess patient for indicators of kidney stone formation: intermittent pain, nausea, vomiting, and hematuria.

NIC Fluid Monitoring; Urinary Elimination Management; Electrolyte Management: Hypercalcemiaz

PHOSPHORUS IMBALANCE
(normal serum level 2.5 to 4.5 mg/dl or 1.7 to 2.6 mEq/L)

Phosphorus, the primary anion ($^-$ or negative ion) of the ICF, has a wide variety of vital functions: formation of energy-storing substances (e.g., adenosine triphosphate [ATP]); formation of red blood cell 2,3-diphosphoglycerate (DPG) (facilitates the release of O_2 from the Hgb to be used by the cells); metabolism of carbohydrates, protein, and fat; and maintenance of acid-base balance. In addition, phosphorus is critical to normal nerve and muscle function and provides structural support to bones and teeth.

Plasma phosphorus levels vary with diet and acid-base balance. Glucose, insulin, or sugar-containing foods cause a temporary drop in phosphorus because of a shift of serum phosphorus into the cells. Phosphorous and calcium have an interdependent effect on each other and share many of the common causes of abnormalities. Alkalosis, particularly respiratory alkalosis, may cause hypophosphatemia as a result of an intracellular shift of phosphorus. Although the exact mechanism for this shift is not fully understood, it may be related to an alkalosis-induced cellular glycolysis, with increased formation of phosphorus-containing metabolic intermediates. Respiratory acidosis may cause a shift of phosphorus out of the cells and contribute to hyperphosphatemia.

Although the level of ECF phosphate is affected by a combination of factors, including dietary intake, intestinal absorption, and hormonally regulated bone resorption and deposition, phosphorus balance depends largely on renal excretion.

HYPOPHOSPHATEMIA (serum phosphate level less than 2.5 mg/dl or less than 1.7 mEq/L)

PATHOPHYSIOLOGY
Hypophosphatemia (serum phosphorus less than 2.5 mg/dl) may occur because of transient intracellular shifts, increased urinary losses (most common), decreased intestinal absorption, or increased utilization (see History and Risk Factors). Severe phosphorus deficiency also may develop because of a combination of factors in conditions such as chronic alcohol abuse and DKA.

HYPOPHOSPHATEMIA ASSESSMENT
Goal of the Assessment
Evaluate the signs, symptoms, and risk factors for hypophosphatemia. Acute, severe hypophosphatemia can be a life-threatening condition. Symptoms can be so profound that care providers focus on extensive workups while sometimes overlooking the hypophosphatemia.

History and Risk Factors
- *Intracellular shifts*: Carbohydrate load, respiratory alkalosis, treatment of DKA
- *Increased utilization because of increased tissue repair*: Total parenteral nutrition (TPN) with inadequate phosphorus content; recovery from protein-calorie malnutrition. Hypophosphatemia is common in the critical care patient largely because of nutritional deficiency.
- *Increased urinary losses*: hypomagnesemia, ECF volume expansion, hyperparathyroidism, use of thiazide diuretics, diuretic phase of ATN, glucosuria
- *Reduced intestinal absorption or increased intestinal loss*: Use of phosphorus-binding medications; vomiting and diarrhea; malabsorption disorders such as vitamin D deficiency; prolonged gastric suction
- *Other conditions*: Chronic alcohol abuse, DKA, severe burns, sepsis
- *Resulting from interventions*: Postoperative patients, patients on mechanical ventilation, postoperative renal transplant patients

Observation
Symptoms may be caused by sudden decreases in serum phosphorus, or they may develop gradually because of chronic deficiency. The majority of symptoms are secondary to decreases in ATP and 2,3 DPG; therefore, the patient will become acutely hypoxic at the cellular level, producing a high lactate and metabolic acid load, resulting in poor coordination, confusion, seizures, and coma. Other acute symptoms include:
- Chest pain as a result of poor oxygenation of the myocardium
- Muscle pain and weakness
- Increased susceptibility to infection
- Numbness and tingling of the fingers
- Numbness of the circumoral region
- Respiratory alkalosis from hyperventilation
- Difficulty speaking due to decreased strength
- Bruising and bleeding because of platelet dysfunction
- Rhabdomyolysis, hemolysis
  Chronic symptoms include memory loss, lethargy, weakness, bone pain, joint stiffness, arthralgia, cyanosis, osteomalacia, and possible pseudo-fractures.

Vital Signs

- Decreased respiratory rate
- Increased PAWP
- Decreased CO
- Decreased BP with decreased response to pressor agents

> **Safety Alert** *Respiratory alkalosis causes phosphorus to move intracellularly, aggravating the existing hypophosphatemia.*

Diagnostic Tests for Hypophosphatemia

Test	Purpose	Abnormal Findings
Serum phosphate level	Determine the severity of hypophosphatemia	*Decreased:* Less than 2.5 mg/dl (1.7 mEq/L) *Mild:* 1–2.5 mg/dl *Severe:* Less than 1 mg/dl
Parathyroid hormone (PTH)	Evaluate if hyperparathyroid	*Elevated:* In hyperparathyroidism to more than 350 pg/ml
Serum magnesium	Evaluate loss of magnesium	Decreased because of increased urinary excretion of magnesium in hypophosphatemia
Skeletal radiographs	Evaluate bone changes	Skeletal changes of osteomalacia

COLLABORATIVE MANAGEMENT

Care Priorities

1. **Discontinue use of phosphate binders** (e.g., aluminum, magnesium, or calcium gels of antacids).
2. **Correct respiratory alkalosis if present** See *Acid-Base Balance*, p. 1.
3. **Increase phosphorus intake** Mild hypophosphatemia may respond to increased intake of foods high in phosphorus, such as milk (Box 1-6).
4. **Administer oral phosphate supplements** Moderate hypophosphatemia is treated with phosphate supplements including Neutra-Phos (sodium and potassium phosphate) or Phospho-soda (sodium phosphate).
5. **Administer IV sodium phosphate or potassium phosphate** Severe hypophosphatemia is treated with sodium phosphate or potassium phosphate. IV infusions are also used for patients with a nonfunctional GI tract.
6. **Monitor for resolution or progression of neurologic and hematologic signs and symptoms.**

CARE PLANS FOR HYPOPHOSPHATEMIA

 Ineffective protection *related to inability to guard self from internal and external threats due to impaired decision making resulting from changes in mental status*

Box 1-6   FOODS HIGH IN PHOSPHORUS

Dried beans and peas
Eggs and egg products (e.g., eggnog, soufflés)
Fish
Meats, especially organ meats (e.g., brain, liver, kidney)
Milk and milk products (e.g., cheese, ice cream, cottage cheese)
Nuts (e.g., Brazil, peanuts)
Poultry
Seeds (e.g., pumpkin, sesame, sunflower)
Whole grains (e.g., oatmeal, bran, barley)

GOALS/OUTCOMES Within 24 to 48 hours of initiating treatment, the patient more consistently verbalizes orientation to time, place, and person. The patient does not exhibit evidence of injury caused by neurosensory changes.
NOC Cognitive Orientation, Distorted Thought Self-Control, Neurologic Status

Neurologic Monitoring
1. Monitor patient for worsening hypophosphatemia: Disorientation to time, place, and person; and deterioration in neurologic status.
2. Note personality changes, hallucinations, paranoia, and memory loss. Inform patient and significant others that altered sensorium is temporary and will improve with treatment. Use reality therapy: clocks, calendars, and familiar objects; keep them at the bedside within patient's visual field.
3. Apprehension, confusion, and paresthesias are signals of developing hypophosphatemia. Assess and document LOC, orientation, and neurologic status with each vital sign check. Reorient patient as necessary. Alert physician or midlevel practitioner to significant changes.
4. Inform patient and significant others that altered sensorium is temporary and will improve with treatment.
5. Keep the side rails up and the bed in its lowest position with wheels locked.
6. Use reality therapy: clocks, calendars, and familiar objects. Keep these articles at the bedside within patient's visual field.
7. If patient is at risk for seizures, pad the side rails and keep an appropriate-size airway at the bedside.

Electrolyte Management: Hypophosphatemia
1. Monitor serum phosphorus levels in patients at increased risk. Consult physician or midlevel practitioner for decreased levels. Monitor for signs of associated electrolyte and acid-base imbalances: hypokalemia, hypomagnesemia, respiratory alkalosis, and metabolic acidosis.
2. When IV phosphorus is administered as potassium phosphate, the infusion rate should not exceed 10 mEq/hr. Monitor IV site for signs of infiltration, because potassium phosphate can cause necrosis and sloughing of tissue.

HIGH ALERT! *Do not administer IV phosphate at a rate greater than that recommended by the manufacturer. Potential complications of IV phosphorus administration include tetany as a result of hypocalcemia (serum calcium levels may drop suddenly if serum phosphorus levels increase suddenly; see Hypocalcemia, p. 57, for additional information); soft tissue calcification (if hyperphosphatemia develops, the calcium and phosphorus in the ECF may combine and form deposits in tissue); and hypotension, caused by a too-rapid delivery.*

3. Encourage intake of foods high in phosphorus (see Box 1-6). Teach patient and significant others the importance of using phosphorus-binding antacids only as prescribed.

NIC Medication Administration

Impaired gas exchange *related to respiratory muscle weakness, coupled with inability of red blood cells to offload O_2 at the cellular level due to decreased 2,3-DPG levels.*

GOALS/OUTCOMES Within 12 hours of initiation of treatment, the patient has increasingly normal gas exchange as evidenced by RR 12 to 20 breaths/min with normal depth and pattern (eupnea); orientation to time, place, and person; Spo_2 at least 92%; and absence of the indicators of hypoxia (e.g., restlessness, somnolence).
NOC Respiratory Status: Gas Exchange

Safety Alert *With decreased 2,3-DPG levels, the oxyhemoglobin dissociation curve will shift to the left. At a given Pao_2 level, more O_2 will be bound to Hgb and less will be available to the tissues.*

Respiratory Monitoring
1. Assess patient for signs of hypoxia: Restlessness, confusion, increased respirations, complaints of chest pain, and cyanosis (a late sign).
2. Monitor Spo_2 as available. Administer O_2 as prescribed to maintain Spo_2 at ≥92%.

3. Monitor rate and depth of respirations in patients with severe hypophosphatemia. Assess for decreased tidal volume or decreased minute ventilation. Consult physician or midlevel practitioner for changes.
4. Monitor ABG values for evidence of hypoxemia or hypercapnia. Consult physician or midlevel practitioner for significant changes.
5. Monitor serum phosphate levels in mechanically ventilated patients; they exhibit a high incidence of hypophosphatemia. Hypophosphatemia may contribute to difficulty in weaning patients from ventilators.

NIC Oxygen Therapy

⚕️ Impaired physical mobility *related to muscle weakness resulting from hypophosphatemia*

GOALS/OUTCOMES Within 24 hours of initiation of therapy, patient is able to move purposefully and has full or baseline ROM and muscle strength.
NOC Mobility, Transfer Performance

Exercise Promotion: Strength Training
1. Monitor all patients with suspected hypophosphatemia for decreasing muscle strength. Perform serial assessments of hand grasp strength and clarity of speech. Consult physician or midlevel practitioner for changes.
2. Monitor serum phosphorus levels if mobility or strength decreases. Consult physician or midlevel practitioner for changes.
3. Assist the patient with ambulation and activities of daily living (ADLs).
4. Medicate for pain as prescribed.

NIC Energy Management; Pain Management

⚕️ Decreased cardiac output *related to cardiac muscle weakness related to hypophosphatemia*

GOALS/OUTCOMES Within 12 hours of initiation of treatment, patient's CO is increasingly adequate as evidenced by CO at least 4 L/min, CI at least 2.5 L/min/m^2, CVP 4–6 mm Hg, PAP 20 to 30/8 to 15 mm Hg, HR ≤100 bpm, BP within patient's normal range, and absence of the clinical signs of heart failure or pulmonary edema.
NOC Cardiac Pump Effectiveness

Cardiac Care
1. Monitor patient for signs of heart failure or pulmonary edema: crackles, rhonchi, SOB, decreased BP, increased HR, increased PAP, or increased CVP.
2. Prevent patient from hyperventilating. Metabolic alkalosis causes increased movement of phosphorus into cells, which will reduce CO.
3. For additional interventions if decreased CO develops, see *Heart Failure*, p. 421.

NIC Cardiac Care: Acute Hemodynamic Regulation; Vital Signs Monitoring

Ineffective protection *related to compromised immunity resulting from hypophosphatemia*

GOALS/OUTCOMES Patient is free of infection as evidenced by normothermia and absence of erythema, swelling, warmth, and purulent drainage at invasive sites.
NOC Immune Status

Infection Protection
1. Monitor temperature every 4h for evidence of infection. Obtain cultures of wounds and drainage as prescribed if infection is suspected.
2. Use meticulous aseptic technique when changing dressings or manipulating indwelling lines (e.g., TPN catheters, IV needles).
3. Provide oral hygiene and skin care at regular intervals. Intact skin and membranes are the body's first line of defense against infection.

NIC Risk Identification

HYPERPHOSPHATEMIA (serum phosphate level greater than 4.5 mg/dl or greater than 2.6 mEq/L)

PATHOPHYSIOLOGY

Hyperphosphatemia is common in patients with renal insufficiency/failure whose kidneys are unable to effectively excrete excess phosphorus. Other causes of hyperphosphatemia include increased intake of phosphates, extracellular shifts (i.e., movement of phosphorus out of the cell and into the ECF), cellular destruction with concomitant release of intracellular phosphorus, and decreased urinary losses that are unrelated to decreased renal function. As serum phosphorus levels increase, serum calcium levels often decrease, leading to hypocalcemia. Hypocalcemia is most likely to occur in sudden, severe hyperphosphatemia (e.g., after IV administration of phosphates) or in patients prone to hypocalcemia (e.g., those with chronic renal failure).

The primary complication of hyperphosphatemia is metastatic calcification (i.e., the precipitation of calcium phosphate in the soft tissue, joints, and arteries). Chronic hyperphosphatemia in the patient with chronic renal failure may contribute to the development of renal osteodystrophy.

Precipitation of calcium phosphate occurs when the product of the serum calcium and serum phosphorus (i.e., calcium $\times$ phosphorus) exceeds 70 mg/dl.

HYPERPHOSPHATEMIA ASSESSMENT

Goal of the Assessment

Evaluate the signs, symptoms, history, and risk factors for hyperphosphatemia.

History and Risk Factors

- *Renal failure:* Acute and chronic; may signal declining glomerular filtration rate
- *Increased intake*
  - Excessive administration of phosphorus supplements
  - Vitamin D excess with increased GI absorption
  - Excessive use of phosphorus containing laxatives or enemas
  - Massive transfusion
- *Extracellular shift:* Respiratory acidosis, diabetic ketoacidosis (prior to treatment)
- *Cellular destruction*
  - Neoplastic disease (e.g., leukemia, lymphoma) treated with cytotoxic agents
  - Increased tissue catabolism
  - Rhabdomyolysis
- *Decreased urinary losses:* Hypoparathyroidism, volume depletion

Observation

- *GI symptoms:* Anorexia, nausea, vomiting
- *Neuromuscular symptoms:* Muscle weakness, hyperreflexia, tetany

Vital Signs

- Hypotension secondary to vasodilation
- Heart failure secondary to decreased myocardial contractility
- Tachycardia

Percussion

- *Positive Trousseau sign:* Ischemia induced carpopedal spasms. Elicited by applying a BP cuff to the upper arm and inflating it past systolic BP for 2 minutes.
- *Positive Chvostek sign:* Unilateral contraction of facial and eyelid muscles. Elicited by stimulating the facial nerve during percussion of the face just in front of the ear.

 Safety Alert   *Usually patients experience few symptoms with hyperphosphatemia. The majority of symptoms relate to development of hypocalcemia or soft tissue (metastatic) calcifications. Indicators of metastatic calcification include oliguria, corneal haziness, conjunctivitis, irregular HR, and popular eruptions.*

Screening

- 12-Lead ECG: Deposition of calcium phosphate in the heart may lead to dysrhythmias and conduction disturbance; prolonged QT interval caused by elongation and elevation of ST segment

Diagnostic Tests For Hyperphosphatemia		
Test	**Purpose**	**Abnormal Findings**
Serum phosphate level	Determine severity of hyperphosphatemia	*Elevated*: More than 4.5 mg/dl (2.6 mEq/L).
Parathyroid hormone (PTH)	Evaluate for hypoparathyroidism	*Decreased*: In hypoparathyroidism
Skeletal radiographs	Assess for bony changes	May show skeletal changes of osteodystrophy

COLLABORATIVE MANAGEMENT
Care Priorities

1. **Reduce severely elevated phosphate level** Hemodialysis may be used for acute, severe hyperphosphatemia accompanied by symptoms of hypocalcemia.
2. **Administer phosphate binders** Aluminum, magnesium, or calcium antacids
3. **Monitor for symptoms of hypocalcemia** Positive Chvostek and/or positive Trousseau sign

 Calcium carbonate and calcium acetate are the preferred preparations for the patient with chronic renal failure. Magnesium antacids are avoided in renal failure because of the risk of hypermagnesemia. Aluminum-containing antacids are contraindicated because they may lead to aluminum accumulation and contribute to the development of bone disease.

CARE PLANS FOR HYPERPHOSPHATEMIA
Deficient knowledge *related to medications that may induce hyperphosphatemia*

GOALS/OUTCOMES Within the 24-hour period before discharge from intensive care unit, patient describes the potential complications of uncontrolled hyperphosphatemia and preventive measures.
NOC Health Promoting Behavior; Knowledge: Medication

 Prevention of long-term complications relies primarily on adequate patient education, because symptoms of hyperphosphatemia may be minimal.

Teaching: Prescribed Medication
1. Teach patients the purpose of phosphate binders. Stress the need to take binders as prescribed with or after meals to maximize effectiveness.
2. Educate patients about possible constipation from phosphate binders. Encourage use of bulk-building supplements or stool softener if constipation occurs. *Phosphate-containing laxatives and enemas must be avoided (i.e., Fleet's Phospho-soda products).*
3. Phosphate binders are available in liquid, tablet, or capsule form. Confer with physician or midlevel practitioner regarding an alternate form or brand for individuals who find binders unpalatable or difficult to take. Phosphate binders vary in aluminum, magnesium, or calcium content. One may not be exchanged for another without first ensuring that the patient is receiving the same amount of elemental aluminum, magnesium, or calcium.

4. Discuss avoiding or limiting foods high in phosphorus (see Box 1-6).
5. Review the importance of avoiding phosphorus-containing over-the-counter medications: certain laxatives, enemas, and mixed vitamin-mineral supplements. Instruct the patient and significant others to read the label for the words "phosphorus" and "phosphate."

NIC Teaching: Prescribed Medication; Electrolyte Management: Hyperphosphatemia

Ineffective protection *related to inability to avoid internal complications related to hyperphosphatemia*

- -

GOALS/OUTCOMES Patient does not develop symptoms of physical injury caused by precipitation of calcium phosphate in the soft tissue or joints, or by hypocalcemic tetany.
NOC Activity Tolerance, Mobility, Energy Conservation

Electrolyte Management: Hyperphosphatemia
1. Monitor serum phosphorus and calcium levels. Calculate the calcium-phosphorus product (calcium $\times$ phosphorus). Values greater than 70 mg/dl are associated with precipitation of calcium phosphate in the soft tissues. Consult physician or midlevel practitioner for abnormal values. *Phosphorus values may be kept slightly higher (4 to 6 mg/dl) to ensure adequate levels of 2,3-DPG in chronic renal failure patients, to minimize effects of chronic anemia on O_2 delivery to the tissues.*
2. Vitamin D products and calcium supplements (taken between meals) may be limited until the serum phosphorus approaches a normal level.
3. Consult physician or midlevel practitioner if patient develops indicators of metastatic calcification: oliguria, corneal haziness, conjunctivitis, irregular HR, and papular eruptions.
4. Monitor patient for symptoms of increasing hypocalcemia that may precede overt tetany: numbness and tingling of the fingers and circumoral region, hyperactive reflexes, and muscle cramps. Positive Trousseau or Chvostek sign may signal latent tetany. Consult physician or midlevel practitioner promptly if these symptoms develop (See Hypocalcemia, see p. 57.)
5. Because hyperphosphatemia can impair renal function, monitor renal function carefully: urine output, BUN, and creatinine values.

NIC Neurologic Monitoring; Energy Management

MAGNESIUM IMBALANCE
(normal serum magnesium level 1.5 to 2.5 mEq/L)

Approximately 60% of the body's magnesium is located in bone, and approximately 1% is located in the ECF. The remaining magnesium is contained within the cells. Mg^{2+} is the second most abundant intracellular cation ($+$ or positive ion) after potassium. Magnesium is regulated by a combination of factors, including vitamin D–regulated GI absorption and renal excretion.

Because magnesium is a major intracellular ion, it plays a vital role in normal cellular function. Specifically, it activates enzymes involved in the metabolism of carbohydrates and protein, and it triggers the sodium-potassium pump, thus affecting intracellular potassium levels. Magnesium also is important in the transmission of neuromuscular activity, neural transmission within the CNS, and myocardial functioning.

HYPOMAGNESEMIA
(serum magnesium level less than 1.5 mEq/L)

PATHOPHYSIOLOGY

Hypomagnesemia usually results from decreased GI absorption, increased urinary loss, or excessive GI loss (e.g., vomiting, diarrhea), and with prolonged administration of magnesium-free parenteral fluids. Chronic alcohol abusers (see History and Risk Factors that follow) and critically ill patients most commonly experience low Mg^{2+}. Hypomagnesemia is associated with increased mortality in the critical care setting. Dysrhythmias and sudden death increase when decreased magnesium levels occur in combination with myocardial infarction, heart failure, or digitalis toxicity. Hypomagnesemia usually is associated with hypocalcemia and hypokalemia (see *Hypokalemia*, p. 52, and *Hypocalcemia*, p. 57 for additional information). Symptoms of hypomagnesemia tend to develop once the serum magnesium level drops below 1 mEq/L. Decreased magnesium intake has been identified as a risk factor for hypertension, cardiac dysrhythmias, ischemic heart disease, and sudden cardiac death.

HYPOMAGNESEMIA ASSESSMENT
Goal of Assessment
Evaluate for the signs, symptoms, and risk factors for hypomagnesemia and further investigate whether patient may also have hypokalemia and/or hypocalcemia.

History and Risk Factors
- *Chronic alcoholism*: Poor dietary intake, decreased GI absorption, increased urinary excretion
- *Decreased GI absorption*: Cancer, colitis, pancreatic insufficiency, surgical resection in the GI tract, use of laxatives, diarrhea
- *Increased GI losses*: From prolonged vomiting or gastric suction
- *Administration of low-magnesium or magnesium-free parenteral solutions*: Especially with refeeding after starvation
- *Poorly controlled diabetes including DKA*: A result of movement of magnesium out of the cell and loss in the urine because of osmotic diuresis
- *Increased urinary excretion*: Use of diuretics, diuretic phase of ATN
- *Medications*: Amphotericin, tobramycin, gentamicin, cisplatin, cyclosporine, or digoxin
- *Protein-calorie malnutrition*
- *Cardiopulmonary bypass*

Observation
- *Behavioral changes*: Mood changes, lethargy, hallucinations, confusion
- *Neuromuscular symptoms*: Weakness, fatigue, paresthesias, tremors, convulsions, tetany
- *GI symptoms*: Anorexia, nausea, vomiting

Vital Signs
- Hypotension
- Tachycardia
- Shallow respirations with respiratory muscle weakness
- Laryngeal stridor

Percussion
- Increased reflexes
- Positive Chvostek sign
- Positive Trousseau sign
- Skeletal muscle weakness

Screening
- 12-Lead ECG: PVCs, possible torsades de pointes, prolonged PR interval, widened QRS complex, prolonged QT interval, depressed ST segment, flattened T wave, prominent U wave, atrial fibrillation, paroxysmal atrial tachycardia (PAT) with variable block, or other heart blocks related to digitalis effect (in those taking digitalis derivatives)

Diagnostic Tests for Hypomagnesemia

Test	Purpose	Abnormal Findings
Serum magnesium level	Evaluate for low magnesium	*Decreased*: Less than 1.5 mEq/L
Magnesium tolerance test	Identify those with or at risk	Results based on the amount of magnesium retained after an infusion of magnesium
Serum potassium level	Evaluate the sodium potassium pump	*Possibly decreased*: Possible failure of the cellular sodium potassium pump to move potassium into the cell and the accompanying loss of potassium in the urine. *This hypokalemia may be resistant to replacement until the magnesium deficit has been corrected*
Serum calcium level	Assess for hypocalcemia	*Possibly decreased*: Magnesium deficit may lead to hypocalcemia because of a reduction in the release and action of parathyroid hormone.

COLLABORATIVE MANAGEMENT
Care Priorities
1. Increase magnesium level
   - *Administer IV or IM magnesium*: To manage severe hypomagnesemia and related symptoms
   - *Administer magnesium supplements*: Chronic loss is treated with magnesium oxide or chloride. Magnesium containing antacids (e.g., Mylanta, Maalox, Milk of Magnesia, Gelusil) may be used.
   - *Encourage food high in magnesium*: See Box 1-7.
2. Monitor for ECG changes and manage changes with IV magnesium.   Check for hypokalemia, and manage hypomagnesemia prior to treating hypokalemia.
3. Monitor for hypotension, shallow respirations, and laryngeal stridor

CARE PLANS FOR HYPOMAGNESEMIA
Ineffective protection *related to inability to control the internal effects of hypomagnesemia*

GOALS/OUTCOMES Within 8 hours of initiation of treatment, patient verbalizes orientation to time, place, and person. Patient does not exhibit evidence of cardiac or brain injury caused by complications of severe hypomagnesemia.
NOC Neurological Status: Consciousness, Neurological Status

Electrolyte Management: Hypomagnesemia
1. Monitor serum magnesium levels in patients at risk for hypomagnesemia and its deleterious effects (e.g., those who are alcohol abusers or experiencing heart failure, cases of recent myocardial infarction or digitalis toxicity). Normal range for serum magnesium is 1.5 — 2.5 mEq/L. Consult physician or midlevel practitioner for abnormal values.

Box 1-7   FOODS HIGH IN MAGNESIUM

Bananas	Molasses
Chocolate	Nuts and seeds
Coconuts	Oranges
Grapefruits	Refined sugar
Green, leafy vegetables (e.g., beet greens, collard greens)	Seafood
Kelp	Soy flour
Legumes	Wheat bran

Safety Alert *Symptoms of hypomagnesemia may be mistakenly attributed to delirium tremens of chronic alcoholism. Be alert to indicators of magnesium deficit in these patients.*

2. Administer IV MgSO$_4$ slowly. Refer to manufacturer's guidelines. Too-rapid administration may lead to dangerous hypermagnesemia, with cardiac or respiratory arrest. Patients receiving IV magnesium should be monitored for decreasing BP, labored respirations, and diminished patellar reflex (knee jerk). An absent patellar reflex signals hyporeflexia (seen with dangerous hypermagnesemia). Should any of these changes occur, stop the infusion and consult physician or midlevel practitioner immediately (see *Hypermagnesemia,* p. 73). Keep calcium gluconate at the bedside in the event of hypocalcemic tetany or sudden hypermagnesemia.

3. For patients with chronic hypomagnesemia, administer oral magnesium supplements as prescribed. All magnesium supplements should be given with caution in patients with reduced renal function because of an increased risk of the development of hypermagnesemia. Caution patient that oral magnesium supplements may cause diarrhea. Administer antidiarrheal medications as needed.

4. When it is appropriate, encourage intake of foods high in magnesium (see Box 1-7). For most patients, a normal diet is usually adequate.

5. Maintain seizure precautions for patients with symptoms (i.e., those who have hyperreflexia). Decrease environmental stimuli (e.g., keep the room quiet; use subdued lighting).

6. For patients in whom hypocalcemia is suspected, caution against hyperventilation. Metabolic alkalosis may precipitate tetany as a result of increased calcium binding.

7. Dysphagia may occur in hypomagnesemia. Test the patient's ability to swallow water before giving food or medications.

8. Assess and document LOC, orientation, and neurologic status with each VS check. Reorient patient as necessary. Notify physician or midlevel practitioner for significant changes. Inform patient and significant others that altered mood and sensorium are temporary and will improve with treatment.

9. See *Hypokalemia* (p. 52), *Hypocalcemia* (p. 57), and *Hypophosphatemia* (p. 63) for nursing care of patients with these disorders.

 Safety Alert *Because magnesium is necessary for the movement of potassium into the cell, intracellular potassium deficits cannot be corrected until hypomagnesemia has been treated.*

NIC Neurologic Monitoring; Electrolyte Management: Hypomagnesemia; Electrolyte Management: Hypokalemia; Electrolyte Management: Hypocalcemia; Seizure Precautions; Medication Administration

Decreased cardiac output *related to abnormal contraction of myocardial tissues resulting in heart failure*

- -

GOALS/OUTCOMES Within 24 hours of initiating treatment, patient's CO is adequate as evidenced by CO at least 4 L/min, CI at least 2.5 L/min/m², normal configurations on ECG, and HR within patient's normal range. Patient has urinary output of at least 0.5 ml/kg/hr.
NOC Cardiac Pump Effectiveness, Circulation Status

Cardiac Care
1. Monitor HR and regularity with each VS check. Consult physician or midlevel practitioner for changes. Be alert to decreased CO and CI.

2. Assess ECG for evidence of hypomagnesemia. Consider hypomagnesemia as a possible cause if a patient develops sudden ventricular dysrhythmias.

3. Because hypomagnesemia (and hypokalemia) potentiate the cardiac effects of digitalis, monitor for digitalis-induced dysrhythmias. ECG changes may include multifocal or bigeminal PVCs, paroxysmal atrial tachycardia with varying AV block, and other heart blocks.

4. Monitor for and report decreased urinary output and delayed capillary refill.

NIC Dysrhythmia Management

Imbalanced nutrition: less than body requirements *related to a diet lacking in magnesium or poor overall food intake*

GOALS/OUTCOMES Within 24 hours of resumption of oral feedings, patient receives diet adequate in magnesium.
NOC Knowledge: Diet, Nutritional Status: Nutrient Intake

Teaching: Prescribed Diet
1. Encourage intake of small, frequent meals.
2. Teach patient about foods high in magnesium content (see Box 1-7), and encourage intake of these foods during meals.
3. Include patient, significant others, and dietitian in meal planning as appropriate.
4. Provide oral hygiene before meals to enhance appetite.
5. As with the other major intracellular electrolyte levels, magnesium depletion may develop with refeeding after starvation. Anticipate hypomagnesemia with refeeding, and ensure increased dietary intake or supplementation.
6. Consult physician or midlevel practitioner for patients receiving magnesium-free solutions (e.g., TPN) for prolonged periods.

NIC Nutritional Monitoring; Nutrition Management; Nutrition Therapy; Nutritional Counseling

HYPERMAGNESEMIA
(serum magnesium level greater than 2.5 mEq/L)

PATHOPHYSIOLOGY

Hypermagnesemia occurs almost exclusively in individuals with renal failure who have an increased intake of magnesium (e.g., those who use magnesium-containing medications). It also may occur in acute cases of adrenocortical insufficiency (Addison disease) or in obstetric patients treated with parenteral magnesium for pregnancy-induced hypertension. In rare cases hypermagnesemia occurs because of excessive use of magnesium-containing medications (e.g., antacids, laxatives, enemas). The primary symptoms of hypermagnesemia are the result of depressed peripheral and central neuromuscular transmission. Symptoms usually do not occur until the magnesium level exceeds 4 mEq/L.

HYPERMAGNESEMIA ASSESSMENT
Goal of Assessment
Evaluate the signs, symptoms, and risk factors for the development of hypermagnesemia

History and Risk Factors
- *Decreased magnesium excretion:* Renal failure or adrenocortical insufficiency
- *Increased intake of magnesium:* Excessive use of magnesium containing antacids, enemas, or laxatives
- *Excessive administration of magnesium sulfate:* In the treatment of hypomagnesemia or pregnancy-induced hypertension

Observation
- *Neurologic/neuromuscular symptoms:* Altered mental status, drowsiness, coma, muscular weakness or paralysis, sensation of warmth, diaphoresis, flushing, thirst
- *Paralysis of respiratory muscles:* When magnesium level exceeds 10 mEq/L
- *Nausea and vomiting*

Vital Signs
- Hypotension
- Bradycardia
- Decreased arterial pressure caused by peripheral vasodilation

Palpation
- Soft tissue calcification (metastatic)
- Decreased deep tendon reflexes
- Loss of patellar reflex when level exceeds 8 mEq/L

Screening
- 12-Lead ECG: Prolonged PR interval, prolonged QRS and QT intervals with levels of greater than 5 mEq/L, complete heart block, cardiac arrest in severe hypermagnesemia

Diagnostic Tests for Hypermagnesemia		
Test	**Purpose**	**Abnormal Findings**
Serum magnesium level	Evaluate severity	*Elevated:* more than 2.5 mEq/L
Electrocardiogram	Assess for presence of abnormalities	*Magnesium levels more than 5 mEq/L:* Prolonged PR, QRS, and QT intervals *Magnesium levels more than 15 mEq/L:* Complete heart block and cardiac arrest

COLLABORATIVE MANAGEMENT
Care Priorities
1. **Discontinue magnesium-containing medications** Especially in patients with renal failure (see Box 1-7).
2. **Administer diuretics and IV fluids** Use loop diuretics and 0.45% NaCl solution to promote magnesium excretion in patients with adequate renal function.
3. **Administer IV calcium gluconate** Use 10 ml of 10% solution to antagonize the neuromuscular effects of magnesium for patients with potentially lethal hypermagnesemia.
4. **Consider use of hemodialysis** A magnesium-free dialysate may be used for patients with severely decreased renal function, who may not respond as readily to other magnesium lowering strategies. Patients must be very closely monitored for other electrolyte changes during treatment.
5. **Monitor ECG for changes and manage dysrhythmias** Manage according to Advanced Cardiac Life Support (ACLS) guidelines, bearing in mind the special considerations related to correcting the hypermagnesemia while using additional recommended strategies.
6. **Monitor hypotension and bradycardia** Manage according to ACLS guidelines, bearing in mind the special considerations related to correcting the hypermagnesemia while using additional recommended strategies.
7. **Monitor for neurologic and neuromuscular status changes** To help gauge efficacy of treatment.

CARE PLANS FOR HYPERMAGNESEMIA
Ineffective protection *related to inability to control internal changes caused by hypermagnesemia*

GOALS/OUTCOMES Within 12 hours of initiation of treatment, patient verbalizes orientation to time, place, and person. The patient does not exhibit evidence of injury as a result of complications of hypermagnesemia, including no symptoms of soft tissue (metastatic) calcifications: oliguria, corneal haziness, conjunctivitis, irregular HR, and papular eruptions. **NOC** Neurological Status

Neurologic Monitoring
1. Monitor serum magnesium levels in the patient at risk for hypermagnesemia (e.g., those with chronic renal failure). Normal range for serum magnesium levels is 1.5 to 2.5 mEq/L.
2. Assess and document LOC, orientation, and neurologic status (e.g., hand grasp) with each vital sign check. Assess patellar (knee jerk) reflex in patients with a moderately elevated magnesium level (greater than 5 mEq/L). With patient lying flat, support the knee in a moderately fixed position and tap the patellar tendon firmly just below the patella. Normally the knee will extend. An absent reflex suggests a magnesium level of greater than 7 mEq/L. Consult physician or midlevel practitioner for significant changes.
3. Reassure patient and significant others that altered mental functioning and muscle strength will improve with treatment.
4. Keep side rails up and the bed in its lowest position with the wheels locked.
5. Assess patient for the development of soft tissue calcification. Consult physician or midlevel practitioner for significant findings.

6. Monitor for cardiopulmonary effects of hypermagnesemia: hypotension, flushing, bradycardia, respiratory depression.

NIC Electrolyte Management: Hypermagnesemia

Deficient knowledge *related to magnesium-containing medications*

GOALS/OUTCOMES Within the 24-hour period before discharge from the intensive care unit, patient verbalizes the importance of avoiding unusual magnesium intake and identifies potential sources of unwanted magnesium.
NOC Knowledge: Medication

Teaching: Individual
1. Caution patients with chronic renal failure to review all over-the-counter medications with physician or midlevel practitioner before use.
2. Provide a list of common magnesium-containing medications (Table 1-9).
3. Caution patients to avoid combination vitamin-mineral supplements because they usually contain magnesium.

NIC Teaching: Prescribed Diet; Teaching: Prescribed Medication

---

Table 1-9	MAGNESIUM-CONTAINING MEDICATIONS
Brand Name Antacids	**Laxatives**
Aludrox Camalox Di-Gel Gaviscon Gelusil and Gelusil II Maalox and Maalox Plus Mylanta and Mylanta-II Riopan Simeco Tempo	Magnesium citrate Magnesium hydroxide (Milk of Magnesia, Haley's M-O) Magnesium sulfate (Epsom salts) Magnesium-containing mineral supplements

HEMODYNAMIC MONITORING

Hemodynamic monitoring refers to the specialized methods used to evaluate cardiovascular performance, which includes information about the CO, tissue perfusion, blood volume, tissue oxygenation, and vascular tone. Hemodynamic readings reflect the efficacy of the pumping action of the heart (stroke volume [SV] or CO), and circulation of blood throughout the body (BP). Hemodynamic monitoring readings encompass a broad array of measurements, depending on the technology used. Understanding the values is important in determining actions used to improve cardiac function and overall circulation. Accurately determined hemodynamic values are used to guide cardiovascular drug– and device-based therapies provided to critically ill patients.

The three overarching assessment parameters provided by hemodynamic monitoring are calculation of *preload* (end-diastolic volume and pressure in both ventricles prior to contraction), *afterload* (pressure created by blood volume and arterial tone which the heart must overcome to open the aortic and pulmonic heart valves), and *contractility* (ability of the heart muscle to pump/contract effectively.) Preload, afterload, contractility, and HR ultimately determine SV, CO, and BP and may be constantly manipulated using drugs and devices. Usage guidelines were developed to outline when use of hemodynamic monitoring provides the most benefit (Box 1-8).

| **Box 1-8** | **OPTIMAL USE OF PULMONARY ARTERY CATHETERS** |

In 2007, the ACC/AHA produced guidelines on perioperative cardiovascular evaluation and care for patients undergoing noncardiac surgery. The following excerpts concern their recommendations on the use of hemodynamic monitoring.

> The use of a PA catheter (PAC) may be helpful in the surgical patient at risk for hemodynamic disturbances detectable using a PAC. The guideline suggests 3 parameters should be assessed prior to use: Patient disease (incidence of fluid shifts), surgical procedure (anticipate fluid shifts), and practice setting (presence of skilled personnel to maintain the PAC and interpret data). Routine use of a PAC perioperatively, especially in patients at low risk of developing *hemodynamic* disturbances, is not recommended.

ACC/AHA 2007 guidelines on perioperative cardiovascular evaluation and care for noncardiac surgery. Retrieved November 12, 2008, from XXXXXXXXXX.

In 2003, *Practice Guidelines for Pulmonary Artery Catheterization: An Updated Report by the American Society of Anesthesiologists Task Force on Pulmonary Artery Catheterization* was published.

> The task force recommended looking at the patient, surgery, and setting prior to making a clinical decision to use hemodynamic monitoring. "Patients at increased risk for hemodynamic disturbances are those with clinical evidence of significant cardiovascular disease, pulmonary dysfunction, hypoxia, renal insufficiency, or other conditions associated with hemodynamic instability (e.g., advanced age, endocrine disorders, sepsis, trauma, burns).
> *Low risk patients*: Include those with American Society of Anesthesiologists (ASA) physical status score of 1 or 2, with hemodynamic disturbances unlikely to cause organ dysfunction. *Moderate risk patients*: Category ASA 3 who have hemodynamic disturbances that occasionally cause organ dysfunction. *High Risk patients*: Category ASA 4 or 5 who have hemodynamic disturbances with a great chance of causing organ dysfunction or death. "The assessment of risk should be based on a thorough analysis of the medical history and physical examination findings, rather than on exclusive consideration of specific laboratory results or other quantitative criteria. Surgical procedures associated with an increased risk of complications from hemodynamic changes, including damage to the heart, vascular tree, kidneys, liver, lungs, or brain, may increase the chance of benefiting from PA catheterization."

American Society of Anesthesiologists Task Force on Pulmonary Artery Catheterization: Practice guidelines for pulmonary artery catheterization: an updated report by the American Society of Anesthesiologists Task Force on Pulmonary Artery Catheterization. *Anesthesiology* 99(4):988-1014, 2003.

In 2000, The National Heart, Lung, and Blood Institute and Food and Drug Administration Workshop developed a consensus statement regarding pulmonary artery catheterization and clinical outcomes.

> The conclusions stated a need exists for collaborative education of physicians and nurses in performing, obtaining, and interpreting information from the use of pulmonary artery catheters. Recommendations include that professional groups develop and disseminate standard education programs to facilitate learning the key points of using hemodynamic monitoring.

JAMA 283(19):2568-2572, 2000.

In one of the most collaborative efforts to date, the Pulmonary Artery Catheter Education Project (PACEP) was developed. www.pacep.org

The following organizations have participated in the education project to promote optimal use of pulmonary artery catheters: American Association of Critical Care Nurses, American Association of Nurse Anesthetists, American College of Chest Physicians, American Society of Anesthesiologists, American Thoracic Society, National Heart Lung Blood Institute, Society of Cardiovascular Anesthesiologists, Society of Critical Care Medicine. The recommendations from the consensus statement are more consistently followed as a result of their ongoing educational efforts.

PATHOPHYSIOLOGY

Changes in any of the four determinants of CO—preload, afterload, contractility, or HR—may produce significant adverse effects on the BP with resulting adverse changes in cellular function and energy production due to altered tissue perfusion. Hemodynamic monitoring helps to assess these parameters in the critically ill so appropriate treatments can be provided.

Determinants of Cardiac Output and Blood Pressure

The most powerful determinant of CO is the metabolic O_2 demand. As metabolism and O_2 consumption increase or decrease, the CO increases or decreases in direct response to increased or decreased need. The heart works as a two-sided pump, with the right side pumping deoxygenated blood into the lower pressure pulmonary circulation (reflected by PA pressure) and the left side pumping oxygenated blood into the higher pressure systemic circulation (reflected by BP). Evaluation of CO requires an assessment of the components that determine SV (*preload, afterload,* and *contractility*) for both sides of the heart and factors affecting the HR.

In the absence of underlying pathology, such as intracardiac right-to-left or left-to-right shunting, the output of the ventricles should be the same. If the output of one of the ventricles changes, the other ventricle should adjust its output to compensate for the difference. The right and left sides of the heart are connected by the pulmonary arteries and veins. Many specialized types of central vessel catheters are available to measure the pressures within the pulmonary circulation and provide a means to calculate CO. The original PA catheter was known as the Swan-Ganz catheter. All PA catheters provide information about the right and left heart, as well as systemic circulation. Options for measurements vary with each uniquely configured catheter. Once the hemodynamic data are evaluated, strategies may be implemented to manipulate preload, afterload, contractility, and HR.

Preload   Understanding Frank Starling's law is fundamental to understanding preload. Starling's law of the heart states, "The greater the ability of the myocardial muscle to stretch at the end of diastole, the greater is the force of myocardial contraction." However, if the stretch becomes consistently excessive, the force of contraction will diminish. Preload is determined by the compliance (ability to stretch) of the ventricles during diastole as the blood volume fills the ventricles. As the blood volume increases, the heart must "stretch" with each heartbeat to accommodate it. As the blood volume decreases, the heart stretches much less but must still generate the force needed to propel the blood volume forward during systole. This mechanism enables the heart to adjust ventricular size to varying blood volumes. Preload coupled with the heart's electrical conduction system coordinates the output of the right and left ventricles.

Factors that affect ventricular blood volume include venous return, circulating blood volume, condition of the heart valves, and atrial contractility. Ventricular compliance is affected by stiffness and thickness of the cardiac muscle. Any stressor that influences one of these factors will result in a change in preload, with a concomitant change in CO. Heart disease affects preload. Patients with biventricular heart failure and/or "stiff ventricles" are not able to handle increased intravascular volume. Their preload is always high because the heart cannot stretch normally to accommodate more volume. The diseased heart has little ability to compensate for volume changes. Patients with a right ventricular (RV) infarction are in a difficult position, as they require a higher preload to maintain a normal CO since the infarct zone cannot stretch. Extra ventricular blood volume, or higher preload, creates more stretch in the normal RV tissues to promote better RV output but can result in excessive work for the left ventricle. All patients with heart disease may develop heart failure, so expert monitoring by the clinician is required to optimize CO (see *Heart Failure,* p. 421).

Clinically, preload is measured as ventricular end-diastolic pressure (VEDP), because pressure in the ventricles correlates closely with volume. For the right side of the heart, RV end-diastolic (filling) pressure (RVEDP) is reflected by the right atrial (RA) pressure (RAP) or the central venous pressure (CVP). Left ventricular (LV) end-diastolic (filling) pressure (LVEDP) is reflected by left atrial (LA), PA diastolic (PAD), or PA occlusive (PAOP) or wedge pressure measurements. If preload begins to increase in a patient with heart disease, appropriate medications, including diuretics, may be given to help decrease the CVP and PAOP. Vasodilating drugs with strong venodilating properties may also be used to decrease venous return so a heart with limited ability to stretch can accommodate and pump the lesser blood volume. An increase in preload signals the ventricles may be unable to eject enough of the end-diastolic volume, causing more blood to be retained in the ventricles.

Afterload Afterload refers to the pressure or force which must be generated within the right and left ventricles/ventricular myocardium during systole to overcome the vascular resistance to ejection. The pressures created by the blood volume and vascular tone within the pulmonary, aortic, and systemic circulation create resistance against the aortic and pulmonic valves, which can impede ventricular ejection. Other resistant forces include increased blood viscosity, reduced distensibility of the vascular system (created by athero-sclerosis or "hardening of the arteries"), and diseased heart valves. The clinician should be aware that diseased ventricles are extremely sensitive to abrupt changes in afterload because the diseased tissue cannot readily generate additional force to overcome additional resistance to ejection. Paying close attention to PA pressures, as well as systemic arterial pressure, is of paramount importance. If blood volume starts to be retained in the ventri-cles, rather than being normally ejected, VEDP increases, followed by increases in PA pressure. When these changes are noticed, measures such as administration of diuretics or vasodilating drugs with strong arterial dilating properties may be initiated to decrease afterload and help improve ventricular ejection. Medications used for management of hypertension are administered to reduce afterload.

Since vascular resistance plays a major role in determining pressures throughout the heart and lungs, RV afterload is evaluated by calculating the pulmonary vascular resistance (PVR) while LV afterload is reflected by SVR. The higher the afterload, the greater the myocardial wall tension/pressure must be to open the aortic and/or pulmonic valves and the greater is the work of the heart to overcome resistance to flow. This explains why hypertension is called "the silent killer," as the constantly increased afterload strains the heart. Increased cardiac work requires increased myocardial blood flow to deliver additional O_2. When blood flowing through the coronary arteries is diminished by atherosclerosis, the demand for the increased blood flow needed to manage energy needs created by increased afterload may not be met, resulting in myocardial ischemia, injury, and possibly infarction.

Contractility This is the inherent capacity of the myocardium to contract during systole. This mechanism functions independently of variations in preload and afterload. Changes in ventricular contractility have a significant effect on tissue perfusion and the shape/slope of the ventricular function curves generated during CO measurement. Although contractility cannot be measured directly, a change in contractility can be inferred when CO is decreased and other variables that affect CO (i.e., preload, afterload, HR) remain the same. Changes in ventricular function curves infer changes in contractility. Several factors positively influence contractility: sympathetic stimulation, calcium, positive inotropic agents such as digitalis, dobutamine, milrinone, and beta-adrenergic drugs. Factors such as acidemia, hypoxia, myocardial ischemia, myocardial infarct, cardiomyopathies, beta-blocker drugs, and antidysrhythmic drugs can decrease contractility.

Heart Rate Changes in HR affect myocardial functioning significantly. Slight increases in HR with a constant SV result in increased CO. Very rapid HRs are associated with a reduction in CO as the duration of diastole is shortened, resulting in decreased coronary perfusion and reduced ventricular filling time. Critically ill patients often manifest sinus tachycardia to maintain a CO that meets demand for O_2 and nutrients at the cellular level. The heart requires more O_2 when the HR increases, and as long as coronary artery perfu-sion is adequate, HR increases provide compensation needed for increased metabolic demands. Tachycardia can, however, reach a critical point where the heart is receiving less O_2 if filling time becomes too brief to provide appropriate coronary artery perfusion. Bradycardia often results in decreased CO unless there are increases in SV during the lon-ger ventricular filling times. Athletes are able to maintain excellent CO with slower HRs, but the critically ill may not be as fortunate when HR decreases. Algorithms have been created for advanced cardiac life support, which include both pharmacologic and electrical therapies to manage HR.

HEMODYNAMIC ASSESSMENT

The goal of hemodynamic monitoring is to obtain accurate measurements, which are used in combination with physical assessment findings to provide appropriate, effective therapies to maintain adequate BP and CO. The hemodynamic measurements listed in Table 1-10 are considered the values needed in a complete hemodynamic profile.

Table 1-10 HEMODYNAMIC NORMAL VALUES AND DERIVED VALUES

Parameter	Formula	Normal Values
Arterial blood pressure (BP) systolic/diastolic		90–130/50–80 mm Hg
Mean arterial pressure (MAP)	$$\frac{\text{Systolic BP} + 2\,(\text{Diastolic BP})}{3}$$	70–100 mm Hg
Central venous pressure (CVP)		2–6 mm Hg
Right atrial pressure (RAP)		4–6 mm Hg
Left atrial pressure (LAP)		8–12 mm Hg
Right ventricular pressure (RVP)		20–30/0–8 mm Hg
Pulmonary artery systolic pressure (PAS)		20–30 mm Hg
Pulmonary artery diastolic pressure (PAD)		8–15 mm Hg
Pulmonary artery occlusive pressure (PAOP) Same as wedge (PCWP) or (PWP)		6–12 mm Hg
Mean pulmonary artery pressure (MPAP, PAM)	$$\frac{\text{PAS} + 2(\text{PAD})}{3}$$	10–20 mm Hg
Cardiac output (CO)	$$\frac{O_2\,\text{consumption}}{A - Vo_2}$$	4–8 L/min
Cardiac index (CI)	$$\frac{CO}{\text{Body surface area (BSA)}}$$	2.5–4 L/min/m^2
Systemic vascular resistance (SVR)	$$\frac{\text{MAP} - \text{RAP}}{CO} \times 80$$	800–1200 dynes•sec•cm^{-5}
Pulmonary vascular resistance (PVR)	$$\frac{(\text{PAM} - \text{PAOP}) \times 80}{CO}$$	150–250 dynes•sec•cm^{-5}
Coronary perfusion pressure (CPP)	Diastolic BP − PAOP	50–70 mm Hg
Stroke volume (SV)	$$\frac{CO}{HR} \times 1000$$	55–100 ml/beat
Stroke volume index (SVI)	$$\frac{SV}{BSA}$$	30–60 ml/beat/m^2
Right ventricular stroke work index (RVSWI)	SVI(PAM − RAP) × 0.0136	4–8 g/m^2/beat
Left ventricular stroke work index (LVSWI)	SVI(MAP − PAOP) × 0.0136	40–75 g/m^2/beat
Arterial oxygen content (Cao$_2$)	(Hgb ×1.34) ×Sao$_2$	18–20 ml/vol%
Venous oxygen content (Cvo$_2$)	(Hgb × 1.34 × Svo$_2$)	15.5 ml/vol%
Oxygen delivery (Do$_2$)	CaO$_2$ × CO × 10	800–1000 ml/min
Oxygen delivery index (Do$_2$I)	CaO$_2$ × CI × 10	500–600 ml/min/m^2

Continued

Table 1-10	HEMODYNAMIC NORMAL VALUES AND DERIVED VALUES—cont'd	
Parameter	**Formula**	**Normal Values**
Arteriovenous oxygen content difference ($C[a-v]O_2$)	$CaO2 \times CvO2$	4–6 ml/vol%
Oxygen consumption ($\dot{V}O_2$)	$CO \times 10 \times C(a-v)O_2$	200–250 ml/min
Oxygen consumption index ($\dot{V}O_2I$)	$CI \times 10 \times C(a-v)O_2$	115–165 ml/min/m^2
Arterial oxygen saturation (SaO_2)		95%–98%
Mixed venous oxygen saturation (SvO_2)	$(CO \times CaO_2 \times 10) - VO_2$	60%–80%

Systemic Arterial Pressure or Blood Pressure May Be Measured Indirectly and/or Directly

- *Indirect measurement*: A "spot check" or "snapshot" of the BP in a moment of time; performed with a manually inflated BP cuff and manometer. Arterial pressure is auscultated over a pulse point using a stethoscope or Doppler ultrasound device. A noninvasive automatic BP cuff (NIBP or NBP) may be used, in lieu of manually inflating the cuff and auscultating the pressure using a stethoscope and manometer. Manual or auscultatory BP readings are wrought with pitfalls that cause false high and false low readings. Proper cuff size, proper cuff position, arm position being level with the heart, and skill in determining the onset of the first Korotkoff sound are imperative components for accurate readings.
- *Direct monitoring*: Continuous monitoring of BP that requires insertion of a hollow, rigid, IV catheter into an artery to create an arterial line (A-line). The BP is a dynamic or ever-changing event. Cardiovascular dynamics are assessed through review of pressure waveforms and analysis of trends in arterial pressure readings. Arterial lines are used to obtain arterial blood samples for labwork, including blood gas determinations, without repeated arterial punctures.

RESEARCH BRIEF 1-1

Mixed venous-arterial P_{CO_2} difference has been shown to be inversely related to cardiac index (CI). A central venous P_{CO_2} may provide similar information. Eighty-three consecutive intensive care unit patients in an urban tertiary care hospital had simultaneous blood gases from arterial, pulmonary artery (PA), and central venous (CV) catheters obtained. Cardiac indices were measured by the thermodilution technique (an average of three measurements) at the same time. The cardiac indices obtained by the venous-arterial differences were compared with those determined by thermodilution. Results revealed the correlation between the mixed venous-arterial P_{CO_2} difference and cardiac index was 0.903 ($p < 0.0001$), while the correlation between the CV-arterial P_{CO_2} difference and cardiac index was 0.892 ($p < 0.0001$). Venous-arterial P_{CO_2} differences obtained from PA and CV circulations are inversely correlated with cardiac index. Using CV rather than mixed venous-arterial P_{CO_2} difference provides an accurate alternative method for calculating cardiac output.

From Cuschieri J, Rivers EP, Donnino MW, et al: Central venous-arterial carbon dioxide difference as an indicator of cardiac index. *Intens Care Med* 31(8):1141, 2005.

Arterial Oxygen Saturation

- The percentage of oxyhemoglobin (Hgb bound with O_2) compared to the total amount of Hgb can be measured directly using blood samples from the arterial line or approximated indirectly by photoelectric technology using an external pulse oximetry probe placed on the patient's finger, ear, or forehead.

Central Venous Pressure or Right Atrial Pressure

- CVP can be monitored continuously or "spot checked" using a central line.
- CVP and RAP may be used interchangeably to assess intravascular fluid volume, efficacy of venous return to the right heart, and RV end-diastolic pressure or preload.
- RAP is obtained using the RA port of a PA catheter.

Pulmonary Artery Pressures

- PAPs are measured continuously using a flow-directed, multilumen catheter placed in the PA. PA catheters vary in technology. More sophisticated catheters provide information about O_2 delivery and O_2 consumption and may provide continuous cardiac output (CCO) measurements. Basic PA catheters provide measurement of RAP, PAP, PA occlusive pressure (PAOP) or "wedge pressures," and CO.
- The RAP, PAP, PAOP, and CO provide information that helps in calculating preload, afterload, and contractility. Waveform analysis helps to identify any pathology or abnormality of the heart valves and other cardiac disorders.

Cardiac Output

CO can be calculated using several methods.

- *Fick Oxygen Consumption Method:* The original, or "gold standard," mathematical method used to calculate CO. The method is based on the principle that total uptake or release of a substance by an organ is the product of the blood flow within the organ and the difference in the amount of the substance in the arterial circulation versus the venous circulation (arteriovenous difference). The formula for CO uses arteriovenous O_2 content difference. A number of technical problems can interfere with getting accurate results, and due to the cumbersome nature of the procedure, the formula is generally used in research laboratories, rather than routinely in clinical practice.

$$CO \text{ (L/min)} = \frac{O_2 \text{ consumption (ml/min)}}{\text{Arteriovenous } O_2 \text{ content difference (ml/dl blood)}}$$

- *Thermodilution method:* Measurement method using a PA catheter to determine the flow rate of a room temperature IV solution (injectate) passing through the heart. The temperature of the injectate is lower than the temperature of the blood in the central circulation. IV solution is injected into a more proximally located port in the PA catheter and travels through the heart to a more distally located port. A temperature sensor is used to track the flow rate of the injectate. The speed of the flow from the proximal to the distal port is used to calculate the cardiac output. It is considered accurate and reliable.
- *CCO measurement:* Performed using a specialized PA catheter using thermal technology which allows the user to obtain readings that are averaged over 3-minute periods and updated every 30 to 60 seconds. The same PA catheter also gives the venous O_2 saturation (Svo_2) via a fiberoptic tip in the PA, and is used for determination of O_2 delivery and O_2 consumption. O_2 delivery is the result of CO multiplied by the arterial O_2 content (Cao_2) (see Table 1-10). The arterial O_2 content is determined by Hgb and arterial O_2 saturation (Sao_2).

Promoting Accuracy of Hemodynamic Values: Setting Up Equipment

Ensuring proper setup and maintenance of the pressure monitoring system will prevent most inaccuracies. Normal waveform configurations must be understood for all readings, so that abnormal waveforms can be readily identified. Abnormal waveforms can sometimes reflect a problem with the system setup or maintenance.

General considerations related to the hemodynamic monitoring setup:

1. Use rigid pressure tubing from the transducer to the patient. Most monitoring kits have the proper set up prepackaged with disposable transducers to assure proper use. Flexible tubing may be used from the flush bag to the transducer.

2. During the initial set up, flush or prime the monitoring system [all tubing and the tranducer(s)] without pressure applied to the flush bag to help prevent formation of air bubbles from turbulent flow within the empty tubing. Slower priming allows for more even fluid dispersion throughout the system.
3. Remove excess air from the flush bag prior to flushing to help prevent an air embolus from entering the patient's vasculature. The excess air can be accidentally introduced into the patient.
4. Flush all stopcocks and apply dead-end caps to seal the system. Vented caps are not recommended, since the venting offers an entry point for organisms and could create a leak in the system.
5. Maintain a minimum of 100 ml in the flush bag and change bag according to institutional guidelines. Many institutions focus on maintaining a closed system to minimize the chance of contamination. The Centers for Disease Control and Prevention (CDC) recommends the tubing be changed every 96 hours.
6. Apply and maintain 300 mm Hg of pressure to the pressure bag enclosing the flush bag.
7. Maintain electrical safety guidelines to avoid microshocks entering the heart via the fluid column created by the monitoring system.
8. Normal saline is the recognized flush solution of choice for hemodynamic monitoring systems. Heparinized saline is no longer recommended for routine use to avoid the risk for inducing heparin-induced thrombocytopenia (HIT positive).

Leveling and zeroing the system:
1. All monitoring systems must be leveled prior to use. To level the system, the transducers are positioned at the phlebostatic axis to provide the most accurate pressure readings. Transducers must remain leveled to provide accurate pressure readings. The phlebostatic axis is located at the intersection of the fourth intercostal space and the line that denotes half the anteroposterior diameter of the chest. Readings are accurate with the head of the bed (HOB) elevated from 0 to 60 degrees. Higher HOB elevation will result in falsely low readings.
2. Transducers must be "zeroed" prior to using the monitoring system. Newer computerized bedside monitors remind the nurse to zero the system. Zeroing the transducer requires opening the transducer to air while possibly pressing a button on the bedside monitor to establish a referenced atmospheric pressure of zero.
3. Leveling and zeroing should be done at least once a shift and when there is any change in patient position and/or question in readings obtained or waveforms.

Square wave testing (also called fast flush or dynamic response test):
1. The test is done to test the compliance of the monitoring system to provide a common measure of accuracy. Hemodynamic systems are constructed differently in each monitoring setting, but minimally, each should have a flush system pressurized at 300 mm Hg and a continuous fluid column contained within rigid tubing between the transducer and the patient. The number of transducers, type and length of tubing may vary. Flaws within the system directly affect the accuracy of pressure readings. The test indicates if the system is normal, overdamped, or underdamped.
2. *Overdamping* causes the systolic pressure to be falsely low and the diastolic pressure to be falsely high. Large air bubbles, loose connections, no or low amount of flush solution in the system, low pressure on the flush bag, or a kinked catheter causes overdamping.
3. *Underdamping* causes the systolic pressure to be falsely high and the diastolic pressure to be falsely low. Small air bubbles, a defective transducer, or pressure tubing that is too long causes underdamping.
4. Testing should be done when the system is set up, once every shift, when the system is opened to air for any reason (including blood sampling), and when waves appear distorted from the usual appearance.
5. To perform the square wave test:
   - Fast flush the monitoring system by pulling the pigtail or pressing the appropriate button for each transducer. The flush should be pressurized to 300 mm Hg.
   - When the system is being flushed, a large, square wave appears on the monitor. Stop flushing and observe the shape of the square wave, and wait for the pressure waveform to normalize.
   - An acceptable response is the waveform normalizing and returning to baseline following one or two oscillations (Figure 1-4A). If the resulting waveform is abnormally shaped, lacks shape, amplitude, or does not return to baseline, the response is abnormal.

Square wave test configuration

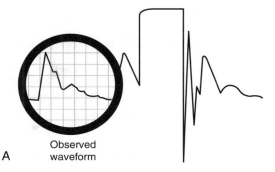

Observed
A   waveform

Square wave test configuration

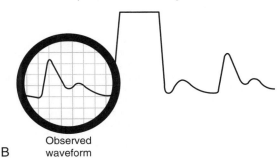

Observed
B   waveform

Square wave test configuration

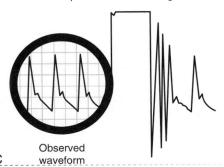

Observed
C   waveform

Figure 1-4 Dynamic response testing (square wave, frequency response testing) using the fast-flush system. *A,* Optimally damped system. *B,* Overdamped system. *C,* Underdamped system.

- In optimally damped systems, one small undershoot (negative deflection) and one small overshoot (exaggerated positive deflection or bounce) are seen, followed by a return of the normal waveform.
- *Overdamped* systems (Figure 1-4*B*) demonstrate an absence of bounces, and a slurring of the square wave down stroke. Waves are blunted, sluggish, and falsely wide.
- *Underdamped* systems (Figure 1-4*C*) generally have multiple, sharp bounces with waves that are exaggerated, narrow, and falsely peaked.

- *If overdamping or underdamping is present,* troubleshoot the monitoring system. If troubleshooting is ineffective, the monitor system should be checked by a biomedical engineer or technician. If these problems cannot be resolved, another monitor may be needed to obtain accurate readings. Also see Troubleshooting (Table 1-11).

Hemodynamic Monitoring: Considerations during Setup, Line Insertion, and Placement
Arterial pressure monitoring:

- The most common sites used for IV catheter insertion are the radial, brachial, or femoral arteries. Arterial catheters are inserted via the radial artery, because this artery is readily accessible and collateral blood flow is usually adequate. The arterial catheter may also be inserted in the femoral or brachial artery. The arterial pressure waveform is displayed on a bedside monitor to provide continuous observation of systolic, diastolic, and mean arterial pressures (Figure 1-5). The appearance of the arterial waveform is

Table 1-11	MECHANICAL PROBLEMS AFFECTING HEMODYNAMIC MEASUREMENTS		
Problem	**Waveform Appearance**	**Cause**	**Corrective Action**
Overdamping	Smaller than usual with a slow rise; diminished or absent dicrotic notch (arterial and pulmonary artery catheters). Square wave test will have less than two deflections.	Tubing too long	Remove extra length of tubing.
		Nonpressure tubing used	Replace with pressurized tubing.
		Air bubbles in system	Flush air out of system.
		Thrombus formation	Consider changing catheter.
		Lodging of catheter against vessel wall	Flush line for at least 10 seconds. Ensure pressure bag inflated to 300 mm Hg.
		Loose connection in tubing or transducer	Tighten all connections on initial setup, and if any leakage is noted, then flush air from system. (Initially flushing lines without pressure will result in fewer air bubbles.)
		Incorrect calibration	Recalibrate (zero) transducer.
		Spontaneous catheter migration into a near-wedged position (PA catheter only)	Flush PA line; if PAC wedges with 0.5 cc of air or less, notify physician or midlevel practitioner for repositioning.
		Kinking or knotting of catheter or tubing	Externally ensure lines are straight; if internal jugular sites tend to kink at insertion site, neck may need to be supported for prevention. If internally PA catheter kink or knot is seen on chest radiograph, notify physician or midlevel practitioner.
Catheter whip or fling Under-dampening	Erratic, "noisy" waveform with highly variable and inaccurate pressures. Square wave test may be hyperdynamic or more than three deflections.	Spurious movement of the catheter tip within the vessel lumen (may require repositioning) Catheter too long for vessel (arterial) Pressure tubing too long	Assess proper position of PAC with chest radiograph and determine if PAC will wedge with 0.5–1.5 cc of air. Minimize length of pressure tubing. Re-zero monitor. Notify physician or midlevel practitioner if improper placement is found or if catheter whip (fling) is uncorrected despite above measures.

Table 1-11	**MECHANICAL PROBLEMS AFFECTING HEMODYNAMIC MEASUREMENTS — cont'd**		
Problem	**Waveform Appearance**	**Cause**	**Corrective Action**
No waveform	Complete absence of waveform	PEA, absence of pulse, with electrical activity	Check patient condition. Check pulse (PEA); begin CPR.
		Stopcock turned to wrong position	Most common; if patient stable, check system; start at patient and work back to transducer.
		Large leak in the system, usually with blood backing up into the tubing Loose or cracked transducer or air in transducer	Turn system off to patient at nearest stopcock until leak can be found and corrected.** If system has been contaminated, you should change setup.
		Catheter tip or lumen totally occluded by clot	Notify physician or midlevel practitioner.
		Inadequate pressure (<300 mm Hg) on pressure bag	Ensure bag is inflated and maintaining pressure. If flush bag has less than 100 cc, you should change bag.
		Defective transducer or amplifier	Assess monitor cable first, then amplifier, and then change transducer.
Inability to obtain a PAOP reading (PA catheter only)	Absence of wedge waveform after balloon inflation of up to 1.5 cc of air. If when instilling air (1.5 cc or less) into the balloon, the waveform goes up and off the screen; this is overwedging.	Retrograde catheter slippage Balloon rupture Migration of PAC into smaller vessel	Assess waveform; ensure it is a PA waveform and not already in wedge position or an RV waveform. If it is a PA waveform, the catheter needs to be repositioned for proper placement. If it is an RV waveform, the catheter should immediately be pulled back to the RA to prevent ventricular dysrhythmias. If when less than 0.5 cc of air is instilled the waveform goes up and is lost at high range, the catheter is overwedging and needs to be repositioned. The catheter level should be assessed to see if it has changed positions since insertion. If in wedge position, notify physician. If unable to wedge, the physician should be notified. If balloon rupture is suspected, notify physician immediately and do not attempt any further PAOP readings; close balloon port.

*Whenever the amplitude of an arterial or PA waveform decreases, the patient first should be assessed for hypovolemia or shock.

**If line has become disconnected or a portion open to air, the patient must be assessed for any potential air embolus; then the line should be changed to prevent sepsis. PA catheters must always be tranduced, as it is necessary to assess catheter migration through waveform analysis. Catheter migration may result in pulmonary infarction if not identified and managed.

influenced by variations in BP, dysrhythmias, and mechanical factors. Mechanical factors that influence the waveform include overdamping, catheter whip, and inaccurate calibration/zeroing (Table 1-12).

- *Potential complications include* decreased perfusion distal to the insertion site, which can cause limb ischemia. Slower blood flow can lead to thrombus formation. If air inadvertently enters the system during line insertion, through a crack or other flaw in the closed system, an air embolus may result, which, if lodged in the hand, can render distal tissues anoxic. Rarely, patients have needed to have fingers amputated due to prolonged lack of perfusion. If the closed system is cracked or becomes disconnected, exsanguination may occur.

Pulmonary artery pressure monitoring:

- The most common sites used for PA catheter insertion are the internal jugular or subclavian veins. Femoral and brachial veins may also be used. The most common PA catheter placement technique is percutaneous insertion of the catheter introducer/introducing

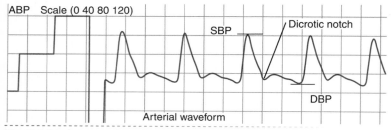

Figure 1-5 Arterial pressure waveform. Redrawn from Daily E, Schroeder J: *Techniques in Bedside Hemodynamic Monitoring,* ed. 4. St. Louis, 1989, Mosby.

Table 1-12	ABNORMAL PULMONARY ARTERY PRESSURES	
Hemodynamic Pressure	**Normal Range**	**Clinical Conditions**
Pulmonary artery systolic pressure (PAS)	20–30 mm Hg	*Increased:* Right ventricular failure, chronic left ventricular failure, constrictive pericarditis, cardiac tamponade, pulmonary hypertension (primary or related to lung disease) *Decreased:* Hypovolemia, preload reduction
Pulmonary artery diastolic pressure (PAD)*	8–15 mm Hg	*Increased:* Left ventricular failure, mitral stenosis, left-to-right shunts, pulmonary hypertension (primary or related to lung disease) *Decreased:* Hypovolemia, preload reduction
Pulmonary artery occlusive pressure (PAOP)†	6–12 mm Hg	*Increased:* Left ventricular failure, cardiac tamponade, mitral valve regurgitation, mitral valve stenosis, acute ventricular septal defect, fluid volume overload *Decreased:* Hypovolemia, afterload reduction

*PAD may exceed PAOP by ≥5 mm Hg in patients with pulmonary hypertension, hypoxemia, acidosis, pulmonary emboli, and other lung disease.
†PAOP > PAD signals a mechanical problem (i.e., overwedging or improper identification of PAD).

needle using the Seldinger technique for insertion, in combination with waveform analysis provided by the hemodynamic monitoring system as the catheter passes through the heart. Waveform analysis and pressure readings provide the practitioner the information needed to know the position of the catheter. Insertion may also be done using a cutdown to expose the vessel but is rarely needed. Catheter placement is occasionally done under fluoroscopy for patients with abnormal cardiac or vasculature structures.

- *Potential complications include* decreased perfusion distal to end of the PA catheter if the catheter is inserted too far or migrates out of position. This can cause pulmonary tissue ischemia or infarction, if it is severe. Slower blood flow can lead to thrombus formation. If air inadvertently enters the system during line insertion, through a crack or other flaw in the closed system, an air embolus may result. If the closed system is cracked or becomes disconnected, exsanguination may occur. The cardiac chambers can be perforated during insertion, resulting in hemorrhage into the mediastinum and cardiac tamponade. The vasculature can be perforated during insertion, resulting in the extravascular catheter tip causing fluid or blood accumulation in the pleural space or the mediastinum and/or a pneumothorax. Dysrhythmias may occur, particularly when the catheter passes through the right ventricle.

RESEARCH BRIEF 1-2

This purpose of this prospective clinical investigation of university hospital patients with pulmonary artery catheters (PAC) was to determine if lower limb (calf) sequential compression devices (SCDs) had a significant effect on thermodilution cardiac output measurements made using the PAC. A total of 43 patients in surgical and neurosurgical intensive care units were included. Cardiac output was measured (three readings averaged) when the SCDs were turned off, during the first 2 to 4 seconds of the inflation cycle, during seconds 4 to 8 of the inflation cycle, and when the SCDs were turned off again. Cardiac output measurements were consistently lower when measured during the SCD inflation cycle. Cardiac output decreased from 7.58% to 49.5%, with a mean reduction of 24.51% in the first 2 to 4 seconds and 20.61% during seconds 4 to 8 ($p < 0.001$). One patient had an increase of 2.78% and the other had an increase of 13.5% during the inflation cycle. Measurements were also made using a pulse contour-analysis cardiac output device on 11 of the study patients. No changes in pulse contour-analysis cardiac output were observed. The study concluded thermodilution cardiac output measurements via a PAC should not be done during the inflation cycle of lower limb SCDs because they produce a falsely low cardiac output.

From Killu K, Oropello JM, Manasia AR, et al: Effect of lower limb compression devices on thermodilution cardiac output measurement. *Crit Care Med* 35(5):1307–1311, 2007.

DIAGNOSTIC TESTS
Factors Affecting Hemodynamic Measurements

Systolic blood pressure: This is determined by (1) the amount of blood ejected by the ventricle per beat (SV), (2) wall compliance of the arterial system, and (3) peripheral resistance. Elevations in systolic pressure produce large, steep waveforms, often reflective of changes in vascular compliance, such as the hypertension seen in patients with atherosclerosis. A decrease in systolic pressure producing smaller, slightly wider waveforms is seen in connection with heart disorders that result in decreased SV. The use of arterial vasodilators such as nitroprusside, hydralazine, and nifedipine will cause a rapid upstroke and steep decline with drop in diastolic pressure related to the potent arterial dilation.

Diastolic blood pressure: This is determined by (1) volume of blood within the arterial system, (2) compliance of the arterial wall, and (3) peripheral resistance. Coronary artery blood flow occurs during diastole, and a drop in diastolic pressure may result in myocardial ischemia as flow is reduced with lower diastolic pressure. Monitoring of diastolic BP is critical, especially when vasodilating drugs are administered, since diastolic BP generally decreases from the effect of these medications.

Diagnostic Tests Associated with PA Catheter Placement for Hemodynamic Monitoring

Test	Purpose	Abnormal Findings
Noninvasive Cardiology		
Continuous cardiac monitoring (ECG): The ECG should be monitored continuously during insertion of pulmonary artery (PA) catheters and throughout use of hemodynamic monitoring using a 5- or 3-lead system.	Assesses for dysrhythmias during PA catheter insertion. ECG tracings are used to correlate pressure waveforms with the cardiac cycle as part of acquiring accurate measurements.	*During insertion:* PVCs may occur as the catheter passes quickly through the ventricle on the way to the pulmonary artery. If ventricular ectopy persists, the catheter should be withdrawn into the RA and refloated. The balloon on the catheter should remain inflated throughout the procedure so the blood flow moves the catheter through the heart.
Radiology		
Chest radiograph (CXR) A CXR should be done upon insertion, and daily to assess central catheter position. *CVP placement:* Tip at the superior venacaval/atrial junction. *PA catheter placement:* Tip should be in the middle third of lung fields within the pulmonary artery and within or barely outside of the sternal border. Most PA catheters are inserted into the right PA.	Assesses for abnormal findings following PA catheter or central venous catheter insertion or manipulation. If catheters are positioned improperly in the blood vessels, ischemia may occur distally from the catheter, or the catheter may cause erosion of vessel walls. Medication administration should not be done until it is confirmed the catheter is in the proper position.	*Pneumothorax or hemothorax:* May occur with central line placement in the internal jugular, external jugular, or subclavian insertion sites. *Widening mediastinum:* Indicative of acute cardiac tamponade, which may indicate rupture of a chamber of the heart during PA catheter insertion. *Subclavian insertion:* If a CVP catheter is not readily seen, inspect upper portion of film to make sure the catheter is not in the internal jugular vein. *RA catheter positioning:* A CVP line positioned in the RA is more likely to cause atrial perforation and cardiac tamponade, although rare. Happens more often with peripherally inserted central catheters (PICC lines) due to arm movement. *Left PA positioning:* PA catheters can be placed in the left PA. On the AP film, the catheter appears to be pointing distally. When seen, assess for knotting or coiling of the PA catheter within the RV, which may have caused the catheter to be directed toward the left PA.
Fluoroscopy radiographic method wherein catheter can be visualized as it passes through the heart and blood vessels	Used during PA catheter insertion to ensure accurate placement. Used at varying frequencies, depending on MD practice patterns. If not used often, may cause a delay insertion.	Some centers use fluoroscopy only for anticipated "difficult" PA catheter insertions, while others use it frequently. Abnormal vasculature or structural abnormality of the heart may be visualized as the catheter passes into position.

Safety Alert *Caution must be used in managing hypertension or decreasing afterload with sodium nitroprusside (e.g., Nipride), as this medication causes both venous and arterial vasodilation and can rapidly decrease the BP, causing hypotension with rapid decrease in delivery of O_2 and nutrients to the cells. Nitroprusside may also induce deterioration in arterial O_2 saturation if ventilation cannot increase enough to "match" the increased blood in the lungs caused by pulmonary vasodilation. If the BP is extremely labile, the patient may be intravascularly volume depleted or hypovolemic. Replacing fluid volume or blood (if hemorrhage is the cause) will help stabilize the BP.*

Mean arterial pressure: The normal MAP value is 70 to 100 mm Hg. MAP is the average pressure within the arterial tree throughout the cardiac cycle, reflecting the average force that pushes blood through the systemic circulation to the tissues. MAP is the product of CO × SVR. An increase in CO or SVR will increase MAP. A decrease in either value will decrease MAP. MAP is the most accurate noninvasive measurement of central aortic pressure. The intra-aortic balloon pump (IABP) provides the most accurate invasive measurement. MAP can be calculated by the following formula:

$$MAP = \frac{\text{Systolic BP} + 2(\text{Diastolic BP})}{3}$$

Central venous pressure: The normal CVP value is 2 to 6 mm Hg. CVP is the measurement of systemic venous pressure at the level of the superior vena cava just before it enters the right atrium. CVP can be measured by a catheter threaded into the jugular, subclavian, or other large vein, by the use of a central venous catheter; often, these are multilumen catheters. *The RA pressure (RAP) correlates to the CVP as the normal values and waveforms (Figure 1-6) are the same and the terms are used interchangeably in practice.* Using a PA catheter, the RAP is measured through the proximal port, which lies in the right atrium. Since 60% of total blood volume resides in the venous system, the CVP is valuable in assessing for fluid volume excess or deficit and venous tone. The CVP also provides indirect information regarding RV function. RV failure, cardiac tamponade, fluid volume overload, pulmonary hypertension, tricuspid valve disease, and chronic LV failure may increase CVP. Decreased CVP is most often caused by hypovolemia. Venous dilation caused by sepsis, drugs, or neurogenic dysfunction also may decrease CVP. Complications of central venous catheters include venous air embolism, dysrhythmias, hemorrhage, infection, vascular erosion, perforation of cardiac chambers, pneumothorax, and thromboembolic problems.

Safety Alert *Be alert for air embolism during central catheter insertion and maintenance of the CVP monitoring system. This is an uncommon but potentially fatal event. As little as 20 ml of air may cause a problem for critically ill patients. Entry of 200 to 300 ml of air into the vessel over a short period of time (seconds) has a 50% mortality rate. Prevention is the key. During insertion, ensure the practitioner inserting the catheter does not allow*

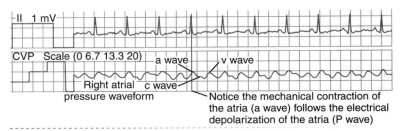

Figure 1-6 **Right atrial pressure waveform with ECG.** Redrawn from Daily E, Schroeder J: *Techniques in Bedside Hemodynamic Monitoring,* ed. 4. St. Lousis, 1989, Mosby.

ports to be uncapped or uncovered (open to air) once inside the vessel. Air can be entrained down the port by the blood flow during inspiration (when intrathoracic pressure is negative), resulting in embolization. If air embolism is suspected, place the patient with HOB down (Trendelenberg position), in the left lateral decubitus position, immediately (see Suspected Air Embolism in the Collaborative Management section.)

Right atrial pressure: The normal mean RAP is 4 to 6 mm Hg. *RAP is measured via the proximal catheter port and is essentially the same as CVP.* With the PA catheter, RAP can be monitored continuously and displayed on a bedside screen (see Figure 1-6). In addition, the catheter lumen can be used for fluid or drug administration.

Right ventricular pressure: The normal RVP is 20 to 30/0 to 8 mm Hg. RVP is measured only during catheter insertion and provides information about the function of the right ventricle and the tricuspid and pulmonic valves. Elevation of RV systolic pressure may be seen in pulmonic stenosis, pulmonary hypertension, or ventricular septal defect (VSD) with left-to-right shunt. Elevation of RV diastolic pressure may occur with RV failure, cardiac tamponade, or constrictive pericarditis.

Safety Alert

It is important for the nurse to identify the normal RV waveform (Figure 1-7) because a complication of the PA catheter is potential displacement of the catheter tip into the right ventricle, causing ventricular ectopy. Immediate action to reposition the PA catheter should be performed. Some institutions may allow nurses to reposition the patient and inflate the PA catheter balloon so blood flow into the PA carries the catheter back into position, while others may be required to immediately pull the PA catheter back into the RA.

Pulmonary artery pressures: Multiple values are measured via the use of a PA catheter (PAC) (see Table 1-10). PA pressure monitoring is used to evaluate heart function and pulmonary vascular status. PA catheters (e.g., Swan-Ganz, Opti-cath, and others) provide valuable information

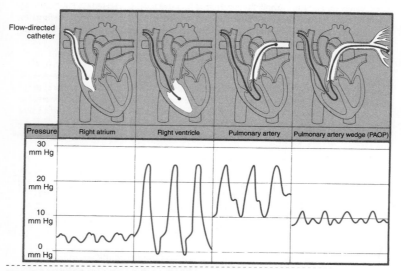

Figure 1-7 Location of catheter tip and waveforms obtained during insertion of pulmonary artery catheter. *PAOP,* pulmonary artery occlusion pressure. (From Urden LD, Stacy KM, Lough ME: *Priorities in critical care nursing,* ed 5. St. Louis, 2008, Mosby.)

used to assess and treat life-threatening illness or injury. Blood volume, heart function, and tissue oxygenation can be assessed using various available pressures. PA catheters are inserted via the jugular, subclavian, brachial, or femoral vein and passed through the right side of the heart into the PA, where the tip of the catheter is positioned in the distal PA. The PA catheter should be positioned in zone 3 of the lung field, below the level of the left atrium to promote maximal accuracy of readings, given the effects of gravity on blood flow through the lungs.

PA pressures are normally one-fifth of systemic BP. PA systolic (PAS), PA mean (PAM), and PA diastolic (PAD) pressures are monitored continuously by the distal port of the PA catheter, after the catheter is passed out of the right heart, through the pulmonic valve, and into the PA. PAOP can be assessed after inflating the balloon on the distal end of the catheter, which allows it to float and "wedge" into a smaller branch of the PA. Once the artery is occluded by the balloon, the filling pressures of the left heart can be indirectly measured. *The PAOP is often referred to as the PA wedge (PAW) pressure or occasionally the pulmonary capillary wedge pressure (PCWP) or, in general conversation, as the "wedge."*

If a more sophisticated Svo_2 PA catheter is used, mixed venous O_2 saturation levels are also continuously monitored. CO can be measured intermittently using thermodilution or, with some PA/Svo_2 catheters, is measured continuously. A full hemodynamic profile can also be calculated for the patient, including SV, stroke work, pulmonary vascular resistance, and SVR (see Table 1-10). All values are helpful in determining how to manage the patient's fluid balance, heart function, and vascular tone and can be individualized to the patient's body size (index values). There is ongoing research on the usefulness of indexing hemodynamic values to body weight in the morbidly obese population; no consensus has been formed. Abnormal PA pressures are discussed in Table 1-12. Complications of PA catheters include ventricular or atrial dysrhythmias, pulmonary ischemia or infarction, valvular damage (tricuspid, pulmonic), PA rupture, infection, emboli (thrombotic, air, balloon), and pneumothorax. The incidence of PA catheter complications is about 3%.

PA systolic (PAS), diastolic (PAD), and mean pressures (PAM)   Normal PA pressures are 20 to 30/8 to 15 mm Hg (PAS/PAD) with PAM 10 to 20 mm Hg (Figure 1-8). The PA pressures are used to evaluate heart function and pulmonary vascular disease. In patients with healthy pulmonary vasculature, the PAD pressure corresponds closely to the PAOP and reflects the LVEDP. A significant difference (i.e., greater than 5 mm Hg) between the PAD and PAOP is seen with pulmonary disease or a pulmonary embolus. When this occurs, PA systolic and diastolic pressures are elevated, whereas the PAOP remains normal. Specific disease states that result in elevated PA pressures include pulmonary hypertension, pulmonary embolism, hypoxia, LV failure resulting from valve disease, myocardial infarction (MI), cardiomyopathy, and left-to-right intracardiac shunt. Decreased PA pressures are seen with hypovolemia and pharmacologic preload reduction.

Pulmonary artery occlusive pressure (PAOP)   Normal mean PAOP is 6 to 12 mm Hg (Figure 1-9). The PAOP reflects the LVEDP and is used to evaluate cardiac performance. PAOP does not accurately reflect LVEDP in patients with severe pulmonary hypertension. An elevated PAOP may be seen with LV failure, acute mitral regurgitation, acute VSD, and acute cardiac tamponade. A decreased PAOP is seen with hypovolemia and afterload reduction. On mechanically ventilated patients, positive end-expiratory pressure (PEEP) or continuous positive airway pressure (CPAP) settings of greater than 10 cm H_2O may result in

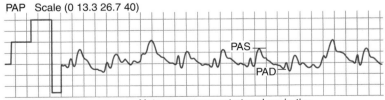

Note: measurement at end expiration with patient receiving positive pressure ventilation

Figure 1-8 Pulmonary artery pressure waveform. Redrawn from Daily E, Schroeder J: *Techniques in Bedside Hemodynamic Monitoring,* ed. 4. St. Lousis, 1989, Mosby.

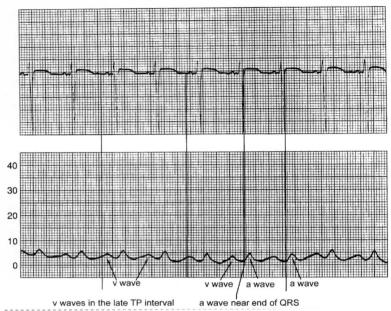

v wave   v wave / a wave | a wave

v waves in the late TP interval   a wave near end of QRS

Figure 1-9 Pulmonary artery occlusive pressure waveform. (From American Association of Critical Care Nurses: *AACN procedure manual for critical care*, ed 5. Philadelphia, 2005, WB Saunders.)

falsely elevated PA pressures and PAOP. Regardless of the inaccuracy, patients should not be disconnected from the ventilator to measure PA pressures, because significant hypoxemia and inaccurate measurements can result. Correlation of measured pressures with the respiratory cycle improves the accuracy of these measurements.

Cardiac Output and Cardiac Index The normal CO value is 4 to 8 L/min. CO is the volume of blood in liters ejected by the heart each minute and is calculated as the product of the SV and the HR (CO = SV × HR). SV is the volume of blood ejected by the heart per beat. Normal SV is 55 to 100 ml/beat. *The CO is commonly individualized in relation to body size by dividing the CO by the body surface area (BSA) to obtain the value known as the cardiac index (CI).* The normal CI is 2.5 to 4 $L/min/m^2$. If continuous CO monitoring is done, an average CO is recorded over 3-minute intervals and updated every 30 to 60 seconds. Continuous CO monitoring closely and accurately monitors a patient's hemodynamic profile. Benefits of continuous CO monitoring may improve response to changes in output, resulting in improved outcomes for severely ill patients (e.g., cardiomyopathy, ejection fractions [EFs] less than 20%). CO reflects the overall management of preload, afterload, contractility, and HR. The presence of intracardiac shunts renders CO measurements invalid, as pulmonary and systemic blood flows are erratic and unequal.

Left atrial pressure The normal value for LAP is 8 to 12 mm Hg. LAP is the most direct measure of the volume within the left ventricle at the end of diastole (LVEDP). A small, rigid catheter is inserted into the left atrium during cardiac surgery and brought through the chest wall or epigastric area. Continuous monitoring of LVEDP may be indicated for the cardiac surgery patient with significant pulmonary hypertension. PAOP is no longer reflective of left heart function when severe pulmonary hypertension is present. Since the catheter enters directly into the left atrium, the patient is at high risk for air or tissue emboli. An in-line air filter should be added to the flush system to reduce the risk of air emboli. If the waveform pattern dampens, the catheter should be aspirated until blood is seen. If there is no blood return, consult the physician. It is not advisable to flush the LA catheter because of the risk of inducing arterial air embolism.

Calculated or Derived Measurements

All hemodynamic readings can be adjusted to body size by dividing the direct reading by the BSA. It is sometimes beneficial to use indexed values to gain a clearer idea of the normalcy of the hemodynamic profile. On first glance, a profile may appear relatively normal, but when indexed, numerous values are found out of normal range (see Table 1-10).

In addition to indexed values, various other calculations are done to help guide therapies:

Systemic vascular resistance   The normal value for SVR is 800 to 1200 dyneslseclcm^{-5}. SVR is the major factor that determines LV afterload or resistance that must be overcome prior to LV ejection. The formula for SVR is the following:

$$SVR = \frac{(MAP - RAP) \times 80}{CO}$$

Any factor that increases SVR will increase the workload of the heart and may reduce cardiac output. Vasodilator therapy is used to reduce SVR to normal limits. A low SVR can indicate systemic vasodilation, commonly seen with septic, anaphylactic, and neurogenic shocks, and seen immediately postoperatively when recovering vascular tone. Vasopressors and IV fluids are administered to manage vasodilatation along with medications directed at the cause. Patients with low SVR often have high CO due to low resistance to ventricular ejection. Medications may affect the SVR: norepinephrine, vasopressin, and phenylephrine (Neo-Synephrine) increase it, whereas isoproterenol, nifedipine, prostaglandins, sodium nitroprusside, and acetylcholine decrease it.

Pulmonary vascular resistance   The normal value is 150 to 250 dyneslseclcm^{-5}. PVR measures RV afterload or the resistance the right ventricle must overcome to eject into the pulmonary circulation. The formula for PVR is the following:

$$PVR = \frac{(PAM - PAOP) \times 80}{CO}$$

PVR may be elevated as a result of primary pulmonary hypertension or secondary pulmonary hypertension due to mitral or aortic valve disease, congenital heart disease, long-standing LV heart failure, hypoxia, chronic obstructive pulmonary disease (COPD), or pulmonary embolus. Medications may affect the PVR: norepinephrine, vasopressin, and phenylephrine increase it, whereas isoproterenol, nifedipine, prostaglandins, sodium nitroprusside, and acetylcholine decrease it.

Mixed venous oxygen saturation   The normal range for Svo$_2$ is 60% to 80%. Svo$_2$ is defined as the average percentage of Hgb bound with O$_2$ in the venous blood, which infers the balance of O$_2$ supply and demand at the tissue level. Traditional belief was that hemodynamic stability and normal arterial blood gas levels meant O$_2$ delivery (Do$_2$) to tissues was adequate to meet and address cellular O$_2$ needs. As technology developed, it became clear conventional methods were not able to measure cellular O$_2$ needs (O$_2$ demand) or use (O$_2$ consumption) by assessing O$_2$ delivery alone. With the development of monitors displaying Svo$_2$ continuously, the onset of O$_2$ supply/demand/consumption imbalance can be more readily identified. Svo$_2$ can be measured intermittently using mixed venous blood samples from the distal port of the PA catheter or continuously using a specialized fiberoptic Svo$_2$ PA catheter. Cardiac output, Hgb level, and arterial O$_2$ saturation impact O$_2$ delivery. Svo$_2$ is reflective of O$_2$ delivery and consumption. If O$_2$ delivery is inadequate, or O$_2$ demand is high, more O$_2$ will be extracted from Hgb. If the patient is anemic, there are fewer red blood cells carrying oxyhemoglobin, so more O$_2$ is extracted. If the patient has pulmonary disease, such as ARDS, O$_2$ saturation is less, so less O$_2$ is delivered. Normal O$_2$ delivery is 600 ml O$_2$/min/m^2 if CO, Hgb level, and O$_2$ saturation (Sao$_2$ or Spo$_2$) are normal. Normal O$_2$ consumption ($\dot{V}O_2$), which should mirror demand, is 150 ml/min/m^2, which means 450 ml/min/m^2 of O$_2$ should be left on the red blood cells returning to the heart. In other words, about 25% of the O$_2$ is used, leaving behind about 75%. The textbook normal value for Svo_2 is 0.75, or 75%. Very low levels (less than 30%) indicate poor perfusion and are often associated with lactic acidosis (see *Acid-Base Balance*, p. 1). If the Svo_2 value changes by more than 10% for longer than 10 minutes, the nurse should evaluate Sao_2, CO, Hgb, and $\dot{V}o_2$. Svo_2 monitoring can be used to evaluate the effects of medical and nursing interventions on tissue O_2 use. By examining the variables involved in tissue oxygenation, the nurse can help determine which parameters may need to be better managed to meet the current metabolic demands (Table 1-13).

Table 1-13   FACTORS AFFECTING MIXED VENOUS OXYGEN SATURATION

Svo_2 is a sensitive indicator of oxygen supply/demand balance. If Svo_2 decreases to less than 50%, the patient should be rapidly assessed for the cause of an increased oxygen demand, or decrease in supply. Anemia, hypoxemia, and decreased CO may result in markedly reduced oxygen delivery. In the presence of the high metabolic demands imposed by critical illness, a reduction in O_2 delivery or further increase in O_2 demand can produce profound instability in the patient. Changes in Svo_2 often precede overt changes reflective of physiologic instability.

Factor	Effect on Svo_2	Clinical Examples
Arterial Oxygen Saturation		
↑Sao_2	↑Svo_2	Supplemental oxygen
↓Sao_2		
	↓Svo_2	Reduced oxygen supply (e.g., ARDS, ET suctioning, removal of supplemental oxygen, pulmonary disease, asthma, respiratory failure, obstructive sleep apnea)
Cardiac Output		
↑CO	↑Svo_2	Administration of inotropes to increase contractility
↓CO	↓Svo_2	Dysrhythmias, increased SVR, MI, hypovolemia, ↑HR, or ↓HR
Hemoglobin		
↓Hgb	↓Svo_2	Hemorrhage, hemolysis, severe anemia in patients with cardiovascular disease
Oxygen Consumption		
↑$\dot{V}o_2$	↓Svo_2	States in which metabolic demand exceeds oxygen supply (e.g., shivering, seizures, hyperthermia, hyperdynamic states)
↓$\dot{V}o_2$	↑Svo_2	States in which there is failure of peripheral tissue to extract or use oxygen: Significant peripheral arteriovenous shunting: cirrhosis, renal failure Redistribution of blood away from beds where oxygen extraction occurs: sepsis, acute pancreatitis, major burns Blockage of oxygen uptake or utilization: cyanide poisoning (including nitroprusside toxicity), carbon monoxide poisoning
Mechanical Problems	↑Svo_2	Wedged PA catheter creates falsely elevated Svo_2

ARDS, acute respiratory distress syndrome; *CO*, cardiac output; *ET*, endotracheal; *Hgb*, hemoglobin; *MI*, myocardial infarction; *PA*, pulmonary artery; *SVR*, systemic vascular resistance.

COLLABORATIVE MANAGEMENT

The need for accuracy of hemodynamic values cannot be stressed enough. Making clinical decisions based on these values and the calculations derived from them, is the reason for using hemodynamic monitoring in critically ill patients.

Care Priorities

1. **Promote patient safety by meticulously managing the monitoring system, assessing the pressure readings/waveforms, and assessing the patient (Table 1-11).**
   - *Ensure proper setup and maintenance of the pressure monitoring system.* Assessment of the PAOP provides information about the blood being pumped from the left heart, as does the CO. In combination with BP readings, the values frame the treatment plan. Configuration of normal waveforms must be understood so abnormalities can be recognized, analyzed, and managed.
   - *Assess for proper system compliance.* Prior to initiating monitoring, and any time over-damping or underdamping is suspected, square wave testing is done to assess proper compliance within the system, which is essential for accurate readings.
   - *Prevent pulmonary infarction.* A continuous PAOP waveform with the balloon deflated indicates the catheter has migrated distally and is lodged in a small pulmonary vessel. The chest radiograph may reveal the catheter is visible beyond the mediastinal structures, which indicates the catheter has passed too far into the distal pulmonary circulation. The catheter should be repositioned immediately according to institutional protocol to avoid damage to the surrounding lung tissues.
   - *Prevent limb ischemia.* Prior to radial artery catheter insertion, the practitioner should perform the Allen test to ensure the ulnar artery is pulsatile. Maintaining all arterial lines should include a neurovascular assessment distal to the catheter.
   - *Prevent RV irritation by the catheter.* RV waveform instead of the PA wave indicates improper positioning. The catheter should be repositioned according to institutional protocol to avoid ventricular dysrhythmias.
2. **Recognize and manage the complications associated with hemodynamic monitoring equipment.**
   - *Complications of arterial catheters:* Arterial thrombosis with ischemia, infection, infiltration, and blood loss caused by disconnection. Continuous observation of the arterial line insertion site for infection and leakage is an essential nursing responsibility. Monitor and document pulses distal to the catheter site every 1 to 2 hours. It is important to note a patient's baseline BP and to compare left and right cuff BPs with arterial BPs. Meticulous care should be taken with setup and maintenance of the arterial pressure monitoring system. If air enters a peripheral arterial catheter, the distal structures (e.g., hand, leg) are at highest risk for ischemic complications caused by air bubbles lodging in smaller arterial vessels.
   - *Suspected air embolus:* Complications are seen more frequently from venous air emboli, which may happen during any central catheter insertion, including PA catheters. Symptoms include acute respiratory distress, apnea, possible wheezing, sudden hypotension, syncope, hypoxia, cyanosis, possible murmur, elevated CVP, neurologic deficits, cardiac arrest with asystole, pulseless electrical activity (PEA), or ventricular fibrillation. Arterial monitoring systems connected to intra-aortic balloon catheters can cause life-threatening air embolism in the central circulation, including the aorta, but this is rarely seen in clinical practice.

HIGH ALERT!   **Suspected Air Embolus**

The patient should immediately be placed in left lateral Trendelenburg (head down) position and 100% O_2 administered. Have the patient try to perform a Valsalva maneuver. Aspirate air from the system: IV tubing, arterial line tubing, or the catheter itself. If severe complications ensue, hyperbaric O_2 treatment using the Diving Accident Protocol (DAP) may be used if available. Perform CPR if necessary. Air can cause stroke or death in the patient.

3. **Recognize the characteristics of normal waveforms and pressure readings.**
   - *Arterial pressure waveform:* The upstroke on arterial pressure waveform represents the rapid ejection phase of ventricular systole. The anacrotic shoulder (rounded peak) is where the systolic pressure is measured. The descent represents slowed ventricular ejection followed by aortic valve closure represented by the dicrotic notch, followed by runoff of flow systemically during diastole. The diastolic pressure is measured as the end-diastolic pressure just prior to the next systole (see Figure 1-5).
   - *PA waveform:* Has the same waveform components as the arterial pressure, except the dicrotic notch represents pulmonic valve closure, followed by runoff flow in the pulmonary vasculature during diastole. The PA pressure measurements are taken at the peak systolic and end diastolic pressures (see Figure 1-8.)
   - *End-expiratory pressures:* Care must be taken to measure and record all end-expiratory pressures. With positive pressure ventilation, these will be at the low point of the wave. With spontaneous ventilation, end-expiratory pressures are higher than pressure during inspiration. One must be careful not to import or just assume that the digital average is an accurate reading. Readings must be done at end expiration; as with respiratory fluctuations, values can be off 10 to 20 mm Hg.
   - *RAP, CVP, and PAOP waveforms:* Are composed of an *a-wave*, followed by an *x descent*; a *c-wave* may look like a notch on the *a-wave* or may be a separate wave, followed by a *v-wave*, and this is followed by the *y* descent (see Figure 1-6). The *a-wave* represents atrial systole, the *c wave* if present represents valvular closure, the *x* descent is atrial relaxation, and the *v-wave* is produced by atrial filling during ventricular systole as the atrioventricular valve bulges toward the atrium when the ventricle contracts. The *c-wave* is not commonly seen in the PAOP waveform due to the time of retrograde transmission (see Figure 1-9).
   - *Timing waveforms with the ECG:* The *a-*and *v-*waves are distinguished by their timing with the ECG. The heart's electrical conduction occurs prior to mechanical contraction. This is why the RAP/CVP *a-wave* is found just prior to the QRS and the *v-wave* is found at the T wave. The PAOP wave has farther to travel to be transmitted; therefore, the *a-wave* follows the QRS and the *v-wave* is found after the T and prior to the next P wave (see Figure 1-6).
   - *Cannon waves and large V waves:* ECG correlations are important diagnostic adjuncts, since *a* waves are absent in an atrioventricular junctional or idioventricular rhythm. Large, abnormal *a* waves called cannon waves are caused by the atria trying to contract against a closed AV valve, which occurs during atrial fibrillation and complete heart block. PAOP with a large *v-wave* is an indication of mitral insufficiency.
   - *Inflating the PAOP balloon:* When obtaining the PAOP, the PA catheter balloon should be inflated slowly with no more than 1.5 ml of air. The PA waveform should be observed changing to a smaller PAOP/wedge waveform. No additional air should be used once the change has begun. Once the PAOP has been obtained, the balloon should be deflated passively; the syringe is removed and emptied of air, and then reattached to prevent accidental balloon inflation (see Figures 1-7 and 1-9).

HIGH ALERT!   **Pulmonary Artery Rupture and Occlusion**

Overwedging or rapid balloon inflation can cause PA rupture. Prolonged balloon inflation or PA catheter migration can lead to balloon rupture, as well as clot formation and pulmonary infarction. PAOP may be assessed less frequently if a strong correlation is established between the PAOP and the PAD to avoid repeated trauma to the pulmonary vessels and to prolong the life of the balloon. The PA waveform must be continually monitored to observe for distal migration of the catheter, or proximal displacement due to pulling on the catheter or movement of the external monitoring system during patient care procedures (see Table 1-11).

CARE PLANS FOR HEMODYNAMIC MONITORING

Deficient knowledge *related to the rationale for hemodynamic monitoring and procedure for catheter insertion*

GOALS/OUTCOMES Prior to and during catheter placement, the patient or significant other states they are comfortable with the rationale for hemodynamic monitoring, procedure for insertion of lines, and sensations that are experienced during and after the procedure.

NOC Knowledge: Treatment Regimen

Teaching: Procedure/Treatment

1. Assess patient's knowledge about hemodynamic monitoring. As indicated, explain to patient/family that hemodynamic monitoring measures the BP within the body and the BP within the heart and lungs and gives information about the pumping action of the heart, which is useful in guiding therapy.

2. Teach the patient about the insertion procedure, emphasizing that a local anesthetic agent will be used, he or she will not be able to move during the procedure, and, following the procedure, a dressing will be applied to the insertion site. For radial arterial lines, explain that an armboard or other device may be used to immobilize the wrist. For PA and central lines, explain that a large drape is placed over the body and face during insertion and a chest radiograph will be obtained following the procedure.

3. Explain that unusual sensations may be felt during the procedure and that a nurse will be present to hold his or her hand, offer support should they have questions, and be able to administer supplemental medications to promote their comfort. Depending on the situation, a clue to the next sensation anticipated is best rendered during the procedure, such as, "You may feel coolness from the cleansing solution" or, "You may feel a 'bee sting' from injection of the local anesthetic" or, "You may feel pressure as the catheter advances."

Risk for ineffective cardiac tissue perfusion *related to complications from PA catheter presence in the pulmonary circulation, including circulatory impairment from migration of PA catheter into a wedged position, "overwedging" of the catheter balloon, PA rupture, pulmonary vascular thrombosis, or other patient safety hazards associated with the monitoring system*

GOALS/OUTCOMES Within 15 minutes of recognizing a complication with the hemodynamic monitoring system, the problem is addressed and resolved.

NOC Tissue Perfusion: Cardiac; Tissue Perfusion: Peripheral; Tissue Perfusion: Pulmonary

Hemodynamic Regulation

1. Monitor the PA waveform continuously. Report any change in configuration, particularly if the waveform becomes decreased in amplitude and flattened in appearance (see Table 1-11).

2. Assess the patient for decreased pulmonary arterial blood flow as evidenced by acute onset of pleuritic chest pain, SOB, tachypnea, and hemoptysis.

3. Evaluate the position of the catheter via chest radiograph according to institutional protocol. Never push the PA catheter forward in the PA to avoid possibility of PA rupture or lodging the catheter in a small vessel.

4. Record the position of the PA catheter when inserted. Assess and record this level every shift. If there is a change in the waveform, catheter position should be reassessed. The physician or midlevel practitioner should be notified for catheters that are out of position or fail to wedge.

5. Exercise care in taking PAOP measurements. Prolonged and repeated readings can cause trauma to the vessel wall. The catheter can also be "overwedged." Proper wedging entails slow injection of enough air to obtain a wedge configuration, but no more than the amount recommended by catheter manufacturer. Never pull back on the plunger of a balloon syringe to remove air; rather, disconnect the syringe and allow passive deflation of the balloon.

6. Verify and document PAD and PAOP every 4 to 8 hours. PAD may exceed PAOP by ≥ 5 mm Hg in patients with acidosis, hypoxemia, pulmonary emboli, lung disease, and pulmonary hypertension. If the PAD approximates the PAOP, the frequency of PAOP readings may be able to be reduced in some practice settings, to preserve the catheter balloon and reduce the possibility of vessel erosion.

7. Consult a physician or midlevel practitioner if the PA waveform remains in wedged position after balloon deflation. This may indicate the catheter has lodged in the vessel, which can lead to pulmonary infarction due to lack of perfusion distal to the lodged catheter.

8. Pay special attention to PA waveform when the patient is moved (e.g., when being taken to the radiology department; getting into a chair, when position is changed or bed is made). The monitoring system may no longer be appropriately leveled with the patient's phlebostatic axis (RA level) after the patient has changed position. Assess the catheter position to ensure the catheter has not moved. Also ensure the catheter is not pulled on when moving the patient.

Ineffective protection *related to inability to control internal responses and external threats posed by the presence of invasive hemodynamic catheters*

GOALS/OUTCOMES Patient is free of infection as evidenced by normothermia, white blood cell (WBC) count ≤11,000/mm³, negative culture results, and absence of erythema, heat, swelling, or purulent drainage at the insertion site.

NOC *SUGGESTED OUTCOMES* Immune Status

Infection Protection
1. Prior to insertion full barrier precautions should be in place per institution protocol. Central line catheter insertion and dressing changes are to be done with strict adherence to sterile technique. Following a central line bundle checklist is recommended.
2. On a daily basis, monitor for temperature elevations ≥37.7°C (100°F) and WBC count elevation.
3. Monitor the catheter insertion site for erythema, tenderness to the touch, local warmth, and purulent drainage.
4. Use normal saline rather than D₅W for hemodynamic flush solution, since dextrose solutions better support bacterial growth.
5. Change hemodynamic tubing, transducer, and flush solution according to hospital protocol.
6. Maintain a closed system from the transducer to the flush solution and the patient. Keep all external openings and stopcocks securely capped at all times.
7. Use a closed system for CO injection fluid.
8. Maintain an occlusive, dry sterile dressing over insertion site. As prescribed, obtain culture of any suspicious drainage and report positive findings.
9. Change the central/PA line dressing per hospital protocol, using aseptic technique.
10. Record the date of catheter insertion: ensure the catheter is changed per agency protocol.
11. If the line becomes infected, notify the physician or midlevel practitioner. The catheter should be removed and the catheter tip cut off and then sent in a sterile container for a culture and sensitivity test.

Safety Alert *CVP monitoring is the recommended monitoring strategy during early goal-directed therapy recommended by the Society of Critical Care Medicine, for patients with sepsis. Line sepsis may be masked as a potential cause of current infection. The lines should be changed only as needed unless reddened, WBCs are increasing, or the patient is febrile. Most central lines are able to remain in place for 7 days.*

Ineffective peripheral tissue perfusion (involved extremity) *related to interrupted blood flow secondary to presence of arterial catheter or thrombosis caused by catheter*

GOALS/OUTCOMES Within 15 minutes of this diagnosis, patient has adequate perfusion to affected extremity as evidenced by brisk capillary refill (less than 2 seconds), natural color, warm skin, normal sensation, and the ability to move the fingers.

NOC Circulation Status

Circulatory Precautions
1. Continuously monitor capillary refill, color, temperature, sensation, pulses, and movement. Be alert to indicators of ischemia and teach them to the patient, stressing the importance of notifying staff members promptly if they occur.
2. Maintain arterial line on continuous flush at 3 ml/hr with normal saline with the pressure bag inflated to 300 mm Hg. Heparinized saline is infrequently used, as it has not shown to be significantly more effective at maintaining patency, when all other measures of pressure monitoring are done.
3. Ensure tight connections of tubing throughout the system.
4. Support patient's wrist or appropriate extremity with armboard or other supportive device to prevent flexion and movement of the catheter.

Ineffective protection *related to potential for insertion complications secondary to ventricular irritability, patient movement during insertion procedure, or difficult anatomy*

 GOALS/OUTCOMES Patient has no complications from PA or CVP catheter insertion as evidenced by normal sinus rhythm on ECG, BP within patient's normal range, HR ≤100 bpm, RR ≤20 breaths/min with normal pattern and depth (eupnea), normal breath sounds, and absence of adventitious breath sounds or muffled heart sounds.

NOC Circulation Status

Risk Identification

1. Use patient safety precautions used for any invasive *procedures to conduct a preprocedure verification process;* mark the correct site and use of "Time Out" to assure patient safety.
2. During preprocedure teaching, caution patient about the importance of remaining still during insertion of catheter. Provide sedation and analgesics as prescribed.
3. Perform a baseline assessment, monitoring BP, HR, RR, breath sounds, heart sounds, and ECG.
4. Be alert to decreased BP, pulsus paradoxus, increased HR or RR, diminished or absent breath sounds, and muffled heart sounds, as well as dysrhythmias on ECG. Report significant findings to the physician or midlevel practitioner.
5. Perform a postprocedure assessment, comparing it with baseline findings. After the procedure, obtain a chest radiograph as prescribed.
6. Monitor for catheter related complications (see Table 1-11).
7. Keep amiodarone or lidocaine at bedside for immediate IV injection if patient has sustained ventricular dysrhythmias. This precaution should be rarely required.

MECHANICAL VENTILATION

There are multiple purposes to provide ventilation, which is generally referred to as the movement of gas in and out of the lungs. The major goals are related to blood-alveolar clearance of CO_2 and the uptake of O_2 into the blood, designed to support O_2 delivery to the tissues. For the ventilatory process to be initiated, the nervous system must be intact, the diaphragm and respiratory muscle groups must contract, the rib cage must be intact, the external fibrous level of the pleural sac must be attached to the rib cage, and there cannot be anything altering the intrapleural or intra-alveolar pressures. All of these conditions exist in order to decrease the alveolar resting pressures, promoting a pressure gradient that facilitates gas movement into the conducting tubes and ultimately distending (recruiting) the alveoli.

Spontaneous ventilation (whether or not supported) depends on the ability to generate alveolar distention, or negative pressure, and therefore increase compliance. This is referred to as either *increasing alveolar compliance (static compliance), a decrease in alveolar pressure (pPlat),* or *negative pressure breathing.* There are other conditions that must be present for patients to generate negative pressure and breathe spontaneously (Box 1-9). When patients are too weak to generate the force (negative pressure) required or too weak to maintain their airway, too sick or sedated to stimulate and contract the diaphragm, or when the conducting airways or the alveolar units are constricted, collapsed, or congested (Box 1-10), the need for ventilator support may be unavoidable. To ensure optimal care of the patient who requires mechanical ventilation, the practitioner must have adequate knowledge of the equipment and processes involved in mechanical ventilation. An exhaustive review of mechanical ventilation is not possible in this chapter; however, basic concepts must be addressed.

REVIEW OF BASIC VENTILATION TERMS
Respiratory Rate (RR or *f* [frequency of breathing])
- Charted as breaths per minute: bpm
- The frequency of breaths enabled by the patient and/or delivered by the ventilator may range from 10 to 50 bpm depending on ventilation strategies, except during weaning, when the frequency of breaths may be less than 10 to augment, rather than fully support, breathing.

Box 1-9	FACTORS AFFECTING NORMAL SPONTANEOUS VENTILATION

1. Having intact phrenic nerve innervation of the diaphragm
2. Ability of the of the diaphragm and external intercostals to maintain the appropriate contractile force
3. Ability to maintain a patent airway
4. Diameter of the airway
5. Ability of the alveoli to open during inspiration

Box 1-10	CONDITIONS THAT MAY REQUIRE VENTILATOR SUPPORT

Acute obstructive disease: acute severe asthma; airway mucosal edema
Altered ventilatory drive: hypothyroidism; intracranial hemorrhage; dyspnea-related anxiety
Atelectatic disease: ARDS; pneumonia
Burns and smoke inhalation: inhalation injury, surface burns
Cancer; malnutrition; infections
Cardiopulmonary problems: congestive heart failure; pulmonary hemorrhage
Chest trauma: blunt injury; flail chest; penetrating injuries
Chronic obstructive pulmonary disease: emphysema, chronic bronchitis, asthma; cystic fibrosis; bronchiectasis
Fatigue/atrophy: muscle overuse; disuse
Head/spinal cord injury: medullary brainstem injury; Cheyne-Stokes breathing; neurogenic pulmonary edema
Neuromuscular disease: ALS; Guillian-Barre; myasthenia gravis
Postoperative conditions: cardiac and thoracic surgeries
Pharmacological agents/drug overdose: muscle relaxants; barbiturates; Ca^{2+} channel blockers; long-term adrenocorticosteroids; aminoglycoside antibiotics

- Depending on the mode total frequency may also include the breaths that the patient takes between mandatory ventilator breaths.
- It is always abnormal for an adult patient to breath above 22 bpm.

Tidal Volume (V_T)
- Volume (amount) of gas delivered with each *preset* breath
- In mechanically ventilated patients V_T is usually set at 8 to 10 ml/kg/ideal body weight [IDBW] (milliliters per kilogram) according to National Heart, Lung, and Blood Institute ARDS Network (www.ardsnet.org).
- V_T decreases to 6 to 8 ml/kg/IDBW if the patient has a noncompliant lung condition.
- Charted as: V_T or tidal volume: (i.e., 375 ml per breath)

Minute Ventilation (V_E V_{TE} or $M\dot{V}$)
- The amount of volume exhaled per minute (V_E or V_{TE})
- Measured as

$$\text{Respirations} \times V_{TE} \text{ (MV)}$$

- Normal is 8 to 10 L/min.

Fraction of Inspired Oxygen (FIO_2)
- Percent of atmospheric pressure (760 mm Hg) that is O_2
- For example, 0.21 or 21% is calculated as

$$0.21 \times 760 \text{ mm Hg} = 159 \text{ mm Hg } P_{atmos} O_2$$

- For simplicity sake, documented as FIO_2, utilize the decimal (0.21) in P/F calculations or the calculated pressure in A-aDO2 calculations.

Peak Inspiratory Pressure (PIP or PawP or PaP)
- Peak pressure measured when the tidal volume is pushed into the airways
- Value used to set high- and low-pressure alarm limits
- In normal lungs (resistance and compliance normal) less than 35 cm H_2O
- In any condition that increases resistance or decreases compliance, may be greater than 35 cm H_2O

Mean Airway Pressure (MAP)
- Average proximal airway pressure during the entire respiratory cycle; a major determinate for oxygenation and a focus for the settings of alternative ventilation

Pressure measured during inspiratory hold ($p_{Plateau}$ or p_{Plat})

- Airway pressure measured during an inspiratory hold after a volume-controlled breath
- Used to determine a patient's static lung compliance
- Normally less than 25 cm H_2O

Flow Rate ($\dot{V}$)

- The delivery method and rate of speed for the tidal volume breath (also affects time spent in inspiration versus exhalation as well as pressure reached)
- Normally 40 to 60 L/min

> **Safety Alert** *All airway pressures including PIP and PawP, as well as p_{Plat}, are measured by changing the tidal volume, airway resistance, and peak inspiratory flow rate and also very significantly by alterations in compliance.*

Trigger: What starts a breath? Inspiratory flow begins.

- Elapsed time: how many breaths per minute?
- Patient effort: negative inspiratory force: The patient's effort can be "sensed" as a change in pressure or a change in flow (in the circuit).

Sensitivity

- A setting on the ventilator that adjusts how much negative inspiratory pressure the patient must generate (effort as above) before the ventilator delivers a breath. Is activated only in Assist control ventilation (ACMV) or SIMV

Cycle: What stops a breath? Inspiratory flow ends.

1. *Pressure cycle:* A predetermined and preset pressure terminates inspiration. Pressure is constant/volume is variable. Used for pressure control ventilation
2. *Volume cycle:* A predetermined and preset volume when delivered terminates the inspiration. Volume is constant/pressure is variable. Used for volume control ventilation
3. *Time cycle:* Delivers air/gas over a set time after which the inspiration ends (affects the I:E)—inspiratory time/exhalation time (I:E).
   - Directly related to how rapidly or slowly the flow of tidal volume occurs
   - Directly related to the pressure achieved when volume is delivered at a certain rate of speed
4. I:E time examples
   - If an assumed tidal volume of 400 ml/breath is delivered at a flow rate (rate of speed) of 80 L/min, either volume or pressure control limits will be reached rapidly and *"inspiratory time" will be shorter and "exhalation time" will be longer.* This strategy is used in compliant lungs when CO_2 retention or ventilator dysynchrony is evaluated.
   - If an assumed tidal volume of 400 ml/breath is delivered at a flow rate (rate of speed) of 40 L/min, either volume or pressure control limits will be reached over a longer period of time and *"I time" will be longer and "E time" will be shorter.* This strategy may be used to recruit alveoli when lungs are noncompliant and hypoxemia is the problem, that is, low oxygen and high pressures are an issue. The expectation is that the pressure generated when the tidal volume flows will be lower.
   - If an assumed tidal volume of 400 ml/breath is delivered at a flow rate (rate of speed) of 100 L/min, either volume or pressure control limits will be reached over a shorter period of time and *"I time" will be shorter and "E time" will be longer.* This strategy may be used to allow for more time to exhale and is generally used if the expectation is that the pressure generated when the tidal volume flows will be lower, but that the patient's major problem is alveolar recoil (i.e., COPD disease).

NEGATIVE PRESSURE VENTILATION

Normal intrapleural pressure ranges from -2 (rest) to -10 cm H_2O (inspiration). Negative pressure ventilators generate subatmospheric pressure to the thorax and trunk (similar to applying an external vacuum) to initiate respiration and do not require intubation for use. The iron lung, chest cuirass shell, and poncho chest shell are examples. Since these devices are noninvasive and do not require intensive monitoring, there has been a resurgence of interest in their use for long-term home therapy. They are not discussed here.

POSITIVE PRESSURE VENTILATION

Today, all external applications of mechanical ventilation largely require a method of administering positive pressure for delivery of a predetermined volume of gas. Positive pressure ventilation is related to the creation of a super atmospheric pressure (greater than 760 mm Hg), which is generated at the upper airway. The resultant pressure gradient between the upper airway and the alveoli then allows for the "pushing" gas volume. This delivery system may be administered via a mask system (noninvasive) or invasively via an ET tube or tracheostomy. The concept, put quite simply, is to decrease the need for the development of a significant negative pressure or force, supplanting that requirement with the super atmospheric pressure.

NONINVASIVE POSITIVE PRESSURE VENTILATION (NiPPV OR NPPV)

Positive pressure support may be administered via a face mask, nasal mask, helmet, or mouth seal. This may also be presented as CPAP or BiPAP. The early application of *NPPV or noninvasive mechanical ventilation (NIMV)* may enhance respiratory rescue and may be applied by trained providers outside of the intensive care unit. The indications for consideration include airway obstruction disorders, chest wall disease, neuromuscular weakness, and sleep-related breathing disorders. Currently NPPV is contraindicated in patients who cannot protect their airway or who cannot clear their secretions and those who present with severe agitation or shock. NPPV allows patients to maintain normal functions, such as speaking and eating, and assists in the avoidance of the risks and complications of intubation and sedation.

1. *CPAP*—A mode of assistance with positive pressure via application of a constant pressure to the airways. This method does not supply any volume breath, rather maintains airway and alveolar opening in order to facilitate inspiration and decrease collapse during exhalation. Very similar in concept and design to methods applied for sleep apnea.
2. *BiPAP*—A mode of ventilatory assistance that uses alternating inspiratory positive pressures (IPAP) and expiratory positive pressures (EPAP) to enhance variable spontaneous tidal volumes. The resistance and compliance of the airways will determine the IPAP "driving pressure" necessary to produce a desired tidal volume. The level of EPAP needed is based on the oxygenation status of the patient. The physician determines a tidal volume goal (usually 8 to 12 ml/kg) and an oxygenation goal the clinician will use to determine the titration range for IPAP, EPAP, and F_{IO_2}. BiPAP (may be referred to as BiLevel) mode can be found on many conventional ventilators and on freestanding units used for NPPV.

INVASIVE MECHANICAL VENTILATION

When intubation is required (Box 1-11), the oral route is generally preferred to reduce incidence of sinusitis. After intubation, the nurse or respiratory therapist should do the following:
1. Confirm the placement of the ET tube using a CO_2 detector and then auscultate for bilateral breath sounds.
2. Mark and chart the centimeter mark on the tube using the teeth as a reference point.
3. Secure the tube to the face and head.
4. Cut/shorten the tube to reduce dead space, taking care not to cut the pilot balloon, so only 4 cm protrudes from the teeth.
5. Over the next 4 hours, monitor for the development of a life-threatening tension pneumothorax, by assessing for hypoxia, bradycardia, tachycardia, and moderate to life threatening hypotension.

Box 1-11	REASONS TO CONSIDER INTUBATION
Severe acidosis or hypoxemia	Aspiration risk
Severe dyspnea	Copious/viscous secretions
Respiratory arrest	Recent facial trauma
CV instability	Extreme obesity

BASIC VENTILATION MODES
Assist-Control Ventilation (A/C or ACV)

This mode can be used with either volume or pressure as the limit. In Assist-control (often labeled "volume control," or pressure control or ACV), patients may receive either controlled or ventilator assisted breaths. The set rate will deliver breaths in a time line (i.e., rate of 12 ventilator delivers breaths 12 times per minute). In addition, when the patient generates his, it own negative pressure event (sensitivity set on the ventilator) triggers the ventilator, the ventilator turns on and delivers a breath of identical duration and magnitude as the mandatory breath. The patient receives a breath regardless of actual minute ventilation requirement. The "interactive" feature of this mode is the patient receives a breath when he or she generates enough negative pressure to turn the ventilator on. The advantage of this mode is patients breathe spontaneously with small amounts of work. Conventional assist-control (A/C) delivers a preset breath based on time intervals (defined by frequency). The inspiratory flow rate is measured in liters per minute, and it determines how quickly the breath is delivered. The time required to complete inspiration is determined by the tidal volume delivered and the flow rate: $T_i = V_T/\text{Flow rate}$. The breath is limited by reaching either the preset volume (volume control [VC]) or pressure (when volume is delivered reaching a predetermined pressure [pressure control (PC)]).

In addition to the mandatory breaths, the patient may initiate a negative pressure respiratory effort (inspiration) and the ventilator will turn on and deliver a ventilator breath, either PC or VC. In this way every breath is controlled (either pressure or volume), but the patient may take more breaths than the mandatory rate determines. In other words, the patient can generate a request for an additional breath between mandatory ventilator breaths and the ventilator will turn on delivering breaths at the preset volume or pressure control levels. See Table 1-14.

ALL breaths in ACMV are ventilator assisted: Set rate plus patient generated request (effort).

Ventilator rate + Patient request rate = Total respiratory rate

EVERY breath, whether ventilator determined or patient requested, is a ventilator breath and predetermined for either pressure or volume control.

Safety Alert   *Control mode should never be deliberately set as ventilators should never be insensitive to a patient's inspiratory effort. New ventilators do not incorporate a pure "control" method, although the rate predetermined by the provider in conjunction with sedation and analgesic management will essentially "control" the patient. Controlling ventilation is related to the context and must be due to the loss of sympathetic and parasympathetic drive (i.e., spinal cord injury) or pharmacologic control.*

Synchronized Intermittent Mandatory Ventilation (SIMV)

Delivers a preset mandatory volume-controlled or pressure-controlled breath at a preset rate. Patient can also breathe spontaneously (at his or her own rate with a variable tidal volume and pressure) between mandatory ventilator breaths from a flow-by circuit. The difference between ACMV and SIMV is that in SIMV the patient may take spontaneous NON-VENTILATED breaths between the required ventilator breaths. In addition, the ventilator is synchronized to deliver the mandatory breath (controlled volume or pressure) when the patient initiates

Table 1-14	VOLUME VERSUS-PRESSURE-CONTROLLED MECHANICAL VENTILATION	
Volume Control	**Pressure Control**
Volume delivery constant	Volume delivery varies
Inspiratory pressure varies	Inspiratory pressure constant
Inspiratory flow constant	Inspiratory flow varies
Inspiratory time determined by set flow and V_T	Inspiratory time set by clinician

inspiration; however, if time is reached when mandatory breath must be administered, it will be done even if the patient has not initiated his or her own negative inspiratory effort. SIMV is generally administered in conjunction with pressure support, which is applied on spontaneous flow-by breaths.

Only set rate breaths in SIMV are ventilator assisted: Set rate plus patient generated request (effort).

Ventilator rate + Patient request rate = Total respiratory rate

ONLY set breath is a ventilator breath and predetermined for either pressure or volume control. All patient breaths are volume/pressure variable.

Safety Alert   *All providers should analyze the methods and modes of ventilation support and consider the use of SIMV and the flow rate prior to administration of sedatives to control the patient and/or reduce their efforts. Frequently, agitation will be present if the flow rate of the gas is too low or if the patient feels like he or she cannot control his or her own breathing. After consideration of flow and mode, sedation may be used to decrease respiratory drive, and machine sensitivity should be adjusted to prevent hyperventilation in patients whose respiratory rate increases because of mild anxiety or neurologic factors. AC ventilation has effectively replaced controlled ventilation, as the control of respiratory efforts must be performed pharmacologically and not mechanically.*

Pressure Support Ventilation (PSV)

PSV augments or supports a patient's spontaneous inspiration with a preselected pressure level. Pressure is applied (via flow of gas) at the initiation of inspiration and ends when a minimum inspiratory flow rate is reached. The patient retains control over inspiratory and expiratory time, frequency, tidal volume, and spontaneous minute ventilation. PSV creates less patient discomfort and diaphragmatic stress than assist-control or SIMV alone. Compensating for resistance created by the demand valve or ET tube size decreases inspiratory work. PSV MUST be combined with SIMV to improve patient tolerance of mechanical ventilation, to overcome the resistance offered by the ET tube (tube compensation), and to decrease the work of breathing through the ET tube. PSV is often used to facilitate weaning from mechanical ventilation.

These two methods are flow triggered/limited and (pressure) and volume-controlled. In ACMV when the patient takes a breath, the controlled method (volume) turns on. In SIMV when the patient takes a breath, the breath may either be a synchronized ventilator breath or a spontaneous volume breath.

Mode and method of ventilation should be determined by patient need and provider expertise rather than by individual bias.

Breath Limit

- *Time limited or cycled*: Relates to time that inspiratory flow is administered and is determined by a preset time or percent of cycle that relates to inspiration. Inspiratory time is increased to deliver a volume-controlled or pressure-controlled breath over a longer time of the breath cycle. Depending on the manufacturer, I and E times or flow rate may be the direct setting to adjust. In either case, one may maintain the tidal volume, minute ventilation-and frequency when adjusting the E time. I time is increased to deliver a volume-controlled or pressure-controlled breath over a longer time of the breath cycle. This will affect the frequency and therefore the tidal volume delivered. This may be used for non compliant lungs and alveolar recruitment to promote better oxygenation and is referred to as inverse I to E.
- *Pressure controlled (PC)*: The peak inspiratory pressure (PIP) is preset based on the estimated tidal volume requirements. A smaller tidal volume may be given if the preset pressure is reached too soon, such as in a state of low compliance or high airway resistance.
- *Volume control (VC)*: Volume is preset and the pressure is variable in order to deliver the preset volume. The PIP seen at the end of inspiration is higher under conditions of low compliance and/or high airway resistance.

Comparison of ventilator strategies and variables is available in Table 1-15.

Table 1-15	MODES OF MECHANICAL VENTILATION			
Type	Volume	Pressure	Flow	Inspiratory Time
Spontaneous (patient dependent)	Variable	Variable	Variable	Variable
VCV	Fixed	Variable or limited	Fixed	Fixed
PCV	Variable or targeted	Fixed	Variable	Fixed
PSV (pt dependent)	Variable	Fixed	Variable	Variable
SIMV				
combination of spontaneous, PS and the mandatory breath type	Any	Any	Any	Any

VCV: Volume-Controlled Ventilation
PCV: Pressure-Controlled Ventilation
PSV: Pressure Support Ventilation
SIMV: Synchronized Intermittent Mandatory Ventilation

Safety Alert *Airway pressure and lung volumes have a DIRECT impact on the intrathoracic pressure, which then may decrease blood flow and BP and INDIRECTLY affect different organ systems.*

BASIC VENTILATION ADJUNCTS
Positive End-Expiratory Pressure (PEEP) and Alveolar Mechanics

The application of trapping of fresh gas (flow) is known as PEEP. PEEP increases functional residual capacity (FRC) and compliance while decreasing dead space ventilation, shunt fraction, and is very effective for recruitment of atelectatic alveoli, as well as for equalizing opening pressures in alveoli that are filled with fluid. PEEP does not improve lung function due to poor perfusion and may affect the perfusion of lung capillaries. As the alveolar pressure rises, the vessels are compressed and pulmonary blood flow is reduced. There may be a decrease in right atrial filling, which also affects overall perfusion.

Generally, PEEP pressures range from 2.5–20 cm H_2O. Higher pressures (greater than 35 cm H_2O) may be used if the patient can tolerate the increase and if the condition is warranted.

The role of PEEP in lung ventilation is to stabilize alveoli, decreasing alveolar collapse and promoting better gas exchange. PEEP is applied when the exhalation valve in the circuit closes, promoting lung trapping of gas (refreshed), which then is measured as pressure sustained at the end of expiration. When PEEP is increased, the valve closes earlier. In lung protective ventilation, PEEP allows for better distribution of gas over a larger open lung surface, while preventing alveolar over distention. Gattinoni et al. showed that injured lungs have less lung surface, which participates in ventilation, and the application of PEEP in this diagnosis can open collapsed alveoli and prevent the shear stresses caused by alveolar recruitment/derecruitment. In the open lung approach, alveoli and small airways are stented open with a constant airway pressure. This allows the breath to reach more functional surface area early in inspiration, as alveolar opening is maintained by the application. PEEP promotes better gas exchange, increases the P/F ratio and allows for reduction of FIO_2, and is frequently used in conjunction with mechanical ventilation to improve oxygenation. Clinical improvements are reflected by increased partial pressure of O_2 in arterial blood (PaO_2) and the ability to decrease FIO_2.

Application of PEEP increases intra thoracic pressure and can compromise the patient's hemodynamic status by compressing the heart and great vessels. Increased intrathoracic pressure decreases venous return, RV filling pressures, and cardiac output, which may cause or potentiate hypotension and shock. Patients with intravascular volume depletion are at higher risk for associated hemodynamic instability. High levels of PEEP can cause pneumothorax, particularly if lung compliance is diminished. The understanding gained through the study of alveolar mechanics would suggest that an open lung approach might minimize shear stress, and improve oxygenation. Multiple modes of ventilation will allow for open lung ventilation: high-frequency oscillatory ventilation (HFOV), airway pressure release ventilation (APRV), and alveolar recruitment maneuvers (high levels of PEEP applied for short times to open collapsed alveoli) followed by the application of PEEP. The decision-making strategies for patient management are discussed in Table 1-16.

 Safety Alert *Clinicians should be prepared for a narrowing pulse pressure, decreasing SV, BP, and CO when PEEP levels are increased. Hemodynamic changes may include volume resuscitation and/or inotropic support to correct the decrease in BP and CO.*

Low Tidal Volume/Protective Lung Ventilation/Permissive Hypercapnia

The strongest evidence-based methods for mechanically supported ventilation are reflected in the work of the ARDS Network. Low tidal volumes used with PEEP levels high enough to open a ? recruitable lung may allow the most injured portions of the lung to "rest" until the resolution of the underlying lung injury.

A methodologic approach to low tidal volume, Fio_2, and PEEP can be accessed at http://www.ardsnet.org/system/files/Ventilator+Protocol+Card.pdf.

Calculation of predicted or ideal body weight can be performed with the automatic calculator at ARDSnet: http://ardsnet.org/node/77460.

Formulas: Males: PBW (kg) = 50 + 2.3(height [in] − 60)

Females: PBW (kg) = 45.5 + 2.3(height [in] − 60)

RESEARCH BRIEF 1-3

The study compared mortality, morbidity, and length of stay in two types of tidal volume strategies.

Traditional: V_T 10 to 15 ml/kg, keep plateau less than 50 cm H_2O

Low tidal volume ventilation: V_T 6 ml/kg, keep plateau less than 30 cm H_2O

Those in the low V_T group needed a high respiratory rate to prevent acidosis.

Permissive hypercapnia was tolerated well. If needed, IV bicarbonate was used to correct acidosis and maintain pH. The researchers added PEEP in the low V_T group to prevent atelectrauma (open-close alveoli leads to alveolar fracture) as well as to promote alveolar recruitment. Results revealed a lower mortality in the low V_T group (31% versus 39.8%, $p < 0.007$), a greater number of days without ventilation use, and lower average plateau pressures compared to the traditional V_T group.

From the Acute Respiratory Distress Syndrome Network: Ventilation with lower tidal volumes as compared with traditional tidal volumes for acute lung injury and the acute respiratory distress syndrome. *N Engl J Med* 1301–1308, 2000.

ADDITIONAL MODES OF MECHANICAL VENTILATION TO PROMOTE ALVEOLAR RECRUITMENT

This discussion is designed to introduce alternative ventilatory methods. It is beyond the scope of this book to perform a substantive manual of alternative techniques.

When Fio_2 is at a toxic level (levels of oxygen that promote radical byproducts which may actually cause alveolar lining destruction), it may be of vital importance to consider alternative strategies designed to increase the functional lung surface available for gas exchange. The following list is a small sample of current and experimental ventilator modes designed to optimize mean airway pressure and alveolar recruitment:

Table 1-16	FACTORS CONSIDERED WHEN CHOOSING MODES OF VENTILATION	
Gas Exchange	**Ventilation Effect**	**Airway Compliance**
Fio_2 of < 0.35	Vital capacity > 10–15 ml/kg BW	Tidal volume > 325 ml
Pao_2 of > 60 mm Hg	Maximal negative insp pressure	Tidal volume/BW > 4 ml/kg
A-a Pao_2 gradient of < 350 mm Hg	< -30 cm H20	Dynamic Compliance > 22 ml/m H20
Pao_2/Fio_2 ratio of > 200	Minute ventilation < 10 l/min	Static compliance > 33 ml/cm H20
	Maximal voluntary ventilation more than twice resting MV	

Inverse Ratio Ventilation (IRV)

During IRV, the inspiratory phase is prolonged (as the flow rate is low for a given volume or pressure) and the expiratory phase is shortened. Normal inspiration/expiration (I/E) ratio is 1:2 to 1:4. During IRV, the inspiratory phase of the I:E ratio is increased to greater than 1:1 (e.g., 2:1), thereby promoting alveolar recruitment through achieving a more constant mean airway pressure (at the level required for alveolar opening), which improves oxygenation by keeping alveoli open for longer periods of time. The patient will require administration of sedation, analgesia, and possibly a paralyzing agent to minimize the discomfort and anxiety associated with this unusual breathing pattern.

Airway Pressure Release Ventilation (APRV or BiVent)

Airway Pressure Release Ventilation (APRV) is basically a set level of CPAP that intermittently releases (valve open) to a lower level using a time-controlled release valve. High CPAP and lung volumes are re-established when the release valve closes. The principle of reducing lung volume distinguishes this technique from other modes of ventilation. APRV always implies a reverse I:E ratio as it utilizes a very short low pressure time (for removal of CO2) for PRESSURE RELEASE. APRV is a mode with two basic methods applied: PC/IRV (via a BiPAP method) and SIMV. First, it appears similar to PC/IRV as it uses a high-pressure time that may be relatively long and a low-pressure time that is profoundly short. The inverse times promote a constant airway pressure and an intrinsic PEEP (auto-PEEP) to optimize oxygenation. An inspiratory time (T HIGH) and an expiratory time (T LOW) are set, as well as inspiratory pressure (P HIGH) and expiratory pressure (P LOW). During the high time, the patient may breath spontaneously as well as receive ventilator breaths, which will be synchronized whenever possible (SIMV). Spontaneous breathing is not required, but facilitated. No breathing occurs during low time until weaning begins.

BiLevel Ventilation

BiLevel is a method of switching between low and high pressure limits based on the patient's inspiration and exhalation. In BiPAP, the circuit switches between a high and low airway pressure in an adjustable time sequence. If the patient is not breathing spontaneously, the I:E ratio and the ventilatory frequency can be adjusted to optimize ventilation and oxygenation. If you reverse the I:E ratio, you have set up APRV, and mandatory breaths can be applied. Breathing is allowed during both high-pressure and low-pressure times. Airway pressure is not as well controlled. BiLevel can be used initially as pressure-controlled ventilation, can be weaned to biPAP, and then weaned to CPAP prior to extubation.

High Frequency Oscillatory Ventilation (HFOV)

Recently, this mode of ventilation has received much more attention for use in the adult population. HFOV uses very small tidal volumes (not really tidal volume, but rather amplitude, termed Delta P: P) usually equal to, or less than, the dead space (150 mL) to maintain a continuously high alveolar opening pressure. "Breaths" are administered at a very fast rate (Hertz-Hz set at 4–5 breaths per second). Given that large tidal volumes in ARDS cause alveolar stress (via continuously opening and closing alveoli), in theory, very small, rapid tidal volumes used in HFOV should be protective because alveoli are no longer fully closing, and are continuously recruited by the higher constant airway pressure.

ADJUNCTS TO MECHANICAL VENTILATION

Auto-flow is a new advance in volume-controlled modes of mechanical ventilation. The ventilator automatically regulates inspiratory flow. This autoregulation works in conjunction with the set tidal volume and the patient's lung compliance.

Mandatory minute ventilation or minimum minute ventilation (MMV) provides a predetermined minute ventilation to augment the patient's spontaneous minute ventilation (breathing efforts). It is used to prevent hypoventilation and respiratory acidosis during ventilator weaning when SIMV is supporting the patient.

In *proportional assist ventilation (PAV)*, the ventilator automatically adjusts airway pressure in response to the patient's ventilatory patterns. The ventilator frequently adjusts needed support based on the patient's inspiratory flow rate, exhaled tidal volume, compliance, and resistance.

Other methods such as tracheal gas insufflation, ECMO, and other methods that may be used for patients with refractory hypoxemia are currently used in less than 5% of institutions and therefore will not be discussed further here.

Diagnostic Evaluation of Appropriate Ventilation		
Test	**Purpose**	**Abnormal Findings**
Noninvasive Pulmonary Volumes and Pressures		
Pulmonary pressures measured during volume control breath	Measures the relationship of volume delivered and the compliance of the surface, which contains it. Normal PawP or PIP when receiving a 10 ml/kg/IDW breath is 35 cm H_2O Normal $p_{Plateau}$ when holding a 10 ml/kg/IDW breath at the end of inspiration is 25 cm H_2O.	Patients presenting with lung injury and distress will have significant increases in $p_{Plateau}$ pressures to >25 cm H_2O. This increase may or may not manifest as a proportional increase in PIP. For example, with a 350 ml breath, the patient with ARDS may have a PIP of 48 and a p_{Plat} of 43.
Static compliance	Measures the distensibility of the lungs and chest wall when gas has been delivered into the lung, but no exhalation has occurred (inspiratory hold). $V_{TE}/p_{Plateau}$ Normal compliance$_{stat}$ 50–80 ml/cm H_2O	Patients presenting with loss of lung compliance will have significant decrease in measures of static compliance as well as increasing $p_{Plateau}$ pressures. Subtract PEEP from p_{Plat} before performing calculation
Blood Studies		
Arterial blood gas analysis	Evaluates the oxygenation of the arterial blood as well as the presence or absence of acid and the effect on the pH (environment of the cells). See ABGs.	Although not always predictable when in the disease process changes will occur, generally patients will develop hypoxemia which may initially be resolved with increasing the Fio_2, but eventually will require great increases in Fio_2 and ultimately will no longer respond to oxygen therapy.

Diagnostic Evaluation of Appropriate Ventilation—cont'd		
Test	**Purpose**	**Abnormal Findings**
Pao2/Fio$_2$ ratio	The Pao2 divided by the Fio$_2$ (Pao2/Fio$_2$ ratio, or more simply P/F) can be used to more simply assess the severity of the gas exchange defect. The normal value for the ratio of the partial pressure of oxygen in arterial blood to Fio$_2$ (Pao2/Fio$_2$) (Fio$_2$ is expressed as a decimal ranging from 0.21 to 1.00) is 300 to 500.	A value of less than 300 indicates gas exchange derangement, and a value below 250 is indicative of severe impairment, and compliance calculations should be performed to encourage alveolar recruitment strategies.
Radiology		
Chest x-ray (CXR)	Assesses size of lungs, presence of fluids, abnormal gas or fluids in the pleural sac, diaphragmatic margins, the pulmonary hilium, as well as integrity of the rib cage	Presence of fluids in the lung parenchyma initially presents as pulmonary edema. The continuous accumulation differentiates this edema formation to one that is not cardiac.
Computed tomography (CT) lung scan	Assesses the three-dimensional lung capacities, fluid load, and the primary displacement of the fluid	Normally a large gas-filled surface, the ALI/ARDS lung when seen on CT is frequently fluffy and white due to fluid that has extravagated through the endothelial deficits (capillary leak).

COMPLICATIONS RELATED TO MECHANICAL VENTILATION
Barotrauma, Volutrauma, and Pneumothorax

Barotrauma can occur when ventilatory pressures increase intrathoracic and intrapleural pressures, causing damage to the lungs, the major vessels, and possibly all organs in the thorax, with referred damage to the abdomen. If severe, barotrauma can lead to pneumothorax; a partially or totally collapsed lung. Symptoms vary depending on the amount of lung collapsed.

Tension Pneumothorax

This develops when pressurized air escapes from the lungs and enters and collects in the thoracic cavity, causing one or both lungs to collapse. High pressure from mechanical positive pressure ventilation may tear diseased or fragile lung tissue, leading to this life-threatening complication. Symptoms include respiratory distress, fluctuations in BP, shifting of the trachea toward the unaffected side, and sudden and sustained increases in peak inspiratory pressure.

HIGH ALERT! If tension pneumothorax is suspected, the patient should be disconnected from the ventilator immediately and ventilated using a bag/valve/tube device (Ambu bag). While the primary nurse/therapist is using tube/mask ventilation, others will facilitate an emergency physician call and set up the patient for immediate chest tube insertion/placement.

Gastrointestinal Complications

Peptic ulcers with profound hemorrhage may develop as a result of physiologic pressures and stress. Histamine H$_2$-receptor antagonists (e.g., ranitidine) or proton pump inhibitors (e.g., Prilosec, Protonix) or sucralfate (Carafate) may be administered to prevent these ulcers from developing. A great deal of controversy surrounds the best strategy for peptic ulcer prevention and the evidence is evolving. In addition, gastric dilation can occur as a result of the large amounts of air swallowed in the presence of an artificial airway. If gastric dilation is left untreated, paralytic ileus, vomiting, and aspiration may develop. Extreme dilation can compromise respiratory effort because of the restriction of diaphragmatic movement. Treatment includes insertion of a gastric tube orally or nasally (oral placement may be preferred) connected to low intermittent suction to remove air from the GI tract.

Hypotension with Decreased Cardiac Output
This develops as a result of decreased venous return secondary to increased intrathoracic pressure caused by positive pressure ventilation. Unless associated with tension pneumothorax, this phenomenon is transient and is seen immediately after the patient has been placed on mechanical ventilation. This may require aggressive volume resuscitation.

Sustained Hypotension with Decreased Cardiac Output
PEEP, especially at levels greater than 20 cm H_2O, and mean airway pressure strategies to open the alveoli (lung) may increase the incidence and severity of the phenomena due to the compression of the heart and large blood vessels from the increased intrathoracic pressure. This produces an arterial hypovolemic state. Aggressive IV fluid therapy and occasionally inotropic support may be used with PEEP to maintain adequate intravascular volume for sufficient CO to perfuse vital organs. HR and BP should be monitored frequently if the patient is unstable.

Increased Intracranial Pressure
Increased ICP occurs as a result of decreased venous return to the heart due to compression of intrathoracic blood vessels when using PEEP greater than 5 cm H_2O or mean airway pressure strategies. This may limit cerebral venous outflow, therefore increasing the ICP. See *Traumatic Brain Injury*, p. 331, for additional information.

Fluid Imbalance
Increased production of ADH occurs as a result of increased pressure on baroreceptors in the thoracic aorta, which causes the system to react as if the body were volume depleted. ADH stimulates the renal system to retain water. Patients may need diuretics if signs of hypervolemia are present. Be alert to new symptoms of dependent edema or adventitious breath sounds.

Ventilator-Acquired Pneumonia
Studies indicate that 70% to 90% of mechanically ventilated patients colonize hospital-acquired bacteria in the oropharynx, trachea, or digestive tract. Aspiration of bacteria from the oropharynx is a leading cause of ventilator-acquired pneumonia. The onset of infection may have several mechanisms:

- Presence of an ET/tracheostomy tube creates a bypass of upper respiratory tract defense mechanisms of cough and mucociliary clearance action.
- Contaminated secretions pool above the ET/tracheostomy tube cuff promoting colonization of bacteria and ultimately leak into the lower respiratory tract.
- Supine positioning, the presence of a nasogastric tube, or reflux of bacteria from the stomach contribute to oropharyngeal colonization. The medications that mechanically ventilated patients may receive to prevent gastrointestinal bleeding also alter the gastric pH. Use of sucralfate, which does not increase gastric pH, decreases the incidence of pneumonia compared with antacids alone or in combination with hydrogen ion antagonists.
- Use of contaminated equipment/supplies, inadequate hand washing, or poor infection control practices may directly inoculate the tracheobronchial tree with pathogens. Consult with your infection control practitioner for additional practice guidelines.

Anxiety
Many individuals experience anxiety related to the discomfort associated with loss of control over their ventilatory process and the perception that their health status is threatened. Hypoxemia and air hunger, if present, contribute to anxiety and prompt rapid, shallow, and often irregular respiratory efforts. The first approach is always to evaluate mode and method of ventilation in order to insure appropriate ventilatory support. The flow rate of the volume must be considered, and can best be evaluated with a volume pressure loop. Coordinated and

effective ventilation may not be possible with severe anxiety and agitation. Diligent administration of anxiolytic drugs and analgesics, along with close monitoring of the patient's response to potent medications, may be necessary to reduce the work of breathing and facilitate effective mechanical ventilation. The use of an approved sedation scale is also recommended (see Sedation and Neuromuscular Blockade, p. 158). In extreme cases, if a patient is unable to tolerate the ventilator mode most appropriate for his or her condition and cannot be managed using high-dose anxiolytic agents, sedatives, and analgesics, the physician may consider use of neuromuscular blockade (induced paralysis) to facilitate more effective ventilation. Neuromuscular blockade should be reserved for only the most extreme situations, wherein the patient's life is threatened by the overall energy expenditure related to fear, anxiety, or inability to attain control over his or her breathing pattern despite other efforts (see Sedation and Neuromuscular Blockade, p. 158).

WEANING THE PATIENT FROM MECHANICAL VENTILATION

Weaning patients from mechanical support requires skill, knowledge, and patience. This goal may take many forms ranging from abrupt cessation to gradual withdrawal from ventilatory support. Successful weaning depends primarily on the patient's overall condition as well as the techniques used. Patients for whom attempts at weaning fail constitute a unique problem in critical care. Physiologic factors (cardiovascular status, fluids and electrolyte balance, acid-base balance, nutritional status, comfort, and sleep pattern) and emotional factors (fear, anxiety, coping skills, general emotional state, ability to cooperate) are important and must be evaluated both before and during the weaning process. Adequate pulmonary function parameters must be attained before the weaning process is begun (Table 1-17). To begin the weaning process, patients must be hemodynamically stable and able to initiate a spontaneous breath. A weaning assessment tool that is chosen for use in critically ill patients should be well designed and supported by evidence, so strategies have a better opportunity for success. The most well evaluated and internationally used is the Burns Weaning Assessment Tool (BWAP). A series of predictors for weaning success is listed in Table 1-17, and a listing of ventilator adjustments during weaning is included on Table 1-18.

Contact the UVA Patents Office for permission to use the BWAP for free:
Christopher M. Harris, PhD
Senior Licensing Associate
UVA Patent Foundation
1224 W. Main Street, Suite 1-110
Charlottesville, VA 22903
UVA P.O. Box 800755
(434) 243-5792
Fax : (434) 982-1583
E-mail: cmh7k@Virginia.EDU

Traditional Weaning Methods

Traditionally, three methods have been used for weaning the patient from mechanical ventilation.

1. **SIMV mode:** The patient is switched to SIMV from assist-control mode, or respiratory rate and pressure support are decreased if the patient is already on SIMV.
Patients with Nonchronic Pulmonary Disease Decrease rate every 30-minute interval. After 2 hours at a mandatory rate of zero with CPAP, if the patient is clinically stable, he or she may be extubated.
Patients with Chronic Pulmonary Disease Begin with an RR of 8 breaths/min and decrease SIMV rate by 2 breaths per hour unless patient experiences clinical deterioration. If stable after at least 1 hour of a mandatory rate zero with CPAP, the patient may be extubated.

2. **Pressure support ventilation (PSV):** Start with 25cm of PS and no mandatory breaths.
Patients with Nonchronic Pulmonary Disease Decrease pressure support every 30 minutes; if the patient is able to tolerate PSV of zero for 2 hours, he or she can be extubated.
Patients with Chronic Pulmonary Disease Decrease PS by 2 to 4 cm H_2O every hour as long as the patient is stable.

When PSV is zero for at least 1 hour, fit the patient with a T-piece or initiate CPAP and observe.

Table 1-17	**PARAMETERS FOR WEANING FROM MECHANICAL VENTILATION**	
Pulmonary Function	**Optimal Parameters**	**Definition**
Minute ventilation	≤ 10 L/min	Tidal volume $\times$ respiratory rate; if adequate, means patient is breathing at a stable rate with adequate tidal volume
Negative inspiratory force	≥ -20 cm H_2O	Measures respiratory muscle strength; maximum negative pressure that patient is able to generate to initiate spontaneous respirations; indicative of patient's ability to initiate inspiration independently
Maximum voluntary ventilation	$\geq 2 \times$ resting minute ventilation	Measures respiratory muscle endurance; indicates patient's ability to sustain maximal respiratory effort
Tidal volume	5–10 ml/kg	Indicates patient's ability to ventilate lungs adequately
Arterial blood gases Fractional concentration of inspired oxygen (Fio_2)	$Pao_2 \geq 60$ mm Hg $Pao_2 \leq 45$ mm Hg pH 7.35–7.45 or patient's baseline ≤ 0.40	

Table 1-18	**COMMON ADJUSTMENTS DURING WEANING TO IMPROVE GAS EXCHANGE**	
Ventilation Strategies		**Oxygenation Strategies**
When CO_2 retention is the problem		When refractory oxygenation is the problem
Increase minute ventilation	Increase f (RR) Increase V_T	Increase Fio_2 When Fio_2 is > 0.40 (40%), consider PEEP
Increase flow rate		When PEEP is >12–15, consider MawP strategies

V_T: Tidal Volume
PEEP: Positive End Expiratory Pressure
MawP: Mean Airway Pressure
RR: Respiratory Rate

3. **T-piece method**: A T-shaped adapter is placed on the end of the ET tube. The patient is taken off the ventilator and allowed to initiate spontaneous breaths for increasingly longer periods of time. The T-piece method may be used by starting with 1 to 2 minutes off the ventilator, followed by 58 to 59 minutes on, with a gradual reversal of this ratio until the patient breathes independently. In this manner, the patient builds strength and endurance for independent respiratory effort.

Spontaneous Breathing Trials
There is a newer approach in which the patient is closely monitored for a period of time while disconnected from the ventilator. Respiratory pattern, gas exchange, hemodynamic stability, and patient comfort should be monitored closely. If the patient tolerates the spontaneous breathing trial (SBT) for 30 to 120 minutes, extubation should be considered.

HIGH ALERT!   Apnea
Frequent patient assessments with vigilant monitoring must be done, as there may not be ventilator backup or an apnea program to support the patient if the patient fails to breathe.

FAILURE TO WEAN

Patients who fail the transition from ventilator support to sustained spontaneous breathing do so primarily because of assessment weakness of the respiratory muscles, including the diaphragm. Considerations regarding the following should be evaluated prior to attempting weaning. The following parameters should be evaluated when patients are unable to be weaned from the ventilator.

- Nutrition and metabolic deficiencies: K, Mg, Ca, phosphate, and thyroid hormone
- Complications related to use of corticosteroids, or need for corticosteroids
- Chronic renal failure which alters capacity for compensation
- Systemic diseases which affect protein synthesis, degradation, glycogen stores
- Hypoxemia and hypercapnia

TROUBLESHOOTING MECHANICAL VENTILATOR PROBLEMS

The most important assessment factor in troubleshooting a mechanical ventilator is the effect on the patient. Regardless of which alarm sounds, always assess the patient first to evaluate his or her physiologic response to the problem. (See Table 1-19 and Box 1-12 for processes that contribute to high-pressure and low-pressure alarm situations.) If at any time the patient is not receiving the proper volumes or the nurse is unable to properly assess and manage the alarm situation, take the patient off the ventilator, ventilate with a bag-valve tube system, and ask someone to contact the respiratory therapist immediately.

Table 1-19	CAUSES OF HIGH-PRESSURE ALARMS DURING MECHANICAL VENTILATION	
Increased airway resistance		Decreased lung compliance
Patient requires suctioning		Pneumothorax
Kinks in ventilator circuitry		Pulmonary edema
Water or expectorated secretions in circuitry		Atelectasis
Patient coughs or exhales against ventilatory breaths		Worsening of underlying disease process
Patient biting ET tube		ARDS
Bronchospasm		
Herniation of airway cuff over end of artificial airway		
Change in patient position that restricts chest wall movement		
Breath stacking		

ARDS, acute respiratory distress syndrome; *ET*, endotracheal.

Box 1-12	CAUSES OF LOW-PRESSURE ALARMS

Patient disconnected from machine
Leak in airway cuff
    Insufficient air in cuff
    Hole or tear in cuff
    Leak in one-way valve of inflation port
Leak in circuitry
    Poor fittings on water reservoirs
    Dislodged temperature-sensing device
    Hole or tear in tubing
    Poor seal in circuitry connections
Displacement of airway above vocal cords
Loss of compressed air source	

CARE PLANS FOR MECHANICAL VENTILATION

Impaired gas exchange *related to altered oxygen supply resulting from an abnormal tidal volume distribution associated with mechanical ventilation*

GOALS/OUTCOMES Patient has adequate gas exchange as evidenced by Pao_2 greater than 60 mm Hg, $Paco_2$ 35 to 45 mm Hg, Spo_2 greater than 92%, Svo_2 greater than 60%, and RR 12 to 20 breaths/min.

NOC Respiratory Status: Gas Exchange

Mechanical Ventilation

1. Observe for, document, and report any changes in patient's condition consistent with increasing respiratory distress (see *Acute Respiratory Failure*, p. 383).
2. Position the patient to allow for maximal alveolar ventilation and comfort. Remember that the dependent lung usually receives more ventilation and more blood flow than the nondependent lung; however, during mechanical ventilation the dependent portion of the lung receives less distribution of tidal volume than do the nondependent areas.
   - Analyze Spo_2, Svo_2, and ABG results with patient in different positions to determine adequacy of ventilation.
   - Use postural drainage principles where appropriate.
   - In unilateral lung disease, position the patient with the healthy lung down.
   - In bilateral lung disease, position the patient in the right lateral decubitus position, inasmuch as the right lung has more surface area. If ABG results show that the patient tolerates left lateral decubitus position, alternate between the two positions. Rotational therapy (rotating patient and/or use of a chest percussion bed) may be effective.
3. Turn patient at least every 2 hours if signs of deteriorating pulmonary status occur.
4. Auscultate the upper chest over the artificial airway to assess for leaks.
5. Assess the ventilator for proper functioning and parameter settings, including Fio_2, tidal volume, rate, mode, peak inspiratory pressure, and temperature of inspired gases. In addition, ensure connections are tight and alarms are set. A thorough ventilator check is generally done every 2 hours in best practice settings. Ventilator checks should be systematically documented in the medical record, by the respiratory care practitioner. Assessing the ventilator for proper function and the patient's response to therapy is most often a collaborative effort between nursing and respiratory therapist.
6. Keep the ventilator circuitry free of condensed water and expectorated secretions. Not all ventilators have a problem with condensation. Fluids present in the circuit may obstruct the flow of gases to and from the patient. Water is a warm, moist environment that is ideal for the growth of microorganisms. Gloves should be worn any time the ventilator circuit is manipulated.
7. Monitor serial ABG results. Be alert for hypoxemia (decreases in Pao_2) or hypercapnia (increases in $Paco_2$) with concomitant decrease in pH (less than 7.35), which can signal hypoventilation and/or inadequate oxygenation. Also observe for decreased $Paco_2$ (less than 35 mm Hg) with increased pH (greater than 7.45), which may signal mechanical hyperventilation.
8. Notify the physician or midlevel practitioner of dysrhythmias, which can occur even with modest alkalosis if the patient has heart disease or is receiving inotropic medications (see Appendix 6).
9. If changes in patient status are noted, note the Spo_2 reading and end-tidal CO_2, if used, or follow institutional protocol for addressing deterioration in the status of a patient receiving mechanical ventilation. An ABG analysis may be warranted.
10. Keep manual resuscitator or bag-valve device at the bedside for ventilation in case of malfunctioning equipment.

Ineffective airway clearance (or risk for same) *related to altered anatomic structure secondary to presence of ET or tracheostomy tube*

GOALS/OUTCOMES Patient maintains a patent airway as evidenced by absence of adventitious breath sounds or signs of respiratory distress, such as restlessness and anxiety.

NOC Respiratory Status: Airway Patency

Airway Management

1. Assess and document breath sounds in all lung fields at least every 2 hours. Note quality and presence or absence of adventitious sounds.
2. Monitor patient for restlessness and anxiety, which can signal early airway obstruction and hypoxia.
3. Avoid routine or scheduled suctioning. Use aseptic technique (including use of sterile gloves) for suctioning based on the needs of the patient. The decision to suction is based on assessment findings, and is done to maintain a

patent airway when the patient is unable to cough out secretions. Document the amount, color, and consistency of tracheobronchial secretions and the patient's tolerance of the procedure. Collaborate with the respiratory care practitioner and report significant changes (e.g., increase in production of secretions, tenacious secretions, bloody sputum) to the physician or midlevel practitioner. Maintain the artificial airway in a secure and proper alignment.

4. Maintain the correct temperature (32° to 36°C [89.6° to 96.8°F]) of inspired gas. Cold air irritates the airways, and hot air may burn fragile lung tissue.

5. Maintain humidification of inspired gas either using the ventilator or an alternative device, to prevent drying of tracheal mucosa. Without humidification, tracheobronchial secretions may become thick and tenacious, creating mucous plugs that place patient at risk for development of atelectasis and infection.

Ineffective breathing pattern (or risk for same) *related to anxiety secondary to use of mechanical ventilation*

GOALS/OUTCOMES Patient exhibits a stable respiratory rate of 12 to 20 breaths/min (synchronized with ventilator) without restlessness, anxiety, lethargy, or sounding of the high-pressure ventilator alarm.
NOC Mechanical Ventilation Response: Adult

Ventilation Assistance

1. Monitor for evidence of ventilator dyssynchrony: Frequent sounding of high-pressure alarm when patient breathes against mechanical inspiration or mismatch of patient's respiratory rate and ventilatory cycle.

2. Monitor the respiratory rate and quality, and for early signs of respiratory distress (e.g., tachypnea, hyperventilation, anxiety, restlessness, lethargy). Cyanosis is a late sign of respiratory insufficiency.

3. Teach the patient the technique for progressive muscle relaxation (see Appendix 7). When the patient becomes anxious, remain at the bedside until the respirations are under control. Reassure the patient they have the best opportunity to synchronize respirations with the ventilator if he/she relaxes.

HIGH ALERT!   **Restlessness Management**

Administer prescribed medication for restlessness only after any physiologic causes, including hypoxia and hypoglycemia, have been ruled out. Restlessness, if due to a nonphysiologic cause such as anxiety or unrelieved pain, should be managed with either sedation or analgesia, since it increases O_2 demand and consumption and can interfere with adequate ventilation.

Ineffective protection *related to increased environmental exposure (contaminated respiratory equipment); tissue destruction (during intubation or suctioning); invasive procedures (intubation, suctioning, presence of ET tube); immunocompromised state, and/or the physiologic stress resulting from a critical illness*

GOALS/OUTCOMES Patient is free of infection as evidenced by normothermia, WBC count $\leq 11,000/mm^3$, clear sputum, and negative sputum culture results.
NOC Immune Status

Infection Protection

1. Assess patient for signs and symptoms of infection, including temperature greater than 38°C (100.4°F), tachycardia (HR greater than 100 bpm), erythema of tracheostomy, and foul-smelling sputum. Document all significant findings.

2. To minimize the risk of cross-contamination, wash hands before and after contact with the respiratory secretions of any patient (even though gloves were worn) and before and after contact with patient who is undergoing intubation.

3. Maintain appropriate seal on artificial airway cuff to prevent aspiration of oral secretions.

4. Keep cuff sealed and, unless contraindicated, HOB elevated 30 to 45 degrees, especially for patients receiving continuous gastric feedings. Monitor patient for reflux of feedings, as well as for signs of intolerance to feedings (absence of bowel sounds, abdominal distention, residual feedings of more than 100 ml), which can precipitate vomiting and result in pulmonary aspiration of gastric contents.

5. Consider use of a post pyloric feeding tube if patient is at high risk for aspiration or is intolerant of conventional feeding strategies.

6. Recognize that bacteria and spores can be introduced easily during suctioning. Follow standard techniques:
   - Use aseptic technique during suctioning process, including use of sterile catheter and gloves. Use of lavage solutions is not recommended.
   - Suction tracheobronchial tree before suctioning the oropharynx if using the same suction catheter, to avoid introducing oral pathogens into tracheobronchial tree. Ideally, a separate tonsil suction device is dedicated to use exclusively in the oropharynx.
   - Never store or reuse a single-use suction catheter. Consider use of closed system for suctioning.
   - Change suction canisters and tubing within the time frame established by agency and/or always when filled. Change canisters and tubing between patients.
7. Wash hands and use sterile gloves when performing tracheostomy care to prevent colonization of stoma with bacteria from practitioner's hands.
8. Provide oral hygiene at least every 4 hours to prevent overgrowth of normal flora and aerobic gram-negative bacilli. Suction oropharynx and posterior pharynx to prevent pooling of secretions. Products are available to provide continuous suctioning of the posterior pharynx. Oral rinse products with chlorhexidine have been used to help control bacteria. Specialized suctioning toothbrushes may be used to brush the teeth and tongue every 12 hours.
   - Change the entire ventilator circuit (ventilator tubing) within the time frame established by policy, or sooner if soiled with secretions or blood.
   - Empty condensed water or expectorated secretions in tubes into attached traps. Avoid disconnecting tubing, and do not allow secretions to drain back into patient.
   - Empty water traps on tubing during each ventilator check.
   - When disconnecting patient from ventilatory circuits, keep ends of connectors clean. Avoid unnecessary disconnection.
   - Keep connectors on manual resuscitator bags clean and free of secretions between uses. Although no data suggest that disposable bags be changed with any frequency, reusable bags should not be used between patients without sterilization.
9. Be aware of special risk factors for patients with tracheostomy tubes, and intervene accordingly:
   - Maintain the tracheostomy tube in a secure and proper alignment to avoid irritation of stoma from too much movement.
   - Change the tracheostomy ties daily, or more frequently if heavily soiled with secretions or wound exudate.
   - Perform stoma care at least every 8 hours, using aseptic technique until stoma is completely healed. Keep area around stoma dry at all times to prevent maceration and infection. Change stoma dressing as needed to keep it dry.
   - Avoid use of cotton-filled gauze or other material that may shed small fibers. Patient may aspirate fibers, which in turn can lead to infection.
   - Use aseptic technique (including use of sterile gloves and drapes) when changing tracheostomy tube.
   - Culture secretions or wound drainage; administer antibiotics as prescribed.

Anxiety *related to actual or perceived threat to health status as a result of need for or presence of mechanical ventilation*

- -

GOALS/OUTCOMES During the interval of mechanical ventilation, patient relates the presence of emotional comfort and exhibits a decrease in irritability, with an HR within patient's normal range.
NOC Anxiety Level

Anxiety Reduction
1. Reassure patient and significant others that ventilatory support may be a temporary measure until the underlying pathophysiologic process has resolved. The patient may be weaned from the ventilator at that time. Some in the general public equate ventilator placement with a hopelessly chronic, vegetative state. Set timelines for reevaluation of patient's progress.
2. Reassure the patient that he or she will not be left alone.
3. Explain all procedures before they are initiated to patient and significant others. Inform patient of his or her progress.
4. Describe and point out the alarm system, explaining that it will alert staff in the event of any problem with the ventilator, including an accidental disconnection.
5. Provide the patient with a mechanism for communication (e.g., picture board, erasable marker board, pen and paper).
6. If aggressive sedation is used, perform a sedation vacation at least every 24 hours to assess if the patient can tolerate mechanical ventilation without sedation. Weaning the patient from sedation is an important step in the weaning from mechanical ventilation process. Sedatives can also mask symptoms of pain.
7. Evaluate the patient's need for pain control; particularly during the daily sedation vacation. Analgesics should be administered to control pain.

Impaired gas exchange (or risk for same) *related to decreasing support or ventilation during weaning from mechanical ventilation*

GOALS/OUTCOMES Patient has adequate gas exchange as evidenced by Pao₂ less than 60 mm Hg, Paco₂ less than 45 mm Hg, Spo₂ greater than 92%, Svo₂ greater than 60%, and pH 7.35 to 7.45 (or values within 10% of patient's baseline).

NOC Mechanical Ventilation Weaning Response: Adult

Mechanical Ventilatory Weaning

1. Maintain patient in a comfortable position to enhance ventilation. Many patients find that semi-Fowler's position, with the head of the bed elevated 30 to 45 degrees, promotes more effective ventilation. Studies support these findings and recommend the head of the bed remains elevated throughout mechanical ventilation, to reduce the risk of aspiration.
2. Observe for indicators of hypoxia, including tachycardia, tachypnea, cardiac dysrhythmias, pain, anxiety, and restlessness.
3. Assess and record VS every 15 minutes for the first hour of weaning, then hourly if patient is stable. Report significant findings to physician or midlevel practitioner, such as increased respiratory effort, hyperventilation, anxiety, lethargy, and cyanosis.
4. Check patient's tidal volume after the first 15 minutes of weaning and as needed. Optimally, it will be within 5 to 10 ml/kg.
5. Obtain a specimen for ABG analysis during weaning as indicated and per hospital protocol. Monitor Spo₂ continuously and, as available, Svo₂ for values outside normal range.

Anxiety *related to perceived threat to health status secondary to weaning process*

GOALS/OUTCOMES During the weaning process, patient expresses the attainment of emotional comfort and is free of the signs of harmful anxiety as evidenced by HR less than 100 bpm, RR less than 20 breaths/min, and BP within patient's normal range.

NOC Anxiety Self-Control

Anxiety Reduction

1. Before weaning process is initiated, discuss plans for weaning with patient and significant others. Explain that patient's condition will be assessed at frequent intervals during the weaning procedure. Provide time for questions and answers about the procedure.
2. Stay with patient during the initial phase of weaning, keeping patient informed of progress being made. Provide positive feedback for positive efforts.
3. Teach patient progressive muscle relaxation technique, which may reduce anxiety and fear and thus relax chest muscles (see Appendix 7).
4. Instruct patient to take deep breaths if he or she is capable of doing so. This may provide the confidence of knowing that he or she can initiate and sustain respirations independently.
5. Encourage patient to sit in the chair or to move about in the bed as much as possible.
6. Leave call light within patient's reach before leaving bedside. Reassure patient that help is nearby.

NIC Acid-Base Management; Acid-Base Monitoring; Airway Management; Airway Suctioning; Anxiety Reduction; Aspiration Precautions; Bedside Laboratory Testing; Infection Control; Laboratory Data Interpretation; Mechanical Ventilation; Mechanical Ventilatory Weaning; Oxygen Therapy; Positioning; Respiratory Monitoring; Vital Signs Monitoring

ADDITIONAL NURSING DIAGNOSES

Also see nursing diagnoses and interventions under *Prolonged Immobility* (p. 149) and *Emotional and Spiritual Support of the Patient and Significant Others* (p. 200).

NUTRITIONAL SUPPORT

The goal of nutritional support therapy is to identify preexisting malnutrition, prevent further protein-calorie deficiencies, optimize the patient's current state, and reduce further morbidity. Outcomes for patients with protein-calorie malnutrition demonstrate increased mortality and morbidity, including weakness, compromised immunity, decreased wound healing, infection, and organ failure. When protein-calorie malnutrition, marasmus, is complicated with stressors, such as burns, trauma, surgery, or sepsis, the neuroendocrine response results in hypermetabolism, hypercatabolism, and depletion of lean body mass. The body adapts to starvation through a series of hormonal changes that compensate for the decreased intake of nutrients. If starvation is prolonged, the body uses its own substrate to optimize survival, with a resulting loss of skeletal muscle and adipose tissue.

NUTRITIONAL ASSESSMENT

Multiple sources of information are used, including medical and nutritional history, anthropometric data (body measurements), biochemical analysis of blood and urine, and type and duration of the disease process. With a critically ill individual, this history may be obtained from significant others.

Medical/Nutritional History

A nutritional history identifies individuals who are or may be at risk for malnutrition. The medical history is included to assess diseases or conditions affecting nutritional status. It should describe the adequacy of both usual and recent food intake, as well as focus on factors which may have impaired adequate selection, preparation, ingestion, digestion, absorption, and excretion of nutrients. Include the following:

- Comprehensive review of usual dietary intake, including food allergies, food aversions, use of nutritional supplements including vitamins, supplements, and alternative/complementary therapies
- Recent weight loss or gain—intentional or unintentional
- Chewing or swallowing difficulties
- Nausea, vomiting, or pain with eating
- Altered pattern of elimination (e.g., constipation, diarrhea)
- Diseases/conditions increasing energy needs (e.g., burns, extensive wounds, decubitus ulcers, sepsis, surgery, trauma)
- Chronic disease affecting utilization of nutrients (e.g., malabsorption, pancreatitis, diabetes mellitus)
- Use of medications (e.g., laxatives, antacids, antibiotics, antineoplastic drugs)
- Who obtains food and prepares meals
- Cultural preferences restricting specific nutrient intake or causing excessive intake
- Alcohol or drug use
- Recent fad or vegetarian diets

Risk Factors

The following factors may place a patient at risk of or indicate the presence of nutritional deficiencies. The patient:

- Is younger than 18 years or older than 65 years (increased risk age at older than 75 years)
- Has had a recent unintentional weight loss of more than 5% in 1 month or more than 10% in 6 months. Weight loss is calculated as follows:
  - Percent weight loss = (UBW − CBW)/UBW, where UBW is usual body weight and CBW is current body weight
- Has excessive alcohol intake or other substance abuse
- Is homeless or living with limited access to food
- Has a limited capacity for oral intake due to physical problems such as dysphagia, odynophagia, stomatitis, or mucositis
- Has been NPO for more than 3 days
- Is experiencing increased metabolic demands induced by extensive burns, major surgery, trauma, fever, infection, draining abscesses or wounds, fistulas, pregnancy
- Has protracted nutrient losses associated with malabsorption syndromes, short gut syndrome, draining abscesses, wounds, or fistulas; effusions, renal dialysis
- Requires intake of catabolic drugs including corticosteroids, immunosuppressants, and antineoplastic agents
- Has experienced protracted emesis from conditions such as anorexia nervosa, bulimia, hyperemesis gravidarum, radiation, or oncologic chemotherapy
- Has a chronic disease such as AIDS, diabetes, cystic fibrosis, stroke, or cancer

PHYSICAL ASSESSMENT

Most physical findings are not conclusive for particular nutritional deficiencies. Compare current assessment findings with past assessments, especially related to the following:

- Loss of muscle and adipose tissue
- Work and muscle endurance, neuromuscular function
- Changes in hair and nails and the presence of skin lesions

Anthropometric Data

Anthropometrics is the measurement of the body or its parts. Pounds and inches are converted to metric measurements using the following formulas:

Divide pounds by 2.2 to convert to kilograms (kg).

Multiply inches by 2.54 to convert to centimeters (cm).

- *Height:* Used to determine ideal weight and body mass index; if unavailable, obtain estimate from family or significant others.
- *Weight:* A readily available and practical indicator of nutritional status that can be compared with previous weight and ideal weight or used to calculate body mass index. Large changes may reflect fluid retention (edema, third spacing), diuresis, dehydration, surgical resections, traumatic amputations, or weight of dressings or equipment. Remember that 1 liter (L) of fluid equals approximately 2 pounds (lb). Use actual body weight to avoid overfeeding in starved patients and ideal body weight in patients who weigh greater than 120% of ideal body weight (Table 1-20).

Table 1-20	HEIGHT AND WEIGHT GUIDELINES FOR MEN AND WOMEN					
	Men (weight in lb)			Women (weight in lb)		
Height	Small Frame	Medium Frame	Large Frame	Small Frame	Medium Frame	Large Frame
4 ft 10 in	...	...	...	102–111	109–121	118–131
4 ft 11 in	...	...	...	103–113	111–123	120–134
5 ft	...	...	...	104–115	113–126	122–137
5 ft 1 in	...	...	...	106–118	115–129	125–140
5 ft 2 in	128–134	131–141	138–150	108–121	118–132	128–143
5 ft 3 in	130–136	133–143	140–153	111–124	121–135	131–147
5 ft 4 in	132–138	135–145	142–156	114–127	124–138	134–151
5 ft 5 in	134–140	137–148	144–160	117–130	127–141	137–155
5 ft 6 in	136–142	139–151	146–164	120–133	130–144	140–159
5 ft 7 in	138–145	142–154	149–168	123–136	133–147	143–163
5 ft 8 in	140–148	145–157	152–172	126–139	136–150	146–167
5 ft 9 in	142–151	148–160	155–176	129–142	139–153	149–170
5 ft 10 in	144–154	151–163	158–180	132–145	142–156	152–173
5 ft 11 in	146–157	154–166	161–184	135–148	145–159	155–176
6 ft	149–160	157–170	164–188	138–151	148–162	158–179
6 ft 1 in	152–164	160–174	168–192	...	...	...
6 ft 2 in	155–168	164–178	172–197	...	...	...
6 ft 3 in	158–172	167–182	176–202	...	...	...
6 ft 4 in	162–176	171–187	181–207	...	...	...

- *Body mass index (BMI):* Used to evaluate adult weight. One calculation and one set of standards apply to both men and women:

$$BMI(kg/m2) = \frac{Weight\ (kg)}{Height\ (m) \times Height\ (m)}$$

BMI values of 20 to 25 are optimal; values greater than 25 indicate obesity. Values less than 20 and greater than 40 indicate significant increase in morbidity and are associated with longer intensive care unit stay, increased postoperative complications, and higher readmission rates.
- *Midarm muscle circumference (MAMC):* Measures muscle mass of the mid-upper arm using a formula.
- *Triceps skinfold thickness (TSF):* Measured at the midpoint of the upper arm by taking half the distance between the olecranon and the acromion process and grasping the skin and subcutaneous tissue at the back of the arm approximately 1 cm from the midpoint. Surgical calipers are used to measure the skinfold. A TSF measurement of less than 3 mm signals severely depleted fat stores.

Specially trained clinicians and dietitians should perform this assessment for more accurate and consistent results. The skill level and technique used vary among clinicians.

DIAGNOSTIC TESTS
No laboratory test specifically measures nutritional status. Status can be estimated, however, using the following parameters:

Visceral Protein Status
Normal values may vary with different laboratory procedures and standards. If the hydration status is normal and anemia is absent, albumin and transferrin levels may be the initial parameters used for a general assessment of nutritional status. The following are all visceral proteins:
- *Serum albumin (3.5 to 5.5 g/dl):* An indicator associated with increased morbidity in critical illness if the level is less than 3.5 gm/dl. It has a long half-life (19 days) and changes slowly in response to nutritional support when protein-calorie malnutrition is present.
- *Prealbumin (20 to 30 mg/dl):* A reliable indicator of response to nutritional therapy. It has a short half-life (24 to 48 hours) and may not be reliable if patient is severely stressed or ill, has an elevated C-reactive protein (CRP) level, is on steroid therapy, or has renal failure.
- *Retinol binding protein (4 to 5 mg/dl):* The indicator with the shortest half-life (10 hours) used to assess the response to nutritional therapy. It is not as reliable if the patient is severely stressed or ill.
- *Transferrin (180 to 260 mg/dl):* The indicator with a longer half-life (9 days), used as a baseline indicator of protein intake and synthesis. Like prealbumin, it may not be reliable when the patient is severely stressed.

Nitrogen Balance
This is used to discern if the patient is anabolic (building body stores or healing) or catabolic (breaking down body stores, deteriorating). If more nitrogen is received than excreted, nitrogen is said to be positive and an anabolic state exists. When nitrogen excretion is higher than intake, a negative balance or catabolic state exists. Most nitrogen loss occurs through the urine, with a small, constant amount lost via skin and feces. Nitrogen balance studies should be performed by specialists, because accurate measurement of 24-hour nitrogen intake and urine output is required. Heavy losses of protein in the presence of ascites, large wounds, malabsorption, and excessive chest tube drainage are difficult to measure but should be considered.

ESTIMATING NUTRITIONAL REQUIREMENTS
Energy Needs
The primary goal of nutritional support is to meet the energy needs for body temperature, metabolic processes, and tissue repair. The nutritional plan should avoid overfeeding and the complications associated with excessive caloric intake. Energy needs can be estimated using

the following options:

Calculation Based on Patient Weight

Estimated energy requirements are 25 to 35 kcal/kg daily for the nonstressed patient. Patients who are highly stressed may require up to 40 kcal/kg daily. Obese patients may require 15 to 25 kcal/kg daily.

Indirect Calorimetry

A test that measures O_2 consumption and CO_2 production as a byproduct of metabolism and gives the resting energy expenditure (REE) or basal energy expenditure (BEE). Older terminology refers to REE or BEE as the basal metabolic rate (BMR.) Specialized personnel and access to a metabolic cart are required to provide accurate results. The BEE is a major component of the total daily energy expenditure.

Harris Benedict Equations

The most common method used to determine the basal energy expenditure (BEE). It is calculated using the following equations developed by Harris and Benedict:

$$BEE\ (male) = 66 + (13.7 \times W) + (5 \times H) - (6.8 \times A)$$
$$BEE\ (female) = 655 + (9.6 \times W)\ (1.7 \times H) - (4.7 \times A)$$

where W = weight (kg), H = height (cm), and A = age (yr).

The BEE is multiplied by a stress factor that is estimated from the degree of stress and the need for weight maintenance or repletion. Multiplying the BEE by 1.2 to 2.5 provides a range appropriate for most patients. The lower factor is appropriate for patients without significant stress, whereas the higher factor is appropriate for patients with higher levels of stress, such as occurs with major trauma, sepsis, or burns.

Provision of Energy and Protein

- *Carbohydrate (CHO):* Carbohydrates should comprise 40% to 60% of the total caloric intake. Dextrose is the carbohydrate source in PN. Increased dextrose loads in PN can lead to hyperglycemia, excessive CO_2 production, hypophosphatemia, fat deposits in the liver, and transient elevated liver enzymes.
- *Protein:* Protein requirements for maintenance therapy are 0.8 to 1.2 g/kg/day. Critically ill patients may need an estimated 1.5 to 2 g/kg/day. Fever, infection, and wounds increase needs to the same range. Severe stress or burns may increase this requirement to 3 g/kg/day.
- *Fat requirements:* Fat requirements range from 25% to 55% of total calories. Fat can be administered in minimal quantities to satisfy needs for essential fatty acids, or it can be provided in larger quantities, as tolerated, to meet energy needs.
- *Abnormal elevations in liver enzymes:* These often occur in patients maintained on TPN for longer than 3 weeks. TPN should be used ONLY when enteral feeding is not possible or not tolerated. If needed, giving cyclic TPN, in which the patient receives TPN for 12 to 16 hours of 24 hours, may prevent enzyme elevation. Usually the enzymes return to normal on cessation of TPN.
- *Including protein in caloric count:* Although controversy still exists as to whether to count protein calories (4 cal/g) in PN, many clinicians do include them based on the rationale that they are included when calculating enteral and oral caloric intake. Also, it is impossible to prevent some protein from being used for energy once it is administered. A protein-sparing regimen in which calories from protein are not counted (only nonprotein calories are counted) is sometimes used to ensure that the patient is receiving enough energy from carbohydrate and fat to ensure that protein is not used for energy but instead is used for repleting protein stores and building muscle mass.

Vitamin and Essential Trace Mineral Requirements

In general, follow the Recommended Dietary Allowances (RDAs) to provide minimum quantities of vitamins, minerals, and essential fatty acids. For specific patients, supplements of specific vitamins or minerals are needed in increased amounts for existing disease states (e.g., zinc and vitamins A and C for burns; thiamine, folate, and vitamin B_{12} for chronic alcohol ingestion).

Fluid Requirements

Many factors affect fluid balance. All sources of intake (oral, enteral, intravenous, and medications), as well as output (urine, stool, drainage, emesis, fluid shifts, and respiratory and evaporative losses), must be considered. Fluid intake is closely associated to energy provided. Approximately 1 ml fluid per calorie is the standard method to calculate fluid requirements. Fever increases fluid needs, and fluid intake should be closely monitored in renal and cardiac dysfunction.

Special Diets or Enteral Formulas for Organ-Specific Pathology

These diets and formulas are costly, and the metabolic advantages of some products remain unproved.

- *Hepatic failure:* Branched-chain amino acids (BCAAs) in combination with reduced aromatic amino acid concentrations may help alleviate encephalopathy associated with hepatic failure. However, data with regard to the efficacy of BCAAs are very limited.
- *Renal disease:* High percentages of high biological value proteins (animal proteins) are used to improve nitrogen use and decrease urea formation.
- *Respiratory disease:* Avoidance of overfeeding any substrate (fat, carbohydrate, or protein) in this patient population prevents an increase in CO_2 production and, consequently, prevents an increase in the work of breathing.
- *Diabetes:* Reduced carbohydrates and higher fiber content are used for glucose intolerance. Fat consists of higher monounsaturated fatty acids to stay within guidelines for the prevention of coronary artery disease.

NUTRITIONAL SUPPORT MODALITIES

Enteral or tube feedings are recognized as the preferred strategy for nutritional support in the critically ill. Studies indicate enteral feedings prevent passage of bacteria from the GI tract into the lymphatic system (bacterial translocation) and other organs, reducing a major source of sepsis and possible organ failure. Cost, safety, and convenience considerations have been the rationale for using enteral over PN support, and comparatively speaking, the potential physiologic benefits justify that every effort be made to avoid the use of PN. Enteral feedings foster wound healing and immunocompetence and preserve gut function. Part of the failure of enteral feedings lies in use of the wrong type of feeding for the patient's ability to digest coupled with the underlying disease. Strategies to evaluate tolerance of feedings are not well understood, including residual volumes and occurrence of diarrhea. If the interdisciplinary team is knowledgeable and takes the time needed for proper evaluation and modification of enteral feedings, the current literature suggests there are few types of patients who should require parenteral feeding.

RESEARCH BRIEF 1-4

Elpern et al. conducted a prospective, descriptive study of a convenience sample of 39 patients admitted during a 3-month period (276 feeding days) to a medical intensive care unit. Patients received a mean of 64% of goal energy intake. Patients received continuous enteral tube feedings for at least 48 hours and were studied until discontinuation of feedings, discharge from the unit, or death. The mean total duration of interruptions in enteral feedings was 5.23 hours per patient per day. The leading three reasons for interruptions were patients being prepared for tests (35.7%), changing body position (15%), and exceeding the acceptable gastric residual volume (11.5%), defined as 150 ml (used as the cutoff point to define high gastric residual volumes). Almost half (36% to 45%) of the interruptions were due to temporary cessation of feeding during other procedures. Patients had diarrhea on 105 (38%) of 276 feeding days. Gastric residual volumes exceeded 150 ml on 28 measurements in 11 patients. Five patients experienced nausea and vomiting. Four patients aspirated feeding. Precautionary interruptions in enteral feedings to decrease the risk of aspiration were common and resulted in underfeeding. Episodes of vomiting and of aspiration were uncommon.

From Elpern EH, Stutz L, Peterson S, Gurka DP, Skipper A: Outcomes associated with enteral tube feedings in a medical intensive care unit. *Am J Crit Care* 13(3):221-227, 2004.

Enteral Formulas

Enteral formulas are composed of a wide variety of standard and modular formulas. See also Table 1-21.

- *Standard*–Consist of intact proteins and a caloric source; most are lactose-free; all are sterile, and suitable for small-bore feeding tubes and have a fixed nutrient composition. Vitamins and trace elements and minerals are included.
- *Modular*–Consist of a single nutrient that may be combined with other modules (nutrients) for a formula tailor-made for an individual's specific deficits (e.g., carbohydrate, fat, protein). Limited use of modular formulas due to concerns for bacterial contamination.
- *Specialty*–Enteral formulas that are disease specific as described in previous section on special diets for organ-specific pathology.

Table 1-21	TYPES OF ENTERAL FORMULATIONS
Enteral Formula	**Description**
Blenderized Diet	
Compleat, Compleat Modified	Nutritionally complete, requiring complete digestive capabilities; composed of natural foods, including meat, vegetables, milk, and fruit
Standard Lactose-Free Formulas	
Ensure, Boost, Nutren, Isosource, Osmolite	Nutritionally adequate, liquid preparation; used for non–disease-specific nutritional support; standard isotonic; low residue formulas
Specialty Formulas	
Hepatic failure	
Nutrihep	Nutritionally complete; has a greater ratio of branched chain to aromatic amino acids while restricting total amino acid concentrations and adding nonprotein calories. Calorie dense to prevent fluid overload.
Renal failure	
Suplena Renalcal	Low-protein, calorie-dense, low-electrolyte (no electrolytes in Renalcal) formulas designed for patients with reduced kidney function but not yet on dialysis; restricted total protein content may reduce or postpone need for dialysis. High in vitamin B_6 and folic acid.
Nepro Novasource Renal Nutren Renal	Calorie-dense, high-protein, low-electrolyte formulas designed for patients on dialysis. High in vitamin B6 and folic acid.
Respiratory insufficiency	
Pulmocare Novasource Pulmonary Nutren Pulmonary	Nutritionally complete; contains a higher proportion of fat to carbohydrates; may help prevent an increase in CO_2 production. Helpful in patients with COPD, cystic fibrosis, or respiratory failure.
Oxepa	Specialized formula with unique blend of patented oils (EPA and GLA) to help modulate the inflammatory response in critically ill and ventilated patients, especially those with ALI, ARDS, and sepsis.
Hypermetabolic and trauma states	
Crucial Pivot	Very high protein, calorically dense, immune enhancing formulas with added arginine for the metabolically stressed, immunosuppressed patient.

Continued

Table 1-21	TYPES OF ENTERAL FORMULATIONS—cont'd
Enteral Formula	**Description**
Impact, Impact glutamine	Specialized nutrition for surgical and trauma patients.
Oxepa	Specialized formula with unique blend of patented oils (EPA and GLA) to help modulate the inflammatory response in critically ill and ventilated patients, especially those with ALI, ARDS, and sepsis
Diabetes or hyperglycemia	
Diabetasource, Glucerna	Reduced carbohydrate, fiber containing formulas to help minimize glycemic response. Lactose free.
Fiber Enhanced	
Ultracal, Boost with Fiber, Compleat, FiberSource, Ensure Fiber, Jevity, Nutren with Fiber	Nutritionally complete; require intact GI function and absorption; hypertonic; milk, soy, or sodium and calcium caseinate protein source; some brands come in standard and high-calorie or high-nitrogen concentrations.
Calorically Dense Products	
Novasource 2.0, Resource 2.0, TwoCal HN, Nutren 2.0, NuBasics, 2.0, Deliver 2.0	Calorie content is 2 calories/ml to provide adequate nutrients in lower volume for volume-restricted patients; some standard products also come in 1.5 calories/ml concentration.
Elemental or Semielemental	
Peptinex, Tolerex, Vivonex, Criticare HN, Crucial, Optimental, Peptamen, Perative, Impact Glutamine, Criticare HN, Vital HN	Designed for easy absorption for patient who has malabsorption or atrophied intestine; protein source is free amino acids or protein hydrolysates (peptides) or both; fat source are oils easily absorbed: MCT, soybean, canola, safflower; some formulas contain fiber; some have flavor packets for oral use.

MCT: Medium Chain Triglycerides
COPD: Chronic Obstructive Pulmonary Disease
EPA: Eicosapentaenoic acid
GLA: Gamma Linolenic acid,
ALI: Acute Lung Injury
ARDS: Acute Respiratory Distress Syndrome
GI: Gastrointestinal

Nutritional composition of enteral formulas

- *Carbohydrates*—The most easily digested and absorbed component in enteral formulas; 80% of all carbohydrates are broken down and absorbed as simple glucose in the normal intestine. Nearly all enteral formulas are lactose-free to avoid problems in individuals with lactase deficiencies.
- *Fiber*—Included in many commercial preparations because it is claimed to be helpful in controlling blood glucose, reducing hyperlipidemia, and controlling bowel disorders, such as diverticulae. Begin the infusion slowly to reduce transient symptoms of gas and abdominal distention.
- *Protein*—Three forms commonly used:
    - *Polymeric*—Protein found in complete and original form (e.g., commercial and blenderized whole food diets that require normal levels of pancreatic enzyme).
    - *Semielemental*—Protein that has been broken down into smaller peptides to assist absorption. It is better absorbed in short bowel syndrome or pancreatic insufficiency.
    - *Elemental*—Protein that requires no further digestion, as proteins are already available as free amino acids, and is ready for absorption. It is most useful in severe malabsorption.
- *Fat*—Two forms are the primary sources:
    - *Long-chain triglycerides (LCT)* —A major source of essential fatty acids, fat-soluble vitamins, and calories.
    - *Medium-chain triglycerides (MCT)*—Foster the absorption of fat but have lower incidence of nausea and vomiting, abdominal distention, and diarrhea.

Types of feeding tubes and sites

- *Stomach*–Easiest site for enteral tube placement; simulates normal GI function; may be used for bolus, intermittent, cyclic, or continuous feedings. The stomach is the site reserved for patients who are alert, with intact gag and cough reflexes. Entry site is nasal, oral, or percutaneous.
  - *Small-bore*–Soft polyurethane or silicone with or without weighted tip; designed for long-term use; size 6 to 12 Fr; length 36 to 45 in. Some nasoenteric feeding tubes have a Y port added, allowing irrigation and medication administration without disconnecting the administration set.
  - *Large-bore*–Stiff, polyvinyl chloride; size 10 to 18 Fr; used for short-term (less than 1 week) feeding after gastric suction is no longer needed.
  - *Surgical gastrostomy*–A soft tube inserted directly into the stomach. Complications may include infections, leakage, catheter occlusion, and expulsion. Placed in operating room at time of other GI surgery or when percutaneous gastrostomy unable to be done for technical reasons.
  - *Percutaneous endoscopic gastrostomy (PEG)*–Soft tube inserted into the stomach via the esophagus and then drawn through the abdominal skin using a stab incision.
- *Small bowel (postpyloric feeding)*–Used for patients with diminished protective pharyngeal reflexes; the small bowel is less affected by postoperative ileus than the stomach and colon. Tube placement is more difficult. Continuous feedings are tolerated better, inasmuch as the continuous drip approximates normal gastric delivery to the small bowel. Entry sites are nasal, oral, duodenal, and jejunal. Nurses and other health care professionals can be taught to insert postpyloric feeding tubes using oral or nasal entry sites.
  - *Dual tubes*–Placed either via gastrostomy or nasally. Have one port for feeding into the jejunum and a second port that allows for aspiration and decompression of the stomach.
  - *Duodenum/jejunum*–Minimizes risk of vomiting and aspiration compared with gastric feedings. Small-bore feeding tubes can be inserted nasally or orally and pushed past the ligament of Treitz into the jejunum (postpyloric feeding). A jejunostomy tube is a soft, small-bore feeding tube inserted directly into the jejunum, via percutaneous endoscopic (PEJ) or open surgical approach. These tubes are not easily dislodged.

Infusion rates: See Table 1-22.
Management of complications: See Table 1-23.

Parenteral Nutrition

The postinjury metabolic stress response is said to peak at 3 to 4 days. Initiating nutritional support within 48 hours by supplying nutrients to prevent catabolism of skeletal and visceral protein stores can decrease morbidity in a previously well-nourished person who is critically ill. Many caregivers remain reticient to use enteral feedings until bowel sounds return. Current literature suggests that for some patients, an enteral feeding provides the stimulus needed for digestion to ensue and, thus, the bowel sounds to return. Absence of bowel sounds is not a reliable predictor of the patient's ability to tolerate enteral feedings and is not sufficient justification to withhold enteral feeding. Parenteral nutrition should be used only when enteral feedings are not well tolerated or when contraindicated. Literature has reflected for many years that use of PN in a well-nourished surgical patient may not improve outcome when used for less than 7 days, so to use a few days of PN as a "bridge" to when bowel sounds return is adding complexity and cost to the care without much benefit for the patient.

Parenteral nutrition provides some or all nutrients using either a peripheral venous catheter (IV) or central venous catheter (CVC). IV nutrition can meet total nutritional needs in patients who cannot be given enteral support safely or whose GI tract cannot be accessed. Parenteral nutrition is also used when the GI tract is unable to function, such as in the case of motility disorders, such as postoperative ileus, or small bowel obstruction.

- **Parenteral solutions**— These solutions are derived from combinations of dextrose, amino acids, fat, electrolytes, water, vitamins, and trace elements. Total nutrient admixtures (TNA) are formulated by combining dextrose, fat, and amino acids in one container; or dextrose and amino acids are combined and a separate delivery device is used for fat.

Table 1-22	METHODS AND RATES OF ADMINISTRATION FOR ENTERAL PRODUCTS	
Type	**Typical Rate of Administration**	**Comments**
Bolus	250–400 ml 4–6 times daily Administer using an open-ended, 60-ml catheter-tipped syringe allowing infusion by gravity. Do not push until feeding tolerance is well established.	Recommended for stable, ambulating patients. May cause cramping, bloating, nausea, diarrhea, aspiration; not recommended for unstable critically ill patients. Higher risk for aspiration.
Intermittent	Bolus feeding infused by pump: Begin with 120 ml isotonic formula at 120 ml/hr over 1 hour, with 30–50 ml H_2O; flush over 30–60 minutes. *Advancement:* Increase formula by 60 mL every 8–12 hours if residual is less than half the volume of the previous feeding to a maximum of 450 ml of feeding.	*Starting regimen* Should not exceed 30 ml/min; may cause cramping, nausea, bloating, diarrhea, aspiration; May need to reduce infusion rate to decrease discomfort and increase tolerance.
Cyclic	Continuous tube feeding generally infused over 12–20 hours daily. Rate to be determined by formula and caloric needs. Full-strength formula should be used to afford the patient the best opportunity to receive maximal support from the feeding.	Recommended for patients who cannot tolerate bolus or intermittent feeding and patients with J-tubes. Allows more time for absorption of nutrients while also allowing time for gut rest and allowing time for patient to ambulate freely.
Continuous	Rate to be determined by formula and caloric needs. Full-strength formula should be used. If not well tolerated, reducing the infusion rate may be warranted. Be mindful of the number of interruptions in feedings, as each interruption reduces the amount of nutritional support the patient receives.	Allows more time for absorption of nutrients. Less risk of aspiration. Recommended for critically ill patients and patients with J-tubes.

A 0.22-micron (μm) in-line filter cannot be used with TNA because it traps lipid molecules. However, a 0.22-micron in-line filter must be used with PN formulas of amino acids and dextrose solutions.

- *Carbohydrates*–Dextrose solutions are used to meet part of the patient's energy needs. With excess CHO intake, insulin demand, CO_2 generation, and O_2 consumption are increased, and may lead to respiratory distress and hypermetabolism.
- *Protein*–Essential and nonessential amino acid formulations are available in concentrations of 3% to 15%. Special amino acid formulations for specific disorders are available (see Estimating Nutritional Requirements, p. 120).
- *Fat*–Lipids are an isotonic solution providing essential fatty acids and a source of concentrated calories. For best use and tolerance, lipids should be infused with carbohydrates and protein over no less than 8 hours. Symptoms of an adverse reaction include febrile response, chills and shivering, and pain in the chest and back. A second type of adverse reaction occurs with prolonged use of IV fat emulsions and may result in a transient increase in liver enzyme levels, kernicterus, eosinophilia, and thrombophlebitis. In addition, IV lipids are contraindicated in patients with an egg allergy as the emulsion contains egg phospholipids. Maintain the infusion rate at 1 ml/min for the first 15 to 30 minutes as a test dose. Subsequent infusions are given over 12 to 24 hours. CDC guidelines recommend that when IV lipids are given as a separate infusion, the IV lipids should be infused over 12 hours (as opposed to a 24-hour infusion) to prevent fungemia. When in a TNA, the admixture may infuse over 24 hours. Patients receiving propofol (Diprivan), which is lipid-based, should receive fat emulsion with caution not to exceed 60% of total calories from fat.

Table 1-23	MANAGEMENT OF COMPLICATIONS IN THE TUBE-FED PATIENT
Complication/Possible Causes	**Suggested Management Strategy**
Nausea and Vomiting	
Fast rate Fat intolerance Fiber content Lactose intolerance Delayed gastric emptying	Decrease rate. Change to a low-fat formula. As prescribed, change to lactose-free product.
Blocked Tube	
Viscous formula/medications; inadequate flushing	Flush tube with 50–150 ml water after each feeding/medication administration. Flush every 4 hours with 30 ml water as ordered. For clogged feeding tubes, flush with warm water (60–100 ml), repeat as necessary. If feeding tube still clogged, may consider enzyme solution to unclog feeding tube. Do not use Coca-Cola or pineapple juice to unclog feeding tube.
Instillation of crushed medications	Do not instill crushed medications in small-bore tubes. Substitute liquid preparations after consulting a pharmacist and prescriber. Some medications may be crushed into a fine powder and dissolved. Check with pharmacist, since crushing can alter medication characteristics. Never crush time-released medications. Incompatibilities between drugs and feeding formulas are possible. Some medications that require that tube feeding be held around administration include phenytoin, Warfarin, and fluoroquinolone antibiotics (ciprofloxacin, levofloxacin, and moxifloxacin)

Parenteral Feeding: Selection of Catheter Insertion Site

Central venous IV catheter (CVC): Used for infusion of large amounts of nutrients or electrolytes with smaller fluid volumes (hypertonic solutions) than those in peripheral PN (PPN). The solution usually is delivered through a large-diameter vein (e.g., superior vena cava via the subclavian vein). The volume of blood flow rapidly dilutes the hypertonic solutions and decreases irritation of vein walls.However, there are more complications with CVC than with the peripheral route (Table 1-24).

Peripheral venous (IV): Generally not as effective as central venous administration: The need for low osmolality of solutions (less than 900 milliosmole [mOsm]/L) reduces efficacy of treatment. Combining solutions of dextrose, amino acids, and lipids with lower osmolality can provide a concentrated energy source that can be delivered through a peripheral vein, usually of the hand or forearm. Reserved for individuals who need partial or total nutritional support for short periods (5 to 7 days) when CVC access is unavailable or not warranted. Adverse reactions to PPN include phlebitis and burning at the infusion site.

Types of catheters: See Table 1-24.

Monitoring infusion rates: PN is given at a constant rate using an infusion pump. When initiated, the infusion rate is gradually increased to avoid hyperglycemia and fluid overload. For example, 1 L is infused the first day. Volume is increased to 2 L on the second day while monitoring tolerance of fluid and dextrose intake. If a higher rate is needed, it is achieved by day 3. Discontinuation of PN is accomplished by reducing the rate by half for 2 to 4 hours, then stopping the PN.

Managing complications: See Table 1-25.

Electrolyte imbalances occurring in both enteral and parenteral nutrition: See Table 1-26.

TRANSITIONAL FEEDING

A period of adjustment is needed before discontinuing nutritional support. Taper enteral and PN as oral intake increases. Patients receiving PN may have some mucosal atrophy of the bowel and need a period of adjustment before the bowel can fully resume its normal function.

Table 1-24   CATHETERS USED IN PARENTERAL NUTRITION

Catheter	Description
Temporary/Short-term Use	
PICC (peripherally inserted central catheter)	May be inserted into a peripheral vein and threaded into a central vein at bedside by physician or specially trained infusion therapy nurse. May be a single or double lumen. May be used for TPN administration at home. Catheter may remain in place for several months. Multiple uses of a single lumen for blood sampling, nutritional support, and medication administration increase the risk of infection, especially in immunocompromised patients.
Multilumen central venous catheter (CVC)	Inserted at bedside. May have up to four lumens. Subclavian or jugular vein accessed. Dedicate one lumen, preferably the most distal, for administration of TPN. Other lumen(s) are used for medication administration and drawing of blood samples.
Permanent/Long-term Use	
Right atrial catheter (e.g., Hickman, Broviac)	Generally placed surgically by a physician into the subclavian or jugular vein with the catheter tunneled and exiting from the skin. The catheter usually includes a Dacron cuff from which the catheter exits the vessel. This type of catheter is associated with the lowest infection rates of all central lines.
Implantable venous access device (IVAD, such as Infuse-a-Port, or Port-a-Cath)	May be placed by a radiologist or surgeon. Designed for repeated access, making the need for repeated venipuncture unnecessary.

Modified from Eisenberg P. In Swearingen PL, editor: *Manual of medical-surgical nursing care*, ed 6, St. Louis, 2007, Mosby Elsevier.

CARE PLANS: PATIENTS RECEIVING ENTERAL AND PARENTERAL NUTRITION

Imbalanced nutrition: less than body requirements *related to inability to ingest, digest, or absorb nutrients*

GOALS/OUTCOMES Within 7 days of initiating parenteral/enteral nutrition, the patient's nutritional status is improving, evidenced by stable weight or steady weight gain of ¼ to ½ lb/day (weight gain is not often seen in the acute care setting); malnutrition is improved indicated by increasing or normal measures of protein stores (serum albumin, transferrin, thyroxine-binding prealbumin, and retinol-binding protein; positive nitrogen balance; presence of wound granulation; and absence of infection (see *Risk for Infection*, p. 134).
NOC Nutritional Status: Biochemical Measures; Nutritional Status: Nutrient Intake; Nutritional Status: Food and Fluid Intake

Nutritional Monitoring
1. Ensure nutritional screening and assessment of patient within 24 hours of admission by nursing staff and within 72 hours by a dietitian; document. See *Nutritional Assessment*, p. 118. Reassess weekly.
2. Monitor electrolytes and blood glucose level daily until stabilized. Ensure that serum albumin, transferrin, or prealbumin and trace elements are monitored weekly.
3. Monitor Hgb and Hct, as patient may be iron deficient.
4. Monitor lymphocytes and other WBC differential indicators of the status of immune protective mechanisms.
5. Weigh patient daily.
6. Monitor for dry, flaky skin with depigmentation.
7. Monitor for pale, reddened, and dry conjunctival tissue.
8. Evaluate energy level for malaise, weakness, and fatigue indicative patient is not receiving adequate nutrition to promote strength and mobility.
9. Monitor for spoon-shaped, brittle, ridged nails.
10. Record I&O carefully, tracking fluid balance trends. Check volume enteral or PN infused and rate of infusion hourly.

Table 1-25	COMPLICATIONS IN PATIENTS RECEIVING PARENTERAL NUTRITION
Potential Complications	**Management Strategy**
Upon Central Line Insertion	
Pneumothorax	Position a rolled towel under the patient's back, parallel to the spine before the temporary catheter is inserted. Ensure that x-ray is done immediately after insertion to determine placement of catheter before initiating TPN. Monitor for diminished or unequal breath sounds, tachypnea, dyspnea, and labored breathing. The greater the number of catheter attempts, the greater the chance for pneumothorax.
Accidental subclavian artery penetration leading to hemothorax	If pulsatile, bright red blood returns into the syringe during central catheter insertion into the subclavian vein, assist with immediate removal of the needle and apply pressure for 10 minutes anteriorly and posteriorly at the point of penetration. If internal bleeding is unable to be controlled, patient will develop a hemothorax and hemorrhagic shock.
During Catheter Maintenance	
Catheter occlusion	If solution is infusing sluggishly, flush line using positive pressure with saline. Check to see if line or tubing is kinked. If line is occluded, try to aspirate clot and contact physician or midlevel practitioner who may pre-scribe a thrombolytic agent, such as Cathflo TPA, TPA (tissue plaminogen activator), or urokinase, per agency protocol.
Leakage or catheter puncture	Do not insert needles into central line port lumen caps to avoid damaging the catheter. If the lumen is accidentally punctured and begins leaking, notify the physician or midlevel practitioner immediately for further actions.
Air embolism (a medical emergency)	If signs of air embolism occur, examine the catheter to determine whether an open port enabled air to enter the infusion system. Clamp the catheter distal to any opening discovered. Turn patient onto their left side and place in Trendelenberg position (head down, feet up) and notify physician or midlevel practitioner immediately while administering oxygen.
Central line–related thrombosis leading to upper extremity DVT	Assess for swelling of the upper extremities, and perform a neurovascular assessment. If limb is swollen, is cool, and has reduced or absent pulses, the physician or midlevel practitioner should be notified and consideration given to removing the CVC. The extremity should be elevated and the thrombosis managed as ordered to address anticoagulation.

11. Ensure that patient receives the prescribed amount of nutrients.
12. Be mindful that residual volumes of gastric feedings include not only feeding but also gastric secretions. The amount of residual feeding is NOT purely feeding. More recent studies indicate caregivers may not need to be concerned about residual volumes of less than 450 ml. Patient positioning also effects the amount of residual volume which may be found by the caregiver.

Ineffective protection resulting in risk for aspiration *related to GI bleeding; delayed gastric emptying or location/type of feeding tube*

GOALS/OUTCOMES Patient is not aspirating as evidenced by auscultation of clear breath sounds; VS within patient's baseline; and absence of signs of respiratory distress.
NOC Nutritional Status: Nutrient Intake

Enteral Tube Feeding
1. Check the radiograph to assess the position of the feeding tube before the first feeding. Mark and secure the tube for future reference. Insufflation with air and aspiration of stomach contents are commonly used to confirm position thereafter but do not guarantee correct position and are no longer recommended by American Association of Critical Care AACN guidelines.

Table 1-26	POSSIBLE ELECTROLYTE IMBALANCES OCCURRING IN ENTERAL AND PARENTERAL NUTRITION

Sodium: Daily requirement is 60–150 mEq. Sodium is the primary extracellular cation in maintaining concentration and volume of extracellular fluid.

Complication	Pathophysiology and Management
Hypernatremia	May result from free water deficit, overdiuresis, excessive water loss, hypertonic TPN solutions, inadequate volume of TPN solutions, or inadequate water flushes via feeding tube. May be due to nephrogenic or central diabetes insipidus, uncontrolled diabetes mellitus, or use of sodium penicillin, heparin sodium, or corticosteroids. *Management* *Parenteral:* Increase free water, decrease sodium in TPN, increase volume of TPN. *Enteral:* All enteral formulas are low sodium. Change tube feeding formula to less concentrated formula and increase water flushes.
Hyponatremia	Most common cause in patients receiving TPN is administration of hypotonic fluids or volume overload. In tube-fed patients, hyponatremia may be caused by excessive fluid administration or excessive water flushes. Other causes of hyponatremia include adrenal insufficiency, renal insufficiency, SIADH (syndrome of inappropriate antidiuretic hormone), cirrhosis, and chronic heart failure. *Management* *Parenteral:* Decrease fluid and/or increase sodium in TPN. *Enteral:* Switch to calorie dense, fluid-restricted tube feeding formula, decrease water flushes via feeding tube or flush with normal saline as directed.

Potassium: Daily requirement is 50–100 mEq. Potassium is the major intracellular cation required for neurotransmission, protein synthesis, cardiac and renal function, and carbohydrate metabolism.

Complication	Pathophysiology and Management
Hyperkalemia	May be caused by excessive parenteral or enteral potassium supplementation, metabolic acidosis, increased tissue catabolism, and renal insufficiency. Medications that can cause elevated potassium levels include ACE inhibitors, angiotensin receptor blockers (ARBS), heparin, cyclosporine, and potassium-sparing diuretics. *Management* *Parenteral and enteral:* Decrease potassium in TPN or switch to low electrolyte tube feeding formula. Decrease other sources of exogenous potassium (in IV fluids, potassium supplementation). Consider stopping or reducing dose of potassium-sparing medications. Correct metabolic acidosis with sodium bicarbonate if present. May require administration of glucose with insulin, IV calcium gluconate, beta$_2$-adrenergic agents (e.g., albuterol) or hemodialysis in severe cases.
Hypokalemia	May occur during anabolism (tissue synthesis) in patients or in refeeding syndrome causing potassium to shift into the intracellular space. Other causes include excessive GI losses, diuretic use, or inadequate potassium intake. In metabolic alkalosis, potassium is also decreased (potassium is decreased by 0.4–1.5 mEq/L for every 0.1 increase in pH). *Management* *Parenteral:* Increase potassium in TPN, provide potassium supplementation in patients receiving tube feeding. Potassium given via a peripheral line can be irritating to the peripheral vein. Administration via a peripheral line should not exceed 10 mEq/hr. *Enteral:* PO potassium supplementation can be irritating to GI mucosa and may cause diarrhea. If hypomagnesemia is present, it should be corrected prior to potassium supplementation. *Both:* Initiate tube feeding or TPN slowly to avoid refeeding syndrome. Correct metabolic alkalosis if present.

Table 1-26	POSSIBLE ELECTROLYTE IMBALANCES OCCURRING IN ENTERAL AND PARENTERAL NUTRITION—cont'd

Phosphorus: Daily requirement is approximately 700 mg. Phosphorus is required for release of oxygen from hemoglobin in the form of 2,3-diphosphoglycerate and for bone deposition, calcium regulation, and synthesis of carbohydrates, fats, and protein.

Complication	Pathophysiology and Management
Hyperphosphatemia	Occurs in catabolic stress, renal failure, and hypocalcemia or excessive exogenous administration of phosphorus. Medications that can cause hyperphosphatemia include phosphorus-rich solutions, antacids, diuretic agents, and steroids. Associated with metabolic acidosis. *Management* *Parenteral:* Decrease phosphate in TPN or other exogenous phosphate administration. *Enteral:* May require treatment with phosphate binders such as sevelamer (Renagel), calcium acetate (PhosLo). Change to a renal tube feeding formula.
Hypophosphatemia	A complication with a high mortality, often found in malnourished patients with refeeding syndrome. As the patient receives fluids containing dextrose, phosphorus shifts rapidly into the intracellular space, causing hypophosphatemia. Refeeding syndrome also affects other intracellular electrolytes, particularly potassium and magnesium. Associated with metabolic alkalosis. *Management* *Parenteral and enteral:* Initiate tube feeding or TPN slowly to avoid refeeding syndrome. *Parenteral:* Increase phosphorus in TPN or provide other sources of phosphorus (sodium phosphate, potassium phosphate) in patients with low phosphorus levels.

Magnesium: Daily requirement is 18–30 mEq. Magnesium is required for carbohydrate and protein metabolism and enzymatic reactions.

Complication	Pathophysiology and Management
Hypermagnesemia	Generally seen with excessive magnesium supplementation including magnesium-containing antacids or renal failure. Medications include Milk of Magnesia and magnesium citrate. *Management* *Parenteral:* Decrease magnesium in TPN or IV fluids. *Parenteral and enteral:* Discontinue any medications that contain magnesium. May require diuresis or hemodialysis in severe cases.
Hypomagnesemia	Low levels commonly occur in patients with severe malnutrition, patients with refeeding syndrome, or in patients with lower GI losses, prolonged NG suctioning, and diabetic ketoacidosis (DKA). Often occurs in alcoholics, malabsorption syndromes, and the critical care population. Medications that can cause hypomagnesemia include diuretics, insulin, and cyclosporine. *Management* *Parenteral:* Increase magnesium in TPN, give supplemental magnesium. Parenteral magnesium should be used to treat moderate to severe hypomagnesemia in patients receiving parenteral and enteral nutrition. *Enteral:* Give oral magnesium supplements.

Calcium: Daily requirement is 1000–1500 mg of elemental calcium. Calcium is a necessary ingredient of the cells that play a major role in neurotransmission and bone formation.

Continued

Table 1-26	POSSIBLE ELECTROLYTE IMBALANCES OCCURRING IN ENTERAL AND PARENTERAL NUTRITION—cont'd
Complication	**Pathophysiology and Management**
Hypercalcemia	Occurs in prolonged immobilization, malignancy, hyperparathyroidism, tumor lysis syndrome, adrenal insufficiency, and renal failure. Medications that can cause hypercalcemia include thiazide diuretics, lithium, calcium supplements, and aluminum- and magnesium-containing antacids. *Management* *Parenteral and enteral:* Volume expansion with normal saline, which disrupts the stimulus for calcium reabsorption in the kidney. Loop diuretics are calcium wasting and may be used in cases of severe hypercalcemia. Bisphosphonates can be used to treat chronic hypercalcemia. *Parenteral:* Decrease calcium in TPN.
Hypocalcemia	Occurs with reduced vitamin D intake, hypoparathyroidism, and hypomagnesemia. Medications that can cause hypocalcemia include loop diuretics, bisphosphonates, calcitonin, phenobarbital, and phenytoin. *Management* *Parenteral and enteral:* Calcium supplementation (parenteral or oral). Ionized calcium level should be used as a guide to replacement, as serum calcium is bound to albumin. If albumin level is low, calcium level will appear falsely low.

2. Assess the respiratory status at least every 4 hours, observing respiratory rate and effort, and presence of adventitious breath sounds.
3. Monitor temperature at least every 4 hours.
4. Auscultate for bowel sounds, and assess abdominal contour and girth every 8 hours. Consult the physician or midlevel practitioner if the abdomen becomes distended or nausea and vomiting occur.
5. Elevate the HOB at least 30 degrees during and for 1 hour after feeding.
6. Notify the physician or midlevel practitioner if gastric residual is more than 450 ml if the patient is uncomfortable. The patient should be positioned on their right side for 20 minutes prior to aspirating the enteral tube for residual volume to ensure the feeding is being directed toward the small bowel. False high volumes may be reported if the feeding has pooled in the body of the stomach in a supine patient. If the caregiver is certain the residual volume was properly obtained, hold feeding for 1 hours, and recheck residual.
7. Stop the enteral feeding ½ to 1 hour before chest physical therapy or lowering the HOB when the patient is supine.
8. Discuss with physician or midlevel practitioner the possibility of placing feeding tube beyond the pylorus to help minimize the risk for severe aspiration.
9. As prescribed for delayed gastric emptying, administer metoclopramide HCl or other agents that promote gastric motility.

Diarrhea *related to intolerance of feeding, bolus feeding; too fast of an infusion rate, lactose intolerance; bacterial contamination; osmolality intolerance; medications; low fiber or high fiber content. Medications may also be a contributing factor, especially those intended to increase gastric motility (metoclopramide [Reglan]) and erythromycin. In addition, many liquid medications contain sorbitol, which can aggravate or cause diarrhea.*

GOALS/OUTCOMES Patient has begun to form normal stools within 24 to 48 hours of intervention.
NOC Bowel Elimination

Diarrhea Management
1. Assess abdomen and GI status, including bowel sounds, distention, consistency and frequency of bowel movements, characteristics of stools, cramping, skin turgor, and indicators of hydration such as skin turgor, thirst, presence or absence of sunken eyes.
2. Obtain daily weights and monitor I&O status carefully.

Specific Problems
3. Cramping or diarrhea associated with bolus feeding: Evaluate whether proper technique is used for bolus feeding, including a slow infusion of a room temperature feeding. If proper technique is used and cramping results, switch to an intermittent, cyclic, or continuous feeding method.

4. Evaluate patient for presence of clostridium difficile if diarrhea is present with any critically ill patient. Diarrhea is often blamed on tube feeding intolerance, when the actual cause is inappropriate use of antibiotics resulting in colitis. Obtain stool sample for *Clostridium difficile* (C Diff) after discussing with the physician or midlevel practitioner.
5. Avoid lactose-containing products.
6. Bacterial contamination
   - Use clean technique in handling feeding tube, enteral products, and feeding sets.
   - Change all equipment every 24 hours.
   - Refrigerate all opened products but discard after 24 hours.
   - Discard feedings according to institutional protocol, or at least every 6 hours.
7. Osmolality intolerance
   - Determine osmolality of feeding formula. Most are isotonic (plasma osmolality 300 mOsm). If hypertonic, change to an isotonic formula.
8. Medications
   - Monitor use of antibiotics, antacids, potassium chloride, and sorbitol in liquid medications. Dilute liquid medications with water. Controversy exists about the use of tap water vs. sterile water for dilution of medication. Since the medications are bypassing the normal mechanisms associated with swallowing, some practitioners believe best practice is to use sterile water for medications.
   - As prescribed, administer *Lactobacillus acidophilus* to restore GI flora or use tincture of opium to decrease GI motility.
   - Low-fiber content: Add bulk-forming agents (psyllium or fiber-enriched enteral formula).

Impaired tissue integrity *related to mechanical irritant presence of enteral tube, intolerance of tube feeding, diarrhea or hyperglycemia*

GOALS/OUTCOMES At time of discharge from critical care, patient's tissue is intact with absence of erosion around orifices, excoriation, skin rash, or mucous membrane breakdown.
NOC Tissue Integrity: Skin and Mucous Membranes

Skin Surveillance
1. Initiate appropriate strategies to manage diarrhea, control blood glucose, and assess tolerance of tube feeding. Changing the site of feeding/feeding tube insertion and type of feeding may assist with tolerance of feedings and diarrhea, which will facilitate improvement of skin integrity. Control of hyperglycemia indicates reasonable cellular uptake of glucose in feedings to facilitate healing.

Nasoenteric Tube/Postpyloric Feeding Tube
2. Assess nares for irritation or tenderness every 8 hours and alter position to avoid pressure. Use hypoallergenic tape to anchor tube.
3. Use a small-bore tube if possible.
4. Provide frequent oral care to maintain integrity of teeth and oral mucosa.
5. If long-term support is needed, discuss using gastrostomy or jejunostomy tube with physician or midlevel practitioner.
6. Give ice chips, chewing gum, or hard candies PRN if permitted.
7. Apply petroleum jelly to lips every 2 hours.
8. Brush teeth and tongue every 8 hours.

Gastrostomy Tube/PEG
9. Assess site for erythema, drainage, tenderness, and odor every 4 hours.
10. Monitor placement of tube every 8 hours.
11. Secure tube so there is no tension on patient's tissue and skin.
12. For first 3 days after insertion, clean skin with 1:1 solution of water and H_2O_2 unless the tissues are granulating, wherein plain soap and water may be used. Wipe with gauze. After day 3, wash skin with soap and water daily; pat dry.

Jejunostomy Tube/PEJ
13. Assess site for erythema, drainage, tenderness, and odor every 4 hours.
14. Secure tube to avoid tension. Coil tube on top of dressing if necessary.
15. Provide frequent oral care to maintain integrity of teeth and oral mucosa.
16. Skin care for a PEG tube is the same as for gastrostomy tube.
17. Avoid large volume water flushes (more than 120 ml) as this may cause small bowel necrosis.

Risk for infection *related to presence of central line for parenteral nutrition*

GOALS/OUTCOMES Patient does not acquire a bloodstream infection as evidenced by temperature and VS within normal limits, total lymphocytes 25% to 40% (1500 to 4500 ml), white blood cell (WBC) count ≤11,000/mm^3, and absence of clinical signs of sepsis, including erythema and swelling at insertion site, chills, fever, and hyperglycemia.
NOC Immune Status

Infection Protection
1. When central line is inserted, ensure the CDC central line insertion guidelines are followed, including use of full barrier precautions.
2. Twice weekly and PRN, monitor total lymphocyte count, WBC count, and differential for values outside normal range.
3. Check blood glucose at least every 6 hours, or using the facility's guidelines for values outside normal range.
4. Examine catheter insertion site(s) every 8 hours for erythema, swelling, or purulent drainage.
5. Use sterile technique when changing central line dressing, containers, or lines.
6. Avoid using the nutritional support port on the central or peripheral IV catheter for blood drawing, pressure monitoring, or administration of medications or other fluids.
7. Change all IV administration sets and rotate insertion site within the time frame per institutional protocol.
8. Do not allow parenteral solutions to hang longer than 24 hours.
9. If sepsis is suspected, take blood specimens for culture and administer antibiotics as prescribed. Remove catheter and culture catheter tip if prescribed.

Altered cardiopulmonary tissue perfusion (or risk for same) *related to interruption of arterial flow from air embolus introduced into central IV line during line insertion or maintenance*

GOALS/OUTCOMES Patient has adequate cardiopulmonary tissue perfusion as evidenced by stable VS, stable ABG values, and arterial oximetry within normal limits, and absence of dyspnea, tachypnea, cyanosis, chest pain, tachycardia, and hypotension.
NOC Circulation Status, Vital Signs

IV Insertion
1. When central line is inserted, place patient in Trendelenberg position.
2. Observe central line insertion procedure and remind practitioner inserting the line to avoid leaving the catheter open to air once blood vessel has been entered.
3. If patient experiences SOB, tachypnea, chest pain, hypotension, or cyanosis during line insertion, place on his or her left side in the head down position to facilitate trapping any air introduced in the right ventricle, and administer high flow O$_2$ by face mask.
4. Check chest radiograph film to determine catheter position following insertion.

IV Therapy
1. Use Trendelenburg position when changing tubing or when central vein catheters are inserted or removed.
2. Teach patient Valsalva maneuver (if possible) for implementation during tubing changes.
3. Use Luer-Lok connectors on all connections.
4. Use occlusive dressing over insertion site for 24 hours after catheter is removed to prevent air entry via catheter-sinus tract.
5. Monitor patient for chest pain, tachycardia, tachypnea, cyanosis, and hypotension.
6. If air embolus is suspected, clamp the catheter and turn patient to left side-lying Trendelenburg position to trap air in the right ventricle. Administer high-flow O$_2$ and contact physician immediately.

Deficient fluid volume (or risk for same) *related to failure of regulatory mechanisms; hyperglycemia; hyperglycemic hyperosmolar nonketotic syndrome (HHNS); diuretic use, prerenal azotemia, diarrhea, fistulas*

GOALS/OUTCOMES Patient's hydration status is adequate as evidenced by baseline VS, glucose less than 300 mg/dl, balanced I&O, urine specific gravity 1.010 to 1.025, and electrolytes within normal limits.
NOC Fluid Balance

Fluid Management
1. Weigh patient daily; monitor I&O hourly.
2. Consult physician or midlevel practitioner for urine output less than 0.5ml/kg/hr.
3. Check urine specific gravity; consult physician or midlevel practitioner for elevated specific gravity according to institutional guidelines.
4. Monitor serum osmolality and electrolytes daily and PRN; consult physician or midlevel practitioner for abnormalities.
5. Monitor for circulatory overload during fluid replacement.
6. Monitor for indicators of hyperglycemia and manage appropriately to avoid osmotic diuresis. Perform point-of-care blood glucose reading at least every 6 hours or using institutional guidelines until blood glucose is stable. Administer insulin according to institutional guidelines to control blood glucose. Targets for blood glucose during critical illness may range from 140 to 180 mg/dl.
7. Assess rate and volume of nutritional support hourly. For HHNS, discontinue infusion until blood glucose and fluid balance is normalized. Reset to prescribed rate as indicated (see *Hyperglycemia*, p. 711).
8. Provide 1 ml water for each calorie of enteral formula provided (or 30 to 50 ml/kg body weight).

ADDITIONAL NURSING DIAGNOSES
For other nursing diagnoses and interventions, see *Fluid and Electrolyte Disturbances* (p. 37), which includes discussion of the electrolyte abnormalities listed in Table 1-26.

PAIN
PATHOPHYSIOLOGY
Critically ill patients endure substantial pain from pathologic conditions, injury, therapeutic interventions such as surgery, and multiple invasive diagnostic procedures. Even seemingly unconscious patients experience pain. The patient's pain experience is compounded by fear, anxiety, and multiple barriers to communication. In addition, pain control frequently assumes a low priority when juxtaposed against respiratory or hemodynamic instability, either of which is common in critical care areas. The presence of pain is a significant stressor for critically ill patients and contributes to and potentiates other problems such as confusion, inadequate ventilation, immobility, sleep deprivation, depression, and immunosuppression, which can lead to extended healing times.

The subjective nature of pain adds to its complexity. *Pain* is defined by the International Association for the Study of Pain as "an unpleasant sensory and emotional experience associated with actual or potential tissue damage or described in terms of such damage." Pain is a warning signal to which the body responds to prevent further injury. Noxious substances that are released in response to damaged tissue initiate the pain (nociceptive) nerve transmission. Afferent nerve fibers such as A delta (Aδ) and C fibers respond to pain stimuli peripherally and relay this information to the spinal cord entering through the dorsal horn. Aδ fibers are small, myelinated, fast-conducting fibers that transmit pain sensation that is well localized. C fibers are small, unmyelinated, slow-conducting fibers that transmit poorly localized, dull, aching pain sensations.

In the dorsal horn, nociceptive neurotransmitters are released in response to the nociceptive input that activates the second-order dorsal horn neurons. The activation of the second-order neurons results in (1) spinal reflex responses such as vasoconstriction, muscle spasm, and increased sensitization and (2) activation of the ascending tracts, which transmits the nociceptive input to several regions within the brain. This is where several responses to pain occur, including the perception of pain and the emotional and behavioral responses.

Uncontrolled Pain: A Widespread Problem
Characteristic pain patterns develop according to the area affected and the underlying pathophysiologic process. Despite the availability of effective analgesics and new pain-control technologies, many critically ill patients continue to be underassessed and treated inadequately for

pain. There are three types of pain: *somatic, visceral*, and *neuropathic*. All three types can be acute or chronic. Somatic, visceral, and neuropathic pain can be felt simultaneously or alone at different times. Somatic pain is caused by the activation of pain receptors in either the body surface (cutaneous tissues) or deep tissues (musculoskeletal tissues). Deep somatic pain is described as dull or aching but localized. Surface somatic pain is sharper and may have a burning or prickling quality.Visceral pain is caused by activation of pain receptors due to compression, infiltration, extension, or stretching of the thoracic (chest), abdominal, or pelvic viscera within their cavities. Visceral pain is not usually localized and is described as pressure-like, deep squeezing. Neuropathic pain is caused by injury to the nervous system, is severe and described as burning or tingling.

Professional and patient-related barriers have contributed to poor pain management. These barriers include (1) societal expectations concerning pain (e.g., unrelieved pain is expected and accepted in certain situations such as during surgical or invasive procedures, treatment for malignant conditions, or as a normal part of aging); (2) professionals' knowledge deficits regarding the pharmacokinetics and equianalgesic dosing; (3) patients' lack of knowledge concerning the side effects of unrelieved pain and the lack of knowledge of pain management in general; (4) inadequate pain assessment techniques by health care professionals; (5) inappropriate professional attitudes and beliefs (e.g., certain patients do not have pain [e.g., neonates], pain management is low priority); (6) inappropriate patients' attitudes and beliefs (e.g., pain builds character, pain is a part of procedures); (7) cultural norms which frame the expected response to pain (e.g., succumbing to pain is a sign of weakness); (8) views of the spiritual significance of enduring suffering (e.g., suffering on earth will entitle the person to more rewards in the afterlife); and (9) fear of tolerance, addiction, and analgesic side effects by both professionals and patients. Patients may report their pain as less than it truly is for fear of addiction or upsetting the nurse. Nurses have an ethical obligation to relieve pain and reduce associated physiologic and psychologic risks of untreated pain, which may be poorly understood by the patient.

Uncontrolled pain has multisystem effects. The cardiovascular effects of unrelieved pain are increased HR, BP, SVR; increased myocardial O_2 consumption; altered regional blood flow; and deep vein thrombosis. The pulmonary effects noted of uncontrolled pain are decreased lung volumes, atelectasis, decreased cough effort, increased sputum retention, and hypoxemia. GI and GU effects are decreased gastric and bowel motility and urinary retention. The neuroendocrine response to uncontrolled pain is to release more of the stress hormones such as catecholamines, cortisol, and glucagon. Psychological effects are anxiety, fear, and sleeplessness.

Pain management must be made a priority and a visible part of daily patient care. Methods which make pain management more visible and a priority include (1) displaying pain assessment tools in patients' rooms, (2) designating pain as the fifth vital sign to signify its importance, and (3) incorporating pain assessment into documentation tools. Continuous assessment and documentation increase awareness and effectiveness of pain intervention. Nurses must be willing to demonstrate patience and perseverance when dealing with pain, which is difficult to manage. It is essential to offer a continuous evaluation of the effectiveness of pain medications to provide the patient the best opportunity to attain pain relief.

ASSESSMENT OF PAIN

A thorough baseline assessment, whenever possible, is important in accurately evaluating and managing pain. Frequent, brief assessments are necessary postoperatively and during acute episodes of pain until the pain is well controlled. Health care professionals need to establish a good rapport with patients and use therapeutic communication skills.

History and Risk Factors

Question the patient regarding previous and current pain, usual ways in which pain is described and expressed; previously used pharmacologic and nonpharmacologic methods of pain control and how effective these methods have been in relieving pain; previous history of chemical dependence, including alcohol use; attitudes and beliefs toward pain and use of opioid, anxiolytic, or other medications; typical coping responses for pain or stress; and expectations regarding pain management.

RESEARCH BRIEF 1-5

Cintron and Morrison reviewed 35 journal articles regarding ethnicity and race and its effect on pain assessment and management. Findings revealed that the majority of studies show disparities in access to effective pain treatment. Minority patients are less likely to have pain scores documented and more likely to have pain underestimated, while African Americans and Hispanics are more likely to have their pain untreated/ undertreated and less likely to receive opioid analgesics. African Americans report they are likely to use prayer/spiritual coping and Hispanics are least likely to visit a doctor or use prescription medications due to concern about: cost, addiction, adverse effects of medications, and doctors not believing or understanding their pain.

From Cintron A, Morrison RS: Pain and ethnicity in the United States: a systematic review. *J Palliat Med* 9(6):1454–1473, 2006.

Subjective Presentation

Because pain is subjective, the mainstay of pain assessment should be patients' self-report. Patients should be asked to describe the nature of the pain, along with their pain relief goal or comfort goal on a scale of 0 to 10 (e.g., onset, location, duration, intensity, quality, aggravating/ alleviating factors, related symptoms, treatments). The nurse should determine how much pain medication the patient is requiring over the past 24 hours, patients' pain ratings over last 24 hours, and frequency of PRN doses. Is the patient taking doses as often as ordered, and is this bringing relief to meet the patient's pain relief goal? One or more of several pain assessment tools should be used to assist the patient in rating pain during rest and activity, during pain, and before and after pain management interventions. Patient teaching should be implemented to stress the importance of patient's honesty and participation so health care personnel can accurately determine appropriate treatments and interventions and evaluate their effectiveness as well as patients' pain intensity levels.

- *Numeric rating scale (NRS) or graphic rating scale (GRS):* Patient ranks pain numerically, usually from 0 to 10. This scale also contains numbers and word descriptors such as *none, mild, moderate,* and *severe.* These scales may be a horizontal or vertical 10-cm line; one version is represented vertically as a thermometer, and the higher the number, the higher is the pain score/intensity.
- *Visual analog scale (VAS):* Patient marks a 10-cm horizontal or vertical line, which contains word anchors "no pain" and "pain as bad as it could be" at each end of the line to indicate pain intensity. The line is then measured in millimeters (mm) to obtain the patient's pain score.
- *Adjective rating scale (ARS):* Patient selects an adjective that best describes the pain intensity. This should be used in addition to a numerical or faces scale.
- *Faces Rating Scales:* Patients view six photographs of children's faces (Oucher Scale) with increasing pain intensity from left to right and choose the face that best represents their current pain level, while the Wong-Baker Faces Scale contains six "cartoon" round faces with increasing severity from smiling on the far left to frowning on the far right. These may be helpful for older adults, culturally diverse populations, patients with language barriers, and children.

Once the nurse determines which scale the patient can use, the same scale should be used for the duration of clinical care so accurate comparisons may be made regarding the patient's pain intensity, effectiveness of pain management strategies, and to guide further alterations in pain relief efforts.

Objective Presentation

The following may be used to supplement self-reports or used exclusively if the patient is unconscious or has other profound communication barriers.

- *Physiologic:* Responses to pain are related to autonomic nervous system stimulation, as seen in increases in HR, BP, and RR, all of which are associated with untreated acute pain. Other physiologic responses associated with autonomic stimulation are listed in Box 1-13.

Box 1-13	AUTONOMIC INDICATORS OF PAIN

Diaphoresis, pallor
Vasoconstriction
Increased systolic and diastolic blood pressure
Increased pulse rate (greater than 100 bpm)
Papillary dilation
Change in respiratory rate (usually increased to greater than 20 breaths/min)
Muscle tension or spasm
Decreased intestinal motility, evidenced by nausea, vomiting, abdominal distention, and possibly ileus
Endocrine imbalance, evidenced by sodium and water retention and mild hyperglycemia

- *Behavioral:* Social, cultural, ethnic, and environmental factors affect a patient's understanding of and attitudes toward pain. Patients respond according to learned attitudes and beliefs. A number of nonverbal indicators are listed in Table 1-27.

Vital Signs and Hemodynamics

Unrelieved pain usually results in autonomic stimulation (e.g., elevated HR, RR, BP, SVR). IV opiate analgesics promptly reduce SVR directly as a result of vasodilation and indirectly as a result of pain relief. The SVR reduction is sometimes misleading, as the patient may continue to have pain despite the change in SVR.

COLLABORATIVE MANAGEMENT
Care Priorities

1. Relieve pain using a combination of pharmacologic and nonpharmacologic therapies.
2. Avoid oversedation and respiratory depression.

Pharmacologic Therapies

Opioid agonists: Centrally acting analgesics that bind with receptors in the CNS and other tissues, thus blocking pain sensation and causing various other effects, including feelings of well-being, peripheral vasodilation, and possibly respiratory depression. They are used to manage moderate to severe acute pain. For the most effective therapy, titrate in small increments to produce the desired analgesia with minimal side effects. "As needed" dosing provides poor pain management because of delays in administration and fluctuations in the patient's analgesic blood levels. Patient-controlled analgesia (PCA) pumps, continuous peripheral or epidural infusions, and small, frequent IV bolus dosing are effective methods

Table 1-27	NONVERBAL INDICATORS OF PAIN	
Skeletal Muscle Tension	**Behavioral Reactions**	
Facial grimace, tension	Short attention span	
Guarding or splinting of the affected part	Irritability	
Restlessness	Anxiety	
Increase in motor activity	Sleep disturbances	
Decrease in motor activity	Anger	
	Crying	
	Fearfulness	
	Withdrawal	

used for patients in critical care areas. Opioid tolerance, physiological or psychological dependence, and addiction are unusual when opioids are used to manage acute pain in patients without a history of chemical dependency. Parenteral opioids may cause hypotension in patients with hypovolemia. Restore fluid volume before or concurrently with administration. Some patients are at a greater risk for respiratory depression. Those at a greater risk are the opioid naïve, those with compromised pulmonary status or neuromuscular disease, the extremely young (neonates), and older adults. Opioid-induced respiratory depression can be prevented with careful titration and monitoring.

Safety Alert *To reduce the risk of respiratory depression, hypotension, and circulatory collapse, dilute opioid agonists (e.g., hydromorphone, meperidine, morphine) for direct IV administration with at least 5 ml sterile water or normal saline; and inject slowly over 5 minutes. A dose reduction of 25% to 50% may be warranted, but initial drowsiness will subside with continued use.*

 Older adults are more sensitive to the therapeutic and toxic effects of analgesics. The distribution of medications is altered by age. With aging, lean body mass decreases and body fat increases. Also, muscle and soft-tissue mass decrease, and body water declines. This results in water-soluble opioid analgesics such as morphine having a lower volume of distribution. This causes an increased rate of the onset of action and raises the peak concentration, which is associated with increased toxicity. Lipid-soluble opioid analgesics (e.g., fentanyl) may be more widely distributed, resulting in a delayed onset of action and accumulation with repeated doses. Because of age-related changes in metabolism and elimination, older adults are also at risk for drug-accumulation toxicity.

 • In treating older adults, it is best to start at lower doses (50% to 75% of recommended younger adult doses). The interval between doses can be increased, using opioids with shorter half-lives (morphine, hydromorphone, oxycodone). All older adults should be monitored for signs of opiate toxicity, including increased sedative effects, inability to awaken patient easily, and respiratory depression. With careful assessment, proper dosing and titration, knowledge of analgesic onset and peak times, and careful monitoring, the risk for respiratory depression is low. However, naloxone (Narcan), an opioid antagonist, should be immediately available to reverse respiratory depression.

Safety Alert *Because of excessive sedation and respiratory depression, older adults and individuals with asthma, COPD, and other respiratory disorders should be monitored closely when receiving opiate analgesics.*

Safety Alert *Naloxone reduces respiratory depression but also reverses analgesia—dilute 0.4 mg ampule in 10 ml 0.9% normal saline and administer 0.5 ml (0.02 mg) by direct IV push every 2 minutes; titrate to effect/patient response to avoid withdrawal, seizures, and severe pain; onset occurs within 1 to 2 minutes with a duration of approximately 45 minutes. Patients can sometimes exhibit aggressive and sometimes violent behavior when the naloxone takes effect. See Table 1-28 for equianalgesic doses of narcotic analgesics and Table 1-29 for uses of opioid and opioid agonist-antagonist analgesia.*

• *Morphine*—Most frequently used opioid; considered "first-line" therapy for moderate to severe acute pain. With its vasodilatory effects and little effect on CO and HR, morphine is beneficial for patients with LV failure, pulmonary hypertension, or pulmonary edema. Rapid IV injection may trigger histamine release with related vasodilation, decreased preload, and decreased BP. Continuous opioid infusion minimizes hemodynamic changes that can occur with bolus dosing. Epidural administration may result in reduced responsiveness of the respiratory center in the brainstem to CO_2. This results in gradual

Table 1-28	EQUIANALGESIC DOSES OF NARCOTIC ANALGESICS		
Class/Name	**Route**	**Equianalgesic Dose (mg)***	**Average Duration (hr)**
Morphine-Like Agonists			
Codeine	IM, SC	130†	3
	PO	180†	3
Hydromorphone (Dilaudid)	IM, SC	1.5	4
	PO	6–7.5	4
Levorphanol (Levo-Dromoran)	IM, SC	2	6
	PO	4	6
Morphine	IM, SC	10	4
Oxycodone (Percodan)	PO	30†	4
Oxymorphone	IM, SC	1	4
(Numorphan)	Rectal	15–20	4
Meperidine-Like Agonists			
Fentanyl (Sublimaze)	IV, IM, SC	0.1	3–4‡
Meperidine (Demerol)	IM, SC	100	3
Methadone-like agonists			
Methadone (Dolophine)	IM, SC	10	6
	PO	10–20	6
Propoxyphene (Darvon)	PO	130–250†	4
Mixed Agonist-Antagonist			
Buprenorphine (Buprenex)	IM	0.3–0.4	4
Butorphanol (Stadol)	IM, SC	2	3
Nalbuphine (Nubain)	IM, SC	10	3–4
Pentazocine (Talwin)	IM	150	3
	PO	60	3

Modified from Hazard V, Hopfer DJ: *Davis' drug guide for nurses*, ed 5. Philadelphia, 1997; FA Davis, Macintyre PE, Ready LBN: *Acute pain management: a practical guide*, London, 1996, Saunders; and Salerno E: Pharmacologic approaches. In Salerno E, Willens JS, editors: *Pain management handbook: an interdisciplinary approach*, St. Louis, 1996, Mosby.

*Recommended starting dose; actual dose must be titrated to patient response.

†Starting doses lower (codeine 30 mg, oxycodone 5 mg, meperidine 50 mg, propoxyphene 65-130 mg, pentazocine 50 mg).

‡Respiratory depressant effects persist longer than analgesic effects.

IM, intramuscular; *IV*, intravenous; *PO*, oral; *SC*, subcutaneous.

decrease in the depth and rate of respiration, increase in $Paco_2$, increase in sedation level, and respiratory acidosis.

- *Hydromorphone (Dilaudid)*—Highly effective opioid; substitute analgesic for patients with morphine allergy or intolerance. Care must be taken to modify the dose of hydromorphone in comparison to morphine, since hydromorphone is approximately 5 times stronger than morphine (see Table 1-28).
- *Meperidine (Demerol)*—Indicated for brief courses (i.e., less than 48 hours, less than 600 mg/24 hr) in patients with allergy or intolerance to morphine, hydromorphone, or other opiates. Morphine is approximately 5 times stronger than meperidine, so meperidine doses are much higher (see Table 1-28). The drug is not well tolerated by older adults. Its toxic metabolite, normeperidine, is a cerebral irritant and may cause seizures, which has decreased its usage in both older adults and the critically ill. Some patients report little pain relief from meriperidine, despite stating a strong feeling of intoxication.

Route	Commonly Prescribed Medications	Advantages	Disadvantages
Table 1-29	**USE OF OPIOID AND OPIOID AGONIST-ANTAGONIST ANALGESIA**		
Continuous IV infusion	Morphine, fentanyl (Sublimaze), hydromorphone (Dilaudid)	Useful for severe, predictable pain Relieves pain with lower doses than IV bolus Avoids peaks and valleys of pain present with IV bolus and IM injections	Requires frequent observation to monitor flow rate VS must be monitored often, especially respiratory status Weaning necessary
IV bolus	Morphine, fentanyl, hydromorphone, meperidine (Demerol)	Useful for severe, intermittent pain (i.e., for procedures, treatments) Rapid onset of action	Relatively short duration of pain relief Fluctuating levels Possibility of excessive sedation as drug levels peak
Patient-controlled, may be delivered IV or SC	Morphine, fentanyl, buprenorphine (Buprenex)	Useful for moderate to severe pain Enables titration by patient for effective analgesia without excessive sedation Relief of pain with lower dosages of medication Immediate delivery of medication Patient's sense of self-control lowers anxiety Less nursing time spent preparing medications	Pumps necessary to analgesia (PCA); Patient must have clear mental status Health care provider resistance to self-administration by patient
Epidural and Intrathecal	Morphine, fentanyl, local anesthetics (e.g., bupivacaine)	Provides greater analgesia with less CNS depression than parenteral narcotics Enables direct binding of narcotics to opioid receptor sites in the spinal cord, thereby minimizing CNS depression Directly blocks pain impulse transmission to central cortex when anesthetics are used	Difficult to assess patency and placement Significant infection risk
IM/SC injection	Meperidine, morphine, pentazocine (Talwin), nalbuphine (Nubain), butorphanol (Stadol), buprenorphine	Useful for moderate to severe pain Longer duration of action than with IV route Faster pain relief than with oral medication SC route useful for patients with poor IV access and little muscle mass	Variable absorption and fluctuating levels, especially in hypotensive and edematous patients Possibility of excessive sedation as drug levels peak Potential delay in administration Demerol's propensity toward seizures decreases its efficacy

CNS, central nervous system; *IV*, intravenous; *IM*, intramuscular; *SC*, subcutaneous; *VS*, vital signs.

Safety Alert *Use of naloxone on patients receiving chronic or high-dose therapy may result in seizures due to predominance of convulsant activity from normeperidine overriding the CNS depressant effects of merperidine.*

- *Fentanyl*—Potent synthetic opioid. IV preparation is especially useful in critical care because of minimal cardiovascular effects, short duration of action, and rapid onset of action. Duration of action increases with repeated doses. Caution must be taken if large doses of fentanyl are given rapidly. This may cause chest wall muscle rigidity requiring ventilatory support and rapid-acting muscle relaxants. Other forms for chronic pain are a transdermal patch, an oral transmucosal lozenge (Actiq), effervescent buccal oralets (Fentora), and fentanyl buccal solution film (Onsolis, a highly potent opiate that will be discussed separately).

HIGH ALERT!   A fentanyl patch may be used for continuous analgesia, usually with supplemental doses of morphine or another opiate titrated to produce analgesia for breakthrough pain but should be used only for patients with opiate tolerance. A fentanyl patch is not recommended for mild pain, acute postoperative pain, or intermittent pain because of its slow onset (12 to 16 hours) and long duration and because it is difficult to reverse its side effects and adverse effects. Respiratory depression with hypoventilation occurs, as with morphine. Transdermal fentanyl absorption can be increased in patients with elevated temperatures.

- *Oxymorphone (Opana)*—Available in immediate- and extended-release formulations and may be given PO, IV, SC, or IM. It is twice as strong as morphine and is indicated for moderate to severe pain.
- *Onsolis (fentanyl buccal soluble film)*—A new dosage form for fentanyl approved by the FDA in July 2009. Onsolis is available under a Risk Evaluation and Mitigation Strategy (REMS). An REMS is required from manufacturers to ensure the benefits of a drug or biological product outweigh the risks. As part of the REMS for Onsolis, the drug is available through a restricted distribution program called FOCUS. The FOCUS Program prescription process includes additional steps that must be completed for the patient to be able to receive the medication both inside the hospital and at home.

Safety Alert *Onsolis is not an extended-release opioid and is only for opioid-tolerant patients. Onsolis is a highly potent opioid designed for a much more limited patient population than extended-release and long-acting opioids. Onsolis cannot be substituted for any other fentanyl product. There are substantial differences in Onsolis absorption compared to other oral transmucosal fentanyl products. Substitution of Onsolis for another oral transmucosal fentanyl product may result in fatal overdose.*

Opioid agonist-antagonists: These stimulate and antagonize opiate receptors to varying degrees, depending on agent and dose. They may precipitate withdrawal in patients receiving opiates on a regular basis (see Tables 1-28 and 1-29).
- *Pentazocine (Talwin)*—Predominantly agonist effects but with weak antagonist activity. It may cause increased MAP, LVEDP, and mean PAP, thus increasing myocardial workload.
- *Butorphanol (Stadol)*—Adverse effects reported in patients with congestive heart failure (CHF) or acute MI. It may be useful in decreasing side effects associated with epidural morphine.

Nonsteroidal anti-inflammatory drugs (NSAIDs): They are used to treat mild to moderate pain and are used as an adjunct with opioids to treat moderate to severe pain. NSAIDs inhibit the synthesis and release of prostaglandins peripherally, rendering afferent receptors less sensitive to bradykinin, histamine, and serotonin, which in turn decreases pain receptor stimulation. Most NSAIDs are given orally (e.g., ibuprofen, aspirin), but injectable NSAIDs such as ketorolac are available. Prostaglandin inhibition leads to decreased renal blood flow and acute renal failure; increased gastric irritation; and decreased platelet adhesiveness, which may result in bleeding complications (Box 1-14).

- *Ketorolac (Toradol)*–Effective for short-term use in relieving mild to moderate pain. The effect on ventilation is minimal, and the drug has been effective when given on an alternate schedule with morphine or another opiate analgesic during ventilator weaning of postoperative patients. Renal toxicity is possible, which limits use to patients with normal renal function. Bleeding complications are more likely with high-dose therapy and in older adults.

Other pharmacologic interventions: Sedatives and anxiolytics (e.g., midazolam [Versed]) are often used to reduce anxiety associated with pain and to promote amnesia when painful procedures are planned. Spinal analgesia with a local anesthetic agent may be used with epidural opiates. Intermittent or continuous local neural blockade, such as intercostal nerve block, is used for specific localized pain.

Nonpharmacologic Interventions
These interventions include sensory, emotional, and cognitive interventions, such as massage, relaxation, distraction, guided imagery, repositioning, and TENS unit; and are used for mild pain and anxiety and as adjuncts to pharmacologic management of moderate to severe pain (Box 1-15).

CARE PLANS FOR PAIN MANAGEMENT
Pain *related to biophysical injury secondary to pathology; surgical, diagnostic, or treatment interventions; or related to trauma*

GOALS/OUTCOMES Within 1 hour of initiating therapy, patient's subjective evaluation of discomfort improves, as documented by a pain scale. Patient does not exhibit nonverbal indicators of pain (see Table 1-27). Autonomic indicators (see Box 1-13) are diminished or absent. Verbal responses, such as crying or moaning, are absent.

NOC Pain Control

Pain Management
1. Develop a systematic approach to pain management for each patient. The primary nurse should collaborate with the physician and patient for optimal management of pain. See Figures 1-10 and 1-11 for pain treatment flow charts for preoperative and postoperative patients.
2. Monitor patient at frequent intervals for the presence of discomfort. Use a formal, patient-specific method of assessing pain. One method is to have the patient rate discomfort on a scale of 0 (no discomfort) to 10 (worst pain imaginable). Other methods may be used, but the method selected should be used consistently and patient's report should be respected and documented as reported.
3. Evaluate patients with acute and chronic pain for nonverbal indicators of discomfort (see Table 1-27).

Box 1-14	COMMON NONNARCOTIC AND NONSTEROIDAL ANTI-INFLAMMATORY ANALGESICS
Acetaminophen (Tylenol, Tempra) Acetylsalicylic acid (aspirin) Ibuprofen (Motrin, Advil, Nuprin)	Indomethacin (Indocin) Ketorolac (Toradol) Naproxen (Naprosyn, Anaprox, Aleve)

Box 1-15   COMMON NONPHARMACOLOGIC METHODS OF PAIN CONTROL

Physical therapies/modalities

- Massage: To relax muscular tension and increase local circulation. Back and foot massage are especially relaxing.
- ROM exercises (passive, assisted, or active): To relax muscles, improve circulation, and prevent pain related to stiffness and immobility.
- Heat/cold applications: To alter pain threshold, reduce muscle spasm, and decrease vascular congestion, particularly in the area of injury. Cold decreases initial tissue injury response. Heat facilitates clearance of tissue toxins and fluids.
- Transcutaneous electrical nerve stimulation (TENS): A battery-operated device used to send weak electric impulse via electrodes placed on the body. The sensation of pain is reduced during and sometimes after treatment.

Emotional interventions

- Prevention and control of anxiety: Limiting anxiety reduces muscle tension and increases the patient's pain tolerance. Anxiety and fear contribute to autonomic stimulation and pain responses. Progressive relaxation exercises and encouraging slow, controlled breathing may be helpful.
- Promoting self-control: Feelings of helplessness and lack of control contribute to anxiety and pain. Techniques such as PCA and promoting self-helping behaviors contribute to feelings of self-control.

Cognitive interventions

- Preparatory information: Preparing the patient by explaining what can be expected, thereby reducing stress and anxiety. Preoperative teaching is an example of this technique.
- Patient education: Teaching methods for preventing or reducing pain. Examples include suggesting comfortable postoperative positions, methods of ambulation, and splinting of incisions when coughing.
- Distraction: Encouraging patient to focus on something unrelated to the pain. Examples include conversing, reading, watching television or videos, listening to music, relaxation techniques (see Appendix 7).
- Humor: Can be an excellent distraction and may help the patient cope with stress.
- Guided imagery: The patient employs a mental process that uses images to alter a physical or emotional state. This technique promotes relaxation and decreases pain sensations.
- Biofeedback: The patient learns conscious control of physiologic processes that normally are controlled unconsciously. Muscle tension and chronic or episodic pain may be reduced.

Many of these techniques may be taught to and implemented by the patient and significant others.

PCA, patient-controlled analgesia; *ROM*, range of motion.

RESEARCH BRIEF 1-6

Owens and Flom indicate family members of patients in intensive care unit are able to predict when their loved one is in pain about 75% of the time, but the severity is usually underestimated.

From Owens D, Flom J: Integrating palliative and neurological critical care. *AACN Clin Issues Adv Pract Acute Crit Care* 16(4):542–550, 2005.

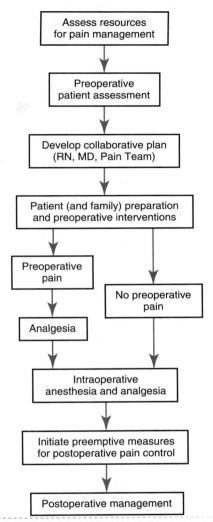

Figure 1-10 Pain treatment flowchart: preoperative and intraoperative phases. (From Agency for Health Care Policy and Research, Public Health Service; Acute Pain Management Guideline Panel: *Acute pain management: operative and medical procedures and trauma, clinical practice guideline.* Rockville, MD, 1992, US Department of Health and Human Services. AHCPR Pub. No. 92-0032.)

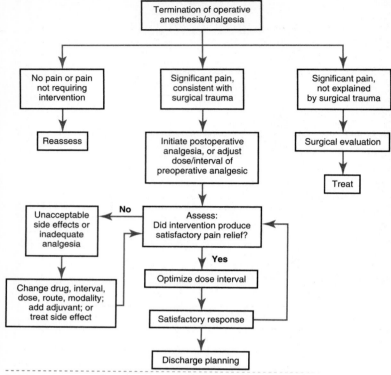

Figure 1-11 Pain treatment flow chart: postoperative phase. (From Agency for Health Care Policy and Research, Public Health Service; Acute Pain Management Guideline Panel: *Acute pain management: operative and medical procedures and trauma, clinical practice guideline.* Rockville, MD, 1992, US Department of Health and Human Services. AHCPR Pub. No. 92-0032.)

RESEARCH BRIEF 1-7

Herr et al. recommend the following guiding principles for assessment of pain in intubated and/or unconscious patients: (1) *Self-report*—use serial assessment since cognition can wax and wane. (2) *Potential causes of pain/discomfort*—pain sources may include medical condition, trauma, invasive procedures, and treatments; assume patients are unable to report pain and experience pain and discomfort. (3) *Observation of patient behavior*—see Table 1-31, Use Behavioral Pain Assessment Tools—e.g., FLACC (Face, Legs, Activity, Cry, Consolability Observational Tool, CPOT—Critical Care Pain Observation—tested in adult intensive care setting. (4) *Surrogate reporting of pain*—One aspect of the pain assessment in a critically ill patient should include a family member's impression of the patient's pain and their response to intervention. (5) *Analgesic trial*—if pain suspected, initiate an analgesic trial to verify presence of pain. Paralyzing agents and sedatives are not substitutes for analgesics.

From Herr K, et al: Pain assessment in the nonverbal patient: position statement with clinical practice recommendations. *Pain Manage Nursing* 7(2):44-52, 2006.

Pain

4. Evaluate patients with acute pain for autonomic indicators of discomfort (see Box 1-13). Be aware that patients with chronic pain (more than 6 months' duration) will not exhibit an autonomic response.
5. Evaluate health history for evidence of alcohol and drug (prescribed and nonprescribed) use. Individuals with a history of chemical dependence may require a higher dose for effective analgesia. Persons with evidence of chronic or acute hepatic insufficiency require a reduced dose and careful selection of appropriate analgesics. Consult pain control team if available. All care providers must be consistent in setting limits while providing effective pain control through pharmacologic and nonpharmacologic methods. Psychiatric consultation may be warranted. Be aware that some opioid agonist-antagonist analgesics (e.g., butorphanol, buprenorphine, pentazocine) have strong narcotic antagonist activity and may trigger withdrawal symptoms in individuals with opiate dependency.

Analgesic Administration
1. Administer opioid and related mixed agonist-antagonist analgesics as prescribed (see Table 1-29). Monitor for side effects, such as excessive sedation, respiratory depression, nausea, vomiting, and constipation.

Safety Alert   *Opioid-induced sedation precedes respiratory depression, so frequent assessment is warranted to determine patient arousability especially in patients who are opioid-naive, or receiving opioids by IV or epidural routes. Opioids should be stopped if the patient is difficult to arouse. Be aware that meperidine (Demerol) may produce excitation, muscle twitching, and seizures, especially in conjunction with phenothiazines. Do not administer mixed agonist-antagonist analgesics concurrently with morphine or other pure agonists, because reversal of analgesic effects may occur. Meperidine is poorly tolerated by older adults.*

2. Assess patients receiving opioid analgesics at frequent intervals for evidence of excessive sedation when awake or respiratory depression (i.e., RR less than 10 breaths/min or Sao_2 less than 92%). In the presence of respiratory depression, reduce the amount or frequency of the dose as prescribed. Have naloxone (Narcan) readily available to reverse severe respiratory depression.
3. If the patient is receiving epidural or intrathecal opioid, monitor closely for side effects and complications.
4. Check patient's analgesia record for the last dose and amount of medication given during surgery and in the postanesthesia care unit. Be careful to coordinate timing and dose of postoperative analgesics with previously administered medication.

Medication Management
1. Administer nonnarcotic and NSAIDs (see Box 1-14) as prescribed for relief of mild-to-moderate pain or on alternating schedule with opiate analgesics for moderate-to-severe pain.

Safety Alert   *Long-term use of acetaminophen is associated with hepatotoxicity and nephrotoxicity. Daily dose restrictions are recommended: 4000 mg/day for short-term use in normal, healthy adults, up to 3600 mg/day for chronic, long-term use, and no more than 2000 mg for older adults. Total daily doses should be calculated on a running 24-hour clock and include all combination products such as hydrocodone (e.g., Lortab, Vicodin) and propoxyphene (e.g., Darvocet). Patient teaching should include attention to products containing acetaminophen and cumulative daily doses (e.g., maximum total number of pills taken per day). NSAIDs are especially effective when pain is associated with inflammation and soft-tissue injury. Ketorolac (Toradol) may be given IM or IV when oral agents are contraindicated. Monitor for excessive bleeding, gastric irritation, and renal compromise in patients receiving all NSAIDs, including all products containing ibuprofen and naproxen.*

2. Administer PRN analgesics before pain becomes severe. Assess pain and offer the patient PRN pain medication around-the-clock (ATC) based on the PRN schedule to achieve better and more even pain relief. Prolonged stimulation of pain receptors results in increased sensitivity to painful stimuli and will increase the amount of drug required to relieve pain.
3. Administer intermittently scheduled or supplemental analgesics before painful procedures (e.g., suctioning, chest tube removal) and ambulation and at bedtime, scheduling them so that their peak effect is achieved at the inception of the activity or procedure.

4. Augment analgesic therapy with sedatives and tranquilizers to prolong and enhance analgesia. Avoid substituting sedatives and tranquilizers for analgesics.
5. Wean patient from opioid analgesics by decreasing dosage or frequency of the drug. When changing route of administration or medication, be certain to use equianalgesic doses of the new drug (see Table 1-28). Remember doses listed on the table are ratios of one drug to another and one route to another; these ratios should be used as estimates for a new starting dose along with pain intensity, patient pain assessment, and patient response to the drug. The current total 24-hour dosage will need to be calculated first, include scheduled and rescue doses.

Self-Responsibility Facilitation
1. Augment action of medication by using nonpharmacologic methods of pain control (see Box 1-15). Many of these techniques may be taught to and implemented by the patient and significant others.
2. Sudden or unexpected changes in pain intensity can signal complications such as internal bleeding or leakage of visceral contents. Carefully evaluate the patient's report of pain, compare to previous pain reports, and consult the surgeon immediately.
3. Educate patients about their medications, including asking for medications when in pain and declining them if offered when not in pain.

Environmental Management: Comfort
1. Maintain a quiet environment to promote rest. Plan nursing activities to enable long periods of uninterrupted rest at night.
2. Evaluate for and correct nonoperative sources of discomfort (e.g., position, full bladder, infiltrated IV site).
3. Position patient comfortably, and reposition at frequent intervals to relieve discomfort caused by pressure and to improve circulation.
4. Document efficacy of analgesics and other pain control interventions, using the pain scale or other formalized method.

NIC Analgesic Administration; Analgesic Administration: Intraspinal; Patient-Controlled Analgesia (PCA) Assistance

Ineffective breathing pattern *related to neuromuscular impairment secondary to central respiratory depression; pain-induced splinting*

GOALS/OUTCOMES Patient exhibits effective ventilation within 30 minutes of this diagnosis as evidenced by relaxed breathing, RR 12 to 20 breaths/min with normal depth and pattern (eupnea), clear breath sounds, normal color, Pao_2 ≥80 mm Hg, pH 7.35 to 7.45, $Paco_2$ 35 to 45 mm Hg, HCO_3^- 22 to 26 mEq/L, and Spo_2 ≥92%.
NOC Respiratory Status: Ventilation

Respiratory Monitoring
1. Assess and document respiratory rate and depth hourly. Note signs of respiratory compromise, including RR less than 10 or greater than 26; shallow or grunting respirations; use of accessory muscles of respiration; prolonged I:E ratio; pallor or cyanosis; decreased vital capacity; and increased residual volume. Consult physician for evidence of respiratory compromise.
2. Monitor Spo_2 and ABG values. Consult physician for decreased Spo_2 (less than 92%) or increased $Paco_2$ (more than 45 mm Hg).
3. Assess and document LOC every 1 to 2 hours.
4. Use apnea monitor as indicated.
5. Keep naloxone (Narcan) at patient's bedside during and for 24 hours after epidural or intrathecal administration.
6. Maintain IV access for immediate administration of naloxone to reverse respiratory depression.
7. Respiratory depression may persist for as long as 24 hours after the last dose of epidural morphine. Monitor for respiratory depression during and for 24 hours after patient's receipt of epidural or intrathecal opioids.

NIC Airway Management; Oxygen Therapy; Aspiration Precautions

Urinary retention *related to inhibition of reflex arc secondary to opioid action*

GOALS/OUTCOMES Within 4 hours of this diagnosis, complete bladder emptying is achieved. Overflow incontinence is absent.
NOC Urinary Elimination

Urinary Retention Care
1. Monitor for symptoms of urinary retention: bladder distention, frequent voiding of small amounts of urine, sensation of bladder fullness, residual urine, dysuria, and overflow incontinence.
2. Monitor I&O precisely.
3. Catheterize bladder intermittently or insert indwelling catheter as prescribed.
4. Administer IV naloxone as prescribed.

NIC Urinary Catheterization

Risk for impaired skin integrity *related to itching secondary to alteration in sensory modulation from opioid effects*

GOALS/OUTCOMES Patient's skin remains intact.
NOC Tissue Integrity: Skin and Mucous Membranes

Medication Management
1. Decrease the opioid dose via epidural or PCA infusion.
2. Administer diphenhydramine or hydroxyzine as prescribed. Monitor sedation when antihistamine added.
3. Maintain comfortably cool environment.
4. Apply cool, moist compresses.
5. If relief from the above measures is inadequate, administer small amounts of IV naloxone as prescribed and until RR is at least 8/min, continue to assess patient closely and frequently since naloxone may need to be repeated since effect of opioid is of longer duration than the effect of naloxone.
   See also Prolonged Immobility in following section.

NIC Skin Surveillance; Positioning; Pressure Ulcer Prevention

PROLONGED IMMOBILITY

Prolonged immobility is a common consequence of prolonged hospitalization for severe and critical illness. Morbidity related to prolonged immobility is often profoundly impacted by nursing care. Nurses attend to patients continuously, providing ongoing, expert assessments and interventions. Significant adverse outcomes of prolonged immobility have been demonstrated to be preventable. These are listed in Box 1-16.

Illnesses or diseases that may necessitate prolonged bed rest include:
- *Neurologic disorders* such as stroke/cerebrovascular accident (CVA) and Guillain-Barré syndrome
- *Cardiovascular disorders* such as severe heart failure and cardiomyopathy
- *Pulmonary disorders* such as chronic obstructive lung disease and pneumonia
- *Musculoskeletal disorders* such as post motor vehicle accident and joint contractures
- Others
  - Complications from surgery
  - Severe sepsis
  - Failure to thrive

The following set of nursing care plans frames the care of those who require prolonged periods of bed rest and/or those who are immobile.

CARE PLANS FOR PROLONGED IMMOBILITY

Activity intolerance *related to prolonged bed rest; generalized weakness; and imbalance between O_2 supply and demand*

| Box 1-16 | PHYSIOLOGIC EFFECTS AND COMPLICATIONS OF BED REST (DECONDITIONING) |

Cardiovascular
- Increased heart rate and blood pressure for submaximal workload
- Decrease in functional capacity
- Decrease in circulating volume
- Orthostatic hypotension
- Reflex tachycardia
- Deep vein thrombosis

Pulmonary
- Modest decrease in pulmonary function
- Atelectasis
- Pneumonia
- Pulmonary embolus

Gastrointestinal
- Ileus
- Deficient protein state
- Negative nitrogen state

Musculoskeletal
- Loss of muscle mass
- Loss of muscle contractile strength
- Bone demineralization
- Joint contractures

Skin
- Decubitus ulcers

GOALS/OUTCOMES Within 48 hours of discontinuing bed rest, patient exhibits cardiac tolerance to low-intensity exercise (defined below) as evidenced by:
- HR $\leq$20 bpm over resting HR
- Systolic BP $\leq$20 mm Hg over or under resting systolic BP
- Sao_2 greater than 90%
- Svo_2 $\geq$60%
- RR $\leq$20 breaths/min
- Normal sinus rhythm
- Skin warm and dry
- Absence of crackles, murmurs, and chest pain

NOC Activity Tolerance, Endurance

Exercise Promotion: Strength Training
- *Perform low-intensity exercise 2, 3, or 4 times daily:* ROM exercises on each extremity. Individualize the exercise plan on the basis of the following guidelines. Depending on the degree of debility of the patient, it may be necessary to begin with passive exercises, moving the joints through the motions of *abduction, adduction, flexion, and extension.*
- *Progress to active-assisted exercises,* in which you support the joints while the patient initiates muscle contraction. When the patient is able, supervise him or her in active exercises and then isotonic exercises, during which the patient contracts a selected muscle group, moves the extremity at a slow pace, and then relaxes the muscle group. Have the patient repeat each exercise 3 to 10 times.

HIGH ALERT! Avoid isometric exercises in cardiac patients. Stop any exercise that causes muscular or skeletal pain. Consult with a physical therapist for necessary modifications to allow for exercise without causing muscular or skeletal pain.

---

1. *Assess exercise tolerance.*
   - Be alert to signs and symptoms that the cardiovascular and respiratory systems cannot meet the demands of the low-level ROM exercises. Excessive SOB may occur if:
     - Transient pulmonary congestion occurs secondary to ischemia or LV dysfunction.
     - Lung volumes are decreased.
     - O_2-carrying capacity of the blood is reduced.
     - There is shunting of blood from the right to the left side of the heart without adequate oxygenation.
   - If CO does not increase to meet the body's needs during modest levels of exercise, look for:
     - A fall in the systolic BP
     - Dysrhythmias

- Crackles that can be auscultated
- A new S_3 or a systolic murmur indicating mitral regurgitation that may occur
- If the patient tolerates the exercise, increase the intensity or number of repetitions each day.
- Ask the patient to rate perceived exertion (RPE) using the scale shown in Table 1-30 (Borg, 1982). The patient should not experience an RPE greater than 3 while performing ROM exercises. Reduce the intensity of the exercise and increase the frequency until RPE of ≤3 is attained.

2. *Monitor the intensity of the activity.*
   - *Begin with three to five repetitions,* as tolerated by the patient.
   - *Assess exercise tolerance* by measuring HR and BP at rest, peak exercise, and 5 minutes after exercise.
     - If HR or systolic BP increases more than 20 bpm or more than 20 mm Hg over the resting level, decrease the number of repetitions.
     - If HR or systolic BP decreases more than 10 bpm or more than 10 mm Hg at peak exercise, this could be a sign of LV failure, denoting that the heart cannot meet this workload.
   - *Plan to increase duration.*
     - Begin with 5 minutes or less of exercise.
     - Gradually increase the exercise to 15 minutes as tolerated.
   - Plan to increase frequency.
     - Begin exercises 2 to 4 times daily.
     - As the duration increases, the frequency can be reduced.

3. *Increase activity as the patient's condition improves.*
   - Progress to sitting in a chair as soon as possible.
     - Assess for orthostatic hypotension, which can occur as a result of decreased plasma volume and difficulty in adjusting immediately to postural change.
   - Prepare the patient by *increasing the amount of time spent in high-Fowler's position* and moving the patient slowly and in stages as follows:
     - *Level I/bed rest:* Allow flexion and extension of extremities 4 times daily with 15 repetitions per extremity. Deep breathing should occur 4 times daily, 15 breaths each time. Reposition the patient every 2 hours.
     - *Level II/out of bed to chair:* Patient sits in the chair 2 or 3 times daily for 20 to 30 minutes as tolerated. ROM exercises may be performed 2 times daily while sitting in the chair.
     - *Level III/ambulate in room:* Patient ambulates for 3 to 5 minutes, 3 times daily as tolerated.
     - *Level IV/ambulate in the hall:* Patient initially walks 50 to 200 feet 2 times daily, and progresses to 600 feet 4 times daily. Slow stair climbing may be incorporated in preparation for hospital discharge.
   - If the patient is able, have him or her independently perform self-care activities such as eating, mouth care, and bathing as tolerated.

Table 1-30	RATING PERCEIVED EXERTION
Rating	**Perceived Exertion**
0	Nothing at all
1	Very weak effort
2	Weak (light) effort
3	Moderate
4	Somewhat stronger effort
5	Strong effort
6	
7	Very strong effort
8	
9	Very, very strong effort
10	Maximal effort

From Borg G: Psychophysical bases of perceived exertion. *Med Sci Sports Exerc* 14(5):377, 1982.

4. Teach and involve significant others in interventions for preventing deconditioning.
5. Provide emotional support to help allay fears of failure, pain, or medical setbacks.

NIC Exercise Therapy: Ambulation; Energy Management; Cardiac Care: Rehabilitative

---

Risk for disuse syndrome *related to mechanical or prescribed immobilization; severe pain; altered LOC*

- -

GOALS/OUTCOMES Patient displays full ROM without verbal or nonverbal indicators of pain.
NOC Mobility

Exercise Promotion
1. Prevent joint contractures by performing ROM exercises. The following areas are at high risk for joint contractures:
   - *Shoulders* can become "frozen," which would limit abduction and extension.
   - *Wrists* can "drop," prohibiting extension.
   - *Fingers* can develop flexion contractures that limit extension.
   - *Hips* can develop flexion contractures that affect the gait by shortening the limb or can develop external rotation or adduction deformities that affect the gait.
   - *Knees* can develop flexion contractures that limit extension and alter the gait.
   - *Feet* can "drop" as a result of plantar flexion, which limits dorsiflexion and alters the gait.
2. Change the patient's position at least every 2 hours. Post a turning schedule at patient's bedside. Position changes will:
   - Maintain all joints in a neutral position
   - Reduce strain on the joints
   - Prevent contractures
   - Minimize pressure on bony prominences
   - Promote maximal chest expansion.
3. Position to achieve proper standing alignment and maintain with pillows, towels, or other positioning aids.
   - Head neutral or slightly flexed on neck
   - Hips extended
   - Knees extended or minimally flexed
   - Feet at right angles to the legs
   - HOB elevated 30 degrees
   - Patient's shoulders and arms extended using pillows for support
   - Fingertips to extend over the edge of the pillows to maintain normal arching of hands
   - Hip flexion contracture prevention. Ensure that when the patient is in the side lying position, the hips are extended for the same amount of time the patient is in the supine position.

HIGH ALERT! Because elevating the HOB promotes hip flexion, ensure that the patient spends equal time with the hips in extension. When patient is in the side-lying position, extend the lower leg from the hip to help prevent hip flexion contracture.

---

4. Maintain the joints in neutral position by using:
   - Pillows, rolled towels, blankets, sandbags, anti-rotation boots, splints, orthotics
   - When using adjunctive devices, monitor the involved skin at frequent intervals for alterations in integrity. Implement measures to prevent skin breakdown.
5. Prevent foot drop.
   - Foot posture naturally in plantar flexion so be alert to the patient's inability to pull the toes up.
   - To prevent foot drop, foam boots or "high top" tennis shoes may be used to support the feet.
   - Document this assessment daily.
   - Teach the patient the rationale and procedure for ROM exercises, and have the patient return the demonstrations, if able.
6. Ensure that patient does not exceed his or her tolerance by performing constant assessment of activity tolerance. Provide passive exercises for patients unable to perform active or active-assistive exercises. Incorporate exercising

all joints with activities of daily living, such as changing position, giving bed baths, using bedpan, and changing the patient's gown.

7. Assess patient's existing muscle mass, strength, and joint motion.
   - Perform and document limb girth measurements.
   - Use dynamography, hand-grip device to measure muscle strength.
   - Establish exercise baseline limits.
   - Perform ROM.
8. Educate the patient. Maintaining or increasing muscle strength and tissue elasticity surrounding joints is imperative. Consult with the physician about the form and extent of the exercise. Muscle atrophy occurs from disuse leading to decrease in muscle mass, decrease in blood supply, and loss of tissue elasticity surrounding joints → pain → further difficulty moving.
9. Reinforce progress.
   - Post the exercise regimen at the bedside to ensure consistency by all health care personnel.
   - Provide a chart to show patient's progress.
   - Provide large amounts of positive reinforcement.
10. Balance rest and activity. Provide periods of uninterrupted rest between exercises/activities to enable patient to replenish energy stores.
11. Consult rehabilitation services. Seek a referral to a physical therapist (PT) or occupational therapist (OT) as appropriate.

NIC Positioning; Pressure Management; Exercise Therapy: Joint Mobility; Exercise Therapy: Muscle Control

---

Impaired skin integrity of the oral mucous membrane *related to ineffective oral hygiene*

GOALS/OUTCOMES Patient's oral mucosa, lips, and tongue are intact within 24 hours before discharge from intensive care unit.
NOC Tissue Integrity: Skin and Mucous Membranes

Oral Health Maintenance
1. Assess patient's oral mucous membrane, lips, and tongue at least every 4 hours, noting presence of dryness, exudate, swelling, blisters, and ulcers.
2. Perform oral care every 2 to 4 hours.
   - Use a soft-bristle toothbrush (premade mouth care kits are available) to cleanse the teeth. This is particularly important for patients who are intubated since evidence shows that pneumonia can be reduced or prevented. Suction mouth continuously during oral hygiene to remove fluid and debris.
   - Use a moistened cloth or sponge-tip applicator to moisten and help remove crusty areas or exudate on tongue and oral mucosa.
3. Offer sips of water or ice chips to prevent dryness if patient is alert and able to take oral fluids.
4. Apply lip balm every 2 hours and as needed to prevent cracking of lips.
5. **Consider** using an artificial saliva preparation to assist in keeping mucous membrane moist.
6. Have patient wear dentures as possible, to improve communication and enhance comfort.
7. Teach family the proper oral hygiene techniques and encourage them to perform oral hygiene.

NIC Self-Care Assistance: Bathing, Hygiene

Self-care deficit *related to cognitive, neuromuscular, or musculoskeletal impairment; activity intolerance secondary to prolonged bed rest*

GOALS/OUTCOMES Patient's physical needs are met by patient, nursing staff, and/or significant others while patient is being encouraged to participate as much as possible.
NOC Self-Care: Activities of Daily Living

Self-Care Assistance: Bathing/Hygiene, Feeding, and Toileting
1. Assess patient's ability to perform self-care on the basis of functional status (e.g., comatose state, hemiplegia, sensory or motor deficit, alterations in vision).
   - *Use assessment criteria for activity tolerance:* If patient experiences a decrease in BP of more than 20 mm Hg, an increase in HR of more than 20 bpm above resting HR, or a HR above 120 bpm in a patient receiving beta-adrenergic drugs, the patient is not fully tolerating the activity.

2. If patient is comatose, meet all patient's physical needs: bathing, oral hygiene, feeding, elimination.
3. Explain all procedures to patient and significant others before performing them.
   - Involve significant others in the plan of care.
   - Invite family and/or significant other in care as feasible.
   - Collaborate with the patient and/or significant other to develop the plan of care.
4. For patient who is not comatose:
   - Promote as much self-care as the patient is capable of providing.
   - Schedule care activities around the periods of time the patient has the most energy.
   - Question the patient about activity intolerance when assessment findings reveal the activity may exceed the patient's tolerance.
5. If patient is alert, keep toiletries and other necessary items within reach.
6. Do not rush patient; allow adequate time for performance of self-care activities and try to schedule activities at a point in the work shift to allow patient to have the time needed.
7. Encourage patient; reinforce the value of progress that is made.
8. Provide assistive devices. Consult with occupational therapy department regarding use of devices such as large handle utensils for eating.
9. If visual impairment exists, place all objects within patient's field of vision. If diplopia is present, apply an eye patch and alternate it between patient's eyes every 2 to 3 hours as prescribed.

NIC Energy Management; Self-Care Assistance: Dressing/Grooming

Nursing diagnosic ineffective peripheral tissue perfusion *related to interrupted arterial and venous flow secondary to prolonged immobility*

GOALS/OUTCOMES By discharge from the intensive care unit, patient has adequate peripheral circulation as evidenced by normal skin color and temperature and adequate distal pulses (more than 21 on a 0 to 41 scale) in peripheral extremities. (Distal pulse scales may vary with facility.)
NOC Circulation Status

Circulatory Care: Venous Insufficiency
1. Identify patients at highest risk for tissue impairment including those with altered LOC, extreme immobility/ inability to assist wth ADLs, hypothermia, hyperthermia, cachexia, hypoalbuminuria, and advanced age.
2. Identify patients at risk for deep vein thrombosis (DVT): Chronic infection, malignancy, peripheral vascular disease, history of smoking, obesity, anemia, prolonged bed rest, and advanced age.
3. DVT/VTE (venous thromboembolism) prophylaxis should be initiated per institutional guidelines (see *Pulmonary Embolus,* p. 396).

 Safety Alert *Note: All patients who are in bed greater than 50% of the time, including at night, should have DVT prophylaxis, either medical (heparin, enoxaparin) or mechanical (Geerts, 2008).*

Embolus Precautions
The following measures are generally a part of a DVT prevention program:
1. Assess for a positive Homan sign. The Homan sign is not very sensitive or specific for DVT but can be elicited by flexing the knee 30 degrees and dorsiflexing the foot. Pain elicited with the dorsiflexion may indicate DVT and may warrant further evaluation by a physician.
2. Assess lab values and VS for risk of DVT.
   - Fever
   - Tachycardia
   - Elevated sedimentation rate (ESR)
   - CRP is a nonspecific marker of inflammation and may be elevated with DVT.
   - "Hypercoagulable" patients are at higher risk for DVT.
   - In patients prone to DVT
     - Acquire bilateral baseline measurements of the midcalf, knee, and midthigh.
     - Record above measurements on patient's initial assessment.

- Monitor above measurements daily.
- Compare measurements with the baseline measurements to rule out extremity enlargement that could be caused by DVT.

3. Teach patient and family the signs of DVT.
   - Pain
   - Swelling and warmth in the involved area
   - Coolness, unnatural color or pallor in involved area
   - Superficial venous dilation distal to the involved area
   - Report signs to a staff member, physician, or midlevel practitioner promptly if they occur.

4. Advise the patient and family to perform only the exercises prescribed by the health care team. Discourage practices such as massaging the legs when swelling and discomfort are noted.

5. Exercises for DVT prevention.
   - Teach patient calf-pumping (ankle dorsiflexion-plantar flexion)
   - Teach patient ankle-circling exercises.
   - Unless symptomatic, instruct patient to repeat each movement 10 times hourly during extended periods of immobility.
   - Help promote circulation by performing passive ROM or encouraging active ROM exercises.
   - Encourage deep breathing, which increases negative pressure in the lungs and thorax to promote emptying of large veins.

6. Provide mechanical venous compression for patients on bed rest.
   - When not contraindicated by peripheral vascular disease, ensure that patient wears antiembolic hose or pneumatic sequential compression stockings.
   - Remove mechanical venous compression device for 10 to 20 minutes every 8 hours.
   - Inspect underlying skin for evidence of irritation or breakdown.
   - Reapply hose after elevating patient's legs at least 10 degrees for 10 minutes.

7. Position for maximal venous circulation. Instruct patient not to cross the feet at the ankles or knees while in bed because doing so may cause venous stasis. If patient is at risk for DVT, elevate the foot of the bed 10 degrees to increase venous return.

8. Reduce the potential for thrombus formation and embolization.
   - Medications that inhibit blood clotting:
     - Heparin
     - Low-molecular-weight heparin
     - Aspirin
     - Platelet inhibitors
     - Sodium warfarin

9. Administer medication as prescribed, and monitor appropriate laboratory values.
   - Prothrombin time (PT)
   - International normalized ratio (INR)
   - Partial thromboplastin time (PTT)
   - Heparin level

10. Educate patient to self-monitor for and report bleeding:
    - Epistaxis
    - Bleeding gums
    - Hematemesis
    - Hemoptysis
    - Melena
    - Hematuria
    - Ecchymoses

Safety Alert   *Note: High-risk patients may have an inferior vena caval (IVC) filter placed to protect against pulmonary embolism.*

 Circulatory Precautions

❧ **Altered cerebral tissue perfusion: (orthostatic hypotension)** *related to interrupted arterial flow to the brain secondary to prolonged bed rest*

GOALS/OUTCOMES When getting out of bed, patient has adequate cerebral perfusion as evidenced by HR less than 120 bpm and BP ≥90/60 mm Hg immediately after position change (or within 20 mm Hg of patient's normal range), nondiaphoretic skin, normal skin color, denial of vertigo, no syncope, and HR and BP to resting levels within 3 minutes of position change.

NOC Neurological Status, Neurological Status: Consciousness

Cerebral Perfusion Promotion
1. Assess patient for factors that increase the risk of orthostatic hypotension.
- Fluid volume changes
  - Recent diuresis
  - Diaphoresis
  - Change in vasodilator therapy
- Altered autonomic control
  - Diabetic cardiac neuropathy
  - Denervation after heart transplant
  - Advanced age
  - Severe LV dysfunction
2. Educate the patient. Explain cause of orthostatic hypotension and measures for prevention.
3. Apply elastic stockings to help prevent orthostatic hypotension. For patients who continue to have difficulty with orthostatic hypotension, it may be necessary to supplement the hose with elastic wraps to the groin when the patient is out of bed. Ensure that these wraps encompass the entire surface of the legs.
4. Prepare patient for getting out of bed. Encourage position changes within necessary confines. Consider using a tilt table to reacclimate patient to upright positions.
5. Follow these guidelines for mobilization:
- *Closely monitor the BP* of any high-risk patient for whom this will be the first time out of bed.
- *Dangle patient's legs at the bedside.* Be alert to indicators of orthostatic hypotension:
  - Diaphoresis
  - Pallor
  - Tachycardia
  - Hypotension
  - Syncope
  - Feeling of lightheadedness or dizziness
- Check VS for indicators of orthostatic hypotension and return the patient to a supine position with:
  - Drop in systolic BP of 20 mm Hg
  - Increased pulse rate
  - Feeling of vertigo
  - Impending syncope,
- *Stand at bedside if leg dangling is tolerated.* Have at least two staff members assisting patient. Progress to ambulation if no adverse signs or symptoms occur.

NIC Energy Management; Surveillance

❧ **Constipation** *related to less-than-adequate fluid or dietary intake and bulk; immobility; lack of privacy; positional restrictions; use of opioid analgesics*

GOALS/OUTCOMES Within 24 hours of this diagnosis, patient verbalizes knowledge of measures that promote bowel elimination. Patient relates the return of his or her normal pattern and character of bowel elimination within 3 to 5 days of this diagnosis. Older adults often experience constipation.

NOC Bowel Elimination

Bowel Management
1. Assess patient's bowel history. Determine normal bowel habits and interventions that are used successfully at home.
2. Monitor and document patient's bowel movements, diet, and I&O. Be alert to the following indications of constipation:

- Fewer than patient's usual number of bowel movements
- Abdominal discomfort or distention
- Straining at stool
- Patient complaints of rectal pressure or fullness
- Fecal impaction, which may be manifested by oozing of liquid stool and confirmed via digital examination.
3. Auscultate each abdominal quadrant for at least 1 minute to determine the presence of bowel sounds. Normal sounds are clicks or gurgles occurring at a rate of 5 to 34/min.

Safety Alert *Bowel sounds are decreased or absent with paralytic ileus. High-pitched rushing sounds may be heard during abdominal cramping, indicating an intestinal obstruction.*

---

4. Remove rectal fecal impaction. Use a gloved, lubricated finger to remove stool from the rectum. Digital stimulation alone may prompt a bowel movement. Oil-retention enemas may soften impacted stool.
5. Encourage a high-fiber/high-fluid diet. Unless contraindicated, a high-roughage diet and a fluid intake of at least 2 to 3 L/day help to promote regular bowel movements. Individualize fluid intake according to physiologic state for patients with renal, hepatic, or cardiac disorders.
6. Promote bowel regularity.
   - Offer the bedpan at intervals and allow for use of bedside commode when safe.
   - Ensure privacy.
   - Time laxatives, enemas, or suppositories to take effect at the time of day the patient normally has a bowel movement.
   - Provide warm fluids before breakfast.
   - Encourage toileting to gain advantage of gastrocolic or duodenocolic reflexes.
7. Promote peristalsis. Encourage as much activity as tolerated.
8. Consult physician for pharmacologic interventions as necessary. To help prevent rebound constipation, make a priority list of interventions to ensure minimal disruption of patient's normal bowel habits. The following is a suggested hierarchy of interventions:
   - Bulk-building additives (e.g., psyllium)
   - Mild laxatives (e.g., apple or prune juice, milk of magnesia)
   - Stool softeners (e.g., docusate sodium or docusate calcium)
   - Potent laxatives and cathartics (e.g., bisacodyl, cascara sagrada)
   - Medicated suppositories
   - Enemas
9. Discuss, with the patient, the role narcotics and other medications have in constipation. Consider alternative methods of pain control (see Box 1-15) in an attempt to reduce narcotic dosage.

NIC Constipation/Impaction Management

Deficient diversional activity *related to prolonged illness and hospitalization*

GOALS/OUTCOMES Within 24 hours of intervention, patient engages in diversional activities and relates the absence of boredom.
NOC Motivation

Self-Responsibility Facilitation
1. Prevent boredom. Provide patient with something to read or do. Explore activities patient enjoys. Assess patient's activity tolerance using the criteria listed in the Activity Intolerance nursing diagnosis on the first care plan in this section.
2. Personalize the patient's environment with favorite objects and photographs. Suggest that significant others bring in a radio or a television, if not part of the standard room furnishings.
3. Tailor activities to attention span. Initiate activities that require little concentration, and proceed to more complicated tasks as patient's condition allows. For example, if reading requires more energy or concentration than patient is capable of, suggest that significant others read to patient or bring in audiotapes of books, such as those marketed for the visually impaired.

4. Remember the pleasant past. Encourage discussion of past activities or reminiscence as a substitute for performing favorite activities during convalescence.
5. Progress activities as patient's endurance improves. Move from reading to other diversions, such as puzzles, model kits, handicrafts, and computerized games and activities.
6. Encourage visitation by significant others within limits of patient's endurance. Involve significant others in patient activities, such as playing cards or backgammon. Encourage significant others to stagger their visits throughout the day.
7. Provide social interaction time. Spend time talking with patient. Arrange for hospital volunteers to visit, play cards, read books, or play board games as appropriate. Consider relocation to a room in an area of high traffic if patient desires more social interaction.
8. Remember the outdoors to promote normalcy. As patient's condition improves, assist him or her with sitting in a chair near a window. When able, provide opportunities to sit in a solarium so patients can interact together. If the physical condition and weather permit, take patient outside for brief periods. Natural sunlight helps to promote a more normal sleep-wake cycle.
9. Support spiritual, mental, and emotional health. Request consultation for interventions as appropriate from social services, occupational therapy, pastoral services, and psychiatric nurse.

NIC Energy Management; Activity Therapy; Art Therapy; Recreation Therapy; Spiritual Support; Family Support; Emotional Support

SEDATION AND NEUROMUSCULAR BLOCKADE

All critically ill patients aware of their environment experience anxiety, restlessness, and/or agitation, which may require use of sedation. Inadequate pain control may manifest as agitation. Unrelieved stress, manifested in the form of anxiety or agitation, retards healing and can increase mortality. Optimally, causes of agitation are identified and managed using nonpharmacologic methods (see *Emotional and Spiritual Support of the Patient and Significant Others*, p. 200).

When nonpharmacologic methods fail, sedating or anxiolytic agents are administered to promote comfort and decrease anxiety. Anxiety and agitation in severely ill patients may be prompted by emotional factors, including fear, loss of physical control, life-threatening illness, inability to communicate (e.g., mechanical ventilation), and feelings of helplessness. Environmental factors such as noise, temperature extremes, and sleep deprivation add to anxiety and agitation. The influence of environmental factors is sometimes more pronounced in those with altered level of consciousness (see *Alterations in Consciousness*, p. 24). Common pathophysiologic factors that contribute to agitation include hypoxemia, impaired cerebral perfusion, infection, alcohol withdrawal, and encephalopathy (Box 1-17). These findings must be ruled out prior to initiating sedation, as the use of the medications may mask a treatable problem. Litigation resulting from patient harm induced by use of sedation to manage hypoxia-induced agitation is not rare in the United States.

Anxiolysis, or *"light sedation,"* is defined by the American Society of Anesthesiologists (ASA) and The Joint Commission as, "Administration of oral medications for the reduction of anxiety" and "a drug-induced state during which the patient responds normally to verbal commands." ASA guidelines state, "Although cognitive function and coordination may be impaired, ventilatory and cardiovascular functions are unaffected." *Moderate*, or *"conscious," sedation* (or analgesia) is a slightly decreased level of consciousness induced by pharmacologic agents wherein the patient is able to maintain protective reflexes, has a patent airway, and responds/awakens by physical or verbal stimulation. *Deep sedation/analgesia* is an induced state of diminished consciousness or unconsciousness from which the patient cannot easily be aroused. Protective reflexes may be partially or completely lost, including the ability to independently maintain a patent airway and purposefully respond to aggressive or painful stimulation. *General anesthesia* is a controlled state of unconsciousness resulting in complete loss of protective reflexes, including ability to independently maintain a patent airway and respond to painful stimulation. Regardless of the intended level of sedation, the procedure is done on a continuum that may result in the loss of the patient's protective reflexes.

When sedating, anxiolytic, or other adjunctive agents fail to help stabilize ventilation and perfusion in mechanically ventilated patients, neuromuscular blocking agents (NMBAs) may be

Box 1-17   PATHOLOGIC CONDITIONS CONTRIBUTING TO AGITATION

Addison crisis
Alzheimer disease
Anxiety disorder
Delirium
Delirium tremens
Developmental disability
Drugs
  Subtherapeutic
  Supratherapeutic (toxic)
  Withdrawal syndromes
  Idiosycratic reactions
  Drug interactions
  Steroid psychosis
Encephalopathy
  Hepatic
  Metabolic
  Uremic
Fear
Hypercarbia
Hyperthyroidism
Hypoglycemia
Hyponatremia

Hypophosphatemia
Hypoxemia
Impaired cerebral perfusion
  Cerebral thrombosis
  Subarachnoid hemorrhage
  Intracranial bleeding
  Cerebral vasospasm
  Cerebral edema
Increased intracranial pressure
  Tumor
  Cerebrovascular accident
  Hydrocephalus
Infection
  Meningitis
  Encephalitis
  Brain abscess
  Sepsis syndrome
Pain, inadequately controlled
Sleep deprivation
Tachyphylaxis to drugs (drug resistance)
Thyroid disease

added. Neuromuscular blockade results in total paralysis of the patient. Paralysis is always done in conjunction with sedation and analgesia. Ineffective pain management should be ruled out as a cause for instability and agitation, as the situation is compounded by use of both sedatives and NMBAs. The patient may be aware but is rendered unable to move, breathe, or communicate while paralyzed. Patients who receive paralytics without sedation and analgesia may experience overwhelming fear due to being completely helpless while unable to move or take a breath.

Patients may inadvertently "fight" treatments. For example, those with severe lung disease may require use of specialized ventilator settings such as reversing the inspiration to expiration time (reverse I:E ratios). This therapy is physiologically unnatural and the patient's neuromuscular responses may resist the change in timing. Successful ventilation may not be possible without use of NMBAs to stop the patient from tensing in response to the treatment. Tensing reduces tidal volume and requires an increased energy expenditure. Care providers must create an anticipatory plan for pain management when the patient is no longer able to voice his or her needs.

The goal of pharmacologic sedation is to reduce anxiety and produce a calm but communicative state, if possible. This is best accomplished by administering frequent, incremental doses of sedatives just until the desired effects are achieved. If large amounts or medication are necessary, careful consideration should be given for consultation with a physician or midlevel practitioner who specializes in the management of critically ill patients using sedation, analgesia, and, if necessary, neuromuscular blockade. Major organ dysfunction, multiple medications, tissue catabolism, and other factors render critically ill patients especially vulnerable to the toxic effects of many sedatives. Oversedation and toxicity should be carefully avoided through close monitoring, individualized dosing, and titration to desired effect. Excessive sedation has been associated with delayed recognition of neurologic events, muscle wasting, and nosocomial complications such as deep vein thrombosis, compression injury, and pneumonia.

ASSESSMENT OF ANXIETY AND AGITATION

A thorough assessment must be done to differentiate the factors related to agitation, so appropriate management strategies can be implemented. Anxiety requires sedation, while pain requires analgesia, and control of energy expenditure from constant muscle tensing requires use of NMBAs. Characteristics of each condition are as follows:

- *Anxiety:* Subjective characteristics include increased tension, apprehension, fear, shakiness, uncertainty, distress, difficulty concentrating, and feelings of helplessness. Objective

findings include cardiovascular excitation, superficial vasoconstriction, pupil dilation, increased perspiration, restlessness, disturbed sleep patterns, tremors, and facial tension.
- *Pain:* Subjective characteristics of pain are described by the patient. Care providers must listen to the patient to provide the appropriate therapy. "Pain is what a patient says it is." Use a visual analog scale, numeric scale, Wong-Baker scale, or other coded method to establish baseline and evaluate analgesic effectiveness. Objective findings include autonomic responses such as changes in BP and HR, increased or decreased RR, pupil dilation, increased perspiration, guarding, moaning, crying, restlessness, facial grimace, furrowing of the brow, and rigid muscle tone. Patients express pain in many different ways, including the effects of their cultural background. (See *Pain*, p. 135.)

RESEARCH BRIEF 1-8

The Critical Care Pain Observation Tool (CCPOT) was developed and tested by critical care nurses in Canada and used to observe postoperative cardiac surgical patients. Patients were assessed at four intervals: immediately following surgery; at rest; during repositioning; and after repositioning. Facial expressions, body movements, muscular tension, and ventilator compliance were evaluated to assess pain behaviors. Results revealed those who were unconscious, those conscious with an endotracheal tube in place, and those conscious who had been extubated had pain scores on the CCPOT that increased during any noxious procedure. The interrater reliability for the CCPOT scale has been moderate to high, criterion validity is strong, and the scale possesses some discriminate validity.

From Gelinas C, Fillion L, Puntillo KA, et al: Validation of the Critical Care Pain Observation tool in adult patients. *Am J Crit Care* 15:420-427, 2006.

- *Energy expenditure:* When a patient is paralyzed using NMBA therapy, it is of paramount importance to be able to evaluate whether the levels of sedation, analgesia, and paralysis are appropriate. An older assessment measure involves the use of a peripheral nerve stimulator to deliver four tiny, sequential shocks to the muscles of the forearm to evaluate if the muscles are able to twitch. If the muscle can twitch, the NMBA is not blocking the shock from eliciting a response. The muscle response is measured to evaluate how many signals are blocked by the NMBA compared with the number perceived. In the absence of neuromuscular blockade, the muscle should move four times equally in response to four signals. As receptors are saturated with neuromuscular blocking agents (NMBAs), fewer muscle contractions are seen (Table 1-31). Nerve stimulators continue to be used in some facilities, but can be uncomfortable for the patient being evaluated on an hourly basis. An alternative strategy is the use of bispectral analysis or "brain wave" monitoring (BIS monitoring). The patient's EEG is constantly monitored to assess their awareness level. Changes in brain waves prompt dose modification in NMBAs, as well as sedatives and analgesics. Another commonly used method for assessment is providing a "drug holiday," to enable return of neuromuscular function to assess muscle strength. This method is sometimes difficult to manage, as the response of the patient to drug

Table 1-31	NERVE STIMULATION IN RELATIONSHIP TO PERCENT BLOCKAGE
Number of Twitches	**Percent Blockage**
4	0–50
3	60–70
2	70–80
1	80–90
None	>90

weaning is unpredictable and may result in profound instability for patients undergoing neuromuscular blockade.

COLLABORATIVE MANAGEMENT
Care Priorities
1. **Ensure agitation is not caused by pathophysiology.** All agitated patients should be evaluated for the presence of hypoxia, impending shock, hypoglycemia, sepsis, electrolyte imbalance, acid-base imbalance, drug reactions, and other common causes of abnormal behavior. History of mental illness and substance abuse should be evaluated, as psychiatric disorders and substance withdrawal often manifest with agitation. Ensure those with psychopathology are receiving appropriate prehospitalization medications, and those withdrawing from substances are placed on the appropriate management plan.
2. **Attempt to manage pain and anxiety simultaneously, using an opiate analgesic with sedative effects** Opiates reliably relieve pain, are easily titrated, and have significant sedative effects. *Morphine* is widely administered using intermittent bolus dosing and as a continuous infusion. Morphine may be helpful in relieving hypoxia as it acts as a venodilator to reduce preload to help promote better circulation in heart failure patients, as well as dilating the pulmonary vasculature to assist with gas exchange. In renal failure, dosing should be reduced by 50% due to the accumulation of an active metabolite of morphine. Other opiates commonly used include *hydromorphone* (Dilaudid) and *fentanyl citrate* (Sublimaze). Fentanyl and hydromorphone are rapidly absorbed by the CNS and therefore are more potent than morphine. Fentanyl is the shortest acting opiate and is best used as a continuous infusion. The Society of Critical Care Medicine (SCCM) recommends that fentanyl be used for rapid onset of analgesia and in hemodynamically unstable patients. *Meperidine* (Demerol) is not recommended as a primary analgesic, particularly in older adults and those with renal failure. Patients often report inadequate pain control, while experiencing euphoria. Merperidine accumulates with repeated doses and causes an increased risk of neurotoxicity (see Table 1-29).
3. **Manage agitation using benzodiazepines, antipsychotics, or anesthetic agents (for mechanically ventilated patients), as appropriate for the patient's condition.** The patient's underlying medical condition(s) or pathophysiology markedly affects the choice of sedative agent. If use of an opiate is ineffective, or inappropriate, additional strategies should be explored. Although benzodiazepines are considered a mainstay of agitation management, not all patients respond well to benzodiazepines. Patients who experience adverse reactions are sometimes given larger doses to correct the agitation associated with what is actually drug intolerance. Constant assessment of the patient's response to sedation is needed so appropriate revisions can be made to drug dosage and selection. When patients are placed on sedation, the care team must keep in mind the goal is not solely effective sedation but rather to manage the problem causing the agitation so the patient can be weaned off the sedation.

Benzodiazepines Benzodiazepines may be used to relieve anxiety, promote sleep, and produce sedation via nonspecific CNS depression or via a specific depressant effect on gamma-aminobutyric acid (GABA). Benzodiazepines produce muscle relaxation, which facilitates using a lesser dose of NMBAs if the patient requires paralysis. Dose-related effects on mental status range from relief of anxiety to sedation and coma. All benzodiazepines promote amnesia by preventing memory consolidation. This effect is particularly useful in patients undergoing unpleasant procedures. *Midazolam* (Versed) is considered superior to other benzodiazepines in preventing recall. Safety, ease of use, lack of paradoxic agitation, and lack of recall make benzo-diazepines an attractive choice for sedation in many critical care situations. They are the primary drugs used to alleviate symptoms of acute alcohol withdrawal, which commonly contribute to agitation in the critically ill. However, benzodiazepines do not have analgesic properties present in opiates, so pain should always be ruled out as a cause of agitation prior to using solely benzodiazepines. If present, pain should be treated with analgesics before these drugs are initiated. Table 1-32 describes specific characteristics of the widely used benzodiazepines.

- *Lorazepam (Ativan)*—Commonly given as an intermittent bolus and sometimes used as a continuous infusion, particularly with alcohol withdrawal syndrome (AWS). *Lorazepam* has the slowest onset and the longest duration of action of all benzodiazepines. Lorazepam is metabolized by glucuronidation, as opposed to oxidation as with the other benzodiazepines. Use with AWS is common because liver impairment does not

Table 1-32	**BENZODIAZEPINE CHARACTERISTICS**			
	Benzodiazepines	**Lorazepam (Ativan)**	**Diazepam (Valium)**	**Midazolam (Versed)**
Dosage	Intermittent	0.5–1 mg every 1–2 hours	2.5–5 mg every 3–4 hours	0.15–0.35 mg/kg every 1–2 hours
	Continuous	0.25–6 mg/hr	N/A	0.03–0.22 mg/kg/hr 0.5–4 mcg/kg/min
Pharmacokinetics	Metabolism	Hepatic (glucuronidation)	Hepatic (oxidation)	Hepatic (oxidation)
	Active metabolites	No	Yes	Yes
	Excretion	Renal	Renal	Renal

significantly affect drug metabolism. Lorazepam has no active metabolites, so it is safer for use in renally impaired patients. However, at high doses for prolonged periods of time, hyperosmolality, acidosis, and ATN can occur due to the propylene glycol diluent in which the drug is delivered. Caution should be used when administering lorazepam to older adults, those who are severely ill, and those with limited pulmonary reserve. Despite possible complications, it is the agent of choice for prolonged sedation. Moderately sedated patients should awaken within 30 minutes during the daily sedation vacation. When patients have difficulty awakening during the daily "wake up" assessment, the dosage should be decreased.

- *Diazepam (Valium)*–An older, inexpensive benzodiazepine with a long half-life, which may result in prolonged sedation due to an active metabolite (up to 200 hours after a given dose). *Diazepam* should be avoided in patients with liver dysfunction or severe heart failure because of reduced hepatic clearance. Limited solubility in water restricts use of standard formulation to intermittent IV bolus injections.
- *Midazolam (Versed)* –Short-acting and rapidly metabolized, the drug is particularly useful for short invasive procedures (e.g., bronchoscopy or endoscopy). Because of its short half-life, continuous infusions are required to maintain sedation for longer periods. Delayed drug metabolism in some critically ill patients may lead to extended sedation, particularly with sepsis or hepatic impairment. *Midazolam* is used with caution in renal patients, because some of the active metabolites are renally secreted.
- *Chlordiazepoxide (Librium)*–Sometimes used to manage agitation associated with AWS. Usage significantly decreased when parenteral *chlordiazepoxide* was removed from the US market. Still available orally, it is sometimes used when a longer acting agent is desirable. The active metabolites and complicated metabolic and excretion pathways make the drug undesirable for use in liver impaired patients.

Antipsychotics These are used to reduce agitation in disoriented patients. A component of delirium or psychosis should be identified before use of these agents is initiated. Patients should be well hydrated to avoid hypotension if given parenterally.

- *Haloperidol lactate (Haldol)*–A butyrophenone antipsychotic that is especially helpful in managing psychosis and during withdrawal of sedatives. Incremental bolus doses or continuous infusions are used. The IV route is considered investigational but has been widely used in critically ill patients because onset of action is rapid and extrapyramidal side effects occur less frequently than with the intramuscular (IM) route. Haldol should be given cautiously to patients with severe cardiovascular disorders because of the possibility of transient hypotension and QT prolongation.
- *Chlorpromazine (Thorazine)*–A phenothiazine sometimes used as a sedative, particularly if the patient also displays evidence of psychosis. Chlorpromazine produces alpha-receptor blockade, and hypotension is likely. For this reason and because it generally is less potent than haloperidol, chlorpromazine is not used frequently in critically ill patients.

Atypical Antipsychotics This is a newer generation of antipsychotics that is used to reduce agitation in disoriented patients. These medications are associated with fewer extrapyramidal side effects than haloperidol. A component of delirium or psychosis should be identified prior to use. These medications may be used as part of management of alcohol withdrawal syndrome.

- *Aripiprazole (Abilify)*—Provides sedation via partial agonist activity at dopamine and serotonin (5-HT1A) receptors and antagonist activity at serotonin (5-HT1B) receptors. Also used to manage patients with schizophrenia and bipolar disorders. It is given in a dose of 9.75 mg IM at most every 2 hours to a maximum of 30 mg/day.
- *Ziprasidone (Geodon)*—A piperazine derivative that antagonizes alpha-adrenergic, dopamine, histamine, and serotonin receptors and inhibits reuptake of serotonin and norepinephrine. It is given as 10 mg IM every 2 hours or 20 mg every 4 hours to a maximum of 40 mg/day to diminish depression, mania associated with bipolar disorders, and the symptoms associated with schizophrenia.
- *Olanzapine (Zyprexa)*—This thienobenzodiazepine derivative antagonizes alpha$_1$-adrenergic, dopamine, histamine, muscarinic, and serotonin receptors. It is given as 5 to 10 mg IM every 2 hours to a maximum of 30 mg/day to prompt CNS depression to decrease symptoms associated with schizophrenia and bipolar mania.

Anesthetic Agents Although there is no absolute definition of *anesthesia*, there are four recognized components or levels accomplished by the use of one or more agents—analgesia, amnesia, absence of pathologic reflexes (e.g., vagal response to pain), and lack of purposeful movement. Once restricted to use under the direct supervision of an anesthesiologist in a surgical setting, use of anesthetic agents has been increasingly used in critical care areas to provide sedation for mechanically ventilated patients.

- *Propofol (Diprivan)*—A lipid-based emulsion administered as a titratable, continuous infusion for short-term (several hours to 5 days) sedation for mechanically ventilated patients (Table 1-33). *Propofol* is considered a caloric supplement, containing 1.1 kcal/ml. This should be taken into account when patients are receiving TPN in addition to propofol. When discontinued, patients usually awaken readily with prompt return to baseline mental function. Hemodynamic changes (e.g., vasodilation, decreased MAP) can be minimized by adequate hydration and slow increases in the infusion rate. Propofol is particularly useful for patients with neurologic impairment, because the short action facilitates daily awakening during the sedation vacation to evaluate underlying mental status. The drug is not an analgesic, so pain medication should be prescribed. Effectiveness of pain management should be assessed during daily awakening. Scheduled doses or a continuous infusion of opiate analgesics provide effective pain control when used in combination with propofol. The drug accumulates more readily in obese patients, so dosing should be based on ideal body weight in obese patients. Obese patients are at increased risk for a more prolonged recovery time. Prolonged recovery time may occur with any patient when the infusion is continued for more than 3 days at high doses. Society of Critical Care Medicine (SCCM) guidelines recommend propofol be infused for no longer than 72 hours.
- *Dexmedetomidine (Precedex)*—A newer, more expensive, novel agent with a mechanism of action similar to clonidine. The drug blocks sympathetic outflow through a central alpha stimulation to produce sedation when used as a continuous infusion. Although not an analgesic, *dexmedetomidine* has been shown to have opiate-sparing properties. Level of awareness may be assessed without downward titration of the drip. The drug

Table 1-33	PROPOFOL (DIPRIVAN) CHARACTERISTICS
Dosage*	1–3 mg/kg/hr 5–50 mcg/kg/min
Pharmacokinetics Metabolism Metabolites Excretion Half-life	Hepatic None Renal 1.5–2 hours
Cardiovascular effects	Minimal: 15% ↓BP and MAP (short lived = 15 minutes) (cause: ↓SVR and [−] inotrope)

*Propofol is a sedative-hypnotic at the above recommended dosages but is classified chemically as an anesthetic.

is effective in managing AWS, delirium, and failed extubation and is safe for more extended use (3.5 days). Dexmedetomidine is not associated with respiratory depression but has resulted in hypotension and bradycardia. The drug should be initiated in well-hydrated patients to avoid hypotension. The recommended initial bolus dose may be omitted in borderline hypovolemic patients. SCCM has been more favorable recently in recommending use, despite not discussing the drug extensively in their last published sedation guidelines. Recent labeling changes allow for a new maximum dose of 1 mcg/kg/hr as well as use in nonintubated patients, primarily for procedures.

Neuromuscular Blocking Agents   NMBAs are used when longer periods of complete paralysis are necessary in mechanically ventilated patients. All possible causes of agitation (e.g., pain, fear, suctioning, hypoxemia) must be investigated thoroughly before neuromuscular blockade is initiated. Outside the operating room and other invasive procedural areas, paralysis should be used as "a last resort" to control energy expediture in unstable patients only when all methods of sedation have failed. NMBAs generally are used in the following situations: (1) to decrease O_2 consumption in patients who otherwise cannot obtain satisfactory O_2 saturation; (2) to alleviate specific medical conditions (e.g., status asthmaticus, tetanus, malignant hyperthermia, status epilepticus, acute respiratory distress syndrome [ARDS]); (3) to immobilize patients for surgical and invasive procedures; and (4) to manage increased ICP. NMBA therapy also provides effective management of shivering when deleterious effects occur during therapeutic hypothermia, a newer therapy used to facilitate neurological recovery in post cardiac arrest patients.

- *Depolarizing NMBAs*—Succinylcholine (Anectine) is the only depolarizing NMBA with widespread clinical use. It is used to produce rapid, brief paralysis, most often during emergent intubation. Long-term blockade is not practical because of rapid tachyphylaxis and desensitization of receptors to blocking effects.
- *Nondepolarizing NMBAs*—The class of NMBAs most commonly used for paralysis in critically ill patients. The most common agents used are pancuronium (Pavulon), vecuronium (Norcuron), and cisatracurium (Nimbex). Pharmacokinetic and pharmacodynamic properties of the three agents are listed on Table 1-34. Cisatracurium is the most expensive of the three agents, but its cost is justified by decreased incidence of prolonged paralysis and weakness in patients with severe hepatic and/or renal impairment. The drug is beneficial in patients who require steroids, because it lacks the steroidal structure of other nondepolarizing agents. Steroid-induced myopathy associated with concomitant use of NMBAs and steroids is considered less likely with cisatracurium and will be less severe if it occurs.

Table 1-34	NEUROMUSCULAR BLOCKING AGENT CHARACTERISTICS (NMBA)			
	Neuromuscular Blocking Agents	Pancuronium (Pavulon)	Vecuronium (Norcuron)	Cisatracurium (Nimbex)
Dosage	Intermittent	0.04–0.1 mg/kg every 1 hr PRN	0.01–0.015 mg/kg every 15 min	0.03 mg/kg every 15 min
	Continuous	1–1.6 mcg/kg/min	0.8–1.2 mcg/kg/min	0.5–10 mcg/kg/min
Pharmacokinetics	Metabolism Excretion	Renal > hepatic renal	Hepatic > renal Renal (15%) Biliary (30%–50%)	Hoffman (organ independent) Elimination
	Metabolites (active or toxic)	Yes	Yes	No
	Half-life (elimination)	132–257 min (2–4 hr)	80–97 min	22–29 min
Cardiovascular effects		Moderate ↑HR, ↓BP, ↑CO	Minimal <1% ↑HR, ↓BP	None on HR and MAP

Numerous medications and several disease states augment or antagonize neuromuscular blockade (Box 1-18). The patient should be monitored throughout therapy for conditions affecting neuromuscular blockade.

Clinicians should determine a therapeutic endpoint or goal for paralysis and titrate neuromuscular blockade to achieve that goal. Examples of therapeutic endpoints are decreases in peak inspiratory pressure or decreases in O_2 consumption. Negative endpoints include development of extreme weakness or inability to move. Monitoring the degree of neuromuscular blockade is essential. *It cannot be overemphasized that NMBAs provide no analgesia or anxiolysis. All patients receiving NMBAs must also have therapy with continuously dosed opiates and anxiolytics.*

CARE PLANS FOR SEDATION AND NEUROMUSCULAR BLOCKADE

Anxiety   *related to actual or perceived threat of death; change in health status; threat to self-concept or role; unfamiliar people or environment; the unknown*

GOALS/OUTCOMES Within 4 to 6 hours of initiating therapy, the patient's anxiety is diminished as evidenced by verbalization of same, HR less than 100 bpm, RR less than 20 breaths/min, and decrease in restlessness and extraneous motor movement.
NOC Anxiety Self-Control

Anxiety Reduction
1. Carefully assess for and correct factors contributing to anxiety (see Box 1-17).
2. Ensure pathophysiology is not overlooked as the cause of anxiety or agitation.
3. Provide emotional and spiritual support for the patient and family, especially if the patient requires neuromuscular blockade (see *Emotional and Spiritual Support of the Patient and Significant Others,* p. 200).
4. Evaluate adequacy of pain control. Administer opiate or other analgesics in appropriate doses on a schedule or through a continuous infusion (see *Pain* p. 135).
5. Initiate nonpharmacologic measures to reduce anxiety (see Box 1-15).
6. Assess patient using a recognized agitation assessment tool (see *Alterations in Consciousness* p. 24).
7. If administering a short-acting benzodiazepine in small doses at frequent intervals, monitor carefully for excessive sedation and respiratory depression. Have flumazenil (Romazicon) immediately available for reversal of drug effects.

| **Box 1-18** | **DRUGS AND PHYSIOLOGIC CONDITIONS THAT AFFECT NMBAs** |

Drugs that augment neuromuscular blockade	**Physiologic conditions that increase neuromuscular blockade**
Aminoglycoside antibiotics	Acidosis
Bretylium	Dehydration
Calcium channel blockers	Hypercalcemia
Clindamycin	Hypermagnesemia
Cyclosporine	Hypocalcemia
Lidocaine	Hypokalemia
Procainamide	Hyponatremia
Propranolol	Hypothermia
Quinidine	Myasthenia gravis
Vancomycin	
Drugs that antagonize neuromuscular blockade	**Physiologic conditions that decrease neuromuscular blockade**
Anticholinesterase agents	Alkalosis
Azathioprine	Decreased peripheral perfusion
Carbamazepine	Hyperkalemia
Corticosteroids	Hypernatremia
Phenytoin	
Ranitidine	
Theophylline	

8. If anxiety is profound and associated with sensory/perceptual alterations (e.g., hallucinations), consider use of an antipsychotic agent. Ensure adequate hydration before use, and monitor closely for hypotension.
9. For patients undergoing neuromuscular blockade, provide careful monitoring of level of blockade, coupled with effectiveness of sedation and pain management. Use either a peripheral nerve stimulator, bispectral analysis, or a drug holiday to help with the assessment.

Impaired gas exchange (or risk for same) *related to decreased O_2 supply secondary to decreased ventilatory drive occurring with sedative use and CNS depression or secondary to decreased chest wall movement occurring with residual neuromuscular blockade*

GOALS/OUTCOMES Within 1 hour of intervention, patient has adequate gas exchange as evidenced by orientation to time, place, and person; $Pao_2 \geq 80$ mm Hg; $Paco_2$ 24 to 30 mm Hg; $Spo_2 \geq 90$; and RR 12 to 20 breaths/min with normal depth and pattern.
NOC Respiratory Status: Gas Exchange

Ventilation Assistance
1. Assess patient's respiratory rate, depth, and rhythm at least hourly when heavily sedated. Fully sedated patients require continuous direct monitoring until VS are stable and protective reflexes (e.g., gag reflexes) are present.
2. Anesthetic agents should only be used as part of sedation on mechanically ventilated patients to avoid the risk of apnea.
3. Provide appropriate care related to mechanical ventilation (see Mechanical Ventilation pp. 99.)
4. If NMBAs are used, assess depth of paralysis using peripheral nerve stimulator or bispectral analysis (BIS monitoring). Titrate dose to maintain desired level of paralysis (see Table 1-31).
5. Provide a daily sedation vacation and/or drug holiday to assess level of consciousness, ability to initiate spontaneous breaths, and ability to remain stable off sedation and/or neuromuscular blockade.
6. Continuously monitor Spo_2 via pulse oximetry.
7. Alternatively, monitor chest wall movement via apnea monitor.
8. Have appropriate antidote (e.g., naloxone for opiates, flumazenil for benzodiazepines, and pyridostigmine and atropine for NMBAs) and airway management equipment immediately available.
9. Position patient to promote full lung expansion, and turn patient to mobilize sputum.

Deficient knowledge *related to lack of recall, related to interrupted memory consolidation secondary to benzodiazepine use*

GOALS/OUTCOMES Within 12 hours of cessation of benzodiazepine therapy, patient recalls information essential to self-protection and self-care.
NOC Knowledge: Treatment Procedures

Teaching: Procedure/Treatment
1. Remind patient and family that recall of unpleasant procedures (e.g., cardioversion, endoscopy) will be diminished and that this is a desired effect of the medication.
2. Reinforce necessary information (e.g., NPO instructions, need to call for assistance when changing positions, need for deep breathing) with patient and family at frequent intervals until comprehension is demonstrated.
3. Review outcome or findings of procedure with patient as necessary until patient expresses satisfactory understanding.

ADDITIONAL NURSING DIAGNOSIS
Additional nursing care plans are available in *Alterations in Consciousness* (p. 24), *Pain* (p. 135), and *Emotional and Spiritual Support of the Patient and Significant Others* (p. 200).

WOUND AND SKIN CARE

A wound is a disruption of tissue integrity caused by trauma, surgery, or an underlying medical disorder. Wound management is designed to promote healing, prevent infection, and/or reduce deterioration in wound status. Renewed emphasis on the role of nurses in prevention of pressure ulcers is evident in the current Centers for Medicare and Medicaid Services (CMS) standards of care.

Government-regulated programs will no longer pay for the occurrence of pressure ulcers that occur after an admission to an acute care hospital. Pressure ulcers are considered "avoidable" problems within the health care system. If a pressure ulcer is "present on admission" documented by a clinician who diagnoses and treats, the hospital will be entitled to more monies for Stage 3 and Stage 4 pressure ulcers.

There are reliable and valid risk assessment tools to be used in the prevention of pressure ulcer–type wounds: the Braden and Norton scales are the two most recognized tools. Due to the emphasis on prevention of avoidable pressure ulcers and the accompanying economic impact through recently mandated fiscal restraints, more effort is being placed on prevention. Norton scores of 14 are indicative of "onset of risk"; ≤12 indicates "high risk." Braden scores of 18 to 16 indicate moderate risk, and 12 is high risk. There is a question as to the prediction of pressure ulcers in older black and Hispanic adults, indicating the need for more research. Braden and the National Guideline written for the Hartford Institute for Geriatric Nursing suggest using ≤18 for older adults and those with skin of color.

WOUNDS CLOSED BY PRIMARY INTENTION

Clean surgical or traumatic wounds whose edges are closed with sutures, clips, sterile tape strips, or wound glue are referred to as wounds closed by *primary intention*. Impairment of healing most frequently manifests as dehiscence, evisceration, infection, or delayed healing. Individuals at high risk for disruption of wound healing include those who are obese, diabetic, older, malnourished, receiving steroids, immunosuppressed, undergoing chemotherapy or radiation therapy, or receiving vasopressors. Coexistent infections at another body site and colonization with microorganisms such as methicillin-resistant *Staphylococcus aureus* (MRSA) are factors that may contribute to the development of infection. There is a continuum of contamination of wounds from colonized to critically colonized to infection. Recognition of biofilms (matrices that envelop and protect microbial growth) that inhibit efficacy of antibiotics and healing have been recognized.

ASSESSMENT
Optimal Wound Healing
Immediately after surgical injury, the incision line is warm, reddened, indurated, and tender. Inflammation normally subsides in 3 to 5 days. A healing ridge, the rete ridge, is a palpable accumulation of downward projections of the epidermis that forms by day 7 to 9 after injury. In patients who undergo cosmetic surgery, a healing ridge is purposely avoided to minimize scar formation (Table 1-35).

Impaired Healing
Impaired healing is recognized by the lack of an adequate inflammatory response surrounding a wound, continued drainage from an incision line 2 days after injury (when no drain is present), absence of a healing ridge by day 9 after injury, and presence of purulent drainage (see Table 1-35). A chronic wound is one that fails to proceed to healing within a reasonable time, usually 3 months. Assessment includes the presence of the wound by anatomic location, measurements, length of time existent, percent of viable tissue versus necrotic tissue, exudate characteristics by amount, color, presence of odor, and condition of the periwound tissue. Inclusion of previous treatments that were unsuccessful is helpful to expedite more appropriate treatments.

Diagnostic Tests During Wound Healing		
Test	Purpose	Abnormal Findings
Complete blood count (CBC) with differential	Assess for discrepancies in red blood cells, white blood cells, and hemoglobin, platelet count	Low red blood cells and hemoglobin will decrease oxygen to the wound. Platelet count: high will increase risk of clot. Low platelets will add to the risk of abnormal bleeding White blood cells that are high indicate infection. Low white blood cells will impede fighting infection.

Continued

Diagnostic Tests During Wound Healing—cont'd

Test	Purpose	Abnormal Findings
Protein levels: total protein, albumin, and prealbumin	Protein levels assist with the regulation of fluid in the body as well as aid in nourishing the cells	Total protein below 6–8.3 g/dl Albumin below 3.5 g/dl predisposes pt to increased risk of pressure ulcer. Prealbumin below 15 needs nutrition consult. Do weekly testing for trends. Low numbers indicate need for nutritional supplementation as long as liver disease does not contraindicate addition of protein.
Gram stain wound/culture	Indicate the presence of microbes and infection	Gram stain indicates the broad class of organism. Culture takes 48 hours, will be more specific to the organism and sensitivity of antibiotics. Infection is measured by 10^5 count of a pathogen.

COLLABORATIVE MANAGEMENT
Care Priorities for Surgical Wounds Healing by Primary Intention

1. *Application of a sterile dressing in surgery or at the time of injury*—To protect wound from external contamination or trauma or provide pressure. Usually, surgeon or advanced practice nurse changes the initial dressing.
2. *Nutrition (oral diet, enteral nutrition, PN)*—To provide sufficient nutrients for wound healing.
3. *Multivitamins (all but especially C) and minerals (especially zinc and iron)*—To correct any deficits and support healing.
4. *Pain control*—To maximize subcutaneous blood flow to the wound to support healing.
5. *Insulin*—As needed to control glucose levels in individuals with diabetes mellitus or hyperglycemia from other causes (e.g., steroid therapy, TPN, enteral nutrition). Hyperglycemia may delay healing. Critically ill patients often develop insulin resistance, resulting in hyperglycemia.
6. *Local or systemic antibiotics*—Given when infection is present and sometimes used prophylactically for a limited period of time.

Safety Alert *To decrease the occurrence of resistant microbes, prophylactic antibiotics are to be discontinued within 24 hours after the time the surgery is completed. Specific orders have to be written for continuation (Source: Centers for Medicare and Medicaid Services [CMS]).*

Table 1-35	ASSESSMENT OF HEALING OF WOUNDS CLOSED BY PRIMARY INTENTION
Expected Findings	**Abnormal Findings**
Edges well approximated	Edges not well approximated
Good inflammatory response (redness, warmth, induration, pain) lasting 3–5 days	Decreased inflammatory response or inflammatory response that lasts more than 5 days after injury
No drainage (without drain present) 2 days after closure	Drainage continues more than 2 days after injury
Healing ridge present by postinjury day 7–9	No healing ridge present by day 9
	Hypertrophic scar or keloid present

7. *Antiseptics*—Dakins at ¼% may be used for a limited time to clean microbes from a wound bed. Dressings with antiseptic capability may also be used such as cadexomer iodine or silver dressings. Commercial products are on the market such as TechniCare, which is a cleanser with antiseptic capability.

8. *Incision and drainage*—To drain pus when infection is present and localized. Healing occurs by secondary intention. The wound may be irrigated to flush out organisms.

CARE PLANS FOR WOUND HEALING BY PRIMARY INTENTION

Impaired tissue integrity: Wound *related to altered circulation; metabolic disorders (e.g., diabetes mellitus); alterations in fluid volume and nutrition; medical therapy (chemotherapy, radiation therapy, steroid administration)*

GOALS/OUTCOMES Patient exhibits the following signs of wound healing: well-approximated wound edges, good initial postinjury inflammatory response (erythema, warmth, induration, pain), no inflammatory response after the fifth day after injury, no drainage (without drain present) 48 hours after closure, and healing ridge present by postoperative day 7 to 9. Tissue integrity is restored.

NOC Tissue Integrity: Skin and Mucous Membranes

Wound Care

1. Assess wound for indications of impaired healing, including absence of a healing ridge, presence of drainage or purulent exudate, and delayed or prolonged inflammatory response. Monitor VS and labwork for signs of infection, including elevated temperature, HR, and WBC. Document findings.

2. Use standard (universal) precautions and follow proper infection-control techniques when changing dressings. If a drain is present, maintain patency, and handle it gently to prevent it from becoming dislodged. If wound care will be necessary after hospital discharge, teach the dressing change procedure to the patient and significant others. Include the use of home health agency nurses to continue care after discharge as needed.

3. For persons with hyperglycemia, perform serial monitoring of blood glucose and administer insulin to keep glucose level in a normal range or the range recommended by the guidelines of the facility.

4. Explain to patient that deep breathing promotes oxygenation, which enhances wound healing. Stress the importance of smoking cessation. Stress the importance of position changes and activity as tolerated to promote ventilation. Splint incision as needed.

5. Monitor volume status by checking BP, HR, and capillary refill time in the tissue adjacent to incision, moisture of mucous membranes, skin turgor, and I&O.

6. For nonrestricted patients, ensure a fluid intake of at least 2 to 3 L/day.

7. To provide nutrients for healing, provide a diet with adequate protein, calories, vitamins, and minerals. Encourage between-meal supplements and give frequent small feedings as needed.

SURGICAL OR TRAUMATIC WOUNDS HEALING BY SECONDARY INTENTION

Wounds healing by *secondary intention* are those with tissue loss or heavy contamination that form granulation tissue and contract to heal. Most often, impairment of healing is caused by increased contamination and impairment of perfusion, oxygenation, and nutrition, which results in a delay in the healing process. Individuals at risk for impaired healing include those who are obese, diabetic, malnourished, older, receiving steroids, immunosuppressed, undergoing radiation therapy or chemotherapy, or receiving vasopressors.

ASSESSMENT
Optimal Healing
Initially, the wound edges are inflamed, indurated, and tender. Pale granulation tissue on the floor and walls progresses to a deeper pink and then to a beefy red; it should be moist. Epithelial cells from the tissue surrounding the wound gradually migrate across the granulation tissue. As healing occurs, the wound edges become pink and wound contraction occurs. When present, a tract or sinus gradually decreases in size as healing occurs. The time frame for healing depends on the size and location of the wound, as well as on the patient's physical and psychological status (Table 1-36).

Table 1-36	ASSESSMENT OF HEALING OF WOUNDS CLOSING BY SECONDARY INTENTION
Expected Findings	**Abnormal Findings**
Granulation tissue initially pale and moist and then becomes pink and beefy red over time	Granulation tissue remains pale or is excessively dry or moist
No odor	Abnormal odor
No slough or necrotic tissue	Slough or necrotic tissue
No tunneling or undermining	Tunneling or undermining Pain Wound breakdown

Impaired Healing

Exudate, slough, and necrotic material appear on the floor and walls of the wound and do not abate as healing progresses. Note their distribution, color, odor, volume, and adherence. The periwound skin is assessed for signs of tissue damage, including disruption, discoloration, and increasing pain. When a drain is in place, the volume, color, and odor of the drainage are evaluated. See Table 1-36.

DIAGNOSTIC TESTS

See discussion on *Wounds Closed by Primary Intention*, p. 167.

Test	Purpose	Abnormal Findings
Culture	Test for the presence of infection	Bacterial pathogen growth greater than 10^5 indicates infection
Biopsy	To rule out the presence of cancer or dermatologic diagnosis	Cancer cells would necessitate oncology consult; dermatologic findings would necessitate a dermatology consult. Incorrect diagnosis of wound etiology can have untoward delay in treatment.

COLLABORATIVE MANAGEMENT
Care Priorities

1. *Débride slough and necrotic tissue:* To remove dead tissue, use surgical or sharp débridement for rapid removal and enzymatic (e.g., Santyl) or autolytic (e.g., hydrocolloid dressing) for slower removal.
2. *Infection:* Use systemic antibiotics specific to the pathogen. Each time wound care is provided, wound cleansing should be performed. This is to remove waste products and to dislodge and remove bacteria, necrotic tissue, foreign bodies, and exudate.
3. *Moisture:* Wound beds must be moist but neither too dry nor too wet. Dressing choices must meet this need; vigilance to changes in a wound is necessary. Dressings are to keep healthy wound tissue moist; some provide an antiseptic agent to decrease wound surface bacterial counts or débride the wound (Table 1-37).
4. *Edges:* Wound edges may curl downward, effectively stalling healing. This is called epiboly. Surgical or chemical irritants such as silver nitrate may be used to correct epiboly.
5. *Fluids (oral/IV):* Ensure adequate intravascular volume to support healing.
6. *Topical or systemic vitamin A:* As needed, use to reverse adverse effects of steroids on healing.
7. *Drain(s):* Remove excess tissue fluid or purulent drainage. Closed end drains are preferable to open drains due to infection control.
8. *Negative pressure wound therapy:* Draw together the edges of the wound, reduce edema, increase blood flow, remove exudate, and stimulate granulation tissue formation.
9. *Skin graft/cultured keratinocytes/cultured skin substitute:* Provide coverage of wound if necessary.

Table 1-37	DRESSINGS USED FOR WOUND CARE	
Dressing	**Advantages**	**Disadvantages**
Transparent dressing (e.g., Op-Site, Tegaderm, Bioclusive)	Transparent so can view wound; prevents loss of wound fluid; protects from external contamination; protects from friction and shear. Can use as secondary dressing over another type.	Nonabsorptive, may result in maceration of periwound tissue.
Hydrocolloid (e.g., Duoderm, Restore, Cutinova)	Maintains moist wound surface while minimizing pooling; facilitates autolytic débridement; easy to apply, reduces pain.	Cannot be used with heavily draining wounds; opaque; exudates present on removal may be confused with infection; some roll.
Hydrogel (e.g., Curasol, Nu-gel, Vigilon, Saf-gel)	Nonadherent; rehydrates wound; minimizes pain; can be used with infected wounds.	Cannot be used with heavily draining wounds; may macerate periwound skin.
Foam (e.g., Mepilex, Allevyn, Hydrosorb, Lyofoam)	Absorptive; nontraumatic; easy to apply and remove.	Not intended for dry wounds; may require tape or secondary dressing to secure. Has no pressure reduction capability.
Alginates (e.g., Kaltostat, Sorbsan)	Highly absorbent; can use on infected wounds; remove without trauma to wound.	Cannot be used for dry wounds; requires secondary dressing; may have foul odor when removed.
Gauze (e.g., 2 × 2, 4 × 4, roller gauze)	Inexpensive; easy to use; ideal for packing wound.	May result in tissue maceration if inserted too moist; may result in tissue disruption if allowed to dry out.
Composites (e.g., Alldress, Telfa Plus)	Use for partial to full-thickness wounds.	Adhesive borders may disrupt surrounding skin. Composite dressings come in a variety of sizes, may be difficult to carry a large supply.
Silver dressings available in all forms of advanced dressings from foam to gels	Antiseptic capability while in the wound. Different manufacturers will identify the length of time their dressing has in continuing to shed silver.	Allergies to silver. Rare cases of issues of tattooing have been noted. Silver ions will be deactivated by some solutions.

10. *Tissue flap:* Fill tissue defect and provide wound closure with its own blood supply. Requires specialty bed surface to minimize pressure on operative flap.
11. *Growth factors:* These are naturally occurring proteins that stimulate new cell formation (e.g., platelet-derived growth factor, insulin).
12. *Hyperbaric O_2:* Use with difficult wounds to support oxidative processes in healing.
13. *Diet to maintain weight at optimal body mass index, multivitamins and minerals, insulin, pain control, supplemental O_2, antibiotics, and incision and drainage:* See discussion on Wounds Closed by Primary Intention, p. 167.

CARE PLANS FOR WOUNDS HEALING BY SECONDARY INTENTION

Impaired tissue integrity *Wound, related to presence of contaminants; metabolic disorders (e.g., diabetes mellitus); medical therapy (e.g., chemotherapy, radiation therapy); altered perfusion; immunosuppression; malnutrition*

- -

GOALS/OUTCOMES Patient's wound exhibits the following signs of healing: initially, postinjury wound edges are inflamed, indurated, and tender; epithelialization begins. In primary healing, there should be no exudate and healing is observed within 48 hours. In secondary healing, edges become pink; granulation tissue develops and there is no odor or necrotic tissue. Exudate is minimal. Patient or significant other successfully demonstrates wound care procedure before hospital discharge, if appropriate.

NOC Wound Healing: Secondary Intention

Wound Care
1. Monitor for the following signs of impaired healing: decreased inflammatory response or inflammatory response that lasts more than 5 days; epithelialization slowed or mechanically disrupted; granulation tissue remains pale or excessively dry or moist; and presence of odor, exudate, necrotic tissue, pain, and/or wound breakdown. The edges of the wound show epiboly or premature skin cells closing the surface edge.
2. Apply prescribed dressings (see Table 1-37). Insert dressing into all tracts to promote gradual closure of those areas. Do not pack the wounds with dressings; fill the wound without pressure. Ensure good hand washing before and after dressing changes, and dispose of contaminated dressings appropriately.
3. When a drain is used, maintain its patency, prevent kinking of the tubing, and secure the tubing to prevent the drain from becoming dislodged.
4. To help prevent contamination, cleanse the skin surrounding the wound with soap and water. Use minimal friction with cleansing if tissue is friable.
5. Wound cleansing requires applying high-pressure irrigation using a 35-ml syringe with an 18-gauge angiocath. Commercial wound cleansers have the necessary pressure between 4 and 15 pounds per square inch (psi) built into the spray nozzle. If the tissue is friable or the wound is over a major organ or blood vessel, use extreme caution with the irrigation pressure. To remove contaminants effectively, use a large volume of irrigant (e.g., 100–150 ml).
6. When topical enzymes are prescribed, follow package directions carefully. Be aware that some agents, such as povidone-iodine, deactivate the enzymes. Protect undamaged skin with zinc oxide, aluminum hydroxide paste, or skin sealant.
7. Teach patient or significant other the prescribed wound care procedure, if indicated.

PRESSURE ULCERS

Pressure ulcers are a disruption in tissue integrity and are caused by excessive tissue pressure or shearing of blood vessels. High-risk patients include older adults and those who have decreased mobility, decreased LOC, impaired sensation, debilitation, incontinence, sepsis/elevated temperature, malnutrition, third-spacing, or interstitial edema or are receiving vasopressors or treatment with invasive devices that restrict mobility. Diseases that impact the occurrence and ability to heal are diabetes, cardiopulmonary disease, hemotologic diseases, obesity, peripheral vascular diseases, GI diseases affecting the ability to absorb nutrients, and cancers.

ASSESSMENT: PRESSURE ULCER RISK AND STAGING ULCERS

High-risk individuals should be identified on admission assessment, with daily assessments during hospitalization, using a standard assessment tool. Daily use of the Braden or Norton scale with special attention to the parameter indicating danger of the development of a pressure ulcer is indicated. Recommended preventive measures should be implemented when the patient at risk is identified.

When pressure ulcers are present, their severity can be staged on a scale of I to IV and unstageable. The following definitions are from the National Pressure Ulcer Advisory Panel amended to meet the criteria set by the CMS.

> **Safety Alert** *The National Pressue Ulcer Advisory Panel separates "deep tissue injury" as a distinct stage of pressure ulcer. CMS incorporates "deep tissue injury" into the "unstageable" category of pressure ulcers.*

Stage I
Nonblanchable erythema of intact skin usually over a boney prominence. In dark-skinned individuals, discoloration of the skin compared with surrounding skin, difference in the temperature of the involved skin compared with the surrounding, edema, and induration (hardness) may be the only indication of a stage I pressure ulcer.

Stage II
Partial-thickness skin loss that involves epidermis and/or dermis; seen as an abrasion, blister, or shallow crater. This stage may present as a blister that is intact with clear contents. There will not be slough or bruising. Correct staging of stage II does not include perineal dermatitis, skin tears, maceration, or rashes.

Stage III

Full-thickness skin loss that involves subcutaneous tissue but does not extend through fascia. Slough, tracts, and/or undermining may be present. The bridge of the nose, ears, ankles, and occiput are more likely to be stage III due to lack of significant subcutaneous tissue. Bone, tendon, or muscle is not involved.

Stage IV

Full-thickness injury that involves muscle, bone, or supporting structures. There may be tracts and/ or undermining. Slough or eschar may be present. Due to proximity when bone is palpable, osteomyelitis must be considered.

See *Surgical or Traumatic Wounds Healing by Secondary Intention*, p. 167, for other assessment data.

Unstageable

The base of the wound is not visible due to the presence of necrotic tissue, eschar, or slough. Until the necrotic tissue is removed, the stage of the ulcer is unknown. Stable, dry eschar on the heel is not to be removed due to its capacity for providing a barrier. CMS considers the occurrence of deep tissue injury to be a form of unstageable pressure ulcers. Deep tissue injury is described as unbroken skin with the appearance of bruising, purple or maroon coloration. A blood-filled blister is considered unstageable.

DIAGNOSTIC TESTS

See *Diagnostic Tests*, p. 158.

COLLABORATIVE MANAGEMENT

See *Collaborative Management* in *Surgical Wounds Healing by Primary Intention* (p. 168) and *Collaborative Management* in *Surgical or Traumatic Wounds Healing by Secondary Intention* (p. 169).

CARE PLANS FOR PREVENTION AND MANAGEMENT OF PRESSURE ULCERS

 Impaired tissue integrity (or risk for same) *related to excessive tissue pressure; shearing forces; altered circulation. Presence of pressure ulcer with increased risk for breakdown, related to altered circulation; presence of contaminants or irritants (chemical, thermal, mechanical)*

- -

GOALS/OUTCOMES High risk: patient's tissue remains intact. After intervention/instructions, patient/caregiver verbalizes causes and preventive measures for pressure ulcers and successfully participates in the plan of care to promote healing and prevent further breakdown if a pressure ulcer is present. Ulcers present are granulating and decreasing in size. There is no slough tissue, necrotic tissue, or odor present.

NOC Tissue Integrity: Skin and Mucous Membranes

Pressure Management
1. Identify individuals at risk, and systematically assess skin over bony prominences daily; document.
2. Establish and post a position-changing schedule.
3. Assist patient with turning every 1 to 2 hours. Use pillows or foam wedges to prevent direct pressure on bony prominences. Patients with a history of previous tissue injury will require pressure relief measures more frequently. Because high-Fowler's position results in increased shearing, use low-Fowler's position and alternate supine position with prone and 30-degree elevated side-lying positions.

> **Safety Alert** *CMS has addressed the problem of ventilator-acquired pneumonia (VAP) as an avoidable condition. The plan of care to avoid pneumonia incorporates the positioning of the patient with elevation of the HOB at 30 degrees or above. The clinician will make a determination as to the need of the individual patient and height of the HOB.*

4. For immobile patients, float the heels using pillows inserted under the length of the calf.
5. Minimize friction on tissue during activity. Lift rather than drag patient during position changes and transferring; use a draw sheet to facilitate patient movement. Ideally, patient should be moved using minimal lift equipment to prevent injury from friction and shearing as friable skin "drags" over the sheets. Do not massage over bony prominences.
6. Minimize skin exposure to moisture. Cleanse at the time of soiling and at routine intervals. Use moisture barriers and underpads with minimization of disposable briefs.
7. Use an overlay or mattress that reduces pressure, such as foam, alternating air, or gel. Make decision based on the weight of the patient, stage of the ulcer(s), and appropriateness of the surface to the patient.

Pressure Ulcer Care
1. Evaluate stage of pressure ulcer. See *Assessment*, p. 172.
2. Maintain a moist physiologic environment to promote tissue repair and minimize contaminants. Change dressings as prescribed.
3. Be sure patient's skin is kept clean with regular bathing, and be especially conscientious about washing urine and feces from the skin. Commercially prepared wipes are available. If soap must be used, then thoroughly rinse from the skin.
4. If the patient has excessive perspiration, ensure frequent cleansing and change bedding as needed.
5. To absorb moisture and prevent shearing when the patient is moved, apply heel and elbow covers as needed. Socks on the feet are appropriate, with removal for hygiene and replacement afterward.
6. Teach patient and significant others the importance of and measures for preventing excess pressure as a means of treating pressure ulcers.
7. Use an overlay or mattress that reduces pressure, such as foam, alternating air, or gel or air fluidized bed. Make decision based on the weight of the patient, stage of the ulcer(s), and appropriateness of the surface to the patient.

NIC Skin Surveillance; Incision Site Care; Wound Care; Pressure Ulcer Care; Pressure Ulcer Prevention; Wound Irrigation

ADDITIONAL NURSING DIAGNOSES
Also see the following:
Impaired tissue integrity under Surgical or Traumatic Wounds Healing by Secondary Intention, p. 169.
Pain Management; Pain decreasing with cutaneous stimulation
Deficient Knowledge related to care of wound/pressure ulcer
Imbalanced Nutrition, less than body requirements for wound healing

SELECTED REFERENCES
Agency for Health Care Policy and Research (AHCPR): *Pressure ulcers in adults: prediction and prevention*. Rockville, MD: US Department of Health and Human services, Public Health Service, May 1992, Clinical practice guideline 3, Pub. No. 92-0047.

Aizawa K, Kanai T, Saikawa Y, et al: A novel approach to post-operative delirium in older adults after gastrointestinal surgery. *Surg Today* 32(4):310–314, 2002.

American Association of Cardiovascular and Pulmonary Rehabilitation: *Guidelines for cardiac rehabilitation and secondary prevention programs*, ed 4. Champaign, IL, 2004, Human Kinetics.

American College of Radiology: ACR practice guideline for adult sedation/analgesia. Retrieved November 15, 2009, from http://www.acr.org/SecondaryMainMenuCategories/quality_safety/guidelines/iv/adult_sedation.aspx

American Society of Anesthesiologists Task Force on Pulmonary Artery Catheterization: Practice guidelines for pulmonary artery catheterization: an updated report by the American Society of Anesthesiologists Task Force on Pulmonary Artery Catheterization, *Anesthesiology* 99(4): 988–1014, 2003.

American Society of Anesthesiology: Practice guidelines for sedation and analgesia by non-anesthesiologists. *Anesthesiology* 96:1004–1017, 2002. http://www.asahq.org/publicationsAndServices/sedation1017.pdf

Arbour R: Continuous nervous system monitoring, EEG, the bispectral index and neuromuscular transmission. *AACN Clin Issues* 14(2):185–207, 2003.

Ayello EA, Sibbald RG: Preventing pressure ulcers and skin tears. In Capezuti E, Zwicker D, Mezey M, Fulmer T, editors: *Evidence-based geriatric nursing protocols for best practice*, ed 3. New York, 2008, Springer, pp. 403–429.

Baranoski S, Ayello EA: *Wound care essentials: practice principles*. Springhouse, PA, 2004, Lippincott Williams & Wilkins, pp. 54–58.

Bednash G, Ferrell BR: *End-of-life nursing education consortium (ELNEC) faculty guide*. Duarte, CA, 2007, American Association of Colleges of Nursing and City of Hope National Medical Center.

Bergeron N, Dubois M-J, Dumont M, Dial S, Skrobik Y: Intensive care delirium screening checklist: evaluation of a new screening tool. *Intens Care Med* 27(5):859–864, 2001.

Bergstom N, Braden B, Kemp M, et al: Predicting pressure ulcer risk: a multisite study of the predictive validity of the Braden Scale. *Nurs Res* 47(5):261–269, 1998.

Bernard G, et al: Pulmonary artery catheterization and clinical outcomes: National Heart, Lung, and Blood Institute and Food and Drug Administration Workshop Report. Consensus statement. *JAMA* 283:2568–2572, 2000.

Borg GA: Psychophysical basis of perceived exertion. *Med Sci Sports Exerc* 14(5):377–381, 1982.

Bourgault AM, Ipe L, Weaver J, et al: Development of evidence-based guidelines and critical care nurses' knowledge of enteral feeding. *Crit Care Nurs* 27:17–29, 2007.

Bryant R, Nix D: *Acute and chronic wounds: current management concepts*, ed 3. St. Louis, 2007, Mosby.

Bulechek GB, Butcher HK, Dochterman JM, editors: *Nursing interventions classification (NIC)*, ed 5. St. Louis, 2008, Mosby.

Cao P, Kimura S, Macias BR, et al: Exercise within lower body negative pressure partially counteracts lumbar spine deconditioning associated with 28 day bed rest. *J Appl Physiol* 99(1):39–44, 2005.

Centers for Medicare and Medicaid Services (CMS): *Guidance for surveyors in long term care: pressure ulcers*. Baltimore, MD, 2004, CMS.

Centers for Medicare and Medicaid Services: Federal Register Part II.42 CFR Parts 411, 412, 413, 489. Changes to the hospital inpatient prospective payment systems and fiscal year 2008 rates. Final rule. *Fed Register* 72(162):47201–47205, 2007.

Chioffi SM, Macy GE, Meek LG, Cook HA: Olson diabetes mellitus. Potential benefits of bispectral index monitoring in critical care. *Crit Care Nurse* 23(4):45–51, 2003.

Cintron A, Morrison RS: Pain and ethnicity in the United States: a systematic review. *J Palliat Med* 9(6):1454–1473, 2006.

Coffin SC, Klompas M, Classen D, et al: Strategies to prevent ventilator associated pneumonia in acute care hospitals. *Infect Control Hosp Epidemiol* 29(suppl 1):S31–S40, 2008.

Critical Care Nutrition: Early vs delayed nutrient intake. January 8, 2007. Retrieved November 10, 2009, from http://ccn.cissec.com/cpg/2.0_early_07.pdf.

Daily E, Schroeder J: *Techniques in bedside hemodynamic monitoring*, ed 4. St. Louis, 1989, Mosby.

Darovic G: *Hemodynamic monitoring, invasive and noninvasive clinical application*, Philadelphia, 2002, Saunders.

Deglin JH, Vallerand AH: *Davis's Drug guide for nurses*, ed 11. Philadelphia, 2009, FA Davis.

Devlin J, Fong J, Schumaker G, O'Connor H, Ruthazer R, Garpestad E: *Crit Care Med* 35(12):2721–2724, 2007.

Diehl T, Ambrose M, Goldgerg K, Howard J, Mayer B, editors: *Fluid and electrolyte in medical surgical nursing made incredibly easy*. Philadelphia, 2004, Lippincott Williams and Wilkins.

Ferrell B, Coyle N: *Textbook of palliative nursing*, ed 2. New York, 2006, Oxford University Press.

Fleisher L, et al: ACC/AHA 2007 guidelines on perioperative cardiovascular evaluation and care for noncardiac surgery. *J Am Coll Cardiol* 50(17):e159–e241, 2007.

Fluid and electrolytes made incredibly easy, ed 2. Pennsylvania, 2002, Springhouse.

Fukagawa M, Kurokawa K, Papadakis M: Fluid and electrolyte disorders. In Tierney L, McPhee S, Papadakis M, editors: *Current medical diagnosis and treatment*, ed 43. New York, 2004, Lange Medical Books/McGraw-Hill.

Geerts WH, Bergqvist D, et al: Prevention of venous thromboembolism. *Chest* 133:6, 2008.

Prevention of Venous Thromboembolism, Supplement, Antithrombotic and Thrombolytic Therapy, 8th Ed: ACCP Guidelines.

Gelinas C: Management of pain in cardiac surgery intensive care unit patients: Have we improved over time? *Intens Crit Care Nursing* 23:298–303, 2007.

Herr K, Coyne PJ, Key T, et al: Pain assessment in the nonverbal patient: position statement with clinical practice recommendations. *Pain Manage Nurs* 7:44–52, 2006.

Herr K, et al: Pain assessment in the nonverbal patient: position statement with clinical practice recommendations. *Pain Manage Nursing* 7(2):44–52, 2006.

Hess DR, Kallstrom TJ, Mottram CD, et al: AARC Evidence based clinical practice guidelines: care of the ventilator circuit and its relation to ventilator associated pneumonia. *Respir Care* 48(9):869–879, 2003.

http://www.cdc.gov/nchs/datawh/ftpser/ftpicd9/icdguide07.pdf

http://www.com.hhs.gov/AcuteInpatientPPS/downloads/CMS-1390-F.pdf

http://www.wocn.org/About_Us/advocacy_and _policy/ipps_guidance/ 9/11/2008

Iglesias C, Nixon J, Cranny G, et al: Pressure Trial Group. Pressure relieving support surfaces. Trial: cost-effectiveness analysis. *BMJ* 332(7555):1416, 2006.

Iglesias C, Nixon J, Cranny G, et al: Pain: the fifth vital sign. In Ignatavicius DD, Workman ML, editors: *Medical-surgical nursing patient-centered collaborative care,* ed 6. Philadelphia, 2010, WB Saunders.

Institute for Healthcare Improvement: Protecting 5 million lives from harm. Retrieved January 15, 2008, from http://www.ihi.org/IHI/Programs/Campaign

Johnson M, Maas M, editors: *Nursing outcomes classification (NOC).* St. Louis, 1997, Mosby.

Kalisvaart K, de Jonghe J, Bogaards M, et al: Haloperidol prophylaxis for elderly hip-surgery patients at risk for delirium: a randomized placebo-controlled study. *J Am Geriatr Soc* 53(10):1658–1666, 2005.

Kane RL, Ouslander JG, Abrass IB. *Essentials of clinical geriatrics,* ed 5. New York, 2003, McGraw-Hill.

Keckeisen M: Monitoring pulmonary artery pressure. *Crit Care Nurse* 24(3):67–70, 2004.

Knape JTA, Adriaensen H, van Aken H, et al: Guidelines for sedation and/or analgesia by non-anaesthesiology doctors. Section and Board of Anaesthesiology, European Union of Medical Specialists. *Eur J Anaesthesiol* 24:563–567, 2007.

Kress JP, Pohlman AS, O'Connor MF, Hall JB: Daily interruption of sedative infusions in critically ill patients undergoing mechanical ventilation. *N Engl J Med* 342(20):1471–1477, 2000.

Kress JP, Pohlman AS, O'Connor MF, Hall JB: Pain. In Kuebler KK, Heidrich DE, Esper P: *Palliative and end-of-life care clinical practice guidelines,* ed 2. Philadelphia, 2007, WB Saunders.

Lonergan E, Britton A, Luxenberg J, Wyller T. Antipsychotics for delirium. *Cochrane Database Syst Rev* (2):CD005594, 2007.

Lyder C, Ayello E. Pressure ulcers: a patient safety issue in patient safety and quality: an evidence-based handbook for nurses. http://www.ahrq.gov/qual/nurseshdbk/nurseshdbk.pdf

Maccioli GA, Dorman T, Brown BR, et al: Clinical practice guidelines for the maintenance of patient physical safety in the intensive care unit: use of restraining therapies. American College of Critical Care Medicine Task Force 2001–2002. *Crit Care Med* 31(11):2665–2676, 2003.

MacIntyre N: Evidence based guidelines for weaning and discontinuing of mechanical ventilatory support. *Chest* 120:375S–396S, 2001.

Marcantonio E, Flaker J, Wright R, Resnick N: Reducing delirium after hip fracture: a randomized trial. *J Am Geriatr Soc* 49(5):516–522, 2001.

Marquis F, Ouimet S, Riker R, Cossette M, Skrobik Y: Individual delirium symptoms: do they matter? *Crit Care Med* 35(11):2533–2537, 2007.

Moore ZE, Cowman S: Wound cleansing for pressure ulcers. *Cochrane Collaboration* 1:1–16, 2007.

National Guideline Clearinghouse (NGC): Guideline synthesis: pressure ulcer prevention. 2006. (revised 2008) http://www.guideline.gov

National Pressure Ulcer Advisory Panel: Support surface standards initiative. http://www.npuap.org/NPUAP_S31_TD.pdf.

National Pressure Ulcer Advisory Panel: http://www.npuap.org/pr2.htm

Nutrition support in adults: oral nutrition support, enteral tube feeding and parenteral nutrition. 2006. Retrieved November 10, 2009, from http://www.nice.org.uk/CG32

O'Leary-Kelley CM, Puntillo KA, Barr J, Stotts N, Douglas MK: Nutritional adequacy in patients receiving mechanical ventilation who are fed enterally. *Am J Crit Care* 14(3):222–231, 2005.

Owens D, Flom J: Integrating palliative and neurological critical care. *AACN Clin Issues Adv Pract Acute Crit Care* 16(4):542–550, 2005.

Payen JF, Chanques G, Mantz J, et al: Current practices in sedation and analgesia for mechanically ventilated critically ill patients. *Anesthesiology* 106:687–695, 2007.

Porter R, editor: Fluid and electrolyte metabolism. In *The Merck manual.* Whitehouse Station, 2006, Merck Research Laboratories.

Registered Nurses Association of Ontario (RNAO): *Risk assessment and prevention of pressure ulcers.* Toronto, 2005, RNAO.

Rose BD, Somers MJ: Physiologic regulation of effective circulatory volume and plasma osmolality. 2007. 2008. www.uptodate.com

Russo CA, Elixhauser A: Hospitalizations related to pressure sores, 2003. Healthcare Cost and Utilization Project. Rockville, MD, 2006, Agency for Healthcare Research and Quality. http://www.hcup_us.ahrq.gov/reprts/statbriefs/sb3.pdf

Sessler CN, Gosnell M, Grap MJ, et al: The Richmond Agitation-Sedation Scale: validity and reliability in adult intensive care patients. *Am J Respir Crit Care Med* 166:1338–1344, 2002.

Siddiqi N, Stockdale R, Britton A, Holmes J: Interventions for preventing delirium in hospitalized patients. *Cochrane Database Syst Rev* 4, 2008.

Slutsky AS, Dos Santos CC: The contribution of biophysical lung injury to the development of bio-trauma. *Annu Rev Physiol* 68:585–618, 2006.

Society of Critical Care Medicine and American Society of Health-System Pharmacists: Sedation, Analgesia, and Neuromuscular Blockade of the Critically Ill Adult: Revised Clinical Practice Guidelines for 2002. *Am J Health Syst Pharm* 59:147–149, 2002.

Stevens R, Nyquist P: Coma, delirium, and cognitive dysfunction in critical illness. *Crit Care Clin* 22:787–804, 2007.

The Acute Respiratory Distress Syndrome Network: Ventilation with lower tidal volumes as compared with traditional tidal volumes for acute lung injury and the acute respiratory distress syndrome. *N Engl J Med* 342(18):1301–1308, 2000.

The Joint Commission: Sentinel Event Alert: Preventing ventilator-related deaths and injuries. February 26, 2005. Retrieved July 22, 2009, from http://www.jointcommission.org/SentinelEvents/ SentinelEventAlert

U.S. hospital errors continue to rise. Retrieved March 31, 2007, from http://news.yahoo.com/s/hsn/20070402/hl_hsn/ushospitalerroscontinuetorise

World Union of Wound Healing Societies: Principles of best practice: minimizing pain at wound dressing-related procedures, a consensus document. 2008. http://www.wuwhs.org

Wound Ostomy and Continence Nurses (WOCN) Society: *Guideline for prevention and management of pressure ulcers.* Glenview, IL, 2003, WOCN.

Managing the Critical Care Environment

BIOTERRORISM

Bioterrorism is the intentional release of a biologic agent, generally aimed at causing as great a number of people as possible to suffer illness and death. A bioterrorism event should be suspected when there is an unusual and unexplained increase in an illness.

The Centers for Disease Control and Prevention (CDC) identified six biological agents of highest concern for use in terrorism: anthrax, botulism, hemorrhagic fever viruses, plague, smallpox, and tularemia. Several factors explain why these agents are more likely to be used:

1. Most people are susceptible to these organisms.
2. They can be aerosolized.
3. They are fairly stable in aerosolized form.
4. Because of reason 3, they can cause disease in a large group of individuals.
5. Resultant diseases are difficult to diagnose and treat.
6. They have high morbidity and/or mortality rates.

BIOTERRORISM ASSESSMENT: SURVEILLANCE
Goal of Surveillance
The goal is to detect a biological event as early as possible to limit the spread of the infection.

Key Signs
Bioterrorism should be suspected when the following situations are seen:
- An outbreak of an illness within a short period of time; similar to one that happens in a healthy population, without a link to explain the transmission such as a similar food source
- An outbreak of an illness that occurs at an unusual time of year
- An outbreak with an unusual age distribution
- A large cluster of patients are affected by an uncommon disease, which is resulting in a higher than expected death rate.
- The severity of the disease is increased with patients having unusual routes of exposure.
- Strains of organisms seen have unusual antibiotic resistance.
- Those indoors are not as affected as or "as are those" those who have been outdoors.
- With some strains, an increased number of dead animals is noted.
- Those presenting within 48 to 72 hours of exposure have likely been exposed to a biological agent, as opposed to those exposed to a toxin, who present within a few hours.

Monitor
- Observe for an unusual or unexplained increase in an illness, especially with the characteristics just listed in *Key Signs.*

Report
- All occurrences of these six diseases must be reported to the CDC, as they are considered *Category A* agents, the highest priority for monitoring.

- CDC also monitors *Category B* organisms (includes Brucellosis [*Brucella* sp.], epsilon toxin of *Clostridium perfringens*, food safety threats [e.g., *Salmonella* sp., *Escherichia coli* O157:H7, *Shigella*], Glanders [*Burkholderia mallei*], melioidosis [*Burkholderia pseudomallei*], psittacosis [*Chlamydia psittaci*], Q fever [*Coxiella burnetii*], ricin toxin from *Ricinus communis* [castor beans], staphylococcal enterotoxin B, typhus fever [*Rickettsia prowazekii*], viral encephalitis [alphaviruses, e.g., Venezuelan equine encephalitis, Eastern equine encephalitis, Western equine encephalitis], and water safety threats [e.g., *Vibrio cholerae, Cryptosporidium parvum*]). These organisms are the second highest priority.
  - *Category C* organisms are the third highest priority agents and include emerging pathogens that could be engineered for mass dissemination in the future because of availability, ease of production and dissemination, and potential for high morbidity and mortality rates and major health impact. The agents include emerging infectious diseases such as Nipah virus and hantavirus.

Contain (Prevent the Spread of the Disease)
- Appropriate personal protective equipment (PPE) and isolation precautions need to be taken to inhibit the spread of the infectious agent.

Labwork
- Appropriate laboratory studies should be done to confirm the presence of the suspected biological agent. Many of these diseases require testing at specialty laboratories since these are uncommon bacteria and most hospital labs are not set up to test for these agents.

ANTHRAX

PATHOPHYSIOLOGY

Anthrax is a serious disease caused by *Bacillus anthracis,* a spore-forming bacterium. A spore is a dormant (inactive) cell that activates under the right conditions. Anthrax spores, once inside the human body, are able to germinate. Once germinated, the replicating bacteria release endotoxins leading to hemorrhage, edema, and necrosis.

There are three types of anthrax: skin (*cutaneous*), lung (*inhalation*), and digestive (*gastrointestinal*). Hemorrhagic mediastinitis is present with the inhalation form, and bloody diarrhea in seen with the intestinal form. When enough endotoxin is released into the bloodstream, the disease can be fatal even if antibiotics eradicate the bacteria. Anthrax infections are usually very rare since it takes thousands of spores to cause an infection. *Inhalation anthrax* is usually fatal even with treatment. *Gastrointestinal anthrax* has a mortality rate of 25% to 60%, whereas 20% of those with untreated *cutaneous anthrax* die. Cutaneous anthrax is rarely fatal unless untreated.

TRANSMISSION

Anthrax has not been known to spread from one person to another. Humans may acquire anthrax by handling products from infected animals or inhaling anthrax spores from infected animal products (e.g., wool). People acquire gastrointestinal anthrax by eating undercooked meat from infected animals. Anthrax in soil may enter the body through open skin. The organism is easy to obtain, produce, and store.

ASSESSMENT

The symptoms (warning signs) of anthrax differ depending on the type of the disease:
- *Inhalation:* The most serious form with the highest mortality rate, this begins 1 to 6 days after exposure with cold or influenza (flu)-like symptoms, with sore throat, mild fever, and muscle aches. Later symptoms include cough, chest discomfort, shortness of breath, fatigue, and muscle aches. Inhalation anthrax quickly progresses to respiratory failure and shock. Chest radiograph reveals a widened mediastinum and pleural effusions.
- *Cutaneous:* The first symptom is a raised, itchy bump that develops into a blister, seen 1 to 7 days after exposure. The blister progresses to a skin ulcer with a blackened center. The sore, the blister, and the ulcer are painless. Fever, headache, and swollen glands may occur.
- *Gastrointestinal:* At 2 to 5 days after exposure, the person exhibits nausea, loss of appetite, bloody diarrhea, and fever, followed by severe stomach pain. If untreated, it can progress to generalized toxemia and sepsis.

DIAGNOSTIC TESTS

Diagnostic tests to isolate anthrax antigen are not widely available. Confirmation of the diagnosis is made by sending a specimen to a national reference laboratory after the treatment begins. Clinicians should begin treatment based on clinical signs and symptoms, since early treatment is imperative to enhance chances of survival from inhalation anthrax. Standard blood culture may be useful if the laboratory is told to look for bacillus species. A Gram stain, enzyme-linked immunosorbent assay (ELISA), and nasal swab check for spores may also be useful.

COLLABORATIVE MANAGEMENT
Care Priorities

1. **Antibiotics:** Used to treat all three types of anthrax. Ideally, the antibiotic should be based on culture and sensitivity results. If those are not available, the antibiotics of choice are doxycycline and ciprofloxacin. Additionally, levofloxacin is recommended for adults. Occasionally, rifampin may also be used. Early identification and treatment are crucial to minimize the amount of endotoxin released.
2. **Intubation and mechanical ventilation (inhalation):** To support gas exchange and help maintain acid-base balance.
3. **Intravenous fluids (inhalation and gastrointestinal):** To prevent dehydration and maintain adequate circulatory volume.
4. **Prevention after exposure:** Treatment differs when a person exposed to anthrax is not yet having symptoms. Health care providers use antibiotics (e.g., ciprofloxacin, doxycycline, penicillin) combined with anthrax vaccine to prevent anthrax infection and, for contact anthrax, instruct exposed person to immediately scrub hands and arms or take a shower (if available) and remove and place their clothes in a plastic bag when apprised of an exposure.
5. **Treatment after infection:** Treatment is usually a 60-day course of antibiotics. Success depends on the type of anthrax, the general health of the individual, and how early treatment begins. A 60-day course is necessary so the antibiotic is in the person's system when the spores activate. Inactive spores are not susceptible to antibiotics.
6. **Vaccination:** A vaccine to prevent anthrax exists, but it is not yet available to the general public. Anyone at risk for anthrax exposure, including certain members of the U.S. armed forces, laboratory workers, and workers who may enter or reenter contaminated areas, may be vaccinated. If anthrax is used as a weapon, a vaccination program will be initiated to vaccinate as many exposed people as possible.

CARE PLANS: ANTHRAX

Gas exchange, impaired *related to respiratory insufficiency from respiratory infection secondary to inhalation of anthrax.*

GOALS/OUTCOMES: Within 12 to 24 hours of treatment, patient has adequate gas exchange as evidenced by Pao_2 at least 80 mm Hg, $Paco_2$ 35 to 45 mm Hg, pH 7.35 to 7.45, presence of normal breath sounds, and absence of adventitious breath sounds. The respiratory rate (RR) is 12 to 20 breaths/min with normal pattern and depth.
NOC Respiratory Status: Gas Exchange

Respiratory Monitoring
1. Monitor rate, rhythm, and depth of respirations.
2. Note chest movement for symmetry of chest expansion and signs of increased work of breathing such as use of accessory muscles or retraction of intercostal or supraclavicular muscles.
3. Monitor for diaphragmatic muscle fatigue.
4. Ensure airway is not obstructed by tongue (snoring or choking type respirations) and monitor breathing patterns. New patterns that impair ventilation should be managed as appropriate for setting.
5. Auscultate breath sounds noting areas of decrease/absent ventilation and presence of adventitious sounds.
6. Note changes in oxygen saturation from arterial blood gases (Sao_2), pulse oximetry (Spo_2), and end-tidal CO_2 ($ETCO_2$) as appropriate.
7. Monitor for increased restlessness or anxiety.

8. If increased restlessness or unusual somnolence occurs, evaluate patient for hypoxemia and hypercapnia as appropriate.
9. Monitor chest x-ray reports as new films become available.

Oxygen Therapy
1. Administer supplemental oxygen using liter flow and device as ordered. Add humidity as appropriate.
2. Restrict patient and visitors from smoking while oxygen is in use.
3. Document pulse oximetry with oxygen liter flow in place at time of reading as ordered. Oxygen is a drug; the dose of the drug must be associated with the oxygen saturation reading or the reading is meaningless.
4. Obtain arterial blood gases (ABGs) if patient experiences behavioral changes or respiratory distress, to check for hypoxemia or hypercapnia.
5. Monitor for changes in chest radiograph and breath sounds indicative of oxygen toxicity and absorption atelectasis in patients receiving higher concentrations of oxygen (more than FIO_2 45%) for longer than 24 hours. The higher the oxygen concentration, the greater is the chance of toxicity.
6. Monitor for skin breakdown where oxygen devices are in contact with skin, such as nares and around edges of mask devices.
7. Provide oxygen therapy during transportation and when patient gets out of bed.

Mechanical Ventilation
1. Monitor for conditions indicating a need for ventilation support.
2. Monitor for impending respiratory failure.
3. Consult with other health care personnel in selection of the ventilatory mode.
4. Administer muscle-paralyzing agents, sedatives, and narcotic analgesics as appropriate.
5. Monitor the effectiveness of mechanical ventilation on the patient's physiologic and psychological status.
6. Provide patient with means of communication.
7. Monitor adverse effects of mechanical ventilation.
8. Perform routine mouth care.
9. Elevate the head of the bed (HOB) up to 45 degrees as tolerated.

BOTULISM

PATHOPHYSIOLOGY

Botulism is a muscle-paralyzing disease associated with respiratory dysfunction caused by a toxin produced from *Clostridium botulinum* bacteria. The toxin is the most potent lethal substance known to humans. Man-made inhalational botulism is brought into being when aerosolized botulinum toxin is inhaled. The bacterium naturally lives for weeks in nonmoving water and food. There are three naturally acquired types of botulism:

- *Foodborne*—A person ingests toxin that leads to illness in a few hours to days.
- *Infant*—Occurs in a small number of susceptible infants each year who harbor *C. botulinum* in their intestinal tracts.
- *Wound*—Occurs when a wound is infected with *C. botulinum*.

Botulinum toxin, once absorbed into the bloodstream, is transported to the peripheral cholinergic synapses, where it binds irreversibly. The toxin then blocks the release of acetylcholine in the neuromuscular junctions, causing paralysis of the muscles.

TRANSMISSION

Botulism is not spread from person to person. Botulinum toxin is absorbed through lung or intestinal mucosa and nonintact skin. Foodborne botulism occurs in all age groups.

ASSESSMENT

- *Foodborne:* Double vision, drooping eyelids, slurred speech, dysphagia, dry mouth, and descending muscle weakness are symptoms. Weakness starts in the shoulders and upper arms, descends to the lower arms and upper thighs, and eventually spreads down to the lower legs and feet. Paralysis of the respiratory muscles leads to respiratory failure unless ventilation is supported with mechanical ventilation. Patients are generally afebrile and alert.
- *Respiratory assessment:* Patients who are not intubated should have their respiratory status monitored closely to detect deterioration in respiratory muscle strength. One of the best assessment tools is periodic measurement of negative inspiratory force (NIF).

If the NIF falls below 20 cm H₂O, the patient is likely to require intubation and mechanical ventilation.

DIAGNOSTIC TESTS

Currently, the CDC and fewer than 25 public health laboratories perform the diagnostic test for botulism. Diagnosis is made clinically, after ruling out other causes of paralysis. Classic botulism paralysis is descending in nature and involves the cranial nerves.

COLLABORATIVE MANAGEMENT
Care Priorities

1. **Antitoxin:** Botulinum antitoxin is available in two forms from the CDC. Since both are equine derivatives, it is important to perform a skin test as directed in the package insert to check for hypersensitivity before administering . Antitoxin helps prevent further nerve damage from the botulinum toxin but cannot reverse the existing paralysis. It is most effective if given within the first 24 hours. The antitoxin is not effective in infant botulism. For infant botulism, botulism immune globulin-intravenous (BIG-IV) is administered.
2. **Antibiotic:** Antibiotics are given to treat wounds infected with *C. botulinum* and secondary infections. Antibiotics have no effect on botulinum toxin.
3. **Vaccine:** Botulism recombinant vaccine is currently under investigation. Botulism toxoid is available but is recommended only for laboratory personnel who work with *C. botulinum* and military personnel who are likely to be exposed.
4. **Supportive care:** Includes mechanical ventilation, nutritional support, care for immobility, and treatment for secondary infections.

CARE PLANS: BOTULISM

Breathing pattern, ineffective *related to respiratory infection*

- -

GOALS/OUTCOMES: Patient demonstrates effective air exchange as evidenced by RR 12 to 20 breaths/min, Pao₂ ≥80 mm Hg, Paco₂ 35 to 45 mm Hg, pH 7.35 to 7.45, Sao₂ greater than 95%, Svo₂ greater than 60%, and ETCO₂ 5% to 6% (35 to 45 mm Hg).
NOC Respiratory Status: Ventilation

Respiratory Monitoring
1. Monitor rate, rhythm, depth, and effort of respirations.
2. Monitor for diaphragmatic muscle fatigue.
3. Auscultate breath sounds, noting areas of decreased/absent ventilation and presence of adventitious sounds.
4. Assess for breathing effectiveness by monitoring Sao₂, Svo₂, ETCO₂, and changes in ABG values, as appropriate.
5. Insert oral or nasopharyngeal airway if patient cannot maintain patent airway; if severely distressed, patient may require endotracheal intubation.

Ventilation Assistance
1. Position patient to alleviate dyspnea and insure maximal ventilation, generally in a sitting upright position unless severe hypotension is present.
2. Assist with incentive spirometer, as appropriate.
3. Clear secretions from airway by having patient cough, or provide nasotracheal, oropharyngeal, or endotracheal tube suctioning as needed.
4. Have patient breathe slowly or manually ventilate with Ambu bag slowly and deeply between coughing or suctioning attempts.
5. Turn patient every 2 hours if immobile. Encourage patient to turn self or get out of bed as much as tolerated if able to do so.

HEMORRHAGIC FEVER VIRUSES

PATHOPHYSIOLOGY

Hemorrhagic fever viruses (HFVs) include many diseases separated into four families of viruses; not all are viewed as risks for bioterrorism. Those that are thought to pose a significant risk include Ebola virus disease, Marburg virus disease, Lassa fever, New World Arenaviridae,

Rift Valley fever, yellow fever, Omsk hemorrhagic fever, and Kyasanur Forest disease. The pathophysiology of these diseases is not well understood. Outbreaks are sporadic and have occurred in areas with very limited health care. Infection with these viruses leads to thrombocytopenia and possibly platelet dysfunction. The effects of these viruses vary, but all lead to coagulation problems, hemorrhage, and shock. Mortality ranges range from less than 1% with Rift Valley fever to 50% to 90% with Ebola virus. Only one of the Arenaviridae viruses has been identified in the United States. Other HFVs have not emerged.

TRANSMISSION

HFVs reside in many animal hosts and arthropod vectors. Humans become infected when bitten by an infected arthropod, by inhaling aerosolized virus from infected rodent excreta, or from direct contact with infected animal carcasses. Humans infected with Ebola, Marburg, Lassa fever, and arenaviruses can spread the disease to close contacts.

Isolation

Strict airborne and contact isolation are required if a patient is suspected of infection.

ASSESSMENT

Clinical scenarios vary depending on the virus. The most common symptom is a fever.

- *Ebola and Marburg:* Maculopapular rash, bleeding, disseminated intravascular coagulation, jaundice.
- *Lassa fever and New World arenaviruses:* Gradual onset of fever, nausea, abdominal pain, conjunctivitis, and jaundice. Severe exudative pharyngitis in Lassa fever.
- *Rift Valley fever:* Fever, headache, photophobia, and jaundice.

DIAGNOSTIC TESTS

Only the CDC and U.S. Army Research Institute of Infectious Diseases laboratories have testing available.

COLLABORATIVE MANAGEMENT
Care Priorities

1. **Supportive care:** Maintain fluid and electrolyte balances, and treat hypotension with early use of vasopressors if fluid therapy is not effective, mechanical ventilation, renal dialysis, and anticonvulsive therapy. Administration of clotting factor concentrates, platelets, fresh-frozen plasma (FFP), and heparin in patients with disseminated intravascular coagulation (DIC).
2. **Antivirals:** These agents are not effective against these diseases.
3. **Ribavirin:** Institute a 10-day course if Lassa fever or New World arenavirus is confirmed.
4. **Control risk for bleeding:** Intramuscular injections, aspirin, nonsteroidal anti-inflammatory drugs (NSAIDs), steroids, and anticoagulant therapies are contraindicated.
5. **Vaccine:** There is a vaccine only for yellow fever, which is only recommended for travelers going to South America or Africa where yellow fever is endemic and for laboratory personnel who are exposed to yellow fever samples. The vaccine is not helpful postexposure because of the short incubation period compared with the time it takes for immunity to develop.

PLAGUE

PATHOPHYSIOLOGY

Plague is an infectious disease caused by the bacterium *Yersinia pestis* that is found in rodents and their fleas. Several forms of plague can occur individually or in combination: bubonic, pneumonic, and septicemic plague. *Bubonic plague* is the most common, occurring when an infected flea bites a human or when infectious materials enter through a break in the skin. *Pneumonic plague* occurs when *Y. pestis* infects lungs through direct or close contact with a person who has pneumonic plague or in untreated patients with bubonic or septicemic plague, allowing bacterial spread to lungs. *Septicemic plague* can occur as a complication of either of the previous types of plague or alone. The bacteria enter the bloodstream and multiply, prompting the systemic effects of sepsis.

The *Y. pestis* bacteria travel to lymph nodes, where they resist defense mechanisms and rapidly multiply, causing destruction of lymph nodes. Bacteria enter the bloodstream and prompt sepsis, septic shock, DIC, and coma. Without treatment, mortality approaches 100%; with treatment, the mortality can be as low as 5%.

TRANSMISSION

Pneumonic plague is spread through direct contact with an infected person. Neither bubonic nor septicemic plagues are transmitted by person-to-person contact.

- *Pneumonic plague:* Droplet precautions until the patient receives antibiotics for 72 hours.
- *Bubonic or septicemic plague:* Standard precautions.

ASSESSMENT

- *Pneumonic plague:* Fever, headache, weakness, and rapidly developing pneumonia with shortness of breath, chest pain, cough, and sometimes bloody or watery sputum. The pneumonia progresses and in 2 to 4 days can cause respiratory failure and shock. Without treatment, patients with pneumonic plague will die.
- *Bubonic plague:* Swollen, tender lymph glands (called buboes), fever, headache, chills, and weakness.
- *Septicemic plague:* Fever and chills, abdominal pain, and shock with bleeding (due to DIC).

DIAGNOSTIC TESTS

- **Gram's stain of sputum or blood:** Reveals gram-negative bacilli. A laboratory may misidentify the bacteria unless notified that *Y. pestis* is suspected.

COLLABORATIVE MANAGEMENT
Care Priorities

1. **Antibiotics:** Given within the first 24 hours of symptoms. Streptomycin, gentamicin, tetracyclines, and chloramphenicol are all effective in treating pneumonic plague. The preferred choice in adults is streptomycin 1 g intramuscularly (IM) twice a day for 10 days or gentamicin 5 mg/kg either IM or IV once a day or 2 mg/kg loading dose followed by 1.7 mg/kg administered IM or IV three times a day for 10 days. In children, the drug of choice is streptomycin 15 mg/kg IM twice a day with maximum dose of 2 g or gentamicin 2.5 mg/kg IM or IV three times a day for 10 days.
2. **Vaccine:** There currently is no vaccine available in the United States. Work is currently under way to develop a vaccine.
3. **Supportive care:** Ventilatory support, pain management, and treatment for shock, DIC, and multiorgan dysfunction syndrome (MODS), as appropriate.

SMALLPOX (VARIOLA)

PATHOPHYSIOLOGY

Smallpox is a serious, contagious, and sometimes fatal infectious disease. It is a member of the orthopoxvirus family, along with monkeypox, vaccinia, and cowpox. Although all of these can cause skin lesions, only smallpox is readily transmitted from person to person. There are two main clinical forms of smallpox—variola major and variola minor—with several additional strains. *Variola major* is the severe and most common form of smallpox, with a more extensive rash and higher fever. Historically, variola major had a 30% mortality rate. *Variola minor* was less common and much less severe. Smallpox was eradicated after a successful worldwide vaccination program. The last case of smallpox in the United States was in 1949. The last naturally occurring case in the world was in Somalia in 1977. There is currently questionable access to the virus since the separation of the Soviet Union, as Moscow and the United States housed the only two storage laboratories at that time.

Smallpox virus enters the body through the mucosa in the oropharyngeal and respiratory tracts. The virus multiplies in the lymph nodes, the spleen, and the bone marrow. Eventually the virus, contained in lymphocytes, localizes in small blood vessels of the dermis and infects adjacent cells, causing the pustules to form.

Smallpox is an excellent agent for bioterrorism because it is easy to both transport and store, because it is very stable and markedly virulent when aerosolized.

TRANSMISSION

Smallpox is transmitted via droplet nuclei or aerosols expelled from an infected person's oropharynx. Usually direct and fairly prolonged face-to-face contact was required to spread smallpox from person to person. Smallpox can be spread through direct contact with infected bodily fluids or contaminated objects (e.g., bedding or clothing). Rarely, the virus spreads through the air in enclosed settings (e.g., buildings, buses, trains). Humans are the only natural hosts of variola (there is no recorded transmissions from animals or insects).

A person with smallpox is sometimes contagious with onset of fever (prodrome phase). Most infected persons become contagious with the onset of rash. At this stage, the person is usually very sick, unable to move around in the community. The person remains contagious until the last smallpox scab falls off.

ASSESSMENT

- *Clinical case definition:* An illness with acute onset of fever ≥101°F (38.3°C), followed by a rash characterized by firm, deep-seated vesicles or pustules in the same stage of development without other apparent cause. These characteristics help differentiate the smallpox from chickenpox. Smallpox may be easily missed in the early stage by health care providers.
- *Incubation period:* Usually 12 to 14 days but can range from 7 to 17 days. During this time, the patient feels fine and is not contagious.
- *Prodromal period:* Begins with a high fever (101° to 104°F), malaise, headache, and backache. The patient may exhibit severe abdominal pains, vomiting, and delirium. This period lasts for 2 to 4 days before a rash develops. The rash begins with small red spots on the tongue and mouth. During this phase, the person is most contagious.
- *Rash development:* Progresses in the mouth and develops on the skin, starting on the face and moving to the arms and legs and then to the feet and hands. It usually spreads to all parts within 24 hours. When rash appears, the patient's fever subsides and the patient starts to feel better. On day 3, the rash consists of raised bumps. On day 4, the bumps fill with thick, cloudy fluid with a possible indent in the center. Indentation is the classic sign of smallpox rash. The bumps become pustules and eventually scab over. During the pustule stage, the patient is again febrile. After 2 weeks, most of the sores have scabs, which begin to fall off, leaving marks that will become pitted scars on the skin.

DIAGNOSTIC TESTS

Laboratory diagnostic testing for variola should be done by a CDC Laboratory Response Network (LRN) laboratory using LRN-approved polymerase chain reaction (PCR) tests and protocols for variola virus. Laboratory testing should be reserved for cases that meet the clinical case definition, thus classified as being a potential high risk for smallpox.

Safety Alert *Initial confirmation of a smallpox outbreak requires additional testing at the CDC.*

Laboratory Criteria for Confirmation of Smallpox

- PCR identification of variola DNA in a clinical specimen
- Isolation of smallpox (variola) virus from a clinical specimen (World Health Organization [WHO] Smallpox Reference Laboratory or laboratory with appropriate reference capabilities) with variola PCR confirmation

COLLABORATIVE MANAGEMENT

There are no approved treatments for smallpox. Currently, treatment consists of supportive care. However, cidofovir, an antiviral, is currently being studied to see if it is effective against the smallpox virus.

Care Priorities

1. Vaccine: A key is to identify smallpox exposure and administer vaccine within 3 days, to prevent or significantly lessen the severity of the disease process. Vaccine administered within 4 to 7 days after exposure may provide some protection and lessen the disease severity.

2. **Isolation:** Patients presenting with symptoms should be isolated immediately in a negative-pressure room. The door should be kept closed at all times. All health care workers entering the room should wear an N-95 respirator mask. Because smallpox is also transmitted via body fluids (contaminating the bedding), health care workers should use contact precautions (i.e., gown, gloves, and shoe covers) when entering the room. Other infection control practices, such as limiting patient transport, designating patient care equipment, and so forth, should follow the institution's policies. Linen should be autoclaved and corpses cremated.

3. **Supportive management**
   - *Provide hydration:* Intravenous fluids to prevent dehydration
   - *Provide nutrition:* To help strengthen the immune system
   - *Initiate mechanical ventilation:* If patient experiences respiratory failure
   - *Hemodynamic monitoring:* If management of fluid balance and blood pressure is difficult
   - *Control fever:* Antipyretics to reduce body temperature if greater than 103°F
   - *Reduce pain and anxiety:* Analgesics and sedatives as indicated

---

CARE PLANS: SMALLPOX

Body image, disturbed *related to numerous skin lesions resulting from infection with smallpox*

- -

GOALS/OUTCOMES Patient will acknowledge change in physical appearance and express a positive self-worth.
NOC Body Image, Self-Esteem

Body Image Enhancement
1. Use anticipatory guidance to prepare patient for predictable changes in body image.
2. Assist patient to discuss changes caused by illness.
3. Assist patient to separate physical appearance from feelings of personal self-worth.
4. Identify the effects of the patient's culture, religion, race, sex, and age in terms of body image.

Emotional Support
1. Discuss with the patient the emotional experience.
2. Make supportive or empathetic statements.
3. Support the use of appropriate defense mechanisms.
4. Encourage the patient to express feelings of anxiety, anger, or sadness.
5. Listen to and encourage expressions of feelings and beliefs.
6. Refer for counseling as appropriate.

TULAREMIA

PATHOPHYSIOLOGY

Tularemia is caused by a bacterial zoonosis called *Francisella tularensis*. One of the most infectious pathogenic bacteria known, it is found in infected water, soil, vegetation, small mammals, ticks, fleas, and mosquitoes. *F. tularensis* is a small, nonmotile, aerobic, gram-negative coccobacillus that targets the lymph nodes, lungs, pleura, spleen, liver, and kidneys. Bacteria enter through skin, mucous membranes, gastrointestinal tract, and lungs to invade cells, causing inflammation and permanent damage if untreated.

TRANSMISSION

Tularemia is transmitted by bites from infected arthropods; handling infectious animal tissues or fluids; direct contact with or ingestion of contaminated water, food, or soil; and inhaling infected aerosols. There is no evidence of person-to-person transmission. Patients should be placed on standard precautions.

ASSESSMENT

- *Disease presentation:* May vary depending on the infecting organism, dose, and site of inoculation. It usually starts abruptly with a fever of 100.1° to 104°F (38° to 40°C), headache, chills, generalized body aches, rhinitis, and a sore throat. Some patients have dry cough, substernal pain, skin or mouth ulcers, swollen painful lymph glands, and swollen and painful eyes.

- *Illness progression:* Progressive weakness, malaise, anorexia, and weight loss. If untreated, symptoms may persist for several weeks to months. Secondary sepsis, pleuropneumonia, and, rarely, meningitis may develop.

DIAGNOSTIC TESTS

Rapid diagnostic testing for *F. tularensis* is not widely available. If tularemia is suspected, specimens of respiratory secretions and blood should be collected and sent to a designated laboratory for microscopic identification using fluorescent-labeled antibodies.

COLLABORATIVE MANAGEMENT
Care Priorities

1. **Antibiotics:** Antibiotic of choice is streptomycin, although gentamicin may be used. The patient should be placed on a 10-day course.
2. **Vaccine:** A vaccine is currently under review by the U.S. Food and Drug Administration (FDA).

EMERGING INFECTIONS

Emerging infectious diseases are a serious problem. Medicine and technology have moved forward to successfully overcome and prevent many infections, yet new infections continue to emerge. The new infections are complex, and their evolution has been challenging for health care personnel to recognize, understand, and treat. Many emerging infections, such as H1N1, H5N1, hantavirus, and "mad cow" disease, originate from different species of animals and have spread to humans.

INFECTION PROTECTION AND INFECTION CONTROL

For several decades, infection prevention and control have focused on the use of barriers (e.g., gloves, masks, and gowns) to interrupt transmission of organisms between patients and health care providers. Barriers are a major component of the various systems of transmission precautions.

Many different systems of transmission precautions have been used in hospitals over the years and are commonly called *isolation precautions*. These recommendations are updated periodically, with the most recent revision (2007) by the CDC and the Healthcare Infection Control Practices Advisory Committee (HICPAC) intended to reflect evidence-based practices and current knowledge. These techniques and procedures designed to interrupt the transmission of infection adhere to five basic principles:

1. To provide infection control recommendations for the entire health care system, including hospitals, long-term care facilities, ambulatory care, home care, and hospice
2. To reaffirm *standard precautions* as the foundation for preventing transmission of organism, during patient care in all settings
3. To reaffirm the importance of implementing transmission-based precautions based on the clinical presentation of the syndrome and likely pathogens until the infectious etiology is known
4. To provide epidemiologically sound and, whenever possible, evidence-based recommendations
5. To provide a unified infection control approach to multidrug-resistant organisms (MDROs)

The 2007 guideline contains two tiers of precautions:

1. *Standard precautions:* Designed for the care of all patients in the health care setting, regardless of diagnosis or infection status
2. *Transmission-based precautions:* Used for patients known to be infected or colonized with epidemiologically important pathogens that can be transmitted by airborne or droplet or contact with dry skin or contaminated surfaces. Isolation techniques that prevent transmission are the following:
   a. *Airborne infection isolation*—For patients known or suspected to be infected with microorganisms transmitted person to person by airborne droplet nuclei that remain suspended in the air and that can be dispersed widely by air currents.
   b. *Droplet*—For patients known or suspected to be infected with microorganisms transmitted by respiratory droplets (more than 5 micrometers [μm] in size), generated by

the patient coughing, sneezing, or talking or during performance of cough-inducing procedures.

c. *Contact*—For patients with known or suspected infections or evidence of syndromes that represent increased risk for contact transmission, including colonization or infection with MDROs according to recommendations in the CDC guidelines (2007).

d. *Protective environment*—For allogenic, hematopoietic stem cell transplantation (HSCT) patients to minimize gunal spore counts in the air. Specific requirements for the protective environment were defined by the CDC in 2000.

Humans are vulnerable, without natural defenses against these infections. Researchers are hard-pressed to develop vaccines and cures. Regardless of sex, age, socioeconomic status, or ethnic background, infectious disease can strike at any time and may lead to significant morbidity and death.

SEVERE ACUTE RESPIRATORY SYNDROME

Severe acute respiratory syndrome (SARS) is a febrile lower respiratory infection that mimics many other respiratory illnesses. To date, there are no specific clinical or laboratory findings that distinguish with certainty SARS-associated coronavirus (CoV) disease from other respiratory illnesses rapidly enough to facilitate management decisions that must be made soon after the patient presents to the health care system. Therefore, early recognition of this disease still relies on a combination of clinical and epidemiologic features.

The virus may have originated from animals and spread to humans. SARS first emerged in the Guandong Province in China during November 2002 through June 2003, where approximately 15,000 probable cases were identified. A worldwide epidemic occurred when a SARS-infected physician contaminated several guests at a hotel in Hong Kong. The guests were the catalyst leading to large outbreaks of SARS in Hong Kong, Vietnam, Singapore, and Canada. Overall, 8000 probable SARS cases were identified during the outbreak, and 800 total deaths occurred from 29 different countries.

A novel CoV has been identified as the cause of SARS and is now labeled SARS-CoV. CoVs are enveloped RNA viruses that cause diseases in both humans and animals. In humans, this group of viruses is implicated in the causes of the common cold and pneumonia. The distinct microscopic appearance of a crown surrounding the viruses has led to its name. Research in China has detected several CoVs closely related to SARS-CoV in two animal species (masked palm civet cat and raccoon-dog). This provided the first link between human SARS-CoV and its presence in other animals. Both are considered delicacies in China and are consumed by humans. One theory states that this CoV mutated and was transmitted to humans through handling of these animals or contact with their saliva and feces.

PATHOPHYSIOLOGY

The pathophysiology of SARS is unclear. It begins much like the common flu, progressing to pneumonia and potentially to acute respiratory distress syndrome (ARDS) and death. Lymphopenia, thrombocytopenia, and leucopenia are noted. SARS-CoV may infect blood cells and/or induce autoantibodies to damage these cells, leading to immunologic dysregulation in response to the SARS-CoV. Poor patient outcomes have been linked to advanced age and elevated total lactate dehydrogenase (LDH greater than 300 U/L). Increased LDH may reflect cell death or leakage of this enzyme from cells, possibly indicating cellular infection by SARS-CoV.

TRANSMISSION

The most common mode of transmission for SARS is close person-to-person contact: kissing, sharing eating or drinking utensils, close conversation (less than 3 feet), physical examination, and any other direct physical contact. Respiratory droplets are expelled by the infected person by a cough or sneeze into the air. Droplets then reach the mucosal membrane of the nose, mouth, or eyes of a nearby person, infecting him or her.

Surfaces contaminated with SARS droplets may serve as a reservoir for the virus. SARS droplets can remain viable up to several days according to the type of surface they are on. If a person contacts a contaminated surface and then touches the mouth, eyes, or nose, he or she may become infected with SARS-CoV. Contact with feces of an infected person has accounted for a few cases. Other modes of transmission are not yet clearly identified.

ASSESSMENT
Goal of Assessment
Evaluate for early clinical and epidemiologic features of SARS.

History and Risk Factors
Evaluation of SARS-CoV disease among persons presenting with community-acquired illness CDC recommends the following approach for the evaluation of SARS-CoV disease among persons presenting with community-acquired illness. Along with clinical features, clinicians should routinely incorporate into the medical history questions that may provide epidemiologic clues to identify patients.

- **In the absence of person-to-person transmission of SARS-CoV anywhere in the world,** the diagnosis of SARS-CoV should only be considered in patients who require hospitalization for radiographically confirmed pneumonia and who have an epidemiologic history that raises suspicion of SARS-CoV disease. The suspicion of SARS-CoV disease is raised if, within 10 days of symptom onset, the patient:
  - Has a history of recent travel to mainland China, Hong Kong, or Taiwan or close contact with ill persons with a history of recent travel to such areas, OR
  - Is employed in an occupation at particular risk for SARS-CoV exposure, including a health care worker with direct patient contact or a worker in a laboratory that contains live SARS-CoV, OR
  - Is part of a cluster of cases of atypical pneumonia without an alternative diagnosis.
- **Once person-to-person transmission of SARS-CoV has been documented in the world, the diagnosis should still be considered** in patients who require hospitalization for pneumonia and who have the epidemiologic history described above. In addition, all patients with fever or lower respiratory symptoms (e.g., cough, shortness of breath, difficulty breathing) should be questioned about whether within 10 days of symptom onset they have had:
  - Close contact with someone suspected of having SARS-CoV disease, OR
  - A history of foreign travel (or close contact with an ill person with a history of travel) to a location with documented or suspected SARS-CoV, OR
  - Exposure to a domestic location with documented or suspected SARS-CoV (including a laboratory that contains live SARS-CoV) or close contact with an ill person with such an exposure history.

Signs and Symptoms
The initial presentation of SARS is similar to that of other lower respiratory tract infections. No specific clinical or laboratory findings are available to rapidly distinguish SARS from other respiratory illness. Early recognition of SARS requires assessment of clinical and epidemiologic features. The incubation period is 2 to 10 days. Many early clinical manifestations are flulike symptoms: fever, myalgias, headache, and rhinorrhea. Fever is a key component and occurs in most cases. As the disease progresses, more respiratory symptoms may arise. On the second day of the fever, a dry, nonproductive cough may develop, progressing to shortness of breath, hypoxemia, and ARDS. The CDC has delineated three different levels of how patients may clinically present with SARS:

Early illness
- Presence of two or more of the following: fever, chills, rigors, myalgia, headache, diarrhea, sore throat, rhinorrhea

Mild-to-moderate respiratory illness
- Temperature of greater than 100.4°F (38°C), and
- One or more of the clinical findings of lower respiratory illness (e.g., cough, shortness of breath, difficulty breathing)

Severe respiratory illness
- Meets clinical criteria for mild-to-moderate respiratory illness including one or more of the following:
  - Chest radiograph illustrating pneumonia
  - ARDS (see *Acute Lung Injury and Acute Respiratory Distress Syndrome*, p. 365)
  - Autopsy findings of pneumonia or ARDS without an identifiable cause

Screening Labwork

Laboratory studies such as bacterial cultures and respiratory viral panels can be used to rule out other potential causes of respiratory tract infection. SARS-CoV reverse transcription (RT)-PCR and enzyme immunoassay (EIA) tests are not typically ordered until after a high index of suspicion by the physician and notification of public health officials.

Diagnostic Tests for SARS		
Test	**Purpose**	**Abnormal Findings**
Laboratory Studies		
SARS-CoV reverse-transcription–polymerase chain reaction (RT-PCR) test: A signed consent should be completed prior to collection of a sample. The sample should be forwarded to a state or local public health laboratory for processing.	Detects SARS-CoV viral RNA in respiratory samples, stool, and blood. The likelihood of detecting infection is increased if multiple specimens are collected at several times during the course of the illness. Has not been licensed by the U.S. Food and Drug Administration (FDA). Currently approved as an FDA investigational device exemption (test).	A positive SARS-CoV RT-PCR test should be considered presumptive until confirmatory testing by a second reference laboratory is performed. A negative test result for SARs-CoV may not rule out SARS-CoV disease and should not affect patient management or infection control decisions.
SARS-CoV enzyme immunoassay (EIA) test: A signed consent should be completed before collection of the sample. The sample should be forwarded to a state or local public health laboratory for processing.	Detects SARS-CoV antibodies in blood samples. CDC considers detection of SARS-CoV antibody to be the most reliable indicator of infection. Has not been licensed by the FDA. Has been allowed for use by the FDA as a result of the SARS outbreak.	Detectable antibodies
SARS-CoV immunofluorescence assay (IFA) for antibody	Gives results identical to SARS-CoV EIA for antibody	Detectable antibodies
Specimen culture for SARS-CoV	Isolation of SARS-CoV from a clinical specimen to confirm the virus	SARS-CoV identified in specimen
Sputum and blood cultures	Test can aid in ruling out bacterial infection.	Positive for bacterial pathogen
Respiratory viral panels for influenza A and B, respiratory syncytial viruses, and specimens for *Legionella* and pneumococcal and urinary antigen	These tests aid in ruling out other potential sources of infection.	Positive for pathogen
CBC and clotting profile	Monitoring WBC counts to assist in evaluation of other bacterial infection	Evaluation for lymphopenia, thrombocytopenia, and leucopenia
Radiology		
Chest radiograph	Assists in identifying the progression of disease and anatomic involvement	Infiltrates suggestive of pneumonia

Diagnostic Tests for SARS—cont'd		
Test	**Purpose**	**Abnormal Findings**
Respiratory Tests		
Arterial blood gases (ABGs)	Determination of patient oxygen saturation of arterial blood	Alkalosis, acidosis (see Acid-Base Imbalances, p. 1)
Pulse oximetry	Measure patient oxygen saturation of arterial blood	Values of <90%

SARS-CoV Laboratory Studies and Interpretation

Laboratory-confirmed SARS-CoV infection requires detection of antibody for SARS-CoV with confirmation in a reference laboratory:

- In a single specimen, OR
- A four-fold or greater increase in SARS-CoV antibiotic titer between active and convalescent-phase serum specimens tested in parallel, OR
- Negative SARS-CoV antibody test result on acute-phase serum and positive SARS-CoV antibody test result on convalescent-phase serum tested in parallel, OR
- Isolation in cell culture of SARS-CoV from a clinical specimen, with confirmation using a test validated by the CDC.
- Detection of SARS-CoV RNA by RT-PCR validated by CDC with confirmation in a reference laboratory from two clinical specimens from different sources or two clinical specimens collected from the same source on 2 different days

A negative serologic test can rule out SARS-CoV infection if the serum specimen is collected more than 28 days after onset of illness. Some patients do not develop an antibody (test positive) until more than 28 days after onset of illness. Patients with a negative antibody test result whose specimens were obtained 28 days before illness onset or earlier should have another serum specimen collected within 28 days after onset of symptoms.

COLLABORATIVE MANAGEMENT

The Centers for Disease Control and Prevention (CDC) provides guidance on the clinical evaluation and management of patients who present with fever and/or respiratory illness. These guidelines focus on identification of cases and infection control management. At the present time, treatment for SARS is primarily supportive.

Management	Goal
Notify facility infection prevention leadership and the public health department.	Communicate suspected community health threat to comply with public health regulation and facilitate collaboration on the control and diagnosis of SARS-CoV.
At initial suspicion, place a mask on the patient and arrange for isolation. Place patient in an (Airborne Infection Isolation Room. [AIIR] negative pressure room) and wear personal protective equipment (PPE), including gowns, gloves, N-95 respirators, and facial protection upon entry to the room. Removal of protective equipment in a manner that prevents contamination of skin and clothing is a priority.	To prevent the transmission of SARS-CoV to other patients and to yourself.
Oxygen therapy	To support gas exchange and circumvent development of hypoxemia. Maintain pulse oximetry of >90%.
Intubation and mechanical ventilation	To support gas exchange and help maintain acid-base balance
Intravenous fluids	To prevent dehydration and maintain adequate circulatory volume

Antibiotics	To prevent secondary infections. Empirical antibiotic therapy should be prescribed for typical and atypical community-acquired pneumonia. Therapy may include a fluoroquinolone or macrolide.
Antiviral	Ribavirin is the antiviral of choice, but has had mixed results. Adverse side effects include hemolytic anemia and electrolyte imbalances (i.e., hypokalemia and hypomagnesemia). Patients must be monitored closely for significant side effects.
Corticosteroids	May be beneficial in patients with pulmonary infiltrates and hypoxemia. Methylprednisone dosage ranges from 40 mg twice daily to 2 mg/kg daily.

Care Priorities for SARS-CoV

1. **Treating the patient with supportive measures** as outlined earlier is recommended. There are no vaccines or specific management for SARS Co-V.
2. **Infection control:** Patients are to be placed in a negative-pressure room under airborne, contact, and standard precautions. Anyone who enters the patient's room must wear gowns, gloves, an N-95 respirator, and eye protection. Hand hygiene should be performed after contact with a patient on precautions. If there is a lack of negative-pressure rooms and/or there is a need to concentrate infection control efforts and resources, patients may be cohorted on a floor or nursing unit designated for the care of SARs patients only if air-handling systems can be modified to allow these areas to operate under negative pressure relative to surrounding areas.
   - Designate "clean" and "dirty" areas for isolation materials. Maintain a stock of clean patient care and PPE supplies outside the patient's room. Decide where contaminated linen and waste will be placed. Locate receptacles close to the point of use and separate from clean supplies.
   - Limit the amount of patient-care equipment brought into the room to that which is medically necessary. Provide each patient with patient-dedicated equipment (e.g., blood pressure cuff, thermometer).
   - Limit patient movement and transport out of the negative-pressure room. Whenever possible, use portable equipment to perform radiographs and other procedures in the patient room. Limit visits to patients to persons who are necessary for the patient's emotional well-being and care.
   - Health care workers who perform aerosol-generating procedures should be alert to the fact that there may be an increased risk of SARS-CoV transmission when these procedures are performed. PPE should fit properly and protect all skin surfaces and clothing. Wear a fluid-repellant gown or full-body suit, eye protection, N-95 respirator, and gloves that fit snuggly over the gown cuff. After an aerosol-generating procedure (e.g., intubation, bronchoscopy), clean and disinfect horizontal surfaces around the patient as soon as possible.

ADDITIONAL NURSING DIAGNOSES

See nursing diagnoses for *Acute Lung Injury and Acute Respiratory Distress Syndrome* (p. 365), *Acute Pneumonia* (p. 373), *Acute Respiratory Failure* (p. 383), *Mechanical Ventilation* (p. 99), *Fluid and Electrolyte Disturbances* (p. 37), and *Emotional and Spiritual Support of the Patient and Significant Others* (p. 200).

CREUTZFELDT-JAKOB DISEASE

PATHOPHYSIOLOGY

Creutzfeldt-Jakob disease (CJD) is a rare, fatal, neurodegenerative disorder, believed to be caused by an abnormal isoform of a glycoprotein known as a prion, a proteinaceous infectious particle. The most common disorder is bovine spongiform encephalopathy, or "mad cow" disease. A new form of CJD has emerged, called new variant CJD (vCJD or nvCJD). This form of CJD is linked to consumption of cattle with mad cow disease. Clinical and epidemiologic evidence supporting this link between "mad cow" disease and vCJD has become stronger. As of May 2004, a total of

153 cases of vCJD had been reported. vCJD generally affects younger people with a mean age of 29 years, whereas CJD occurs in the age group between 65 and 69 years.

CJD is classified as a transmissible spongiform encephalopathy, a category that includes other diseases (e.g., fatal familial insomnia, Gerstman-Sträussler-Scheinker syndromes). *Prion disease* occurs in animals, particularly cattle, sheep, and goats. CJD is endemic around the world and its estimated incidence report is 1 case per 1 million population. Three forms of "classic" CJD have been identified. *Sporadic* CJD affects older adults with rapid-onset dementia and neurologic symptoms of unknown cause. *Familial CJD* is an inherited disease and generally strikes younger individuals. It has a longer course in comparison to sporadic CJD. *Iatrogenic* CJD occurs through contact with infected tissue via medical procedures or treatments.

Prion proteins are normal proteins in the body and brain. In CJD, these proteins become abnormally shaped, as a result either of genetics or of contamination from an outside source. This leads to surrounding normal prion proteins taking on the abnormal shape. Central nervous system (CNS) function is disrupted, leading to cognitive impairment and cerebellar dysfunction. As the process continues, the abnormal prions accumulate in the brain, causing neuronal dysfunction, neuron death, gliosis (proliferation of neuroglial tissue in the CNS), and ultimately death.

TRANSMISSION

CJD can spread via infectious or hereditary means. Prion infections are transmitted via the peripheral route, either orally or transcutaneously. They may be introduced to lymphatic organs, particularly the spleen and lymph nodes, where initial replication of the infected prions occurs. Either infections enter the circulatory system and are hematogeneously spread to the brain, or infected prions may travel via the vagus nerve to the brain. Genetic mutation of the human prion gene *PrP* on chromosome 20 leads to the dysfunction of the prion protein. More than 20 reported mutations of this chromosome have been reported. All mutations influence the onset and duration of CJD. vCJD is theorized to be caused by the consumption of meat from cattle that is infected with bovine spongiform encephalopathy or mad cow disease (a prion disease). Once ingested, the infected prions follow the same neuroinvasion route of CJD.

ASSESSMENT: CREUTZFELDT-JAKOB DISEASE
Goal of Assessment
Evaluate for clinical signs of CJD.

Risk Factors and History
- Family history of CJD
- Exposure to contaminated tissue. People who have received human growth hormone derived from human pituitary glands or who have had dura mater grafts

Sporadic CJD
- Reported as having "come out of the blue"
- Early symptoms are memory loss, loss of interest, and mood changes that progress quickly (within a few weeks) to confusion and memory problems. Complaints of clumsiness, with jerky and stiff limbs, are also seen.
- Median age at death is 68 years old in patients who are initially seen with dementia and neurologic deterioration.
- Course of illness is often 4 months.
- Blurred eyesight and incontinence follow.
- At end stage, patients are unable to move or speak and need 24-hour care.
- Death occurs approximately 6 months after the onset of the disease.

Familial CJD
- Symptoms vary between different people, depending in part on the type of gene mutation responsible.
- In some cases, the illness is similar to sporadic CJD in type, duration, and progression, while in others, it is a more slowly developing dementia that progresses over a few years.

vCJD
- The incubation period is unknown and may take up to several years before manifesting.
- vCJD affects younger people, with a mean age of 29 years.
- Initial symptoms are more psychiatric than neurologic.
- Patients are anxious and depressed and display withdrawal or other behavioral changes.

- Persistent pain and odd sensations in the face and extremities are common. As disease progresses, the patient develops ataxia, sudden erratic movements, and progressive dementia with marked memory loss.
- Ultimately, the patient will lose the ability to move or speak and will require 24-hour care. Death soon follows.

DIAGNOSTIC TESTS

CJD is diagnosed based on typical signs, symptoms, and progression of disease.

Diagnostic Tests for CID		
Test	**Purpose**	**Abnormal Findings**
Radiology		
Magnetic resonance imaging (MRI): T1-, T2-, and diffusion-weighted and FLAIR sequences should be ordered with MRI.	Identify abnormalities of the brain consistent with CJD	Images will show abnormalities (hyperintensities and cortical ribboning) in specific areas of the brain (e.g., basal ganglia and medial and pons).
Neurophysiology		
Electroencephalogram (EEG)	For sporadic CJD cases Identify alteration in brain waves	Consistent slowing of brain waves and/or presence of periodic sharp wave complexes, generally late in the course of the disease
Laboratory Studies		
Lumbar puncture: cerebrospinal fluid (CSF) examination	Assess for protein levels consistent with CJD	Elevated CSF protein levels. A 14-3-3 CSF protein test should be highly sensitive and specific to CJD.
Brain biopsy	Assess region of brain that appears abnormal on MRI. Only means of confirming CJD besides autopsy.	Deposits or plaques of abnormal bundles of prion protein, spongiform encephalopathy

COLLABORATIVE MANAGEMENT

There is no known treatment or cure for CJD. Management of these patients is supportive and palliative in nature. There is no vaccine for CJD.

Care Priorities

1. **Supportive care:** Ventilatory support, pain management, patient safety, intensive skin care, assessment, nutritional support, care for immobility, and treatment for secondary infections.
2. **Infection control:** Standard precautions are used to care for patients with CJD. If a brain biopsy or other procedure is performed on a patient with CJD or suspected CJD, inform the central sterile department so that stringent chemical and autoclave sterilization methods can be used to reprocess instruments.

ADDITIONAL NURSING DIAGNOSES

See nursing diagnoses and interventions in *Nutritional Support* (p. 117), *Mechanical Ventilation* (p. 99), *Alterations in Consciousness* (p. 24), *Wound and Skin Care* (p. 167), *Prolonged Immobility* (p. 149), *Emotional and Spiritual Support for the Patient and Significant Others* (p. 200), and *Ethical Considerations in Critical Care* (p. 215).

WEST NILE VIRUS

PATHOPHYSIOLOGY

West Nile virus (WNV) is a single-stranded positive RNA virus from the Japanese encephalitis virus serogroup of the genus *Flavivirus*, family Flaviviridae, which is known for Japanese encephalitis and St. Louis encephalitis. In rare cases, WNV may lead to encephalitis or meningitis and death. WNV has an incubation period of 3 to 14 days. It also can be divided into two lineages. Lineage I strains are more widely distributed and linked to human infections.

TRANSMISSION
WNV is a disease that has spread worldwide. Initially, WNV was a disease that only occurred in bird species. Approximately 146 different species of birds have been reported to acquire this disease. This disease is spread among the bird population by 29 different species of mosquitoes (vectors). The natural cycle is from bird 1 to mosquito 1 to bird 2 to mosquito 2, and so forth. Due to a complex intensification of this natural cycle, bridge vectors (mosquitoes that bite both birds and humans) became infected with the WNV and spread the disease to humans. Only birds and humans in the United States and Israel have been known to die from WNV.

ASSESSMENT: WEST NILE VIRUS
Goal of Assessment
Evaluate for signs and symptoms of WNV.

History and Risk Factors
Exposure to mosquitoes where WNV exists increases risk. WNV is common in areas such as Africa, West Asia, and the Middle East. It first appeared in the United States in the summer of 1999 and since then has been found in all 48 contiguous states. Older age is associated with a higher risk for developing more serious CNS disease.

Incubation Period
- Two to 14 days, although longer incubation periods have been documented in immunosuppressed persons.

Mild Infection/West Nile Fever
- Symptoms last 3 to 6 days.
- Sudden onset of a fever with malaise, anorexia, nausea, vomiting, eye pain, headache, myalgia, rash, and lymphadenopathy.

Severe Infection/WNV Meningitis, WNV Encephalitis, and WNV Poliomyelitis
- When the CNS is affected, clinical syndromes ranging from febrile headache to aseptic meningitis to encephalitis may occur, and these are usually indistinguishable from similar syndromes caused by other viruses.
- WNV encephalitis or meningoencephalitis is characterized by altered mental status or focal neurologic findings.
- WNV meningitis involves fever, headache, and nuchal rigidity (stiff neck). Pleocytosis (abnormal increase in WBC count in cerebrospinal fluid) is present. Changes in consciousness are not usually seen and are mild when present.
- WNV encephalitis also involves fever and headache and more global symptoms. There is typically an alteration of consciousness, which may be mild and result in lethargy but may progress to confusion or coma. Focal neurologic deficits, including limb paralysis and cranial nerve palsies, may be observed. Tremor and movement disorders also have been identified.
- WNV poliomyelitis is characterized by the acute onset of asymmetric limb weakness or paralysis in the absence of sensory loss. Pain sometimes precedes the paralysis. The paralysis can occur in the absence of fever, headache, or other common symptoms associated with WNV infections. Involvement of the respiratory muscles, leading to acute respiratory failure, can occur.
- Clinical features
  - Fever
  - Gastrointestinal (GI) disturbances
  - Change in mental status
  - Development of a maculopapular or morbilliform rash (infrequent) involving the neck, trunk, arms, or legs
  - Seizures
  - Myelitis
  - Polyradiculitis

- Optic neuritis
- Cranial nerve abnormalities
- Severe weakness
- Flaccid paralysis sometimes
- Ataxia/extrapyramidal signs
- Myocarditis, pancreatitis, and fulminant hepatitis have been noted in outbreaks before 1990.

Labwork

Certain findings are seen in patients with severe disease.
- Total leukocyte count is mostly normal but can be elevated with lymphocytopenia and anemia.
- Hyponatremia is sometimes present, particularly among patients with encephalitis.
- CSF examination shows pleocytosis, usually with a predominance of lymphocytes. Protein is universally elevated. Glucose is normal.

Diagnostic Tests for West Nile Virus		
Test	**Purpose**	**Abnormal Findings**
Laboratory Studies		
WNV IgM antibody capture enzyme-linked immunosorbent assay (MAC ELISA) of serum or CSF	To diagnose WNV Most efficient diagnostic test. Best to collect 8 to 21 days after the onset of symptoms.	Positive MAC ELISA Patients who have been vaccinated or infected with other flaviviruses (e.g., Japanese encephalitis) may have positive results.
Complete blood count (CBC)	Identify abnormalities associated with WNV	Elevated leukocyte counts with lymphocytopenia and anemia. CBC can be normal with WNV.
Serum chemistry	To assess for hyponatremia which can be seen in WNV	Hyponatremia
Radiology		
Magnetic resonance imaging (MRI)	Identify possible abnormalities associated with WNV	One-third of patients show enhancements of the leptomeninges and the periventricular areas.

Testing for WNV can be obtained through local or state health departments. WNV is on the list of designated nationally notifiable arboviral encephalitides, and the proper authorities should be informed. Check your local or state health department for guidance.

COLLABORATIVE MANAGEMENT

Treatment of WNV infection is supportive. High-dose ribavirin and interferon alfa-2b have some activity against WNV in vitro. There is no specific antibiotic or antidote for the viral infection. There also is no vaccine.

Care Priorities

Supportive care: Includes intravenous fluids to prevent dehydration, antipyretics for fever management, oxygen therapy and ventilatory support, patient safety, nutritional support, and treatment for secondary infections. Standard precautions should be taken at all times; follow organization's policy for appropriate personal protection category.

ADDITIONAL NURSING DIAGNOSES

See nursing diagnoses and interventions in *Nutritional Support* (p. 117), *Mechanical Ventilation* (p. 99), *Alterations in Consciousness* (p. 24), *Wound and Skin Care* (p. 167), *Prolonged Immobility* (p. 149), *Emotional and Spiritual Support for the Patient and Significant Others* (p. 200), and *Ethical Considerations in Critical Care* (p. 215).

PANDEMIC FLU

An epidemic occurs when there are an unusually high number of people affected by a disease. A pandemic is an international epidemic. An influenza pandemic may occur when a new influenza virus is detected and the human population has no immunity. With the increase in global travel and transportation, and urban development with areas of overcrowding, epidemics that result from a new influenza virus are likely to be disseminated around the world and rapidly become a pandemic. The WHO has defined the phases of a pandemic to create a global framework to aid countries in pandemic preparedness and response planning. Pandemics can be either mild or severe in the illness and death they cause. The severity of a pandemic can change during the time the illness continues to spread.

WHO has developed a global influenza preparedness plan that outlines the responsibilities of WHO and national authorities in the event of an influenza pandemic. WHO also offers guidance tools and training to assist in the development of national pandemic preparedness plans (http://www.who.int/csr/disease/influenza/A58_13-en.pdf).

Two strains of flu—seasonal flu and the H1N1 (swine) flu—were circulating in North America during 2009. A third, highly lethal H5N1 (Avian) flu is circulating outside the United States. Healthy people generally recover from the flu without difficulty, but there is a subset of people at higher risk for serious complications. Efforts are under way to monitor the spread of all flu viruses.

AVIAN INFLUENZA ("BIRD FLU")

PATHOPHYSIOLOGY

Avian influenza is an infection caused by avian (bird) flu viruses, type A strains. These viruses occur naturally among birds. Wild birds carry the viruses in their intestines but usually do not get sick from them. However, domesticated birds such as poultry can become very ill and die from avian influenza viruses.

Fifteen subtypes of type A strain influenza have been identified based on their surface proteins. Two proteins, hemagglutinin (H) and neuraminidase (N), are used to delineate the subtypes. All subtypes have been recognized in birds; only three subtypes of H (H1, H2, and H3) and two subtypes of N (N1 and N2) have been known to infect humans.

It is theorized that certain subtypes of avian influenza mutated, crossed species, and infected humans. Three subtypes of avian influenza are linked to human infections: H5N1, H7N7, and H9N2. The H5N1 subtype is of particular concern to humans because of its ability to mutate and its tendency to acquire genes from viruses from other animal species. It has demonstrated high pathogenicity and causes severe disease in humans.

TRANSMISSION

Avian influenza is most commonly spread from infected birds to humans. The virus is harbored in birds (in the intestine), which shed the virus through their saliva, nasal secretions, and feces. The most common means of transmission among birds is fecal to oral. Humans who come in direct contact with infected poultry are susceptible to infection. Avian influenza survives on inanimate objects. Items contaminated with secretions/excretions of infected birds can be a vector for transmission to humans. The spread of avian influenza from one sick person to another has been reported very rarely, and transmission has not been observed to continue beyond one person.

ASSESSMENT
History and Risk Factors

- Direct or close contact with H5N1-infected poultry or H5N1-contaminated surfaces. In outbreaks, most cases have occurred in previously healthy children and young adults.
- A Health Safety Alert will be sent out by the CDC to all hospitals if there are avian influenza outbreaks that lead this federal organization to recommend heightened surveillance and diagnostic testing of targeted patients. In this situation, the CDC will outline triage guidelines, which will likely include travel to the outbreak location within the past 10 days and hospitalization with a severe respiratory illness.

Signs and Symptoms
- Similar to the "common flu": fever, cough, sore throat, muscle aches, and eye infections.
- In more severe cases of avian influenza, when assessed, the patient may display signs and symptoms of viral pneumonia (see *Acute Pneumonia*, p. 373) and ARDS (see *Acute Lung Injury and Acute Respiratory Distress Syndrome*, p. 365).
- These symptoms can be accompanied by nausea, diarrhea, vomiting, and neurologic changes.

DIAGNOSTIC TESTS

Diagnostic Tests For Avian Influenza		
Test	**Purpose**	**Abnormal Findings**
Laboratory Studies		
CBC	Assess for changes suggestive of other bacterial infections	Elevated white blood cell count
Influenza A/H5 (Asian lineage) virus real-time reverse transcription—polymerase chain reaction (RT-PCR) assay: Must consult with and have authorization from local or state health departments. Test is conducted only in designated labs.	To identify causative agent	Positive
Rapid bedside tests: Available but results are not confirmatory	Conduct for rapid screening for virus	Positive Confirmatory tests should be performed.
Viral culture: Must be conducted in biosafety Level 3 laboratory	Identify causative agent	Positive for pathogen
Radiology		
Chest radiograph	Identify progression of lung disease, and anatomic involvement	Infiltrates, atelectasis
Respiratory Tests		
ABG (if patient is in respiratory distress)	Determination of oxygen saturation and blood gases	Acidosis, alkalosis
Pulse oximetry	Measure oxygen saturation	< 90%

COLLABORATIVE MANAGEMENT

At present, the primary medication therapy option is oseltamivir (Tamiflu). An alternative is zanmivir (Relenza); however, there is concern that viruses may become resistant to both of these drugs. Treatment is supportive according to the clinical status of the patient.

Care Priorities

1. **Supportive management:** Includes intravenous fluids to prevent dehydration, antipyretics for fever management, oxygen therapy and ventilatory support, patient safety, nutritional support, and treatment for secondary infections.
2. **Infection control:** Place patient in a negative-pressure room under airborne, contact, and standard precautions. An N-95 respirator should be worn by everyone who enters the room. Gowns and gloves are to be worn for all patient contact, and eye protection should be worn when within 3 feet of the patient. Good hand hygiene should be practiced. Precautions should be continued for 14 days after onset of symptoms or until either an alternative diagnosis is established or diagnostic test results indicate that the patient is not infected with influenza A virus. Restricted visitation should be implemented and an ongoing log kept of all persons entering the patient's room.

Minimize the number of health care personnel caring for the patient. All equipment and other items should remain in patient's room and should not be used with other patients or outside the isolation room.

3. **Vaccination of health care workers:** Health care workers caring for patients with documented or suspected avian influenza should be vaccinated with the most recent seasonal influenza vaccine. This allows for protection against the predominant circulating strain and reduces the likelihood of health care workers becoming co-infected with human and avian strains, which could lead to the emergence of a pandemic strain. There is no vaccine for avian influenza at the present time.

ADDITIONAL NURSING DIAGNOSES

See nursing diagnoses for *Acute Lung Injury and Acute Respiratory Distress Syndrome* (p. 365), *Acute Pneumonia* (Chapter 4), *Acute Respiratory Failure* (p. 383), *Mechanical Ventilation* (p. 99), and *Emotional and Spiritual Support of the Patient and Significant Others* (p. 200).

THE 2009 H1N1 INFLUENZA ("SWINE" FLU)

The 2009 H1N1 ("swine flu") is a new influenza virus causing illness in humans that was first detected in the United States in April 2009. This virus continues to spread between and among humans internationally, in a similar fashion to the spread of seasonal influenza viruses. On June 11, 2009, the WHO raised the influenza alert level to Phase 6, the highest level, indicating a *global pandemic* of 2009 H1N1 flu was under way.

TRANSMISSION

Transmission is the same as for regular flu—via coughing, sneezing, and sometimes touching objects contaminated with the virus.

ASSESSMENT: H1N1
History and Risk Factors

Those at highest risk of contracting H1N1 are pregnant women, people who live with or care for infants younger than 6 months of age, health care and emergency medical services personnel, anyone from 6 months through 24 years of age, and anyone from 25 through 64 years of age with certain chronic medical conditions or a weakened immune system. Those in these groups are given the highest priority for administration of the H1N1 vaccine.

Signs and Symptoms
• Fatigue, fever, sore throat, muscle aches, chills, coughing, and sneezing

COLLABORATIVE MANAGEMENT

At present, the primary medication therapy option is oseltamivir (Tamiflu). Another alternative is zanmivir (Relenza); however, there is concern that viruses may become resistant to both of these drugs. Treatment is supportive according to the clinical status of the patient.

Care Priorities

For information on how to provide care for hospitalized patients, see Avian flu care priorities, p. 197.

1. **Prevention: Administer H1N1 vaccine**
   • Inactivated vaccine (vaccine containing dead virus) is injected into the muscle, like the annual flu shot.
   • A live intranasal vaccine (the nasal spray vaccine) is also available.

Safety Alert *Patients who should not receive the 2009 H1N1 flu vaccine include those with a severe (life-threatening) allergy to eggs or to any other substance in the vaccine. Patients who need advice from an expert practitioner on whether to receive the vaccine include those who have had a life-threatening allergic reaction after a dose of seasonal flu vaccine or Guillain-Barré syndrome. Patients who are moderately or severely ill should be advised to wait until recovered before getting the vaccine. Pregnant or breastfeeding women can get inactivated 2009 H1N1 flu vaccine. Inactivated 2009 H1N1 vaccine may be given at the same time as other vaccines, including seasonal influenza vaccine.*

2. **High-risk populations:** When the vaccine was first available, the CDC Advisory Committee on Immunization Practices (ACIP) recommended the 2009 H1N1 vaccine for the following five **target** groups:
   - Pregnant women
   - Household and caregiver contacts of children younger than 6 months of age (e.g., parents, siblings, and daycare providers)
   - Health care and emergency medical services personnel
   - Persons aged 6 months through 24 years
   - Persons aged 25 through 64 years who have medical conditions associated with a higher risk of influenza complications
3. **Reactions to vaccination:** Should be reported through the Vaccine Adverse Event Reporting System (VAERS) website at http://www.vaers.hhs.gov, or by calling 1-800-822-7967.
4. **Further information:** *To learn more about flu and vaccinations, advise patients to call* the local or state health department or to contact the CDC:
   - Call 1-800-232-4636 (1-800-CDC-INFO).
   - Visit the CDC website at http://www.cdc.gov/h1n1flu or http://www.cdc.gov/flu.
   - Visit the web at http://www.flu.gov.

EMOTIONAL AND SPIRITUAL SUPPORT OF THE PATIENT AND SIGNIFICANT OTHERS

Nurses must be acutely aware of the need to assess objectively and carefully, to avoid imposing personal views on others. Caregivers may feel they are in the best position to assign significance to an event or to decide the most appropriate response to an event. When faced with challenging situations, in order to facilitate therapeutic interactions, the nurse must assess both the patient's and significant others' understanding and perception of the situation prior to implementing a plan of care. Assessment requires active listening, being fully present in the interaction, and investing quality time by an interdisciplinary team to assist with problem solving. Given the resource intensity and possible inconsistency of caregiver assignments or coverage by other disciplines, time constraints may prompt dysfunctional situations not to be handled in the best manner to produce a sustainable solution or, in the worst case scenario, not to be noticed at all.

It is of paramount importance that nurses are familiar with how to provide both emotional and spiritual support to patients and families, to help guide them through the challenges posed by critical illness and hospitalization. Complex support system issues may include identification of high-risk dependent relationships between older adults, family members, domestic partners, children, or religious leaders. Actions required may include steps to prevent further infliction of physical, emotional, or sexual harm, including neglect of the basic necessities of life or exploitation.

Communication must be valued by all caregivers. Time must be invested to develop skills, enhance cognition, and learn to control emotions. Effective exchange of information is foundational for collaboration between the health care team and the patient. Accurate and timely information should be shared throughout the hospitalization to ensure the delivery of holistic patient care. Successful communication results from the development and implementation of strong relationships. In today's fast-paced, dynamic health care environment, relationships among health care professionals vary and change over time. With less opportunity to establish relationships, trusting the clinical knowledge, decisions, and judgment of unknown colleagues may be difficult. In large metropolitan teaching hospitals, the problem is compounded as the monthly rotation of multiple levels of physician house staff ensues.

Nursing care is often delivered in various time frames on a dynamic schedule and includes increasing numbers of contract and per diem clinical staff. Stabilizing the team and taking the time needed to provide effective communication can be challenging. The larger the number of either health care team members involved or family/significant others involved, the greater is the challenge. Emotionally charged events are common in the critical care environment, and to provide care of the whole patient and family system, emotional support is necessary to assist with coping. Occasionally, the caregivers are also in need of emotional support to cope with difficult situations.

Emotional support is defined as support for emotions the patient feels that will help provide the best outcomes for that patient. Key elements of holistic care include providing encouragement, reassurance, and acceptance during the times of stress. Mental, emotional, and spiritual interventions are needed to help with coping and decision making during critical illness. Emotional responses may be closely associated with mental processes. Thoughts or perceptions drive feelings about life events. Knowledge affects perception, so keeping patients and families informed and up-to-date is of paramount importance to their emotional well-being, as knowledge will promote them having more perceived control of the situation. Frequent, repetitive, simple explanations are often needed, because during emotional upset, ability to remember the information given is often impaired.

Nurses provide assistance to patients to facilitate adaptation to perceived stressors, changes, or threats that interfere with meeting the demands present in their lives, including the role they play when interacting with others. Coping techniques that are used vary with individuals, including the care providers, and are affected by culture. Counseling or family-centered care team conferences may be provided, using an interactive, helping approach, to focus on the needs, problems, or feelings of the patient, significant others, and health care team members. Actions are designed to enhance or support coping, crisis management, problem solving, and interpersonal relationships.

Emotionally charged ethical issues, particularly end-of-life decision making, frequently arise in the critical care environment, prompting care providers to address do-not-resuscitate issues, withdrawal of care, and whether the family desires to be present if resuscitation is needed. Despite countless benefits having been noted, sociology studies have concluded family presence during resuscitation will not be an acceptable practice until all care providers shift to a more holistic perspective. Involvement of the interdisciplinary team, including pastoral care, mental health professionals including the psychologist and/or social worker, palliative medicine or palliative care, and the ethicist, may be warranted on admission to the critical care unit, and throughout the stay if complex end-of-life issues arise.

RESEARCH BRIEF 2-1

A large percentage of the U.S. general public has stated they would like to remain with a loved one during resuscitation. Despite the countless benefits reported, family presence during resuscitation is a controversial, highly debated issue among health professionals in adult critical care units. The authors designed an exploratory, descriptive, and correlational study to determine the relationship between spirituality of health care professionals and support for family presence during invasive procedures and resuscitation. A holistic Spirituality Assessment Scale (SAS) developed by Howden was used to glean information regarding a more comprehensive meaning of spirituality—not focused exclusively on religious beliefs and feelings of patients, but rather, inclusive of feelings of health care providers. Data were collected from 73 nurses, 31 physicians, and 4 physician assistants. Results suggested a link between a holistic perspective and support for family presence. The higher the scores of spirituality for health care providers, the greater was the likelihood that they supported family presence as patient's right and part of holistic care. The study helps to fill the gap in current literature regarding certain demographic characteristics affecting whether health care providers are willing to allow families to be present during invasive procedures and resuscitation. Further analysis of extraneous variables is needed before the results of this study can be generalized.

From Baumhover N, Hughes L: Spirituality and support for family presence during invasive procedures and resuscitations in adults. *Am J Crit Care* 18(4):357–367, 2009.

Promoting psychological peace in the final phase of life is of paramount importance to the patient and involves exploration of the spiritual beliefs of all those involved in decisions. Disagreement on the appropriate course of action among health care team members stems from many factors, including their spirituality. Confusion among significant others regarding the wishes of the patient, their own views on death and dying, or vacillating patient views may create a dysfunctional care environment. The problem is compounded when various subgroups of decision makers share perspectives in isolation, rather than discussing them openly in a group composed of all key decision makers.

In extreme cases, anger and confusion may result in violent behavior, and the lines of communication may deteriorate if appropriate avenues are not initiated to repair damages. The American College of Critical Care Medicine has developed patient and family guidelines that help widen perspectives, open new options, and suggest different ideas for health care providers to help abate situations escalating to the point of physical violence.

Spiritual support is a part of providing holistic care. Several authors describe spirituality as a variable of holism. Spirituality is not to be confused with religion. Although the vast majority of nurses believe spiritual care is a part of providing patient-centered, holistic care, over half feel inadequate to perform spiritual care interventions. Spirituality has been described as values, beliefs, and behaviors of an individual related to purpose and meaning in life; connectedness to self, others, and life and universal dimensions; and innerness or inner resources and capacity for transcendence. Using these characteristics, Howden developed the Spirituality Assessment Scale (SAS) (Box 2-1). The 28 items on the SAS provide a strong operational framework for evaluating the ability of all involved with patient care and decision making to connect or to be sensitive to the spiritual dimensions of others and possibly frame how to approach the emotional needs of others. If a care provider has not developed the capacity to connect with others, providing care that requires embracing a viewpoint outside of his or her personal sphere of perception is extremely difficult. Behavior modification of the patient, significant others, or health care team members may be necessary as part of facilitating compliance with life changes for the patient and significant others resulting from the hospitalization. Values may collide, based on the past experiences of all involved. Staying focused on the present can assist all involved in remaining objective when approaching the situation.

Box 2-1	**ELEMENTS OF THE HOWDEN SPIRITUAL ASSESSMENT SCALE (SAS)**
Has a Sense of Belongingness	Feels Part of the Community Lived In
Has Capacity to Forgive	Feels Reconciling Relationships Is Important
Can Rise Above or Go Beyond Mental and Physical Problems	Can Rise Above or Go Beyond Body Changes or Body Losses
Is Concerned about Environmental Destruction	Feels Responsible for Preserving the Planet
Can Find Peace during a Devastating Event	Has Inner Resources for Dealing with Uncertainty
Has a Sense of Kinship to Others	Has Found Inner Strength during Past Struggles
Has a Connection to All of Life	Possesses Life Goals and Aims
Relies on Inner Strength When Struggling	Possesses Inner Strength
Enjoys Serving Others	
Has a Sense of Inner Spiritual Guidance	Feels a Sense of Fulfillment in Life
	Trusts Life Is Good Despite Discouraging Events
Perceives Ability for Self-Healing	Feels Good About Themselves
Perceives Meaning of Life Provides Peace	Has the Sense Life Has Meaning and Purpose
Feels a Sense of Balance Within Life	Feels Inner Harmony and Peace
Boundaries of Personal Universe Extend Beyond Space and Time	Inner Strength Is Related to Belief in a Higher Power or Supreme Being

Items are rated 1 (Strongly disagree) through 6 (Strongly agree) on a Likert scale after reading statements about the elements listed here.

ASSESSMENT OF NEED FOR EMOTIONAL AND SPIRITUAL SUPPORT

Goal of Assessment

To determine the ability of the patient and significant others to maintain a healthy response to changes brought forth by critical illness, so appropriate emotional and spiritual support can be provided to facilitate appropriate decision making as part of patient and family-centered care. Providing family-centered care requires the creation of mutually beneficial partnerships among patients, families, and health care providers. The patient is a part of a larger support system, and each caregiver is a part of a larger care system. Intense effort may be needed to create one voice for the right course of action in every situation that arises.

History and Risk Factors

Innumerable variables affect coping and decision making. The factors listed in Box 2-1 have been demonstrated by various studies to affect how decisions are made and may adversely affect coping because of a difference in beliefs related to spirituality. Difficulty coping may be more likely if the patient or any member of the decision-making team has a poor self-image, is unfulfilled in life, has significant financial problems, has developed unhealthy dependent relationships with others, is extremely resistant to change, has no sense of meaning or purpose in their life, has difficulty learning, has unrepaired significant relationships, has a poor sense of belongingness, does not feel inner peace or inner strength, is unable to forgive others for past offenses, has difficulty relating to others, cannot feel a sense of connectedness to others, or is unclear about life goals.

CARE PLANS: EMOTIONAL AND SPIRITUAL SUPPORT OF THE PATIENT, FAMILY, AND SIGNIFICANT OTHERS

Anxiety *related to actual or perceived threat of death; change in health status; threat to self-concept or role; unfamiliar people and environment; the unknown*

GOALS/OUTCOMES: Within 12 hours of intervention, anxiety is absent or reduced as evidenced by patient's verbalization of same, heart rate (HR) less than or equal to 100 beats/min, RR less than or equal to 20 breaths/min, and an absence of or decrease in irritability and restlessness. Family members are calmer.

NOC Anxiety Level, Anxiety: Self-Control, Concentration, Coping

Anxiety Reduction

1. Engage in honest communication with the patient and family; empathize. Actively listen, and establish an atmosphere that enables free expression. Express to patient that you care about his or her health.
2. Assess level of anxiety with patient and family. Be alert to verbal and nonverbal cues:
   a. *Mild:* Restless, irritable, asks more questions, focuses on the environment
   b. *Moderate:* Inattentive, expresses concern, narrowed perceptions, disturbed sleep pattern, increased HR
   c. *Severe:* Expressing feelings of doom; rapid speech; tremors; poor eye contact; preoccupation with the past; inability to understand the present; possible presence of tachycardia, palpitations, nausea, and hyperventilation
   d. *Panic:* Cannot concentrate or communicate, distorting reality, increased motor activity, vomiting, tachypnea
3. For severe anxiety or panic state, refer to appropriate psychiatric health care team member.
4. If hyperventilation occurs, encourage slow, deep breaths by having patient or significant other mimic your own breathing pattern.
5. Validate the nursing assessment of anxiety with the patient or significant other. ("You seem distressed; are you feeling anxious or overwhelmed?")
6. After an episode of anxiety, review and discuss the thoughts and feelings that led to the episode.
7. Identify coping behaviors currently being used (e.g., denial, anger, repression, withdrawal, daydreaming, drug or alcohol dependence). Review coping behaviors used in the past. Assist in using adaptive coping to manage anxiety.
8. Encourage expression of fears, concerns, and questions. ("I know this room looks like a maze of wires and tubes; please let me know when you have any questions.")
9. Reduce sensory overload by providing an organized, quiet environment. See *Alterations in Consciousness*, p. 24.
10. Introduce self and other health care team members; explain each individual's role as it relates to the plan of care or care map.
11. Teach relaxation and imagery techniques. See Sample Relaxation Technique, Appendix 7.
12. Enable support persons to be in attendance whenever possible.

13. Consult palliative care services if available and appropriate.
14. Engage in and promote awareness of touch to significant others when appropriate. Kinds of touch are described in Box 2-2.

NIC Coping Enhancement; Calming Technique, Active Listening, Presence

Social isolation *related to altered health status; inability to engage in satisfying personal relationships; altered mental status; altered physical appearance*

GOALS/OUTCOMES Within 24 hours of this diagnosis, patient demonstrates interaction and communication with others.
NOC Loneliness Severity, Mood Equilibrium, Personal Well-Being

Socialization Enhancement
1. Assess factors contributing to social isolation.
   - Restricted visiting hours
   - Absence of or inadequate support system
   - Inability to communicate (e.g., presence of endotracheal (ET) tube/tracheostomy)
   - Physical changes that affect self-concept
   - Denial or withdrawal
   - Critical care environment
2. Recognize patients at higher risk for social isolation: the older adult, disabled, chronically ill, economically disadvantaged.
3. Assist patient with identification of feelings associated with loneliness and isolation. ("You seem very sad when your family leaves the room. Can you tell me more about your feelings?")
4. Determine need for socialization, and identify available and potential support systems. Explore methods for increasing social contact (e.g., tapes of loved ones, more frequent visitations/hospital volunteers, scheduled interaction with nurse or support staff).
5. Provide positive reinforcement for socialization that lessens feelings of isolation and loneliness. ("Please continue to call me when you need to talk to someone. Talking will help both of us to better understand your feelings.")
6. Facilitate patient's ability to communicate with others (see Alterations in Consciousness, p. 24).

NIC Support System Enhancement, Mood Management

Compromised family coping *related to situational crisis (patient's illness)*

GOALS/OUTCOMES After intervention, family/significant others demonstrate effective adaptation to change/traumatic situation as evidenced by seeking external support when necessary and sharing concerns.
NOC Family Coping, Family Normalization

Box 2-2	KINDS OF TOUCH

Instrumental touch
- Task or procedure related
- May be negatively perceived but accepted as impersonal

Affective touch
- Expressive, personal
- Caring
- Comforting
- May be positively or negatively perceived
- Influenced by cultural patterns

Therapeutic touch
- Deliberate intervention to accomplish a purpose
- Acupressure
- Use of space around the individual to mobilize energy fields

Coping Enhancement

1. Assess character of family/significant others: social, environmental, ethnic, and cultural factors; relationships; and role patterns. Identify developmental stage. Be aware that other situational or maturational crises may be ongoing, such as an older parent or teenager with a learning disability.
2. Assess previous adaptive behaviors. ("How do you react in stressful situations?") Discuss observed conflicts and communication breakdown. ("I noticed that your brother would not visit your mother today. Has there been a problem we should be aware of? Knowing about it may help us better care for your mother.")
3. Acknowledge the family's/significant others' involvement in patient care, and promote strengths. ("You were able to encourage your wife to turn and cough. That is very important to her recovery.") Encourage participation in patient care conferences. Promote frequent, regular patient visits.
4. Provide information and guidance related to the patient. Discuss the stresses of hospitalization, and encourage discussions of feelings, such as anger, guilt, hostility, depression, fear, or sorrow. ("You seem to be upset since having been told that your husband is not leaving the hospital today.") Refer to clergy, case manager, clinical nurse specialist, social services, or palliative care specialist as appropriate.
5. Evaluate interactions among patient and family/significant others. Encourage reorganization of roles and priority setting as appropriate. ("I know your husband is concerned about his insurance policy and seems to expect you to investigate it. I'll ask the financial counselor to talk with you.")
6. Encourage family/significant others to schedule periods of rest and activity outside the critical care unit and to seek support when necessary. ("Your neighbor volunteered to stay in the waiting room this afternoon. Would you like to rest at home? I'll call you if anything changes.")

NIC Family Support; Family Process Maintenance; Normalization Promotion, Financial Resource Assistance

---

Fear *related to patient's life-threatening condition; lack of information*

GOALS/OUTCOMES After intervention, patient and family/significant others relate that fear has been lessened or is manageable.
NOC Fear Level, Fear Self-Control

Security Enhancement

1. Assess fears and understanding related to the patient's clinical situation. Evaluate verbal and nonverbal responses.
2. Acknowledge the fears. ("I understand these tubes must frighten you, but they are necessary to help nourish your son.")
3. Assess history of coping behavior. ("How do you react to difficult situations?") Determine resources and significant others available for support. ("Who/what usually helps during stressful times?")
4. Provide opportunities for expression of fears and concerns. Recognize that anger, denial, withdrawal, and demanding behavior may be adaptive coping responses during initial period of crisis.
5. Provide information at frequent intervals about patient's status and the therapies and equipment used. Demonstrate a caring attitude.
6. Encourage use of positive coping behaviors by identifying the fear(s), developing goals, identifying supportive resources, facilitating realistic perceptions, and promoting problem solving.
7. Be alert to maladaptive responses to fear: potential for violence, withdrawal, severe depression, hostility, and unrealistic expectations of staff or of patient's recovery. Provide referrals to psychiatric clinical nurse specialist or palliative care specialist as appropriate (see Box 2-3 for ways to reduce the risk of violence).
8. Assess your own feelings about the patient's life-threatening illness. Acknowledge that your attitude and fear may be reflected to the family/significant others.

NIC Coping Enhancement; Calming Technique; Support System Enhancement

---

Grieving *related to perceived potential loss of physiologic well-being (e.g., expected loss of body function or body part, changes in self-concept or body image, terminal illness)*

Box 2-3   SAFETY PRECAUTIONS IN THE EVENT OF VIOLENT BEHAVIOR

Patient safety

- Remove harmful objects from the environment, such as heavy objects, scissors, tubing.
- Apply padding to side rails according to agency protocol if patient is acting out.
- If available, use bed alarms. Ensure all unit staff members are aware of potential for violence.
- Use physical or chemical restraints as necessary and prescribed. Monitor patient's neurovascular status at frequent intervals.
- Set limits on patient's behavior, using clear and simple commands.
- As prescribed, consider chemical sedation when unable to control patient's behavior with other means.
- Explain safety precautions to patient and family/significant others.

Caregiver safety

- Place patient in bed closest to nursing station. Maintain visibility at all times by keeping door open.
- Alert hospital security department when risk of violence is present from patient or family.
- Do not approach a violent patient or family member without adequate assistance from others.
- Never turn your back on a violent patient or family member.
- Maintain a calm, matter-of-fact tone of voice. Set limits on family's behavior.
- Monitor security measures at frequent intervals.
- Remain alert.

Bureau of Labor Statistics (BLS), U.S. Department of Labor, for the National Institute for Occupational Safety and Health (NIOSH), Centers for Disease Control and Prevention: Survey of Workplace Violence Prevention, 2005. http://www.bls.gov/iif/home.htm

GOALS/OUTCOMES After interventions, patient and significant others/family express grief, participate in decisions about the future, and communicate concerns to health care team members and to one another.
NOC Adaptation to Physical Disability, Body Image Enhancement

Acceptance Health Status
1. Assess whether perceived sense of loss is real or unreal to patient or significant other.
2. Assess factors contributing to anticipated loss.
3. Assess and accept patient and family's behavioral response. Expect reactions such as disbelief, denial, guilt, anger, and depression. Determine stage of grieving as described in Table 2-1.
4. Assess spiritual, religious, and sociocultural expectations related to loss. ("Is religion an important part of your life? How do you and your family/significant others deal with serious health problems?") Refer to the clergy or community support groups as appropriate.

Emotional Support
1. Encourage patient and family/significant others to share their concerns. ("Is there anything you'd like to talk about today?") Also, respect their desire not to speak, and actively listen.
2. Demonstrate empathy. ("This must be a very difficult time for you and your family.") Touch when appropriate (see Box 2-2).
3. In selected circumstances, provide an explanation of the grieving process. This approach may assist in better understanding and acknowledging feelings.
4. Assess grief reactions of patient and family/significant others, and identify a potential for dysfunctional grieving reactions (e.g., absence of emotion, hostility, avoidance). If the potential for dysfunctional grieving is present, refer to case manager, psychiatric clinical nurse specialist, clergy, or palliative care specialist as appropriate.
5. When appropriate, assess patient's wishes about tissue donation.

NIC Active Listening; Dying Care; Grief Work Facilitation

Table 2-1	STAGES OF GRIEVING
Protest stage	Denial: "No, not me" Disbelief: "But I just saw her this morning" Anger Hostility Resentment Bargaining to postpone loss Appeal for help to recover loss Loud complaints Altered sleep and appetite
Disorganization	Depression Withdrawal Social isolation Psychomotor retardation Silence
Reorganization	Acceptance of loss Development of new interests and attachments Restructuring of lifestyle Return to preloss level of functioning

Spiritual distress *related to separation from spiritual/religious/cultural supports; challenged belief and value system*

GOALS/OUTCOMES Within 72 hours of this diagnosis, patient and family verbalize spiritual or religious beliefs and express hope for the future, the attainment of spiritual or religious support, and the availability of what is required to resolve conflicts.
NOC Spiritual Health, Dignified Life Closure

Spiritual Support
1. Assess spiritual or religious beliefs, values, and practices. ("Do you have a religious preference? How important is it to you? Are there any religious or spiritual practices you wish to participate in while in the hospital?")
2. Inform patient and family/significant others of the availability of spiritual aids, such as a chapel, religious services, or pastoral care service. Discuss advance directives.
3. Present a nonjudgmental attitude toward religious or spiritual beliefs and values. Create an environment conducive to free expression and invite sharing of beliefs. Identify available support systems that may assist in meeting the patient's religious or spiritual needs (e.g., clergy, patient's fellow church members, support groups).
4. Be sensitive to comments related to spiritual concerns or conflicts. ("I don't know why God is doing this to me." "I'm being punished for my sins.")
5. Use active listening and open-ended questioning to assist in resolving conflicts related to spiritual issues. ("I understand that you want to be baptized. We can arrange to do that here.")
6. Provide privacy and opportunities for religious practices, such as prayer and meditation.
7. If spiritual beliefs and therapeutic regimens are in conflict, provide honest, concrete information to encourage informed decision making. ("I understand that your religion discourages receiving blood transfusions. Do you understand that by refusing blood your condition is more difficult to treat?")

NIC Coping Enhancement, Conflict Mediation, Presence

Ineffective individual coping and ineffective denial *related to health crisis; sense of vulnerability; inadequate support systems*

GOALS/OUTCOMES Within 24 hours of this diagnosis, patient verbalizes feelings, identifies strengths, and begins using positive coping behaviors.
NOC Coping, Acceptance Health Status, Personal Well-Being, Adaptation to Physical Disability

Emotional and Spiritual Support

Coping Enhancement
1. Assess patient's perceptions and ability to understand current health status.
2. Establish honest communication. ("Please tell me what I can do to help you.") Assist with identifying strengths, stressors, inappropriate behaviors, and personal needs.
3. Support positive coping behaviors. ("I see that easy listening music seems to help you relax.")
4. Provide opportunities for expression of concerns; gather information from nurses and other support systems. Provide explanations about prescribed routine, therapies, and equipment. Acknowledge feelings and assessment of current health status and environment.
5. Identify factors that inhibit ability to cope (e.g., unsatisfactory support system, knowledge deficit, grief, fear).
6. Recognize defensive and maladaptive coping behaviors (e.g., severe depression, drug or alcohol dependence, hostility, violence, suicidal ideations). Confront these behaviors. ("You seem to be requiring more pain medication. Are you experiencing more physical pain, or does it help you to remove yourself from reality?") Refer patient to case manager, psychiatric liaison, clinical nurse specialist, clergy, or palliative care specialist as appropriate (see Box 2-3 for ways to reduce the risk of violence).

Support System Enhancement
1. Encourage regular visits by significant others. Encourage them to engage in conversation with patient to help minimize patient's emotional and social isolation.
2. Assess significant others' interactions with patient. Attempt to mobilize support systems by involving them in patient care whenever possible.
3. As appropriate, explain to significant others that increased dependency, anger, and denial may be adaptive coping behaviors used by patient in early stages of crisis until effective coping behaviors are learned.

NIC Socialization Enhancement; Resiliency Promotion, Self-Awareness Enhancement

Disabled family coping *related to inadequate or incorrect information or misunderstanding; temporary family disorganization and role change; exhausted support systems; unrealistic expectations; fear; anxiety*

GOALS/OUTCOMES After interventions, family/significant others verbalize feelings, identify ineffective coping patterns, identify strengths and positive coping behaviors, and seek information and support from the nurse or other support systems.
NOC Caregiver-Patient Relationship, Caregiver Performance: Direct Care, Caregiver Performance: Indirect Care

Caregiver Support
1. Have the family designate one member as the primary point of contact for the nurse. Explain how this will allow the nurse to spend more time taking care of the patient and less time on the telephone explaining the patient's status to each family member separately.
2. Establish open, honest communication. Assist in identifying strengths, stressors, inappropriate behaviors, and personal needs. ("I understand your mother was very ill last year. How did you manage the situation?" "I know your loved one is very ill. How can I help you?")
3. Assess for ineffective coping (e.g., depression, substance abuse, violence, withdrawal), and identify factors that inhibit effective coping (e.g., inadequate support system, grief, fear of disapproval by others, knowledge deficit). ("You seem to be unable to talk about your husband's illness. Is there anyone with whom you can talk about it?") (See Box 2-3 for ways to reduce the risk of violence.)
4. Assess knowledge regarding patient's current health status and therapies. Provide information frequently, and allow sufficient time for questions. Reassess understanding at frequent intervals.
5. Provide opportunities in a private setting to talk and share concerns with nurses or other health care providers. If appropriate, refer to psychiatric clinical nurse specialist for therapy.
6. Offer realistic hope. Help family/significant others develop realistic expectations for the future and identify support systems that will assist them with planning for the future.
7. Reduce anxiety by encouraging diversionary activities (e.g., period of time outside of hospital) and interaction with outside support systems. ("I know you want to be near your son, but if you would like to go home to rest, I will call you if any changes occur.")
8. Establish open, honest communication and rapport. ("I am here to care for your mother and to help you, as well.")
9. Identify ineffective coping behaviors (e.g., violence, depression, substance abuse, withdrawal). ("You seem to be angry. Would you like to talk to me about your feelings?") Refer to psychiatric clinical nurse specialist, clergy, or support group as appropriate.

10. Identify perceived or actual conflicts. ("Are you able to talk freely among yourselves?" "Are your brothers and sisters able to help and support you during this time?")
11. Encourage healthy functioning. For example, facilitate open communication and encourage behaviors that support cohesiveness. ("Your mother enjoyed her last visit. Would you like to see her now?")
12. Assess knowledge about patient's current health status. Provide opportunities for questions; reassess understanding at frequent intervals.
13. Assist with developing realistic goals, plans, and actions. Refer to clergy, case manager, psychiatric nurse, social services, financial counseling, and family therapy as appropriate.
14. Encourage family/significant others to spend time outside of the hospital and to interact with support individuals. Respect the need for occasional withdrawal.
15. Include the family/significant others in the patient's plan of care. Offer them opportunities to become involved in patient care, for example, range-of-motion (ROM) exercises, patient hygiene, and comfort measures (e.g., back rub).

NIC Family Involvement Promotion; Family Mobilization; Family Support

---

Powerlessness *related to health care environment; treatment regimen*

GOALS/OUTCOMES Within 24 hours of this diagnosis, assess patient and family's preferences, needs, values, and attitudes. The patient makes decisions about self-care and therapies and relates an attitude of realistic hope and a sense of self-control and family accepts decisions.

NOC Depression Self-Control, Family Participation in Professional Care, Health Beliefs: Perceived Control

Self-Responsibility Facilitation
1. Explain the *Patient and Family Rights and Responsibilities* information the hospital provides. Help the patient understand their rights and responsibilities, and responsibilities of the hospital with regard to patient care.
2. Ensure the patient and family know who is taking care of the patient. Tell the patient and family if a staff member does not have an ID badge visible, it is alright to ask for their name and their role in patient care.
3. Before providing information, assess patient's and family's understanding of health condition, prognosis, and plan of care.
4. Recognize expressions of fear, lack of response to events, and lack of interest in information, any of which may signal a sense of powerlessness.
5. Evaluate medical and nursing interventions, and adjust them, as appropriate, to support patient's and/or caregiver's sense of control. For example, if the patient always bathes in the evening to promote relaxation before bedtime, modify the care plan or map to include an evening bath rather than follow the hospital routine of giving a morning bath.
6. Assist patient to identify and demonstrate activities that can be performed independently.
7. Encourage the patient and/or family to keep a notebook with them at all times, which can serve as a helpful tool to remember questions or write down information which will be shared with other family members during this stressful time.
8. Whenever possible, offer alternatives related to routine hygiene, diet, diversion activities, visiting hours, or treatment times.
9. Encourage patient and family to ask to speak with the charge nurse, nurse manager, nurse supervisor, or patient advocate/patient representative if there is a problem with any member of the health care team.
10. Ensure privacy and preserve territorial rights whenever possible. For example, when distant relatives and casual acquaintances request information about the patient's status, refer them to the patient or a family member who can provide acceptable amounts of information.
11. Discourage patient's dependency on staff. Avoid overprotection and parenting behaviors.
12. Assess support systems; enable significant others to be involved in care whenever possible.
13. Offer realistic hope for the future. If appropriate, encourage direction of thoughts beyond the present.
14. Provide referrals to clergy, palliative care specialists, and other support systems as appropriate.

NIC Emotional Support; Family Involvement Promotion, Support Group

---

Sleep pattern, disturbed *related to environmental changes; illness; therapeutic regimen; pain; immobility; psychological stress*

GOALS/OUTCOMES After discussion, patient identifies factors that promote sleep. Within 8 hours of intervention, patient attains 90-minute periods of uninterrupted sleep and verbalizes satisfaction with ability to rest.

NOC Personal Well-Being, Sleep

Sleep Enhancement
1. Assess usual sleeping patterns (e.g., bedtime routine, hours of sleep per night, sleeping position, use of pillows and blankets, napping during the day, nocturia).
2. Explore relaxation techniques that promote rest/sleep (e.g., imagining relaxing scenes, listening to soothing music or taped stories, using muscle relaxation exercises).
3. Identify causative factors and activities that contribute to sleep pattern disturbance, adversely affect sleep patterns, or awaken patient. Examples include pain, anxiety, depression, hallucinations, medications, underlying illness, sleep apnea, respiratory disorder, caffeine, fear, and medical and nursing interventions.
4. Organize procedures and activities to allow for 90-minute periods of uninterrupted rest/sleep. Limit visiting during these periods.
5. Whenever possible, maintain a quiet environment by providing ear plugs or decreasing alarm levels. The use of "white noise" (e.g., low-pitched, monotonous sounds; electric fan; soft music) may facilitate sleep. Dim the lights for a period of time every 24 hours by drawing the drapes or providing blindfolds.
6. If appropriate, limit daytime sleeping. Attempt to establish regularly scheduled daytime activity (e.g., ambulation, sitting in chair, active ROM), which may promote nighttime sleep.
7. Investigate and provide nonpharmacologic comfort measures that are known to promote sleep (Table 2-2).

NIC Environmental Management; Environmental Management: Comfort

Table 2-2	NONPHARMACOLOGIC MEASURES TO PROMOTE SLEEP
Activity	**Example(s)**
Mask or eliminate environmental stimuli	Use eye shields, ear plugs Play soothing music Dim lights at bedtime Mask odors from dressings/drainage; change dressing or drainage container as indicated
Promote muscle relaxation	Encourage ambulation as tolerated throughout the day Teach and encourage in-bed exercises and position change Perform back massage at bedtime If not contraindicated, use a heating pad
Reduce anxiety	Ensure adequate pain control Keep patient informed of his or her progress and treatment measures Avoid overstimulation by visitors or other activities immediately before bedtime Avoid stimulant drugs (e.g., caffeine)
Promote comfort	Encourage patient to use own pillows, bedclothes if not contraindicated Adjust bed; rearrange linens Regulate room temperature
Promote usual presleep routine	Offer oral hygiene at bedtime Provide warm beverage at bedtime Encourage reading or other quiet activity
Minimize sleep disruption	Maintain quiet environment throughout the night Plan nursing activities to allow long periods (at least 90 minutes) of undisturbed sleep Use dim lights when checking on patient during the night

Body image disturbance *related to loss of or change in body parts or function; physical trauma*

GOALS/OUTCOMES Before hospital discharge, patient acknowledges body changes and demonstrates movement toward incorporating changes into self-concept. Maladaptive responses, such as severe depression, are absent.
NOC Body Image, Adaptation to Physical Disability
NOC Self-Esteem, Psychosocial Adjustment: Life Change

Body Image Enhancement
1. Establish open, honest communication. Promote an environment that is conducive to free expression. ("Please feel free to talk to me whenever you have any questions.") Assess indicators suggesting body image disturbance as listed in Box 2-4.
2. When planning care, be aware of interventions that may influence body image (e.g., medications, procedures, monitoring).
3. Assess knowledge of patient's pathophysiologic process and current health status. Clarify any misconceptions.
4. Discuss the loss or change with the patient. Recognize that what may seem to be a small change may be of great significance to the patient (e.g., arm immobilizer, catheter, hair loss, ecchymoses, facial abrasions).
5. Explore expressions of concern, fear, and guilt. ("I understand that you are frightened. Your face looks very different now, but you will see changes and it will improve. Gradually you will begin to look more like yourself.")
6. Encourage patient and family/significant others to interact with one another. Help family/significant others to support the patient's feelings related to the changed body part or function. ("I know your son looks very different to you now, but it would help if you speak to him and touch him as you would normally.")
7. Encourage gradual participation in self-care activities as the patient becomes physically and emotionally able. Allow for some initial withdrawal and denial behaviors. For example, when changing dressings over traumatized part, explain what you are doing but do not expect the patient to watch or participate initially.
8. Discuss the potential for reconstruction of the loss or change (i.e., surgery, prosthesis, grafting, physical therapy, cosmetic therapies, organ transplant).
9. Recognize manifestations of severe depression (e.g., sleep disturbances, change in affect, change in communication pattern). As appropriate, refer to case manager, psychiatric clinical nurse specialist, clergy, or support group.
10. Help patient attain a sense of autonomy and control by offering choices and alternatives whenever possible. Emphasize strengths, and encourage activities that interest patient.
11. Offer realistic hope for the future.

NIC Self-Esteem Enhancement; Emotional Support; Grief Work Facilitation, Suicide Prevention

Complicated grieving *related to loss of physiologic well-being; fatal illness*

GOALS/OUTCOMES Within 48 hours of this diagnosis, patient and family express grief, explain the meaning of the loss, and talk with each other. The patient completes necessary self-care activities.
NOC Mood Equilibrium, Grief Resolution, Depression Self-Control

| **Box 2-4** | **INDICATORS SUGGESTING BODY IMAGE DISTURBANCE** |

Nonverbal indicators
- Missing body part—internal or external (e.g., splenectomy, amputated extremity)
- Change in structure (e.g., open, draining wound)
- Change in function (e.g., colostomy)
- Avoiding looking at or touching body part
- Hiding or exposing body part

Verbal indicators
- Expression of negative feelings about body
- Expression of feelings of helplessness, hopelessness, or powerlessness
- Personalization or depersonalization of missing or mutilated part
- Refusal to acknowledge change in structure or function of body part

Emotional and Spiritual Support

Grief Work Facilitation
1. Assess grief stage (see Table 2-1) and previous coping abilities. Discuss feelings of patient and family, the meaning of loss, and goals. ("How do you feel about your condition/illness or your loved one's condition? What do you hope to accomplish in these next few days/weeks? Are you afraid your family will not be taken care of if you pass away?")
2. Acknowledge and permit anger; set limits on the expression of anger to discourage destructive behavior. ("I understand that you must feel very angry, but for the safety of others, you may not throw equipment.")
3. Identify suicidal behavior (e.g., severe depression, statements of intent, suicide plan, previous history of suicide attempt). Ensure safety, and refer to case manager, psychiatric clinical nurse specialist, psychiatrist, clergy, or palliative care specialist.
4. Encourage patient and family/significant others to participate in ADLs and diversion activities. Identify physiologic problems related to loss (e.g., eating or sleeping disorders), and intervene accordingly.
5. Collaborate with care team about a visit by another individual with the same disorder, if appropriate.

Hope Instillation
1. Provide opportunities for the patient to feel cared for, needed, and valued by others. For example, emphasize importance of relationships. ("Tell me about your grandchildren." "It seems that your family loves you very much.")
2. Support significant others who seem to spark or maintain patient's feelings of hope. ("Your husband's mood seemed to improve after your visit.")
3. Recognize factors that promote sense of hope (e.g., discussions about family members, reminiscing about better times).
4. Promote anticipation of positive events (e.g., mealtime, grandchildren's visits, bath time, extubation, removal of traction).
5. Help patient recognize that although there may be no hope for returning to original lifestyle, there is hope for a new but different life.
6. Avoid insisting that the patient assume a positive attitude. Encourage hope for the future, even if it is the hope for a peaceful death.
7. Set realistic, attainable goals, and reward achievement.

NIC Suicide Prevention, Family Integrity Promotion

Risk for self-directed violence or risk for other-directed violence by patient or family
related to sensory overload; suicidal behavior; rage reactions; neurologic disease; perceived threats; toxic reaction to medications; substance withdrawal

- -

GOALS/OUTCOMES Patient or family does not harm themselves or others.
NOC Aggression Self-Control, Abusive Behavior Self-Restraint, Abuse Cessation

Environmental Management: Violence Prevention
1. Assess factors that may contribute to or precipitate violent behavior (e.g., medication reactions, inability to cope, suicidal behavior, confusion, hypoxia, substance withdrawal, preictal and postictal states), or dysfunctional family behaviors such as arguing, pushing, and shoving.
2. Attempt to eliminate or treat causative factors. For example, provide patient teaching, assess the family for homicidal behavior, reorient patient, and reduce sensory overload (see Alterations in Consciousness, p. 24). Facilitate mental health consults as appropriate.
3. Approach patient and family in a positive manner, and encourage verbalization of feelings and concerns. ("I understand that you are upset and frightened. I will be here from 3 PM to 11 PM to care for you, or for your family member.")
4. Help patient distinguish reality from altered perceptions, including hallucinations, delusions, and illusions. Orient to time, place, and person. Alter the environment to promote reality-based thought processes (e.g., provide clocks, calendars, pictures of loved ones, familiar objects).
5. For acute confusion that becomes aggressive, do not attempt to reorient patient and avoid arguing. Instead, provide support by stating, "I believe that you (see, hear) that; however, I do not (see, hear) that." Use nonthreatening mannerisms, facial expressions, and tone of voice.
6. Initiate measures that prevent or reduce excessive agitation for patient or family:
   - Reduce environmental stimuli (e.g., alarms, loud or unnecessary talking).
   - Before touching patient/family, ask for permission. Provide concise explanations.

- Speak quietly (but firmly, as necessary), and project a caring attitude. ("We are very concerned for your comfort and safety. Can we do anything to help you feel more relaxed?")
- Avoid crowding (e.g., of equipment, visitors, health care personnel) in patient's personal environment.
- Avoid direct confrontation.

7. Explain and discuss patient's behavior with family/significant others. Acknowledge frustration, concerns, fears, and questions. Review safety precautions with family/significant others (see Box 2-3).

Abuse Protection Support

1. Assess for history of physical aggression, family violence, extreme dependence in relationships (including religious leaders), and substance abuse as maladaptive coping behaviors (see Box 2-3).
2. Discuss the need for Adult Protective Services involvement to protect the patient or family caregiver(s) with the medical team, case manager, and social worker if pathologic relationships are identified.
3. Monitor for early signs of increasing anxiety and agitation (e.g., restlessness, verbal aggressiveness, inability to concentrate). Assess for body language that is indicative of violent behavior: clenched fists, rigid posture, increased motor activity.

NIC Delusion Management, Anger Control Assistance, Anxiety Reduction, Surveillance: Safety, Crisis Intervention

Readiness for enhanced family coping: potential for growth *related to use of support systems and referrals; choosing experiences that optimize wellness*

GOALS/OUTCOMES At the time of the patient's diagnosis, family/significant others express their intent to use support systems and resources and identify alternative behaviors that promote communication and strengths. Family/significant others express realistic expectations and decrease use of ineffective coping behaviors.
NOC Family Functioning, Family Normalization, Respite Care

Normalization Promotion

1. Assess relationships, interactions, support systems, and individual coping behaviors. Permit movement through stages of adaptation. Encourage further positive coping.
2. Acknowledge expressions of hope, future plans, and growth among family members/significant others.
3. Encourage development of open, honest communication. Provide opportunities in a private setting for interactions, discussions, and questions. ("I know the waiting room is very crowded. Would you like some private time together?")
4. Refer the family/significant others to community or support groups (e.g., ostomy support group, head injury rehabilitation group).
5. Encourage exploration of outlets that foster positive feelings, for example, periods of time outside the hospital area, meaningful communication with the patient or support individuals, and relaxing activities (e.g., showering, eating, exercising).

NIC Support Group, Resiliency Promotion, Anticipatory Guidance

Deficient knowledge *related to disease process, diet, medication, prescribed activity, fall prevention, infection control, health resources, treatment procedures, treatment regimen, substance use control, personal safety*

GOALS/OUTCOMES Patient and family/significant others verbalize understanding of current diet, disease process, health resources, medication, prescribed activity, treatment procedures, and treatment regimen prior to discharge from the critical care unit.
NOC Knowledge: Disease Process, Diet, Fall Prevention, Health Behavior, Illness Care, Infection Control, Medication, Personal Safety, Substance Use Control

Teaching Individual and Family Support

1. Assess current level of knowledge about all aspects of disease process and illness management, including health resources, medication, prescribed activity, treatment procedures, and treatment regimen.
2. Assess cognitive and emotional readiness to learn.
3. Recognize barriers to learning, such as impaired verbal communication, altered thought processes, confusion, impaired memory, sensory alterations, fear, anxiety, and lack of motivation.

Emotional and Spiritual Support

4. Assess learning needs, and establish short- and long-term goals.
5. Use individualized verbal or written information to promote learning and enhance understanding. Give simple, direct instructions. If indicated, use audiovisual tools to supplement information.
6. Encourage significant others to reinforce correct information rendered by health care providers.
7. Encourage interest about health care information by involving patient in planning care. Explain rationale for care.
8. Interact frequently with patient to evaluate comprehension of information given. Ask patient and family to repeat what has been explained. Individuals in crisis often need repeated explanations before information can be understood. Also be aware that many individuals may not understand seemingly simple medical terms (e.g., "terminal," "malignant," "constipation").
9. As appropriate, assess understanding of informed consent. Assist patient to use information received to make informed health care decisions (e.g., about invasive procedures, surgery, resuscitation).
10. Assess understanding of right to self-determination; provide information as indicated. If requested, assist patient with mechanism for executing an advance directive for health care.
11. At frequent intervals, inform the family/significant others about the patient's current health status, therapies, and prognosis. Use individualized verbal, written, and audiovisual strategies to promote understanding.
12. Evaluate family/significant others at frequent intervals for understanding of information that has been provided. Adjust teaching as appropriate. Some individuals in crisis need repeated explanations before comprehension can be assured. ("I have explained many things to you today. Would you mind summarizing what I've told you so that I can be sure you understand your husband's status and what we are doing to care for him?")
13. Encourage family/significant others to relay correct information to the patient. This also reinforces comprehension for family/significant others and patient.
14. Ask if needs for information are being met. ("Do you have any questions about the care your mother is receiving or about her condition?")
15. Help family/significant others use the information they receive to guide health care decisions (e.g., regarding patient's surgery, resuscitation, organ donation).
16. Promote active participation in patient care when appropriate. Encourage family/significant others to seek information and express feelings, concerns, and questions.

NIC *Teaching:* Disease Process, Prescribed Medication, Procedure/Treatment, Health System Guidance, Fall Prevention; Health Education; Patient Rights Protection; Infection Protection, Learning Facilitation; Learning Readiness Enhancement

Impaired verbal communication *related to neurologic or anatomic deficit (e.g., hearing impairment, visual impairment); psychological or physical barriers (e.g., tracheostomy, intubation); cultural or developmental differences*

GOALS/OUTCOMES At the time of intervention, patient communicates needs and feelings and relates decrease in or absence of frustration over communication barriers.
NOC Communication: Expressive, Communication: Receptive, Information Processing

Communication Enhancement: Speech, Hearing, and/or Visual Deficit
1. Assess etiology of impaired communication (e.g., tracheostomy, stroke, cerebral tumor, Guillain-Barré syndrome).
2. With patient and significant others, assess patient's ability to hear, see, speak, read, write, and comprehend English. If patient speaks a language other than English, collaborate with English-speaking family member or interpreter to establish effective communication.
3. When communicating, use eye contact; speak in a clear, normal tone of voice; and face the patient.
4. If patient cannot speak because of a physical barrier (e.g., tracheostomy, wired mandibles), provide reassurance and acknowledge frustration. ("I know this is frustrating for you, but please do not give up. I want to understand you.")
5. Provide slate, word cards, pencil and paper, alphabet board, pictures, or other communication device to assist patient. Adapt the call system to meet the patient's needs. Document the meaning of the patient's signals in response to questions.
6. Explain to significant others the source of the communication impairment; demonstrate effective communication alternatives (see preceding intervention).
7. Be alert to nonverbal messages, such as facial expressions, hand movements, and nodding of the head. Validate meanings of nonverbal cues with the patient.

8. Recognize that the inability to speak may foster maladaptive behaviors. Encourage patient to communicate needs; reinforce independent behaviors.
9. Be honest; do not relate understanding if you cannot interpret patient's communication.

NIC Active Listening; Communication Enhancement: Hearing Deficit, Speech Deficit, Visual Deficit

Disturbed sensory perception *related to therapeutically or socially restricted environment; psychological stress; altered sensory reception, transmission, or integration; chemical alteration*

GOALS/OUTCOMES At the time of intervention, patient verbalizes orientation to time, place, and person; relates the ability to concentrate; and expresses satisfaction with the degree and type of sensory stimulation being received.
NOC Distorted Thought Self-Control, Neurological Status: Cranial/Sensory Motor Function, Vision Compensation Behavior

Environmental Management
1. Assess factors contributing to the sensory/perceptual alteration.
   - Environmental: Excessive noise in the environment; constant, monotonous noise; restricted environment (immobility, traction, isolation); social isolation (restricted visitors, impaired communication); therapies.
   - Physiologic: Altered organ function; sleep or rest pattern disturbance; medication; history of altered sensory perception.
2. Determine the appropriate sensory stimulation needed; plan care accordingly.
3. Control factors that contribute to environmental overload. For example, avoid constant lighting (maintain day/night patterns); reduce noise whenever possible (e.g., decrease alarm volumes, avoid loud talking, keep room door closed, provide ear plugs).
4. Provide meaningful sensory stimulation:
   - Display clocks, large calendars, and meaningful photographs and objects from home.
   - Depending on patient's preferences, provide a radio, music, reading materials, and tape recordings of family and significant others. Earphones help block out external stimuli.
   - Position patient toward window when possible.
   - Discuss current events, time of day, holidays, and topics of interest during patient care activities.
   - As needed, orient patient to surroundings. Direct patient to reality as necessary.
   - Establish personal contact by touch to help promote and maintain contact with the real environment.
   - Encourage significant others to communicate with patient frequently, using a normal tone of voice.
   - Convey concern and respect. Introduce yourself, and call patient by name.
   - Stimulate vision with mirrors, colored decorations, and pictures.
   - Stimulate sense of taste with sweet, salty, and sour substances if appropriate.
   - Encourage use of appropriate eyeglasses and hearing aids.
5. Inform patient before initiating interventions and using equipment.
6. Encourage participation in health care planning and decision making whenever possible by asking patient first.
7. Provide patients with choices when possible.
8. Assess sleep-rest pattern to evaluate its contribution to the sensory/perceptual disorder. Ensure that patient attains at least 90 minutes of uninterrupted sleep as frequently as possible. For more information, *see Sleep Pattern, Disturbed, P. 209*

NIC Environmental Management; Cognitive Restructuring; Cognitive Stimulation

ETHICAL CONSIDERATIONS IN CRITICAL CARE

More controversy surrounds health care decisions made by and for critical care patients than in any other health care area. These decisions have been debated vigorously in the literature, and although some of these issues have been resolved, others continue to be argued. Here we will examine what is currently considered morally acceptable practice.

Health care providers must develop a clear understanding of ethical issues to ensure that the care they provide is morally and legally acceptable. Ethical reasoning enables the health care professional to examine the moral principles involved in decision making and determine what he or she ought to do. There are four predominant principles used in health care ethics for decision making: (1) respect for autonomy (recognizing that each patient has a right to make decisions for him/herself), (2) nonmaleficence (not harming a patient), (3) beneficence (helping a patient), and (4) justice (treating patients equally). Ethical dilemmas occur when one of these principles conflicts with another. When a patient refuses needed treatment, the principles of autonomy and beneficence are in conflict. Other processes and documents related to decision making are discussed next.

INFORMED CONSENT

Without adequate knowledge, patients and their significant others cannot make good decisions. Part of a nurse's obligation is to inform patients and families, in a caring manner, what is to be expected of different treatment options. Informed consent serves not only to protect the health care provider from liability; its primary purpose is to support the ethical principle of respect for autonomy. Informed consent is instrumental to a patient's right to accept, continue, or reject all or part of health care interventions of any sort. The elements of informed consent should be used as a guide but are not absolutely necessary for all nursing or medical interventions (Box 2-5).

If a patient is unsure, does not understand, or feels pressured about consenting to the treatment plan, nurses are responsible to advocate for the patient and communicate this to the physician, other health care professionals, and to the hospital or health care agency administration if necessary.

ADVANCE DIRECTIVES

Advance directives refer to a patient's directions on how to provide care in the event that the patient becomes unable to make decisions on his or her own behalf. An advance directive can be written or verbal and can be in the form of a living will or a durable power of attorney for health care (DPAHC).

A living will specifies what treatment a patient wants or does not want in the event that the condition is terminal and the patient cannot make health care decisions. A DPAHC appoints a person to make decisions for a patient when the patient cannot make decisions.

A surrogate decision maker is someone named in the DPAHC. When no DPAHC exists, the legal next of kin becomes the surrogate decision maker for the patient. If the patient does not have family or a DPAHC, a court-appointed guardian becomes the surrogate decision maker. This person is obligated to make choices that the patient would make. If those choices are unknown, the surrogate decision maker must try to determine, based on the patient's values, what the patient would want.

Advance directives appeal to the ethical principle of respect for autonomy. When no advance directive is available, we then turn to the ethical principle of beneficence by making decisions in the patient's best interest. Advance directives are supported by the Patient Self-Determination Act, which encourages their use as well as prompts health care providers and institutions to honor them. Interpretation of advance directives can be problematic. Although

---

Box 2-5	ELEMENTS OF INFORMED CONSENT

Threshold elements (preconditions)
1. Competence (to understand and decide)
2. Voluntaries (in deciding)

Information elements
3. Disclosure (of material information)
4. Recommendation (of a plan)
5. Understanding (of items 3 and 4)

Consent elements
6. Decision (in favor of a plan)
7. Authorization (of the chosen plan)

From Beauchamp TL, Childress JF: *Principles of biomedical ethics*, ed 6. New York, 2009, Oxford University Press.

many patients express a desire for no "extraordinary measures," the meaning of this term can vary. For example, a ventilator can be considered "extraordinary," but it is also part of quite common temporary treatments regularly used in critical care. Despite problems with interpretation, caregivers must responsibly deal with their ambiguities and seek to honor their spirit.

CONFIDENTIALITY

Confidentiality in a relationship between a health care provider and a patient means that we do not identify or expose information that is not relevant to care. Also, we do not communicate information gained from a patient except with providers and decision makers identified by the patient. Confidentiality appeals to the ethical principles of respect for autonomy, beneficence, and nonmaleficence. Almost all nursing and medical codes provide for keeping all information about a patient confidential. Any disclosure of patient information should be considered very carefully.

The Health Insurance Portability and Accountability Act of 1996 (HIPAA) was mandated by the U.S. Congress to establish a federal standard regarding confidentiality of specific electronic medical information. Individual states may have stricter privacy laws. HIPAA sets the lowest acceptable standard for privacy. State laws apply over HIPAA.

There are situations in which we are legally obligated to breach patient confidentiality. These situations include public welfare risks, sexually transmitted diseases, gunshot wounds, and suspected abuse and/or neglect of children, older adults, or developmentally disabled individuals. HIPAA supports the disclosure of protected health information when required by law.

QUALITY OF LIFE

Most quality-of-life dilemmas in health care appeal to the ethical principle of justice. A person's quality of life is based on physical, intellectual, emotional, and social components. Although improving quality of life is a primary focus of health care, assessing quality of life is difficult at best. Numerous studies have demonstrated that health care providers consistently rate patients' quality of life lower than the patients do themselves. Studies also reveal that such judgments by health care providers do affect care. Nurses in critical care should be aware they are seeing only a minuscule part of a patient's entire life. Quality-of-life assessments may be based on a patient's medical condition during this time. Patients take into account things such as family, relationships, and finances when assessing their own quality of life.

A patient's assessment of quality of life may be compromised when that patient becomes depressed or newly disabled (e.g., stroke, paraplegia, quadriplegia). Although critical care nurses care for many patients in such situations, it is usually the first time that this patient or family has faced such life-altering circumstances. The stress of the situation makes evaluation of quality of life difficult for them. It is important to provide the patient and family with support and time before making critical decisions.

Studies indicate that health care providers not only base quality of life on the patient's medical condition but also have social prejudices that affect care. These include prejudices against older adults, persons with alternative lifestyles, those with alcohol and/or other substance abuse, and patients with a history of criminal activity. Judgments may be passed on to others during nursing reports. This promotes prejudice rather than good care. Our justice system, not our health care system, determines what behaviors to punish and how they should be punished.

WITHHOLDING AND WITHDRAWING TREATMENT

The acts of withholding (not starting) and withdrawing (stopping) treatment are considered to have no moral or legal difference. However, health care providers and patients' family members are misguidedly more comfortable withholding than withdrawing treatment. Once a treatment has been started and is determined to be of no benefit to the patient, the reasons used to justify withholding treatment can be used when stopping or withdrawing care. The decision can be reinforced by appealing to the principles of nonmaleficence and beneficence along with the knowledge that the treatment has not benefited the patient.

It has been noted that when decisions to withhold resuscitation (do not resuscitate [DNR]) have been made, it seems unclear what other care should be provided. DNR does not mean do not treat. Many patients with DNR orders receive critical care interventions, surgery, and other treatments and then survive to discharge. Once a decision has been made to withhold resuscitation, it is important to clearly define treatments to be withheld or provided.

ASSISTED SUICIDE

Assisted suicide occurs when someone provides a means for a patient to commit suicide (such as deliberately providing enough medicine for an overdose) but the patient actually performs the act that results in death. Although controversy surrounds assisted suicide, the American Nurses Association (ANA), the American Association of Critical Care Nurses (AACN), the American Medical Association (AMA), and the National Hospice Organization (NHO) explicitly oppose it. Most states have laws that make assisted suicide a criminal act. In 1994, Oregon became the first and only state to allow physician-assisted suicide for terminally ill patients. The Oregon law continues to face legal challenges. In the summer of 1997, the U.S. Supreme Court determined that there is no constitutional right to physician-assisted suicide.

EUTHANASIA

Euthanasia refers to one person killing another person without causing pain. Several studies reveal a significant number of nurses believe euthanasia is justifiable and should be legalized. This indicates a serious conflict of interest by health care providers. Euthanasia is illegal, is opposed by nursing and medical codes, and is morally unacceptable to persons with certain ethical or religious convictions. Even if the intent of euthanasia is "compassion" and the patient requests it, if the health care provider intentionally kills a patient, that health care provider is morally and legally responsible for that patient's death.

COMFORT CARE

Patients who are chronically ill, debilitated, or dying are generally isolated from and by society as well as by health care providers. Health care providers now recognize pain and depression may be undertreated in the routine care of patients and while caring for those who are chronically ill or dying. Concerns center around fears of causing dependence, unresponsiveness, and even death. When faced with a dying patient, it is unreasonable to worry about potential dependence on medication. The benefits of analgesics far outweigh the risks of dependence. Health care providers should try to provide the maximal pain relief possible while preserving responsiveness. When that is not possible, most patients and families choose to accept a decreased responsiveness to ensure that adequate pain relief is provided for the dying patient.

Many health care providers voice concerns that giving potent opioids or opiates to a dying patient may actually kill the patient. This concern is magnified when decisions to withdraw and withhold treatments have been made simultaneously. Opioid and opiate analgesics afford a broad therapeutic index and have a long history of safe use in medically frail patients. Patients can tolerate increasing doses of these drugs without adverse respiratory or cardiovascular effects.

Even though it is very difficult to determine what amount of opioid or opiate will cause a person's death, such medicines can still be given by appealing to the principle of double effect. Simplified, this principle explains that giving narcotics to relieve pain is morally acceptable, even while knowing that it may also cause the patient to die sooner. When narcotics and sedatives are given to a patient at the end of life, the intent is to provide comfort until death; the health care provider does not intend to cause the patient to die. If the health care provider gives a medicine with the primary intent of killing a patient, the health care provider is euthanizing that patient and the action is immoral and illegal.

ETHICAL REASONING

When nurses find themselves in a situation in which they think something is "wrong," they should first consider the situation logically and systematically. By doing this, nurses can defend their positions rationally and provide ethically as well as medically sound care.

1. Identify the problem. Is the care provided inappropriate?
2. Determine the relevant facts of the case. These facts include the patient's medical, mental, and emotional condition, as well as the current plan of care.
3. Evaluate personal biases. The nurse must consider his or her personal values and ethical position regarding the situation as it may affect care. Nurses should consider the values and ethical positions of all of the decision makers involved.
4. Check for advance directives. If the patient is incompetent, does he or she have an advance directive?

5. Explore options and their consequences. Explore all plausible options for resolving the dilemma. Consider the consequences of each option.
6. Discuss the relevant ethical principles in the situation. For example, a question asked may be "Will continued aggressive treatment respect the patient's autonomy by following the advance directive?"
7. Rank the acceptable options in order of importance. Develop and implement a plan for choosing options, including timelines for choices.
8. Clarify the expectations and wishes of those involved. Box 2-6 outlines steps used to begin clarifying our understanding of the situation so appropriate decisions can be made.

If direct communication with those involved does not resolve the issue, the bedside nurse should then involve the charge nurse or unit manager. The medical director's involvement may be beneficial also. If assistance is still needed in resolving the dilemma, The Joint Commission (TJC; formerly, the Joint Commission on Accreditation of Healthcare Organizations [JCAHO]) requires that health care providers have access to institutional means for resolving ethical dilemmas (such as an ethics consultant or committee). If a nurse strongly believes that unethical care is being provided and an acceptable resolution to the issue is not found, the nurse should withdraw from caring for that patient. Before withdrawing from that patient, however, the nurse must be replaced by another equally competent nurse who does not oppose the plan of care.

PREVENTIVE ETHICS

Just as it is easier to prevent heart disease than it is to cure it, it is easier to prevent an ethical conflict than it is to resolve one. When evaluating actions taken to resolve a dilemma, nurses should consider how those actions can provide help with future dilemmas. When the bedside nurse first sees signs of a problem, strategies used in previous, similar situations should be employed to prevent this situation from developing into a conflict. Many seemingly ethical problems are actually communication deficits. Such problems may be resolved after gathering information and coordinating a patient care conference involving all relevant persons. All professionals should refrain from speculation or gossip and instead openly communicate with the patient, family, and other members of the care team about the plan of care. The nurse should promote discussions in advance of all possible outcomes. Last and most important, nurses should respect each patient as a person and treat that patient accordingly.

CARE PLANS FOR ETHICAL CONSIDERATIONS

Deficient knowledge *related to medical/nursing interventions related to end-of-life care*

- -

GOALS/OUTCOMES Before any medical or nursing intervention, the patient and significant others will know, understand, and agree to or refuse the intervention.
NOC Knowledge: Treatment Procedure(s)

Box 2-6	**COMPONENTS OF ETHICAL REASONING**

1. Identify the actual problems.
2. Determine the relevant facts of the case.
3. Consider the values and ethical positions of everyone involved.
4. Determine possible options for resolving the dilemma.
5. Consider consequences of each option identified.
6. Apply relevant ethical principles to each option identified.
7. Prioritize acceptable options.
8. Develop and implement a plan to resolve the dilemma.
9. Evaluate the resolution of the dilemma.

Ethical Considerations in Critical Care

Teaching: Procedure/Treatment
1. Determine appropriate decision maker.
2. Assess decision-making capacity.
3. Assess decision maker's understanding of intervention; provide information as indicated.
4. Determine voluntariness.
5. Accept patient's/significant others' permission for or refusal of the intervention.

NIC *Teaching:* Procedure/Treatment; *Teaching:* Disease Process; Learning Facilitation

Deficient knowledge *related to end-of-life decisions related to available documents*

GOALS/OUTCOMES Patient will know and understand options regarding living wills and DPAHC.
NOC Knowledge: Disease Process

Decision-Making Support
1. Provide patient with information regarding living wills and DPAHC.
2. Assess understanding of living wills/DPAHC; provide information as indicated.
3. Determine who is legally empowered as a surrogate decision maker.

NIC Health System Guidance; Patient Rights Protection

Grieving *related to withholding/withdrawal of treatment; anticipation of loss*

GOALS/OUTCOMES After intervention, patient and significant others communicate feelings and participate in decisions regarding death and dying.
NOC Grief Resolution

Anticipatory Guidance
1. Assess patient's/significant others' understanding of medical prognosis and planned interventions.
2. Provide specific information regarding what to expect, what care/interventions will be given, and what will be withheld/discontinued; answer questions openly.
3. Allow for significant others to be with patient during the dying process.
4. Provide all comfort measures possible for patient/significant others.

NIC Grief Work Facilitation; Support System Enhancement; Active Listening; Family Support; Environmental Management: Comfort; Spiritual Support; Decision-Making Support

PATIENT SAFETY

In 1999, the Institute of Medicine (IOM) released the report *To Err Is Human: Building a Safer Health Care System*, which focused national attention on patient safety. The IOM estimated that between 44,000 and 98,000 persons die annually as a result of medical error and that more than 1 million patients sustain injury as a result of medical errors. Since its release, regulatory agencies, health care facilities, and consumers have joined together to enhance patient safety. The report emphasized that individual clinicians' competency, hard work, and good intentions were not the cause of these errors but the complex health care system with complicated processes were leading to these errors.

Shifting the goal from eliminating individual errors to reducing or eliminating the *potential* for patients to be harmed is significant. A proactive approach generally yields more globally successful outcomes. Nurses can contribute significantly to keeping patients safe by focusing on system-wide improvements, rather than reacting to events that could have been prevented. Nurses spend extensive periods of time with patients and are placed in roles that require interdisciplinary care coordination. The coordinative role prompts familiarity with a variety of hospital processes that may place the patient at risk for harm. Although it is not an easy journey, health care facilities now focus attention on designing systems where errors are prevented, and when they occur, practitioners can easily recognize and recover from actual and possible errors.

PATIENT SAFETY STANDARDS

Patient safety standards are set by a variety of organizations, including TJC, which is recognized as the primary group responsible for setting the standard. Other organizations provide information to support a culture of patient safety, including the Agency for Healthcare Research and Quality (AHRQ), the National Quality Forum (NQF), the Institute for Healthcare Improvement (IHI), and the National Patient Safety Foundation (NPSF). All four agencies have done extensive research related to health care quality and provide extensive materials to support health care providers in performance improvement efforts that will help to improve patient safety. The web addresses for these agencies are as follows:

AHRQ (www.AHRQ.gov)
The AHRQ mission is to improve the quality, safety, efficiency, and effectiveness of health care for all Americans. The agency's research assists both consumers and professionals to make more informed decisions about health care and facilitate quality improvement in health care services. AHRQ was formerly known as the Agency for Health Care Policy and Research.

IHI (www.ihi.org)
The IHI is an independent, nonprofit organization that strives to lead the improvement of worldwide health care. The IHI facilitates improvement by augmenting the desire or will for change, developing concepts for improving patient care, and helping health care systems put those ideas into action.

NQ F (www.qualityforum.org)
TheNQF is a not-for-profit organization focused on improving the quality of health care for all Americans. Their three-part mission includes setting priorities for performance improvement, supporting national consensus standards for performance measurement and public reporting of this information, and facilitating attainment of national goals by offering education and outreach programs.

NPSF (www.npsf.org)
The NPSF is an independent, not-for-profit organization founded in 1997, with a mission to improve safety of patients and families within the health care system. NPSF is committed to a collaborative, multistakeholder approach, to include and unite disciplines and organizations across the continuum of care.

TJC (www.jointcommission.org)
The mission of TJC is to continuously improve the safety and quality of care provided to patients through the provision of health care accreditation. The organization has set standards that include National Patient Safety Goals and Sentinel Event Alerts. The 2007 Joint Commission Annual Report on Quality and Safety revealed inadequate communication between health care providers, or between providers and the patient and family members, was the main or root cause of at least half the serious adverse events in hospitals. Other causes included inadequate assessment of the patient's condition, and poor leadership or training. TJC has launched several patient safety initiatives including the "Do Not Use Abbreviation" list, Infection Control, "Speak Up," and Universal Protocol ("Time Out"). Many of these initiatives have risen as a result of sentinel events that have occurred across the United States.

Web sites for additional resources are listed in Table 2-3.

Sentinel Event Alerts In 1996, TJC established the *sentinel event policy*, which called for the identification, reporting, evaluation, and prevention of sentinel events, defined as any unexpected occurrence involving death or serious physical or psychological injury or risk thereof (Boxes 2-7 and 2-8). One of the fundamental aspects of the sentinel event policy is the publication of sentinel event alerts by TJC. Sentinel event alerts consolidate experiences and "lessons learned" by accredited health care organizations with the goal of preventing medical errors in the future.

National Patient Safety Goals In July 2002, TJC launched the National Patient Safety Goal (NPSG) program in all accredited facilities. NPSGs are identified and prioritized by the Patient Safety Advisory Group, which consists of physicians, nurses, pharmacists, and other clinicians with expertise in patient safety for all accredited bodies (i.e., acute care facilities, ambulatory health care, behavioral health, etc.). The Patient Safety Advisory Groups use data from sentinel events and other authoritative sources to define NPSGs from year to year.

Table 2-3	RESOURCES ON PATIENT SAFETY
Agency for Healthcare Research and Quality	www.ahrq.gov
American Hospital Association	www.aha.org
Centers for Medicare and Medicaid Services	www.cms.hhs.gov
Emergency Care Research Institute	www.ecri.org
Institute for Safe Medication Practices	www.ismp.org
National Patient Safety Foundation	www.npsf.org
National Priorities Partnership	www.nationalprioritiespartnership.org
Texas Medical Institute of Technology (TMIT)	www.safetyleaders.org
The Institute for Health Care Improvement	www.ihi.org
The Joint Commission	www.jointcommission.org
The Just Culture Community	www.justculture.org
WHO Collaborating Centre for Patient Safety Solutions	www.ccforpatientsafety.org

Box 2-7	SENTINEL EVENT POLICY

A sentinel event is an unexpected occurrence involving death or serious physical or psychological injury, or the risk thereof. The terms "Sentinel Event" and "Medical Error" are not synonymous. Not all sentinel events are due to a medical error, nor do all medical errors result in a sentinel event. All accredited organizations are required to define "sentinel event" for its own purpose and establish how all sentinel events will be identified and managed. Accredited organizations' response to a "sentinel event" includes conducting a timely, thorough, and credible root cause analysis, and development of an action plan.

From The Joint Commission. www.jointcommission.org

Box 2-8	OCCURRENCES THAT ARE SUBJECT TO REVIEW BY THE JOINT COMMISSION UNDER THE SENTINEL EVENT POLICY

- Event has resulted in an unanticipated death or major permanent loss of function, not related to the natural course of the patient's illness or underlying condition
  OR
- Suicide of any patient receiving care, treatment, and services in a staffed around-the-clock care setting or within 72 hours of discharge
- Unanticipated death of a full-term infant
- Abduction of any patient receiving care, treatment, and services
- Discharge of an infant to the wrong family
- Rape
- Hemolytic transfusion reaction involving administration of blood or blood products having major blood group incompatibilities
- Surgery on the wrong patient or wrong body part
- Unintended retention of a foreign object in a patient after surgery or other procedure
- Severe neonatal hyperbilirubinemia (bilirubin >30 mg/dl)
- Prolonged fluoroscopy with cumulative dose >1500 rads to a single field or any delivery of radiotherapy to the wrong body region or >25% above the planned radiotherapy dose

NPSGs are evaluated each year, and a decision is made to continue current goals, add to the goal, delete the goal, and/or add additional goals (Box 2-9). Some of the patient safety goals may be moved from the NPSG chapter to the main body of standards in the TJC standards manual over time. Patient safety goals evolve into the standard of care.

"Never Events" In 2002, the National Quality Forum (NQF) endorsed a list of 21 adverse events that were defined as serious and largely preventable. These events are concerning to both the public and health care providers for the purpose of health care accountability: the responsibility of health care providers to assure the public efforts are underway to prevent errors. Over the years, the list has expanded to encompass 28 events (Box 2-10). In 2008, the Centers for Medicare and Medicaid Services (CMS) announced the new Medicare and Medicaid payment policies designed to use reimbursement as an incentive to improve safety for all hospitalized patients. Effective October 2008, health care facilities no longer receive payment from CMS for any patient who suffers a "Never Event" while in the care of the facility. The condition lists included on the CMS "Never Events" and the NQF "Never Events" overlap but are not identical. Refer to the CMS website (www.cms.hhs.gov) for current regulations surrounding payment structure for "Never Events."

To receive reimbursement for the conditions included on the "Never Events" listing, the hospital must have evidence in the documentation of physicians indicating presence of one or more "Never" conditions such as a pressure ulcer or a urinary tract infection at the time of hospital admission. CMS will pay for care rendered for "Never" conditions acquired outside the hospital but not those acquired inside the hospital. Documentation on nursing admission assessments is sometimes reviewed by physicians as a "check and balance" to ensure their documentation is complete. It is imperative all health care providers familiarize themselves with the listing of CMS "Never Events," including ongoing revisions, to remain attuned to key areas to be assessed.

Box 2-9   THE 2009 JOINT COMMISSION NATIONAL PATIENT SAFETY GOALS

- Improve the accuracy of patient identification.
  - Use at least two patient-specific identifiers whenever administering medications or performing any invasive procedure (standard identifiers: patient name and birth date).
  - Follow the blood transfusion procedure for patient identification.
  - When involvement of patient is not possible, involve the family.
- Improve the safety of using medications.
  - Look-alike/sound-alike medications
  - Label all medications and medication containers, including syringes or other solutions on and off the sterile field.
  - Reduce the risk of harm associated with anticoagulation therapy.
- Reduce the risk of health care–acquired infections.
  - Comply with hand hygiene guidelines.
  - Practice to prevent central bloodstream infections, multidrug-resistant infections, and surgical site infections.
  - Follow Surgical Care Infection Prevention (SCIP) core measure indicators.
- Reduce the risk of patient harm resulting from falls.
- Improve recognition and response to changes in a patient's condition.
- Improve the effectiveness of communication among caregivers.
  - Read-back process with all verbal orders and critical diagnostic results.
  - Do not use unapproved abbreviations.
  - Use a standard approach to "hand off" patient information from one caregiver to the next.
- Reconcile medications across the continuum of care.
- Engage the patient as an active partner.
  - Communicate with the patient/family all aspects of his or her care, treatment, or services, and encourage patient involvement.
- Identify safety risks inherent in the patient population.
  - Inpatient: identify patients at risk for suicide.
  - Educate patients receiving oxygen therapy at home on fire safety.

Box 2-10 | NATIONAL QUALITY FORUM "NEVER EVENTS"

- Artificial insemination with the wrong donor sperm or donor egg
- Unintended retention of a foreign object in a patient after surgery or other procedure
- Patient death or serious disability associated with patient elopement (disappearance)
- Patient death or serious disability associated with a medication error (e.g., errors involving the wrong drug, wrong dose, wrong patient, wrong time, wrong rate, wrong preparation, or wrong route of administration)
- Patient death or serious disability associated with a hemolytic reaction due to the administration of ABO/HLA-incompatible blood or blood products
- Patient death or serious disability associated with an electric shock or elective cardioversion while being cared for in a health care facility
- Patient death or serious disability associated with a fall while being cared for in a health care facility
- Surgery performed on the wrong body part
- Surgery performed on the wrong patient
- Wrong surgical procedure performed on a patient
- Intraoperative or immediately postoperative death in an ASA Class I patient
- Patient death or serious disability associated with the use of contaminated drugs, devices, or biologics provided by the health care facility
- Patient death or serious disability associated with the use or function of a device in patient care, in which the device is used or functions other than as intended
- Patient death or serious disability associated with intravascular air embolism that occurs while being cared for in a health care facility
- Infant discharged to the wrong person
- Patient suicide, or attempted suicide resulting in serious disability, while being cared for in a health care facility
- Maternal death or serious disability associated with labor or delivery in a low-risk pregnancy while being cared for in a health care facility
- Patient death or serious disability associated with hypoglycemia, the onset of which occurs while the patient is being cared for in a health care facility
- Death or serious disability (kernicterus) associated with failure to identify and treat hyperbilirubinemia in neonates
- Stage 3 or 4 pressure ulcers acquired after admission to a health care facility
- Patient death or serious disability due to spinal manipulative therapy
- Any incident in which a line designated for oxygen or other gas to be delivered to a patient contains the wrong gas or is contaminated by toxic substances
- Patient death or serious disability associated with a burn incurred from any source while being cared for in a health care facility
- Patient death or serious disability associated with the use of restraints or bedrails while being cared for in a health care facility
- Any instance of care ordered by or provided by someone impersonating a physician, nurse, pharmacist, or other licensed health care provider
- Abduction of a patient of any age
- Sexual assault on a patient within or on the grounds of the health care facility
- Death or significant injury of a patient or staff member resulting from a physical assault (i.e., battery) that occurs within or on the grounds of the health care facility

PATIENT SAFETY CULTURE

Health care organizations have identified that 95% of medical errors are directly related to system flaws, whereas only 5% of medical errors are caused by incompetent or poorly intended care (Sexton and Thomas, 2004). System flaws are largely related to flawed communication, which may lead to disjointed or uncoordinated care. Not all members of the team are consistently aware of key information that, if omitted, may cause harm to the patient. Therefore, to improve patient safety and address medical errors, health care organizational culture must value communication and team collaboration. Focus on these two factors will result in improved clinical effectiveness and job satisfaction among health care professionals (Box 2-11).

Communication

Despite years of training, coaching, and experience, communication among health care professionals remains a challenge and a leading root cause of sentinel events in many facilities. In a meta-analysis of research studies, Seago (2008) found that the evidence remains mixed on a preferred format for communication strategies. In the AACN Standards for Establishing and Sustaining a Healthy Work Environment, Skilled Communication is the first standard addressed and is the one standard that weaves its way into the five other standards. The emphasis by AACN on healthy work environment standards is a testimony to the importance of excellent communication skills in critical care (Table 2-4).

Nurses and physicians are trained to deliver and receive communication in different strategies that often lead to a communication gap between these highly skilled health care professionals. Nurses tend to communicate in a lengthier manner, unfolding patient conditions in narrative and highly descriptive style (e.g., patient has an alteration in comfort versus a patient is in pain). Physicians are taught in medical school to present "highlights" to their attending physician, giving them only the needed data to make a clinical decision. Therefore, when a nurse communicates with a physician or midlevel practitioner and does not provide a focused report, the physician sometimes loses concentration in the conversation and may not hear key patient care data.

The power of structured communication methods has been successfully used in many industries including the airline industry, nuclear power, and the U.S. Department of Defense. One such method of structured communications is the Situation-Background-Assessment-Recommendation (SBAR) documentation format. Using SBAR is helpful to those who have

Box 2-11	COMPONENTS OF SUCCESSFUL TEAMWORK

- Trust
- Respect
- Collaboration
- Open communication
- Nonpunitive environment
- Clear direction
- Methods to evaluate outcomes and amend processes as needed
- Defined roles and responsibilities of team members
- Atmosphere of respect
- Flattening of caregiver hierarchy
- Methodologies to resolve conflict
- Defined decision-making procedures

From O'Daniel M, Rosenstein AH: Professional communication and team collaboration. In: Hughes RG, editor: *Patient safety and quality: an evidence-based handbook for nurses*. Rockville, MD, 2008, AHRQ.

Table 2-4	AACN STANDARDS FOR ESTABLISHING AND SUSTAINING HEALTHY WORK ENVIRONMENTS
Skilled communication	Nurses must be as proficient in communication skills as they are in clinical skills.
True collaboration	Nurses must be relentless in pursuing and fostering true collaboration.
Effective decision making	Nurses must be valued and committed partners in making policy, directing and evaluating clinical care, and leading organizational operations.
Appropriate staffing	Staffing must ensure effective match between patient needs and nurse competencies.
Meaningful recognition	Nurses must be recognized and must recognize others for the value each brings to the work of the organization.
Authentic leadership	Nurse leaders must fully embrace the imperative of a healthy work environment, authentically live it, and engage others in its achievement.

From AACN Advanced Critical Care Nursing, 2008, p. 7.

difficulty with focused, concise communications. AHRQ and others across the United States have advocated for SBAR as a form of standardized communication (Table 2-5).

TJC recognizes the importance of communication and has woven communication throughout many of the NPSGs. In particular, TJC calls for each accredited facility to define a methodology for which staff communicates information about patient care in a consistent manner when moving a patient from one practitioner to the care of a different practitioner. A report at the time of transition of caregivers is called "hand-off communication" (Box 2-12).

Several national programs have been developed to enhance both intradisciplinary and interdisciplinary communication among health care providers:

TeamSTEPPS™

The AHRQ and the Department of Defense have partnered together to develop an evidence-based curriculum and training program with the goal of promoting patient safety through improving communication and teamwork skills among health care professionals (Table 2-6).

The focus of TeamSTEPPS™ is to develop competency in four primary trainable teamwork skills. These skills are leadership, communication, situation monitoring, and mutual support. When all individuals of a team possess competency in these skills, research has demonstrated that the team can enhance three types of teamwork outcomes: performance, knowledge, and attitudes.

Table 2-5	STRUCTURED COMMUNICATION: SBAR	
Prior to initiating an SBAR conversation, nurses should assess the patient; review medical record for appropriate physician or other care provider to call; know the patient's diagnoses, procedures, and medical history; read all recent physician progress notes (especially from the last 12 hours); have available the following clinical data — chart, allergies, medications recently given, recent diagnostic tests, and patient code status — and, last, take a moment to organize all data, thoughts, and requests.		
S Situation	Give your name and unit you are calling from, the patient's full name, room number, and attending physician name if calling the on-call physician. If the problem is urgent, please notify the provider at the beginning of the call. Patient's code status if appropriate.	"Dr. James, I'm Susie, a critical care RN. Mr. Smith is a 42-year-old currently in radiology for a CT of the head after a motor vehicle crash (MVC). I am the rapid response nurse and was called to see him for anxiety and shortness of breath."
B Background	Patient's admission diagnosis, admission date, and *pertinent* medical history. Provide a brief synopsis of the treatments and plan of care thus far.	"Mr. Smith was the driver and sustained blunt chest trauma during the MVC approximately 3 hours ago. There is no significant medical history."
A Assessment	Provide a brief description of the problem or primary concern. If uncertain of the problem, acknowledge the uncertainty. Provide clinical data such as most recent vital signs, physical assessment findings, and clinical changes specific to the problem you are calling about. Provide update of all *pertinent* therapies (IVs, O$_2$, etc.).	"I think Mr. Smith has a right pneumothorax. Breath sounds are absent in the right middle and lower lobes. He is short of breath, anxious, and tachypneic with an oxygen saturation of 88% on 4 liters of oxygen."
R Recommendation	Express what you think the patient needs to address the problem. If unclear on what interventions are needed, acknowledge uncertainty. If requesting the practitioner to come and assess the patient, clarify with the practitioner the exact time-frame to expect their arrival.	"I think Mr. Smith needs more oxygen and a chest tube right away. I have asked the radiology technician to obtain the supplies for chest tube placement. Can you come to radiology to assess the patient for chest tube placement, or is there someone else we should call?"

Box 2-12	HAND-OFF COMMUNICATION

Elements of hand-off communication
- Standardized to the situation to which it applies
- When to use certain techniques (i.e., read-back or repeat-back)
- *Interactive*—Allow for questioning between giver and receiver of the patient information.
- Contain the most recent information regarding patient care, treatment, services, condition, and any recent or anticipated changes.
- Interruptions during hand-offs are limited.

Strategies to improve hand-off communication
- Use clear language and avoid all abbreviations or terms that can be misinterpreted.
- Use effective communication techniques.
  - Limit interruptions and distractions.
  - Provide adequate time for interaction.
- Standardize utilization of tools facilitate the interaction, especially during high-volume high-distraction times such as shift-to-shift, unit-to-unit.
- Use technology to enhance communications—electronic medical records, portable computers, handheld devices, etc.

Table 2-6	THREE PHASES OF THE TeamSTEPPS™ IMPLEMENTATION
Phase 1 Assess the Need	Determine the organizational readiness for undertaking a TeamSTEPPS™-based initiative. • Establish an organizational change team. • Conduct a site assessment. • Define the problem, challenge, or opportunity for improvement. • Define the goal of the intervention.
Phase 2 Planning, Training, and Implementation	TeamSTEPPS™ is designed to be customized to the organization. Implementation options inclued utilization of all tools and strategies across the entire organization or a phased-in approach that targets specific units or departments, or selected individual tools can be introduced at specific intervals. • Define the intervention. • Develop a plan for determining the interventions and effectiveness. • Develop an implementation plan. • Gain leadership commitment to the plan. • Develop a communication plan. • Prepare the facility. • Implement training.
Phase 3 Sustainment	Sustain and spread improvements in teamwork performance, clinical processes, and outcomes. Continual learning and reinforcement of skills on the unit or within the facility: • Provide opportunities for clinicians to practice skills. • Ensure leaders emphasize new skills. • Provide regular feedback and coaching. • Celebrate and measure successes. • Update the plan.

Patient Safety

"Just Culture"

The creation of a "Just Culture" has been advocated as a means to enhance the patient safety culture of an organization. A culture of learning must exist that encourages the reporting of adverse events and near misses without the fear of retribution. The practitioner must be offered protection from disciplinary action when they report injuries, errors, and near misses when personally involved. This implies that errors are most often not intentional, nor are they caused by human failures alone. Most are often a series of system failures that come together at an intersection involving the patient.

The creation of a "Just Culture" does acknowledge there are exceptions where health care workers do not have protection. Protection should not be granted for criminal behavior, for active malfeasance, or in cases are in which an injury is not reported in a timely manner (Box 2-13).

PATIENT/FAMILY INVOLVEMENT

Patient and family involvement in the plan of care can be a crucial element of patient safety, since both are familiar with key information that, if known, may prevent harm. Understanding of medications, the health history, and proposed plan of care is vital to a safe patient care experience. Patients and families may feel reluctant to challenge, remind, or question their health care providers. There has been a recent shift within all patient safety organizations, as well as professional organizations to include the patient in daily rounds, to provide time for daily goal setting, and to ensure all parts of the treatment plan have been communicated and are understood. Several national programs have been developed and promoted to facilitate the involvement of patients and families in the plan of care (Box 2-14).

Speak Up™
- In March 2002, TJC along with CMS launched a national campaign urging patients to partner with their health care provider to prevent health care errors by becoming involved in their care. The campaign offers facilities a variety of tools (brochures, artwork, etc.) to educate patients on steps they can take to partner with health care workers to enhance the safe delivery. Topics include but are not limited to "Help Avoid Mistakes with Your Medication," "Five Things You Can Do to Prevent Infection," and "What You Should Know about Pain Management" (Box 2-15).

Nothing about Me, without Me
- In 2001, the NPSF established a Patient and Family Advisory Council to provide guidance and expertise on all NSPF's activities. One of the fundamental principles advocated by this council is the philosophy of "Nothing about Me, without Me." This phrase was suggested in 1998 by an English midwife at a seminar advocating that patients should be

Box 2-13	"JUST CULTURE"

Creation of a culture where clinicians are willing to report errors so that the process can be analyzed and solutions found, but clinician responsibility for events is maintained. The culture is not "blame free" but blame appropriate.

From Marx D: *Patient safety and the "just culture": a primer for health care executives.* 2001, R01 HI53772. http://www.psnet.ah rq.gov/resource.aspx?resourceID-1582.

Box 2-14	STEPS TO INVOLVING PATIENTS IN PATIENT SAFETY

Obtain patient feedback through a variety of sources such as patient satisfaction, focus groups, community groups, hotlines, etc.

Review patient plan of care and daily goals with patients and their families.

Never separate a patient from their family unless that is desired; allow patient access 24 hours per day.

Never deny a patient information; a variety of tools can be utilized to enhance communication and sharing of information such as reviewing the medical record, orientation to the unit, equipment, and team members, wipe boards, sharing clinical pathways, patient conferences with interdisciplinary team, customized discharge instructions.

Encourage patient's and family's involvement in care by inviting them to participate through creative campaigns; staff wearing buttons asking "Ask me if I've washed my hands"; tent cards in patient rooms; brochures and pamphlets educating patients on how to be involved in their care.

From http://www.jointcommission.org/GeneralPublic/smart_patient.htm

Box 2-15 SPEAK UP™

Speak up if you have questions or concerns. If you still don't understand, ask again. It's your body and you have a right to know.

Pay attention to the care you get. Always make sure you're getting the right treatments and medicines by the right health care professionals. Don't assume anything.

Educate yourself about your illness. Learn about the medical tests you get and your treatment plan.

Ask a trusted family member or friend to be your advocate (advisor or supporter).

Know what medicines you take and why you take them. Medicine errors are the most common health care mistakes.

Use a hospital, clinic, surgery center, or other type of health care organization that has been carefully checked out. For example, The Joint Commission visits hospitals to see if they are meeting The Joint Commission's quality standards.

Participate in all decisions about your treatment. You are the center of the health care team.

From http://www.jointcommission.org/GeneralPublic/Speak + Up/about_speakup.htm

involved in every step of their health care. This phrase has now been quoted by key patient safety leaders such as but not limited to Delbanco, Berwick, Tye, and IOM's *Crossing the Quality Chasm* report. (Table 2-7 outlines the NPSF recommendations.)

HIGH RELIABILITY ORGANIZATIONS

High reliability organizations (HROs) are those that are known to be complex and risky yet maintain safety and effectiveness. Key characteristics of HROs include preoccupation with failure and safety, deference to expertise, sensitivity to operations, commitment to resilience, and reluctance to simplify. HROs are continually analyzing and asking questions to prevent failures within the systems and analyzing how to minimize effects from failures when and if they occur. The utilization of the prospective tool of a failure mode and effects analysis (FMEA) and the utilization of a retrospective tool such as a root cause analysis (RCA) have proven valuable to health care organizations (Table 2-8).

Patient safety is an ever-changing specialty within health care; new resources and knowledge are constantly being defined as research is completed. The provision of safe care delivery is demanded by regulators, payers, health care providers, and, most important, the patient. Therefore, it is critical that every clinician accept accountability for the provision of a health care environment that both supports and provides a culture of safe care delivery.

Table 2-7	NATIONAL AGENDA FOR ACTION: PATIENTS AND FAMILIES IN PATIENT SAFETY: ROAD MAP FOR ACTION
Education and Awareness	• Raise public awareness on the definition and frequency of medical error and patient safety.
	• Educate the public on how to aid in safeguarding their own care.
	• Educate health care professionals and leadership about the importance of the patient/family perspective.
	• Raise health care providers' awareness of the experiences of patients and their families.
	• Raise awareness in the behavioral health community on medical errors.
	• Educate the media.
	• Build patient safety and medical error prevention into all health care professional education curricula.
	• Build interactive, interdisciplinary education programs.
	• Develop a central clearinghouse and interactive resource center.

Continued

Table 2-7	NATIONAL AGENDA FOR ACTION: PATIENTS AND FAMILIES IN PATIENT SAFETY: ROAD MAP FOR ACTION—cont'd
Build a Culture of Patient- and Family-Centered Patient Safety	• Teach and encourage effective communication skills. • Engage leadership in promoting and training providers in open communication about medical error. • Empower hospital patient representatives to effectively advocate. • Establish patient and family advisory councils. • Represent patients' interests on boards and trustees. • Establish patient safety task forces. • Create a national forum for state coalitions.
Research	• "Bridging the gap" • Disclosure • Short- and long-term effects of incorporating patients and families into the system • Current patient safety information and resource landscape for patients and families • Posttraumatic stress specific to medical error • Team relationships
Support Services	• National resource center and information line • Emergency hotline • Peer resource counseling • Support groups for families and individuals who have suffered due to a medical error • Disclosure and communication programs • National training programs for hospitals implementing any of the above programs

From *Nothing about Me, without Me:* http://www.npsf.org/pdf/paf/AgendaFamilies.pdf

Table 2-8	FMEA VERSUS RCA
Failure Mode and Effects Analysis (FMEA)	**Root Cause Analysis (RCA)**
• Proactive analysis of a process or equipment to anticipate any potential process or product failure	• Retrospective analysis of an event that has already occurred; actual failure
• Looks forward through a process to identify any potential failure points	• Looks back chronologically after a process has failed
• Multidisciplinary team involvement key to success	• Multidisciplinary team involvement by all who were involved in the failure a key to the success

• Three key questions are addressed:
  • How likely is the equipment or process to fail?
  • What is the significance of the failure?
  • How likely it is that someone will be able to detect this failure?
	• Three key questions are addressed:
	  • What happened?
	  • Why did it happen?
	  • What can be done to prevent it from happening again?

• Analytical tools used:
  • Flow diagrams of all main and subprocesses
  • Brainstorm
  • Cause-and-effect diagrams
	• Analytical tools used:
	  • Timeline
	  • Cause-and-effect diagrams
	  • Frequency plots
	  • Scatterplots

SELECTED REFERENCES

Agency for Health Care Research and Quality: TeamSTEPPS™: National implementation. Retrieved February 2, 2009, from http://teamstepps.ahrq.gov/index.htm

American Association of Critical Care Nurses: AACN standards for establishing and sustaining healthy work environments: a journey to excellence. Am J Crit Care 14(3): 187-197, 2005.

Aron SS, et al: Botulinum toxin as a biological weapon: medical and public health management. JAMA 285(8):1059-1070, 2001.

Bagian JP, Gosbee J, Lee Z, et al: The Veterans Affairs root cause analysis system in action. Jt Comm J Qual Improve 28(10):531-545, 2002.

Baumhover N, Hughes L: Spirituality and support for family presence during invasive procedures and resuscitations in adults. Am J Crit Care 18(4):357-367, 2009.

Beauchamp TL, Childress JF: Principles of biomedical ethics, ed 6. New York, 2009, Oxford University Press.

Belay ED, Schonberger LB: Variant Creutzfeldt-Jakob disease and bovine spongiform encephalopathy. Clin Lab Med 22:849-862, 2002.

Benner P: Seeing the person behind the disease. Am J Crit Care 13(1):75-78, 2004.

Berghs M, et al: The complexity of nurses' attitudes toward euthanasia: a review of the literature. J Med Ethics 31(8):441-446, 2005.

Borio L, et al: Hemorrhagic fever viruses as biological weapons: medical and public health management. JAMA 287(18):2391-2405, 2002.

Centers for Disease Control and Prevention: Avian influenza (bird flu) fact sheet, June 30, 2006. Retrieved October 12, 2008, from http://www.cdc.gov/flu/avian/gen-info/facts.htm

Centers for Disease Control and Prevention: Avian influenza A virus infections of humans, May 23, 2008. Retrieved November 2, 2008, from http://www.cdc.gov/flu/avian/gen-info/avian-flu-humans.htm

Centers for Disease Control and Prevention: Avian influenza: current situation, June 15, 2007. Retrieved November 2, 2008, from http://www.cdc.gov/flu/avian/outbreak/pdf/current.pdf

Centers for Disease Control and Prevention: Clinical guidance on the identification and evaluation of possible SARS-CoV disease among persons presenting with community-acquired illness, May 3, 2005. Retrieved November 2, 2008, from http://www.cdc.gov/ncidod/sars/clinicalguidance.htm

Centers for Disease Control and Prevention: Consent form (SARS-CoV EIA laboratory testing), May 3, 2005. Retrieved November 2, 2008, from http://www.cdc.gov/ncidod/sars/lab/eia/consent.htm

Centers for Disease Control and Prevention: Creutzfeldt-Jakob disease, classic questions and answers, CJD infection control practices, June 2008. Retrieved October 21, 2008, from http://www.cdc.gov/ncidod/dvrd/cjd/qa_CJD_infection_control.htm

Centers for Disease Control and Prevention: Fact sheet: variant Creutzfeldt-Jakob disease, June 2008. Retrieved October 21, 2008, from http://www.cdc.gov/ncidod/dvrd/vcjd/factsheet_nvcjd.htm

Centers for Disease Control and Prevention: Guidance for persons who may have been exposed to severe acute respiratory syndrome (SARS), May 2005. Retrieved November 2, 2008, from http://www.cdc.gov/ncidod/sars/exposuremanagement.htm

Centers for Disease Control and Prevention: Guideline for isolation precautions: preventing transmission of infectious agents in healthcare settings, June 2007. Retrieved October 12, 2008, from http://www.cdc.gov/ncidod/dhqp/pdf/guidelines/Isolation2007.pdf

Centers for Disease Control and Prevention: Health alert: update on Avian influenza A (H5N1), February 2005. Retrieved October 12, 2008, from http://www2a.cdc.gov/HAN/ArchiveSys/ViewMsgV.asp?AlertNum=00221

Centers for Disease Control and Prevention: In the absence of SARS-CoV transmission worldwide: guidance for surveillance, clinical and laboratory evaluation, and reporting version 2, January 2004. Retrieved November 2, 2008, from http://www.cdc.gov/ncidod/sars/absenceofsars.htm

Centers for Disease Control and Prevention: Interim recommendations for infections control in health-care facilities caring for patients with known or suspected avian influenza, May 21, 2004. Retrieved Novembser 2, 2008, from http://www.cdc.gov/flu/avian/professional/infect-control.htm

Centers for Disease Control and Prevention: Severe acute respiratory syndrome (SARS), May 3 2005. Retrieved October 12, 2008, from http://www.cdc.gov/ncidod/sars/

Centers for Disease Control and Prevention: Severe acute respiratory syndrome (SARS); public health guidance for community-level preparedness and response to severe acute respiratory syndrome (SARS) version 2/3, May 3, 2005. Retrieved October 12, 2008, from http://www.cdc.gov/ncidod/sars/guidance/

Centers for Disease Control and Prevention: Severe acute respiratory syndrome (SARS); public health guidance for community-level preparedness and response to severe acute respiratory syndrome (SARS) version 2, Supplement F: Laboratory guidance, January 2004. Retrieved November 2, 2008, from http://www.cdc.gov/ncidod/sars/absenceofsars.htm.

Centers for Disease Control and Prevention: Supplement I: Infection control in health care, home, and community settings, January 8 2004. Retrieved November 2, 2008, from http://www.cdc.gov/ncidod/sars/guidance/i/pdf/i.pdf

Centers for Disease Control and Prevention: West Nile virus (WNV) infection: information and guidance for clinicians, September 29, 2004. Retrieved October 24, 2008, from http://www.cdc.gov/ncidod/dvbid/westnile;clinicians;clindes.htm

Centers for Medicare and Medicaid Services. Details for: CMS improves patient safety for Medicare and Medicaid by addressing Never Events. Retrieved February 2, 2009, from http://www.cms.hhs.gov/apps/media/press/factsheet.asp

Cheng VC, Lau SK, et al: Severe acute respiratory syndrome coronavirus as an agent of emerging and reemerging infection. *Clin Microbiol Rev* 20(4):660–694, 2007.

Davidson JE, Powers K, Hedayast KM, et al: Clinical practice guidelines for the support of the family in the patient centered intensive care unit. American College of Care Medicine Task Force 2004-2005. *Crit Care Med* 35(2):605–622, 2007.

Delgado C: Meeting clients' spiritual needs. *Nurs Clin N Am* 42(2):279–293, 2007.

Dennis DT, et al: tularemia as a biological weapon: medical and public health management. *JAMA* 285(21):2763–2773, 2001.

Dreher H, et al: What you need to know about SARS now. *Nursing* 34(1):58–64, 2004.

Edgman-Levitan S: Involving the patient in safety efforts. In Leonard A, Frankel A, Simmonds T, editors: *Achieving safe and reliable health care: strategies and solutions,* Chicago, 2004, ACHE Health Administration Press.

Frankel A: Accountability: Defining the Rules. In Leonard A, Frankel A, Simmonds T, editors: *Achieving safe and reliable health care: strategies and solutions.* Chicago, 2004, ACHE Health Administration Press.

Friesen MA, White SV, Byers JF: Handoffs: implications for nurses. In Hughes RG, editor: *Patient safety and quality: an evidence-based handbook for nurses.* Rockville, MD, 2008, AHRQ.

Fry ST, Johnstone M: *Ethics in nursing practice: a guide to ethical decision making,* ed 3. Chichester, UK, 2008, Wiley-Blackwell.

Grace PJ, Hardt E: Ethics Column: I don't trust hospitals and I don't want strangers in my home! Should Mrs. Rosario be permitted to refuse assistance? *Am J Nurs* 2008.

Grace PJ: *Nursing ethics and professional responsibility in advanced practice.* Sudbury, MA, 2009, Jones & Bartlett.

Haggerty LA, Grace PJ: Clinical wisdom: the essential component of 'good' nursing care. *J Prof Nurs* 24(4):235–240, 2008.

Health Canada: Learning from SARS, October 2003. Retrieved October 24, 2008, from http://www.phac-aspc.gc.ca/publicat/sars-sras/naylor/

Henderson DA, et al: Smallpox as a biological weapon: medical and public health management. *JAMA* 281(22):2127–2137, 1999.

http://www.publichealth.va.gov/documents/SARS_lab/lab_guide.pdf

http://www.usatoday.com/news/health/bioterrorism/2002-03-20-smallpox.htm. Retrieved June 30, 2008.

Huhn GD, Sejvar JD, et al: West Nile virus in the United States: an update on an emerging infectious disease. *Am Fam Phys* August 2003. Retrieved November 13, 2008, from http://www.aafp.org/afp/20030815/653.html

Inglesby TV, et al: Anthrax as a biological weapon: medical and public health management. *JAMA* 283(17):2281–2290, 2000.

Inglesby TV, et al: Anthrax as a biological weapon, 2002: updated recommendations for management. *JAMA* 287(17):2236–2252, 2002.

Institute of Medicine: *Keeping patients safe: transforming the work environment of nurses.* Washington, DC, 2004, National Academies Press.

Institute of Medicine: *Patient safety: achieving a new standard for care.* Washington, DC, 2004, National Academies Press.

Institute of Medicine: *To err is human: building a safer health system.* Washington, DC, 2000, National Academies Press.

Jonsen AR, et al: *Clinical ethics: a practical approach to ethical decisions in clinical medicine,* ed 6. New York, 2006, McGraw-Hill, Medical Pub Division.

Karwa, M, et al: Bioterrorism: preparing for the impossible or the improbable. *Crit Care Med* 33(1):S75–S95, 2005.

Leonard M, Frankel A: Focusing on high reliability. In Leonard A, Frankel A, Simmonds T, editors: *Achieving safe and reliable health care: strategies and solutions.* Chicago, 2004, ACHE Health Administration Press.

Leonard M, Graham S Taggart B: The human factor: effective teamwork and communication in patient strategy. In Leonard A, Frankel A, Simmonds T, editors: *Achieving safe and reliable health care: strategies and solutions.* Chicago, 2004, ACHE Health Administration Press.

Marx D: *Patient safety and the "just culture": a primer for health care executives.* New York, NY, 2001, Trustees of Columbia University. [Funded by a grant from the National Heart, Lung, and Blood Institute, National Institutes of Health (grant R01-HL-53772, Harold S. Kaplan, MD, principal investigator).]

Maze CD: Registered nurses' personal rights vs. professional responsibility in caring for members of underserved and disenfranchised populations. *J Clin Nurse* 14(5):546–554, 2005.

Mazur MA, Cox LA, Capon JA: The public's attitude and perception concerning witnessed cardiopulmonary resuscitation. *Crit Care Med* 4(12):2925–2928, 2006.

Meade C, Bursell A, Ketelsen L: Effects of nursing rounds on call light use, satisfaction and safety. *Am J Nursing* 106:58–70, 2006.

Nance JJ: *Why hospitals should fly: the ultimate flight plan to patient safety and quality care.* Bozeman, MT, 2008, Second River Healthcare Press.

National Institute of Neurological Disorders and Stroke: Creutzfeldt-Jakob disease fact sheet, October 15, 2008. Retrieved October 21, 2008, from http://www.ninds.nih.gov/disorder/cjd/detail_cjd.htm

National Patient Safety Foundation: National agenda for action: patients and families in patient safety: Nothing about Me, without Me. 2003. Retrieved February 10, 2009, from http://www.npsf.org/pdf/paf/AgendaFamilies.pdf

National Quality Forum: National Quality Forum updates endorsement of serious reportable events in health care. Retrieved February 2, 2009, from http://www.qualityforum.org/pdf/news/prSeriousReportableEvents10-15-06.pdf

O'Daniel M, Rosenstein AH: Professional communication and team collaboration. In Hughes RG, editor. *Patient safety and quality: an evidence-based handbook for nurses.* Rockville, MD, 2008, AHRQ.

Petersen LR, Marfin AA: West Nile virus: a primer for the clinician, *Ann Intern Med* 137(3):173–179, 2002.

Reason J, Hobbs A: *Managing maintenance error: a practical guide.* Burlington, VT, 2003, Ashgate.

Rosenblum A, et al: Opioids and the treatment of chronic pain: controversies, current status and future directions. *Exp Clin Psychopharmacol* 16(5):405–416, 2008.

Sampathkumar P, et al: SARS: epidemiology, clinical presentation, management, and infection control measures. *Mayo Clin Proc* 78:882–890, 2003.

Scholtes PR, Joiner BL, Streibel BJ: *The team handbook,* ed 3. Madison, WI, 2003, Oriel.

Seago JA: Professional communication. In Hughes RG, editor: *Patient safety and quality: an evidence-based handbook for nurses.* Rockville, MD, 2008, AHRQ.

Sexton B, Thomas E: Measurement: assessing a safety culture. In Leonard A, Frankel A, Simmonds T, editors: *Achieving safe and reliable health care: strategies and solutions.* Chicago, 2004, ACHE Health Administration Press.

Simmonds T, Whittington J: *Analytical tools.* In Leonard A, Frankel A, Simmonds T, editors: *Achieving safe and reliable health care: strategies and solutions.* Chicago, 2004, ACHE Health Administration Press.

Solomon T, et al: West Nile encephalitis. *BMJ* 326:865–869, 2003.

The Joint Commission: *Hand-off communications.* Retrieved February 8, 2009, from http://www.jointcommission.org/AccreditationPrograms/HomeCare/Standards/09_FAQs/NPSG/Communication/NPSG.02.05.01/hand_off_communications.htm

The Joint Commission: *National patient safety goals.* Retrieved February 2, 2009, from http://www.jointcommission.org/PatientSafety/NationalPatientSafetyGoals/09_hap_npsgs.htm

The Joint Commission: *Patient safety.* Retrieved January 30, 2009, from http://www.jointcommission.org/PatientSafety/

The Joint Commission: *Sentinel event policy.* Retrieved January 30, 2009, from http://www.jointcommission.org/NR/rdonlyres/F84F9DC6-A5DA-490F-A91F-A9FCE26347C4/0/SE_chapter_july07.pdf

The Joint Commission: *Speak Up initiatives.* Retrieved February 7, 2009, from http://www.jointcommission.org/GeneralPublic/Speak+Up/about_speakup.htm

Van Rynen JL, Rega PP, Budd C, Burkholder-Allen KJ: The use of negative inspiratory force by ED personnel to monitor respiratory deterioration in the event of a botulism-induced MCI. *J Emerg Nurs* 32(2):114–117, 2009.

Wainwright P, Gallagher A: Ethical aspects of withdrawing and withholding treatment. *Nurs Stand* 21(33):46–50, 2007.

Watson J: *Nursing. The philosophy and science of caring.* Boulder, 2008, University Press of Colorado.

Weick KE, Sutcliffe KM: *Managing the unexpected: assuring high performance in an era of complexity.* San Francisco, 2001, Jossey-Bass.

Wheeler DJ: *Understanding variation: the key to managing chaos,* ed 2. Knoxville, TN, 2000, SPC Press.

Willis DG, Grace PJ, Roy C: A central unifying focus for the discipline: Facilitating humanization, meaning, choice, quality of life, and healing in living and dying. *Adv Nurs Sci* 31(1):E28–E40, 2008.

Wolf ZR, Hughes RG: Error reporting and disclosure. In Hughes RG, editor. *Patient safety and quality: an evidence-based handbook for nurses.* Rockville, MD, 2008, AHRQ.

World Health Organization: Avian influenza, January 2008. Retrieved November 2, 2008, from http://www.who.int/topics/avian_influenza/en/

www.bt.cdc.gov/index.asp (Accessed April 5, 2009)

www.cidrap.umn.edu/cidrap/ (Accessed April 5, 2009)

www.upmc-biosecurity.org/website/focus/agents_diseases/index.html (Accessed April 5, 2009)

MAJOR TRAUMA

PATHOPHYSIOLOGY

Traumatic injuries account for over 5 million deaths worldwide. In the United States, traumatic injuries are the leading cause of death for patients between the ages of 1 and 44 years. Traumatic injuries also account for over 2.6 million hospitalizations each year. Major trauma occurs when energy is applied to body tissues in excess of what the tissues are able to absorb. The energy can be in the form of kinetic, thermal, chemical, electrical, and radiant energy. Trauma can also occur when the body is deprived of an essential element such as oxygen or heat. Kinetic energy is the most common cause of trauma and includes mechanisms such as motor vehicle collisions, falls, and gunshot wounds. Thermal, chemical, electrical, and radiation energy cause burns. Lack of oxygen occurs in drownings and hanging injuries. The amount of damage to the tissue will depend on the amount of force applied, the length of time the force is applied, and the resiliency of the tissue. Hollow organs tend to absorb more energy and are injured less frequently than are solid organs since the organ tissue has more flexibility to withstand the forces.

The primary pathophysiologic process that occurs with major trauma is shock. Major trauma patients are at risk for all types of shock, but the most common type is hypovolemic shock due to hemorrhage. Hypovolemic shock is usually broken down into four stages that are used to describe the physiologic response to hemorrhage and are useful in estimating the amount of blood loss.

All body systems require both oxygen and glucose for cellular energy production. The classic signs of hypovolemic shock occur from activation of the central nervous system (CNS). Following major injury, the CNS triggers a series of reactions to increase delivery of oxygen and glucose to the cells. Catecholamines (epinephrine and norepinephrine) and glucocorticoids are released from the adrenal glands to preserve perfusion to vital organs, mobilize glycogen stores, increase available glucose and oxygen, suppress pancreatic insulin secretion, and enhance glucose uptake. Hyperglycemia is common following major trauma. Glycogen stores are rapidly depleted (within 24 hours). Without nutrition, energy is generated from the breakdown of the body or catabolism. Breakdown of muscle tissue, fat, and viscera creates a negative nitrogen balance. Subclinical adrenal insufficiency may become clinically apparent after severe injury.

The posterior pituitary release of antidiuretic hormone (ADH) promotes water absorption in the distal renal tubules. Intravascular volume increases as urinary output decreases. Blood pressure (BP) is increased by the renin-angiotensin-aldosterone system. Aldosterone promotes sodium and water resorption to increase intravascular volume, and angiotensin II causes vasoconstriction.

Several factors must also be considered that can alter the patient's response to blood loss and must be considered in the resuscitation of these patients. These include the patient's age, location, type and severity of the injury, the amount of time that has elapsed since the injury, prehospital interventions to address blood loss, and medications taken for chronic conditions, especially anticoagulants and beta-blockers. Since the patient has many other injuries, the classic signs of shock may be altered.

The source of the bleeding must be identified and stopped and the patient must be adequately resuscitated or the patient is at risk of developing acidosis, coagulopathy, and hypothermia, which are considered the deadly triad of trauma. Once these conditions occur, they tend to promote each other and become a vicious cycle that is hard to break.

Acidosis occurs when the number of red blood cells is reduced from blood loss and cellular oxygen supply is reduced, resulting in end-organ hypoxia due to inadequate tissue perfusion. Anaerobic metabolism may ensue if blood and volume replacement is inadequate to maintain perfusion. As anaerobic metabolism continues, lactic acid builds up, leading to an increase in the base deficit and decrease in the pH.

After initial restoration of circulating fluid volume, the body may develop a hyperdynamic circulatory state to help compensate for the cellular oxygen debt incurred. This phase should peak at 48 to 72 hours and diminish within 7 to 10 days. The hyperdynamic state is evidenced by an increased cardiac index (CI), oxygen delivery (Do_2), and oxygen consumption ($\dot{V}o_2$). Inability to achieve and maintain a hyperdynamic state is associated with higher mortality and shock-related organ failure.

Coagulopathy develops from both the consumption of clotting factors as the body forms clots in an attempt to stop the bleeding of injured tissues and due to dilution of the blood from infusion of crystalloids and massive transfusion of packed red blood cells when clotting factors are not replaced. If coagulopathy is not reversed, disseminated intravascular coagulopathy (DIC) can occur. Factors contributing to development of DIC include hypotension, impaired tissue perfusion, and capillary dysfunction leading to stasis, hypoxemia, and hypothermia.

Multiple factors increase the likelihood of hypothermia in major trauma. Exposed body surface area or viscera may occur at the scene of injury or during the initial resuscitation. If blood and resuscitation fluids are infused without warming, the core body temperature can drop. Prolonged exposure to cool temperatures in resuscitation or operative areas can also lower the body temperature. When present, central thermoregulatory failure caused by CNS injury, intoxication, or hypoperfusion contributes to hypothermia. Mild hypothermia can help preserve the function and viability of major organs, particularly when tissue perfusion is diminished as a result of injury, shock, or surgical clamping of arteries. Severe hypothermia creates significant physiologic alterations, including CNS depression, dysrhythmias, acidosis, and significant electrolyte imbalances. Catecholamine infusions are often ineffective until body temperature approaches 93°F.

In patients who sustain major trauma, a widespread inflammatory response known as *systemic inflammatory response syndrome* (SIRS) may be triggered by massive tissue injury and the presence of foreign bodies such as road dirt, missiles, and invasive medical devices. Inflammatory mediators activate the coagulation cascade, increased catecholamines stimulate the production and release of white blood cells, and endothelial dysfunction ensues. The hemodynamic response and clinical findings are similar to those with sepsis. (See Chapter 11 for information on SIRS.)

The overwhelming inflammation associated with SIRS may lead to *multiple organ dysfunction syndrome* (MODS). MODS is a major cause of late mortality in multitrauma patients, accounting for about 10% of trauma deaths. Inadequate initial resuscitation or inability to achieve and maintain a compensatory hyperdynamic state contributes to the development of organ failure in trauma patients. Presence of endotoxin, tumor necrosis factor (TNF), interleukin-1, and other inflammatory mediators causes vasodilation, leading to hypotension. Capillary dysfunction results in poor cellular circulation and subsequent tissue destruction. Acidosis, pulmonary compromise, and circulatory collapse may result. Clinical trials are under way for therapies to help control inflammatory mediators. Activated protein C (Drotrecogin alfa) is the only approved medication to help control SIRS leading to MODS; however, its use is contraindicated in many patients since it causes clot lysis.

Psychological Response

Victims of major trauma sustain life-threatening injuries. The patient often is aware of the situation and fears death. Even after the physical condition stabilizes, the patient may have a prolonged and severe psychological reaction triggered by the trauma called posttraumatic stress disorder (PTSD).

MAJOR TRAUMA ASSESSMENT: PRIMARY
Goal of System Assessment
Evaluate and treat life-threatening injuries.

Airway Assessment
Determine airway patency.
- Is the airway open?
- Can the patient maintain the open airway?
- Is there potential for airway obstruction?
- Inspect the face and neck for signs of trauma.
- Look in the mouth for secretions, blood, vomitus, or loose teeth.
- Palpate the neck for crepitus.

Breathing Assessment
- Is there adequate air exchange?
- Inspect the chest for signs of trauma that could interfere with chest excursion.
- Inspect the neck for tracheal deviation and jugular vein distention (JVD).
- Palpate the chest for crepitus, tenderness over the ribs or sternum.
- Auscultate breath sounds.
- What is the oxygen saturation?

Circulatory Assessment
- Observe skin color.
- Is there any obvious bleeding?
- Palpate for pulses, and note strength and rate.
- Palpate skin for temperature.
- Auscultate heart sounds and BP.

Disability Assessment
- Observe the patient's responsiveness.
- If not alert, does patient respond to shout or pain?
- Determine patient's Glasgow Coma Scale (GCS) score.
- Assess pupils for size, equality, and responsiveness.

Exposure
Expose the patient to observe for signs of trauma.
- Institute measures to keep the patient warm.

MAJOR TRAUMA ASSESSMENT: SECONDARY
Goal of System Assessment
Identify all the injuries the patient has incurred.

Vital Signs
- Pulse rate may be elevated if the patient has experienced blood loss or stimulation of the sympathetic nervous system (SNS) or be decreased in response to elevated intracranial pressure (ICP) from a severe head injury.
- Respiratory rate may also be increased due to SNS stimulation or hypoxia or may be decreased secondary to decreased level of consciousness.
- BP will be elevated with SNS stimulation or increased ICP or decreased due to hemorrhage.
- Temperature may be decreased from exposure to cold environment and development of hemorrhagic shock.

History
- AMPLE (Allergies, Medications, Past surgeries and pertinent medical conditions, Last meal, Events leading up to incident)
- Last menstrual period for women of child-bearing age
- Determine the mechanism of the trauma.
  - Determine any injury modifiers.
  - Identify safety devices used.

- Determine the use of intoxicants.
- Tetanus status

Head-to-Toe Assessment

- Observe each area for signs of trauma including bruising, abrasions, lacerations, and contusions.
- Palpate each area to feel for crepitus and swelling.
- Auscultate for lung sounds, heart sounds, bowel signs, and bruits.

Head and Neck
- Observe head for Battle signs (temporal bruising) and raccoon eyes (periorbital bruising).
- Observe the neck for tracheal alignment, JVD, and expanding hematomas.

Chest
- Observe for symmetrical chest wall movement.
- Percuss chest for dullness or hyperresonance.
- Palpate over ribs and sternum for tenderness.
- Listen to breath sounds, noting equality and for any abnormal breath sounds.

Abdomen and Pelvis
- Observe the abdomen for distention.
- Palpate for tenderness and guarding.
- Auscultate for bowel sounds.

Extremities
- Observe for deformities.
- Palpate for crepitus.
- Check neurovascular status of all four extremities.

Posterior Surface
- Inspect the posterior surface; if the patient's spine has not been cleared, the patient must be log-rolled, maintaining spinal precautions.

Labwork

Blood studies can reveal indications of hypoxia and/or continued bleeding and developing shock as well as identify special circumstances such as pregnancy and intoxication.

- Blood typing and screening or cross-matching
- Complete blood counts: hemoglobin (Hgb), increased white blood cell (WBC) count
- Coagulation studies including platelets, prothrombin time (PT), partial thromboplastin time (PTT), and international normalized ratio (INR)
- Serial arterial blood gases (ABGs)
- Electrolytes
- Urine or serum beta human chorionic gonadotropin (hCG) for pregnancy
- Blood alcohol levels and toxicology screens

Diagnostic Tests for Major Trauma		
Test	**Purpose**	**Abnormal Findings**
Blood Studies		
Type and screen/ type and cross-match	To have type-specific and cross-matched blood available for resuscitation	Inability to cross-match if specimen is collected after multiple units of blood are transfused.
Arterial blood gas (ABG)	Assess for adequacy of oxygenation and ventilation and to determine the level of anaerobic metabolism.	pH <7.35 with increased $PaCO_2$ (>45 mm Hg) indicates respiratory acidosis. Serum bicarbonate <22 mEq/L with a pH <7.35 can indicate metabolic acidosis. Decreased PaO_2 indicates hypoxemia. Increased $PaCO_2$ indicates inadequate ventilation. Base deficit <-2.0 mEq/L indicates increased oxygen debt.

Diagnostic Tests for Major Trauma —cont'd		
Test	**Purpose**	**Abnormal Findings**
Complete blood count (CBC) Hemoglobin (Hgb) Hematocrit (Hct)	Assess for blood loss.	Decreased Hgb and Hct indicate blood loss. Often Hgb and Hct are within normal range initially, especially if the patient has not received a significant amount of fluid to replace the blood loss. The Hgb and Hct should be repeated after the patient has a fluid challenge if there is any indication of significant bleeding.
Electrolytes Potassium (K$^+$) Glucose Creatinine	Provide a baseline and assess for possible alterations.	Potassium may be elevated with crush injuries. Glucose is usually elevated after injury. Decreased glucose indicates hypoglycemia and may cause decreased level of consciousness. Elevated creatinine indicates decreased renal functioning, and care should be taken when administering contrast for radiologic studies.
Coagulation profile Prothrombin time (PT) with international normalized ratio (INR) Partial thromboplastin time (PTT) Fibrinogen D-dimer	Assess for causes of bleeding, clotting and disseminated intravascular coagulation (DIC) indicative of abnormal clotting present in shock or ensuing shock.	Decreased PT with low INR promotes clotting; elevation promotes bleeding; elevated fibrinogen and D-dimer reflect abnormal clotting is present.
Blood alcohol	To determine the level of alcohol in the patient's blood	>10 mg/dl indicates the presence of alcohol in the patient's blood. The higher the level, the more chance the patient has of showing signs of intoxication, but an absolute value will depend on the patient's tolerance. This may interfere with neurologic assessment.
Carbohydrate deficient transferring (CDT)	To identify patients who have had excessive drinking for the past few weeks and may be at risk for alcohol withdrawal	>20 units/L for males and >26 units/L for females indicate excessive drinking.
Drug screen	To identify the presence of drugs in the patient's system	Positive value indicates recent use of the substance.
Radiology		
Chest radiograph (CXR)	Assess thoracic cage (for fractures), lungs (pneumothorax, hemothorax); size of mediastinum, size of heart.	Displaced lung margins will be present with pneumothoraces and hemothoraces. Cardiac enlargement may reflect cardiac tamponade.
Pelvic radiograph	Assess the integrity of the pelvic ring to indentify fractures and determine stability of the pelvis.	Fracture lines through any of the bones in the pelvis, widening of the symphysis pubis, and widening of the sacroiliac joint(s)
Computerized tomography head, neck, chest, abdomen, and/or pelvis	Assess for internal injuries.	Any findings of skeletal fractures, misalignment, organ damage, or abnormal collections of blood indicates injury to the organ/tissue involved.
Ultrasound: FAST Focused Assessment with Sonography for Trauma	Assess for fluid around the heart, liver, spleen and bladder.	Abnormal collection of fluid

Major Trauma

Continued

Diagnostic Tests for Major Trauma — cont'd		
Test	**Purpose**	**Abnormal Findings**
Invasive Studies		
Diagnostic peritoneal lavage (DPL)	Assess for blood or in the peritoneal cavity or abnormal substrates in the peritoneal lavage fluid.	The presence of red or white blood cells, bile, food fibers, amylase, or feces in the lavage fluid suggests injury to the abdominal organs. Lavage fluid coming from the Foley catheter indicates bladder rupture. Lavage fluid coming from the chest tube, if present, indicates diaphragm rupture.

COLLABORATIVE MANAGEMENT

The primary goals of initial assessment in major trauma are to identify life-threatening injuries, stop bleeding, and restore adequate oxygenation to the tissues. Once life-threatening injuries have been addressed, a secondary assessment is performed to indentify all injuries the patient may have sustained. It is important to perform a thorough organized head-to-toe assessment to minimize the chance of missing injuries. The following treatments may be required:

Care Priorities

1. **Secure a patent airway:** A patent airway must be secured when a GCS score less than 8 or potential for airway compromise is possible and/or the patient has respiratory failure requiring mechanical ventilation. The airway is secured by intubation using a rapid sequence intubation protocol to prevent patient movement during the procedure. If the patient is unable to be intubated, a surgical airway must be performed. The surgical airway of choice in an emergency situation is a cricothyroidotomy. If the cervical spine has not been cleared, the spine must be stabilized during the procedure by maintaining constant in-line positioning with gentle traction.

2. **Support ventilation:** If the patient is not adequately ventilating to maintain oxygen saturations above 95%, the patient should be placed on supplemental oxygen. Most major trauma patients will require supplemental oxygen. Blood loss creates reduced oxygen-carrying capacity, and tissue demand for oxygen is greatly increased during the hypermetabolic phase. High-flow oxygen by mask is indicated initially. Oxygen therapy can be titrated according to ABG and pulse oximetry values. Mechanical ventilation may be required if the patient is not ventilating well enough to remove CO_2. If the patient does not have equal breath sounds, a pneumothorax or hemothorax should be suspected and a tube thoracotomy may be indicated.

3. **Manage hemorrhage and hypovolemia:** Stopping blood loss and restoring adequate circulating blood volume are imperative. Lack of resuscitation will lead to increasing oxygen debt and eventually to MODS and death. The goal of resuscitation in any trauma patient should be to restore adequate tissue perfusion. Two or more large-bore ($\geq$16-gauge) short catheters should be placed to maximize delivery of fluids and blood. Use of intravenous (IV) tubing with an exceptionally large internal diameter (trauma tubing), absence of stopcocks, and use of external pressure are techniques used to promote rapid fluid volume therapy when indicated. In some cases the patient may require large central venous access, such as an 8.5 Fr introducer. When rapid infusion of large amounts of fluid is required, all fluid should be warmed to body temperature to prevent hypothermia. Rapid warmer/infuser devices are available to facilitate rapid administration of blood products. Fluid resuscitation should be used more judiciously in pediatric and older patients, as well as patients with significant craniocerebral trauma, who have precise fluid requirements (see Traumatic Brain Injury, p. 341).
   - *Crystalloids:* Initial fluid used for resuscitation should be an isotonic electrolyte solution such as 0.9% normal saline (NS), or lactated Ringer's (LR). Other balanced electrolyte solutions, such as Normosol-R pH 7.4 (Hospira) or Plasmalyte-A 7.4 (Baxter) may be used after initial fluid resuscitation has been completed.

- *Rapid bolus*: From 1 to 2 L of rapid IV fluid infusion for adults and 20 ml/kg for pediatric patients should be initiated in the prehospital setting. If the patient continues to show signs of shock after the bolus is complete, blood transfusions should be considered.
- *Packed red blood cells (PRBCs)*: Typed and cross-matched blood is ideal, but in the immediate resuscitation period, if cross-matched blood is not available, type O blood may be used. Once the patient has been typed, type-specific blood can be used. Those patients requiring continuous blood transfusions need reassessment to identify the source of bleeding and definitive treatment to stop ongoing blood loss. A massive transfusion protocol may also need to be initiated.
- *Massive transfusion* is defined as replacement of one half of the patient's blood volume at one time or complete replacement of the patient's blood volume over 24 hours. A massive transfusion protocol ensures the patient receives plasma, platelets, and cryoprecipitate in addition to the packed red blood cells to prevent the complications related to coagulopathy. Another concern with massive transfusion is hypocalcemia caused by calcium binding with citrate in stored PRBCs, resulting in depressed myocardial contractility, particularly in hypothermic patients or in those with impaired liver function. One ampule of 10% calcium chloride should be considered for administration after every 4 units of PRBCs.

Safety Alert   *Only O-negative packed cells should be transfused into prepubescent females and women in childbearing status to prevent sensitization and future complications during pregnancy.*

- *Autotransfusion*: Shed blood from the patient can be collected, filtered, and reinfused. Shed blood is captured from chest tube drainage or the operative field and reinfused immediately. Various techniques are used to capture and reinfuse the blood. Advantages of autotransfusion include reduced risk of disease transmission, absence of incompatibility problems, and availability. Disadvantages include risk of blood contamination and presence of naturally occurring factors that promote anticoagulation.
- *Colloids*: Resuscitation with colloids has not been shown to reduce mortality and is not used in the initial resuscitation of trauma patients.
- *Recombinant factor VIIa (rFVIIa)*: The standard use of rFVIIa in the resuscitation of trauma patients is still controversial. Some studies have shown a decrease in the number of units of PRBCs required for patients in hemorrhagic shock but have not shown a decrease in mortality. More studies are needed to determine the appropriate indications, contraindications, dosage, and timing of rFVIIa administration in trauma patients experiencing hemorrhagic shock.

 4. **Identify, prevent, and/or manage hypothermia:** Warmed blankets, forced warm air blankets, and warmers for IV fluids and blood should be used to prevent hypothermia. If the patient is already hypothermic, more aggressive measures to rewarm the patient may be necessary. Warming lights are useful for pediatric patients. Core rewarming measures can include irrigation of the peritoneal and/or thoracic cavities with warmed saline, use of heated humidified oxygen, and extracorporeal blood rewarming.

5. **Provide gastric decompression:** *Gastric intubation* permits gastric decompression, aids in removal of gastric contents, and helps to prevent vomiting or possible aspiration. The nasal route is contraindicated in patients with basilar skull fractures (BSFs) because of the need to prevent tubes entering the cranial vault via abnormal openings in the fractured skull. In patients with facial trauma or suspected or known BSF, gastric tubes should be placed orally.

6. **Ensure urinary drainage:** An indwelling catheter is inserted to obtain a specimen for urinalysis and to monitor hourly urine output. See Renal and Lower Urinary Tract Trauma, p. 317, for precautions.

7. **Prevent infection with antibiotics:** Broad-spectrum antibiotics are used initially to prevent infections if there are open wounds or compound fractures. More specific antimicrobial agents are used when results from culture and sensitivity tests are available.

8. **Control pain and anxiety with analgesics and anxiolytics:** Relief of pain and anxiety are accomplished using IV opiates and anxiolytics. All IV agents should be carefully titrated to desired effect, while avoiding respiratory depression, masking injury, or disguising changes in physiologic parameters. Use of the World Health Organization (WHO) ladder for pain management and a pain-rating scale are essential for the trauma population.

9. **Provide tetanus prophylaxis:** Tetanus immunoglobulin and tetanus-toxoid are considered on the basis of Centers for Disease Control and Prevention (CDC) recommendations (Table 3-1).

10. **Initiate nutritional support therapy:** Infection and sepsis contribute to the negative nitrogen state and increased metabolic needs. Prompt initiation of nutrition therapy is essential for rapid healing and prevention of complications. Parenteral nutrition or postpyloric (jejunal) feedings may be used if postoperative ileus or injury to the gastrointestinal (GI) tract is present. For more information, see Nutritional Support, p. 117.

11. **Facilitate evaluation for surgery:** Need for surgery depends on the type and extent of injuries. The surgical team is coordinated by the trauma surgeon. When several specialty surgeons are required for various injuries, the order of surgeries is coordinated carefully to preserve life and limit the potential for disability.

CARE PLANS: MAJOR TRAUMA

Ineffective tissue perfusion, cardiopulmonary *related to significant blood loss/volume*

GOALS/OUTCOMES Within 24 hours of this diagnosis, patient exhibits adequate tissue perfusion, as evidenced by BP within normal limits for patient, heart rate (HR) 60 to 100 beats per minute (bpm), normal sinus rhythm on electrocardiogram (ECG), peripheral pulses greater than 2+ on a 0-to-4+ scale, warm and dry skin, hourly urine output ≥0.5 ml/kg, base deficit between +2 and −2 mmol/L, serum lactate less than 2.2 mmol/L, measured cardiac output (CO) 4 to 7 L/min, pulmonary artery wedge pressure (PAWP) 6 to 12 mm Hg, and patient awake, alert, and oriented.

NOC Blood Loss Severity

Shock Management: Volume
1. Monitor for sudden blood loss or persistent bleeding.
2. Prevent blood volume loss (e.g., apply pressure to site of bleeding).
3. Monitor for fall in systolic BP to less than 90 mm Hg or a fall of 30 mm Hg in hypertensive patients.
4. Monitor for signs/symptoms of hypovolemic shock (e.g., increased thirst, increased HR, increased systemic vascular resistance (SVR), decreased urinary output [urine output], decreased bowel sounds, decreased peripheral perfusion, altered mental status, or altered respirations).

Table 3-1	**GUIDE TO TETANUS PROPHYLAXIS IN ROUTINE WOUND MANAGEMENT**			
	Clean Minor Wounds		**All Other Wounds***	
History of Adsorbed Tetanus Toxoid (Doses)	**Tdap or Td†**	**TIG§**	**Tdap or Td†**	**TIG§**
<3 or unknown	Yes	No	Yes	Yes
≥3 Doses¶	No**	No	No††	No

* Such as (but not limited to) wounds contaminated with dirt, feces, soil, and saliva; puncture wounds; avulsions; and wounds resulting from missiles, crushing, burns, and frostbite.

† For children younger than 7 years, DTaP is recommended; if pertussis vaccine is contraindicated, DT is given. For persons 7–9 years of age or 65 years or older, Td is recommended. For persons 10–64 years, Tdap is preferred to Td if the patient has never received Tdap and has no contraindication to pertussis vaccine. For persons 7 years of age or older, if Tdap is not available or not indicated because of age, Td is preferred to TT.

§ TIG is human tetanus immune globulin. Equine tetanus antitoxin should be used when TIG is not available.

¶ If only three doses of fluid toxoid have been received, a fourth dose of toxoid, preferably an adsorbed toxoid, should be given. Although licensed, fluid tetanus toxoid is rarely used.

** Yes, if it has been 10 years or longer since the last dose.

†† Yes, if it has been 5 years or longer since the last dose. More frequent boosters are not needed and can accentuate side effects.

From Centers for Disease Control and Prevention: Manual for the surveillance of vaccine-preventable diseases. Atlanta, GA, 2008, Centers for Disease Control and Prevention.

5. Position the patient for optimal perfusion.
6. Insert and maintain large-bore IV access.
7. Administer warmed IV fluids, such as isotonic crystalloids, as indicated.
8. Administer blood products (e.g., PRBCs, platelets, plasma, and cryoprecipitate) as appropriate.
9. Administer oxygen and/or mechanical ventilation, as appropriate.
10. Draw arterial blood gases and monitor tissue oxygenation.
11. Monitor Hgb/hematocrit (Hct) level.
12. Monitor coagulation studies, including INR, PT, PTT, fibrinogen, fibrin degradation/split products, and platelets.
13. Monitor lab studies (e.g., serum lactate, acid-base balance, metabolic profiles, and electrolytes).
14. Monitor fluid status, including intake and output, as appropriate.
15. Monitor for clinical signs and symptoms of overhydration/fluid excess.

Vital Signs Monitoring
1. Monitor BP, pulse, temperature, and respiratory status, as appropriate.
2. Note trends and wide fluctuations in BP.
3. Auscultate BPs in both arms and compare, as appropriate.
4. Initiate and maintain a continuous temperature monitoring device, as appropriate.
5. Monitor for and report signs and symptoms of hypothermia and hyperthermia.
6. Monitor the presence and quality of pulses.
7. Monitor cardiac rate and rhythm.

Acid-Base Monitoring
1. Examine the pH level in conjunction with the $PaCO_2$ and HCO_3 levels to determine whether the acidosis/alkalosis is compensated or uncompensated.
2. Monitor for an increase in the anion gap (greater than 14 mEq/L), signaling an increased production or decreased excretion of acid products.
3. Monitor base excess/base deficit levels.
4. Monitor arterial lactate levels.
5. Monitor for elevated chloride levels with large volumes of NS.

Impaired gas exchange *related to airway obstruction, inadequate oxygenation*

GOALS/OUTCOMES Within 12 to 24 hours of treatment, patient has adequate gas exchange as evidenced by PaO_2 ≥80 mm Hg, $PaCO_2$ 35 to 45 mm Hg, pH 7.35 to 7.45, presence of normal breath sounds, and absence of adventitious breath sounds. RR is 12 to 20 breaths/min with normal pattern and depth (eupnea).
NOC Respiratory Status: Gas Exchange; Respiratory Status: Ventilation

Airway Management
1. Assess for patent airway; if snoring, crowing, or strained respirations are present, indicative of partial or full airway obstruction, open airway using chin-lift or jaw-thrust and maintain cervical spine alignment.
2. Insert oral or nasopharyngeal airway if patient cannot maintain patent airway; if severely distressed, patient may require endotracheal intubation.
3. When spine is cleared, position patient to alleviate dyspnea and ensure maximal ventilation, generally in a sitting inclined position unless severe hypotension is present.
4. Clear secretions from airway by having patient cough vigorously, or provide nasotracheal, oropharyngeal, or endotracheal tube suctioning as needed.
5. Have patient breathe slowly or manually ventilate with bag-valve-mask device slowly and deeply between coughing or suctioning attempts.
6. Assist with use of incentive spirometer as appropriate.
7. Turn patient every 2 hours if immobile. Encourage patient to turn self, or get out of bed as much as tolerated if patient is able.
8. Provide chest physical therapy as appropriate, if other methods of secretion removal are ineffective.

Oxygen Therapy
1. Provide humidity in oxygen.
2. Administer supplemental oxygen using liter flow and device as ordered.
3. Restrict patient and visitors from smoking while oxygen is in use.
4. Document pulse oximetry with oxygen liter flow in place at time of reading as ordered. Oxygen is a drug; the dose of the drug must be associated with the oxygen saturation reading or the reading is meaningless.

5. Obtain arterial blood gases if patient experiences behavioral changes or respiratory distress to check for hypoxemia or hypercapnia.
6. Monitor for changes in chest radiograph and breath sounds indicative of oxygen toxicity and absorption atelectasis in patients receiving higher concentrations of oxygen (FiO_2 greater than 45%) for longer than 24 hours. The higher the oxygen concentration, the greater is the chance of toxicity.
7. Monitor for skin breakdown where oxygen devices are in contact with skin, such as nares and around edges of mask devices.
8. Provide oxygen therapy during transportation and when patient gets out of bed.

Respiratory Monitoring
1. Monitor rate, rhythm, and depth of respirations.
2. Note chest movement for symmetry of chest expansion and signs of increased work of breathing such as use of accessory muscles or retraction of intercostal or supraclavicular muscles.
3. Ensure airway is not obstructed by tongue (snoring or choking-type respirations) and monitor breathing patterns. New patterns that impair ventilation should be managed as appropriate for setting.
4. Note that trachea remains midline, as deviation may indicate patient has a tension pneumothorax.
5. Auscultate breath sounds following administration of respiratory medications to assess for improvement.
6. Note changes in oxygen saturation (SaO_2), pulse oximetry (SpO_2), end-tidal CO_2 ($ETCO_2$), and ABGs as appropriate.
7. Monitor for dyspnea and note causative activities/events.
8. If increased restlessness or unusual somnolence occurs, evaluate patient for hypoxemia and hypercapnia as appropriate.
9. Monitor chest x-ray reports as new films become available.

Acute pain *related to physical injury*

GOALS/OUTCOMES Within 30 minutes of intervention, patient's subjective evaluation of discomfort improves, as documented by a pain scale. Nonverbal indicators, such as grimacing, are absent. Vital signs return to baseline. ECG changes present during event resolve.
NOC Comfort Status: Physical, Pain Level

Pain Management
1. Assess and document the location and intensity of the pain. Devise a pain scale with patient, rating discomfort from 0 (no pain) to 10 or any system that assists in objectively reporting pain level. If intubated, use a physiologic scale such as adult nonverbal pain scale or the FLACC scale.
2. Determine the needed frequency of making an assessment of patient comfort and implement monitoring plan.
3. Provide the patient with optimal pain relief with prescribed analgesics.
4. Ensure pretreatment analgesia and/or nonpharmacologic strategies prior to painful procedures.
5. Evaluate the effectiveness of the pain control measures used through ongoing assessment of the pain experience.

Hypothermia *related to altered temperature regulation*

GOALS/OUTCOMES Patient will maintain a normal body temperature above 36°C (96.8°F).
NOC Thermoregulation

Temperature Regulation
1. Monitor temperature at least every 2 hours, as appropriate.
2. Institute a continuous core temperature monitoring device, as appropriate.
3. Monitor BP, pulse, and respirations, as appropriate.
4. Monitor skin color and temperature.

Treatment for Hypothermia
1. Cover with warmed blankets, as appropriate.
2. Administer warmed (37° to 40°C) IV fluids, as appropriate.
3. Administer heated oxygen, as appropriate.
4. Infuse all whole blood and PRBCs through a warmer.
5. Institute active core rewarming techniques (e.g., colonic lavage, hemodialysis, peritoneal dialysis, and extracorporeal blood rewarming), as appropriate.
6. Minimize exposure of the patient.
7. Keep the room temperature comfortable for the patient.

❧• Posttrauma Syndrome *related to inadequate coping ability due to major physical and emotional stress*

GOALS/OUTCOMES Patient exhibits appropriate coping mechanism and reduced anxiety as evidenced by decreased restlessness, pulse rate 60 to 100 bpm, respiratory rate 12 to 20 breaths/min, and decrease in the amount of pain medication requested.

NOC Anxiety Level; Coping

Anxiety Reduction
1. Explain all procedures, including sensations likely to be experienced during the procedure.
2. Provide factual information concerning diagnosis, treatment, and prognosis.
3. Encourage family to stay with patient, as appropriate.
4. Create an atmosphere to facilitate trust.
5. Control stimuli as appropriate, for the patient needs.
6. Determine the patient's decision-making ability.
7. Administer medications to reduce anxiety, as appropriate.
8. Assess for verbal and nonverbal signs of anxiety.
9. Support the use of appropriate defense mechanisms.

Coping Enhancement
1. Provide an atmosphere of acceptance.
2. Provide the patient with realistic choices about certain aspects of care.
3. Acknowledge the patient's spiritual/cultural background.
4. Encourage the use of spiritual resources, if desired.
5. Encourage verbalization of feelings, perceptions, and fears.
6. Assist the patient to identify available social supports.
7. Encourage family involvement, as appropriate.

Emotional Support
1. Make supportive and empathetic statements.
2. Encourage the patient to express feelings of anxiety, anger, or sadness.
3. Refer for counseling, as appropriate.

ADDITIONAL NURSING DIAGNOSES
Also see nursing diagnoses and interventions as appropriate in Nutritional Support (p. 117), Mechanical Ventilation (p. 99), Hemodynamic Monitoring (p. 75), Prolonged Immobility (p. 149), and Emotional and Spiritual Support of the Patient and Significant Others (p. 200).

ABDOMINAL TRAUMA

PATHOPHYSIOLOGY
The patient with abdominal injury can be the most challenging and difficult to manage. Forces may be blunt or penetrating and the organs are either solid (pancreas, kidneys, adrenal glands, liver, and spleen) or hollow (stomach, small bowel, and colon). This patient may have subtle signs of internal hemorrhage, which can be a major contributor to the increase in mortality and morbidity noted after the initial injury has been managed. The severity of abdominal injury is related to the type of force applied to the organs suspended inside the peritoneum. Motor vehicle collision (MVC), either auto-auto or auto-pedestrian, is the most common cause of blunt abdominal trauma worldwide.

Blunt Trauma
There are three mechanisms of action with blunt trauma.
1. Rapid deceleration: On impact, the different organs that reside inside abdominal cavity move at different speeds depending on their density. This creates what is known as shear force, that is, two different directions applied to the organ, usually at the point of attachment, causing injury to other organs such as the aorta.

2. Crush of contents between the walls: Solid viscera are exceptionally affected when the compression occurs from the anterior abdominal wall and the spine or posterior cage.
3. External compression force: The force of external traumatic impact may increase the organ and abdominal pressures to such a degree that the hollow organs rupture.

Mechanisms of Action with Penetrating Injury

External penetration to the abdominal cavity can be caused by any missile or object that intrudes into the abdominal cavity. Penetrating forces injure the organ(s) in the direct path of the instrument or missile, while shock waves from high-velocity weapons (e.g., high-powered rifles) may also injure adjacent organs. Stab wounds are generally easier to manage than gunshot wounds but may be fatal if a major blood vessel (aorta) or highly vascular organ (liver) is penetrated. The three most common injuries associated with penetrating abdominal trauma are those to the small bowel, liver, and colon. With blunt trauma, injuries to the liver, spleen, and kidney are more common. Undetected mesenteric damage may cause compromised blood flow, with eventual bowel infarction. Perforations or contusions result in release of bacteria and intestinal contents into the abdominal cavity, causing serious infection.

The abdomen can be divided into four areas: (1) intrathoracic abdomen, (2) pelvic abdomen, (3) retroperitoneal abdomen, and (4) true abdomen.

Intrathoracic abdomen: The upper abdomen resides beneath the rib cage and includes the diaphragm, liver, spleen, and stomach.
- *Diaphragm:* Commonly injured at the left posterior portion after blunt trauma, the tear is best visualized by chest radiograph, which reveals an elevation of the left hemidiaphragm and air under the diaphragm.
- *Spleen:* The organ most frequently injured after blunt trauma, massive hemorrhage from splenic injury is common. Damage to the spleen may occur with the most trivial of injuries, so index of suspicion should be high. Splenic injury is often associated with hepatic or pancreatic injury due to close proximity of these organs. Splenectomy is the treatment of choice for major spleen injuries. Minor splenic injuries may be managed with direct suture techniques
- *Liver:* Most frequently involved in penetrating trauma (80%) because of its large size and location, the liver is less often affected by blunt injury (20%). Control of bleeding and bile drainage is the priority with hepatic injury. Mortality from liver injuries is about 10%. In most patients, bleeding from a liver injury can be controlled, such as with perihepatic packing. About 5% of injuries require packing for bleeds. Major arterial bleeding from the liver parenchyma will require further attention. Biliary tree injuries may require surgical repair and should be suspected with liver injury. The patient may be asymptomatic or have mild to moderate abdominal discomfort with biliary tree injury.

Pelvic abdomen: As defined by bony pelvis, this includes the urinary bladder, urethra, rectum, small intestine, and, in females, the ovaries, fallopian tubes, and uterus. Diagnosis is difficult becauses many of these injuries are extraperitoneal (outside the peritoneal cavity).

Retroperitoneal abdomen: This includes the kidneys, ureters pancreas, aorta, and vena cava. Evaluation may require a computed tomography (CT) scan, angiography, and an IV pyelogram.
- *Retroperitoneal vessels:* Tears in retroperitoneal vessels associated with pelvic fractures or damage to retroperitoneal organs (pancreas, duodenum, and kidney) can cause bleeding into the retroperitoneum.
- Although the retroperitoneal space can accommodate up to 4 L of blood, detection of retroperitoneal hematomas is difficult and sophisticated diagnostic techniques may be required.

True abdomen: This includes the small and large intestines, uterus (when enlarged), and bladder (when distended). Perforation usually presents with peritonitis such as pain and tenderness.
- *Colon:* Injury is most frequently caused by penetrating forces, although lap belts, direct blows, and other blunt forces cause a small percentage of colonic injuries. Because of the high bacterial content, infection is even more a concern than it is with small bowel injury. Most patients with significant colon injuries require a temporary colostomy.
- *Undetected mesenteric damage:* May cause compromised blood flow, with eventual bowel infarction. Perforations or contusions result in release of bacteria and intestinal contents into the abdominal cavity, causing serious infection.
- *Pelvis:* See Renal and Lower Urinary Tract Trauma, p. 317.

Occasionally the **lower portion of the esophagus** is involved in penetrating trauma. The stomach is usually not injured with blunt trauma since it is flexible and readily displaced, but it may be injured by direct penetration. Injury to either the esophagus or stomach results in the escape of irritating gastric fluids due to gastric perforation and the release of free air below the level of the diaphragm. Esophageal injuries often are associated with thoracic injuries. Once hemorrhage has been controlled, attention is turned to prevention of further contamination by controlling spillage of gut contents.

Traumatic **pancreatic or duodenal** injury is uncommon but is associated with high morbidity and mortality. These injuries are difficult to detect and may be associated with massive injury to nearby organs, prompting spillage of irritating fluids, activated enzymes, and bile, which augments the inflammatory response. Pancreatic injury is rare; however, the pancreas can be contused or lacerated. Clinical indicators of injury to these retroperitoneal organs may not be obvious for several hours.

Injuries to **major vessels** such the abdominal aorta and inferior vena cava most often are caused by penetrating trauma but also occur with deceleration injury. Hepatic vein injuries frequently are associated with juxtahepatic vena caval injury and result in rapid hemorrhage. Blood loss after major vascular injury is massive. Survival depends on rapid transport to a trauma center and immediate surgical intervention.

ASSESSMENT: ABDOMINAL TRAUMA
Goal of System Assessment
Rapidly evaluate for significant primary and secondary injuries (for all systems) while performing basic and advanced trauma life support. **Airway, breathing, circulation, disability, and exposure are the structural components of all trauma assessment.**

Safety Alert *In an unstable patient, immediate identification of free intra-abdominal fluid by Focused Assessment with Sonography for Trauma (FAST) examination or a diagnostic peritoneal lavage (DPL) is imperative and supports decisions to move straight to the operating room.*

In the traditional perspective of the "Golden Hour of Trauma" (period of time immediately after traumatic injury in which rapid intervention may prevent death), the American College of Surgeons (ACS) guideline recommends that rapid assessment of hemorrhage includes aggressive volume resuscitation.

History and Risk Factors
First and foremost, it is essential to establish issues involved with the injury event (Box 3-1). These details regarding circumstances of the accident and mechanism of injury are invaluable in detecting the presence of specific injuries. Second, allergies, medications, and last meal eaten will play an important role in the maintenance of good resuscitation. Other information, previous abdominal surgeries, and use of safety restraints (if appropriate) should be noted. Hollow viscous injury is often missed but should always be suspected with a visible contusion on the

Box 3-1	INITIAL HISTORY TAKING OF MOTOR VEHICLE COLLISION PATIENTS (BYSTANDERS, PASSENGERS, AND RESCUE PERSONNEL)

- Extent of damage to the vehicle
- Approximate speed
- Did the airbag deploy?
- Were they wearing a seat belt?
- Were they ejected?
- Was prolonged extrication required?
- Was there a "T-bone" type of occurrence (intrusion into the passenger/or driver side)?
- Alcohol or drugs?
- Possible psychiatric problems/suicide attempts?

All patients in MVC are suspected as having dual diagnosis of head and spine until cleared.

abdomen. Medical information including current medications and last tetanus-toxoid immunization should be obtained. The history is sometimes difficult to obtain because of alcohol or drug intoxication, head injury, breathing difficulties, or impaired cerebral perfusion. Family members and emergency personnel may be valuable sources of information.

Vital Signs

Assess for impending hemorrhagic shock: Pulse greater than 100 bpm, decreased pulse pressure, oliguria: blood loss 750 to 1500 ml; pulse greater than 120, hypotension, oliguria, confusion: blood loss 1500 to 2000 ml; pulse greater than 140, severe oliguria, lethargy: blood loss greater than 2000 ml .

HIGH ALERT! **Persistent Tachycardia**

Persistent tachycardia should always be considered a clue to tissue hypoxia. As the neuroendocrine response ensues, persistent tachycardia should warn all observers that there is response to tissue signals of hypermetabolism and inadequate resuscitation.

- *Hypotension*: Presence of hypotension is a sign of impending doom, but the absence of hypotension does not always accurately reflect an absence of hemorrhage. After an injury, a profound neuroendocrine response ensues to activate the beta receptors (sinus node and ventricular contractile tissue), the alpha receptors (smooth muscle in the arteries), and the renal tubules (promoting preservation of fluid), resulting in significant tachycardia, profound vasoconstriction, and progressive oliguria. These responses may mask the severity of hemorrhage. Patients on alpha or beta antagonists or those with acute spinal cord injuries (above C5) will not manifest these responses and therefore will have few compensatory mechanisms.
- *Pulse pressure*: This measure may be effectively used to determine the amount of volume in the arteries (systolic minus diastolic BP, normal greater than 40 mm Hg). Pulse pressure generally correlates with the volume ejected by the left ventricle and therefore is a valuable tool for indication of volume in the vascular bed. Presence of pulsus paradoxus (Box 3-2) may be visualized with either the invasive arterial pressure trace or the plethysmograph of the pulse oximeter and is an invaluable tool in evaluating arterial volume.

Observation and Subjective/Objective Symptoms

- Inspection of all surfaces of trunk, head, neck, and extremities, including anterior lateral and posterior exposure, with notation of all penetrating wounds, contusions, tenderness, ecchymosis, or other marks and indicators. Multiple wounds may represent entrance or exit wounds but do not eliminate the possibility of objects that may remain internally.
- *Kehr* sign (left shoulder pain caused by splenic bleeding) also may be noted, especially when the patient is recumbent.
- Nausea and vomiting may occur, and the conscious patient who has sustained blood loss often complains of thirst—an early sign of hemorrhagic shock.
- Preoperative pain is anticipated and is a vital diagnostic aid. The nature of postoperative pain also can be important. Incisional and some visceral pain can be anticipated, but intense or prolonged pain, especially when accompanied by other peritoneal signs, can signal bleeding, bowel infarction, infection, or other complications.

Box 3-2 **MEASURING PARADOXICAL PULSE**

- After placing BP cuff on patient, inflate it above the known systolic BP. Instruct patient to breathe normally.
- While slowly deflating the cuff, auscultate BP.
- Listen for the first Korotkoff sound, which will occur during expiration with cardiac tamponade.
- Note the manometer reading when the first sound occurs, and continue to deflate the cuff slowly until Korotkoff sounds are audible throughout inspiration and expiration.
- Record the difference in millimeters of mercury between the first and second sounds. This is the pulsus paradoxus.

Safety Alert	*It is important to note that damage to retroperitoneal organs such as the pancreas and duodenum may not cause significant signs and symptoms for 6 to 12 hours or longer. Relatively slow bleeding from abdominal viscera may not be clinically apparent for 12 hours or longer after the initial injury. In addition, the nurse should be aware that complications such as bowel obstruction caused by adhesions or narrowing of the bowel wall from localized ischemia, inflammation, or hematoma may develop days or weeks after the traumatic event. The need for vigilant observation in the care of these patients cannot be overemphasized.*

Inspection

- Abrasions and ecchymoses may indicate underlying injury. The absence of ecchymosis does not exclude major abdominal trauma and massive internal bleeding. In the event of gunshot wounds, entrance and exit (if present) wounds should be identified.
- Ecchymosis over the left upper quadrant (LUQ) suggests splenic rupture, and erythema and ecchymosis across the lower portion of the abdomen suggest intestinal injury caused by lap belts.
- *Grey-Turner sign*, a bluish discoloration of the flank, may indicate retroperitoneal bleeding from the pancreas, duodenum, vena cava, aorta, or kidneys.
- *Cullen sign*, a bluish discoloration around the umbilicus, may be present with intraperitoneal bleeding from the liver or spleen. Ecchymosis may take hours to days to develop, depending on the rate of blood loss.

Auscultation

It is important to auscultate before palpation and percussion, because these maneuvers can stimulate the bowel and confound assessment findings.

- *Bowel sounds*: These are likely to be decreased or absent with abdominal organ injury or intraperitoneal bleeding. The presence of bowel sounds, however, does not exclude significant abdominal injury. Immediately after injury, bowel sounds may be present, even with major organ injury. Bowel sounds should be auscultated in each quadrant every 1 to 2 hours in patients with suspected abdominal injury. Absence of bowel sounds is expected immediately after surgery. Failure to auscultate bowel sounds within 24 to 48 hours after surgery suggests ileus, possibly caused by continued bleeding, peritonitis, or bowel infarction.

Palpation

- Tenderness to light palpation suggests pain from superficial or abdominal wall lesions, such as that occurring with seatbelt contusions.
- Deep palpation may reveal a mass, which may indicate a hematoma. Internal injury with bleeding or release of GI contents into the peritoneum results in peritoneal irritation and certain assessment findings. Box 3-3 describes signs and symptoms that suggest peritoneal irritation.
- Subcutaneous emphysema of the abdominal wall is usually caused by thoracic injury but also may be produced by bowel rupture.
- Measurements of abdominal girth may be helpful in identifying increases in girth attributable to gas, blood, or fluid. Visual evaluation of abdominal distention is a late and unreliable sign of bleeding.
- Peritoneal signs (pain, guarding, rebound tenderness) or abdominal distention in an unconscious patient requires immediate evaluation in either case.

Box 3-3	**SIGNS AND SYMPTOMS THAT SUGGEST PERITONEAL IRRITATION**

- Generalized abdominal pain and tenderness
- Involuntary guarding of the abdomen
- Abdominal wall rigidity
- Rebound tenderness
- Abdominal pain with movement or coughing
- Decreased or absent bowel sounds

HIGH ALERT! Flank (*Grey-Turner sign*) or umbilical (*Cullen sign*) ecchymosis may be delayed several hours to days in patients with retroperitoneal hemorrhage. Based on index of suspicion, persistent hypotension is always investigated with ultrasound or radiography.

- Mild tenderness to severe abdominal pain may be present, with the pain either localized to the site of injury or diffuse.
- Blood or fluid collection within the peritoneum causes irritation that results in involuntary guarding, rigidity, and rebound tenderness.
- Fluid or air under the diaphragm may cause referred shoulder pain.

Percussion
- Unusually large areas of dullness may be percussed over ruptured blood-filled organs. For example, a fixed area of dullness in the LUQ suggests a ruptured spleen. An absence (or decrease in the size) of liver dullness may be caused by free air below the diaphragm, a consequence of hollow viscous perforation, or, in unusual cases, displacement of the liver through a ruptured diaphragm.
- The presence of tympany suggests gas; dullness suggests that the enlargement is caused by blood or fluid.

HIGH ALERT! Massive intestinal edema is common following laparotomy and prolonged shock. Inflammatory response, neuroendocrine stimulation, aggressive crystalloid resuscitation, bowel handling, intra-abdominal packing, and retroperitoneal hematomas may cause a delay in abdominal closure. If the abdomen is closed, the intra-abdominal volume may compress arteries, capillaries, the bladder, and the ureters. This compartment hypertension (abdominal compartment syndrome) may cause a significant hypotension, oliguria, and base deficit that will be difficult to combat. (See *Abdominal Hypertension and Abdominal Compartment Syndrome*, p. 861).

Diagnostic Evaluation of Abdominal Trauma		
Test	**Purpose**	**Abnormal Findings**
FAST: focused assessment with sonography for trauma	Rapid, portable, noninvasive method to detect hemoperitoneum. Uses four views to evaluate	Based on the assumption that all clinically significant abdominal injuries are associated with hemoperitoneum. If positive for blood, may require CT. If negative, but suspicious, proceed to DPL.
CT scan	Used to evaluate integrity of cavities and organs	Wound tract outlined by hemorrhage, air, bullet or bone fragments that clearly extend into the peritoneal cavity; the presence of intraperitoneal free air, free fluid, or bullet fragments; and obvious intraperitoneal organ injury
Rectal examination	Evaluate for bony penetration	Blood in the stool (gross or occult) and/or the presence of a high riding prostate (indicates genitourinary or bowel injury)
Chest radiograph (CXR)	Assess size and integrity of heart, thoracic cage and lungs; rules out chest cavity penetration	Hemothoraces or pneumothoraces; air under diaphragm indicates peritoneal penetration.

Diagnostic Evaluation of Abdominal Trauma — cont'd		
Test	Purpose	Abnormal Findings
Blood Studies		
Complete blood count (CBC) Hemoglobin (Hgb) Hematocrit (Hct) RBC count (RBCs) WBC count (WBCs)	Assess for occult bleeding or effects of gross bleeding	Decreased Hgb or Hct reflects blood loss, may be false negative when patient has lost significant volume. Repeat after 2 L of isotonic fluid resuscitation.
Electrolytes Potassium (K^+) Magnesium (Mg^{2+}) Calcium (Ca^{2+}) Sodium (Na^+)	Assess for possible causes of dysrhythmias and/or heart failure	Decrease in K^+, Mg^{2+}, or Ca^{2+} may cause dysrhythmias. Elevation of Na^+ may indicate dehydration.
Coagulation profile Prothrombin time (PT) with international normalized ratio (INR) Partial thromboplastin time (PTT) Fibrinogen D-dimer	Assess for causes of bleeding, clotting, and disseminated intravascular coagulation (DIC) indicative of abnormal clotting present in shock or ensuing shock	Decreased PT with low INR promotes clotting; elevation promotes bleeding; elevated fibrinogen and D-dimer reflects abnormal clotting is present.

COLLABORATIVE MANAGEMENT

The initial focus should be stabilization and supporting hemodynamics, but the highest priority is to diagnose and repair causes of hemorrhage. Timely provision of needed surgery, preferably in a trauma center, is the critical factor impacting survival. Prolonged hypovolemia and shock result in organ ischemia and ultimately failure (see *Major Trauma* [p. 235], *Acute Respiratory Distress Syndrome* [p. 365], *Cardiogenic Shock* [p. 472], *Acute Renal Failure* [p. 584], *Hepatic Failure* [p. 785]).

Care Priorities

1. **Identify and manage hypothermia:** Trauma patients are often profoundly hypothermic on arrival in the emergency department as a result of inadequate protection, IV fluid administration, ongoing blood loss, and environmental exposure. Hemorrhagic shock leads to decreased cellular perfusion and oxygenation and impoverished heat production. Hypothermia interferes with coagulation and platelet aggregation, and therefore exacerbates hemorrhage.
Remove all wet clothing and make sure the patient is dry. The patient should be actively warmed with blankets, air-warming devices, or possibly continuous arteriovenous warming techniques. A simple method is to cover all extremities and the abdomen with plastic (e.g., blue side of underpads or trash bags) to trap all heat produced.

2. **Provide oxygen therapy to manage hypoxia:** Abdominal injury may result in poor ventilatory efforts caused by pain or compression of thoracic structures. High-flow supplemental oxygen is indicated initially and then titrated according to ABG values. Mechanical ventilation may be necessary.

3. **Manage hypovolemia and anemia:** Because massive blood loss is associated with most abdominal injuries, immediate volume resuscitation is critical. Initially, LR or a similar balanced salt solution is given. Colloid solutions may be helpful in the postoperative period if there are low filling pressures and evidence of decreased plasma oncotic pressure. Typed and cross-matched fresh blood is the optimal fluid for replacement of large blood losses. However, since fresh whole blood is rarely available, a combination of packed cells and fresh frozen plasma often is used. Overaggressive use of colloids and PRBCs may increase third spacing and SIRS. (See Major Trauma, p. 235, for more information.)

   - *Indication for immediate blood transfusion:* Ongoing blood loss indicates hemodynamic instability despite the administration of 2 L of fluid to adult patients.
   - *Acidosis:* Hemorrhagic shock reduces perfusion, resulting in hypoxemia, anaerobic metabolism, and lactic acidosis. The compensatory vasoconstrictive response shunts blood to the heart, lungs, and brain from the skin, muscles, and abdominal organs. Base deficit or lactate levels should be used to guide fluid resuscitation, ventilation, and BP support.

- *Coagulopathy*: Hypothermia, acidosis, and massive blood transfusion all lead to coagulopathy. The top priority is to stop the bleeding. Coagulopathy is treated by the administration of fresh frozen plasma, factor VII, cryoprecipitate, and platelets and correcting the hypothermia and acidosis. If bleeding persists, consider vasopressin infusion, which causes vasoconstriction and calcium chloride.

4. **Consider surgery for penetrating abdominal injuries:**
   - Indication for emergency laparotomy:
     - Signs of peritonitis
     - Uncontrolled shock or hemorrhage
     - Clinical deterioration during observation
     - Positive hemoperitoneum findings with FAST or DPL examinations
   - Removing penetrating objects can result in additional injury; thus attempts at removal should be made only under controlled situations with a surgeon and operating room immediately available.
   - If evisceration occurs initially or develops later, do not reinsert tissue or organs. Place a saline-soaked gauze over the evisceration, and cover with a sterile towel until the evisceration can be evaluated by the surgeon.
   - The issue of mandatory surgical exploration versus observation and selective surgery, especially with stab wounds, remains controversial. There is a trend toward observation of patients without obvious injury or peritoneal signs.
   - *Indications for laparotomy include one or more of the following:* (1) penetrating injury suspected of invading the peritoneum (e.g., abdominal gunshot wound or abdominal stab wound with evisceration, hypotension, or peritonitis); (2) positive peritoneal signs (e.g., tenderness, rebound tenderness, involuntary guarding); (3) shock; (4) GI hemorrhage; (5) free air in the peritoneal cavity as seen on x-ray film; (6) evisceration; (7) massive hematuria; and (8) positive findings on DPL.

| **Safety Alert** | *The patient should be evaluated for peritoneal signs at least hourly by the same examiner. Consult surgeon immediately if the patient shows peritoneal signs, evidence of shock, gastric or rectal bleeding, or gross hematuria.* |

---

5. **Consider an appropriate surgical intervention based on type of injury:**
   - **Blunt, nonpenetrating abdominal injuries:** Physical examination is important in determining the necessity for surgery in alert, cooperative, nonintoxicated patients. Additional diagnostic tests such as abdominal ultrasound, DPL, or CT are necessary to evaluate the need for surgery in the patient who is intoxicated or unconscious or who has sustained head or spinal cord trauma.
     - *Immediate laparotomy for blunt abdominal trauma is indicated under the following circumstances:* (1) clear signs of peritoneal irritation (see Box 3-3); (2) free air in the peritoneum; (3) hypotension caused by suspected abdominal injury, or persistent and unexplained hypotension; (4) positive DPL findings; (5) GI aspirate or rectal smear positive for blood; and (6) other positive findings in diagnostic tests such as CT or arteriogram.
     - Carefully evaluated, stable patients with blunt abdominal trauma may be admitted to a critical care unit for observation. These patients should be evaluated in the same manner as that described in the section Surgical Considerations for Penetrating Abdominal Injuries.
    - **Need for immediate surgery vs. triad of failure:** Once in the operating room, it may become apparent that the patient cannot survive a long procedure, or that the *triad of failure* (acidosis, hypothermia, and coagulopathy) may cause death. At this point the surgeon may do limited repair and packing, choosing to delay major surgical repair.
     - Transfer patient to the ICU, where the triad may be corrected. Survival from abdominal trauma and surgery requires an integrated team effort.
     - Focus is to limit the effects of hemorrhage, acidosis, and coagulopathy and to promote perfusion of all organs.

6. **Considerations regarding closure of the abdominal surgical incision:** During closure after surgery, if the bowel (intestines) can be visualized with an abdominal horizontal view, the abdomen fascia should not be closed. If the abdomen has been closed, it may become necessary to open it again either in the ICU or the operating room. There are multiple methods discussed in the literature to supplement closure.

1. *Silo bag closure:* A 3-L sterile plastic irrigation bag is emptied and cut to lie flat. The edges are trimmed and sutured to the skin.
2. *Vacuum pack:* A 3-L sterile plastic irrigation bag is emptied and cut to lie flat, then placed into the abdomen, and the edges are placed under the sheath. Two suction drains are placed on top of the bag, and a large adherent steridrape is then placed over the whole abdomen. The catheters are placed to suction, providing continuous drainage.
3. *Vacuum-assisted closure:* This consists of a sterile sponge dressing with an adherent dressing and a continuous negative pressure; it promotes closure, blood flow, and collagen formation.

HIGH ALERT! Sudden release of the abdominal pressure may lead to further injuries such as ischemia-reperfusion, acute vasodilatation, and cardiac dysfunction and arrest. The nurse should hydrate the patient with at least 2 L of volume. IV fluids and vasopressors should be immediately available in case severe hypotension occurs.

7. **Provide nutritional support:** Patients with abdominal trauma have complex nutritional needs because of the hypermetabolic state associated with major trauma and traumatic or surgical disruption of normal GI function. Often infection and sepsis contribute to a negative nitrogen state and increased metabolic needs. Prompt initiation of parenteral or postpyloric feedings, as appropriate, in patients unable to accept conventional enteric feedings and the administration of supplemental calories, proteins, vitamins, and minerals are essential for healing. For additional information, see Nutritional Support, p. 117.
8. **Prevention infection with antibiotics:** Abdominal trauma is associated with a high incidence of intra-abdominal abscess, sepsis, and wound infection, particularly with injury to the terminal ileum and colon. Persons with penetrating or blunt trauma and suspected intestinal injury are started on parenteral antibiotic therapy immediately. Broad-spectrum antibiotics are continued postoperatively and stopped after approximately 72 hours unless there is evidence of infection.
9. **Manage pain using analgesics:** Because opiates alter the sensorium, frequent assessment of level of consciousness is important. Analgesics are used in the immediate postoperative period to relieve pain and promote ventilatory excursion. Nonsteroidal anti-inflammatory drugs (NSAIDs) can increase risk of bleeding and should be used cautiously.

CARE PLANS: ABDOMINAL TRAUMA

Deficient fluid volume *related to active loss of blood volumes or secondary to management of fluids*

GOALS/OUTCOMES Within 12 hours of this diagnosis, patient becomes normovolemic as evidenced by mean arterial pressure (MAP) greater than 70 mm Hg, HR 60 to 100 bpm, normal sinus rhythm on ECG, central venous pressure (CVP) 2 to 6 mm Hg, PAWP 6 to 12 mm Hg, cardiac index (CI) greater than 2.5 L/min/m^2, SVR 900 to 1200 dynes/sec/cm^{-5}, urinary output greater than 0.5 ml/kg/hr, warm extremities, brisk capillary refill (less than 2 seconds), and distal pulses greater than 2+ on a 0-to-4+ scale. Although hemodynamic parameters are helpful to determine adequacy of resuscitation, serum lactate and base deficit are essential to evaluate cellular perfusion.
NOC Fluid Balance; Electrolyte and Acid-Base Balance

Fluid Management
1. Monitor BP every 15 minutes, or more frequently in the presence of obvious bleeding or unstable vital signs. Be alert to changes in MAP of greater than 10 mm Hg.

Abdominal Trauma

Safety Alert *Even a small but sudden decrease in BP signals the need to consult the physician, especially with the trauma patient in whom the extent of injury is unknown.*

2. Monitor HR, ECG, and cardiovascular status every 15 minutes until volume is restored and vital signs are stable. Check ECG to note HR elevations and myocardial ischemic changes (i.e, ventricular dysrhythmias, ST-segment changes), which can occur because of dilutional anemia in susceptible individuals.
3. In the patient with evidence of volume depletion or active blood loss, administer pressurized fluids rapidly through several large-caliber (16-gauge or larger) catheters. Use short, large-bore IV tubing (trauma tubing) to maximize flow rate. Avoid use of stopcocks, because they slow the infusion rate.
4. Fluids should be warmed to prevent hypothermia.

HIGH ALERT! Evaluate patency of IV catheters continuously during rapid-volume resuscitation.

5. Measure central pressures and thermodilution CO every 1 to 2 hours or more frequently if blood loss is ongoing. Calculate SVR and pulmonary vascular resistance (PVR) every 4 to 8 hours or more often in unstable patients. Be alert to low or decreasing CVP and PAWP.

HIGH ALERT! An elevated HR, along with decreased PAWP, decreased CO/CI, and increased SVR, suggests hypovolemia (see Table 5-10 for hemodynamic profile of hypovolemic shock). Anticipate slightly elevated HR and CO caused by hyperdynamic cardiovascular state in some patients who have undergone volume resuscitation, particularly during the preoperative phase. Also anticipate mild to moderate pulmonary hypertension, especially in patients with concurrent thoracic injury, such as pulmonary contusion, smoke inhalation, or early acute respiratory distress syndrome (ARDS). ARDS is a concern in patients who have sustained major abdominal injury, inasmuch as there are many potential sources of infection and sepsis that make the development of ARDS more likely (see Acute Respiratory Distress Syndrome, p. 365).

6. Measure urinary output every 1 to 2 hours. Be alert to output less than 0.5 ml/kg/hr for 2 consecutive hours. Low urine output usually reflects inadequate intravascular volume in the patient with abdominal trauma.
7. Monitor for physical indicators of arterial hypovolemia: (1) cool extremities, (2) capillary refill greater than 2 seconds, (3) absent or decreased amplitude of distal pulses, (4) elevated serum lactate, and (5) base deficit.
8. Estimate ongoing blood loss. Measure all bloody drainage from tubes or catheters, noting drainage color (e.g., coffee grounds, burgundy, bright red [Table 3-2]). Note the frequency of dressing changes as a result of saturation with blood to estimate amount of blood loss by way of the wound site.

NIC Electrolyte Management; Fluid Monitoring; Hypovolemia Management

Acute Pain *related to physical injury secondary to trauma or surgical intervention*

GOALS/OUTCOMES Patient's subjective evaluation of discomfort improves, as assessed by use of a pain scale and/or assessed by nonverbal indicators of discomfort, such as grimacing, restlessness, and/or physiologic indicators.
NOC Pain Control; Comfort Level

Pain Management
1. Medicate appropriately for pain relief. It is important to note that opiate analgesics can decrease GI motility, causing nausea, vomiting, and delay of bowel activity. These factors are especially significant if the patient has had a recent laparotomy.
2. Provide comfort measures, maintain proper positioning of affected extremities while turning patient and supporting incisional areas.
3. Explain procedures to patient and include education regarding pain relief measures.

Risk for infection *related to inadequate primary infection defenses secondary to physical trauma or surgery; inadequate secondary defenses caused by decreased Hgb or inadequate immune response;*

tissue destruction and environmental exposure (especially to intestinal contents); multiple invasive procedures

---

GOALS/OUTCOMES Patient is free of infection as evidenced by core or rectal temperature less than 37.7°C (100°F); HR less than 100 bpm, CI less than 4 L/min/m²; SVR greater than 900 dynes/sec/cm⁻⁵; orientation to time, place, and person; and absence of unusual redness, warmth, or drainage at surgical incisions and drain sites.
NOC Risk Control

Infection Protection
1.   Note color, character, and odor of all drainage from any surgical site, orifice, drain, or site of invasive catheters.
2.   Report the presence of foul-smelling or abnormal drainage. See Table 3-2 for a description of the usual character of GI drainage.
3.   Monitor temperature, hemodynamics, and vital signs closely.

Safety Alert   *Administer pneumococcal vaccine to patients with total splenectomy to minimize the risk of postsplenectomy sepsis.*

---

4.   For more interventions, see this diagnosis in Major Trauma, p. 235.
NOC Infection Control; Infection Protection

Ineffective tissue perfusion: gastrointestinal *related to interruption of arterial or venous blood flow or episodes of hypovolemia resulting in decreased perfusion to gastrointestinal organs*

GOALS/OUTCOMES Patient has adequate GI tract tissue perfusion as evidenced by normoactive bowel sounds; soft, nondistended abdomen; and return of bowel elimination.
NOC Tissue Perfusion: Abdominal Organs

Circulatory Precautions
1.   Auscultate for bowel sounds hourly during the acute phase of abdominal trauma and every 4 to 8 hours during the recovery phase. Report prolonged or sudden absence of bowel sounds during the postoperative period, because these signs may signal bowel ischemia or mesenteric infarction.

Table 3-2	CHARACTERISTICS OF GASTROINTESTINAL DRAINAGE
Source	**Composition and Usual Character**
Mouth and oropharynx	Saliva; thin, clear, watery; pH 7
Stomach	Hydrochloric acid, gastrin, pepsin, mucus; thin, brown to green, acidic
Pancreas	Enzymes and bicarbonate; thin, water, yellowish brown; alkaline
Biliary tract	Bile, including bile salts and electrolytes; bright yellow to brownish green
Duodenum	Digestive enzymes, mucus, products of digestion; thin, bright yellow to light brown, may be green, alkaline
Jejunum	Enzymes, mucus, products of digestion; brown, watery with particles
Ileum	Enzymes, mucus, digestive products, greater amounts of bacteria; brown, liquid, feculent
Colon	Digestive products, mucus, large amounts of bacteria; brown to dark brown, semi-formed to firm stool
Postoperative (gastrointestinal surgery)	Initially, drainage expected to contain small amounts of fresh blood appearing bright to dark; later, drainage mixed with old blood appearing dark brown ("coffee grounds"); and then approaches normal composition
Infection present	Drainage cloudy, may be thicker than usual; strong or unusual odor, drain site often erythematous and warm

It is important to know the normal in order to recognize the abnormal.

Abdominal Trauma

2. Evaluate patient for peritoneal signs (see Box 3-3), which may occur initially as a result of injury or may not develop until days or weeks later, if complications caused by slow bleeding or other mechanisms occur.
3. Ensure adequate intravascular volume (see Deficient Fluid Volume, p. 253).
4. Evaluate laboratory data for evidence of bleeding (e.g., serial Hct) or organ ischemia (e.g., AST, ALT, lactic dehydrogenase [LDH]). Desired values are as follows: Hct greater than 28% to 30%, AST 5 to 40 IU/L, ALT 5 to 35 IU/L, and LDH 90 to 200 U/L.
5. Document amount and character of GI secretions, drainage, and excretions.
6. Assess and report any indicators of infection or bowel obstruction (e.g., fever, severe or unusual abdominal pain, nausea and vomiting, unusual drainage from wounds or incisions, change in bowel habits).

HIGH ALERT! Note changes that suggest bleeding (presence of frank or occult blood), infection (e.g., increased or purulent drainage), or obstruction (e.g., failure to eliminate flatus or stool within 3 to 4 days after surgery).

NIC Circulatory Care: Arterial Insufficiency; Bowel Management

Impaired skin integrity *related to mechanical factors (including physical injury); increased metabolic needs secondary to trauma/stress response; altered circulation secondary to hemorrhage or direct vascular injury; exposure to irritants (gastric secretions)*

GOALS/OUTCOMES Patient has adequate tissue integrity by the time of hospital discharge as evidenced by wound healing within an acceptable time frame (according to extent of injury) and absence of skin breakdown caused by GI drainage.
NOC Tissue Integrity: Skin and Mucous Membranes

Skin Surveillance
1. Protect the skin surrounding tubes, drains, or fistulas, keeping the areas clean and free from drainage. Gastric and intestinal secretions and drainage are highly irritating and can lead to skin excoriation. If necessary, apply ointments, skin barriers, or drainage pouches to protect the surrounding skin. If available, consult ostomy nurse for complex or involved cases.
2. For other interventions, see this diagnosis in Major Trauma, p. 235.

NIC Wound Care; Tube Care

Imbalanced nutrition: less than body requirements *related to decreased intake secondary to disruption of GI tract integrity (traumatic or surgical); increased need secondary to hypermetabolic posttrauma state*

GOALS/OUTCOMES Patient has adequate nutrition as evidenced by maintenance of baseline body weight and state of nitrogen balance on nitrogen studies.
NOC Nutritional Status: Food and Fluid Intake; Nutritional Status

Nutrition Management
1. Collaborate with physician, dietician, and pharmacist to estimate patient's metabolic needs on the basis of type of injury, activity level, and nutritional status before injury.
2. Consider patient's specific injuries when planning nutrition. For example, expect patients with hepatic or pancreatic injury to have difficulty with blood sugar regulation.
3. Patients with trauma to the upper GI tract may be fed enterally, but feeding tube must be placed distal to the injury. Disruption of the GI tract may require a feeding gastrostomy or jejunostomy. Patients with major hepatic trauma may have difficulty with protein tolerance.
4. Ensure patency of gastric or intestinal tubes to maintain decompression and encourage healing and return of bowel function. Avoid occlusion of the vent side of sump suction tubes, because this may result in vacuum occlusion of the tube.

Safety Alert	*Use caution when irrigating gastric or other tubes that have been placed in or near recently sutured organs.*

- For additional information, see Nutritional Support (p. 117) and Major Trauma (p. 235).

NIC Electrolyte Management; Feeding; Nutrition Therapy; Tube Feeding

Disturbed body image *related to creation of stoma (often without the patient's prior knowledge); as part of management of penetrating physical injury to internal organs*

GOALS/OUTCOMES Patient able to acknowledge body changes, views and touches affected body part, and demonstrates movement toward incorporating changes into self-concept and able to verbalize some level of coping.
NOC Body Image; Self-Esteem

Body Image Enhancement
1. Evaluate the patient's reaction to the stoma or missing/mutilated body part by observing and noting evidence of body image disturbance (see Box 2-4).
2. Anticipate feelings of shock and disbelief initially. Be aware that trauma patients usually do not receive the emotional preparation for ostomy, amputation, and other disfiguring surgery that the patient undergoing elective surgery receives.
3. Anticipate and acknowledge normalcy of feelings of rejection and isolation (and uncleanliness in the case of fecal diversion).
4. Offer patient opportunity to view stoma/altered body part. Use mirrors if necessary.
5. Encourage patient and significant others to verbalize feelings regarding altered/missing body part.
6. Offer patient the opportunity to participate in care of ostomy, wound, or incision.
7. Confer with surgeon regarding advisability of a visit by an ostomate or a patient with similar alteration in body part.
8. Be aware that most colostomies are temporary in persons with colonic trauma. This fact can be reassuring to the patient, but it is important to verify the type of colostomy with the surgeon before explaining this to the patient.

NIC Ostomy Care

ADDITIONAL NURSING DIAGNOSES
Also see Major Trauma for Hypothermia (p. 244) and Posttrauma syndrome (p. 245). For additional information, see other diagnoses under Major Trauma, as well as nursing diagnoses and interventions in the following sections, as appropriate: *Hemodynamic Monitoring* (p. 75), *Prolonged Immobility* (p. 149), *Emotional and Spiritual Support of the Patient and Significant Others* (p. 200), *Peritonitis* (p. 805), *Enterocutaneous Fistula* (p. 778), *SIRS, Sepsis, and MODS,* (p. 924), and *Acid Base Imbalances* (p. 1).

ACUTE CARDIAC TAMPONADE
PATHOPHYSIOLOGY
Cardiac tamponade is a condition that results in a low CO state caused by decreased filling of the chambers of the heart from pressure exerted by fluid, blood, purulent liquid, or gas in the pericardial space. Cardiac tamponade is classified as acute, subacute, occult, or regional. Acute cardiac tamponade occurs when there is a rapid accumulation of fluid, which results in sudden hemodynamic instability that can be life threatening.
    Potential causes of cardiac tamponade include the following:
- *Trauma:* blunt or penetrating cardiac trauma
- *Iatrogenic:* cardiac surgery, cardiac catheterization, pacemaker implant
- *Nontraumatic hemorrhage:* dissecting aortic aneurysm, anticoagulation therapy
- *Left ventricular rupture:* following extensive myocardial infarction

- *Infection*: viral, bacterial, or fungal
- *Neoplasms/carcinoma*: most commonly breast and lung
- *Other*: connective tissue disease, pleural effusions, radiation therapy, uremic states

Acute cardiac tamponade is usually the result of trauma, iatrogenic causes, and hemorrhage. Subacute tamponade causes are related to the slower accumulation of fluids seen with infections, neoplasms, and tissue disease. Occult or low pressure tamponade is seen in hypovolemic settings. Regional tamponade can occur with large pleural effusions or with any loculated fluid within the pericardial space. Pericardial effusions can be described using the Horowitz classification system based on the echo-free space seen with echocardiograms (Box 3-4). One must be aware that any nonacute tamponade may become acute when rapid deterioration in patient condition related to low CO occurs and requires emergent care.

Acute cardiac tamponade results in inadequate CO and decreased tissue perfusion and potential death. The rapid detection and treatment of acute tamponade are the key to patient survival. The pericardial sac contains 20 to 50 ml of fluid to protect and provide a friction-free surface for the beating heart. The pericardial sac has a fibroelastic quality, which allows limited stretching ability. A sudden addition of 50 to 100 ml of fluid can markedly increase intrapericardial pressure. Conversely, a slowly accumulating tamponade can result in 2000 ml of fluid collection without life-threatening cardiac compromise.

When there is a rapid rise in intrapericardial pressure, the heart is compressed causing a decrease in intraventricular filling. The compliance of the right side of the heart is limited, as it is competing for the fixed volume within the pericardium. The right atrium (RA) as a low pressure heart chamber is the most susceptible to collapse, which decreases filling of the right ventricle. This decreased filling results in the JVD. As the pressure continues to increase, the right ventricle (RV) has partial collapse during early diastole. The decreased RV free wall compliance causes a right-to-left shift of the septum, which is pronounced during inspiration, causing the pulsus paradoxus seen with cardiac tamponade. An unresolved tamponade puts pressure on all chambers of the heart, pulmonary vessels, and coronary arteries, causing hemodynamic instability. Hemodynamically, pulmonary artery pressures increase, an equalization of pressures of the right and left atria are seen, and decreased ventricular filling occurs. This hemodynamic compromise is the result of decreased CO and hypotension with decreased tissue perfusion.

ASSESSMENT: ACUTE CARDIAC TAMPONADE
Goal of System Assessment
Determine rapid diagnosis and treatment of acute cardiac tamponade to prevent cardiac collapse and irreversible shock.

HIGH ALERT! Pulseless electrical activity (PEA) may be the presenting sign of cardiac tamponade. Have a high suspicion of tamponade if presenting rhythm is narrow-complex tachycardia without a pulse. Cardiopulmonary resuscitation (CPR) must be initiated immediately.

- IV insertion and advanced airway placement as soon as possible
- Epinephrine 1 mg IVP or vasopressin 40 units IVP with ongoing CPR
- Fluid administration: LR or NS bolus
- Emergent pericardiocentesis
- Prepare for emergent thoracotomy if qualified surgeon is present

---

Box 3-4	HOROWITZ CLASSIFICATION OF PERICARDIAL EFFUSIONS

Grade 1: Small: Echo-free space in diastole less than 10 mm
Grade 2: Moderate: Echo-free space at least greater than 10 mm posteriorly
Grade 3: Large: Echo-free space greater than 20 mm
Grade 4: Very Large: Echo-free space greater than 20 mm and compression of heart is present

Observation

- *Early signs and symptoms*: Muffled or distant heart tones, distended neck veins, hypotension (*Beck triad*), pulsus paradoxes, and unwillingness to lay flat/supine, anxiety, dyspnea, change in sensorium
- *Early hemodynamic changes*: Decreased BP, increase in RA pressure (RAP) or CVP. Pulsus paradoxus of greater than 10 mm Hg (see Box 3-2); low CO
- *Late signs and symptoms*: Signs of cardiogenic shock including decreased BP, weak or thready pulse, confusion, restlessness, cold clammy skin, pallor
- *Late-stage hemodynamic changes*: Continued hypotension, low CO, right and left atrial pressures equalize, and pulmonary artery pressure (PAP) increases

Vital Signs

- Sinus tachycardia, commonly seen as compensatory response to decreased stroke volume
- Monitor BP; assess for significant hypotension, narrow pulse pressure, systolic BP less than 90, and pulsus paradoxus. Pulsus paradoxus is a drop of greater than 10 mm Hg in the systolic BP during inspiration and results from the decreased stroke volume with increased intrathoracic pressure.
- Exertional dyspnea early progressing to dyspnea and orthopnea
- Hoarseness and hiccups may be present due to laryngeal and phrenic nerve involvement.
- Low urine output is the result of low CO and taken with other signs should be viewed as a signal for intervention in the absence of hemodynamic monitoring.

Auscultation

- *Beck triad* of muffled or distant heart tones, distended neck veins, and hypotension, although described as classic, are seen in 10% to 33% of patients. Muffled heart tones may not be apparent with the patient sitting upright, depending on the volume of tamponade. JVD is not always present in acute tamponade, as it is commonly seen in constrictive pericarditis. In the presence of hypovolemia, blood flowing toward the RA during inspiration makes the finding of JVD less likely. Pericardial friction rub may be heard with pericarditis.

Percussion

- Dullness to percussion under the left scapula posteriorly, related to compression of the left lower lobe, Bamberger-Pins-Ewart sign

Hemodynamic Monitoring

If hemodynamic monitoring is not already in progress, do not delay other treatments, but prepare for appropriate monitoring, according to the hemodynamic system used. This may include insertion and monitoring of an arterial line and pulmonary artery catheter or another system capable of cardiac output measurement.

- *Decreased BP*: SBP less than 90 mm Hg requires intervention
- *Increased CVP*: Greater than 12 mm Hg
- *Pulsus paradoxus*: Greater than 10 mm Hg; easily seen in arterial waveform with lower systolic BP during inspiration
- *Absence of Kussmaul sign*: Kussmaul sign is the absence of a decline in jugular venous pressure during inspiration. Because the RV can accommodate increased volume with inspiration in tamponade, a decline in the jugular venous pressure can be seen. This is significant as to differentiate tamponade from constrictive pericarditis.
- *Low CO*: CI less than 2.2
- *Pulmonary artery pressure (PAP)*: Increased
- CVP equalizes with left atrial pressure (LAP) or pulmonary artery occlusive pressure (PAOP).
- BP, CO, and CI continue to decrease, requiring fluid and vasopressor and inotropic support until definitive treatment is provided.
- If untreated, tamponade can lead to PEA or total cardiac arrest.

Safety Alert *Abnormally elevated CVP, PAP, and pulsus paradoxus may not be seen with hypovolemic patient until fluid administration is begun.*

Acute Cardiac Tamponade

- Pulsus paradoxus related to hypovolemia will resolve with fluid administration.
- Pulsus paradoxus will not resolve in acute cardiac tamponade with fluid administration alone.

Screening Diagnostic Tests
- Echocardiogram is indicated as a quick diagnostic tool for assessment.

Diagnostic Tests for Acute Cardiac Tamponade		
Test	**Purpose**	**Abnormal Findings**
Noninvasive Cardiology		
Electrocardiogram (ECG): 12 lead	Assess for any ischemia or infarct, underlying rhythm disturbances, or pericarditis.	Electrical alternans is a beat-to-beat change in the QRS, from swinging of the heart within the pericardium. It is rare and seen with very large volume effusions. Presence of ST-segment depression or T-wave inversion (myocardial ischemia), ST elevation (acute myocardial infarction), new bundle branch block (especially left bundle branch block), or pathologic Q waves (resolving/resolved myocardial infarction) in two contiguous or related leads. Pericarditis shows ST-segment and T-wave changes, which are often confused with ischemic changes but are more diffuse and follow a four-stage pattern (Table 5-9). Low voltage of QRS highly indicative of tamponade
Radiology		
Chest radiograph (CXR)	Assess for a widening mediastinum. Assess size of heart, thoracic cage (for fractures), thoracic aorta (for aneurysm), and lungs (pneumonia, pneumothorax); assists with differential diagnosis of chest pain.	Widening mediastinum is indicative of acute cardiac tamponade, especially important for trauma, postprocedural, and postsurgical patients. Cardiac silhouette enlargement with clear lung fields is indicative of pericardial effusion; but >200 ml of fluid must be present for this finding to be apparent.
Echocardiography (2D or Doppler ECHO)	It is the most definitive test for diagnosing early cardiac tamponade. Assessment of thoracic aneurysms that might have dissected into the valve or coronary arteries causing tamponade. Determine type of fluid within the pericardial space. Assess for mechanical abnormalities related to effective pumping of blood from both sides of the heart.	Pericardial effusions with and without tamponade. Aortic dissections and aneurysms. Abnormal ventricular wall movement or motion, low ejection fraction, incompetent or stenosed heart valves, abnormal intracardiac chamber pressures

Diagnostic Tests for Acute Cardiac Tamponade — cont'd		
Test	**Purpose**	**Abnormal Findings**
Transesophageal ECHO	Post cardiac surgery effusions often accumulate at the posterior wall with compression of RA. Useful for assessment of regional cardiac tamponade. Also can be done without delay while patient is being prepped in operating room for emergent thoracotomy or can be done in operating room. Assess for mechanical abnormalities related to ineffective pumping of blood from both sides of the heart using a transducer attached to an endoscope.	Same as above but can provide enhanced views, particularly of the posterior wall of the heart.
Blood Studies		
Complete blood count (CBC) Hemoglobin (Hgb) Hematocrit (Hct) RBC count (RBCs) WBC count (WBCs) Erythrocyte sedimentation rate (ESR)	Assess for anemia, inflammation, and infection; assists with differential diagnosis of cause of tamponade.	Decreased RBCs, Hgb, or Hct reflects hemorrhage or anemia. Elevated WBC and or ESR indicative of infection or inflammatory pericarditis unless secondary to uremia.
Coagulation profile Prothrombin time (PT) with international normalized ratio (INR) Partial thromboplastin time (PTT) Fibrinogen D-dimer	Assess for causes of bleeding, clotting, and disseminated intravascular coagulation (DIC) indicative of abnormal clotting present in shock or ensuing shock. Anticoagulated patients are at higher risk for tamponade with procedures.	Elevated PTT, PT with high INR promotes bleeding; elevated fibrinogen and D-dimer reflect abnormal clotting is present.
Electrolytes Potassium (K^+) Magnesium (Mg^{2+}) Calcium (Ca^{2+}) Sodium (Na^+)	Assess for possible causes of dysrhythmias and/or heart failure.	Decrease in K^+, Mg^{2+}, or Ca^{2+} may cause dysrhythmias. Elevation of Na^+ may indicate dehydration (blood is more coagulable). Low Na^+ may indicate fluid retention and/or heart failure.
Other C-reactive protein (CRP) Anti–streptolysin O (ASO)	Assess for cause of pericarditis.	CRP can be indicative of inflammation unless patient has uremia. ASO elevated with immunologic cause.

COLLABORATIVE MANAGEMENT

Guidelines on the Diagnosis and Management of Pericardial Disease from the Task Force on the Diagnosis and Management of Pericardial Diseases of the European Society of Cardiology

In 2004, findings were published from the Task Force on the Diagnosis and Management of Pericardial Diseases in the European Heart Journal. These findings included specific recommendations for various forms of pericardial disease to include cardiac tamponade. The treatment guidelines have been widely cited in the worldwide medical literature. The following are limited to the recommendations for the treatment of acute (surgical) cardiac tamponade.

Intervention	Rationale
The diagnostic tests as presented reflect these guidelines with the addition of CT, spin-echo, and cine MRI.	To assess the size and extent of simple and complex pericardial effusions. These are also helpful to measure the size of very large effusions.
Pericardiocentesis (Class I)	Absolute indication for cardiac tamponade with hemodynamic instability
Surgical drainage with bleeding suppression (Class I)	For wounds, ruptured ventricular aneurysm, or dissecting aorta aneurysm with hemorrhage or any tamponade in which needle clotting would make needle evacuation impossible
Thoracoscopic drainage, subxiphoid window, or open surgery	Indicated for loculated tamponade

In 2003, the American College of Cardiology (ACC), the American Heart Association (AHA), and the American Society of Echocardiography (ASE) presented a task force recommendation for the use of echocardiography for all patients with pericardial disease. This recommendation would include the cardiac tamponade patient unless an emergent surgical procedure was needed prior to evaluation.

From www.acc.org/qualityandscience/clinical/statements.htm

Care Priorities

1. **Stabilize ventilation with oxygen, intubation, and mechanical ventilation:** Oxygen is administered using the equipment that most effectively corrects each patient's hypoxia. Devices used range from nasal cannula to 100% nonrebreather masks to mechanical ventilators. If patient presented in cardiac arrest, chest compressions may be in progress while ventilation is being stabilized.

2. **Facilitate providing pericardiocentesis:** Needle aspiration of the pericardium can be performed using a subxiphoid or left parasternal approach to drain excess fluid from the pericardial space. The blood removed often will not clot, since the heart action can cause clotting factors within the pericardial sac to break down (defibrination).
   Pericardiocentesis alone may not suffice to manage acute pericardial tamponade. Surgical exploration with pericardial window is recommended because of the high incidence of recurrent bleeding if surgery is not performed. A drain may stay in place until fluid output decreases or ceases.

3. **Anticipate the need to provide a surgical procedure:** Subxiphoid pericardiostomy is a resection of the xiphoid process to drain the pericardial sac. It is performed using either local or general anesthesia. Other, more extensive surgical procedures, including a pericardiectomy, can be used for cardiac decompression. An immediate thoracotomy can be done in the ICU or emergency department if the patient becomes suddenly bradycardic (HR less than 50 bpm) or severely hypotensive (systolic BP less than 70 mm Hg) or has a PEA or cardiac arrest. Thoracotomy allows for pericardial sac evacuation, hemorrhage control, and internal cardiac massage if needed.

4. **Provide fluid resuscitation:** IV fluid infusion is used to increase ventricular filling pressures during diastole and may result in increased CO and BP. Blood products, colloids, or crystalloids may be used.

5. **Administer vasopressors:** Medications used to increase the BP by stimulating vasoconstriction in the peripheral vasculature include neosynephrine or norepinephrine. These medications are less effective in a setting of hypovolemia.

6. **Administer inotropic agents:** Medications used to increase myocardial contractility and CO include dopamine, dobutamine, and milrinone (see Appendix 6).
7. **Stabilize BP with ongoing titration of medications and fluids:** This must be done with hemodynamic monitoring and goal-directed therapy derived at by the entire critical care team.

CARE PLANS: ACUTE CARDIAC TAMPONADE

Decreased cardiac output (CO) *related to decreased preload secondary to compression of ventricles by fluid in the pericardial sac*

GOALS/OUTCOMES Within 4 to 6 hours after fluid resuscitation or evacuation of tamponade, patient has adequate CO as evidenced by CVP 4–6 mm Hg, CO 4 to 7 L/min, CI $\geq$2.5 L/min, systolic BP at least 90 mm Hg (or within patient's normal range), HR 60 to 100 bpm, normal sinus rhythm on ECG, and absence of new murmurs or gallops, distended neck veins, and pulsus paradoxus.
NOC Cardiac Pump Effectiveness

Cardiac Care: Acute Hemodynamic Regulation
1. Assess cardiovascular function by evaluating heart sounds and neck veins hourly. Consult physician for muffled heart sounds, new murmurs, new gallops, irregularities in rate and rhythm, and distended neck veins.
2. Monitor all patients with blunt or penetrating trauma to the chest and abdomen for physical signs of acute cardiac tamponade, persistent hemodynamic instability, and shock symptoms more severe than expected for the blood loss.
3. Evaluate patient for pulsus paradoxus: an abnormal decrease in arterial systolic BP during inspiration compared with that during expiration of greater than 10 mm Hg difference (see Box 3-2).
4. Measure and record hemodynamic parameters. Consult physician or midlevel practitioner for sudden abnormalities or changes in trend. Early signs of tamponade include elevated CVP with normal BP and pulsus paradoxus. Later signs include equalization of CVP and LAP (PAOP) and elevated PAP in the presence of hypotension and low CO and CI (see Box 3-4).
5. Evaluate ECG for ST-segment changes, T-wave changes, rate, and rhythm. The optimum is sinus rhythm or sinus tachycardia. Maintain continuous cardiac monitoring.
6. For patients presenting with PEA and narrow-complex tachycardia on ECG, have a high suspicion of acute cardiac tamponade as the cause and follow ACLS guidelines.
7. Administer blood products, colloids, or crystalloids as prescribed. For trauma patients, use large-bore IV lines in the periphery, if possible. Use pressure infusers and rapid-volume/warmer infusers for patients who require massive fluid resuscitation.
8. Be prepared to administer vasopressor agents (e.g., norepinephrine, phenylephrine, dopamine) if fluid resuscitation does not support patient's BP. Positive isotropic agents (e.g., milrinone) may be used to support CO in short-term management. The underlying problem is decreased ventricular filling, so these are temporizing measures for hemodynamic support until correction of the tamponade occurs.
9. Have emergency equipment available for immediate pulmonary artery catheterization, central line insertion, arterial line insertion, pericardiocentesis, or thoracotomy.
10. Assess heart rate and monitor ECG: sinus tachycardia, commonly seen as compensatory response to decreased stroke volume.

NIC Cardiac Care; Cardiac Care: Acute; Emergency Care; Hemodynamic Regulation; Invasive Hemodynamic Monitoring; Fluid Monitoring; Fluid Management; Blood Product Administration; Medication Administration; Oxygen Therapy; Resuscitation; Shock Management: Cardiac; Vital Signs Monitoring; Dysrhythmia Management

Ineffective tissue perfusion: pulmonary, peripheral, and cerebral *related to interruption of arterial and venous flow secondary to compression of the myocardium, by the collection of fluid within the pericardial sac.*

GOALS/OUTCOMES Within 4 to 6 hours after management with fluids or evacuation of tamponade, patient has adequate perfusion as evidenced by orientation to time, place, and person; systolic BP at least 90 mm Hg (or within patient's normal range); RR 12 to 20 breaths/min with normal depth and pattern (eupnea) and ease of respirations; Sao$_2$ at least 95%; peripheral pulses at least 2+ on a 0-to-4+ scale; equal and normoreactive pupils; warm and dry skin; brisk capillary refill (less than 2 seconds); and urine output at least 0.5 ml/kg/hr.
NOC Circulation Status

Acute Cardiac Tamponade

Shock Management: Cardiac

1. Assess tissue perfusion by evaluating the following at least hourly: level of consciousness (LOC), BP, pulses, pupillary response, skin temperature, and capillary refill.
2. Evaluate urine output hourly to ensure that it is at least 0.5 ml/kg/hr.
3. Maintain tissue perfusion by delivering prescribed blood products, colloids, crystalloids, vasopressors, and positive inotropes.
4. If hypotension occurs: ensure hypovolemia is treated, with fluid administration, prior to or simultaneously with vasopressors for treatment of hypotension. Administer vasopressors via central line whenever possible. Frequently assess peripheral IV lines for evidence of infiltration. If vasopressor agents infiltrate subcutaneous tissues, necrosis occurs. Follow appropriate management protocol for your institution.
5. Have emergency oxygen and intubation and mechanical ventilation equipment available.
6. Anticipate and prepare for emergent surgery and pericardiocentesis evacuation, if needed.

Safety Alert *Vasopressors (e.g., norepinephrine, phenylephrine, dopamine) should be infused through a central line.*

 Cardiac Care: Acute; Circulatory Care; Emergency Care; Invasive Hemodynamic Monitoring; Respiratory Monitoring; Shock Management; Vital Signs Monitoring; Cerebral Perfusion Promotion; Neurologic Monitoring; Medication Administration; Medication Management; Oxygen Therapy; Intravenous Therapy; Fluid/Electrolyte Management

---

ADDITIONAL NURSING DIAGNOSES

For other nursing diagnoses and interventions see also Major Trauma (p. 235), Chest Trauma (p. 238), Hemodynamic Monitoring (p. 75), and Emotional and Spiritual Support of the Patient and Significant Others (p. 200).

ACUTE SPINAL CORD INJURY

PATHOPHYSIOLOGY

Injury to the spinal cord can be a devastating event initiating a cascade of physical and psychological changes that may last a lifetime. Spinal cord injury (SCI) affects 7800 to 10,000 people each year. The average age at injury is 37.6 years; this number depicts an increasing trend across all injury categories (MVCs, sports, and falls). The rising trend reflects an increase in the number of injuries in those who are 60 years and older. Female injuries now account for 21.8% of new SCIs, but young white males continue to lead the injury profile. Cervical injuries occur most frequently at a rate of 56% over lumbar and thoracic injuries. MVCs cause 44% of injuries, followed by acts of violence (24%), falls (22%), sports injuries (8%), and other causes (2%). Persons living with an SCI are estimated as between 250,000 and 400,000, and approximately 85% of SCI patients who survive the initial 24 hours live at least 10 years.

The spinal cord is approximately 18 inches in length running from the base of the brain to the lumbar (L) spine area between L1-2 where the cord tapers to form the conus medullaris, a bulbous end that terminates into a collection of nerve roots known as the cauda equina (horse's tail). The spinal nerve roots exit the spinal cord at corresponding levels below the vertebral body of the spinal column and are the anatomical connection between the central and peripheral nervous system. Since the spinal cord ends at L1-2, the nerves descending from the conus medullaris making up the cauda equina are considered peripheral nerves. The brain and spinal cord communicate sensory and motor information along a complex system of tracts, some descending from the brain (motor) and others ascending from the periphery (sensory). Damage to pathways along this communication system results in unique but quite distinguishable syndromes that include upper motor neurons (UMNs), which carry messages between the brain and the periphery along the spinal cord, and lower motor neurons (LMNs), those nerves that branch out from the vertebrae (peripheral nerves). Damage to UMNs results in muscle spasticity and hyperreflexia, while damage to LMNs results in muscle flaccidity and areflexia.

Mechanisms of injury to the spinal cord can be traumatic or nontraumatic. Traumatic injuries include MVCs, falls, sports injuries, or acts of violence (e.g., gunshot wounds or stabbings). These injuries are the result of mechanical forces that result in sudden flexion, hyperextension, vertebral fracture, compression of the cord, rotation of the cord, or direct injury to the cord as in a stabbing or gunshot wound. Nontraumatic injuries may be a result of vascular injury (aortic disruption or spinal artery occlusion), degenerative diseases (spondylosis), inflammatory events, neoplasms, or autoimmune diseases (multiple sclerosis). Injuries to the spinal cord regardless of mechanism of injury include concussion, contusion, laceration, transsection, hemorrhage, ischemia, and avascularization. See SCI classifications and terminology in Table 3-3.

Fractures Involving the Vertebral Bodies

These fractures may or may not cause SCI. Severe SCI can occur without damage to the vertebrae. With severe fractures, such as the "burst" fracture (fragmentation of a vertebral body with penetration of the spinal cord), paralysis almost always occurs. Penetration of the spinal cord with bony fragments may cause hemorrhage, infection, and leakage of cerebrospinal fluid (CSF).

Spinal Shock

Spinal shock occurs following both complete and partial transsection of the cord. It is a temporary loss of reflex function in all segments below the level of injury that occurs immediately after SCI, lasting several hours to weeks.

Neurogenic Shock

Neurogenic shock occurs in patients who injure the cervical or upper thoracic cord, disrupting sympathetic innervation to the vasculature, and the heart is impaired, causing dilation of blood vessels and bradycardia, often causing hypotension. The loss of sympathetic innervation also causes venous pooling in the extremities and splanchnic vasculature. Venous return to the heart is decreased, resulting in decreased CO and poor tissue perfusion.

Spinal Shock with Neurogenic Shock

Patients who injure the cervical or upper thoracic cord may experience neurogenic shock and spinal shock simultaneously.

> **Safety Alert** *Although spinal shock is seen in SCIs at any level, the loss of central control of peripheral vascular tone (neurogenic shock) occurs most dramatically in high cervical spine injuries, with interruption of the sympathetic nervous system. Profound bradycardia and hypotension are possible. With SCIs lower than the midthoracic area, the patient will experience a phase of neurogenic shock, with loss of sympathetic innervation to vasculature below the level of the lesion; however, the effects of that loss are not as dramatic.*

Table 3-3	SPINAL CORD INJURY CLASSIFICATIONS AND TERMINOLOGY
Type	Closed (blunt) Open (gunshot wound or stabbing)
Cause	Motor vehicle crashes, falls, sports-related injury, acts of violence
Site	Level of injury involved (cervical thoracic, lumbar, sacral)
Mechanism	Flexion (deceleration injury, backward fall, diving injury) Extension (whiplash or fall with hyperextension of neck)
Stability	Integrity of supporting anatomy including vertebral bodies, ligaments, articulating processes, and facet joints
Complete	Tetraplegia (quadraplegia) or paraplegia (absence of motor, sensory, and vasomotor function below the level of the injury) More frequently seen in cervical injuries
Incomplete	Sparing of some motor and sensory function below the level of the lesion More frequently seen in lumbar injuries

Acute Spinal Cord Injury

Autonomic Dysreflexia

A life-threatening condition affecting victims with lesions at or above T6, stemming from stimulation of the SNS by relatively minor events. The resultant uncompensated cardiovascular response may cause seizures, subarachnoid hemorrhage, fatal cerebrovascular accident, and myocardial infarction if not immediately recognized and treated. *Once spinal shock resolves, autonomic dysreflexia (AD) may occur at any time from the acute phase to several years following the injury.*

Causes: Most commonly, stimuli to the bladder, including distention, infection, calculi, cystoscopy; or from the bowel with fecal impaction, rectal examination, suppository insertion; or from the skin, such as tight clothing or sheets, temperature extremes, sores, or areas of broken skin.

Cord Syndromes

Anterior cord syndrome, central cord syndrome, lateral cord (Brown-Sequard) syndrome, conus medullaris syndrome, and cauda equina syndrome are discussed under *Acute Phase Assessment, Cord Syndromes* p. 266.

ACUTE PHASE ASSESSMENT
Goal of Assessment
Identify and initiate management of fractures, spinal shock, and cord syndromes.

Observation and Physical Assessment Findings
Spinal shock Initial symptoms include:
- Flaccid paralysis below the level of injury of all skeletal muscles with absence of deep tendon reflexes (DTRs)
- Loss of cutaneous sensation
- Loss of temperature control with development of anhidrosis (absence of sweating)
- Loss of vasomotor tone
- Loss of proprioception (position sense)
- Loss of visceral and somatic sensation, and loss of the penile reflex
- Bowel and bladder paralysis resulting in urinary retention and fecal retention occurring along with GI shutdown resulting in paralytic ileus

Recovery phase of spinal shock As spinal shock subsides, the patient may experience:
- Flexor spasms evoked by cutaneous stimulation
- Reflex emptying of the bowel and bladder
- Extensor or flexor rigidity
- Hyperreflexic DTRs, and reflex priapism or ejaculation in the male, evoked by cutaneous stimulation.

Neurogenic shock Symptoms include:
- Vasodilation
- Hypotension
- Bradycardia

Autonomic dysreflexia Symptoms include:
- Pounding headache
- Paroxysmal hypertension (up to 300 mm Hg systolic)
- Flushing of the skin with sweating above the level of the lesion
- Nasal congestion
- Blurred vision
- Nausea
- Bradycardia (30 to 40 bpm)
- Chest pain
- Below the level of the lesion, pilomotor erection (goose bumps), pallor, chills, and vasoconstriction will be present (Table 3-4).

Cord syndromes

Anterior cord syndrome: This syndrome involves injury to the anterior two-thirds of the spinal cord supplied by the anterior spinal artery and may be caused by an acute burst fracture, herniation of an intervertebral disk, or a vascular injury or occlusion due to trauma, clot, or surgical procedure such as aortic aneurysm repair.

Table 3-4	LEVELS OF CORD INJURY
Level of Injury	**Manifestation**
C4 and above	Loss of muscle function, including respiratory function; fatal outcome unless ventilation is provided immediately
C4-C5	Same as above; phrenic nerve may be spared; assisted ventilation; quadriplegia/tetraplegia
C6-C8	Diaphragm and accessory muscles or respiration retained; movement of neck, shoulders, chest, and upper arms; quadriplegia
T1-T3	Neck, chest, shoulder, arm, hand, and respiratory function retained; difficulty maintaining a sitting position; paraplegia
T4-T10	More stability of trunk muscles; paraplegia
T11-L2	Use of upper extremities, neck, and shoulders; some function of upper thigh; reflex emptying of bowel; males may have difficulty achieving and maintaining an erection; decreased seminal emission
L3-S1	Reflex emptying of bowel/bladder; decreased/lack of ability to have an erection; decreased seminal emission; all muscle groups in upper body function; most muscles of lower extremities function
S2-S4	Flaccid bowel and bladder; lower extremity weakness; all muscle groups function; no ability to have a reflex erection

The prognosis varies with each patient and depends on the degree of structural damage and edema.

Symptoms include:

- Loss of varying degrees of motor function below the level of the injury
- Loss of pain and temperature sensation below the level of the injury
- Position, pressure, and vibration sensations remain intact.

Central cord syndrome: Most common SCI affecting the central gray matter of the spinal cord. Primary causes of injury include compression of the cord, low-velocity injuries, fractures and dislocations, and interruption of blood supply to the central spinal cord. In older persons with underlying conditions such as cervical spondylosis, a hyperextension injury related to a fall may result in central cord injury. Vertebral injury may be noted on the radiograph. Motor and sensory deficits are less severe in the lower extremities than in the upper extremities because of the central arrangement of cervical fibers in the spinal cord. Incomplete injuries carry a relatively good prognosis. Many patients can ambulate with an assistive device and may regain bowel and bladder function. There is a less favorable prognosis regarding regaining useful function in the hands.

Symptoms include the following:

- Motor and sensory deficits are usually severe in the upper extremities and profound in the hands and fingers.
- With sparing of sacral and some lumbar fibers, there will be some motor and sensory function in the perineum, genitalia, and lower extremities.
- Bladder dysfunction varies with each patient.

Lateral cord (Brown-Séquard) syndrome: Results from a horizontal hemisection of the spinal cord (e.g., from a gunshot or stab wound). Patients usually have bilateral motor and sensory impairment, with a relative difference in function from one side to the other. Prognosis is usually good for recovery of upper and lower extremity function.

Symptoms include:

- Ipsilateral weakness
- Decrease in light touch, vibratory, and position senses
- Contralateral pain (hypalgesia) and temperature loss
- Usually there are bilateral motor and sensory deficits, but motor activity will be better on the contralateral side and sensory activity will be better on the ipsilateral side.

Conus medullaris syndrome: This injury is a result of a lumbar burst fracture, lateral disc herniation, lumbar stenosis (multilevel), ankylosing spondylitis, neoplasm, infection (abscess), spinal anesthesia, congenital anomalies (tethered cord, arteriovenous malformations), spinal hemorrhage, and multiple sclerosis. Since the injury is at the junction of the conus medullaris and the cauda equina, the lower cord as well as individual peripheral nerves of the cauda equina may be injured, presenting a confusing clinical picture of UMN and LMN lesions.

Symptoms include:
- Mixed UMN and LMN paralysis
- Variable sensory loss
- Preserved (UMN) or areflexive bladder (LMN)
- Erectile dysfunction (UMN) or anesthesia to sacral dermatomes (LMN)
- May exhibit hypertonicity, especially if the lesion is isolated and primarily UMN
- Muscle stretch reflex (deep tendon reflexes) demonstrate hyperreflexive and muscle tone is increased, causing spasticity.

Differentiation from cauda equina may be difficult because signs and symptoms are very similar except for the bilateral presentation in conus medullaris, and sacral segments including bulbocavernosus reflexes and sphincter tone are preserved or normal.

Cauda equina syndrome: This is an injury associated with a central disc fracture of lumbar disk below the level of the spinal cord and those causes as addressed under *Conus Medullaris Syndrome.*

Symptoms include:
- Pattern of LMN responses (flaccid paralysis, areflexia, and loss of muscle tone with muscle fasciculations)
- Diminished muscle strength in the lower extremities consistent with the involved nerve root (see later).
- Greater involvement in the lower lumbar and sacral roots based on the muscle group distribution innervated by the spinal nerve involved
- Sensation is diminished or lost to pinprick and light touch along the dermatome pattern of the nerve; often there is saddle anesthesia with diminished or absent sensation to the glans penis or clitoris.
- Anal sphincter tone may or may not be present.
- There may be a history of urinary retention or loss of bladder tone and incontinence.
- Diminished or absent muscle strength in the muscles listed next assists in localizing the injury.
    - L2 iliopsoas (hip flexion)
    - L3 quadriceps (knee extension)
    - L4 tibialis anterior (ankle dorsiflexion)
    - L5 extensor hallucis longus (big toe extension)
    - S1 gastrocnemius/soleus (ankle plantarflexion)

DIAGNOSTIC TESTS
Spinal radiograph
CT scans and anteroposterior (AP) and lateral radiographic studies provide insight into the bony anatomy of the spine, thereby delineating fractures, dislocations, and subluxations of the vertebral bodies, as well as demonstrating narrowing of the spinal canal and level of hematomas, neoplasms, or abscesses. Additional views such as open-mouth, bilateral oblique, or flexion-extension films also aid in diagnosis.

 Safety Alert   *Films must be obtained with extreme caution in the evaluation of the patient with a possible SCI because any sudden or incorrect movement of the injured area could cause further trauma to the spinal cord or cause injury in a neurologically intact patient. Flexion-extension films should only be obtained when a patient is alert and able to describe pain on manipulation.*

Spinal MRI Scans
More definitive in evaluating SCI, providing location, degree of compression, extent of contusion, degree of ligament involvement, and other related soft tissue injuries. MRI is also the best method to differentiate between swelling/edema and ischemia.

COLLABORATIVE MANAGEMENT
Care Priorities

1. **Immobilize the injured site:**   Additional injury to the spinal cord as a result of inadequate stabilization after injury is sustained by 10% to 25% of SCI patients. Decompression and surgical fixation may be needed.

Cervical spine injury:

Cervical collar and/or head blocks and backboard: The initial treatment for a suspected cervical spine injury.

Cervical traction: Once the injury has been diagnosed, cervical traction to immobilize and reduce the fracture or dislocation can be achieved in several ways including application of a cervical-thoracic orthotic (CTO), a halo device with vest, or a traction system using Gardner-Wells, Vinke, or Crutchfield tongs. In traction therapy, the tongs are inserted through the outer table of the skull and attached to ropes and pulleys with weights to achieve bony reduction and proper alignment. Cross-table lateral radiographs should be obtained until desired realignment of the vertebral bodies is achieved. Another alternative is a special frame or bed (e.g., RotoRest kinetic treatment table). The use of the CTO or halo device for skeletal fixation of the head and neck allows for earliest mobilization and rehabilitation if no surgery is needed.

Surgical intervention: During the immediate postinjury phase, surgery is controversial, and immediate or early surgery postinjury may have little effect on the neurologic outcome and the benefit-to-harm ratio is uncertain. Surgery may be performed (1) if the neurologic deficit is progressing—for example, if cord compression is imminent, in the presence of an expanding hematoma or neoplasm, (2) in the presence of compound fractures, (3) if there is a penetrating wound of the spine, (4) if bone fragments are localized in the spinal canal, or (5) if there is acute anterior spinal cord trauma. Surgeries may include decompression laminectomy, closed or open reduction of the fracture, or spinal fusion for stabilization. Once stabilization of the spine occurs, the patient can be mobilized unless contraindicated for other reasons.

Thoracic and lumbar spine injuries: May require surgical stabilization with laminectomy with or without fusion and insertion of Harrington or Cotrel-Dubousset (CD) rods. If the injury is stable, it may be treated with closed reduction using a thoracic-lumbar-spine orthotic (TLSO) (turtle shell–like immobilizer). If the fracture is unstable and the patient is unable to go to surgery for repair because of medical instability, bed rest with the use of the TLSO should be a priority.

2. **Prevent secondary injury:**   Although administration of methylprednisolone within 8 hours of injury is still the practice in most trauma centers, the use of steroids in the treatment of acute SCI is under scrutiny. Due to methodologic flaws in the original study that demonstrated improved neurologic outcomes with methylprednisolone as well as increasing evidence of deleterious effects of steroid use, the standard of acute care for SCI management is changing and **high dose methylprednisolone is now one of several treatment options, not a standard of care.** More recent studies are emphasizing arterial oxygenation and spinal cord perfusion. Modulating postinjury inflammation may arrest the secondary injury cascade.

   Other promising therapies that are emerging include thyrotropin-releasing hormone, neuroprotection with minocycline (a semisynthetic second-generation tetracycline derivative), use of calcium channel blockers to aid in axonal conduction, use of Cethrin (a Rho antagonist) for neuroregeneration and neuroprotection, and the use of anti-Nogo monoclonal antibodies to augment plasticity and regeneration. Cell-mediated repair is being investigated using stem cells and bone marrow stromal cells.

   Methylprednisolone protocol is as follows: Within 8 hours of injury, a loading dose (30 mg/kg) is administered by IV bolus over a 15-minute period. After a 45-minute wait, 5.4 mg/kg/hr is then administered in a continuous IV infusion over a 23-hour period and then stopped. If the infusion is interrupted for any reason, it must be recalibrated so that the entire dose can be completed within the original 23-hour time frame.

3. **Support ventilation:**   Respiratory insufficiency is a hallmark in SCI, and the more rostral the injury, the more likely it is that the injury will affect ventilation. The need for assisted ventilation is based on level of injury, ABG values, and the results of pulmonary function tests, pulmonary fluoroscopy, and physical assessment data. The need for mechanical ventilation is likely with injuries at C4 and above, patients older than 40, smokers, and patients with associated chest trauma and immersion injuries. Initially, the patient may require intubation and, later, tracheotomy. Persons with high cervical

injury who survive the initial injury but have paralysis of the muscles of respiration may require permanent tracheostomy and mechanical ventilation.

 4. **Provide aggressive pulmonary care:** Respiratory complications are the most common cause of morbidity and mortality in cervical SCI patients, accounting for up to 80% of deaths with pneumonia occurring in 50% of these deaths. Prevention, detection, and treatment of atelectasis, pulmonary infection, and respiratory failure must be priorities. Chest physiotherapy and noninvasive positive pressure ventilation (NPPV) using bilevel continuous positive airway pressure (BiPAP) may provide support, but intubation with mechanical ventilation is sometimes required.

5. **Manage vasodilation-induced hypovolemia:** In patients with neurogenic shock, blood volume is normal but the vascular space is enlarged, causing peripheral pooling, decreased venous return, and decreased CO. Careful fluid repletion, usually with crystalloids, is indicated. Pressor therapy is initiated for patients unresponsive to fluid volume replacement (see discussion under *Pharmacotherapy*, which follows). For fluid management in patients with multisystem trauma, see *Major Trauma*, p. 235.

6. **Prevent aspiration using gastric decompression:** Place a gastric tube to decompress the stomach, prevent aspiration of gastric contents, and manage paralytic ileus (often seen within 72 hours of injury in patients with lesions higher than T6).

7. **Prevent spinal shock by decompressing the bladder:** Insert an indwelling or intermittent catheter to decompress an atonic bladder in the immediate postinjury phase (spinal shock). With the return of the reflex arc after spinal shock subsides, a reflex neurogenic bladder that fills and empties automatically will develop in patients with lesions above T12. Patients with lesions at or below T12 generally may have an atonic, areflexic neurogenic bladder that overfills, distending the bladder and causing overflow incontinence. Intermittent catheterization may be necessary. Use of a Foley catheter for urinary drainage is recommended while the patient is unstable. Once the stability of the patient is ensured, a bladder program using an intermittent straight catheterization procedure is recommended.

8. **Consider gastric ulcer prevention:**
Proton-pump inhibitors (e.g., pantoprazole, omeprazole): To reduce the production of acid in the stomach by blocking the enzyme in the stomach that produces the acid.
Histamine H$_2$-receptor antagonists (e.g., cimetidine, ranitidine): To suppress secretion of gastric acid and to prevent or treat ulcers in the patient with increased production of gastric acid and an increased susceptibility to gastric ulceration and perforation.

9. **Provide bowel retraining:**
Stool softeners (e.g., docusate sodium): Prevent fecal impaction and distention of the bowel, which could stimulate an episode of AD.
Hyperosmolar laxatives (e.g., glycerin suppository): To facilitate movement of the bowels on a regular basis and prevent fecal impaction.
Irritant or stimulant laxatives (e.g., senna bisacodyl): To stimulate bowel movements as part of a bowel training program.

10. **Relieve pain and anxiety:**
Analgesics (e.g., acetaminophen or acetaminophen with codeine): To decrease pain associated with the injury or surgery.
Sedatives (e.g., midazolam, lorazepam): To decrease anxiety caused by the injury, hospitalization, or fear of the prognosis. May be needed when patient is being mechanically ventilated.
Antihypertensives (e.g., hydralazine hydrochloride, methyldopa, nitroprusside sodium): To treat the severe hypertension that occurs in AD.

Safety Alert *Orthostatic hypotension may be a lifelong problem, especially in patients with cervical and high thoracic injuries. Caregivers should move the patient slowly into the upright position (slow elevation of head of bed prior to 90 degrees) to avoid a sudden drop in BP, prompting cerebral hypoxia and loss of consciousness. Abdominal binders and Ace bandages or thigh-high antiembolic stockings also may help prevent orthostatic hypotension.*

Vasopressors (e.g., vasopressin, norepinephrine): To treat the hypotension during the immediate postinjury stage caused by loss of vasomotor control below the level of injury, with resultant vasodilation and a relative hypovolemia (see Appendix 6).

11. Prevent pneumonia:

 Bronchodilators (e.g., albuterol, theophylline): To dilate bronchioles and facilitate removal of secretions. Early use of theophylline is recommended in patients who have a history of COPD or smoking and who show evidence of difficulty moving secretions.

Mucolytic agents (e.g., guaifenesin, acetylcysteine): To reduce tenacity and viscosity of purulent and nonpurulent secretions.

12. Prevent infection, control inflammation and coagulation:

Antibiotics: To prevent or treat respiratory or urinary tract (UTI) infections.

Anticoagulants (heparin or low-molecular-weight heparins such as dalteparin (Fragmin) or enoxaparin [Lovenox]): To prevent thrombophlebitis, DVT, and pulmonary emboli.

> **Safety Alert** *Patients with SCI are at high risk for development of vascular complications because they are immobilized, have lost vasoconstrictive capabilities below the level of injury, and cannot constrict the muscles in the lower extremities to facilitate venous flow. Patients who are not candidates for anticoagulation therapy may have an inferior vena cava umbrella or Greenfield filter inserted to trap emboli traveling from the lower extremities to the lungs.*

CARE PLANS: ACUTE SPINAL CORD INJURY

Impaired gas exchange *related to altered oxygen supply associated with hypoventilation secondary to paresis or paralysis of the muscles of respiration (diaphragm, intercostals) and/or inability to maintain clear airway occurring with high cervical spine injury or ascending cord edema*

GOALS/OUTCOMES Patient has adequate gas exchange as evidenced by orientation to time, place, and person; Pao_2 ≥80 mm Hg; and $Paco_2$ ≤45 mm Hg. RR 12 to 20 breaths/min with normal depth and pattern, HR 60 to 100 beats/min, BP stable and within patient's normal range, and vital capacity (depth or volume of inspiration) is ≥1 L. Motor and sensory losses remain at the same spinal cord level as the initial findings.

> **HIGH ALERT!** Patients with cervical injuries usually arrive in the ICU already intubated. However, with some high thoracic or low cervical lesions, patients who ventilate independently in the emergency department may arrive in the ICU without assisted ventilation. This patient is at risk for an increasingly higher level of cord damage because of hemorrhage and edema, which can result in a higher level of dysfunction and a change in respiratory status that requires assisted ventilation. Before attempting oral intubation with neck flexion, ensure that cervical x-ray studies have confirmed the absence of cervical involvement. Use either nasal intubation or orotracheal intubation with manual cervical spine immobilization if cervical spine injury is not ruled out. Fiberoptic intubation may also be considered.

NOC Respiratory Status: Ventilation

Respiratory Monitoring
1. Assess for signs of respiratory dysfunction: shallow, slow, or rapid respirations; poor cough; vital capacity less than 1 L; changes in sensorium; anxiety; restlessness; tachycardia; pallor; adventitious breath sounds (i.e., crackles, rhonchi), decreased or absent breath sounds (bronchial, bronchovesicular, vesicular), decreased tidal volume (less than 75% to 85% of predicted value) or vital capacity (less than 1 L).
2. Monitor ABG studies; report abnormalities. Be particularly alert to Pao_2 less than 60 mm Hg, $Paco_2$ greater than 50 mm Hg, and decreasing pH, inasmuch as these findings indicate the need for assisted ventilation possibly caused by atelectasis, pneumonia, or respiratory fatigue.
3. Monitor vital capacity at least q8h. If it is less than 1 L, Pao_2/Pao_2 ratio is ≤0.75, or copious secretions are present, intubation is recommended.
4. If patient does not require intubation with mechanical ventilation, implement the following measures to improve airway clearance:
    * Place patient in semi-Fowler's position unless it is contraindicated (e.g., patient is in cervical tongs with traction).
    * Turn patient from side to side at least every 2 hours to help mobilize secretions.

- Keep room humidified to help loosen secretions.
- Unless contraindicated, keep patient hydrated with at least 2 to 3 L fluid per day.
- Teach coughing and deep-breathing exercises, which should be performed at least every 2 hours.
5. Suction secretions as needed, and hyperoxygenate before suctioning.

HIGH ALERT!   Be alert for bradycardia associated with tracheal suctioning. If patient's cough is ineffective, implement the following method, known as *quad coughing*: Place palm of hand under patient's diaphragm, and push up on the abdominal muscles as patient exhales. Be aware that using the quad cough maneuver in patients with intracaval filters to prevent pulmonary emboli has been reported to have significant complications, including bowel perforation and filter migration and deformation.

---

6. Monitor patient for evidence of ascending cord edema: increasing difficulty with swallowing secretions or coughing, presence of respiratory stridor with retraction of accessory muscles of respiration, bradycardia, fluctuating BP, and increased motor and sensory loss at a higher level than the initial findings.
7. If patient has cranial tongs or traction with a halo apparatus in place, monitor patient's respiratory status every 1 to 2 hours for the first 24 to 48 hours and then every 4 hours if patient's condition is stable. Be alert to absent or adventitious breath sounds, and inspect chest movement to ensure that the vest is not restricting diaphragmatic movement.

Safety Alert   *Have a plan to remove the vest if CPR is needed.*

---

8. If intubation via endotracheal tube or tracheostomy becomes necessary, explain the procedure to patient and significant others.

NIC Airway Management; Oxygen Therapy; Respiratory Monitoring; Mechanical Ventilation

---

Autonomic dysreflexia (AD) (or risk for same)   *related to abnormal response of the autonomic nervous system to a stimulus*

GOALS/OUTCOMES Patient has no symptoms of AD as evidenced by dry skin above the level of injury, BP within patient's normal range, HR ≥60 bpm, and absence of headache and other clinical indicators of AD. ECG demonstrates normal sinus rhythm.
NOC Risk Detection

Dysreflexia Management
1. Assess for the classic triad of AD: throbbing headache, cutaneous vasodilation, and sweating above the level of injury. In addition, extremely elevated BP (e.g., ≥250 to 300/150 mm Hg), nasal stuffiness, flushed skin (above the level of the injury), blurred vision, nausea, bradycardia, and chest pain can occur. Be alert to the following signs of AD that occur below the level of injury: pilomotor erection, pallor, chills, and vasoconstriction.
2. Assess for cardiac dysrhythmias, via cardiac monitor during initial postinjury stage (2 weeks).
3. Implement measures to prevent factors that may precipitate AD: bladder stimuli (i.e., distention, calculi, infection, cystoscopy); bowel stimuli (i.e., fecal impaction, rectal examination, suppository insertion); and skin stimuli (i.e., pressure from tight clothing or sheets, temperature extremes, sores, areas of broken skin).
4. If indicators of AD are present, implement the following measures:
   - Elevate HOB, or place patient in a sitting position. This will decrease BP by promoting cerebral venous return.
   - Monitor BP and HR every 3 to 5 minutes until patient stabilizes.
   - Determine and remove offending stimulus. If the patient's bladder is distended, catheterize cautiously, using sufficient lubricant containing a local anesthetic. If patient has an indwelling urinary catheter, check for obstruction, such as granulation in catheter or kinking of tubing; as indicated, irrigate catheter, using no more than 30 ml NS. If UTI is suspected, obtain a urine specimen for culture and sensitivity once the crisis stage has passed. Check for fecal impaction; perform the rectal examination gently, using an ointment containing a local anesthetic (e.g., Nupercainal). Check for sensory stimuli, and loosen clothing, bed covers, or other constricting fabric as indicated.

5. Consult physician for severe or prolonged hypertension or other symptoms that do not abate. Severe or prolonged elevations of BP may result in life-threatening consequences: seizures, subarachnoid or intracerebral hemorrhage, fatal cerebrovascular accident.
6. As prescribed, administer antihypertensive agent and monitor its effectiveness.
7. Remain calm and supportive of patient and significant others during these episodes.
8. Upon resolution of the immediate crisis, answer patient's and significant others' questions regarding cause of the AD. Provide patient and family teaching regarding signs and symptoms and methods of treatment of AD. This is particularly critical for the patient with SCI who has sustained injury above T6, because these patients are at risk for AD for life.

NIC Dysreflexia Management

Decreased cardiac output (CO) *related to relative hypovolemia secondary to enlarged vascular space occurring with neurogenic shock*

GOALS/OUTCOMES Patient has adequate CO as evidenced by orientation to time, place, and person; systolic BP ≥90 mm Hg (or within patient's normal range); HR 60 to 100 bpm; RAP 4 to 6 mm Hg; PAP 20 to 30/8 to 15 mm Hg; PAWP 6 to 12 mm Hg; SVR 900 to 1200 dynes/sec/cm^{-5}; normal amplitude of peripheral pulses (greater than 2+ on a 0-to-4+ scale); urinary output ≥0.5 ml/kg/hr; and normal sinus rhythm on ECG.
NOC Circulation Status

Hemodynamic Regulation
1. Monitor patient for indicators of decreased CO: drop in systolic BP less than 20 mm Hg, systolic BP greater than 90 mm Hg, or a continuous drop of 5 to 10 mm Hg with each assessment; HR greater than 100 bpm, irregular HR, lightheadedness, fainting, confusion, dizziness, flushed skin; diminished amplitude of peripheral pulses; change in BP, HR, mental status, and color associated with a change in position. Monitor input and output; urine output less than 0.5 ml/kg/hr for 2 consecutive hours should be reported. Assess hemodynamic measurements. In the presence of neurogenic shock, anticipate decreased RAP, PAP, PAWP, and SVR (see Table 1-13).
2. Continuously assess cardiac rate and rhythm; report changes in rate and rhythm.
3. Prevent episodes of decreased CO caused by orthostatic hypotension:
   • Change patient's position slowly.
   • Perform range-of-motion (ROM) exercises every 2 hours to prevent venous pooling.
   • Apply elastic antiembolic hose as prescribed to promote venous return.
   • Avoid placing pillows under patient's knees, "gatching" the bed, or allowing patient to cross the legs or sit with legs in a dependent position.
   • Collaborate with physical therapy personnel in progressing patient from a supine to upright position, using a tilt table.
4. As prescribed, administer fluids to control mild hypotension.
5. Administer and monitor for therapeutic effects of vasopressors (see Appendix 6).
6. Ensure adequate volume repletion before or concurrent with pressor therapy.

NIC Cardiac Care; Fluid Management

Risk for injury: gastric *related to risk of development of gastric ulcer (Cushing) or gastritis secondary to increased gastric acid production*

GOALS/OUTCOMES Result of patient's gastric pH test is greater than 5, and patient has no symptoms of gastric ulcer as evidenced by gastric aspirate and stool culture that are negative for blood; BP within patient's normal range; HR ≤100 bpm; and absence of midepigastric or referred shoulder pain.

HIGH ALERT! Patients sustaining major trauma are at high risk for development of gastritis/gastric ulcers caused by increased production of gastric acid. Although ulceration can occur at any time in the patient with SCI, it is most likely to occur within 3 weeks of the injury.

NOC Risk Control

Bleeding Precautions

1. Assess for indicators of GI ulceration or hemorrhage: midepigastric pain (dull, gnawing, burning ache) if patient has sensation; and hematemesis, melena, constipation, anemia, pallor, decreased BP, increased HR, and complaints of shoulder pain.
2. Test gastric aspirate and stools for blood q8h. Promptly consult physician if blood is present.
3. Monitor CBC for signs of anemia: decreases in Hct, Hgb, and RBCs.
4. As prescribed, implement measures to treat or prevent ulceration and hemorrhage:
   - Administer proton-pump inhibitors or histamine H_2-receptor antagonists to suppress secretion of gastric acids, decrease irritating effects of gastric secretions, and facilitate healing.
   - Insert gastric tube and attach to low, intermittent suction to remove gastric contents.
   - Prepare patient for surgery as indicated.
5. For the patient with GI ulceration and hemorrhage, bowel perforation is an added risk. Be alert to the following indicators: pallor, shock state, abdominal distention, vomiting of material that resembles coffee grounds, absent bowel sounds, elevated WBC count (greater than 11,000/mm^3), and presence of air on abdominal x-ray view. In some cases the only indicators are tachycardia and shoulder pain. Bowel perforation is an emergency situation, requiring immediate surgical intervention.

NIC Surveillance; Medication Administration; Bleeding Precautions; Risk Identification

---

Ineffective tissue perfusion (or risk for same): peripheral and cardiopulmonary *related to interruption of blood flow associated with thrombophlebitis, DVT, and pulmonary emboli (PE) secondary to venous stasis, vascular intimal injury, and hypercoagulability occurring as a result of decreased vasomotor tone and immobility*

GOALS/OUTCOMES Patient is free of symptoms of thrombophlebitis, DVT, and PE as evidenced by absence of heat, swelling, discomfort, and erythema in the calves and thighs; HR ≤100 bpm; RR ≤20 breaths/min with normal pattern and depth; BP within patient's normal range; Pao$_2$ ≥80 mm Hg; and absence of chest or shoulder pain.

NOC Tissue Perfusion: Pulmonary

Cardiac Care: Acute

1. The high-risk interval for this diagnosis is the 6- to 12-week period after injury. Assess for indicators of thrombophlebitis and DVT: unusual heat and erythema of calf or thigh, increased circumference of calf or thigh, tenderness or pain in extremity (depending on patient's level of injury and whether injury is complete or incomplete), pain in the calf area with dorsiflexion (positive reaction for Homan sign).
2. Assess for indicators of pulmonary emboli: sudden chest or shoulder pain, tachycardia, dyspnea, tachypnea, hypotension, pallor, cyanosis, cough with hemoptysis, restlessness, increasing anxiety, and low Pao$_2$.
3. Implement measures to prevent development of thrombophlebitis, DVT, and PE:
   - Change patient's position at least every 2 hours to prevent venous pooling.
   - Perform ROM exercises on all extremities every 1 to 2 hours to promote venous return and prevent stasis.
   - Avoid use of knee gatch or pillows under the knees, which can compromise circulation.
   - If patient is out of bed and in a chair, do not allow patient to cross legs at the knee or sit with legs dependent for longer than 0.5 to 1 hour. For the patient experiencing some return of spinal reflexes below the lesion with spasticity of lower extremities, instruct patient to alert nurse should legs become crossed.
   - Apply sequential compression devices or antiembolic hose as prescribed.
   - Maintain adequate hydration of at least 2 to 3 L/day, unless contraindicated, to prevent dehydration and concomitant increase in blood viscosity, which can promote thrombus formation.
   - Administer prophylactic low-dose, low-molecular-weight heparin as prescribed.

HIGH ALERT! Patients with SCI who are not candidates for anticoagulation therapy may require surgical intervention (insertion of intracaval filter) to prevent pulmonary emboli as a result of thrombophlebitis or DVT.

NIC Circulatory Care: Arterial Insufficiency; Circulatory Care: Venous Insufficiency; Peripheral Sensation Management; Cardiac Care: Acute; Respiratory Monitoring; Shock Management: Cardiac

Risk for impaired skin integrity *related to prolonged immobility secondary to immobilization device or paralysis*

GOALS/OUTCOMES Patient's skin remains intact without areas of breakdown or irritation.
NOC Tissue Integrity: Skin and Mucous Membranes

Pressure Management
1. Perform a complete skin assessment at least every 8 hours. Pay close attention to skin that is particularly susceptible to breakdown (i.e., skin over bony prominences and around halo vest edges). Be alert to erythema, warmth, open or macerated tissue, and foul odors (indicative of infection with tissue necrosis).
2. Turn and reposition patient and massage susceptible skin at least every 2 hours. Post a turning schedule and include patient in the planning and initiating of this schedule.

 Safety Alert *Do not turn patient until the injury has been stabilized; moving the patient will require approval from the neurosurgery trauma team. If turning is allowed before immobilization with tongs, halo, or surgery, use log-rolling technique only, using at least three people to turn patient: one to support the head and neck and keep them in alignment during the procedure, and two to turn the patient.*

---

3. Keep skin clean and dry.
4. Pad halo vest edges (e.g., with sheepskin) to minimize irritation and friction.
5. Provide pressure-relief mattress most appropriate for patient's injury.
6. For more information related to the maintenance of skin and tissue integrity, see *Wound and Skin Care*, p. 167.

NIC Pressure Management; Pressure Ulcer Prevention; Skin Surveillance

Imbalanced nutrition: less than body requirements, *related to decreased oral intake secondary to anorexia, difficulty eating in prone position, fear of choking and aspiration, and inability to feed self because of paralysis of upper extremities; decreased GI motility secondary to autonomic nervous system dysfunction*

GOALS/OUTCOMES Patient has adequate nutrition as evidenced by balanced nitrogen state per nitrogen balance studies, serum albumin 3.5 to 5.5 g/dl, thyroxine-binding prealbumin 20 to 30 mg/dl, and retinol-binding protein 4 to 5 mg/dl.
NOC Nutritional Status

Nutrition Management
1. Perform a complete baseline assessment of nutritional status.
2. Assess patient's readiness for oral intake: presence of bowel sounds, passing of flatus, or bowel movement.
3. If unable to receive proper oral nutrition; prepare to insert a Dobhoff tube for enteral feeding or a PICC line for total parenteral nutrition (TPN).
4. When the patient begins an oral diet, progress slowly from liquids to solids as tolerated.
5. Monitor and record percentage of each meal eaten by patient.
6. Implement measures to maintain or improve patient's intake.
   - Obtain dietary consultation to provide patient with his or her favorite foods, as well as those that are highly nutritious.
   - Provide oral hygiene before and after meals, and decrease external stimuli (which also will help patient concentrate on chewing and swallowing and thus minimize the risk of aspiration).
   - Provide small, frequent feedings, feed patient slowly, providing small, bite-size pieces, which facilitate digestion and help prevent choking; also less likely to cause abdominal distention, which may compromise respiratory movement; and less fatiguing.
   - Feed patient in a position to minimize aspiration risk, and if patient is in a halo device or has been stabilized, feed in high-Fowler's position.
7. Once patient's condition has been stabilized, consult with occupational therapy personnel for selection of assistive devices that will enable patient to feed himself or herself.

NIC Fluid/Electrolyte Management; Swallowing Therapy; Self-Care Assistance: Feeding

Urinary retention or reflex urinary incontinence *related to inhibition of the spinal reflex arc secondary to spinal shock after SCI or related to loss of reflex activity for micturition and bladder flaccidity secondary to cord lesion at or below T12*

GOALS/OUTCOMES Patient has urinary output without incontinence.

HIGH ALERT! Urinary retention with stretching of the bladder muscle may trigger AD. Therefore, it is critical to assess for retention and to treat it promptly.

NOC Urinary Elimination

Urinary Retention Care
1. Assess for indicators of urinary retention: suprapubic distention and intake greater than output.
2. Assess for effects of medications that can cause urinary retention such as tricyclic antidepressants.
3. Catheterize patient as prescribed. Patients usually have an indwelling catheter for the first 48 to 96 hours after injury. Then, intermittent catheterization is used to try to retrain the bladder. If intermittent catheterization is used and episodes of urinary incontinence occur, catheterize more frequently. If more than 400 ml of urine is obtained, catheterize more often and reduce fluids.
4. Measure the amount of residual urine, and attempt to increase the length of time between catheterizations, as indicated by decreased amounts (i.e., less than 50 to 100 ml of urine).
5. Ensure continuous patency of the drainage system to prevent reflux of urine into the bladder or blockage of flow, which could lead to urinary retention or UTI, which may cause AD. Tape the catheter over the pubis to prevent traction on the catheter, which can lead to ulcer formation in the urethra and erosion of the urethral meatus.
6. Maintain a fluid intake of at least 2.5 to 3 L/day to prevent early stone formation caused by mobilization of calcium.
7. Teach patient and significant others the procedure for intermittent catheterization. Alert them to the indicators of UTI (restlessness, incontinence, malaise, anorexia, fever, and cloudy or foul-smelling urine) and the importance of adequate fluid intake, regular urine cultures, good hand-washing technique, and cleansing of the urinary catheter before catheterization.

HIGH ALERT! UTI is one of the leading causes of morbidity and mortality in the patient with SCI. This patient may not be aware of the presence of UTI until he or she is severely ill as a result of pyelonephritis (calculi, infection, septicemia).

8. Monitor and record input and output. Distribute fluids evenly throughout the day to prevent overdistention, which can cause incontinence and increase the risk for AD.
9. Decrease fluid intake before bedtime to prevent nighttime incontinence.
10. For other treatment interventions, see *Autonomic Dysreflexia (or risk for same)*, p. 272.

NIC Urinary Catheterization; Urinary Retention Care

Ineffective thermoregulation *related to inability of the body to adapt to environmental temperature changes secondary to poikilothermic reaction occurring with SCI*

GOALS/OUTCOME Within 2 to 4 hours of this diagnosis, patient becomes normothermic.

HIGH ALERT! With SCI the patient may become poikilothermic, meaning that the patient adapts his or her own body temperature to that of the environment and cannot control core body temperature by means of vasodilation to lose heat or vasoconstriction to conserve heat.

NOC Thermoregulation

Temperature Regulation
1. Monitor patient's temperature at least every 4 hours, and assess patient for signs of ineffective thermoregulation: complaints of being too warm, excessive diaphoresis, warmth of skin above level of injury, complaints of being too cold, pilomotor erection (goose bumps), or cool skin above the level of injury.
2. Implement measures to attain normothermia: regulate room temperature, provide extra blankets to prevent chills, protect patient from drafts, provide warm food and drink if patient is chilled; provide cool drinks if patient is warm, remove excess bedding to facilitate heat loss, provide a tepid bath or cooling blanket to facilitate cooling.

NIC Temperature Regulation; Environmental Management

Constipation *related to atonic bowel, paralytic ileus with concomitant AD or loss of anal sphincter control*

GOALS/OUTCOMES Patient remains free of symptoms of constipation and/or paralytic ileus, as evidenced by auscultation of normal bowel sounds, and free of symptoms of AD, and patient has bowel elimination of soft and formed stools.

HIGH ALERT! Paralytic ileus occurs most often in patients with SCI at T6 and above and usually within the first 72 hours after injury.

NOC Bowel Elimination

Constipation/Impaction Management
1. Obtain history of patient's preinjury bowel elimination pattern.
2. Assess for indicators of paralytic ileus: decreased or absent bowel sounds, abdominal distention, anorexia, vomiting, and altered respirations as a result of pressure on the diaphragm. Report significant findings promptly.
3. Until bowel sounds are present and paralytic ileus has resolved, maintain patient on nothing by mouth (NPO) status, with gastric suction.
4. If indicators of paralytic ileus appear, implement the following, as prescribed:
   • Restrict oral or enteral intake.
   • Insert gastric tube to decompress the stomach; attach to suction.
   • Insert a rectal tube if prescribed.
5. Perform a gentle digital examination for fecal impaction and check for rectal reflexes. Before the return of rectal reflexes, manual removal of feces may be needed. If a fecal impaction is present in an atonic bowel, administration of a small-volume enema may be necessary.
6. Observe closely for signs of AD, which can be triggered by distention of the abdomen (for assessment and treatment of AD, see interventions with *Autonomic Dysreflexia* (or risk for same), p. 266).
7. Monitor patient for indicators of constipation (nausea, abdominal distention, and malaise) and fecal impaction (nausea, vomiting, increasing abdominal distention, palpable colonic mass, or presence of hard fecal mass on digital examination).

HIGH ALERT! Be aware that overdistention of the bowel or stimulation of the anal sphincter caused by impaction, rectal tube, rectal examination, or enema may precipitate AD. Use generous amounts of anesthetic lubricant when performing a rectal examination or administering an enema.

8. If patient has a rectal tube in place, he or she may not have sensation in the rectal area. Therefore, special care is necessary to prevent damage to the rectal mucosa and anal sphincter. Remove the tube as soon as possible.
9. Administer stool softeners (e.g., docusate sodium) daily.
10. If possible, avoid enemas for long-term bowel management, because the patient with SCI cannot retain the enema solution. However, if impaction occurs, a gentle, small-volume cleansing enema may be necessary, followed by manual removal of fecal material.

11. Assess patient's readiness for bowel retraining program, including neurologic status and current bowel patterns, noting frequency, amount, and consistency. Bowel retraining is initiated when the patient is neurologically stable and can resume a sitting position.
12. If patient has upper extremity function, teach him or her how to perform digital rectal stimulation, insert suppository, and massage abdomen to facilitate bowel movement.

NIC Surveillance: Bowel Management; Dysreflexia Management; Tube Care; Constipation/Impaction Management

Risk for infection *related to inadequate primary defenses (broken skin) secondary to presence of invasive immobilization devices*

GOALS/OUTCOMES Patient is free of infection at insertion site for tongs or halo device as evidenced by normothermia; negative culture results; and absence of erythema, swelling, warmth, purulent drainage, or tenderness at insertion site.
NOC Risk Control

Infection Protection
1. Assess insertion sites every 8 hours for indicators of infection: erythema, swelling, warmth, purulent drainage, and increased or new tenderness. Note pin migration. If the pin appears to be loose, consult physician and instruct patient to remain still until the pin can be secured.
2. Perform pin care as prescribed. Cleanse the site with soap and water or NS; the area may be left open to air. Monitor for drainage or infection.

NIC Infection Control; Infection Protection; Skin Surveillance

Disturbed sensory perception: visual *related to presence of immobilization device; use of therapeutic bed*

GOALS/OUTCOME After intervention(s), patient expresses satisfaction with visual capabilities.
NOC Vision Compensation Behavior

Environmental Management
1. Assess for factors that limit the patient's visual capabilities: presence of tongs, cervical traction, halo device, and use of specialty beds.
2. Provide for increased visualization of patient's surroundings:
   - Obtain prism glasses or hand mirror for patient who must remain supine or cannot turn his or her head because of halo traction device.
   - Position mirrors to increase the amount of area that can be visualized from patient's position.
   - Approach patient and converse within patient's visual field.
   - Keep clocks, calendars, and other personal objects within patient's visual field.

NIC Positioning

Sexual dysfunction or ineffective sexuality patterns *related to trauma associated with SCI*

GOALS/OUTCOMES Patient verbalizes sexual concerns before discharge from ICU.
NOC Sexual Functioning

Sexual Counseling
1. Assess patient's level of sexual function or loss from a neurologic and psychological perspective. The general rule for men is that the higher the lesion, the greater is the chance of maintaining the ability to have an erection, but with less chance for ejaculation. For women, ovulation may stop for several months because of stress after the injury. Ovulation usually returns, however, and the woman can become pregnant and have a normal pregnancy. Both men and women with high lesions may experience feelings of excitement similar to a preinjury orgasm.

2. Allow patient to speak about his or her concerns or consult with a counselor.
3. Check level of patient's knowledge, and elicit questions about his or her sexual function after the SCI.
4. It is normal for men to experience a reflex erection upon resolution of the spinal shock, particularly for individuals with lesions in the cervical and thoracic areas. Reassure patient that this is normal and therefore nothing to be embarrassed about.
5. Expect acting-out behavior related to the patient's sexuality. This is a normal response to the patient's concern regarding his or her sexual prognosis.
6. Provide accurate information regarding expected sexual function in an open, interested manner, based on your assessment of the patient's readiness for information.
7. Facilitate communication between the patient and his or her partner.
8. Refer patient and his or her partner to a sex therapist or other knowledgeable rehabilitation professional upon resolution of the critical stages of SCI.
9. Also provide patient with information on the following organizations that can be accessed through the internet: National Spinal Cord Injury Association and Spinal Cord Injury Network International.

NIC Sexual Counseling; Anxiety Reduction; Body Image

ADDITIONAL NURSING DIAGNOSES

Also see nursing diagnoses and interventions as appropriate under *Nutritional Support* (p. 117), *Mechanical Ventilation* (p. 99), *Prolonged Immobility* (p. 149), and *Emotional and Spiritual Support of the Patient and Significant Others* (p. 200).

BURns

PATHOPHYSIOLOGY

Burn injuries involve damage to the skin and underlying tissues, but other organ systems may be affected, especially with extensive burn injuries. The cause of injury may be thermal (flame/flash; contact with hot liquids, semiliquids, or objects), electrical, chemical, or radiation. Relative risk of injury differs by age, gender, occupation, and recreational activities. Estimates for the number of burn injuries in the United States range from 1.4 to 2 million injuries annually, and of those, approximately 500,000 seek medical treatment. Of these, it is estimated that 40,000 require hospitalization. For those who survive their injury, the average length of stay is slightly greater than 1 day per 1% total body surface area (TBSA) burn. The number of fire and burn deaths each year is approximately 4000, of which 75% occur at the scene of the injury. In the United States, the two most common reported etiologies are fire/flame and scalds; electrical burn injuries account for 6.5% of all admissions to burn centers and for approximately 1000 fatalities each year. The burning agent, intensity and duration of exposure, location and depth of burn, and percentage of body exposure determine injury severity. Age of the patient, concomitant injury, and preinjury health—in combination with injury severity—impact mortality, length of hospitalization, and, ultimately, rehabilitation outcomes.

Burn injuries are categorized based on depth and extent (size of injury). The longer and more intense the exposure to the burning agent, the greater is the depth of injury. A burn injury is described as either a partial-thickness or full-thickness injury, relative to the layer(s) of skin and tissues injured. A *superficial injury,* commonly referred to as "first-degree" burn (e.g., sunburn), damages only the epidermis. These burns typically heal within 3 to 5 days and without permanent scarring. *Partial-thickness injury,* called a "second-degree" burn, involves varying levels of the dermis, which contain structures essential to skin function (e.g., sweat and sebaceous glands, hair follicles, sensory nerves, capillary network). These burns heal within 14 to 21 days, depending on the depth. *Full-thickness injury,* a "third-degree" burn, exposes the poorly vascularized fat layer, which contains adipose tissue, roots of sweat glands, and hair follicles; this injury destroys all epidermal elements. These wounds may heal by granulation and migration of healthy epithelium from the wound margins (small wounds only); if wounds require longer than 21 days to heal, surgical excision of the dead tissue and skin grafting are required to improve functional and cosmetic outcomes. When full-thickness injuries include destruction of tendon and bone, clinicians often describe these injuries as "fourth-degree" burns. These injuries are the deepest and require excision, possibly amputation of extremities, and skin grafting to heal. Refer to Table 3-5 for detailed burn wound classification and descriptions.

In patients admitted to burn centers, approximately 10% to 20% have an associated inhalation injury. Inhalation injury commonly occurs with flame injuries, particularly if the victim is trapped in an enclosed, smoke-filled space, and is an important determinant of survival (60% to 70% of patients who die in burn centers have inhalation injuries). The associated pathophysiology can be divided into three types of injury: inhalation of carbon monoxide and other noxious gases, injury above the glottis, and injury below the glottis. Most fatalities occurring at the scene of a fire are due to asphyxiation and/or carbon monoxide inhalation (poisoning). Carbon monoxide binds to Hgb with an affinity that is 200 times greater than oxygen, resulting in tissue hypoxia. Injury above the glottis (nasopharynx, oropharynx, and larynx) can be thermal or chemical in nature. The heat exchange capability of the respiratory tract is very efficient such that tissue damage from breathing in heated air occurs most often above the vocal cords. Heat damage to the pharynx can be severe enough to cause upper airway obstruction. Injury below the glottis is almost always chemical, causing direct damage to

Table 3-5	BURN WOUND DESCRIPTION AND CHARACTERISTICS			
	Cause of Injury	Depth	Characteristics	Treatment and Recovery
First-degree burn	Prolonged ultraviolet light exposure (sun); brief exposure to hot liquids	Limited damage to epithelium; skin remains intact	Erythematous, hypersensitive, no blister formation	Complete healing within 3–5 days without scarring
Superficial partial-thickness (second degree) burn	Brief exposure to flash, flame, or hot liquids	Epidermis destroyed; minimal damage to superficial layers of dermis; epidermal appendages intact	Moist and weepy, pink or red, blisters, blanching, hypersensitive	Complete healing within 21 days with minimal to no scarring
Deep partial-thickness (second degree) burn	Intense radiant energy; scalding liquids, semiliquids (e.g., tar), or solids; flame	Epidermis destroyed; underlying dermis damaged; some epidermal appendages remain intact	Pale; decreased moisture; blanching absent or prolonged; intact sensation to deep pressure but not to pinprick	Prolonged healing (often longer than 21 days); may require skin graft to achieve complete healing with better functional outcome
Full-thickness (third degree) burn	Prolonged contact with flame, scalding liquids; steam; hot objects; chemicals; electrical current	Epidermis, dermis, and epidermal appendages destroyed; injury through dermis	Dry, leather-like; pale, mottled brown, or red; thrombosed vessels visible; insensate	Requires skin grafting
Full-thickness (fourth degree) burn	High-voltage electrical injuries; prolonged contact with flame (often in an unconscious victim)	Epidermis, dermis, epidermal appendages, fat, muscle, and bone can be destroyed	Dry, leather-like eschar; color variable; charring visible in deepest area; insensate; extremity movement limited	Requires skin grafting; may require amputation of extremities involved

Modified from Carrougher GJ, editor: *Burn care and therapy*, St. Louis, 1998, Mosby.

airway epithelium from inhalation of the noxious chemicals (e.g., aldehydes, sulfur oxides, phosgenes) of smoke.

Care for the patient with a major burn injury is based on the patient's stage of recovery from the pathophysiologic changes resulting from the cutaneous burn and inhalation injury. The initial resuscitative period lasts from the time of injury until capillary membrane integrity is restored, typically 48 to 72 hours after the burn occurs. The second stage, or acute phase, may last for days to months following injury. It begins with resolution of the fluid shifts and continues until all wounds are closed or until open wound areas are less than 10% of the TBSA. The last stage, or rehabilitative stage, can continue for many months to years and is seldom a focus for critical care nurses. However, early rehabilitative efforts such as patient positioning, splinting, exercise, and patient and family teaching begin on admission to the hospital.

MAJOR BURN ASSESSMENT

The American Burn Association (ABA) has developed an injury severity classification system that categorizes burn injuries as minor, moderate, and major (Table 3-6). The ABA advocates that patients with major burns be treated in a burn center or a facility with expertise in burn care. Moderate burns usually require hospitalization, although not necessarily in a burn center, and minor burns are often treated on an outpatient basis. Box 3-5 outlines the ABA criteria for patients who should be referred to a recognized burn center.

History and Risk Factors

Several factors affect survival after a major burn injury. The patient's age is a determining factor with those at the extremes of age (less than 2 years and greater than 65 years of age) being at highest risk of death. Patients who sustain a thermal injury in a confined area may have a concomitant inhalation injury and are also at increased risk. Preexisting cardiac or lung disease (e.g., COPD) or history of smoking increases susceptibility to respiratory distress. Patients with preexisting cardiac, vascular, renal, or respiratory conditions may not tolerate aggressive fluid resuscitation therapy and may experience complications. Conditions such as immunosuppression, diabetes, collagen vascular disease, invasive procedures, history of cardiopulmonary or vascular disease, and delayed antimicrobial therapy contribute to the likelihood of infection, sepsis, and prolonged healing. Those patients with a history of drug and/or alcohol abuse have an increased mortality risk and often have longer hospital stays. Burn injury can be associated with a concomitant traumatic injury from a blast, motor vehicle crash, or fall. Careful evaluation for secondary injury is essential.

Table 3-6	AMERICAN BURN ASSOCIATION INJURY CLASSIFICATION SCHEME
Severity Classification	**Criteria**
Major	>25% total burn surface area (TBSA) burn in adults <40 years >20% TBSA burn in adults >40 years and children <10 years *Or* >10% TBSA full-thickness burn in all age groups *or* Injuries involving the face, eyes, ears, hands, feet, or perineum that may result in functional or cosmetic disability; high-voltage electrical injury; all injuries with concomitant inhalation injury or major trauma
Moderate	15%–25% TBSA burn in adults <40 years 10%–20% TBSA burn in adults >40 years and children <10 years *and* <10% TBSA full-thickness burn without cosmetic or functional risk
Minor	<15% TBSA burn in adults <40 years <10% TBSA burn in adults >40 years and children <10 years *and* <2% TBSA full-thickness burn without cosmetic or functional risk

Modified from Carrougher GJ, editor: *Burn care and therapy*, St. Louis, 1998, Mosby.

Burns

Box 3-5	AMERICAN BURN ASSOCIATION BURN CENTER REFERRAL GUIDELINES

- Partial-thickness burns greater than 10% TBSA burn in patients younger than 10 years or older than 50 years
- Partial-thickness burns greater than 20% TBSA burn in patients 11 to 50 years of age
- Burns that involve the face, hands, feet, genitalia, perineum, or major joints
- Full-thickness burns in any age group
- Electrical burns (to include lightning injuries)
- Chemical burns
- Burn injuries with associated inhalation injury
- Burn injury in patients with preexisting medical disorders that could complicate management, prolong recovery, or affect mortality
- Any patient with burns and concomitant trauma in which the burn injury poses the greatest risk of morbidity/mortality
- Burn injury in children at hospitals without qualified personnel or equipment for the care of children
- Burn injury in patients who will require special social, emotional, or long-term rehabilitative interventions

Excerpted from guidelines for the Operation of Burn Centers (PP. 79–86), Resources for Optimal Care of the Injured Patient 2006, Committee on Trauma, American College of Surgeons.

Goal of System Assessment
- Trauma assessment to identify concomitant injury
- Assess for size and depth of burn injury
- Assess for decreased tissue perfusion
- Assess for concomitant inhalation injury
- Assess for pain and anxiety

Vital Sign Assessment
Heart rate, heart rhythm, BP to evaluate cardiac output and perfusion
- Take BP on uninjured extremity if possible. Arterial line may be necessary for BP monitoring if burn injury to bilateral extremities is extensive and/or patient exhibits hemodynamic instability.
- Compare cuff BP to arterial line BP if arterial line is in place; decide which pressure is deemed the most accurate.

Respiratory rate
- Count respiratory rate for full minute, noting signs of accessory muscle use for respirations.
- If intubated tracheally, verify tube placement, work of breathing, and appropriate ventilator settings.
- Pain as fifth vital sign. Assess for location; intensity; cause and associated increase in other vital signs.

Observation
The primary patient survey should include the basic ABCs, with the addition of D and E: A—airway and cervical spine immobilization (based on mechanism of injury), B—breathing, C—circulation, D—disability or neurologic deficit, and E—exposure and evaluation. The secondary survey includes a detailed head-to-toe assessment, exploration of the circumstances of the injury, and the patient's medical history. Injury severity is assessed according to TBSA burned, burn depth and location, potential for inhalation injury, patient's age, past medical history, and concomitant trauma.

The extent of the burn wound is reported as a percent of the TBSA injured. In adults, this is easily estimated by using the rule of nines (Figure 3-1). In children, this rule is altered slightly, reflecting the different body proportion in infants and children. The rule of nines technique is used in prehospital settings and emergency departments when a quick assessment is necessary. For very small and/or irregularly shaped or scattered burns, it helps to remember that the surface area of the patient's palm (palm plus fingers) equals 1% of the TBSA. A more

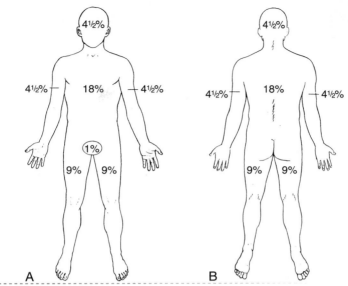

Figure 3-1 Estimation of adult burn injury: rule of nines. A, Anterior view. B, Posterior view.
(From Thompson M, et al: *Mosby's clinical nursing,* ed 4, St. Louis, 1997, Mosby.)

accurate assessment tool is the Lund-Browder chart (Figure 3-2), which is more detailed and accounts for changes in body areas according to age. This chart may be used for both children and adults and is frequently used in critical and acute care settings.

Electrical burn injuries reveal only cutaneous injuries on initial inspection, but extensive damage may occur to deep and underlying tissues, nerves, blood vessels, and muscles along the conduction path and at the electrical current contact sites. Careful assessment determines the full extent of these injuries. Review the ECG for changes secondary to this type of injury. At the time of admission, documentation of injuries is important, not only for resuscitation calculation estimates but also medicolegally. A high percentage of electrical injuries involve litigation for negligence, product liability, or worker compensation.

- Evaluate for wound size (TBSA burn) and depth (partial- or full-thickness burn injury).
- Evaluate for distal tissue perfusion, appearance of uninjured skin, color of nail beds, capillary refill, and temperature of extremities.
- Evaluate for respiratory distress.

Palpation

- Pulse assessment to evaluate for decreased tissue perfusion:
  - Pulse quality and regularity bilaterally (scale 0 to 4+)
  - Edema (scale 0 to 4+): unburned tissue of extremities
  - Evaluate all peripheral pulses to assess for tissue perfusion.
- Turgor assessment of unburned extremities
- Temperature of extremities

Auscultation

- Heart sounds to evaluate for contributors to decreased cardiac output (note changes with body positioning and respirations):
  - S1 and S2: quality, intensity, pitch
  - Extra sounds: S3 (after S2), S4 (before S1) indicative of heart failure
- Respiratory sounds to assess for adventitious breath sounds; confirm for bilateral breath sounds
- Bowel sounds: presence or absence; location

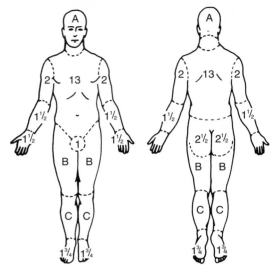

Relative percentages of areas affected by growth
(age in years)

	0	1	5	10	15	Adult
A: Half of head	$9\frac{1}{2}$	$8\frac{1}{2}$	$6\frac{1}{2}$	$5\frac{1}{2}$	$4\frac{1}{2}$	$3\frac{1}{2}$
B: Half of thigh	$2\frac{3}{4}$	$3\frac{1}{4}$	4	$4\frac{1}{4}$	$4\frac{1}{2}$	$4\frac{3}{4}$
C: Half of leg	$2\frac{1}{2}$	$2\frac{1}{2}$	$2\frac{3}{4}$	3	$3\frac{1}{4}$	$3\frac{1}{2}$

Second degree_____and
Third degree_____=
Total percent burned___

Figure 3-2 Estimation of burn injury: Lund and Browder chart. Areas represent percentages of body surface area that vary according to age. The accompanying table indicates the relative percentages of these areas in various stages of life. (From Sabeston DC Jr, editor: *Textbook of surgery: the biographical basis of modern surgical practice*, ed. 11, Philadelphia, 1977, Saunders.)

Respiratory System

Respiratory compromise may occur due to upper airway swelling, inhalation injury, carbon monoxide poisoning, or infection.

- Secure and protect airway; check for any cervical injuries and need to stabilize neck area for appropriate airway protection positioning.
- Progressive swelling of the upper airway may lead to airway obstruction.
- Pulmonary excursion is limited by full-thickness wounds of the neck and torso.
- Check for airway obstruction as a result of swelling caused by heat, smoke, or chemical injury to nasopharyngeal mucosa or by constriction around the neck or chest caused by eschar (burned, devitalized tissue) formation.
- Assess for singed nasal hairs, perioral burns, change in voice, or coughing, especially if productive for soot (mucus will have gray or black particles).
- The upper airway is injured when hot air causes heat injury to the respiratory mucosa. The lower respiratory tract can be damaged by contact with products of combustion and inhalation of vaporized caustic substances, such as sulfur, hydrogen cyanide, ammonia, acrolein, aldehydes, and hydrochloric acid. These noxious gases are produced from the combustion of common household items, such as carpeting, furniture, and decorations.

- Airway injury or respiratory distress may not occur immediately.
- Epithelial sloughing with bronchitis and respiratory distress may occur 6 to 72 hours after the burn occurs.
- Carbon monoxide (CO), a byproduct of combustion, displaces oxygen from Hgb, resulting in hypoxia. Headache, decreased visual acuity, tinnitus, vertigo, confusion, unresponsiveness, and convulsions are signs of CO poisoning. Refer to Table 3-7 for signs and symptoms of CO poisoning.

  Unresponsiveness is not normally associated with burn injuries; patients who are difficult to arouse at the scene or in the emergency department should be evaluated for CO exposure.
- Stridor, severe hoarseness, hacking cough, labored breathing, dyspnea, tachypnea, and possible altered LOC caused by hypoxia

---

Safety Alert *Physical and radiographic evidence of respiratory compromise may be absent initially, despite pulmonary injury. Progression to airway obstruction and acute respiratory distress can occur rapidly, especially in the presence of injury above the glottis or secondary to large fluid volume resuscitation for burns greater than 40% TBSA.*

- Circumferential full-thickness burns of the torso often cause inadequate pulmonary excursion, leading to inadequate ventilation. When pronounced, a chest wall escharotomy should be performed.
- Low blood oxygen content, respiratory distress, impaired chest wall excursion, increased peak pressures, and decreased compliance. Abnormal ABG values.
- Patients with inhalation injury are at risk for pneumonia. On average, 50% of all burn patients with inhalation injury who require mechanical ventilation will develop pneumonia. The frequency of pneumonia and respiratory failure is greatest in those patients who require ≥4 days of mechanical ventilation. Recent data suggest that patients with inhalation injury receiving bronchoscopy have a decreased number of ventilator days and ICU days compared with those who do not receive bronchoscopy.
- Assess for bronchial breath sounds over areas of consolidation, crackles.

Cardiovascular System

Circulatory compromise results from the fluid shifts that occur following a significant burn injury. Increased capillary permeability caused by the inflammatory response results in a shift of intravascular fluid into the interstitial spaces in the first 72 hours postburn. This causes a decrease in circulating volume and increased blood viscosity. Other systemic responses include increases in catecholamines, cortisol, renin-angiotensin, ADH, and aldosterone production as the body attempts to retain sodium and water to replenish intravascular fluid. Rapid fluid shifts can result in massive edema in unburned and burned areas, hemoconcentration, and thrombus formation.

- Signs of shock, such as thirst, pallor, dry mucous membranes, decreased LOC, and cool skin temperature; tachycardia, hypotension, and decreased filling pressures (CVP, PAP, PAWP); decreased or absent peripheral pulses and delayed capillary refill; impaired

Table 3-7	CARBON MONOXIDE POISONING
Carboxyhemoglobin Saturation (%)	**Signs and Symptoms**
<10	Impaired vision
11–20	Headache, facial flushing
21–30	Nausea, trouble with dexterity
31–40	Nausea, vomiting, dizziness, syncope
41–50	Tachypnea, tachycardia, loss of consciousness
>50	Coma, death

Burns

peripheral perfusion with possible obstruction caused by vascular compression with circumferential full-thickness burns or thrombus formation
- Cardiac dysrhythmias caused by direct cardiac damage (electrical burns)
- Electrolyte imbalance (e.g., hyperkalemia caused by cellular hemolysis)
- Peripheral edema as a result of fluid shifts and hypoproteinemia

Gastrointestinal System

Initially, blood flow is shunted away from the GI tract and peristalsis is slowed or stopped completely, causing a gastric ileus (usually resolves within 72 hours after burn injury).
- Prior to the initiation of early enteral feedings, life-threatening stomach and intestinal ulcerations (Curling ulcers) and hemorrhage (associated with a gastric pH of ≤5) often occur. Prophylaxis should be initiated with the use of proton pump inhibitors or H2-receptor antagonists.
- Large fluid volume resuscitation that exceeds 250 ml/kg poses a significant risk for abdominal compartment syndrome.
- Diminished or absent bowel sounds; presence of nausea and vomiting; abdominal distention

Renal System

Hemoconcentration and reduced circulatory volumes result in decreased renal blood flow and low urinary output. Dark concentrated urine in the presence of muscle injury implies myoglobinuria or hemoglobinuria. Continued poor renal perfusion results in acute tubular necrosis and renal failure. Urine output guides fluid resuscitation measures, and recognition of renal compromise or poor cardiac output is essential.

 Target urinary output (UOP) is 30 to 50 ml/hr for adults (up to 100 ml/hr with hemaglobinuria or myoglobinuria) during the initial 24 to 48 hours of resuscitation. Urinary output greater than 50 ml/hr increases risk of compartment syndrome.

- Urine output less than 30 ml/hr in adults and ≤0.5 ml/kg/hr in children; dark-colored, concentrated urine

 Bladder pressures exceeding 20 mm Hg may constitute an emergency, so it is important for the nurse to monitor any increases in trending of bladder pressures.

- Consider bladder pressure monitoring every 4 hours during excessive fluid administration.

Integumentary System

Loss of skin integrity results in increased fluid loss through evaporation; hypothermia, pain, and increased risk of infection. Evaporative fluid losses can be significant, especially in patients with large surface area burns and in burn-injured pediatric patients who have larger surface area/kg of body weight. Significant hypothermia can result in patients with large surface area burns, long transports to the hospital, and long surgeries and in those who require prolonged wound care.
Burn-injured patients have two distinct types of pain:
- Procedural pain is experienced during painful procedures (e.g., wound debridement, dressing changes, staple removal, active physical therapy), and background pain, which is experienced at rest or while doing minimal physical activities.
- Procedural pain is often described as pain that is of short duration and high intensity.
- Background pain is described as constant and of low intensity.
Circumferential full-thickness burns can cause constriction of underlying tissue, blood vessels, and muscles with circulatory compromise to underlying muscles and distal extremities. Healed skin may result in some scar formation which can lead to contractures that limit joint ROM.

See Table 3-5 for a complete description of partial-thickness and full-thickness burn wound injuries.

Wound Infection

Loss of skin integrity means that the body's first line of defense against infection is compromised. Ongoing evaluation for burn wound infection is imperative as a significant infection may lead to delayed healing, tissue loss, and sepsis. Typically, the larger the wound or delay in definitive grafting, the greater is the risk for wound infection.

- Early signs of wound infection include fever, redness, increased wound pain, change in exudate or wound appearance, and loss of previously healed skin grafts.
- Invasive wound infection is indicated by rapid eschar separation (invasive fungal infections); focal, dark red, brown, or black discolorations in the eschar; rapid conversion of an area of partial- to full-thickness injury; and hemorrhagic fat necrosis.

Systemic Inflammatory Response Syndrome/Septic Shock

All severely burned patients display signs and symptoms of systemic inflammatory response syndrome (SIRS); therefore, this term is not used to describe the inflammatory processes in the burn patient. However, if more than three signs and symptoms of SIRS (modified slightly for the burn-injured patient) are present along with a documented source of infection, then sepsis is preset.

Signs of burn sepsis include:
- Tachycardia: HR greater than 110 bpm
- Tachypnea: respiratory rate greater than 25/min
- Decreased BP with low SVR
- Labile core body temperature (may fluctuate by more than 3°, as low as 36.5°C)
- Low platelet count
- Changes in level of consciousness (confusion, disorientation, agitation)
- Hyperglycemia or increasing insulin requirements
- Feeding intolerance; increased enteral feeding residuals; loss of appetite
- Gastric distention or gastric ileus

Diagnostic Tests for Major Burn Injury		
Test	**Purpose**	**Abnormal Findings**
Noninvasive Cardiology		
Electrocardiogram (ECG): 12-lead ECG on admission	To assess cardiac health. A baseline ECG should be completed on patients with a history of cardiac disease and those with a major burn injury (to include electrical injury).	Presence of ST-segment depression or T-wave inversion (myocardial ischemia), ST elevation (acute myocardial infarction), new bundle branch block (especially left BBB) or pathologic Q waves (resolving/resolved myocardial infarction), arrhythmias
Invasive Pulmonary		
Bronchoscopy: Technique of visualizing the inside of the airways for both diagnostic and therapeutic purposes	To assess for evidence of inhalation injury and/or to obtain fluid specimen (bronchoalveolar lavage)	Presence of carbonaceous particles, erythema, edema, and bronchial casts; presence of microorganisms $>10^5$
Noninvasive Metabolic Study		
Indirect calorimetry: Provides the most accurate measurement of energy expenditure	To measure resting energy expenditure (REE). With this data, calories used during the testing period can be extrapolated as well as providing the respiratory quotient (RQ) — the ratio of carbon dioxide produced to oxygen consumed.	RQ values greater than 1.0 may indicate overfeeding of total calories or excessive carbohydrate infusion. RQ values less than 0.6 may indicate ketosis.

Burns

Continued

Diagnostic Tests for Major Burn Injury —cont'd		
Test	**Purpose**	**Abnormal Findings**
Noninvasive Blood Study		
Pulse oximetry: Noninvasive method allowing the monitoring of the oxygenation of the patient's hemoglobin	To assess oxygenation. Not reliable in patients who are profoundly hypovolemic, in shock, or hypothermic.	Below 92% may indicate impaired oxygenation and need for oxygen therapy. Unreliable in the presence of carbon monoxide (CO) poisoning. False readings may occur when hemoglobin is bound to CO that may delay the recognition of hypoxemia (low blood oxygen levels).
End-tidal CO_2: Noninvasive reflection of $Paco_2$	To assess ventilation	Levels above or below normal (35–45 mm Hg) reflect ventilatory problems.
Blood Studies		
Complete blood count (CBC) Hemoglobin (Hgb) Hematocrit (Hct) RBC count (RBCs) WBC count (WBCs) Platelet count	To assess for polycythemia, anemia, inflammation, infection, sepsis, coagulation disorders, dehydration	Increased or decreased RBCs, Hgb, or Hct reflects concentration (secondary to under resuscitation) or anemia. Increased RBCs, Hgb, or Hct may reflect dehydration. Infection or inflammation may increase WBCs. Sepsis may increase or decrease WBCs. Thrombocytopenia (decreased platelet count) may reflect coagulation disorders or sepsis.
Metabolic Panel		
Glucose	Determine whether glucose control is necessary; glucose levels in response to concomitant injuries or secondary conditions. To assess for changes resulting from large-volume fluid shifts	Hyperglycemia may indicate stress response or sepsis. Hypoglycemia may indicate depletion of glycogen stores. Hypoglycemia or hyperglycemia may indicate sepsis or adrenal insufficiency.
Potassium (K^+) Magnesium (Mg^{2+}) Calcium (Ca^{2+})		Decrease in K^+, Mg^{2+}, or Ca^{2+} may cause dysrhythmias.
Sodium (Na^+)		Elevation of Na^+ may indicate dehydration; low Na^+ may indicate fluid retention.
Lactate Base deficit		Increase in lactate and base deficit levels may indicate inadequate fluid resuscitation or shock state (first 12–24 hours post burn), or infection.
Coagulation profile Prothrombin time (PT) with international normalized ratio (INR) Partial thromboplastin time (PTT) Fibrinogen D-dimer	To assess for bleeding, clotting, and disseminated intravascular coagulation (DIC) indicative of abnormal clotting present in shock or ensuing shock or coagulation disorder	Severe burn injury results in a post-burn hypercoagulation — characterized by the activation of coagulation, decreased fibrinolytic activity, and decreased natural anticoagulant activity.

Diagnostic Tests for Major Burn Injury — cont'd		
Test	**Purpose**	**Abnormal Findings**
Arterial Blood Gas Analysis		
pH	To assess for acid-base disorders by measuring the concentration of gases (carbon dioxide and oxygen), bicarbonate, and the pH of the blood. Early ABGs may be normal. Early acidemia may reflect inadequate fluid resuscitation. Later studies may reflect hypoxemia secondary to respiratory failure, with progressive metabolic acidosis in patients with impending shock or SIRS.	pH range: 7.35–7.45; The pH indicates if a patient is acidemic (pH < 7.35) or alkalemic (pH > 7.45).
Po_2		Po_2: 80–100 mm Hg; A low O_2 indicates that the patient is not respiring properly and is hypoxemic.
Pco_2		Pco_2: 35–45 mm Hg; A high Pco_2 indicates underventilation; a low Pco_2 indicates hyperventilation or overventilation. Pco_2 levels can also become abnormal when the respiratory system is working to compensate for a metabolic issue.
HCO_3		HCO_3 range: 22–26 mmol/L. A low HCO_3 indicates metabolic acidosis; a high HCO_3 indicates metabolic alkalosis. HCO_3 levels can also become abnormal when the kidneys are working to compensate for a respiratory issue.
Carboxyhemoglobin (CO) analysis	To assess for carbon monoxide (CO) poisoning. Carbon monoxide, a byproduct of combustion, displaces oxygen from hemoglobin, resulting in hypoxia.	CO levels above 5%–10% in individuals not routinely exposed to CO. Smokers and those routinely exposed to heavy traffic (truckers, taxi drivers) may routinely have nonsignificant CO levels of 5%–15%.
Radiology		
Chest radiograph (CXR)	To aid in the assessment of pulmonary status upon admission and serially for any progression of lung involvement. Done serially.	Chest radiographs are often normal on admission and then progressively worsen within 24–48 hours with significant smoke inhalation and development of ARDS. Pneumonia exhibits a "white out" picture demonstrating pulmonary infiltrates.
Skeletal radiographs	To assess for potential injuries in at-risk patients. Patients with known high-voltage electrical contact should be evaluated for long bone or spinous process fractures due to prolonged muscle tetany.	Fractures, foreign objects

DIAGNOSTIC TESTS
Bronchoscopy
The ABA Consensus Conference on Burn Sepsis and Infection Group has determined that bronchoscopy is the best and most reliable test for diagnosis of smoke inhalation injury below the glottis. Signs of injury below the glottis that can be observed with bronchoscopy include carbonaceous material, edema, and ulceration. Therapeutic bronchoscopy facilitates removal of carbonaceous material and nonviable tissue.

Fluorescein Examination

This procedure uses orange dye (fluorescein) and an ultraviolet light (Wood's lamp) to detect foreign bodies in the eye and/or damage to the cornea. This examination should occur in all patients with possible eye injury and should be performed early (first 24 hours after burn injury), before swelling prevents a thorough examination.

Culture and Sensitivity Studies

This diagnostic test evaluates sputum (pneumonia), blood (bacteremia or septicemia), urine (urinary tract infection), and wound tissue for evidence of colonization and infection.

Burn wound infection is defined as more than 10^5 microorganisms/g of burn wound tissue with active invasion of adjacent, viable, unburned skin. Gram-negative organisms include *Pseudomonas aeruginosa, Klebsiella, Serratia, Acinetobacter, Escherichia coli,* and *Enterobacter cloacae.* Gram-positive organisms (*Staphylococcus* and *Streptococcus*) and fungal pathogens (*Candida and Aspergillus*) may also be present. Colonization of burn wounds is common and not treated with systemic antimicrobial therapy. Topical agents are used to reduce microbes. Surveillance cultures are often collected on admission for screening of multidrug-resistant organisms and methicillin-resistant *Staphylococcus aureus* (MRSA). An epidemiologic investigation may be needed to evaluate infection trends.

Urine Collections

Perform urinalysis and culture and sensitivity early to detect urinary tract infection. A 24-hour urine collection to measure total nitrogen, urea nitrogen, creatinine, and amino acid nitrogen values may indicate return of capillary integrity (3 to 5 days after burn occurrence) and mobilization of third spaced fluids, the degree of catabolism present, and the onset or resolution of acute renal failure. Myoglobinuria can result from muscle injury sustained from an electrical injury or deep full-thickness burn.

Hematology

Elevated Hct due to hemoconcentration during initial resuscitation. Hgb will be decreased secondary to surgical burn wound excision, hemolysis, or multiple lab draws. During the first 24 hours post burn, neither the Hgb level nor the Hct is a reliable guide to fluid resuscitation. WBCs may be elevated due to systemic inflammatory response or sepsis. Burn patients will typically be leukopenic initially as WBCs migrate to areas of burned tissue.

Glucose

Hyperglycemia is common in patients related to the normal stress response of injury. Hyperglycemia is common in patients with sepsis and multiple organ failure. Sodium shifts occur during resuscitation; carefully monitor and adjust type of resuscitation fluid 24 hours post injury. Potassium may be elevated as a result of cell lysis, fluid shifts, or renal insufficiency. Blood urea nitrogen (BUN) is elevated because of hypovolemic state, increased protein catabolism, or possible acute renal failure. Persistent elevation of BUN and creatinine signals inadequate fluid intake or acute renal failure. Total protein and albumin are decreased secondary to leakage of plasma proteins into interstitial spaces. Creatine kinase (CK) is sometimes used as index of muscle damage, but a burn injury that damages even a small quantity of muscle tissue will result in markedly elevated CK levels in the first 24 hours. Troponin levels are more indicative of cardiac damage. Increase in lactate may indicate inadequate fluid resuscitation (first 12 to 24 hours post-burn), infection, or shock state from decreased tissue perfusion, or sepsis.

ECG

Evaluate for tachycardia secondary to hypovolemia or pain. Tachycardia of 100 to 120 bpm is common in the adult patient who appears adequately resuscitated. Myocardial damage secondary to high-voltage electrical burn injury may be evident (e.g., dysrhythmias, prolonged QT interval). Dysrhythmias related to electrolyte imbalance may occur.

COLLABORATIVE MANAGEMENT
Care Priorities

1. **Manage hypoxemia and protect the upper airways by using humidified oxygen therapy:** Treats hypoxemia and prevents drying and sloughing of the mucosal lining of the tracheobronchial tree. If patient is awake, oxygen administration by nonrebreathing

face-mask may be sufficient; intubation may be required if the patient is stuporous, unconscious, or with significant burn injuries to the face or upper airway area. Any patient with suspected carbon monoxide poisoning/inhalation injury should receive humidified 100% oxygen by nonrebreather face-mask or be intubated immediately until the carboxyhemoglobin level falls below 10%. If inhalation injury is suspected, consider intubation with mechanical ventilatory support.

2. **Support ventilation by providing intubation and mechanical ventilation:** Endotracheal intubation is indicated if respiratory failure is present, airway obstruction is imminent (e.g., progressive hoarseness and/or stridor), or the patient cannot protect their airway (impaired level of consciousness). Large burn injury (more than 40% TBSA) may result in global edema even in the absence of inhalation injury, requiring prophylactic intubation for airway protection. Because laryngeal edema typically resolves in 3 to 5 days after burn occurrence, tracheostomy is avoided for upper airway distress unless there is acute obstruction or prolonged need for ventilatory support.

For patients requiring intubation and mechanical ventilation, implementation of measures (e.g., Ventilator Bundle) to prevent ventilator-associated pneumonia (VAP) are instituted. VAP is a new or progressive airway infection that develops more than 48 hours after endotracheal intubation. Current criteria state that there is no minimum period that the ventilator must be in place to diagnose VAP. VAP is the leading cause of death among patients with hospital-acquired infections; it prolongs times spent on the ventilator, in the ICU, and the total hospital length of stay.

The key components of the Ventilator Bundle are:
- Elevation of the head of the bed
- Daily "sedative interruptions" and assessment of readiness to extubate [may need to be individually determined to be appropriate in the burn patient]
- Peptic ulcer disease (PUD) prophylaxis
- Deep venous thrombosis prophylaxis (unless contraindicated)

3. **Thin secretions with bronchodilators and mucolytic agents:** Aid in promoting gas exchange and in loosening of pulmonary secretions.

4. **Relieve constriction of circumferential burns with escharotomy:** An incision through eschar to relieve constriction caused by circumferential, full-thickness burns. Escharotomies of the chest wall relieve respiratory distress secondary to circumferential, full-thickness burns of the trunk. Escharotomies of the extremities lessen pressure created by underlying edema to restore adequate tissue perfusion. The procedure may be performed at the bedside or in the emergency department by trained personnel. Indicated when patients have cyanosis and cold temperature of distal unburned skin, prolonged capillary filling, decreased sensation and movement, or weak or absent peripheral pulses (mimics compartment syndrome), and for burns of thorax, when respiratory excursion is restricted.

5. **Hydrate using large-bore IV access:** Peripheral veins should be used to establish IV access using two large-bore short catheters (≥16 gauge in the adult). Veins underlying unburned skin are preferred; however, veins beneath burned skin can be used if necessary. If peripheral IV access is not possible, obtain central venous line access (preferably through nonburned skin) for IV administration and measurement of CVPs for fluid management.

6. **Fluid resuscitation:** The goal of fluid resuscitation is to maintain tissue perfusion and organ function while avoiding the complications of inadequate or excessive fluid therapy (Advanced Burn Life Support). Fluid replacement protocols are based on body weight and percentage of TBSA burned and provide an estimate for resuscitation. The consensus formula recommends administration of 2 to 4 ml fluid × kg body weight × percent TBSA burned (adult) and 3 to 4 ml fluid × kg body weight × percent TBSA burned (infants and young children). The initial infusion rate is calculated using the consensus formula and subsequent hourly titration is guided by urinary output (30 to 50 ml/hr for adults and 1 ml/kg/hr in children weighing less than 30 kg). LR solution is used in the first 24 hours, with small amounts of colloid fluids added during the second 24 hours after injury. Colloids are generally avoided during the first 12 to 24 hours after injury because increased capillary permeability allows leakage of protein into the interstitial tissues. The greater surface area–to–body mass ratio of children necessitates the

administration of relatively greater amounts of resuscitation fluid. In addition, infants and young children should receive fluid with 5% dextrose (e.g., $D_5 \frac{1}{4}$ NS or $D_5 \frac{1}{2}$ NS) at a maintenance rate in addition to the LR resuscitation fluid. Patients who are particularly sensitive to excessive fluid resuscitation include children, older adults, and those with preexisting cardiac disease.

Safety Alert *Calculate fluid infusion from the time of injury, not the time of hospital admission. Fluid resuscitation and maintenance formulas should be modified, based on individual patient responses and needs. Hourly urine output serves to guide infusion rates. Patients with electrical injuries, very deep burns, inhalation injury, prior dehydration, ethanol intoxication, and concomitant trauma (e.g., crushing injuries) may have greater fluid needs than suggested by their cutaneous burn injury alone.*

---

7. **Maintain an accurate record of the fluid balance:** Insertion of an indwelling urinary catheter may be essential for accurate hourly measurement of urine output and evaluation of renal status in patients with a major burn injury.

8. **Facilitate core body temperature regulation:** For patients with extensive burn injuries, the body's response to injury is to increase core and skin temperatures by 2°C above normal. Increasing the ambient room temperature to 33°C (91.4°F) helps to attenuate the hypermetabolic response. Limit body exposure during wound care and dressing changes.

9. **Prevent aspiration of gastric contents by nasogastric intubation:** Permits gastric decompression, reducing risk of aspiration. Aids in the removal of gastric contents, which may be necessary during the resuscitative phase because of the potential for gastric ileus in patients with a ≥20% TBSA burn and in patients with intubated airway.

10. **Provide proper patient positioning to decrease the potential for further injury.** Burn injured extremities should be elevated to reduce dependent edema formation. Patients with burns of the head or ears should be positioned without a pillow (to prevent the incidence of neck flexion contractures and ear chondritis). Patients should be routinely positioned to reduce contracture formation with frequent position changes to reduce the incidence of pressure sores.

 11. **Provide aggressive nutritional support:** High metabolic activity and increased protein catabolism related to burn injury result in dramatic increases in energy requirements and nutritional needs. Additional injury (e.g., long bone fractures) or poor nutritional status before the burn injury may further increase nutritional needs. This hypermetabolic response to injury typically continues beyond the acute phase of recovery and may last up to 1 year for those with extensive burn injuries (i.e., ≥40% TBSA burn). Energy requirements are estimated using one of several predictive formulas based on body size and extent of burn, with adjustment for age, and are calculated by nutritionists. Indirect calorimetry is also used to measure energy expenditure, thus providing a measure of calories needed. However, the equipment required for indirect calorimetry is expensive and requires trained personnel to administer the test.

Although nutritional practices vary, nutritional support should be initiated early in the recovery process. The appropriate mix of protein, fat, and carbohydrates to be provided is not standardized, but a positive nitrogen state can be achieved with patients who are administered high-protein, moderate-carbohydrate, and low-fat diets.

Oral, enteral, or parenteral methods of delivery are used, based on patient tolerance. Many critically ill burn patients are unable to meet their increased nutritional requirements with oral intake alone. Enteral feedings are preferred in these patients and have the added benefit of decreasing GI acidity and ulcer formation. Either gastric or postpyloric jejunal feedings may be used. Elemental jejunal feedings may be tolerated when conventional feedings are not. TPN may be initiated for the patient with gastric ileus or inability to tolerate an adequate amount of enteral feedings.

For patients who are difficult to wean from the ventilator, it has been suggested that the use of higher-fat, lower-carbohydrate diets may be beneficial since excess carbohydrate increases CO_2 production.

- **Support nutritional status with multivitamin and mineral supplements:** Many vitamins and minerals affect immune function, protein synthesis, and wound healing. Vitamins A and C and zinc are especially important for promoting wound healing. Multivitamins are commonly prescribed for burn-injured patients.

12. **Perform wound care:** Wound cleansing is accomplished with use of mild soap and water. Burns are débrided using manual, enzymatic, or surgical techniques. Topical antimicrobial agents, such as silver sulfadiazine (Silvadene) and mafenide acetate (Sulfamylon), are used to control bacterial proliferation. Burn wounds may be covered and ultimately closed with various temporary and permanent coverings as in the following list. Care of the patient with these coverings depends on the type of wound closure technique used.

Wound coverage and closure techniques:

- **Cutaneous autograft**—includes split-thickness skin graft (STSG) and cultured epithelial autograft (CEA); provides permanent wound coverage
- **Cutaneous allograft**—fresh or preserved donated adult cadaver skin; provides temporary wound coverage until the wound bed is ready for autografting
- **Cutaneous xenograft**—harvested adult porcine epidermis (pigskin); provides temporary wound coverage until the wound bed beneath is healed or is ready for permanent autografting
- **Biosynthetic coverings**—artificial dermis (e.g., Integra); provides a permanent dermal tissue layer that requires a thin autograft for permanent coverage
- **Synthetic coverings**—various dressings often used to cover partial-thickness burns and/or donor sites; provide temporary wound coverage until the wound bed beneath is healed or is ready for permanent autografting

13. **Prepare for surgery as needed:** Need for surgery depends on the depth and extent of the burn injury. The surgical team is coordinated by the burn surgeon.

Pharmacotherapy

 1. **Provide tetanus prophylaxis:** Tetanus immunoglobulin (TIG) or tetanus-toxoid (Tt) should be provided based on the patient's previous immunization for tetanus prophylaxis. Obtain a history of tetanus immunization from medical records so that appropriate tetanus prophylaxis can be accomplished. Individuals with risk factors for inadequate tetanus immunization status should be treated as tetanus immunization – unknown. The tetanus prophylaxis administered should be consistent with the recommendations of the American College of Surgeons (see http://www.facs.org/trauma/publications/tetanus.pdf). Burn injuries are considered 'tetanus-prone wounds.' Tetanus prophylaxis is given intramuscularly.

2. **Manage pain with IV analgesics and anxiolytics:** Morphine sulfate and fentanyl are common agents used for pain management. They are administered in small, frequent IV doses, as needed for comfort and before painful procedure. Consider adjunctive treatment using benzodiazepines (e.g., Ativan, Versed, and Valium) to decrease anxiety. Anxiety increases the perception of pain.

> **Safety Alert**
> *During the resuscitative phase of care, all medications, except tetanus-toxoid, are administered intravenously to avoid sequestration of medication, which then would "flood" the vascular system with the return of capillary integrity and the diuresis of third-spaced fluids.*

3. **Consider gastric acid suppression therapy:** Maintain gastric pH greater than 5.0 and prevent development of Curling ulcer. Early initiation of enteral tube feedings and use of IV proton-pump inhibitors and H_2 blocking agents assist with maintenance of gastric pH and the prevention of ulcers.

4. **Administer antibiotics for known infections:** Antibiotics are not routinely prescribed unless a known or suspected infection exists. Broad-spectrum antibiotics may be used

Burns

initially to treat a suspected infection. More specific antimicrobial agents are used when results from culture and sensitivity tests are available. Burn wound colonization is treated with topical antimicrobial agents only.

5. **Provide DVT prophylaxis:** Prophylactic measures may include the selective use of sequential compression devices on unburned extremities, subcutaneous heparin, low-molecular-weight heparin, or IV heparin drip. The incidence of DVT in the burn population is unknown; however, it is logical to assume this patient population is at high-risk because of hypercoagulability, altered vascular integrity from the burn injury, imposed immobilization, and multiple operative procedures.

CARE PLANS: BURNS

Impaired gas exchange (or risk for same) *related to inhalation injury with tracheobronchial swelling and carbonaceous debris; competition of carbon monoxide (CO) with oxygen for Hgb; hypoventilation associated with constricting circumferential burns to the thorax or large fluid volume resuscitation*

GOALS/OUTCOMES Patient exhibits adequate gas exchange as evidenced by $PaO_2 \geq 80$ mm Hg, oxygen saturation $\geq 95\%$, $PaCO_2$ 35 to 45 mm Hg, age-appropriate RR with a normal pattern and depth, and absence of adventitious breath sounds and other signs of respiratory dysfunction. These outcomes should be adjusted for those individuals with preinjury respiratory disease (e.g., COPD).
NOC Respiratory Status: Gas Exchange

Respiratory Monitoring

1. Assess and document respiratory status, noting rate and depth, breath sounds, and LOC. Identify deteriorating respiratory status as evidenced by indicators of upper airway distress (e.g., severe hoarseness, stridor, dyspnea) and lower airway distress (e.g., crackles, rhonchi, hacking cough, labored or rapid breathing). Infants and young children have relatively smaller airways, thus placing them at greater risk for airway occlusion. Consult physician or mid level practitioner promptly for all significant findings.
2. Administer humidified oxygen therapy, mechanical ventilation, or bronchodilator treatment as prescribed.
3. Unless contraindicated, place patient at a minimum of 30° head elevation to limit upper airway edema formation and to enhance respiratory excursion and prevent aspiration.
4. Monitor for hypoxemia and hypercapnia. Serial ABG values, pulse oximetry, and end-tidal CO_2 monitoring provide critical information concerning arterial oxygen and CO_2 levels. Declining vital capacity, tidal volume, and/or inspiratory force indicates respiratory insufficiency (mechanically ventilated patients only).
5. Teach the nonintubated patient the necessity of coughing and deep-breathing exercises every 2 hours, including use of incentive spirometry while awake.
6. Prepare equipment and patient for intubation and mechanical ventilation, if needed. Note that the position of the patient's head is critical for successful intubation.

NIC Airway Management; Respiratory Monitoring; Oxygen Therapy; Bedside Laboratory Testing; Cough Enhancement: Laboratory Data Interpretation

Ineffective airway clearance (or risk for same) *related to increased pulmonary secretions and inflammation, swelling of nasopharyngeal mucous membranes secondary to smoke irritation or impaired cough; potential of constricting neck and thorax burns and decreased expansion of alveoli secondary to circumferential thorax burns, or pneumonia*

GOALS/OUTCOMES Patient maintains a clear airway as evidenced by auscultation of normal breath sounds over the lung fields and a state of eupnea.
NOC Respiratory Status: Airway Patency

Airway Management

1. Assess and document respiratory status, noting breath sounds and rate and depth of respirations. Identify deteriorating respiratory status as evidenced by crackles, rhonchi, stridor, labored breathing, dyspnea, tachypnea, restlessness, and decreasing LOC. Consult physician promptly for all significant findings.
2. Assess and document character and amount of secretions after each coughing and deep-breathing exercise.

3. Reposition patient from side to side every 1 to 2 hours to help mobilize secretions; position patient head of bed at a 30° elevation. Consider the use of a specialized rotation bed.
4. As prescribed, administer percussion and postural drainage to facilitate airway clearance (this is contraindicated with fresh skin grafts over thorax). Perform oropharyngeal or endotracheal suctioning as indicated by the presence of adventitious breath sounds and the patient's inability to clear the airway effectively by coughing.
5. Administer bronchodilating medications, if prescribed.

NIC Airway Management; Airway Suctioning; Artificial Airway Management; Aspiration Precautions; Cough Enhancement; Mechanical Ventilation

Deficient fluid volume *related to active loss through the burn wound and leakage of fluid, plasma proteins, and other cellular elements into the interstitial space*

GOALS/OUTCOMES   Patient fluid volume status stabilizes as evidenced by MAP greater than 60 mm Hg, BP 110 to 130/70 mm Hg (or lower diastolic and/or within patient's normal preinjury/age-appropriate baseline level), peripheral pulses greater than 2+ on a 0-to-4+ scale, and urine output 30 to 50 ml/hr (adult). Outcomes for urine output should be adjusted for those patients with preexisting renal failure/compromise. In the presence of myoglobinuria (red pigmented urine indicative of myoglobin or Hgb in the urine), a urinary output of 1 to 1.5 ml/kg/hr (approximately 75 to 100 ml/hr in the adult) is the desired outcome until the heme pigments clear from the urine.
NOC Fluid Balance

Fluid Management
1. Monitor patient for evidence of fluid volume deficit, including tachycardia, decreased MAP, decreased amplitude of peripheral pulses, urine output less than 30 ml/hr (adult), urine output less than 1 ml/kg/hr (child weighing less than 30 kg), thirst, and dry mucous membranes.
2. Monitor intake and output; administer fluid therapy using formula or as prescribed. Adjust infusion to maintain desired urine output at the desired resuscitation hourly rate. Do not exceed 50 ml/hr during initial 48 hours of resuscitation (unless heme pigments are present in the urine). Avoid colloids during first 12 to 24 hours following the burn injury.

Safety Alert   *Evaluate patency of IV catheters continuously during rapid-volume resuscitation.*

3. Monitor weight daily during fluid resuscitation; report significant gains or losses. A significant weight gain will occur with large volume fluid resuscitation. A significant weight loss may also occur due to catabolism, an increased metabolic rate, and with extensive removal of burn tissue (e.g., large body fascial excisions).
4. Monitor serial Hct, and Hgb values. During the first 24 hours post-burn, neither the Hct nor Hgb levels are reliable guides to fluid resuscitation. As the circulating volume is restored, hemoconcentration is no longer present and Hct returns to within normal limits (WNL). Consult physician for significant anemia.
5. Monitor patient for signs and symptoms of large volume fluid administration (shortness of breath, tachypnea, excessive urine output). Central hemodynamic monitoring is recommended for patients who have preexisting heart or lung disease.
6. In the presence of myoglobinuria (associated with high voltage electrical injuries or significant soft tissue injury from mechanical trauma), confer with physician regarding the need to increase the rate of fluid administration and to consider urine alkalinization. On occasion, the use of mannitol to promote osmotic diuresis and prevent renal tubular sludging is considered. Other diuretics are avoided because they further deplete an already compromised intravascular volume. Administration of a diuretic precludes the subsequent use of hourly urine output as a guide to fluid resuscitation.
7. With the onset of spontaneous diuresis (48 to 72 hours post-burn), decrease infusion rates as prescribed. Continue to reduce rates gradually according to intake/output ratio and clinical status.

NIC Fluid/Electrolyte Management; Fluid Monitoring; Hypovolemia Management; Shock Prevention; Venous Access Devices Maintenance

Burns

✒ Ineffective tissue perfusion: peripheral *related to thermal injury; circumferential burns; edema; hypovolemia*

- -

GOALS/OUTCOMES Patient maintains adequate tissue perfusion.
Note: Tissue perfusion in burned extremities is adequate when peripheral pulses are greater than 2+ on a scale of 0 to 4+, capillary refill is brisk (less than 2 seconds), and uninjured and healing skin is warm to the touch.
NOC Tissue Perfusion: Peripheral; Circulation Status

Circulatory Precautions
1. Monitor tissue perfusion hourly in burned extremities during the resuscitation phase of care. Note capillary refill, temperature, and peripheral pulses. Report signs of impaired tissue perfusion to the physician immediately, including coolness of the extremity, weak or absent peripheral pulses, pain or paresthesias, and delayed capillary refill.
2. Elevate burned extremities at or above heart level to promote venous return, prevent excessive dependent edema formation, and reduce risk for compartment syndrome.

✒ Hypothermia *related to exposure at the scene of injury; large body surface area burns, administration of large volumes of unwarmed fluid*

- -

GOALS/OUTCOMES Patient's temperature returns to normal (smaller burn injuries) or is slightly elevated (38.5°C; extensive burn injuries) within 24 hours of this diagnosis. Complications of hypothermia have been avoided when the patient remains oriented to time, place, and person; $Pao_2 \geq 80$ mm Hg; and absence of prolonged bleeding from wounds, incisions, and venipuncture sites.
NOC Thermoregulation

Temperature Management
1. Warm fluids administered during the initial resuscitation phase and until the patient approaches desired core temperature. Keep room temperature as warm as possible. Goal is 33°C (91.4°F) ambient room temperature.
2. Avoid unnecessary exposure of the body. Keep patient covered with warmed or warming blanket.
3. Monitor core temperature via rectal or esophageal probe, urinary catheter attachment, or PA catheter.
4. Be aware that vasodilation during rewarming can result in further intravascular fluid volume deficit.
5. Monitor for and promptly report serious dysrhythmias (i.e., atrial fibrillation with rapid ventricular response, ventricular dysrhythmias, atrial ventricular [AV] conduction block), associated with severe or prolonged hypothermia.
6. Monitor ABG values for evidence of hypoxemia. Hypothermia causes a shift to the left in the oxyhemoglobin dissociation curve and may impair oxygen unloading to peripheral tissue.

Risk for infection *related to inadequate primary and secondary defenses secondary to traumatized tissue, bacterial proliferation in burn wounds, presence of invasive IV lines or urinary catheter, and immunocompromised status*

- -

GOALS/OUTCOMES Patient is free of infection as evidenced by core temperatures of 38.5°C (101.3°F) for those with extensive burn injuries, WBC count ≤11,000/mm³, negative culture results, and absence of purulent matter and other clinical indicators of burn wound infection.
NOC Risk Control

Infection Prevention
1. Practice universal precautions to reduce the risk of transmission of microorganisms. Contact isolation measures as appropriate.
2. Recommend sequestration of patients with MRSA, vancomycin-resistant enterococci (VRE), or other resistant organisms.
3. Administer tetanus immunoglobulin or tetanus-toxoid as prescribed.
4. Assess burn wound daily for signs of infection. Report to the physician fever above 39°C (102.2°F), elevated WBC count, change in color or odor of wound exudate, and purulent material. Also report signs of wound deterioration: loss of previously healed wounds, disappearance of a well-defined burn margin with edema formation, and hemorrhagic discoloration.
5. Wash burn wound with a mild soap and rinse thoroughly with water.
6. Monitor temperature every 2 hours. Report temperatures greater than 39°C (102.2°F).
7. Except for eyebrows, shave all hair within burn wound to prevent wound contamination on a daily basis. This practice continues until wound closure.
8. Administer antipyretic and antimicrobial agents as prescribed. Ensure aseptic technique when administering care to burned areas and performing invasive techniques.

9. Assess appearance of grafted site, including adherence to recipient bed, appearance, color, and odor. Be alert to erythema, hyperthermia, increasing tenderness, purulent drainage, and swelling around the grafted site.

10. Assess all invasive lines and devices (e.g., urinary catheters) daily. Review necessity with prompt removal of unnecessary lines and devices.

11. For patients with a central line, implement the central line bundle:
    • Hand hygiene
    • Maximal barrier precautions upon insertion
    • Chlorhexidine skin antisepsis
    • Optimal catheter site selection, with subclavian vein as the preferred site for nontunneled catheters

12. Observe for clinical indicators of sepsis: tachypnea, hypothermia, hyperthermia, ileus, subtle disorientation, unexplained metabolic acidosis, low platelet count, feeding intolerance, and glucose intolerance. If sepsis is suspected, obtain wound, blood, sputum, and urine culture specimens as prescribed.

NIC Environmental Management; Infection Control; Infection Protection; Surveillance; Wound Care; Shock Management

---

Acute pain *related to burn injury and treatment*

GOALS/OUTCOMES Within 30 minutes of treatment/intervention, patient's subjective evaluation of discomfort improves and/or nonverbal indicators of discomfort are absent or diminished.
NOC Pain Control

Pain Management
1. Assess patient's level of discomfort at frequent intervals. Patients with partial-thickness burns may experience severe pain because of damage and exposure of sensory nerve endings. Pain tolerance often decreases with prolonged hospitalization, multiple painful procedures, and sleep deprivation.
2. Monitor patient for clinical indicators of pain: increased BP/MAP, tachypnea, shivering, rigid muscle tone, or guarded position.
3. If possible, avoid wound care procedures during sleeping hours.
4. Administer opioid analgesia and anxiolytics as prescribed. Time dosage for optimal effectiveness before painful procedures.
5. Provide simple explanations of all procedures.
6. Employ adjunctive nonpharmacologic interventions as indicated (relaxation breathing, guided imagery, distraction, music therapy).
7. Ensure that patient receives periods of uninterrupted sleep by grouping care procedures when possible.

NIC Analgesic Administration; Anxiety Reduction; Environmental Management: Comfort; Pain Management

---

Impaired tissue integrity *related to burn injury; edema*

GOALS/OUTCOMES Patient's wound exhibits evidence of healing. Wound healing occurs without hypertrophic scarring (late outcome finding).
Note: Healing time varies with the extent and depth of injury.
NOC Tissue Integrity: Skin and Mucous Membranes

Healing
1. Assess and document extent and depth of burn wound (see Table 3-5).
2. Cleanse and débride wound as prescribed.
3. Apply topical antimicrobial treatments as prescribed, using aseptic technique.
4. Elevate burned extremities at or above heart level to facilitate venous return and reduce risk for compartment syndrome.

For patients with skin grafts:
5. Help prevent graft loss if fluid collection beneath graft occurs. Notify burn surgeon. Small fluid collections can be removed if caught early, allowing for graft re-adherence.
6. Monitor type and amount of drainage from wounds. Promptly report the presence of bright red bleeding, which would inhibit graft take, or purulent exudate, which indicates infection.

Burns

7. Maintain immobility of grafted site for 3 to 5 days or as prescribed. This is achieved with a combination of positioning, splinting, or light pressure and sedation. In some instances, restraints, stents, bulky dressings, or occlusive dressings may be required to maintain immobilization and promote hemostasis of graft.
8. Apply elastic wraps as prescribed to legs that have grafts and/or donor sites to promote venous return and to promote graft adherence when out of bed.
9. Use of a bed cradle may prevent bedding from coming in contact with burned or grafted areas.
10. Provide donor site care as prescribed, and be alert to signs of donor site infection.
11. Teach patient about need for compression to prevent bleeding and to promote graft adherence.

NIC Infection Protection; Positioning; Wound Care

Ineffective tissue perfusion: gastrointestinal *related to hypovolemia and interruption in blood flow associated with splanchnic vasoconstriction secondary to fluid shifts and catecholamine release*

GOALS/OUTCOMES Patient has adequate GI tissue perfusion as evidenced by auscultation of bowel sounds within 48 to 72 hours after burn injury; bowel elimination and appetite within patient's normal pattern; and absence of nausea and vomiting.

Safety Alert	*Be aware that prolonged impaired perfusion to GI organs increases the likelihood of such complications as impaired gastric motility, adynamic ileus, gastritis, and Curling ulcer.*

NOC Tissue Perfusion: Abdominal Organs

Gastrointestinal Intubation
1. Assess bowel function every 2 to 4 hours. Identify abdominal distention and decreasing or absent bowel sounds, which occur with adynamic ileus or abdominal compartment syndrome. Consider bladder pressure monitoring; notify physician as pressures reach 20 mm Hg.
2. During period of absent bowel sounds, maintain gastric tube to intermittent low suction as prescribed. Check at intervals to ensure patency and position of the tube. Before removing tube, clamp for several hours to be certain patient has sufficient GI motility. Abdominal distention, nausea, vomiting, or return of a large volume of gastric contents when tube is reconnected indicates insufficient motility to tolerate tube removal.
3. Maintain NPO status until return of bowel sounds. Provide mouth care for comfort and hygiene.
4. Administer proton pump inhibitors, H_2-receptor antagonists, and other agents prescribed to reduce formation of gastric acids. If prescribed, start enteral feedings.
5. Test gastric aspirate for occult blood as indicated and report to physician.

NIC Gastrointestinal Intubation; Hemodynamic Regulation; Nutritional Management; Tube Care: Gastrointestinal

 Imbalanced nutrition: less than body requirements of protein, vitamins, and calories *related to hypermetabolic state*

GOALS/OUTCOMES Patient has adequate nutrition as evidenced by stable weight (following resuscitation period), balanced nitrogen state per nitrogen studies, serum albumin ≥3.5 g/dl, thyroxine-binding prealbumin 20 to 30 mg/dl, retinol-binding protein 4 to 5 mg/dl, and evidence of continued burn wound healing and graft take.
NOC Nutritional Status

Nutrition Management
1. Collaborate with physician and dietitian to estimate patient's metabolic needs on the basis of injury extent, dry weight, and nutritional status before injury.
2. Consider patient's specific injuries, ability to consume diet, and preexisting medical condition when planning nutrition.
3. Provide diet as prescribed. When patient can take foods orally, promote supplemental feedings/snacks between meals.

4. Consider placement of a soft Silastic feeding tube for provision of enteral tube feedings for those who are unable to meet their caloric and protein requirements orally.
5. Recognize that opioids decrease GI motility and may cause nausea and vomiting.
6. Administer medications to prevent/treat opioid-associated GI complications (constipation, decrease in GI motility).
7. Recognize that patients with an ileus that persists for longer than 4 days or those unable to meet caloric needs enterally may require TPN.
8. Record all intake for daily calorie counts.
9. Monitor patient's weight. Minimize error by weighing patient without dressings or splints, if possible.
10. Monitor markers of nutritional status: serum albumin, thyroxine-binding prealbumin, retinol-binding protein, and urine nitrogen measurements. Long periods of catabolism cause these serum values to decrease. Be alert to measures of protein deficiencies, weight loss, and poor wound healing, all of which are signals that nutritional needs are not being met.

NIC Nutrition Management; Nutrition Therapy; Nutritional Monitoring

Fear *related to potentially threatening situation (e.g., serious injury, hospitalization) and supported by presence of pain, unfamiliarity, and noxious environmental stimuli present in critical care area; communication barrier (e.g., intubation); sensory impairment from direct injuries*

GOALS/OUTCOMES Patient exhibits decreased symptoms of fear: apprehension, tension, nervousness, tachycardia, aggressiveness, and withdrawal.
NOC Fear Control

Anxiety Reduction
1. Assess level of fear and understanding of present condition.
2. Plan care to provide as restful an environment as possible.
3. Provide information regarding nursing care, treatment plan, and progress. It is often necessary to repeat information because injury, stress, and fear can interfere with comprehension.
4. Promote visits by family members and significant others.
5. Offer to consult hospital spiritual care or patient's clergy as desired by patient.
6. Assess and promote patient's usual coping strategies. Consult with psychology for assistance.
7. Provide referral to burn survivor support groups.

NIC Coping Enhancement; Security Enhancement; Support System Enhancement

Disturbed sensory perception: tactile and visual *related to altered reception secondary to medications, sleep pattern disturbance, pain, swollen eyelids, and full-thickness burn wound*

GOALS/OUTCOMES Patient verbalizes orientation to time, place, and person and describes rationale (age appropriate understanding) for necessary treatments.
NOC Vision Compensation Behavior: Cognitive Orientation

Sensory Perception Management
1. Assess patient's orientation to time, place, and person.
2. Answer patient's questions simply and succinctly, providing information regarding immediate surroundings, procedures, and treatments. Anticipate the necessity of having to repeat information at frequent intervals.
3. For patient with cutaneous burn injury, explain why tactile sensation is decreased or absent. If patient's eyelids are swollen shut because of facial edema, reassure patient that he or she is not blind and that swelling will resolve within 3 to 5 days. Apply eye lubricant as prescribed for those patients with excessive swelling and/or inhibited blink.
4. Touch patient on unburned skin to provide nonpainful tactile stimulation.
5. Explain that alterations in perception can be related to opioids and other medications commonly prescribed during the acute phase of burn recovery.

NIC Peripheral Sensation Management; Surveillance: Safety; Communication Enhancement: Visual Deficit; Environmental Management

Burns

Risk for disuse syndrome *related to immobilization from pain, splints, or scar formation*

GOALS/OUTCOMES Patient displays complete ROM without verbal or nonverbal indicators of discomfort.
NOC Risk Control

Positioning
1. Provide ROM exercises every 4 hours while awake. When possible, combine when medicated with analgesics for other procedures and during activities of daily living (ADLs).
2. Apply splints as prescribed to maintain extremities in functional position and to prevent contracture formation.
3. For patient with grafts, institute ROM exercises and ambulation on prescribed postgrafting day (often 3 to 7 days postgrafting). Premedicate with analgesic to aid in mobility and reduce discomfort.

NIC Exercise Therapy: Ambulation; Exercise Therapy: Joint Mobility; Exercise Promotion; Nutrition Management

Disturbed body image *related to biophysical changes secondary to burn injury*

GOALS/OUTCOMES Patient begins to acknowledge body changes and demonstrates movement toward incorporating changes into self-concept.
NOC Body Image

Body Image Enhancement
1. Assess patient's perceptions and feelings about the burn injury and changes in lifestyle and relationships, especially those with significant others.
2. Involve significant others in as much care as possible to maintain bond with patient.
3. Respect patient's need to express anger over body changes.
4. Consider consultation with rehabilitation psychology and/or child life therapy.
5. Provide information concerning eventual appearance of grafts and donor sites.
6. Provide names and telephone numbers of local and national support groups for burn survivors: The American Burn Association, National Headquarters Office, website: www.ameriburn.org, (312) 642-9260; The Phoenix Society for Burn Survivors, Inc, National Headquarters Office, website: www.phoenix-society.org, (800) 888-2876.

NIC Anxiety Reduction; Coping Enhancement; Grief Work Facilitation; Self-Esteem Enhancement; Support System Enhancement

Deficient knowledge *related to lack of knowledge regarding ability for self-care management and/or use of resources for supportive care*

GOALS/OUTCOMES Within 24 hours of transfer to acute care, patient and significant others verbalize knowledge about prescribed medications and techniques that facilitate continued wound healing and limb mobility.
NOC Knowledge: Medication; Knowledge: Treatment Regimen

Teaching: Disease Process
1. Review the splinting and exercise program for contracture prevention, as directed by physical therapist.
2. Teach patient and significant others to monitor for pain or pressure caused by improperly applied splint and to assess splinted extremity for coolness, pallor, cyanosis, decreased pulses, and impaired function.
3. Discuss current skin and wound care plan.
4. Explain indicators of wound infection.
5. Review nutritional needs.
6. Review current pain and anxiolytic medications.

NIC Learning Facilitation; Learning Readiness Enhancement; Teaching: Individual

ADDITIONAL NURSING DIAGNOSES

For other nursing diagnoses and interventions, see the following, as appropriate: *Nutritional Support*, p. 117; *Mechanical Ventilation*, p. 99; *Prolonged Immobility*, p. 149; *Compartment Syndrome/Ischemic Myositis*, p. 301; *Emotional and Spiritual Support of the Patient and Significant Others*, p. 200.

COMPARTMENT SYNDROME/ISCHEMIC MYOSITIS

PATHOPHYSIOLOGY

Compartment syndrome is caused by pathologic elevation of intercompartmental pressures within nonexpansible tissue envelopes. The pressure increase may come from either an increase in volume within a tissue compartment or externally applied pressure compressing a tissue compartment. As pressure within the anatomic space rises, local perfusion is compromised leading, if untreated, to irreversible damage of the tissues within the compartment. Compartment syndrome is a surgical emergency that requires rapid intervention to prevent permanent cosmetic or functional deformity or loss of limb. Compartment syndrome may be acute or chronic (exercise-related forms); this section focuses on the acute peripheral type.

Most compartment syndromes are associated with trauma, but the condition may also occur from multiple other etiologies including reperfusion injuries, ischemia, burns, prolonged limb compression, drug abuse, or poor positioning during prolonged surgical procedures (Table 3-8). The incidence of compartment syndrome in those younger than 35 years is increased probably secondary to the larger muscle mass contained within the osteofascial space.

Any muscle may be affected as long as the pressure within a muscle is sustained for a prolonged period of time. Most often the muscles affected are those that are contained within an osteofascial space in the upper or lower extremity. The most common site in the upper arm is the forearm. The forearm contains two compartments: the volar and dorsal. The volar compartment contains the flexors of the wrist and fingers and the dorsal compartment contains the extensors. The lower extremity contains a total of seven compartments: three in the thigh and four in the calf. The three compartments of the thigh are the anterior, posterior, and medial. The calf compartments are the anterior, lateral /peroneal, deep posterior, and superficial posterior. The tibial nerve lies within the posterior compartment and provides sensation to the plantar surface of the foot and flexion of the toes. The anterior compartment contains the peroneal nerve providing sensation to the first web space and motor function of the extensors of the calf and foot. The anterior compartment of the calf is the most common site of compartment syndrome.

Table 3-8	CAUSES OF COMPARTMENT SYNDROME		
Localized Compartmental Trauma	**Tissue Reaction/ Edema Formation**	**Coagulation Defects**	**Other**
Fractures	Prolonged used of	Hemophilia	Compression during obtundation
Surgery	operative tourniquets	Anticoagulant	(anesthesia, drug overdose)
Hematoma	Arterial or venous	therapy	Infiltrated IV therapy
Venomous bites	obstruction		Constrictive dressings, inflatable
(snake, spider)	Limb reimplantation		splints or casts
Vascular injury	Burns (especially		Closure of fascial defects
Postischemic	when circumferential)		Hypothermia or hyperthermia
swelling	Excessive exercise		*Clostridium perfringens* infections
Crush injuries	(e.g., march gangrene)		Rocky Mountain spotted fever
Electrical injuries	Nephrotic syndrome		Use of pneumatic antishock
			garment (PASG)
			Hypovolemia
			Hypotension

Modified from Callahan J: Orthop Nurs 4(4):11–15, 1985.

Increased and sustained pressure within a muscle compartment can develop because of increased volume in the compartment from a hematoma or edema. A second etiology is prolonged ischemia, which may be due to external compression or arterial compromise. Finally, compartment syndrome may be caused by decreased overall size of the muscle compartment from scar formation, especially following circumferential burns (see Table 3-8).

Regardless of the etiology or location, ischemia begins when the metabolic demands of the tissues cannot be met. The normal pressure in muscle compartments is below 10 to 12 mm Hg. Whitesides' theory states that the development of compartment syndrome depends on both the intracompartmental pressure and the systemic BP. The diastolic BP minus the compartmental pressure should be above 30 mm Hg to avoid ischemia in the tissues. Thus, increasing the compartmental pressure or decreasing the perfusion pressure can each lead to a compartment syndrome.

When injury occurs, the depletion of intracellular energy stores causes cellular swelling and increasing venous pressures, allowing edema to develop and local blood flow to decrease. Lymphatic drainage initially increases and then decreases due to congestion from the growing tissue edema. Compartmental tissue pressure increases compromising capillary blood flow. Histamine is released, producing vasodilation and increased capillary permeability. Rising compartmental pressure further increases venous congestion and results in reduction in the arteriovenous pressure gradient, reducing local tissue perfusion and further increasing capillary pressure. Fluids and proteins escape from the capillaries and contribute to even higher tissue pressures. The higher tissue pressures eventually exceed both capillary and venous pressures, stopping nutrient blood flow and promoting further ischemia. Local blood flow to muscles is severely compromised when the interstitial tissue pressure equals or exceeds the diastolic pressure. As a result of impaired venous return, anaerobic metabolism creates more lactic acid, which stimulates vasodilation further, decreasing BP and elevating tissue pressure. The pressure within the compartment continues to increase, equaling or exceeding the capillary pressure and leading to arteriolar compression, causing further ischemia of the muscle and nerves.

Sustained hypotension and shock are associated with greater incidence of compartment syndrome due to the lowered pressure gradient. Less compartmental pressure is needed to result in arteriolar spasm and ischemic changes in the muscles.

The earliest signs of compartment syndrome are often subtle but are primarily neurologic due to the susceptibility to hypoxia of the nonmyelinated sensory fibers. Sensory changes in the extremity begin with paresthesias or hyperesthesias within 30 minutes of the onset of ischemia and may become functionally irreversible after 12 to 24 hours. The average interval between the initial injury to the compartment and the beginning symptoms of compartment syndrome is 2 hours. Compartmental tissue ischemia that lasts longer than 6 hours results in muscle necrosis and irreversible tissue changes.

Late-onset compartment syndrome is seen in comatose or confused patients unable to communicate symptoms. Late-onset compartment syndrome is often more difficult to recognize and manage, sometimes worsening following treatment with fasciotomy. The late syndrome may occur in compartments already treated with fasciotomy. Healthy granulation tissue may cover necrotic muscle within partially opened compartments. With sufficient muscle tissue injury (e.g., after crush injuries) or undiagnosed compartment syndrome, rhabdomyolysis may develop with the release of metabolic toxin and intracellular components, especially myoglobin. The release of toxins can result in secondary myoglobinemia, leading to acute tubular necrosis (ATN), which may progress to acute kidney injury and multisystem failure.

COMPARTMENT SYNDROME ASSESSMENT
Goal of Assessment
The goals are to prevent ischemia and reduce long-term sequelae by earlier diagnosis and treatment through reduction in internal or external pressure.

History and Risk Factors
- Any patient with a peripheral injury listed in Table 3-8 is at risk for compartment syndrome.
- Patients admitted for acute renal failure after treatment for crush injuries or compartment syndrome should be suspected of having late-onset or continuing compartment syndrome.
- Patients with profound shock who receive aggressive fluid resuscitation are at risk for acute compartment syndrome.

Vital Signs
- Hypotension potentiates compartment syndrome.

Observation and Subjective Symptoms
Early indicators:
- Unusually severe pain for an injury is a cardinal symptom. Passive stretch of an involved muscle group significantly increases the pain.

Late-onset syndrome indicators:
- Persistent peripheral edema or continued elevation of tissue pressures even after fasciotomy.
- If compartment syndrome is not treated, the necrosing muscles become fibrotic and contract and can no longer function (e.g., Volkmann ischemic contracture).
- Late decompression fasciotomy seldom restores lost myoneural function. Early recognition is the key to successful management and preservation of function.
- Extreme pain is out of proportion to the injury.
- Increased pain occurs on passive ROM (stretch) of the affected extremity.

Late findings:
- Paresthesias (early loss of vibratory sensation)
- Pallor of the extremity
- Paralysis

Palpation
- Feel for temperature of affected area; polar (coolness) of affected area is a late sign.
- Palpation of the compartment reveals tension and slowed capillary refill.
- Assess pulses in all extremities; pulselessness is a late sign.

Diagnostic Tests for Compartment Syndrome		
Test	**Purpose**	**Abnormal Findings**
Blood Chemistry: Creatine phosphokinase (CPK)	Elevated is caused by the release of the enzyme by injured muscle tissue.	Continued elevation in the course of treatment may indicate late-onset compartment syndrome. Extensive muscle necrosis may lead to myoglobinemia and myoglobinuria, and may lead to rhabdomyolysis. Blood urea nitrogen and creatinine levels will be elevated if acute renal failure results from rhabdomyolysis.
Serum creatine kinase (CK)-MM	CK-MM isoenzyme is most specific for skeletal muscle damage. Serum CK levels begin increasing 2–12 hours after the onset of muscle injury. They peak within 1–3 days and decrease 3–5 days after muscle injury ceases.	In compartment syndrome CK levels may rise as high as 100,000 IU. Levels above 2000 IU raise the possibility of muscle damage. CK values more than 2000 units/L after surgery can be a warning sign of acute compartment syndrome in ventilated and sedated patients.
Intracompartmental pressure monitoring	Compartment pressure and associated critical values may be monitored intermittently by inserting needles (pressure within 10–30 mm Hg of diastolic blood pressure), which get obstructed by muscle tissue. Continuous infusion catheters (pressure >45 mm Hg) and wick or slit catheters (>30–35 mm Hg) monitor continuously via fluid-filled catheters and pressure monitors. In hypotensive patients at higher risk for compartment syndrome, the delta pressure should be calculated. Delta pressure equals mean arterial pressure minus compartmental pressure.	Delta pressures of ≤30 mm Hg for 6 hr or ≤40 for 8 hr require prompt consultation with the physician. Pressures warranting fasciotomy vary with clinical indicators, the patient's systemic condition, and measurement technique.

Continued

Diagnostic Tests for Compartment Syndrome — cont'd		
Test	**Purpose**	**Abnormal Findings**
Near-infrared spectroscopy (NIRS)	Based on the different light absorption properties, NIRS can measure the local changes in concentration of oxygenated and deoxygenated hemoglobin and perfusion in different tissues including muscle.	More studies are needed, but NIRS may provide the benefit of a rapid, continuous, noninvasive, sensitive, and specific tool for early detection of acute compartment syndrome.
Ultrasound: pulsed phase–locked loop (PPLL)	More investigation is needed to determine effectiveness. The PPLL ultrasound locks on to a characteristic reflection that comes from a specific tissue and can detect the very subtle movements of fascia that correspond to local arterial pulsation.	Increased intracompartmental pressure during compartment syndrome causes a reduction in normal fascial displacements in response to arterial pulsation.
Scintigraphy	Radionuclide imaging that shows the physiologic function of the system being investigated as opposed to its anatomy	Can study all compartments of an extremity at once but limited usefulness because of inability to study over time
Pulse oximetry	Assesses perfusion of distal tissues. Readings should be compared with readings from a contralateral, uninvolved extremity.	Decreased perfusion will result in lower pulse oximetry results but may not be decreased until significant time and injury has occurred. Pulse oximetry cannot measure intracompartmental tissue oxygen saturation and requires adequate pulsatile flow.
Magnetic resonance imaging (MRI)	MRI is useful in detecting soft tissue edema on T1 images.	MRI **cannot** differentiate the edema from trauma with edema from a compartment syndrome so is of limited value in diagnosis in the acute phase. MRI is useful in identifying the tissue changes in an established compartment syndrome in a very late stage.
Arteriograms and venograms	Radiologic examination of blood vessels may be performed when embolus, thrombus, or other vascular injury is suspected.	

Compartmental Pressure Monitoring

Compartmental pressure monitoring continues to be the preferred method of definitive diagnosis of acute compartment syndrome. Several methods of direct compartment measurement exist including the needle manometer, the wick catheter, and the slit catheter. Continuous readings are not possible with the needle manometer method and may result in falsely high levels due to the injection of saline into the muscle. Pressures within compartments may be continuously monitored with either the wick method or the slit catheter method by attaching a pressure transducer to an implanted catheter within a muscle compartment. Indications for continuous or intermittent pressure monitoring are in the unconscious patient, children or other patients difficult to assess, patients with nerve injury, and those with multiple orthopaedic traumas. Regardless of technique, compartmental pressures greater than 30 mm Hg above the systemic diastolic pressure indicate the need for a compartment fasciotomy.

Early indicators:

- Palpation of the compartment reveals tension and slowed capillary refill.
- Tissue pressures vary with the method of measurement. Generally, normal tissue pressures vary from 10 to 12 mm Hg, and sustained pressures greater than 30 mm Hg above the systemic diastolic pressure result in tissue necrosis.
- The thin-walled lower extremity veins may collapse at lower pressures, further contributing to the pathogenesis.

COLLABORATIVE MANAGEMENT
Care Priorities

1. **Eliminate external pressure on the affected compartment:** *Identify and relieve circumferential constriction:* Loosen or remove circumferential casts and padding or dressings; escharotomy for circumferential burns or frostbite.
2. **Manage pain:** *Analgesia:* Parenteral opiates often with sedative adjuncts
3. **Reduce internal compartmental pressure:** *Intravenous hypertonic mannitol:* Used as a preventive measure to reduce compartmental pressure via systemic diuresis and to help the kidneys excrete the large molecules of myoglobin if extensive tissue necrosis is present. This diuresis may potentiate more ischemia if the patient is hypovolemic.
4. **Provide surgical intervention:** *Fasciotomy of myofascial compartment:* The goal of treatment of acute compartment syndrome is to decrease tissue pressure, restore blood flow, and minimize tissue damage.
   - Treatment of choice to accomplish these goals is a surgical fasciotomy to allow unrestricted swelling. The affected compartment alone may be opened but, more commonly, adjacent or all tissue compartments in the area are prophylactically incised. In the forearm, a volar aspect fasciotomy is most common. In the thigh, a lateral incision can decompress at three compartments, and in the calf, a lateral fasciotomy expansible to release all compartments or medial and lateral incisions is generally adequate.
   - Persistent peripheral edema with elevated CPK, or the presence of acute renal failure, may justify reexploration and wide excision of all necrotic muscle in involved and adjacent compartments.
   - Complications of fasciotomy include wound infection, the potential for osteomyelitis, and large scars.
   - Secondary wound closure may be accomplished after 3 to 4 days once the compartmental pressure has returned to normal. Multiple methods of wound closure have been used, including mechanical closure devices, dynamic skin sutures, vacuum-assisted closure, and healing by secondary intention.
   - Skin grafting may be needed to ensure complete coverage of the exposed compartments.
5. **Provide vascular surgical intervention if blood vessel injury caused the compartment syndrome.** *Treat vascular injury:* The involved blood vessel is explored and treated.
   - Papaverine, a vasodilating drug that relaxes smooth muscle, can be injected in a bolus of fluid to reestablish normal internal artery dynamics.
   - Blood vessel lacerations can be repaired or severely damaged vessels can be resected.

CARE PLANS: COMPARTMENT SYNDROME

Ineffective tissue perfusion (or risk for same): peripheral (compartment) *related to interruption of capillary blood flow secondary to increased pressure within the anatomic compartment*

GOALS/OUTCOMES Throughout hospitalization, patient has adequate perfusion to compartment tissues as evidenced by brisk (less than 2 seconds) capillary refill, peripheral pulses greater than 2+ on a 0-to-4+ scale, normal tissue pressures (0 to 10 mm Hg), and absence of edema or tautness. Within 2 hours of admission, patient verbalizes understanding of reporting symptoms of impaired neurovascular status.

NOC Circulation Status

Circulatory Precautions

1. Monitor neurovascular status of injured extremity at least every 2 hours.
2. Assess for increased pain on passive extension or flexion of the digits.
3. Monitor for sluggish capillary refill, decrease in or loss of two-point discrimination, increasing limb edema, and tautness over individual compartments.
4. Use pulse oximetry to help assess distal tissue perfusion, and report significant differences from oximetry readings taken from the uninvolved contralateral extremity.
5. Assess for the *six Ps*:
   a. *Pain* (especially on passive digital movement and with pressure over the compartment)
   b. *Pallor*
   c. *Polar* (coolness)
   d. *Pulselessness*
   e. *Paresthesia*
   f. *Paralysis*
6. Report deficits in neurovascular status promptly.
7. Loosen circumferential dressings as indicated.
8. Teach patient the symptoms to be promptly reported: severe, unrelieved pain, paresthesias (diminished sensation, hyperesthesia, or anesthesia), paralysis, coolness, or pulselessness.
9. Monitor tissue pressures continuously, with an intracompartmental pressure device if needed.
10. Consult physician if pressures exceed normal or preestablished levels.

HIGH ALERT! Pressures greater than 10 mm Hg may reflect significant elevation.

---

11. Monitor closely for additional tissue injury if the patient becomes hypotensive.

NIC Cast Care: Maintenance; Heat/Cold Application; Peripheral Sensation Management; Shock Management; Skin Surveillance; Teaching: Disease Process

Acute pain *related to physical factors (tissue ischemia) secondary to compartment syndrome*

GOALS/OUTCOMES Throughout the hospitalization, the patient's pain is controlled, as reflected by a pain scale. Nonverbal indicators of discomfort (e.g., grimacing) are reduced or absent. Within 2 hours of admission, patient verbalizes understanding of the need to report uncontrolled or increasing pain.
NOC Pain Control; Comfort Level

Pain Management

1. Assess for pain: onset, duration, progression, and intensity. Devise a pain scale with patient, rating discomfort "0" for no pain to "10" for unbearable pain. Noncommunicative or low-level intellect patients may require a simpler or different pain scale.
2. Determine if passive stretching of digits and pressure over limb compartments increases the pain. Both may indicate early compartment syndrome.
3. Adjust the medication regimen to the patient's needs; document medication effectiveness.
4. Promptly report uncontrolled pain.
5. Prevent pressure being applied on involved compartment and neurovascular structures.
6. Following a fasciotomy, pain that remains unrelieved may indicate that the fasciotomy is incomplete.
7. Pain that increases several days after a fasciotomy may signal compartmental infection.
8. Continue to monitor neurovascular function with each vital sign check to assess for recurring compartment syndrome or infection.

NIC Analgesic Administration; Anxiety Reduction; Coping Enhancement; Progressive Muscle Relaxation; Simple Guided Imagery

Risk for infection *related to inadequate primary defenses secondary to necrotic tissue, wide-excision fasciotomy, and open wound*

GOALS/OUTCOMES Throughout the hospitalization, patient is free of infection as evidenced by normothermia; WBC count less than 11,000/mm^3 and absence of wound erythema and other clinical indicators of infection. Within 24 hours of admission, patient verbalizes understanding of the need to report promptly any indicators of infection. **NOC** Risk Control; Wound Healing: Primary Intention

Infection Protection
1. Monitor patient for fever, increasing pain, and laboratory data indicative of infection (e.g., increased WBC count or erythrocyte sedimentation rate).
2. Assess exposed wounds for erythema, increasing wound drainage, purulent wound drainage, increasing wound circumference, edema, and localized tenderness.
3. Assess neurovascular deficits, which may signal infection or pressure in adjacent inflamed tissues.
4. After primary closure or grafting of wound, assess for signs of infection beneath the closure.
5. Assess for chronic infection and osteomyelitis — key complications of compartment syndrome.
6. Instruct patient to report the following indicators of infection: fever, localized warmth, increasing pain, increasing wound drainage (especially if purulent), swelling, and redness.
7. Consult with physician or mid level practitioner promptly regarding significant findings.

NIC Environmental Management; Medication Management; Surveillance; Vital Signs Monitoring; Wound Care; Wound Care: Closed Drainage

Disturbed body image *related to physical changes secondary to large, irregular fasciotomy wound and skin-grafted scar; loss of function in or change in appearance of an extremity; or amputation*

GOALS/OUTCOMES Within the 24-hour period before discharge from ICU, patient acknowledges body changes and demonstrates movement toward incorporating changes into self-concept. Patient does not exhibit maladaptive response (e.g., severe depression) to wound or functional loss.
NOC Body Image; Self-Esteem

Body Image Enhancement
1. Discuss compartment syndrome, therapeutic interventions, and long-term effects.
2. Provide time for the patient to share feelings about his or her changed appearance and function. Encourage questions and discussion of these feelings with patient's significant others.
3. Help patient set realistic goals for recovery.
4. Facilitate progression through the grieving process, as appropriate.
5. Recognize when each patient is ready to view or discuss the injury. Adjustment time varies.
6. Encourage self-care. Provide necessary adjunctive aids (e.g., built-up utensils, button hooks, orthotics) to facilitate independence in activities of daily living.
7. Collaborate with physician or mid level practitioner for patients with functional loss or amputation, introduce use of orthotics and adjunctive devices to facilitate self-care.

NIC Active Listening; Amputation Care; Anxiety Reduction; Coping Enhancement; Emotional Support; Self-Care Assistance; Wound Care

DROWNING

PATHOPHYSIOLOGY

Drowning was defined as a process of experiencing respiratory impairment from submersion/ immersion in a liquid by the 2002 World Congress on Drowning. The terms *drowning* and *near drowning* are often used to distinguish between those individuals who die within 24 hours of the drowning incident and those who live 24 hours or longer following the incident (termed "near drowning"). This is an arbitrary distinction since the individuals classified as near drownings may eventually die from the drowning and health care providers cannot always determine who will die within the first 24 hours, so the treatment will be the same.

The main effects of drownings are from hypoxemia and decreased oxygen delivery to the tissues, which can lead to failure of multiple organs, most importantly the CNS. Hypotension, pulmonary edema, hypothermia, and respiratory and metabolic acidosis occur after near drowning, compounding the detrimental effects of the hypoxemia. In addition to the neurologic deficits from cerebral anoxia, acute lung injury or acute respiratory distress syndrome (ALI or ARDS), pneumonia, acute renal failure secondary to acute tubular necrosis, and DIC can occur. Any aspirated contaminants (e.g., algae, chemicals, sand) may cause or contribute to obstruction and lead to asphyxiation. Bacterial pneumonia can develop, depending on the type of contaminant in the aspirant, and chemical pneumonitis can occur if gastric contents were aspirated.

Drownings are categorized by the type of water (fresh versus salt water) and whether the person aspirated fluid into the lungs (wet versus dry drowning).

Wet versus Dry Drowning

A drowning person goes through a stage of gasping and possible aspiration. Once submersed, hyperventilation is stimulated followed by apnea and some degree of laryngospasm leading to hypoxemia. Wet drowning is more common, wherein the asphyxia allows the airways to relax resulting in aspiration of fluid into the lungs. Dry drowning occurs in 15% of patients whose laryngospasm is maintained until cardiac arrest ensues, so minimal to no fluid is aspirated. Prolonged hypoxemia results in acidosis, which may prompt myocardial dysfunction and, eventually, cardiac arrest and CNS ischemia.

Freshwater Drowning

Freshwater (hypotonic) aspiration results in a rapid absorption of aspirated fluid from the lungs leading to hypervolemia and hypotonicity. The increased intravascular volume leads to dilution of serum electrolytes and hemolysis of RBCs. Surfactant in the alveoli is lost and the pulmonary capillary membranes are damaged, leading to noncardiogenic pulmonary edema. The loss of surfactant causes an increase in the surface tension of the lung tissue, resulting in collapse of the alveoli. Lung compliance also decreases. The atelectasis and pulmonary edema lead to a ventilation-perfusion mismatch, adding to the hypoxia and acidosis.

Saltwater Drowning

Saltwater (hypertonic) aspiration results in a rapid shift of water and plasma proteins from the circulation into the alveoli. The fluid-filled alveoli are not ventilated, while continued perfusion leads to ventilation-perfusion mismatch and hypoxia. Hemolysis is not an issue in saltwater drownings.

Hypothermia, defined as a drop in core temperature to 33°C (91.4°F) or below, may also occur. Its progression can cause muscle activity and vital functions to cease, resulting in ventricular fibrillation (occurs at about 28°C [82.4°F]). Hypothermia may protect the brain from permanent anoxic damage by decreasing cerebral metabolism by as much as 50%. The hypothermic protection is dependent on the temperature dropping to the point of slowing cerebral metabolism prior to the ischemic injury occurring in the brain. This occurs most often with drownings in icy waters or where the victim has been able to stay afloat for a period of time while the temperature drops before being submersed. Since these factors are not often known about the victim, all drowning victims should receive aggressive initial resuscitation. Resuscitation should be continued until the victim is rewarmed to at least 32°C (89.6°F), since the heart may start beating at that temperature. Resuscitation remains possible after 30 minutes of submersion. Resuscitation efforts frequently should be continued for at least 1 hour.

ASSESSMENT: DROWNING
Goal of System Assessment

Evaluate for respiratory and neurologic functioning, as well as determining if concurrent injuries were sustained such as head and/or spinal trauma.

History and Risk Factors

Age of the victim, inability to swim, submersion time, temperature of the water, degree of water contamination, use of alcohol and/or drugs, associated injuries such as head and spine injuries, underlying medical conditions, and prehospital resuscitation received should all be considered.

Vital Signs
- Temperature may be low if drowning occurred in a cold body of water.
- Respiratory rate may be elevated or absent if the patient is in arrest.
- Hypotension
- Heart rate may be increased or decreased depending on the temperature and respiratory status. The patient may also present with asystole or in ventricular tachycardia/ fibrillation.
- Respiratory rate may be increased with dyspnea or may be absent if arrest has occurred. Absent respiratory effort may indicate a high cervical spinal cord injury.

Observation
Evaluate for signs of trauma to head and neck, skin coloring as an indication of hypoxia, signs of neurologic functioning including pupil size and equality and response to stimuli.
- Pink, frothy sputum may indicate pulmonary edema.

Palpation
- Evaluate skin for temperature, neck for deformities, and head for signs of trauma including swelling.

Auscultation
Evaluate lung fields to identify abnormal breath sounds.
- Decreased breath sounds may indicate a pneumothorax or hemothorax.
- Sucking sound on inspiration may indicate an open pneumothorax.
- Crackles, rhonchi, wheezing

Diagnostic Tests for Drowning		
Test	**Purpose**	**Abnormal Findings**
Noninvasive		
Pulse Oximetry	Continuous monitoring of oxygen saturation	$Sao_2 < 95\%$
Capnometry	Continuous monitoring of ventilation	Increased
Blood Studies		
Arterial Blood Gas Analysis	Assess for adequacy of oxygenation and ventilation	pH < 7.35 with increased $Paco_2$ (> 45 mm Hg) indicates respiratory acidosis. Serum bicarbonate < 22 mEq/L with a pH < 7.35 can indicate metabolic acidosis. Decreased Pao_2 indicates hypoxemia.
Complete Blood Count (CBC) WBC Count (WBCs)	Assess for inflammation and infection	WBCs may be elevated due to the inflammatory process that occurs following injury to the tissues and/or infection from exposure to dirty water.
Electrolytes, glucose	Assess for abnormalities due to water aspiration	Electrolyte changes are unusual, will depend on amount of water aspiration. Glucose level may be low.
BUN & Creatinine	Assess for renal function	Increased BUN and creatinine can indicate acute tubular necrosis from the severe hypoxemia that can accompany near drownings.
Toxicology screen	Determine the degree of alcohol and/or drug usage that can interfere with an accurate neurological assessment	Presence of high alcohol level or drug/ substance abuse

Continued

Drowning

Diagnostic Tests for Drowning — cont'd		
Test	**Purpose**	**Abnormal Findings**
Radiology		
Chest radiograph (CXR)	Assess lung fields	Presence of infiltrates, atelectasis, and pulmonary edema
Skull radiograph	Assess for fractures	Linear skull fracture, depressed skull fracture
Spinal radiographs	Assess for fractures	Fracture in any bony structure or misalignment of the spinal column
Head CT	Assess for head injury	Presence of blood in the brain matter or dural spaces indicates a head injury. Blurring of the gray and white matter indicates anoxic brain injury.

COLLABORATIVE MANAGEMENT
Care Priorities
The primary goal of treatment is to restore ventilation and correct hypoxemia and acidosis. Once ventilation is normal, hypoxemia and acidosis may resolve without further treatment; however, many patients, especially those submersed for more than a few minutes may require additional measures. The following treatments may be required:

1. **Provide oxygen therapy:** Oxygen (100%) is initiated immediately to treat hypoxia and is continued. All patients, including those who are alert with spontaneous ventilation, are at risk for hypoxia and acidosis. Warmed oxygen 40° to 43°C (104° to 109.4°F) may be used as part of the rewarming process for patients with hypothermia.
2. **Correct hypothermia with rewarming:** Warm, moist oxygen 40° to 43°C (104° to 109.4°F) may be used to elevate core temperature. Peritoneal lavage also is used for rewarming. Fluid for lavage is warmed to 37°C (98.6°F). The goal is quick rewarming to achieve a normal core temperature. Intravenous fluids should also be warmed to prevent further exacerbation of the hypothermia.
3. **Manage ventilation and acid-base balance:** Profound metabolic acidosis is treated with sodium bicarbonate, aggressive ventilation, and careful monitoring of arterial pH. If bronchospasm is present, aerosolized bronchodilators such as epinephrine, albuterol, or isoproterenol HCl may be used.
4. **Assess for need for endotracheal intubation and mechanical ventilation:** Intubation provides a patent airway for patients who are unable to manage secretions. Mechanical ventilation is used to manage respiratory failure due to reduced lung compliance, or if for any reason the patient is unable to maintain effective respiratory effort. Patients with freshwater aspiration require 1.5 to 2 times normal tidal volume at slower rates to allow optimal lung expansion and ventilation of alveoli.
5. **Initiate positive end-expiratory pressure (PEEP):** If the patient is unresponsive to high levels of oxygen ($Fio_2 \geq 0.50$ to maintain a $Pao_2 \geq 60$ mm Hg), PEEP improves oxygenation by preventing the collapse of alveoli during expiration. The pressure keeps alveoli open despite inadequate surfactant. PEEP should be removed cautiously, since levels of surfactant can remain low for 48 to 72 hours after freshwater aspiration.
6. **Consider bronchoscopy:** To remove aspirated contaminants, if necessary.
7. **Assess for the need of extracorporeal membrane oxygenation (ECMO):** ECMO, if available, may be useful when the patient is unable to maintain good oxygenation despite intubation and mechanical ventilation.
8. **Promote neurologic/brain recovery:** Depends on the severity of the neurologic impairment. Severe impairment may require ICP monitoring, steroids, osmotic diuretics (e.g., mannitol), mechanical ventilation, barbiturate coma, and deep hypothermia (core temperature less than 30°C).
9. **Manage fluid and electrolyte imbalance:** Although uncommon, fluid and electrolyte abnormalities may occur. Usually no specific therapy is required for minor disturbances. Fluid volume may be replaced with crystalloid solutions (LR or NS).

10. **Prevent and/or control infection:** Temperature elevation up to 38°C (100.4°F) during the first 24 hours can be a normal response to injury. Antibiotics may be prescribed if fever greater than 38°C (100.4°F) persists for longer than 24 hours after the submersion or the patient develops pneumonia. Use of steroids and prophylactic antibiotics is not recommended.

11. **Identify and manage the event that precipitated the drowning:** Conditions such as substance abuse, seizure, myocardial infarction, or cervical spine fracture.

CARE PLANS: DROWNING

Impaired gas exchange *related to asphyxiation and aspiration*

GOALS/OUTCOMES Within 12 hours of initiation of treatment, patient has adequate gas exchange as evidenced by the following ABG values: PaO_2 greater than 80 mm Hg and $PaCO_2$ less than 45 mm Hg. Within 3 days of treatment, respiratory rate is less than 20 breaths/min with normal depth and pattern; breath sounds are clear and bilaterally equal; and patient is oriented to time, place, and person (depending on degree of permanent neurologic impairment).

NOC Respiratory Status: Gas Exchange

Respiratory Monitoring
1. Monitor rate, rhythm, and depth of respirations.
2. Note chest movement for symmetry of chest expansion and signs of increased work of breathing such as use of accessory muscles or retraction of intercostal or supraclavicular muscles.
3. Auscultate breath sounds, noting areas of decrease/absent ventilation and presence of adventitious sounds.
4. Determine the need for suctioning by auscultating for crackles and rhonchi over major airways.
5. Monitor patient's respiratory secretions.
6. Note changes in oxygen saturation (SaO_2), pulse oximetry (SpO_2), end-tidal CO_2 ($ETCO_2$), and ABGs as appropriate.
7. Monitor for increased restlessness or anxiety.
8. If patient is restless or has unusual somnolence occur, evaluate for hypoxemia and hypercapnia as appropriate.
9. Monitor chest x-ray reports as new films become available.

Oxygen Therapy
1. Administer supplemental oxygen using liter flow and device as ordered.
2. Add humidity as appropriate.
3. Restrict patient and visitors from smoking while oxygen is in use.
4. Document pulse oximetry with oxygen liter flow in place at time of reading as ordered. Oxygen is a drug; the dose of the drug must be associated with the oxygen saturation reading or the reading is meaningless.
5. Obtain arterial blood gases if patient experiences behavioral changes or respiratory distress to check for hypoxemia or hypercapnia.
6. Monitor for changes in chest radiograph and breath sounds indicative of oxygen toxicity and absorption atelectasis in patients receiving higher concentrations of oxygen (greater than FiO_2 45%) for longer than 24 hours. The higher the oxygen concentration, the greater is the chance of toxicity.
7. Monitor for skin breakdown where oxygen devices are in contact with skin, such as nares and around edges of mask devices.
8. Provide oxygen therapy during transportation and when patient gets out of bed.

Mechanical Ventilation
1. Monitor for conditions indicating a need for ventilation support.
2. Monitor for impending respiratory failure or signs of pneumonia.
3. Consult with other health care personnel in selection of the ventilatory mode.
4. Administer muscle paralyzing agents, sedatives, and narcotics analgesics as appropriate.
5. Monitor for activities that increase oxygen consumption (fever, shivering, seizures, pain or basic nursing activities), which may supersede ventilator support settings and cause O_2 desaturation.
6. Monitor the effectiveness of mechanical ventilation on the patient's physiologic and psychological status.
7. Provide patient with means of communication, if he or she is alert.
8. Monitor adverse effects of mechanical ventilation.
9. Perform routine mouth care.
10. Elevate the head of the bed minimally at 30 degrees.

Hypothermia *related to immersion in cold water*

GOALS/OUTCOMES Within 24 hours of initiating therapy, patient's core temperature increases to 35° to 37°C (95° to 98.6°F). BP, respiratory rate, and HR are normalizing for patient.
NOC Thermoregulation

Hypothermia Treatment
1. Monitor patient's temperature using low-recording thermometer, if necessary.
2. Institute a continuous core temperature–monitoring device, as appropriate.
3. Monitor for and treat ventricular fibrillation.
4. Minimize stimulation of the patient to avoid precipitating ventricular fibrillation.
5. Institute active external rewarming measures (e.g., warming lights, warmed baths, warmed blankets, forced air warming blankets) as appropriate. Do not attempt surface or external warming until core temperature is within acceptable limits (i.e., 35° to 37°C [95° to 98.6°F]). Premature surface rewarming can lead to the return of cold blood to the heart and precipitate an "after-drop" in core temperature.
6. Institute active core rewarming techniques (e.g., colonic lavage, hemodialysis, peritoneal dialysis, and extracorporeal blood rewarming) as appropriate.
7. Monitor for rewarming shock.

Risk for infection *related to aspiration*

GOALS/OUTCOMES Patient is free of infection as evidenced by body temperature less than 37.5°C (99.5°F) after the first 24 hours, WBC count within normal limits for patient, clear sputum, and negative culture results.
NOC Infection Severity

Infection Protection
1. Monitor for signs and symptoms of infection (fever, changes in sputum).
2. Monitor absolute granulocyte count, WBC, and differential results.
3. Obtain cultures, as needed.
4. Encourage deep breathing and coughing, as appropriate.
5. Use aseptic technique when suctioning the patient.

ADDITIONAL NURSING DIAGNOSES
Also see *Posttrauma Syndrome* in *Major Trauma*, p. 245; See other nursing diagnoses and interventions and *Emotional and Spiritual Support of the Patient and Significant Others*, p. 200.

PELVIC FRACTURES
PATHOPHYSIOLOGY
The pelvis is composed of three bones: two innominate bones and the sacrum. The innominate bones are each composed of three bones (ilium, pubis, and ischium) that fuse after childhood. The two innominate bones are joined by the symphysis pubis, a fibrous cartilage joint that connects the two pubic bones anteriorly; they are attached posteriorly to a third bone, the sacrum, by a system of ligaments termed the *posterior osseous ligamentous* structures. Many blood vessels run through the pelvis and join to form the large venous plexus.

MVCs and auto-pedestrian trauma cause approximately two-thirds of all pelvic fractures, which have a mortality rate of up to 50% in some studies. A large force is needed for a pelvic fracture to occur, because these bones are stabilized by a strong network of ligaments. Pelvic fractures have been classified by several systems, but perhaps the most helpful are the systems that classify fractures by their stability and the mechanism of injury (Table 3-9). Pelvic fractures are considered stable fractures when the posterior osseous ligamentous structures are intact. An unstable pelvic fracture occurs when the osseous ligamentous structures are disrupted posteriorly and portions of the pelvis can move in any direction.

The most serious complications from a pelvic fracture are hemorrhage and exsanguination, which cause up to 60% of the deaths. The pelvis receives a rich supply of blood from a complex system of interconnected collateral arteries and the venous plexus of the iliac system, often called the vascular sink. The aorta and internal iliac artery are close to the pelvis. This

Table 3-9	CLASSIFICATION OF PELVIC FRACTURES	
Classification of Injury	**Mechanism of Injury**	**Description**
Anteroposterior compression	External rotation is caused by a crushing force on the posterior superior iliac spines.	"Open book injury"; the force causes the symphysis pubis to spring open. Rupture of anterior sacroiliac and sacrospinous ligaments occurs, but posterior ligaments are intact. Stable vertically but can rotate externally. May be associated with ruptured bladder (intraperitoneal) if injury occurs when bladder is full.
Lateral compression	Internal rotation from a high-energy injury that causes direct pressure to crush anterior sacrum. Pressure on the greater trochanter causes the femoral head to displace the anterior pubic rami.	Most common type of injury. Often does not affect posterior ligamentous complex. Partially unstable fracture that is rotationally unstable but vertically stable. May have extensive soft tissue injury. May be associated with ruptured bladder (extraperitoneal).
Vertical shear (Malgaigne fracture)	Excessive force from trauma such as falls and crush injuries in a vertical plane leads to unstable disruption of the anterior and posterior ring.	Most severe injury with the highest mortality rates. Very unstable. Complete disruption of the posterior osseous ligamentous system. Often accompanied by injuries of the skin and subcutaneous tissues or injuries to the gastrointestinal, genitourinary, vascular, and neurologic systems.
Complex fracture	Excessive and powerful forces from many directions.	Pelvic ring disruptions resulting in bizarre fractures or dislocations in a combination of injury patterns. Usually very unstable.

vascular network can easily be damaged or disrupted by the same forces that injure the pelvis. Pelvic fragments can damage vascular structures. The retroperitoneal space can hold as much as 4 L of blood before spontaneous tamponade occurs. Acute blood loss is difficult to identify until systemic symptoms, such as those occurring with shock, appear. In addition, damage to the sciatic and sacral nerves may occur with sacral and sacroiliac disruption.

The most common cause of pelvic fractures in older adults is falls, as opposed to MVCs in younger people. Older adults have more problems related to preexisting conditions. Cardiovascular disease often causes insufficient compensatory function to manage the stress of injury. Despite a less severe mechanism of injury, rates of sepsis and death are higher in older adults than in trauma patients younger than 65 years with similar injuries.

ASSESSMENT: PELVIC FRACTURES
Goal of System Assessment
Evaluate for stability of the pelvis and the probability of significant blood loss.

History and Risk Factors
Most common mechanisms of injuries are MVCs, motorcycle collisions, pedestrians struck by motor vehicles, and falls. Up to 15% of patients with a pelvic fracture have associated renal and lower urinary tract (LUT) injuries. Fifty percent of patients with both pelvic fractures and urologic injuries also have abdominal injuries.
    Risk factors include:
- Age
- Smoking
- History of bone disease including osteoporosis
- Prior hysterectomy
- Use of anticoagulants
- Concomitant injuries including intra-abdominal organ injuries and bladder and urethral injuries

Stable pelvic fracture
- Can withstand normal physiologic forces without abnormal deformation

Unstable pelvic fracture
- Fracture of the pelvic ring in more than one place that results in displacement

Vital Signs
- Temperature may be low if patient is developing shock.
- Respiratory rate may be elevated as a compensatory mechanism in hypovolemic shock.
- BP may be decreased in response to significant blood loss.
- HR will be increased with significant blood loss.

Observation
Evaluate for signs of trauma to the abdominal and pelvic regions.
- Groin, genitalia, and suprapubic swelling may be present.
- Lower extremity shortening and abnormal internal or external rotation of the leg
- Lacerations of the vagina, peritoneum, groin, or anus may indicate an open pelvic fracture.
- Blood at the meatus, signifying urethral trauma, which often accompanies pelvic fractures

Palpation
The pelvis is palpated by placing inward and posterior compression on the iliac crests.
- Assess for pain with palpation.
- Feeling of movement of the pelvic bones upon palpation
- Neurovascular status of the lower extremities should be checked.
- Palpate for pulses in lower extremities, femoral.
- Check for sensation bilaterally.

Diagnostic Tests for Pelvic Fractures		
Test	**Purpose**	**Abnormal Findings**
Blood Studies		
Complete blood count (CBC) Hemoglobin (Hgb) Hematocrit (Hct)	Assess for blood loss.	Decreased Hgb and Hct indicate blood loss. Often Hgb and Hct are within normal range initially, especially if the patient has not received a significant amount of fluid to replace the blood loss. The Hgb and Hct should be repeated after the patient has a fluid challenge if there is any indication of significant bleeding.
Coagulation profile Prothrombin time (PT) with international normalized ratio (INR) Partial thromboplastin time (PTT) Fibrinogen D-dimer	Assess for causes of bleeding, clotting, and disseminated intravascular coagulation (DIC) indicative of abnormal clotting present in shock or ensuing shock.	Decreased PT with low INR promotes clotting; elevation promotes bleeding; elevated fibrinogen and D-dimer reflect abnormal clotting.
Radiology		
Pelvic radiograph	Assess bony integrity of the pelvis.	Fractures that disrupt the pelvic ring
Pelvic CT scan	Assess bony integrity of the pelvis and presence of retroperitoneal hemorrhage.	Fractures within the pelvic ring, retroperitoneal bleeding

Diagnostic Tests for Pelvic Fractures — cont'd		
Test	Purpose	Abnormal Findings
Interventional Radiology		
Angiography	Indicted when the patient has evidence of hemodynamic instability with an ongoing need for blood transfusion where there is no evidence of other bleeding source besides the pelvic fracture. If contrast extravasation or a false aneurysm is identified, then embolization can be done. Angiography is current the gold standard for diagnosis of arterial bleeding secondary to pelvic fracture.	Extravasation of dye from torn blood vessels

COLLABORATIVE MANAGEMENT
Care Priorities
1. Stabilize the pelvis:

External immobilization: Defined as any device that is applied to immobilize the pelvis either externally or percutaneously through the skin into the bone. Noninvasive external fixation can be accomplished in several ways and can be applied at the scene of injury to preserve function and prevent further orthopedic and neurovascular injury. When an unstable pelvis is identified, the pelvis should be stabilized. Stabilization can be achieved with several methods including

- A sheet wrapped around the pelvis and secured with towel clips
- Commercially available devices such as the T-POD™, SAM Sling®, and PelvicBinder
- Internal rotation and taping the lower extremities, which is referred to as *IRTOTLE*

With all these methods, care should be taken to limit the amount of pressure and time the pressure is applied to prevent skin damage. Most of these devices/techniques should not be used for longer than 24 hours. These are temporary measures to limit the amount of hemorrhaging until more definite treatment can be initiated.

Invasive emergency external fixation device, consisting of one pin in each iliac wing connected by a bar, can be inserted to provide pelvic stability. If an emergency laparotomy is performed, more complex fixation devices may be applied.

If abnormal shortening or rotation has occurred with the injury, the lower extremities should be supported and stabilized in the position in which they were found. A wooden backboard supported by pillows, towels, or blankets taped in place with cloth tape are used until a traction splint can be applied.

> **Safety Alert**
> *Use of an external fixation device is not sufficient for maintaining reduction in the posterior pelvis or for stabilizing the pelvic posterior elements. As long as the patient is on bed rest or in traction, however, it can be used to manage the acute phase of the fracture.*

Internal immobilization: Surgical open reduction and immobilization of unstable pelvic ring disruptions with surgically implanted plates, screws, or other devices. Permanent fixation requires closed reduction for final pelvic stabilization.

2. **Initiate surgical exploration:** Done to identify blood vessels in need of ligation or repair for ongoing hemorrhage. Inflow of blood to the pelvic circulation can be limited by ligation of the internal iliac artery to control bleeding. Since many collateral vessels exist in the pelvic circulation, infarction rarely occurs with this procedure. Surgical exploration is not always recommended. When the peritoneal space is entered, the tamponade is released and bleeding can increase. The extensive vascular sink makes identification of bleeding vessels difficult. Some patients may undergo angiography and selective embolization of bleeding points with either an autologous blood clot or particulate gel foam instead of surgery.

Pelvic Fractures

3. **Replace blood loss with massive transfusion:** Patients who continue to exhibit signs of shock after receiving 2 L of crystalloids should receive blood transfusions. Blood replacement is best given according to established massive transfusion protocols (MTPs), which have been shown to decrease mortality by eliminating the deadly triad of acidosis, hypothermia, and coagulopathy. See Major Trauma, p. 235, for further discussion of MTPs. Some studies have supported withholding aggressive fluid resuscitation until after operative or embolic repair since an increase in MAP will increase intravascular hydrostatic pressure and may increase bleeding from torn vessels.

4. **Initiate pharmacotherapy for the following:**
   a. *Manage infection with antibiotics:* Initial use for prophylaxis against infection is controversial in patients with open fractures. Used later for positive cultures of wounds, blood, or urine.
   b. *Manage pain with analgesics:* IV morphine sulfate usually relieves pain and can be readily reversed with naloxone if hypotension or respiratory insufficiency is noted.
   c. *Control blood pressure with vasopressors:* For hypotension *only* after sufficient volume replacement has occurred (see Appendix 6).
   d. *Provide protection from disease with tetanus immunization:* Booster is given if history is unknown or if a booster is needed (see Table 3-1).

CARE PLANS: PELVIC FRACTURES

Decreased cardiac output *related to blood loss from severity of fracture(s) and/or concomitant injuries*

GOALS/OUTCOMES Within 24 hours of injury, patient demonstrates adequate perfusion as evidenced by the following ABG values: pH between 7.35 and 7.45 and base deficit level above -2.0 mmol/L, regular HR ≤100 bpm, bilaterally strong and equal peripheral pulses, warm and dry extremities, brisk (less than 2 seconds) capillary refill, systolic BP ≥90 mm Hg (or within 10% of patient's normal range), and urine output ≥0.5 ml/kg/hr. If hemodynamic monitoring is present, PAWP is ≥6 mm Hg and CI is ≥2.5 L/min/m^2. Patient is awake, alert, and oriented to time, place, and person without restlessness or confusion.

NOC Tissue Perfusion: Peripheral; Blood Loss Severity

Hemorrhage Control
1. Apply compression device or sheet to pelvic area or tape feet in an internal rotation position to align broken pelvis and decrease bleeding.
2. Note Hgb/Hct levels before and after blood loss.
3. Monitor trends in BP and hemodynamic parameters, if available (e.g., CVP and pulmonary capillary/artery wedge pressure).

Hypovolemia Management
1. Monitor fluid status on an hourly basis, including intake and output.
2. Maintain patent large-bore IV access.
3. Monitor coagulation studies, including INR, PT, PTT, fibrinogen, fibrin degradation/split products, and platelet counts, as appropriate.
4. Monitor the determinants of the adequacy of tissue oxygen delivery (e.g., pH and base deficit).
5. Prepare patient for definitive care of pelvis (e.g., angiography or surgery).
6. Ensure patient has current type and cross-match.
7. Administer blood and blood products, as appropriate. Always use a warming device to deliver large volumes of blood to prevent hypothermia.
8. Monitor for signs of impending renal failure (e.g., increased BUN and creatinine levels, myoglobinemia, and decreased urine output), as appropriate.

Risk for infection *related to impaired wound healing*

GOALS/OUTCOMES Within 24 hours after injury, soft tissues begin to heal without purulent drainage or erythema; WBC count is $\leq11,000$/mm^3; cultures of blood and wounds are negative; pin insertion sites, if present, are free of erythema, edema, or purulent drainage; and surgical wounds are well approximated and without erythema, edema, or purulent drainage.

NOC Wound Healing: Primary Intention; Wound Healing: Secondary Intention

Incision Site Care
1. Inspect the incision for redness, swelling, or signs of dehiscence.
2. Note the characteristics of any drainage.
3. Monitor the healing process at the incision site.
4. Change the dressing at appropriate intervals.
5. Perform pin care as prescribed. Current evidence does not support any one method of pin care.

Infection Prevention
1. Monitor for systemic and localized signs and symptoms of infection.
2. Monitor vulnerability to infection.
3. Monitor absolute granulocyte count, WBC, and differential results.
4. Promote sufficient nutritional intake.
5. Encourage rest.
6. Obtain cultures as needed.

 Impaired physical mobility *related to limitation in movement of pelvis needed to stabilize fracture with fixation device and other loss of joint movement or ability to ambulate independently*

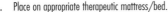

GOALS/OUTCOMES Patient will not develop complications of impaired mobility such as skin breakdown on any dependent areas or areas involved with fracture stabilization; venous thromboembolism; or constipation.
NOC Immobility Consequences: Physiological

Bed Rest Care
1. Place on appropriate therapeutic mattress/bed.
2. Keep bed linen clean, dry, and wrinkle free.
3. Apply devices to prevent foot drop, as needed.
4. Attach a trapeze bar to the bed, as appropriate.
5. Turn immobilized patients every 2 hours, according to a specific schedule.
6. Perform passive and active ROM exercises.
7. Apply antiembolism devices (e.g., stocking, sequential compression devices, foot pump).
8. Monitor for constipation, urinary function, and pulmonary status.

Positioning
1. Premedicate patient before turning as appropriate.
2. Position in proper body alignment.
3. Support the legs during turning to minimize movement of the pelvis.
4. Monitor fixation/traction devices for proper setup, and maintain position and integrity of traction when repositioning patient.
5. Minimize friction and shearing forces when positioning and turning the patient.
6. Place call light within reach.
7. Place frequently used items within reach.

RENAL AND LOWER URINARY TRACT TRAUMA

PATHOPHYSIOLOGY

The genitourinary tract is divided into upper and lower tracts. The upper tract consists of the kidney and the ureters, and the LUT involves the external genitalia, urethra, and bladder.

Injuries to the genitourinary tract occur in approximately 10% of patients with injuries severe enough for admission to a trauma service. Approximately 80% of these injuries are the result of blunt trauma. Common causes include MVCs, falls from heights, and blows to the torso or external genitalia. Pelvic fractures are most commonly associated with injury to the female genital tract.

These injuries are often overlooked in the initial trauma assessment because they frequently accompany life-threatening injuries that require aggressive and immediate management.

Genitourinary tract injury is rarely life threatening. However, shattered kidney, major renal vascular laceration with hemorrhage or renal artery dissection, or pedicle avulsion usually is the result of a significant deceleration injury that may be life threatening or a threat to the kidney itself. These can be seen as the result of a high-speed MVC or a fall from a significant height.

Renal and LUT trauma can occur with penetrating injuries (stab and gunshot wounds). Other mechanisms of injury include physical or sexual assault and consensual intercourse. Injury to the vulva is uncommon and should alert one for prompt screening for interpersonal violence. Penile injury is also uncommon, which results from rupture of the tunica albuginea with concomitant urethral injury in about 20% of patients. Urethral disruption is seen with pelvic fracture in about 5% of women and 25% of men. Pathophysiology for renal and LUT trauma is shown in Table 3-10.

Urethral injury may cause males long-term problems with sexual intercourse and voiding. Sexual dysfunction may be the result of damage to neural and vascular structures. Incontinence may result from damage to the sphincters or their innervations. In patients with complete urethral disruption, approximately 20% have voiding dysfunction and 25% have sexual dysfunction.

RENAL AND LOWER URINARY TRACT ASSESSMENT
Goal of System Assessment
Identify specific location of physical injuries and presence of signs and symptoms indicating injury to organs affected by the renal system or surrounding organs.

History and Risk Factors
- Ask about allergies, current medications, preexisting medical conditions, and factors surrounding the injury.
- Patients with preexisting renal diseases such as polycystic kidney disease and pyelonephritis are at higher risk for renal injury.
- Ask about any suprapubic tenderness.
- Ask about inability to void spontaneously or any past bloody urine.
- Ask about flank pain, pain at the costovertebral angle, back tenderness, and colicky pain with the passage of blood clots.

Observation and Subjective Symptoms
- **Renal trauma:** Abdominal or flank pain, back tenderness, colicky pain with passage of blood clots, pallor, diaphoresis, gross hematuria, restlessness, confusion, obvious wounds, contusions, or abrasions in the flank or abdomen; abdominal distention; *Grey-Turner* sign (bruising over the lower portion of the back and the flank caused by a retroperitoneal hemorrhage); pain at the costovertebral angle

---

HIGH ALERT!   Gross hematuria is present in only slightly more than half of patients with renal trauma and is considered an unreliable diagnostic sign.

- **Ureter trauma:** Gross hematuria may be present; if the ureter is transected, normal urine from the unaffected kidney may still be voided. Late signs may include fever and flank or abdominal discomfort. Urine may be found at the entrance or exit sites of penetrating wound.
- **Bladder trauma:** Inability to void spontaneously, gross hematuria (present in approximately 95% of patients), and abdominal discomfort. Perineal or scrotal edema and hematoma, abnormal position of prostate, abdominal distention, palpable suprapubic mass, palpable and overdistended bladder.
- **Uretheral trauma:** Blood at the meatus, inability to void spontaneously, urethral bleeding, prostate tenderness, microscopic or gross hematuria, pain and tenderness of genitalia, and perineal hematoma. Tracking of urine into tissues of the thighs or abdominal wall, bruised to discolored genitalia.

HIGH ALERT!   Physical signs may be masked because the kidneys are located beneath abdominal organs, back muscles, and bony structures.

Table 3-10	PATHOPHYSIOLOGY FOR RENAL AND LOWER URINARY TRACT TRAUMA		
Type of Injury	Anatomic Considerations	Pathophysiology and Mechanism of Injury	Result of Injury
Renal trauma	Kidneys are well protected from injury posteriorly by muscles of the back, anteriorly by organs of the gastrointestinal tract, and by a tough outer capsule and adipose tissue. Kidneys are fixed in retroperitoneal space only by renal pedicle (vascular system in renal helium) and ureters Blunt renal injury is often caused by compression of kidney by the twelfth rib, which rotates inwardly and squeezes kidney into lumbar spine.	Renal trauma can be divided into three classifications: **Minor trauma:** Incidence 85% Bruising of renal parenchyma; superficial lacerations of renal cortex without rupture of renal capsule **Major trauma:** Incidence 10%—15% Major lacerations through cortex and medulla; continuation of laceration through renal capsule **Critical trauma:** Incidence <5% Renal vascular trauma in which kidney is shattered and renal pedicle is injured; fragmentation (renal fracture)	**Minor trauma:** Hematuria and flank tenderness that will usually result in a full recovery with rest and observation **Major trauma:** Hematuria, flank pain, and possible hypotension that may require surgical intervention **Critical injury:** Severe blood loss and shock requiring immediate surgical intervention
Ureteral trauma	Injury to upper part of ureter is uncommon because of its location deep in retroperitoneum. Ureteral lacerations are most common at ureteropelvic junction, where upper ureter joins renal pelvis.	Ureteral injury is most commonly associated with iatrogenic injuries during gynecologic, colonic, and vascular surgery. Blunt injury may occur when ureter becomes crushed against spinal column. When ureteral injury is not associated with iatrogenic injury, it usually occurs in the setting of severe abdominal compression or significant penetrating abdominal injury.	Extravasation of urine or blood may lead to infection, abscess formation, hemorrhage, or shock; late complications include prolonged voiding time, ureteral strictures, and fistula formation.
Bladder trauma	When bladder is distended, it extends above umbilicus and has less protection from trauma; the bladder ruptures at its point of least resistance (the dome), and blood and urine extravasate into the peritoneal cavity (intraperitoneal rupture). Extraperitoneal rupture occurs most often in conjunction with pelvic fractures; sharp bone fragments perforate bladder at its base, leading to extravasation of blood and urine into space surrounding bladder base.	Motor vehicle crashes are the most common cause of bladder rupture; bladder contusion often results from a direct blow or the cavitational effect of missiles (outward tissue acceleration away from the tract of the bullet); bladder rupture does not require extensive force, which may be a blunt blow to the lower abdomen.	Bladder lacerations or rupture can lead to blood or urine extravasation outside of the peritoneal cavity (80%) and into the peritoneal cavity (20%); infection or hemorrhage can follow.
Urethral trauma	Urethral injury is more common in males than in females because the male urethra is 5 times longer; the male urethra is also rigidly fixed at the urogenital diaphragm (bulbous urethra), whereas the female urethra is short and mobile.	Perineal trauma, straddle injuries, and pelvic fractures are often the causes of urethral injury; vehicular collisions with deceleration and shearing may also lead to injury of the posterior urethra.	Urethral injury may lead to extravasation of blood and/or urine within penis; if disruption to Buck's fascia occurs, extravasation into upper thighs and peritoneum follows; hemorrhage or infection may also occur.

Vital Signs
- Hypotension
- Tachycardia
- Bladder trauma: Late signs may include fever.

Palpation
- Flank or abdominal mass
- Bladder trauma: suprapubic tenderness
- Renal trauma: hematoma over the flank of the eleventh or twelfth ribs
- Ureter trauma: enlarging retroperitoneal mass

Inspection
- Digital rectal examination to check for rectal tone, gross blood, and the position of the prostate. Posterior urethral disruption may result in a "high riding" prostate in males.
- A meticulous vaginal examination should be performed in all women with pelvic fractures to assess for bone fragments or lacerations that could result in hemorrhage and infection.

Diagnostic Tests for Renal and Lower Urinary Tract Trauma		
Test	**Purpose**	**Abnormal Findings**
Urinalysis	To rule out blood in urine; cloudiness, odor	Hematuria; sediment, malodor
Urine culture and sensitivity	Rule out infection or injury	Urethral injury: microscopic ($>3–5$ RBCs/HPF); presence of microorganisms
Imaging		
Safety Alert *Check patient's history for allergy to iodine, iodine-containing foods, or contrast material. Hydration and sometimes diuretics are needed to facilitate excretion of contrast material after testing. Evaluate blood urea nitrogen/creatinine level before use of dye to determine renal functioning.*		
CT scan	CT is the method of choice to assess patients with severe renal trauma.	May reveal hematomas, renal lacerations, renal infarcts, or extravasation of urine. Contrast-enhanced CT detects kidney laceration and arterial occlusion. Delay images are necessary to assess for extravasation of contrast and determination of injury.
Retrograde urethrogram	Diagnose urethral tears or rupture. A small urinary catheter is inserted, and the balloon is inflated in the distal anterior urethra. Contrast material is injected, and a single radiograph film is taken to outline the inner size and shape of the urethra.	In urethral rupture, extravasation of the contrast material occurs. With a partial disruption, extravasation is accompanied by contrast appearing in the bladder. Contrast does not appear in the bladder with complete disruption. This procedure is deferred, however, if there is an indication for pelvic angiography.
Cystogram	If no urethral tear is found on retrograde urethrogram, a catheter is inserted into the bladder. The bladder is filled with 400 ml of contrast material. It is important to fill the bladder to the point of contraction and then forcefully instill another 50 ml of contrast. It is necessary to distend the bladder adequately to ensure extravasation and a meaningful study.	If intraperitoneal or extraperitoneal extravasation of contrast material occurs, the bladder is drained and repeat radiographs are taken to check for small posterior ruptures.

Diagnostic Tests for Renal and Lower Urinary Tract Trauma —cont'd		
Test	**Purpose**	**Abnormal Findings**
CT cystography	Assess for bladder injuries.	Abnormal filling of bladder
Excretory urogram/ intravenous pyelogram (IVP)	Visualize the normal or injured structures of the kidneys, ureters, or bladder. This study has been supplanted with the use of CT imaging. It may, however, be used and is useful in instances when there is a suspected urethral injury and delayed CT images prove nondiagnostic.	Abnormal passage of contrast through the structures of the urinary system
Renal ultrasound	The test is rarely used for early identification of injury because it is too imprecise. The ultrasound is not sensitive enough for diagnosis and exclusion of a significant renal injury.	
Radionuclide imaging	Evaluates for injured lower urinary tract structures and alterations in renal blood flow. After IV injection of a radionuclide, a radioactivity-detecting device scans and records the radioactive uptake. The substance is excreted in 6–24 hr following the test.	Injury to structures of the urinary tract
Kidney-ureter-bladder (KUB) radiography	Evaluates position, size, structure, and defects of the urinary tract	May reveal foreign bodies, retroperitoneal hematoma, fracture of the lower ribs or pelvis, organ displacement, or fluid accumulation
Renal angiography	Arterial injection of a contrast medium, permitting identification on radiograph film of renal vasculature and functional tissue. Identification of any renal injury.	Renal pedicle injury, renal infarct, intrarenal hematoma, lacerations, and shattered kidney
MRI	Used to identify the best surgical approach for more difficult injuries, such as traumatic posterior urethral injury. Identifies severity of injury and may help estimate time needed for recovery.	Localized injury to specific organ or surrounding structures

Blood Studies

HIGH ALERT! If an intraperitoneal bladder rupture has occurred, hyperkalemia, hypernatremia, uremia, and acidosis may occur as a result of reabsorption of urine from the peritoneal cavity.

Hemoglobin, hematocrit	Evaluate for low level or trend.	Below normal level may indicate bleeding, hemorrhage, and should lead to further examination for hematuria or other areas of potential internal hemorrhage.
Blood urea nitrogen (BUN)	Evaluate for elevation denoting level of effect.	Renal dysfunction causes insufficient excretion of urea, elevating nitrogenous wastes in the blood. In renal trauma, BUN level may increase because of body catabolism, dehydration, or from absorption of peritoneal extravasation of urine. When the BUN is elevated as a result of urine absorption, the serum creatinine levels remain normal. Normal BUN is 10–20 mg/dl.

Continued

Diagnostic Tests for Renal and Lower Urinary Tract Trauma — cont'd		
Test	**Purpose**	**Abnormal Findings**
Serum creatinine	Most accurate measure of renal damage	Renal impairment is virtually the only cause of elevated serum creatinine. Creatinine production is fairly constant, since production is proportional to muscle mass. Creatinine is freely filtered at the glomerulus and minimally resorbed, so creatinine excretion is proportional to glomerular filtration rate. Normal value is 0.7–1.5 mg/dl.
Clearance tests	Clearance is the volume of plasma that can be cleared of a specific substance during a specified period of time. Clearance tests evaluate the extent of injury by assessing renal filtration, reabsorption, secretion, and renal plasma flow. Creatinine, inulin (a plant starch), and urea may be tested.	Currently most laboratories will provide an estimated glomerular filtration rate (eGFR) determination in addition to other renal function parameters. This provides a more practical estimation of clearance for the clinician.

COLLABORATIVE MANAGEMENT
Care Priorities

1. Identify and manage bleeding complications, including hypovolemic or hemorrhagic shock.
   - *Hemorrhage shock:* Volume resuscitation with crystalloids, colloids, or blood products as indicated.
2. Manage pain.
   - *Analgesics:* IV morphine sulfate is used to relieve pain and is easily reversed with naloxone if hypotension or respiratory depression is noted. Phenazopyridine (Pyridium) as a urinary analgesic to relieve burning and frequency.
3. Prevent and/or manage infection.
   - *Antibiotics:* Initiate for positive urine culture results, penetrating injuries, or peritonitis.
   - *Infections:* As indicated, obtain blood and urine cultures and initiate appropriate antibiotics and other infection control measures.
4. Support renal function.
   - *Renal dysfunction:* Fluid restriction; dietary restrictions for renal impairment; peritoneal dialysis (not treatment of choice for those with abdominal trauma and those who are hemodynamically unstable); continuous renal replacement therapy; or hemodialysis. See *Acute Renal Failure*, p. 584, for more information.

> **Safety Alert** *If renal function is impaired, may need to adjust dosages of medications metabolized through the renal system.*

---

 5. Manage urinary elimination without causing further injury.
Catheterization:
   - *If patient is unable to void:* Catheter should be passed only as far as it will progress without undue force. If any resistance is met during catheterization, a urethrogram is indicated.
   - *If blood is present at the urethral meatus:* The patient should not be catheterized until a urethrogram is obtained, since the blood may signal urethral injury. In the presence of urethral injury, an improperly placed catheter can cause subsequent incontinence, impotence, and urethral strictures.
     - *Urethral trauma:* A suprapubic catheter may be used to manage severe urethral lacerations and urethral disruption.

- *Renal trauma:* Diversion of urine may be required by nephrostomy tube, depending on location of injury or in cases of coexisting pancreatic and duodenal injury.
- *Ureteral trauma:* Internal ureteral catheters (ureteral stents) may be indicated for ureteral trauma, particularly for gunshot wounds, to maintain ureteral alignment, ensure urinary drainage, and provide support during anastomosis.

6. **Facilitate a timely surgical intervention.**
   - *Surgical correction:* Indicated for transected ureter, partial ureteral tears of more than a third of the circumference of the ureter, bladder perforation with associated abdominal injuries or intraperitoneal rupture, and injuries accompanied by rapidly expanding, pulsating hematomas. See Table 3-11 for examples of procedures for the various types of renal and LUT injuries.
   - *In the incidence of multiple trauma:* The collaboration of the trauma surgeon and the urologist is paramount in the effort to decrease morbidity and mortality.
   - *Organ Injury Scale:* The American Association for the Surgery of Trauma Organ Injury (AAST) has developed an Organ Injury Scale of solid organs including the kidney. This scale was designed to provide a system to describe injuries by a common nomenclature and severity of injury. The severity score for the kidney is described in Table 3-12.

CARE PLANS: RENAL AND LOWER URINARY TRACT TRAUMA

Impaired urinary elimination *related to mechanical trauma secondary to injury to the kidney and lower urinary tract structures*

GOALS/OUTCOMES Within 6 hours after immediate trauma management, patient has a urinary output of ≥0.5 ml/kg/hr with no evidence of bladder distention.
NOC Urinary Elimination

Urinary Elimination Management
1. Monitor urinary outflow. Encourage patient to void. If patient is unable to void, assess for full bladder. Urinary catheterization or suprapubic drainage may be needed. Report findings to the physician. Monitor for the following signs of kidney or LUT trauma:
- Urge but inability to void spontaneously despite adequate volume replacement
- Blood at the urethral meatus
- Difficult or unsuccessful urinary catheterization
- Anuria after urinary catheterization
- Hematuria

Table 3-11	SURGICAL PROCEDURES FOR RENAL AND LOWER URINARY TRACT TRAUMA
Type of Injury	**Surgical Indications/Surgical Management**
Minor renal trauma	None needed. Rest and observation with careful follow-up to prevent progressive deformity and to evaluate blood pressure
Major renal trauma	Surgical intervention if hypotension and hemodynamic instability occur
Critical renal trauma	Immediate surgical exploration; low rates of renal salvage
Proximal ureteral injury	Primary ureterostomy with end-to-end anastomosis
Distal ureteral injury	Ureteral stenting or percutaneous nephrostomy, depending on location and extent of injury
Bladder injury	Use of suprapubic drainage versus indwelling urethral catheter drainage is controversial. Use of suprapubic catheter avoids complications of prolonged urethral catheterization, particularly in males who are prone to the development of urethral strictures.
Urethral injury	Suprapubic cystostomy and drainage for temporary urinary evacuation. Urethral splinting and surgical reconstruction usually are delayed for 3–6 mo to allow reduction in bruising and swelling, which could delay healing of urinary structures.

Table 3-12	AAST TRAUMA ORGAN INJURY SEVERITY SCORE FOR THE KIDNEY	
Grade	Type	Description
1	Contusion or subcapsular hematoma nonexpanding and without parenchymal laceration	Gross hematuria and normal urologic studies. Hematoma without expansion
2	Perirenal hematoma without expansion or laceration to renal cortex without extravasation of urine	Hematoma confined to the retroperitoneum. Depth of laceration <1.0 cm. No extravasation
3	Laceration of renal cortex without urinary extravasation	Depth of renal cortex laceration >1.0 cm without rupture of the collection system or urinary extravasation
4	Laceration of the renal cortex extending into the collecting system or the renal vasculature	Laceration extending through the cortex, medulla, and collections system with urine extravasation. Vascular injury to the main renal artery or vein with contained hemorrhage
5	Shattered kidney, renal pedicle avulsion, or main renal artery thrombosis	Completely shattered kidney Renal hilum avulsion that devascularizes the kidney

2. Do not catheterize patient if there is blood at the urethral meatus. Call physician or mid level practitioner for consultation if urethral injury is suspected.
3. Monitor serum BUN and creatinine.
4. Document input and ouput hourly. Consult physician if urine output is less than 0.5 ml/kg/hr.
5. Assess whether clots may be occluding the drainage system. If indicated, obtain prescription for catheter irrigation or call physician to irrigate catheter. Sudden cessation of urine flow through the collection system (particularly if past output was greater than 50 ml/hr) indicates possible catheter obstruction. If catheter irrigation does not resume urine drainage, consider changing the urinary catheter after discussion with physician.
6. Ensure nephrostomy tubes are not occluded by patient's weight or external pressure. Irrigate the nephrostomy tube *only* if prescribed with ≤5 ml of fluid. The renal pelvis holds less than 10 ml of fluid.
7. Assess entrance site of the nephrostomy tube for bleeding or leakage of urine. Catheter blockage or dislodging causes a sudden decrease in urine output. Inspect urine color and for blood clots. Hematuria is normal for 24 to 48 hours after nephrostomy tube insertion. Consult physician if gross bleeding (with or without clots) occurs.
8. Hydrate to allow for clearing of contrast material from patient's system after diagnostic testing.

NIC Urinary Catheterization; Fluid Management; Fluid Monitoring; Tube Care: Urinary

Risk for infection *related to inadequate primary defenses and tissue destruction secondary to bacterial contamination of the urinary tract system occurring with penetrating trauma, rupture of the bladder into the perineum, or instrumentation*

GOALS/OUTCOMES Patient is free of infection as evidenced by normothermia, WBC count ≤11,000/mm³, and negative results of urine and wound drainage testing for infective organisms.
NOC Immune Status; Risk Control

Infection Protection
1. Use aseptic technique when caring for drainage systems. Keep catheters and collection container at a level lower than the bladder to prevent reflux; ensure that drainage tubing is not kinked.
2. Record the color and odor of urine each shift. Culture urine specimen when infection is suspected.
3. Monitor patient's WBC count daily and temperature every 4 hours for elevations.
4. Assess for signs of peritonitis: abdominal pain, abdominal distention with rigidity, nausea, vomiting, fever, malaise, and weakness.

5. Assess catheter exit site each shift for the presence of erythema, swelling, or drainage.
6. Assess thigh, groin, and lower portion of abdomen for indicators of urinary extravasation: swelling, pain, mass(es), erythema, and tracking of urine along fascial planes.
7. Assess surgical incision for approximation of suture line and evidence of wound healing, noting presence of erythema, swelling, and drainage. Note color, odor, and consistency of drainage. Notify physician of purulent or foul-smelling drainage. Consider obtaining a culture.
8. Assess skin at invasive sites for indicators of irritation: erythema, drainage, and swelling.
9. Cleanse catheter insertion sites with antimicrobial solution. Manage catheter exit sites per protocol.
10. Consider dressing changes every 24 hours or as soon as noted they are wet. If skin is irritated from contact with urine, consider use of a pectin wafer skin barrier for extra protection.

NIC Incision Site Care; Wound Care; Infection Control; Surveillance; Tube Care: Urinary

Acute pain (acute tenderness in lower abdomen) *related to physical injury associated with LUT structural injury, procedures for urinary diversion, or surgical incisions*

GOALS/OUTCOMES: Within 2 hours after giving analgesic agent, patient's subjective evaluation of discomfort improves, as documented by a pain scale. Nonverbal indicators of discomfort, such as grimacing, are absent.
NOC Pain Control; Comfort Level

Pain Management
1. Assess patient for pain at least every 4 hours.
2. Be alert to shallow breathing in the presence of abdominal pain, which can cause inadequate pulmonary excursion. Medicate promptly, and document patient's response to analgesic agent, using the appropriate pain scale. IV narcotics may be indicated if the injury is severe.
3. Explain the cause of the pain to the patient.
4. Assist patient into a position of comfort. Often knee flexion will relax lower abdominal muscles and help reduce discomfort.
5. Implement nonpharmacologic measures for coping with pain: diversion, touch, and conversation.

NIC Analgesic Administration; Positioning; Presence

THORACIC TRAUMA

PATHOPHYSIOLOGY

Thoracic trauma may be caused by blunt or penetrating injuries to the chest, back, flanks, and upper abdomen region. The thoracic cavity contains many vital organs, and thoracic trauma accounts for 25% of all trauma-related deaths. Careful assessment is needed to quickly identify life-threatening injuries to the heart, lungs, and great vessels. Close monitoring is required to prevent complications secondary to injuries that develop over the first 24 hours, such as pulmonary contusions.

Thoracic injuries can result from both direct and indirect forces. Direct force such as direct impact involving an object can result in bony fractures, tissue bruising, and ruptured organs. Indirect forces can cause tissues to stretch beyond their limits and can result in tears leading to rupture of blood vessels and disruption of organs, such as the bronchus and esophagus. Thoracic injuries often lead to problems with ventilation, oxygenation, and perfusion, causing a decrease in the delivery of oxygen and nutrients to the tissues.

The lungs are often affected by space occupying lesions, such as hemothoraces, pneumothoraces, and hemopneumothoraces, which compress lung tissue, interfering with lung expansion, thereby limiting the amount of ventilation and decreasing oxygen exchange at the alveoli level. The most serious of these is a tension pneumothorax where the pressure in the chest is so high that not only is oxygenation impaired, but the venous return to the heart is diminished, leading to decreased cardiac output and shock.

One of the most common thoracic injuries is contusions to the lungs. When the lung tissue is bruised, alveolar hemorrhage and parenchymal destruction occur leading to both local and systemic consequences. The reduced compliance impairs ventilation and causes an increase in shunting with decreased pulmonary blood flow. Hypoxemia and hypercarbia develop and are usually worst at 72 hours.

Blunt thoracic trauma can cause injury to the heart muscle by one or more of the following four mechanisms: compression of the heart between the sternum and vertebrae, bruising of heart tissue by bony structures, rupture or compression of coronary arteries by the blow, or cardiac rupture caused by intrathoracic or intra-abdominal pressure. Causes of blunt cardiac injury (BCI) are MVCs, direct blows to the chest, falls from great heights, sporting and industrial injuries, and kicks from animals. There are no reliable diagnostic tests to identify BCI. Cardiac injury is considered significant when the patient has new findings, such as new dysrhythmias, abnormal cardiac wall motion, or injury to the heart.

Penetrating thoracic trauma is caused by gunshot wounds, stab wounds, or foreign bodies entering the chest or upper abdomen. Open chest injuries can result in an open pneumothorax or lacerations to the lung tissue or the airways, heart, great vessels, and/or the esophagus. Penetrating injuries to the heart are the most common cause of intrapericardial hemorrhage.

ASSESSMENT: THORACIC TRAUMA
Goal of System Assessment
Evaluate for traumatic injuries of the heart, lung, great vessels, and bony thorax.

History and Risk Factors
Age, smoking history, mechanism of injury; chronic lung disease

Vital Signs
- Respiratory rate may be increased if hypoxia is present.
- BP may be decreased.
- HR may increase due to the hypoxia or hemorrhage.

Observation
Check chest for signs of trauma and chest excursion.
- Bruising, abrasions, contusions, and lacerations indicate the thoracic area of the body received some of the force.
- Carefully observe chest wall for signs of penetrating injuries since the skin may close up, masking the entry, especially with low-velocity injuries such as stabbings.
- Logroll the patient to inspect the back of the chest.
- Observe position of the trachea.
- Observe for neck vein distention.

Percussion
- Over the lung fields to identify areas of hyperresonance indicating a collection of air in the pleural space or dullness, which may indicate a collection of blood in the pleural space or atelectasis

Palpation
- Over the ribs, sternum, and scapula to identify areas of tenderness and step-offs
- Feel chest for crepitus.

Auscultation
- Lung fields to identify abnormal breath sounds
- Decreased breath sounds may indicate a pneumothorax or hemothorax.
- Sucking sound on inspiration may indicate an open pneumothorax.
- Heart to identify abnormal heart sounds
- Muffled heart sounds may indicate a pericardial tamponade.

The Nurse and Interdisciplinary Team Are Assessing for the Following Common Problems:
Pneumothorax/Tension Pneumothorax
- Chest pain
- Respiratory distress
- Decreased chest wall excursion

- Hypoxia
- Decreased breath sounds on the affected side
- Tachycardia
- Additionally, with a tension pneumothorax, tracheal deviation, jugular vein distention, hypotension, and cyanosis (late sign) may be present.

Hemothorax
- Chest pain
- Respiratory distress
- Decreased breath sounds on the affected side
- Signs/symptoms of blood loss up to and including shock

Flail Chest
- Paradoxical chest wall movement
- Pain over affected chest wall on palpation
- Hypoxia
- Decreased chest excursion due to pain
- Decreased breath sounds

Pulmonary Contusion
- Hypoxia
- Respiratory distress

Blunt Cardiac Injury
- Arrhythmias

Aortic Trauma
- Hypo/hypertension
- Tachycardia
- Unequal pulses, absent pulses below the level of injury
- Mottling below the level of injury

Diagnostic Tests for Thoracic Trauma		
Test	**Purpose**	**Abnormal Findings**
Non invasive		
Pulse oximetry	Continuous monitoring of oxygen saturation	$Sao_2 < 95\%$
Capnometry	Continuous monitoring of ventilation	Increased
Electrocardiogram (ECG)	Assess for dysrhythmias, which can occur from blunt cardiac injury.	The most common findings with blunt cardiac injury: Multiple premature ventricular contractions Unexplained sinus tachycardia Atrial fibrillation Bundle branch block, usually on the right ST-segment changes
Blood Studies		
Arterial blood gas analysis	Assess for adequacy of oxygenation and ventilation.	$pH < 7.35$ with increased $Paco_2$ indicates respiratory acidosis. Decreased Pao_2 indicates hypoxemia. Increasing base deficit indicates inadequate delivery of oxygen to the tissues and an increase in anaerobic metabolism.
Serial cardiac enzymes Myoglobin CK-MB isoform CK-MB Troponin I Troponin T	Assess for enzyme changes indicative of myocardial tissue damage.	Elevated enzymes reflect muscle damage; if CK-MB and troponins are elevated, the patient may have suffered an acute myocardial infarction. Not useful in diagnosing blunt cardiac injury

Continued

Diagnostic Tests for Thoracic Trauma — cont'd		
Test	**Purpose**	**Abnormal Findings**
Complete blood count (CBC) Hemoglobin (Hgb) Hematocrit (Hct) WBC count (WBCs)	Assess for blood loss, inflammation, and infection.	Decreased Hgb and Hct reflect amount of blood loss. WBCs will be elevated due to the inflammatory process that occurs following injury to the tissues.
Radiology		
Chest radiograph (CXR)	Assess thoracic cage for fractures, pleural space for the presence of air or fluids, size of heart, thoracic aorta and diaphragm, or displacement of organs, structures.	Displaced lung margins indicate a pneumothorax or hemothorax. Cardiac enlargement reflects possible cardiac tamponade. Widened mediastinum and blurring of the aortic knob indicate possible aortic injury. Deviation of the trachea could indicate tension pneumothorax or aortic injury. Intestinal gas pattern in chest may indicate a ruptured diaphragm. Irregular, nonlobular opacifications in the pulmonary parenchyma indicate pulmonary contusions but are not usually seen on CXR for the first 24 hr.
Computed tomography Thoracic CT scan CT angiography (CTA)	Assess pulmonary and vascular structures for damage.	Air or blood in the pleural space (pneumothorax or hemothorax) Mediastinal hematoma on CTA can indicate an aortic injury.
Ultrasound echocardiography (ECHO)	Assess for mechanical abnormalities related to effective pumping of blood and for collection of fluid in the pericardial sac.	Abnormal ventricular wall movement or motion, low ejection fraction, damaged valves, collection of fluid in the pericardial sac
Transesophageal ECHO (TEE)	Assess for mechanical abnormalities related to effective pumping of blood from both sides of the heart using a transducer attached to the endoscope.	Same as above but can provide enhanced views, particularly of the posterior wall of the heart
Aortogram	Useful as an adjunct to spiral CT in diagnosing thoracic aorta injuries; may be able to delineate the exact location and extent of the injury	Hematoma formation and extravasation of fluid around the aorta indicate injury.
Flexible or rigid esophagoscopy	To identify esophageal injuries	Laceration or bruising to the esophageal wall
Flexible or rigid bronchoscopy	To identify tracheobronchial injuries	Tear in the wall of the trachea or bronchus

COLLABORATIVE MANAGEMENT

Collaborative management should start with addressing the ABCs as outlined in Major Trauma including oxygen, IV fluids, and blood as indicated. During the initial assessment, several conditions involving injuries to the thoracic organs may warrant immediate intervention. These include the following:

- Open pneumothorax
- Tension pneumothorax

- Massive hemothorax
- Flail chest
- Cardiac tamponade
- Torn aorta or great vessels

Care Priorities

With pulmonary injuries, interventions are directed toward managing acute respiratory compromise while correcting the underlying injuries that may cause deterioration in the patient's condition. Intervention should be aimed at correcting and preventing hypoxia. With cardiac and great vessel injuries, the care priorities are focused on stopping hemorrhage, restoring perfusion, and supporting cardiac function.

1. **Ensure patent airway.**
   - When the patient is unable to maintain a patent airway either due to trauma or a decreased level of consciousness, an artificial airway is inserted through oral intubation or via emergent tracheostomy.
   - *Intubation:* Maintains patent airway, decreases airway resistance and respiratory effort, provides route for easy removal of airway secretions, and allows for manual or mechanical ventilation, as necessary.
2. **Restore intrathoracic negative pressure.**
   - Interventions are aimed at restoring the negative pressure in the thoracic cavity to allow for adequate ventilation.
   - *Pleural decompression:* Relieves life-threatening tension pneumothorax. A 14-gauge needle or IV catheter is inserted into the second intercostal space at the midclavicular line to relieve the pressure in the chest cavity.

Safety Alert *If a tension pneumothorax is suspected, pleural decompression should not be delayed for a confirmation chest radiograph.*

   - *Tube thoracostomy:* Chest tubes are used to remove fluid or trapped air from the chest cavity as in a hemothorax or pneumothorax. A thoracic catheter is inserted, usually through the second intercostal space, the midclavicular line, or the fifth lateral intercostal space, midaxillary line. Placement depends on the location and extent of the hemothorax, effusion, or pneumothorax. The catheter can be connected to a one-way flutter valve (for air evacuation only) or to a closed chest drainage system. Tension pneumothorax is a life-threatening emergency requiring pleural decompression.
3. **Enhance oxygenation and ventilation.**

   - *Oxygen therapy:* Device is determined by patient's response to therapy and may range from nasal cannula to 100% nonrebreathing mask, depending on extent of hypoxemia.
   - *Pulmonary toileting:* Use of incentive spirometer, chest percussion, and suctioning to prevent atelectasis.
   - *Analgesia:* Manages pain to minimize splinting and improve breathing. Opioid analgesics are used cautiously to avoid respiratory depression. An epidural patient-controlled analgesia (PCA) pump or an intercostal nerve block may help to relieve local rib pain.
   - *Mechanical ventilation:* Must be implemented for extreme respiratory distress or ventilatory collapse.
   - *Stabilization and fixation of flail chest:* Most flail chest injuries stabilize within 10 to 14 days without surgical intervention. Stabilization of fractures is achieved using a volume-cycled ventilator. During surgery, a flail segment can be externally fixated by wiring or otherwise attaching the segment to the intact bony structures.
4. **Restore perfusion and oxygen-carrying capacity.**
   - *Volume replacement:* A high priority in the trauma victim. Blood loss is replaced with PRBCs or whole fresh blood, if available. Blood replacement via autotransfusion is widely accepted. Use of colloid versus crystalloid fluids for volume replacement remains controversial. Volume is more often replaced with crystalloid fluids (e.g., NS, LR) rather than colloidal IV fluids (e.g., plasma, albumin). Colloids increase the risk of developing ARDS and acute renal failure and are more expensive; furthermore, research has failed to demonstrate significant benefit.

- **Thoracotomy:** Consider in patients with penetrating injuries to the chest who arrive in PEA or develop PEA shortly after arrival. This should only be done if a qualified surgeon is present. Opening the chest allows the surgeon to gain control over bleeding and restore intravascular volume in order to get the patient to the operating room for more definitive care.
- **Repair of thoracic aortic injuries:** If the patient is stable, repair should be delayed until the other injuries have been addressed and the patient is over the critical period. Repair may even occur on an elective basis after the patient is discharged from the hospital. Repair using endovascular stenting has been shown to decrease patient morbidity.

5. Support cardiac function.

- **Monitoring of hemodynamic status:** If major cardiac or pulmonary involvement, use pulmonary artery monitoring and cardiac output determinations, with direct arterial pressure monitoring if indicated.
- **Treatment of dysrhythmias:** Use the Advanced Cardiac Life Support protocols of the American Heart Association. If rhythm disturbances do not appear in the first 5 days after trauma, they rarely occur later.
- **Immediate corrective surgical repair:** For ruptured valve, torn papillary muscle, or torn intraventricular septum accompanied by hemodynamic instability.
- **Treatment of shock:** Initially shock should be treated with fluid resuscitation to ensure adequate intravascular volume. Once intravascular volume has been restored, vasopressor drugs (i.e., norepinephrine, dopamine, vasopressin) may be necessary to enhance BP.
- **Treatment of myocardial failure:** Oxygen, diuretics, positive inotropic agents, and monitoring with a pulmonary artery catheter for right- and left-sided heart pressures.

Safety Alert   *Because of the potential for hemorrhage, never remove a penetrating object until the surgeon is present and studies have been completed to determine what the object has penetrated.*

CARE PLANS: THORACIC TRAUMA
Ineffective breathing pattern *related to pulmonary and/or cardiac injury*

GOALS/OUTCOMES Within 24 hours of this diagnosis, respiratory rate stabilizes to 12 to 20 breaths/min with normal work of breathing; lung injuries are managed to provide expanded lungs with minimal fluid/blood accumulation in the thoracic cavity; sources of bleeding are identified and managed to provide adequate Hgb level for adequate oxygenation; lost intravascular volume is replaced to reflect a CVP of 6 to 12 mm Hg; oxygen saturation is at least 95%, with Pao_2 at least 80 mm Hg with oxygen and $Paco_2$ less than 45 mm Hg with (or without) mechanical ventilation; and HR is 60 to 100 bpm with BP stable (at least 100 mm Hg systolic and 60 mm Hg diastolic).
NOC Respiratory Status: Ventilation

Airway Management
1. Monitor for sudden blood loss or persistent bleeding.
2. Prevent blood volume loss (e.g., apply pressure to site of bleeding).
3. Administer oxygen and/or mechanical ventilation, as appropriate.
4. Draw ABGs and monitor tissue oxygenation.

Ventilation Assistance
1. Monitor fluid status, including intake and output, as appropriate.
2. Maintain patent IV access.

Respiratory Monitoring
1. Monitor BP, pulse, temperature, and respiratory status.
2. Note trends and wide fluctuations in BP and auscultate BPs in both arms and compare.
3. Initiate and maintain a continuous temperature-monitoring device.

Decreased cardiac output *related to cardiac injury or ineffective cardiac compensatory response to oxygenation or perfusion deficits*

GOALS/OUTCOMES Within 24 hours of this diagnosis, patient exhibits adequate cardiac output, as evidenced by BP within normal limits for patient; HR 60 to 100 bpm; normal sinus rhythm on ECG; peripheral pulses at least 2+ on a 0-to-4+ scale; warm and dry skin; hourly urine output at least 0.5 ml/kg; measured CO 4 to 7 L/min; CVP 2 to 6 mm Hg; PAP 20 to 30/8 to 15 mm Hg; PAWP 6 to 12 mm Hg; and patient awake, alert, oriented, and free from anginal pain.

NOC Blood Loss Severity, Cardiac Pump Effectiveness

Hemorrhage Control
1. Apply manual pressure and/or pressure dressing as indicated.
2. Identify the cause of the bleeding.
3. Monitor the amount and nature of the blood loss.
4. Monitor Hgb and Hct levels.
5. Monitor clotting status via PT/PTT and INR values.

Shock Management
1. Monitor vital signs, mental status, and urinary output.
2. Use arterial line monitoring to improve accuracy of BP readings, as appropriate.
3. Monitor ABG results and tissue oxygenation.
4. Monitor trends in hemodynamic parameters (e.g., CVP, MAP, pulmonary capillary/artery wedge pressure).
5. Monitor determinants of tissue oxygen delivery (e.g., Pao_2, Sao_2, Hgb levels, CO), if available.
6. Insert and maintain large-bore IV access.
7. Administer crystalloids, as appropriate.
8. Administer blood and blood products, as appropriate.
9. Monitor fluid status, including daily weights and hourly urine output.
10. Administer inotropes, as appropriate.
11. Administer DVT and stress ulcer prophylaxis, as appropriate.

ADDITIONAL NURSING DIAGNOSES

For other nursing diagnoses and interventions, see also *Major Trauma* (p. 235), *Acute Cardiac Tamponade* (p. 257), *Pain* (p. 135), and *Emotional and Spiritual Support of the Patient and Significant Others* (p. 200).

TRAUMATIC BRAIN INJURY

PATHOPHYSIOLOGY

Traumatic brain injury (TBI), also known as acquired brain injury, occurs as a result of either blunt or penetrating forces to the head. Approximately 1.5 million TBIs occur each year with 52,000 resulting in death. Males are twice as likely to suffer a TBI as are females. Blunt injuries to the head are caused by acceleration, deceleration, and rotational forces (e.g., vehicular collisions, falls, high-impact sports). Penetrating injuries occur from piercing forces that traverse the skull and damage underlying brain tissue and support structures.

The initial impact (force) results in widespread injury due to tissue stresses and strain, which activate biomolecular processes within the cells. Injury results from structural and neuronal damage, vascular insufficiency, and inflammation. The cerebral vasculature and skull are often damaged. Tissue stresses result in contusions, diffuse axonal injuries, and compression injuries. Biomolecular processes cause neuroexcitation and deafferentation of the neurons. The neuroexcitatory injury activates excitatory neurotransmitters (glutamate and aspartate), which depolarize neurons. This neurotransmitter surge causes aberrant cell signaling, leading to long-lasting or permanent neuronal dysfunction. Deafferentation destroys the neurofilament of the axon, and the axon swells and retracts. Reduced blood flow augments cell death.

Outcome after TBI can be predicted to some extent based on the type of lesion, severity of injury, and length of coma. Age, preinjury medical status, mechanism of injury, ICP, and brainstem integrity are important factors influencing outcome.

Changes in Intracranial Pressure Dynamics

Intracranial pressure dynamics (IPD) is based on the volume-pressure relationship within the cranium (Monro-Kellie hypothesis). Three volumes exist within the fixed, rigid cranial vault: the brain, the blood, and the cerebrospinal fluid (CSF). Under normal conditions these volumes exert a pressure that is less than 15 mm Hg. The brain requires a constant blood supply to maintain normal function and when volume increases, pressure increases and compensatory mechanisms (shunting of CSF into the intrathecal space or vasoconstriction to reduce blood volume) are activated to reduce the volume. In brain injury, when the intrinsic compensatory mechanisms are damaged or overwhelmed, the functions that serve to maintain cerebral perfusion are compromised. Extrinsic measures are necessary to maintain the normal pressure-volume relationship and preserve CPP. Box 7-1 lists indicators of IICP. Treatment of derangements in IPD is based on the relationship between ICP and CPP and is stated simply: CPP=MAP−ICP

MAP is calculated using the following equation:

$$(\frac{1}{3} \times \text{systolic pressure}) + (\frac{2}{3} \times \text{diastolic pressure}) = \text{MAP}$$

The goal of treatment is to maintain CPP greater than 50 to 70 mm Hg and reduce ICP to less than 20 mm Hg.

Primary Brain Injuries

When the skull and brain are subjected to mechanical forces, a host of injuries in the cerebral cortex, brainstem, or cerebellum may change cerebral perfusion pressure. Severity of brain injuries is classified using the Glasgow Coma Scale (GCS): mild (GCS score = 13 to 15), moderate (GCS score = 9 to 12), and severe (GCS score = ≤8). Specific injuries arising from the mechanical forces are as follows:

- **Contusion:** Bruising that occurs as a result of mechanical forces to the head. Surface (scalp) contusions are focal bruises, lacerations, and capillary hemorrhages found with contact forces. Contusions may or may not be associated with fractures. Coup (brain injury is directly beneath the site of impact) or contrecoup (brain injury is opposite the site of impact) injuries, herniation contusions (parahippocampal structures and cerebellar tonsils forced against the tentorium), and gliding contusions (from rotational forces in the parasagittal areas) can result in focal hemorrhage of the cortex and adjacent white matter.
- **Diffuse axonal injuries (DAI):** Mild to severe injuries that occur when diffuse areas of white matter have been torn or sheared or when axons have been stretched. Injury evolves over time. Initial CT scan may not demonstrate a pathologic condition.
- **Concussion:** Neuroexcitatory injury sometimes associated with diffuse, axonal brain injuries. Classified as mild (no loss of consciousness, possible brief episodes of confusion or disorientation); moderate (brief loss of consciousness, transient focal neurologic deficits); or severe (prolonged loss of consciousness with sustained neurologic deficits lasting less than 24 hours).

Secondary Brain Injuries

Secondary injuries such as inflammation, edema, and changes in blood flow occur after the primary processes and further contribute to brain damage. They may be intrinsic or extrinsic. Secondary injury, despite the underlying cause, compromises the supply-demand ratio for cerebral oxygenation. Failure to manage secondary injury can result in irreversible neuronal damage superimposed on the already compromised injured brain.

- **Intrinsic:** Injuries that result from primary brain injury including intracranial hypertension, hypotension, hypovolemia, impaired autoregulation (causes reduced cerebral blood flow), reperfusion injury, brain edema, hemorrhage, herniation, cerebral vasospasm, hypoxia, inflammation, seizures, shivering, agitation, and hyperthermia.
- **Extrinsic:** Injuries unrelated to primary brain injury resulting from inadequate resuscitation, poor oxygenation, extreme hyperventilation, substance abuse, or nosocomial factors such as infections (meningitis), pneumonia, atelectasis, pulmonary edema, respiratory insufficiency, ventilatory associated lung injury, or anesthetic agents used for surgical repair of injuries (see *Meningitis*, p. 644).

Associated Skull Fractures

Skull fractures occur as a result of blunt or penetrating impact force. Primary and secondary brain injuries are usually present.

- **Linear skull fractures:** Nondisplaced, associated with low-velocity impact
- **Basilar skull fractures:** Linear, involving the base of the cranium's anterior, middle, and posterior fossae
- **Depressed skull fractures:** Depression of the skull over the point of impact; may be comminuted (usually closed without direct brain penetration), compressed, or compound (open)

Vascular Injuries

Vascular injuries are intrinsic brain injuries resulting from impact force that causes bleeding of cerebral arteries or veins. These injuries usually accompany moderate and severe primary injuries.

- **Epidural hematomas:** Commonly occur after a temporal linear skull fracture that lacerates the middle meningeal artery below it or from fractures of the sagittal and transverse sinuses. The hematoma develops rapidly in the space between the skull and dura and represents a life-threatening emergency.
- **Subdural hematomas:** Bleeding from veins between the dura and the arachnoid spaces; may be acute, subacute, or chronic. With the increased use of therapeutic anticoagulation for cardiac, stroke, and vascular problems, may be increasing the incidence of subdural hematoma from falls.
- **Subarachnoid hemorrhage:** Bleeding in the subarachnoid space seen over convexities of the brain or in the basal cisterns.
- **Intracranial hematomas:** Blood collection from injury to the small arteries and veins within the subcortical white matter of the temporal and frontal lobes; usually associated with petechiae, contusions, and edema.

Neurologic Complications

Herniation syndromes: Displacement of a portion of the brain through openings within the intracranial cavity that result from increased ICP. Herniation occurs when there is a pressure difference between the supratentorial and infratentorial compartments within the skull. When herniation occurs, significant portions of the cerebral vasculature are compressed, destroyed, or lacerated, resulting in ischemia, necrosis, and ultimately death.

- *Cingulate herniation:* Occurs because of an increase in ICP in one brain hemisphere. The affected high-pressure side shifts toward the low-pressure side causing compression of the anterior cerebral artery and internal cerebral vein. Reduced blood flow results in development of cerebral ischemia, edema, and IICP. Neurologic deficits include decreased LOC, with unilateral or bilateral lower extremity weakness or paralysis.
- *Uncal herniation:* Life-threatening, emergent situation that occurs when an expanding lesion (blood, edema, tumor) of the middle or temporal fossa forces the tip (uncus) of the temporal lobe toward the midline. The uncus protrudes over the edge of the tentorium cerebelli and compresses the oculomotor (third cranial) nerve and posterior cerebral artery. The uncus may be lacerated in the process and the midbrain is compressed against the tentorial edge. The patient manifests with an irregularly shaped pupil that may become fixed and dilated on the side of herniation, a change in respiratory pattern, marked deterioration in LOC, and further elevation in ICP.
- *Central (transtentorial) herniation:* Life-threatening, emergent situation that occurs with expanding lesions of the frontal, parietal, or occipital lobes or with severe, generalized cerebral edema. Often, cingulate and uncal herniation precede this life-threatening process. Table 3-13 describes the clinical features of uncal and central herniation syndromes. Subcortical structures, including the basal ganglia and diencephalon (thalamus and hypothalamus), herniate through the tentorium cerebelli, causing compression of the midbrain and posterior cerebral arteries bilaterally. Symptoms of increased ICP often occur too rapidly to be observed. Changes in respiratory patterns may not be seen in critically ill patients who are mechanically ventilated, depending on mode of ventilation.

Table 3-13 ASSESSMENT OF CENTRAL AND UNCAL HERNIATIONS

Criteria	Diencephalic		Midbrain/Upper Pons	Lower Pons/Upper Medulla
	Early	Late		
Central Herniation				
Respiratory pattern	Deep sighs, yawning	Cheyne-Stokes	Hyperventilation that is sustained and regular	Shallow, rapid, irregular
Pupils: size/reaction	Small; react to bright light; small range of contraction	Small; react to bright light; small range of contraction	Midpositioned; irregularly shaped; fixed reaction to light	Midpositioned; fixed
Oculocephalic/oculovestibular responses (doll's eyes phenomenon/ice water caloric)	Full conjugate or slightly roving eye movements; full conjugate lateral; ipsilateral response to ice water ear irrigation	Same as early; nystagmus absent	Impaired; may be dysconjugate	No response
Motor Responses				
At rest	Contralateral paresis, which may worsen	Motionlessness	Abnormal extension posturing	Flaccidity
To stimulus	Bilateral Babinski	Abnormal flexion posturing	Rigidity	Bilateral Babinski
	Early third nerve		Late third nerve	
Uncal Herniation				
Respiratory pattern	Normal		Hyperventilation that is regular and sustained	
Pupils: size/reaction	Moderate dilation; ipsilateral to primary lesion; sluggish constriction; brisk contralateral papillary reaction	Present or dysconjugate, full conjugate, slow ipsilateral eye movement or dysconjugate caused by contralateral eye not moving medially	Widely dilated and fixed ipsilateral pupil	
Oculocephalic/oculovestibular responses (doll's eyes phenomenon/ice water caloric)			Impaired or absent Full lateral movement with contralateral eye; absence of medial movement with ipsilateral eye	
Motor response to stimulus	Contralateral extensor plantar reflex		Ipsilateral hemiplegic; abnormal posturing; absence of all responses	

Modified from Plum F, Posner J: *Diagnostic of stupor and coma*, ed 3, Philadelphia, 1980, Davis.

- *Transcranial (extracranial) herniation:* Occurs when intracranial contents under pressure are forced through an open wound, surgical site, or cranial vault fracture. Although the resultant loss of brain volume lowers ICP and may prevent intracranial herniation, this is an ominous sign and the patient is at risk for infection, further brain injury, and death.

ASSESSMENT: TRAUMATIC BRAIN INJURY

Baseline physical examination data should include assessment of:
- Mental status
- Cranial nerves
- Motor status
- Sensory status
- Reflexes

Thereafter, ongoing neurologic assessment should be based on the clinical status of the patient. Ideally, a complete neurologic assessment should be performed. However, many components of the examination require patients to follow commands. For patients unable to follow commands, the neurologic assessment should be tailored individually to the patient's abilities and redesigned as necessary. The Glasgow Coma Scale (see Appendix 2) is applicable for use in the acute phase, and the Rancho Los Amigos cognitive functioning scale (see Cognitive Rehabilitation Goals, Table 1-6) can be used for recovery/rehabilitation assessment and should be part of the neurologic assessment.

The following are assessment findings related to specific types of brain injuries.

Epidural Hematoma/Linear Skull Fracture
- Assess for scalp lacerations, swelling, tenderness, and ecchymosis.
- Classic epidural signs are loss of consciousness, followed by a lucid interval and then rapid deterioration.
- Ipsilateral pupil dilation and contralateral weakness, followed by brainstem compression, occur if treatment is not initiated emergently.

Basilar Skull Fracture
- Dural tears resulting in rhinorrhea and otorrhea are common.
- Anterior fossa injuries are associated with periorbital ecchymosis (raccoon eyes), epistaxis, damage to cranial nerves I and II, and meningitis.
- Middle and posterior fossa injuries may damage cranial nerves VII and VIII and are associated with tinnitus, hemotympanum, and destruction of the cochlear vestibular apparatus.
- Ecchymosis of the mastoid process (*Battle sign*) is common.

Compound Depressed Skull Fracture
- Changes in LOC, pupillary changes
- Headache
- Increased ICP (if measured invasively)
- CSF leaks if the dura has been torn, tympanum rupture

Concussion
- Headache, although there are no overt signs of injury
- Dizziness
- Vomiting
- Memory loss
- Decreased attention and concentration skills

HIGH ALERT! Moderate and severe injuries require close observation because cerebral edema and IICP can develop.

Contusion
- Loss of consciousness is common.
- Neurologic deficits may be generalized or focal, depending on the site and severity of injury.

Diffuse Axonal Injury

- May occur with other injuries and is characterized by an immediate loss of consciousness. Duration of coma varies, depending on the severity of the injury, but often, coma is prolonged and recovery of function is minimal to moderate.
- Edema and unstable ICP dynamics are common.

Subdural Hematoma

- With acute subdural hematoma, neurologic deterioration is seen within 24 to 72 hours (or earlier), changing LOC, ipsilateral dilated pupil, and contralateral extremity weakness.
- Subacute hematoma may present within 48 hours to weeks after injury and manifests initially as a headache as LOC begins to deteriorate, and focal neurologic deficits ensue.

HIGH ALERT!   Neurologic signs associated with a chronic subdural hematoma may occur weeks or months after injury.

- Progression of elusive, fluctuating deficits, such as personality changes, memory loss, headache, extremity weakness, and incontinence, may signal chronic subdural hematoma, especially in high-risk groups such as older adults or chronic alcohol users.

Subarachnoid Hemorrhage (SAH)

- Headache
- Changes in LOC
- Meningeal signs: nuchal rigidity, elevated temperature, and positive *Kernig* sign (loss of ability to extend leg when thigh is flexed on abdomen)

Intracranial Hematoma

- Neurologic deficits are based on the site and severity of injury.

Diagnostic Tests for Traumatic Brain Injury		
Test	**Purpose**	**Abnormal Findings**
Skull radiograph	Detect structural deficits	Skull fractures, facial bone destruction, air-fluid level in sinuses, unusual intracranial calcification, pineal gland location (normally midline), and radiopaque foreign bodies
Cervical spine radiograph	Evaluate for structural deficits of the spine. Cervical spine immobilization is mandated in all trauma patients until the cervical spine (C1-T1) is visualized completely and fractures are ruled out.	Cervical spine injuries, including fractures, dislocations, and subluxations
Computed tomography (CT) Spiral CT can be used for angiographic imaging.	Fast diagnostic tool to evaluate for primary and secondary brain injuries and structural changes secondary to injury	Gray and white matter, blood, and CSF are identified by their different radiologic densities. CT is used to diagnose cerebral hemorrhage, infarction, hydrocephalus, cerebral edema, and structural changes.
Magnetic resonance imaging (MRI)	Identify type, location, and extent of injury	Spatial resolution can follow metabolic processes and detects structural changes.

Diagnostic Tests for Traumatic Brain Injury — cont'd		
Test	**Purpose**	**Abnormal Findings**
Cerebral angiography	Examine the cerebral vasculature	Abnormalities in cerebral circulation, filling defects, diminished blood flow
Electroencephalography (EEG)	Measure spontaneous brain electrical activity via surface electrodes. Drug therapy, especially with narcotics, sedatives, and anticonvulsants, alters brain activity. Use of these drugs should be documented if the drug cannot be withheld 24–48 hr before performing EEG.	Abnormal brain activity (irritability) associated with seizures and generalized brain activity related to drug overdose, coma, or suspected brain death
Evoked responses	Evaluates the electrical potentials (responses) of the brain to an external stimulus (i.e., auditory, visual, somatosensory). Evoked potentials are used to determine the extent of injury in uncooperative, confused, or comatose patients.	Abnormal or delayed expected response levels indicating lesions of the cortex or ascending pathways of the spinal cord, brainstem, or thalamus
CSF analysis	Evaluate for infection	Abnormal color, turbidity/cloudiness, red blood cell (RBC) and WBC counts, protein, glucose, electrolytes, gram stain, culture, and sensitivity.
Labwork WBCs Hemoglobin, hematocrit Electrolyte panel Osmolality	Evaluate for metabolic imbalance, shift, infection	Can indicate infection, anemia, nutritional deficits, sodium imbalance, all of which need to be monitored closely during acute phase

COLLABORATIVE MANAGEMENT
Care Priorities
1. **Surgical intervention**
   - Performed to evacuate mass lesions (epidural, subdural, and intracranial hematomas), place an ICP monitoring system, elevate depressed skull fractures, débride open wounds and brain tissue, and repair dural tears or scalp lacerations. Decompressive craniectomies and frontal and/or temporal lobectomies may be necessary to control severe increases in ICP.
2. **Preoperative and postoperative management of coagulopathies**

   - Home medication history is imperative along with preoperative PT/INR and PTT evaluation in all patients with TBI.
   - Suspect subdural hematomas or intracerebral hemorrhage in patients on clopidogrel (Plavix), aspirin, or Warfarin.

> **Safety Alert**
> *Stop all anticoagulation medication including heparin. If patient is to have an emergent craniotomy for evacuation of a subdural hematoma or other injury, PT/INR and PTT must be normalized.*

- For patients on Warfarin with INR greater than 1.2, infuse fresh frozen plasma (FFP), or factor VII, and administer vitamin K until INR is in ***nontherapeutic range*** (less than 1.2). Monitor PT/INR daily and continue infusion of FFP and administration of vitamin K based on results.
- For patients on Plavix (clopidogrel), infuse platelets to achieve homeostasis. Platelet counts will appear normal, but their coagulation function has been altered by the clopidogrel or aspirin, and a daily regimen of platelet replacement should continue for up to 5 postoperative days.

HIGH ALERT! There are no evidence-based studies for reversing coagulopathies as patients' response to medication is very individual. These strategies are aimed at monitoring the coagulopathy as they wax and wane over the postoperative course.

3. Management of intracranial pressure dynamics
   - ICP monitoring is performed by a variety of techniques (Table 3-14). All monitoring systems provide a digital display of ICP, but CPP must be calculated (see p. 326).
   - The goal is to maintain CPP greater than 50 to 70 mm Hg. Intraventricular catheters and parenchymal catheters are recommended for monitoring ICP over subarachnoid and epidural monitoring systems.

Table 3-14	TYPES OF INTRACRANIAL MONITORING			
System	**Type**	**Placement**	**Advantages/ uses**	**Disadvantages**
Fluid-filled or fiberoptic	Intraventricular cannula	Lateral ventricle in nondominant hemisphere through burr hole	CSF measurement CSF drainage Drug administration Volume-pressure response testing	Rapid CSF drainage can result in collapsed ventricles or subdural hematoma Cannula tip may catch on ventricular wall Risk of intracerebral bleeding and infection May become plugged with debris Possible difficult insertion because of shifting or collapse of ventricle
Fluid-filled	Subarachnoid screw	Subarachnoid space through twist drill hole	Pressure monitoring Less risk of infection than with cannula Useful with small ventricles Does not penetrate brain	Compliance testing may be unreliable No CSF drainage Some risk of infection Risk of hemorrhage or hematoma during insertion Brain may be herniated into bolt, making recording unreliable
Electrical sensor	Epidural sensor	Epidural space Burr hole Fiberoptic sensor	Lowest risk of infection Easy to insert Dura not penetrated	No direct measurement of CSF No CSF drainage Inability to recalibrate to zero Cannot measure volume-pressure response
Fiberoptic	Intraparenchymal	Intraparenchymal via twist drill Fiberoptic sensor	Easy to insert Direct pressure Compliance testing One-time zero and calibration before insertion	Risk of intracerebral bleeding and infection No CSF drainage

CSF, cerebrospinal fluid.

RESEARCH BRIEF 3-1

The *Guidelines for Management of Severe Traumatic Brain Injury* suggest that intracranial pressure (ICP) monitoring is indicated for patients with a Glasgow Coma Scale (GCS) score less than 9 after resuscitation and an abnormal admission computed tomography (CT) scan. Placement of an ICP monitor is also suggested in patients who have a GCS less than 9 with a normal CT scan and two or more of the following are noted on admission: (1) the patient is older than 40 years, (2) the patient has unilateral or bilateral abnormal posturing, or (3) the patient's systolic blood pressure is less than 90 mm Hg. Physician discretion may also determine the use of ICP monitoring. (Brain Trauma Foundation: Guidelines for the management of severe head injury. J Neurotrauma 24(81): 1–106, 2007.)

4. **Reduction of ICP by CSF drainage**
   - Performed using intraventricular or ventriculostomy systems
   - To prevent overdraining, the drainage collection bags must be maintained at the level of the tragus of the ear or higher, thereby preventing excessive CSF flow caused by a higher-to-lower pressure gradient.
5. **Hyperventilation via mechanical ventilation**

Safety Alert *Hyperventilation is no longer recommended as a first-line treatment and should be used only with cerebral oxygen monitoring to reduce ICP. Hyperventilation should be avoided during the first 24 hours after injury.*

   - Prophylactic hyperventilation ($Paco_2$ greater than 25 Hg) is recommended for short periods until more definitive therapies are initiated or increased ICP is reduced to avoid herniation. Maintaining $Paco_2$ within a normal range is now considered optimal ventilation. However, recent evidence reveals hyperventilation may cause neurologic dysfunction as a result of decreased cerebral perfusion.
6. **Monitoring jugular venous oxygen saturation (Sjo_2)**
   - Used to measure cerebral oxygenation by determining oxygen content of cerebral venous blood as a global measurement of oxygen supply and demand. Three types of blood flow can be discriminated:
     - Normal ($Sjo_2 = 55\%$ to 70%)
     - Oligemic (Sjo_2 less than 55%)
     - Hyperemia (Sjo_2 greater than 70%).
   - Treatment should be aimed at maintaining normal range.
7. **Monitoring brain tissue oxygenation ($Pbto_2$)**
   - Used to monitor the partial pressure of regional brain tissue oxygenation at catheter tip in order to detect cerebral ischemia and hypoxia. Cerebral hypoxia, a secondary brain injury event, has been associated with poor patient outcomes.
   - $Pbto_2$ levels greater than 20 are recommended.

HIGH ALERT! Optimal management of a severe TBI should include monitoring of CPP, ICP, and $Pbto_2$ as well as ventilation management. ICP threshold should be less than 20 mm Hg, optimal CPP is 50 to 70 mm Hg, and optimal $Pbto_2$ is greater than 20 mm Hg. As ICP rises and $Pbto_2$ falls, it may be necessary to adjust the Fio_2 to keep $Pbto_2$ greater than 20. It is not uncommon for Fio_2 to be .1 or 100% to maintain adequate cerebral oxygenation. Pao_2 less than 60 mm Hg should be avoided.

   - Other ways to improve $Pbto_2$ include raising BP, treating anemia, and adjusting Pco_2.
8. **Hyperosmolar therapy**
   - Reduces cerebral brain volume by removing fluid from the brain's extracellular compartment.
   - Mannitol, an osmotic diuretic, and hypertonic saline are generally used. Mannitol may be given in 0.25 to 1.0 g/kg body weight doses as needed to reduce ICP or may be

given as a scheduled dose every 4 to 6 hours. While there is no Level 1 evidence supporting the use of hypertonic saline, TBI patients who received hypertonic saline in a small study of polytrauma patients had improved survival and restoration of hemodynamic stability. It may be useful as an adjunct therapy in refractory increased ICP.
- Dehydration is a major complication with the continued use of hyperosmolar therapies. Serum electrolyte and osmolality values should be closely monitored.
- Fluid balance is maintained with fluid therapy (75 to 100 ml/hr). Replacement of urine losses may be prescribed based on the volume of urine collected 1 hour after giving hyperosmolar agents. Given either ml for ml or 0.5 ml for ml over a 3- to 4-hour period.

9. **Maintenance of blood pressure to maintain cerebral perfusion pressure**
   - Hypotension and hypertension can contribute to cerebral edema, which compresses blood vessels. Hypotension can result in decreased oxygen delivery to brain cells. The pH is reduced by elevated $Paco_2$, causing cerebral vessels to vasodilate. Hypotension reduces MAP and thus CPP.
   - Vasoconstrictive medications (phenylephrine, norepinephrine) or inotropic medications (dobutamine) may be used. Aim is to avoid systolic BPs less than 90 mm Hg.
   - Effects of hypertension (elevated CPP and increased cerebral edema) are unclear, but increased capillary permeability and petechial hemorrhage are seen. Antihypertensive medications, such as labetalol HCl (Normodyne) or nitroprusside sodium (Nipride), may be required.

10. **Reduction of metabolic demand**
    - Important strategy when treating ICP problems, because cerebral blood supply must match demand to maintain cerebral function.
    - *Sedating agents:* Use of individual or combined continuous infusions of sedatives, analgesics, and paralytic drugs to reduce metabolic demand. Midazolam HCl (Versed), opiate analgesics such as fentanyl citrate (Sublimaze), sufentanil, or morphine sulfate, and anesthetic agents such as propofol (Diprivan) are used. Dosing recommendations are given in Table 3-15. Nondepolarizing neuromuscular blocking agents, including vecuronium bromide (Norcuron) or atracurium, are used but must be used with sedation and can mask seizure activity. (See also *Sedation and neuromuscular blockade*, p. 158.)
    - *Seizure control:* Anticonvulsants are recommended to prevent early posttraumatic seizures (PTS) (within 7 days of injury) despite the fact that early PTS is not associated with worse outcomes. PTS may occur with all TBIs but, there is a higher incidence in patients with focal brain injuries such as depressed, comminuted, or compound skull fractures, contusions, lacerations, and penetrating injuries. Seizure activity increases the metabolic demand of the brain.
    - Seizure prophylaxis with anticonvulsant agents such as phenytoin sodium (Dilantin) or, less often, levetiracetem (Keppra) is often prescribed. When using phenytoin, a weight-based loading dose of 15 to 20 mg/kg is given slowly at 50 mg/min, followed

Table 3-15	ANALGESICS AND SEDATIVES RECOMMENDATIONS FOR USE IN TRAUMATIC BRAIN INJURY	
Agent	**Dose**	**Comments**
Morphine sulfate	4 mg/hr continuous infusion	Titrate PRN Reverse with Narcan
Midazolam	2 mg test dose; then 2–4 mg/hr continuous infusion	Reverse with flumazenil
Fentanyl	2 mcg/kg test dose; then 2–5 mcg/kg/hr continuous infusion	
Sufentanil	10–30 mcg test dose; then 0.05–2 mcg/kg continuous bolus	
Propofol	0.5 mg/kg test bolus; then 20–75 mcg/kg/min continuous infusion	Do not exceed 5 mg/kg/hr Monitor closely, especially young adults

From Brain Trauma Foundation: Guidelines for the management of severe brain trauma. *J Neurotrauma* 24(suppl 1):S-73, 2007.

by a daily dose of 100 mg three times daily. Phenytoin cannot be administered with a dextrose solution. Therapeutic levels are reported to be between 10 to 20 mg/ml, but dosing should be done to maintain *free dilantin levels* between 1 and 2 mg/ml. Dosing should be patient-specific (higher levels may be necessary to prevent breakthrough seizures, whereas lower levels may be acceptable if seizures are controlled).

 Safety Alert *In a person with normal albumin levels, the free level correlates closely with the therapeutic level, but in people who are hypoalbuminemic, such as patients with acute traumatic brain injury, the free level can be significantly higher and more accurately represents the patient's "true" phenytoin (Dilantin) level.*

- *Barbiturate coma:* A less often used method of reducing metabolic demand, barbiturate administration is recommended to control ICP refractory to standard medical and surgical treatment.
    - High doses of barbiturates should not be used without continuous ICP and hemodynamic monitoring and controlled mechanical ventilation. Barbiturates may induce profound cardiac and cerebral depression. Pentobarbital sodium (Nembutal) is the drug of choice.
    - A loading dose between 5 to 10 mg/kg is given (discontinue if MAP falls to less than 70 mm Hg), followed by a maintenance dose of 1 to 3 mg/kg/hr.
    - Clinically significant hypotension is usually seen with barbiturate coma. It is not responsive to fluid resuscitation and requires the use of vasopressors such as dopamine or phenylephrine.
    - Barbiturates are withdrawn gradually as the patient improves. Patients with barbiturate coma require intensive physical care and physiologic monitoring.
    - Assessment of brain death criteria, if appropriate, cannot be initiated until barbiturate levels return to zero.
- *Maintaining body temperature:* For every 1°C in temperature elevation, there is a 10% to 13% increase in metabolic rate. Body temperature should be normal to control metabolic demand.

HIGH ALERT! Normal temperatures range from 35.8° to 37.5°C (96.4° to 99.5°F) with a diurnal variation of 1°C. Rectal temperatures are 0.2° to 0.6°C higher than oral and can be 0.8°C higher than right atrial, esophageal, and oral temperatures. Evaluation of the etiology of fever is important with brain injury, as it influences treatment choice.

- Fever may be caused by brain injury (central fever), an infectious process (peripheral fever), or drugs (drug fever). Central fever reflects disturbance in the hypothalamic thermoregulatory mechanism. It is characterized by lack of sweating, no diurnal variation, plateaulike elevation patterns, elevations up to 41°C (105.8°F), absence of tachycardia, persistence for days or weeks, and temperature reduction with external cooling rather than with antipyretic agents.
- Peripheral fever is associated with wound infections, meningitis, sepsis, pneumonia, and other bacterial invasion. Sweating, diurnal variation, response to antipyretic agents, and tachycardia are present.
- Drug fever occurs in response to certain medications including antibiotics. External cooling with a hypothermia blanket may cause shivering, the body's mechanism to increase heat production.

HIGH ALERT! Shivering increases metabolic demand and may increase ICP. Shivering may be controlled by wrapping distal extremities in bath towels before initiating hypothermia or using chlorpromazine (Thorazine), which, however, must be used with caution because it may cause hypotension. Research on use of hypothermia in treatment of acute brain injury is evolving. If used, follow a strict hypothermia protocol. At this time there is no support for prophylatic hypothermia.

Traumatic Brain Injury

11. **Modifying nursing care activities that raise ICP**
   - Transient brief and rapid elevations in ICP, which cannot always be avoided, are commonly seen during position changes or other nursing care activities. Generally, the ICP returns to resting baseline within a few minutes.

HIGH ALERT! All nursing care activities that increase ICP should be spaced to enable a return of ICP to baseline and maximizing of CPP. Clustering nursing care such as bathing, turning, and suctioning creates a stair-step rise in ICP. Sustained increases (longer than 5 minutes) should be avoided.

   - *Suctioning:* Causes a significant rise in ICP. To minimize adverse effects associated with suctioning, implement the guidelines found in Box 3-6.
   - *Neck positioning:* Flexion, extension, and lateral movements of the neck can significantly raise ICP. Maintaining the neck in a neutral position at all times is important. In patients with poor neck control, stabilize the neck with towel rolls or sandbags.
   - *Elevating head of bed (HOB):* Although HOB elevation at 30 degrees is believed to improve venous drainage and contribute to ICP reduction, ICP may be improved at higher or lower elevations. Adjust HOB elevation to optimize the patient's CPP and P_{BTO_2} and minimize ICP.
   - *Turning:* Turning the patient with IICP is not contraindicated but should be based on the patient's response to turning. Initially, turning from side to side will elevate pressure, but ICP should return to resting baseline after a few minutes. If the ICP does not return to resting baseline within 5 minutes, CPP may be compromised and the patient should be returned to a position that reduces ICP and maximizes CPP.
   - *Bathing:* Although bathing itself has not been documented as raising ICP, the rapid turning from side to side associated with linen changes raises ICP. These "turn procedures" are actually clustered activities because the length of the procedure does not allow sufficient time for the ICP to return to baseline. Evaluation of the patient's response may necessitate performing the linen change in stages or allowing adequate time for ICP to return to resting baseline.
   - *Sensory stimulation:* A sensory stimulation program may be implemented safely in comatose patients early after injury when ICP is stable. This rehabilitative technique may be an important adjunct to traditional care and improve admission to an active rehabilitation program (Table 3-16).
12. **Nutritional support: Feeding should be initiated as early as possible to achieve full caloric replacement within 7 days of injury**
   - Enteral nutrition helps to maintain the integrity of the gut mucosa and should be initiated as early as possible after injury.
   - When postpyloric (duodenum or jejunum) feeding tubes are used, enteral feedings can be initiated before bowel sounds return to normal.
   - In some cases, gastric tubes for decompression are used simultaneously with the postpyloric tubes. See *Nutritional Support*, p. 117, for documentation of proper placement and checking of residual volumes. If enteral feedings are contraindicated or not tolerated by the patient, parenteral feedings are started.

Box 3-6	**GUIDELINES FOR SUCTIONING PATIENTS AT RISK FOR INCREASED INTRACRANIAL PRESSURE**

   - Suction only if the clinical status of the patient warrants.
   - Precede suctioning with preoxygenation using 100% oxygen.
   - Limit each suctioning pass to ≤10 seconds.
   - Limit suction passes to two.
   - Follow each pass with 60 seconds of hyperventilation using 100% oxygen.
   - Use negative suction pressure less than 120 mm Hg.
   - Keep patient's head in a neutral position.
   - Use a suction catheter with an outer-to-inner diameter ratio of 2:1.

Table 3-16	MANAGEMENT OF SEVERE BRAIN INJURY	
Treatment	**Level of Evidence***	**Recommendation**
Blood pressure	Level II	Avoid early postinjury episodes of hypotension <90 mm Hg.
Oxygenation	Level III	Avoid Pao$_2$ <60 mm Hg and O$_2$ saturation <90%.
ICP treatment threshold	Level II	Treatment to lower ICP should be initiated at 20 mm Hg.
CPP treatment	Level III	CPP should be maintained at >50 mm Hg. Maintain MAP >90 mm Hg.
Cerebral oxygenation	Level III	Keep Pbto$_2$ >20.
Hyperventilation	Level II	Avoid prophylactic hyperventilation (<25 mm Hg); hyperventilate for short duration for refractory increased ICP.
	Level III	Avoid hyperventilation in the first 24 hours postinjury.
Hyperosmolar therapy	Level II	Mannitol: use intermittent boluses of 0.25–1 mg/kg.
	Option	Hypertonic saline (3%). No recommended dose
Barbiturates	Level II	May be considered in patients with hemodynamic stability refractory to other methods to reduce ICP.
Propofol	Level II	Use for control of ICP.
Glucocorticoids	Standard	Use is not recommended.
Nutrition	Level II	Full caloric replacement by postinjury day 7
Seizure prophylaxis	Level II	Anticonvulsants can be considered an option for high-risk patients early after injury.
		Not recommended for preventing late posttraumatic seizures.

Data from Brain Trauma Foundation: Guidelines for the management of severe head injury.
J Neurotrauma 24:S1–106, 2007.
Standard = high level of certainty; *Level II* = moderate clinical certainty; *Level III/Option* = unclear clinical certainty. Level of evidence is based on scientific literature where the highest degree of certainty is drawn from prospective randomized clinical trials.
*Level of evidence denotes the degree that the recommendation represents clinical certainty.
CCP, cerebral perfusion pressure; ICP, intracranial pressure; MAP, mean arterial pressure.

13. **Prevention of aspiration**
    - Prevalent complication after brain injury
    - Aspiration may occur at the time of injury or as an iatrogenic complication of intubation, enteral feedings, or prolonged use of artificial airways.
    - Tracheobronchial secretions should be checked for glucose (a sign that tube feedings have been aspirated).
    - Follow enteral feeding protocols initiated.
    - Initial and ongoing swallowing assessments

14. **DVT prophylaxis**
    - TBI patients are at risk for developing DVT as well as pulmonary emboli as a result of prolonged bed rest. There is concern for the use of anticoagulation therapies as there is risk for expansion of intracranial hemorrhage. There is Level 3 support for the prophylactic use of low-molecular-weight heparin or unfractionated heparin along with mechanical measures to prevent DVT; however, there is no evidence to support optimum dosing or time when to begin therapy. Clinical practice guidelines for TBI also support the use of graduated compression stockings, unless the lower extremity injuries prevent their use. However, there are no recommendations for the therapeutic treatment of DVTs or pulmonary emboli. Management must be determined by the attending physician based on the risk/benefit ratios.

15. **Management of cardiac dysrhythmias**
    - Commonly seen in brain-injured patients and probably related to autonomic (sympathetic and parasympathetic) derangement or compression of midbrain and brainstem structures
    - ECG changes seen with elevated ICP are prominent U waves, ST-segment changes, notched T waves, and prolongation of the QT interval.
    - Bradycardia, supraventricular, tachycardia, and ventricular dysrhythmias
16. **Rehabilitation**
    - Brain injury often results in physical (paralysis, spasticity, and contractures) and cognitive impairments.
    - Consult with physical, occupational, and speech therapists early to minimize deficits and prepare the patient for an acute rehabilitative program.
    - National Institutes of Health (NIH) Consensus Development Conference Recommendations on Rehabilitation of Persons with Brain Injury are available. Support also is available through the Brain Injury Association of America (www.biausa.org).

CARE PLANS: TRAUMATIC BRAIN INJURY

Impaired gas exchange *related to decreased oxygen supply and increased CO_2 production secondary to decreased ventilatory drive occurring with pressure on respiratory center, imposed inactivity, pneumonia, ARDS, and possible neurologic pulmonary edema*

GOALS/OUTCOMES: $Paco_2$ values remain greater than 35 mm Hg and Pao_2 greater than 60 mm Hg. By the time of discharge from ICU or transfer to rehabilitation unit, patient has adequate gas exchange as evidenced by appropriate mental status and orientation; $Pao_2 \geq 60$ mm Hg; respiratory rate 12 to 20 breaths/min with normal depth and pattern; and absence of adventitious breath sounds.
NOC Respiratory Status: Gas Exchange

Respiratory Monitoring
1. Assess patient's respiratory rate, depth, and rhythm. Auscultate lung fields for breath sounds every 1 to 2 hours and as needed. Monitor for respiratory patterns described in Table 3-13. Be alert to IICP (see Box 7-1).
2. Assess patient for signs of hypoxia, including confusion, agitation, restlessness, and irritability. Remember that cyanosis is a late indicator of hypoxia.
3. Ensure a patent airway via proper positioning of neck and frequent assessment of the need for suctioning. Ensure hyperoxygenation of patient before and after each suction attempt to prevent dangerous, suction-induced hypoxia or $PBTO_2$ less than 20.
4. Monitor ABG values; consult physician for significant findings or changes. Be alert to levels indicative of hypoxemia (Pao_2 less than 80 mm Hg) and to $Paco_2 \geq 35$ mm Hg, inasmuch as levels higher than this range may increase cerebral blood flow and thus ICP.
5. Ensure that oxygen is delivered within prescribed limits.
6. Assist with turning every 2 hours, within limits of patient's injury, to promote lung drainage and expansion and alveolar perfusion. Unless contraindicated, raise HOB 30 degrees to enhance gas exchange.
7. Encourage deep breathing at frequent intervals to promote oxygenation. Avoid coughing exercises for patients at risk for IICP.
8. Evaluate the need for an artificial airway in patients unable to maintain airway patency or adequate ventilatory effort.

NIC Airway Management; Oxygen Therapy; Respiratory Monitoring

Risk for infection: CNS *related to inadequate primary defenses secondary to direct access to the brain in the presence of skull fracture, penetrating wounds, craniotomy, intracranial monitoring, or bacterial invasion caused by pneumonia or iatrogenic causes.*

GOALS/OUTCOMES Patient is free of infection as evidenced by normothermia, WBC count $\leq 11,000$/ml, negative culture results, HR ≤ 100 bpm, BP within patient's normal range, and absence of agitation, purulent drainage, and other clinical indicators of infection.
NOC Risk Identification

Infection Protection
1. Assess vital signs at frequent intervals for indicators of CNS infection. Be alert to elevated temperature and increased HR and BP.
2. Monitor patient for signs of systemic infection, including discomfort, malaise, agitation, and restlessness.
3. Inspect cranial wounds for the presence of erythema, tenderness, swelling, and purulent drainage. Obtain prescription for culture as indicated.
4. Monitor CSF fluid from intraventricular catheter for cloudy appearance or increase blood. Analysis of CSF fluid should be done on a routine basis.
5. Apply a loose sterile dressing (sling) to collect CSF drainage from nose. Do not pack the nose or ears if there is CSF drainage. Record amount, color, and character of drainage.
6. Caution patient against coughing, sneezing, nose blowing, or Valsalva or similar maneuvers, because these activities can further damage the dura. Use orogastric tubes if basilar skull fractures or severe frontal sinus fractures are present.
7. Ensure timely administration of prescribed antibiotics.
   - Apply basic principles for care of any invasive device used with ICP monitoring:
     - Use good hand-washing technique before caring for patient.
     - If patient is not comatose, encourage him or her not to touch device; apply restraints only if necessary to keep patient from harm. Restraints can increase ICP by causing straining and agitation.
     - Maintain aseptic technique during care of device, following agency protocol.

NIC Infection Control

Decreased intracranial adaptive capacity *related to decreased cerebral perfusion pressure or infections that can occur with secondary head injury*

GOALS/OUTCOMES Within 12 to 24 hours of treatment/interventions, patient has adequate intracranial adaptive capacity as evidenced by equal and normoreactive pupils; respiratory rate 12 to 20 breaths/min with normal depth and pattern (eupnea); HR 60 to 100 bpm; ICP 0 to 15 mm Hg; CPP greater than 50 mm Hg; and absence of headache, vomiting, and other clinical indicators of IICP. Optimally, by the time of discharge from ICU or transfer to rehabilitation unit, patient is oriented to time, place, and person and has bilaterally equal strength and tone in the extremities.
NOC Neurologic Status

Neurologic Monitoring
1. Assess neurologic status at least hourly. Monitor pupils, LOC, and motor activity; also perform cranial nerve assessments (see Appendix 3). A decrease in LOC is an early indicator of IICP. Changes in the size and reaction of the pupils, a decrease in motor function (e.g., hemiplegia, abnormal flexion posturing), and cranial nerve palsies.
2. Monitor vital signs at frequent intervals. Be alert to changes in respiratory pattern, fluctuations in BP and pulse, widening pulse pressure, and slow HR.
3. Monitor patient for indicators of IICP (see Box 7-1).
4. Monitor hemodynamic status to evaluate CPP and ensure that it is greater than 50 mm Hg. Be alert to decrease in mean systolic arterial BP (less than 80 mm Hg) or increase in MAP. Perform ongoing assessment of ICP, CPP, and P_{BTO_2} recording levels hourly until stable. Consult physician if pressure changes significantly (e.g., ICP greater than 20 mm Hg; P_{BTO_2} less than 20 or other preestablished ranges). Perform ongoing calibration and zeroing of transducer to ensure accuracy of readings.
5. Maintain a patent airway, and ensure precise delivery of oxygen to promote optimal cerebral perfusion.
6. Facilitate cerebral venous drainage by maintaining neck in neutral position.
7. To help prevent fluid volume excess, which could add to cerebral edema, ensure precise delivery of IV fluids at consistent rates.
8. Ensure timely administration of medications that are prescribed for the prevention of sudden increase or decrease in BP, HR, or respiratory rate.
9. Treat elevations in ICP immediately (Box 3-7).

NIC Cerebral Edema Management; Cerebral Perfusion Management; Intracranial Pressure (ICP) Monitoring; Neurologic Monitoring

Box 3-7	NURSING INTERVENTIONS FOR PATIENTS WITH INCREASED INTRACRANIAL PRESSURE

- Maintain head of bed elevation at level that keeps ICP less than 20 mm Hg and CPP greater than 50 mm Hg.
- Loosen constrictive objects around neck to facilitate venous blood flow from the head.
- With position changes, ensure ICP and CPP return to baseline or stay within acceptable parameters within 5 minutes of turn.
- Maintain head in neutral position.
- Correct factors that may increase ICP such as hypoxia, pain, anxiety, fear, and abdominal or bladder distention.
- Evaluate activities that increase ICP (e.g., suctioning, bathing, dressing changes) and reorganize care to minimize elevations.

ICP, intracranial pressure; *CPP*, cerebral perfusion pressure.

Ineffective thermoregulation *related to trauma associated with injury to or pressure on the hypothalamus*

GOALS/OUTCOMES Patient becomes normothermic within 24 hours of this diagnosis.
NOC Thermoregulation

Temperature Regulation
1. Monitor for signs of hyperthermia: temperature greater than 38.3°C (101°F), pallor, absence of perspiration, torso that is warm to the touch.
2. As prescribed, obtain blood, urine, and sputum specimens for culture to rule out underlying infection.
3. Be alert to signs of meningitis: fever, chills, nuchal rigidity, Kernig sign, Brudzinski sign (see *Meningitis*, p. 644).
4. Assess wounds for evidence of infection, including erythema, tenderness, and purulent drainage.
5. If patient has hyperthermia, remove excess clothing and administer tepid baths, hypothermic blanket, or ice bags to axilla or groin, but avoid inducing shivering.
6. As prescribed, administer antipyretics such as acetaminophen.
7. As prescribed, administer chlorpromazine to treat or prevent shivering, which can cause further increases in ICP.
8. Keep environmental temperature at optimal range.
9. Assess for possible drug fever reaction, which can occur with antimicrobial therapy.

NIC Fever Treatment

Risk for disuse syndrome *related to immobilization and prolonged inactivity secondary to brain injury, spasticity, or altered LOC*

GOALS/OUTCOMES Patient has baseline/optimal ROM without verbal or nonverbal indicators of pain.
NOC Mobility Level: Muscle Function

Positioning
1. Begin performing passive ROM exercises every 4 hours on all extremities as soon as patient's acute condition stabilizes. Monitor ICP during exercise, being alert to dangerous elevations outside of the established parameters. Consult with physical therapist accordingly.
2. Teach passive ROM exercises to significant others. Encourage their participation in patient exercise as often as they are able.
3. Reposition patient every 2 hours within restrictions of the head and other injuries, using log-rolling technique as indicated.
4. Ensure proper anatomic position and alignment. Support alignment with pillows, trochanter rolls, and wrapped sandbags.

5. For patient with spasticity, use foot cradles to keep linens off the feet. To maintain dorsiflexion, provide patient with shoes that are cut off at the toes, with the shoes ending just proximal to the head of the patient's metatarsal joints. Because there is no contact of the balls of the feet with a hard surface, the risk of spasticity will be minimized. Consult occupational therapist for use of splints or other supportive device.
6. For patient without spasticity, use foot supports to prevent plantar flexion and external hip rotation.
7. To maintain anatomic position of the hands, provide spastic patient with a splint or a cone that is secured with an elastic band. Either device will limit spasticity by pressing on the muscles, while the elastic band will stimulate the extensor muscles, thereby promoting finger extension.

NIC Exercise Therapy: Joint Mobility

Impaired tissue integrity: corneal (or risk for same) *related to irritation associated with corneal drying and reduced lacrimal production secondary to altered consciousness or cranial nerve damage*

GOALS/OUTCOMES Patient's corneas are moist and intact.
NOC Tissue Integrity: Skin and Mucous Membranes

Risk Identification
1. Assess for indicators of corneal irritation: red and itching eyes, ocular pain, sensation of a foreign object in the eye, scleral edema, and blurred vision.
2. Avoid exposing patient's eyes to irritants such as baby powder or talc.
3. Lubricate patient's eyes every 2 hours with isotonic eye drops or ointment.
4. Facilitate an ophthalmology consultation as indicated.

NIC Medication Administration: Eye

ADDITIONAL NURSING DIAGNOSES
Also see *Decreased Adaptive Capacity: Intracranial* in *Cerebral Aneurysm and Subarachnoid Hemorrhage* (p. 629). As appropriate, see nursing diagnoses and interventions under *Alterations in Consciousness* (p. 24), *Care of the Patient after Intracranial Surgery* (p. 638), and *Meningitis* (p. 644). See *Risk for Trauma* in *Status Epilepticus* (p. 672). Also see nursing diagnoses and interventions under *Nutritional Support*, (p. 117), *Mechanical Ventilation* (p. 99), *Hemodynamic Monitoring* (p. 75), *Prolonged Immobility* (p. 149), *Emotional and Spiritual Support of the Patient and Significant Others* (p. 200). The patient with craniocerebral trauma is at risk for diabetes insipidus and syndrome of inappropriate antidiuretic hormone. See *Diabetes Insipidus* (p. 703) and *Syndrome of Inappropriate Antidiuretic Hormone* (p. 734).

SELECTED REFERENCES
Alsikafe NF, McAninch JW, Elliott SP, Garcia M: Nonoperative management outcomes of isolated urinary extravasation following renal lacerations due to external trauma. *J Urol* 176:2494–2497, 2006.
American Burn Association Consensus Conference on Burn Sepsis and Infection Group: American Burn Association Consensus Conference to define sepsis and infection in burns. *J Burn Care Res* 28(6):776–790, 2007.
American College of Surgery Committee on Trauma: *Textbook on advanced trauma life support for doctors: ATLS student course manual.* Chicago, IL, 2008, American College of Surgeons.
American Heart Association: *ACLS: Principles and practice.* Dallas, TX, 2003, American Heart Association.
American Heart Association: *Handbook of emergency cardiovascular care for healthcare providers.* Dallas, TX, 2006, American Heart Association.
American Spinal Injury Association: *International standards for neurological classification of spinal cord patients.* Chicago, 2002, American Spinal Injury Association.
Baptiste D, Fehlings M: Emerging drugs for spinal cord injury. *Exp Opin Emerging Drugs* 13 (1):63–80, 2008.
Baptiste D, Fehlings M: Update on the treatment of spinal cord injury. *Progr Brain Res* 161:217–233, 2007.

Traumatic Brain Injury

Bartal CA, Yitzhak AB: The role of thromboelastometry and recombinant factor VIIa in trauma. *Curr Opin Anaesthesiol* 22(2):281–288, 2009.

Basta AM, Blackmore CC, Wessells H: Predicting urethral injury from pelvic fracture patterns in male patients with blunt trauma. *J Urol* 177:571–575, 2007.

Berlly M, Shem K: Respiratory management during the first five days after spinal cord injury. *J Spinal Cord Med* 30(4): 309–318, 2007.

Blackmore CC, et al: Predicting major hemorrhage in patient with pelvic fracture. *J Trauma* 61(2):346–352, 2006.

Bodden J: Treatment options in the hemodynamically unstable patient with a pelvic fracture. *Orthop Nursing* 28(3):109–116, 2009.

Bongiovanni MS, Bradley SL, Kelley DM: Orthopaedic trauma: critical care nursing issues. *Crit Care Nursing* 28(1):60–71, 2005.

Brain Trauma Foundation: Guidelines for the management of severe head injury. *J Neurotrauma* 24(S1): 1–106, 2007.

Brain Trauma Foundation, American Association of Neurological Surgeons, Congress of Neurological Surgeons: Guidelines for the management of severe traumatic brain injury. Deep vein thrombosis prophylaxis. *J Neurotrauma* 24(Suppl 1):S32–S36, 2007.

Brain Trauma Foundation, American Association of Neurological Surgeons, Congress of Neurological Surgeons: Guidelines for the management of severe traumatic brain injury. Indications for intracranial pressure monitoring. *J Neurotrauma* 24(Suppl 1):S37–S44, 2007.

Brasel KJ, et al: Significance of pelvic extravasation in patients with pelvic fracture. *J Trauma* 62(5):1149–1152, 2007.

Brewer ME, Strnad BT, Daley BJ, et al: Percutaneous embolization for the management of grade 5 renal trauma in hemodynamically unstable patients: initial experience. *The Journal of Urology* 181:1737–1741, 2009.

Bruch C, et al: Changes in QRS voltage in cardiac tamponade and pericardial effusion: reversibility after pericardiocentesis and after anti-inflammatory drug treatment. *J Am Coll Cardiol* 38:219, 2001.

Carr JA, Phillips BD, Bowling WM: The utility of bronchoscopy after inhalation injury complicated by pneumonia in burn patients: results from the National Burn Repository. *J Burn Care Res* 30(6):967–974, 2009.

Carrougher GJ: Burn wound assessment and topical treatment. In Carrougher GJ, editor: *Burn care and therapy*, St. Louis, 1998, Mosby.

Carrougher GJ, et al: Self-reports of anxiety in burn injured hospitalized adults during routine wound care. *J Burn Care Res* 27(5):676–681, 2006.

Cheatham ML, White MW, Sagraves SG, et al: Abdominal perfusion pressure: a superior parameter in the assessment of intra-abdominal hypertension. *J Trauma* 49:621–627, 2000.

Cheitlin MD, et al: *ACC/AHA/ASE 2003 guideline for the clinical application of echocardiography.* Retrieved January 2008 from www.acc.org/qualityandscience/clinical/statements.htm

Cirocchi R, Abraha I, Montedori A, et al: Damage control surgery for abdominal trauma. *Cochrane Database Syst Rev* 20(1):CD007438, 2010.

Como JJ, Bokhari F, Chiu WC, et al: Practice management guidelines for selective nonoperative management of penetrating abdominal trauma. *J Trauma* 68(3):721–733, 2010.

Cothren CC, et al: Preperitoneal pelvic packing for hemodynamically unstable pelvic fractures: a paradigm shift. *J Trauma* 62(4):834–842, 2007.

Criddle LM: Recombinant factor VIIa and the trauma patient. *JEN* 32(5):404–408, 2006.

Davis KA, Reed L II, Santaniello J, et al: Predictors of the need for nephrectomy after renal trauma. *J Trauma Inj Infect Crit Care* 60(1):164–170, 2006.

Davis JW, et al: Western trauma association critical decisions in trauma: management of pelvic fracture with hemodynamic instability. *J Trauma* 65(5):1012–1015, 2008.

Demetriades D, et al: Blunt traumatic thoracic aortic injuries: Early or delayed repair—results of an American Association for the Surgery of Trauma prospective study. *J Trauma* 66(4):967–973, 2009.

Demetriades K, Hadjizacharia P, Constantinou C, et al: Selective nonoperative management of penetrating abdominal solid organ injuries. *Ann Surg* 244(4):620–628, 2006.

Dente CJ, et al: Improvements in early mortality and coagulopathy are sustained better in patients with blunt trauma after institution of a massive transfusion protocol in a civilian level I trauma center. *J Trauma* 66(6):1616–1624, 2009.

Drowning, Part 10.3 in Circulation 2005. http://circ.ahajournals.org/cgi/content/full/112/24_suppl/IV-133

Eastridge BJ, et al: The importance of fracture pattern in guiding therapeutic decision-making in patients with hemorrhagic pelvic ring disruptions. *J Trauma* 53(3):446–451, 2002.

Elie MC: Blunt cardiac injury. *Mount Sinai J Med* 73(2):542–552, 2006.

Emergency Nurses Association: *Textbook of trauma nursing core course*. Des Plaines, IL, 2007, Emergency Nurses Association.

Fangio P, et al: Early embolization and vasopressor administration for management of life-threatening hemorrhage from pelvic fracture. *J Trauma* 58(5):978–984, 2005.

Faucher L, Furukawa K: Practice guidelines for the management of pain. *J Burn Care Res* 27(5): 659–668, 2006.

Faucher LD, Conton KM: Practice guidelines for deep venous thrombosis prophylaxis in burns. *J Burn Care Res* 28(5):661–663, 2007.

Final Recommendations of the World Congress on Drowning, Amsterdam, June 26-28, 2002. www.cslsa.org/events/ArchiveAttachments/Spr03minutes/AttachmentsG2.pdf

Fox CJ, et al: Effect of recombinant factor VIIa as an adjunctive therapy in damage control for wartime vascular injuries: a case control study. *J Trauma* 66(4): S112–S119, 2009.

Frakes MA, Evans T: Major pelvic fractures. *Critical Care Nurse* 24(2):18–30, 2004.

Gardner MJ, et al: Internal rotation and taping of the lower extremities for closed pelvic reduction. *J Orthop Trauma* 23(5):361–364, 2009.

Gentilello LM, Sanzone A, Wang L, et al: Near-infrared spectroscopy versus compartment pressure for the diagnosis of lower extremity compartment syndrome using electromyography-determined measurements of neuromuscular function. *J Trauma* 51:1–9, 2001.

Gonzales EA: Fluid resuscitation in the trauma patient. *J Trauma Nursing* 15(3):149–151, 2008.

Gordon MD, Gottschlich MM, Helvig EI, et al: Review of evidence-based practice for the prevention of pressure sores in burn patients. *J Burn Care Res* 25:388–410, 2004.

Gourgiotis S, Villias C, Germanos S, et al: Compartment syndrome: a review. *J Surg Educ* 64(3): 178–186, 2007.

Gourlay D, et al: Pelvic angiography for recurrent traumatic pelvic arterial hemorrhage. *J Trauma* 59(5):1168–1174, 2005.

Greenhalgh DG, Saffle JR, Holmes JH, et al: American Burn Association Consensus Conference to Define Sepsis and Infection in Burns. *J Burn Care Res* 28:776–790, 2007.

Harvey CA: Complications. *Orthop Nursing* 26(6):410–412, 2006.

Heetveld MJ, et al: Hemodynamically unstable pelvic fractures: recent care and new guidelines. *World J Surg* 28(9):904–909, 2004.

Hemmila MR, Wahl WL: Management of the injured patient. In GM Doherty and LW Way, editors: *Current surgical diagnosis and treatment*. New York, 2006, Lange.

Ho C, Wuermser L, Priebe M, et al: Spinal cord injury medicine. 1. Epidemiology and classification. *Arch Phys Med Rehabil* 88(S1):S49–S54, 2007.

Honari S: Topical therapies and antimicrobials in the management of burn wounds. *Crit Care Nurs Clin N Am* 16:1–11, 2004.

Hurlbert R: Strategies of medical intervention in the management of acute spinal cord injury. *Spine* 32(11): S16–S21, 2006.

Husain FA: Serum lactate and base deficit as predictors of mortality and morbidity. *Am J Surg* 185(5):485–491, 2003.

Ibsen LM, Koch T: Submersion and asphyxial injury. *Crit Care Med* 30(11):S402–S408, 2002.

Inova Fairfax Hospital, Inova Regional: Trauma Center, Falls Church, VA USA. christopher.michetti@inova.org

Kaplan LJ: *Critical care considerations in trauma*. 2008. www.emedicine.com

Kirshblum S, Priebe M, Ho C, et al: Spinal cord injury medicine. 3. Rehabilitation phase after acute spinal cord injury. 2007.

Kobziff L: Traumatic pelvic fractures. *Orthop Nursing* 25(4):235–241, 2006. www.westerntraumaassociation.org/algorithms/PelvicFractureNotes/NoteD.html

Konstantakos EK, Dalstrom DJ, Nelles ME, et al: Diagnosis and management of extremity compartment syndromes: An orthopaedic perspective. *Am Surg* 73(12):1199–1210, 2007.

Kosir R, Moore FA, Selby JH, et al: Acute lower extremity compartment syndrome (ALECS): Screening protocol in critically ill trauma patients. *J Trauma* 63(2):268–275, 2007.

Köstler W, Strohm PC, Südkamp NP: Acute compartment syndrome of the limb. *Injury* 36(8):992–998, 2005.

Kramer G, et al: Pathophysiology of burn shock and burn edema. In Herndon DN, editor: *Total burn care*, ed 3. London, 2007, Saunders.

LaBorde P: Burn epidemiology: The patient, the nation, the statistics, and the data resources. *Crit Care Nursing Clin N Am* 16:13–25, 2004.

Legome E: Blunt cardiac injury (BCI) in adult trauma. UpToDate 16.3, 2008. www.uptodate.com

Legome E: General approach to blunt thoracic trauma in adults. UpToDate 16.3, 2008. www.uptodate.com

Lettieri CJ: Nonsurgical management of thoracic trauma. *Medscape Pulm Med* 10(2), 2006.

Littlejohns L, Bader M, March K: Brain tissue oxygen monitoring in severe brain injury, I. *Crit Care Nurse* 23(4):17–27, 2003.

Maisch B, Seferovic PM, Ristic AD, et al: Guidelines on the diagnosis and management of pericardial diseases. *Eur Heart J*: 1–28, 2004.

Malbrain ML: Abdominal perfusion pressure as a prognostic marker in intra-abdominal hypertension. In Vincent JL, editor: *Yearbook of intensive care and emergency medicine*. Berlin, 2002, Springer-Verlag, pp. 792–814.

Malbrain ML, et al: Intra-abdominal hypertension in the critically ill: It is time to pay attention. *Curr Opin Crit Care* 11(2):156–171, 2005.

McCall JE, Cahill TJ: Respiratory care of the burn patient. *J Burn Care Res* 26:200–206, 2005.

McGahan PJ, Richards JR, Bair AE, Rose JS: Ultrasound detection of blunt urological trauma: a 6-year study. *Injury Int J Care Injured* 36: 762–770, 2005.

McQueen M: Acute compartment syndrome in tibial fractures. *Curr Orthop* 13:113–119, 1999.

Michetti CP, Sakran JV, et al: Physical examination is a poor screening test for abdominal pelvic injury in adult blunt trauma patients. *J Surg Res* 159(1):456–461, 2010.

Mitropulos D, Pappas P, Banias C, et al: Delayed presentation of posttraumatic internal pudendal artery-urethral fistula treated by selective embolization. *J Trauma Inj Infect Crit Care* 63:1388–1390, 2007.

Moeller MS: Indications for use of recombinant factor VII: a case study with implications for research. *J Trauma Nursing* 13(4):190–192, 2006.

Moltzan CJ, et al: The evidence for the use of recombinant factor VIIa in massive bleeding: development of a transfusion policy framework. *Transfusion Medicine* 18(2):112–120, 2008

Moore KM: Controversies in fluid resuscitation. *J Trauma Nsg* 13(4):168–172, 2006

Mosier MJ, Pham TN: American Burn Association Practice Guidelines for prevention, diagnosis, and treatment of ventilator-associated pneumonia (VAP) in burn patients. *J Burn Care Res* 30(6):910–928, 2009.

Patanwala AE: Factor VIIa (recombinant) for acute traumatic hemorrhage. *Am J Health System Pharmacy* 65(17):1616–1623, 2008.

Patterson DR, et al: Optimizing control of pain from severe burns: a literature review. *Am J Clin Hypertens* 47(1):43–54, 2004.

Perel P, Roberts I: Colloids versus crystalloids for fluid resuscitation in critically ill patients. *Cochrane Database Syst Rev* 17(4):CD000567, 2007.

Pham TN, Cancio LC, Gibran NS: American Burn Association practice guidelines: burn shock resuscitation. *J Burn Care Res* 29:257–266, 2008.

Quagliano PV, Delair SM, Malhotra AK: Diagnosis of blunt bladder injury: a prospective comparative study of computed tomography cystography and conventional retrograde cystography. *J Trauma Inj Infect Crit Care* 61(2):410–422, 2006.

Raza A, Byrne D, Townell N: Lower limb compartment syndrome after urological pelvic surgery. *J Urol* 171:5–11, 2004.

Review: fluid resuscitation with colloids does not reduce mortality more than crystalloids in critically ill patients. *ACP Journal Club* 148(3), 2008. http://online.statref.com/document.aspx?fxid=173anddocid=350

Ross J: Near drowning. *RN* 68(7):36–41, 2005.

Runyon MS: Blunt genitourinary trauma. UpToDate September 24, 2008. *http://uptodateonline.com*.

Ruttmann E, et al: Prolonged extracorporeal membrane oxygenation-assisted support provides improved survival in hypothermic patients with cardiocirculatory arrest. *J Thorac Cardiovasc Surg* 134(3):594–600, 2007.

Sagrista-Sauleda J, et al: Low-pressure cardiac tamponade: clinical and hemodynamic profile. *Circulation* 114:945, 2006.

Salcido R, Lepre SJ: Compartment syndrome: wound care considerations. *Adv Skin Wound Care* 20(10):559–565, 2007.

Schecter SC, Schecter WP, McAninch JW: Penetrating bilateral renal injuries: principles of management. *J Trauma Inj Infect Crit Care* 67(2):E25–E28, 2009.

Seiler JG, Casey PJ, Binford SH: Compartment syndrome of the upper extremity. *J South Orthop Assoc* 9(4), 2000.

Shadgan B, Menon M, O'Brien PJ, Reid WD: Diagnostic techniques in acute compartment syndrome of the leg. *J Orthop Trauma* 22(8):581–587, 2008.

Shariat SF, Roehrborn CG, Karakiewicz PI, Dhami C: Evidence-based validation of the predictive value of the American Association for the Surgery of Trauma Kidney Injury Scale. *J Trauma Inj Infect Crit Care* 62(4):933–939, 2007.

Shariat SF, Trinh QD, Morey A, et al: Development of a highly accurate nomogram for prediction of the need for exploration in patients with renal trauma. *J Trauma Inj Infect Crit Care* 64(6): 1451–1458, 2008.

Shepherd SM: Drowning. 2008. http://www.emedicine.com/emerg/TOPIC744.htm

Simon B, et al: Practice management guideline for "pulmonary contusion-flail chest." June 2006. EAST Practice Management Workgroup for Pulmonary Contusion-Flail Chest. http://east. org/tpg/pulmcontflailchest.pdf

Singisetti K: Postoperative acute compartment syndrome in the nonoperated "well leg": implications to orthopaedic nursing. *Orthop J Neurosurg* 28(2):91–93, 2009.

Spahn DR, Cerny V, Coats TJ, Duranteau J, et al: Task Force for Advanced Bleeding Care in Trauma. Management of bleeding following major trauma: a European guideline. *Crit care* 11(1):R17, 2007.

Spaniol JR: Fluid resuscitation therapy for hemorrhagic shock. *J Trauma Nursing* 14(3):152–160, 2007.

Spodick DH: Acute cardiac tamponade. *N Engl J Med* 349:648, 2003.

Stiefal M, Spiotta A, Gracias V, et al: Reduced mortality rate in patients with severe traumatic brain injury treated with brain tissue oxygen monitoring. *J Neurosurg* 103:805–811, 2005.

Styl J: *Compartment syndromes: Diagnosis, treatment and complications.* Boca Raton, FL, 2004, CRC Press.

Tator C: Review of treatment trials in human spinal cord injury. *Neurosurgery* 59(5): 982–987, 2006.

Thalmann M, et al: Resuscitation in near drowning with extracorporeal membrane oxygenation. *Ann Thorac Surg* 72:607–608, 2001.

The American Burn Association, National Headquarters Office: www.ameriburn.org

The Phoenix Society for Burn Survivors, Inc, National Headquarters Office: www.phoenix-society.org

Tinkoff G, Esposito TJ, Reed J, et al: American Association for the Surgery of Trauma Organ Injury Scale, I: spleen, liver, and kidney, validation based on the National Trauma Data Bank. *J Am Coll Surg* 207(5):646–655, 2008.

Tisherman SA, et al: Clinical practice guideline: endpoints of resuscitation. *J Trauma* 57(4):898–912, 2004.

Tremblay LN, Feliciano DV, Schmidt J, et al: Skin only or silo closure in the critically ill patient with an open abdomen. *Am J Surg* 182:670, 2001.

Van Houtte S, Vanlandewijck Y, Gosselink R: Respiratory muscle training in persons with spinal cord injury: a systematic review. *Respir Med* 100(11):1886–1895, 2006.

Verive M: Near drowning. 2007. http://www.emedicine.com/ped/TOPIC2570.htm

Voelzke B, McAninch JW: Renal gunshot wounds: clinical management and outcome. *J Trauma Inj Infect Crit Care* 66(3):593–601, 2009.

Ward RS: Physical rehabilitation. In Carrougher GJ, editor: *Burn care and therapy.* St. Louis, 1998, Mosby.

Weber JM: Epidemiology of infections and strategies for control. In Carrougher GJ, editor: *Burn care and therapy.* St. Louis, 1998, Mosby.

Wilensky E, Bloom S, Leichter D, et al: Brain tissue oxygenation practice guidelines using the LICOX® CMP Monitoring System. *J Neurosci Nursing* 37(5):278–288, 2005.

Williams FN, Jeschke MG, Chinkes DL, et al: Modulation of the hypermetabolic response to trauma: temperature, nutrition, and drugs. *J Am Coll Surg* 208(4):489–502, 2009.

World Society on Abdominal Compartment Syndrome. *Consensus definitions and recommendations.*

Wuermser L, Ho C, Chiodo A, et al: Spinal cord injury medicine, 2. Acute care management of traumatic and nontraumatic injury. *Arch Phys Med Rehabil* 88(S1):S55–S61, 2007.

Yarlagadda C: Cardiac tamponade. 2008. eMedicine. www.emedicine.com

Zimmer M, Nantwi K, Goshgarian H: Effect of spinal cord injury on the respiratory system: basic research and current clinical treatment options. *J Spinal Cord Med* 30(4):319–330, 2007.

Ziran BH, Chamberlin E, Shuler FD, Shah M: Delays and difficulties in the diagnosis of lower urologic injuries in the context of pelvic fractures. *J Trauma Inj Infect Crit Care* 58(3):533–537, 2005.

RESPIRATORY ASSESSMENT: GENERAL

GOAL OF SYSTEM ASSESSMENT
Evaluate for ineffective breathing patterns, impaired gas exchange, and airway obstruction.

VITAL SIGN ASSESSMENT
- Respiratory rate (RR) and depth to evaluate for tachypnea, bradypnea, and work of breathing
- Pulse oximetry to help identify low readings reflective of impaired gas exchange
- Heart rate (HR) to evaluate for tachycardia or bradycardia; generally associated with respiratory rate changes

CONTINUOUS PULSE OXIMETRY (SPO$_2$ MONITORING)
- Evaluate for changes over time and/or since the last recorded reading. Results should be correlated with the arterial oxygen saturation (Sao$_2$) readings derived from arterial blood gases.
- Pulse oximetry accuracy is dependent on the presence of an adequate pulse in the area in which the measurement probe has been applied.
- Ensure readings are done using an appropriate probe placed on the anatomical location with the best pulse and least interference. Probes are available for the finger, forehead, or ear lobe.
- Readings must be correlated with physical assessment findings and can remain normal despite signs of impending deterioration. Physical assessment findings such as use of accessory muscles or presence of tachypnea are indicative of respiratory distress but may not be reflected in a change in Spo$_2$. If an increasing amount of oxygen (O$_2$) is needed to maintain Spo$_2$, this is also indicative of impending deterioration of the patient.

OBSERVATION
- Evaluate for use of accessory muscles, shortness of breath, and air hunger.
- Ensure the patient is evaluated for the presence of chronic obstructive pulmonary disease (COPD) prior to applying O$_2$ therapy so appropriate liter flow is determined to prevent respiratory impairment.
- Evaluate facial and lip color for pallor or cyanosis indicative of hypoxemia.

AUSCULTATION
- Listen to breath sounds to evaluate for presence of adventitious sounds that reflect factors contributing to respiratory distress, including those related to both airway obstruction and impaired gas exchange.
- Adventitious sounds: *crackles* (rales) indicative of fluid in alveoli, *bubbles* (rhonchi) indicative of secretions in bronchioles, wheezing (inflammation), *inspiratory stridor*

(narrowing of airways due to massive inflammation or obstruction by secretions or foreign body), or *pleural friction rub* (inflammation)
- Lungs must be auscultated anteriorly and posteriorly in all three lobes of the right lung, the two lobes of the left lung, over the right and left main bronchi, and over the trachea.

SCREENING LABWORK
- Arterial blood gas analysis can reveal increases or decreases in pH; levels of O_2, O_2 saturation, CO_2, and bicarbonate; base excess or base deficit indicative of impending respiratory failure; hyperpnea/tachypnea; and metabolic derangements affecting breathing patterns. Blood gas analysis may be done using either arterial blood or mixed venous blood samples. Mixed venous blood samples are available only using a pulmonary artery catheter and can be used to calculate efficacy of both O_2 delivery and O_2 consumption. Arterial blood gases cannot be used to calculate O_2 consumption.

CARE PLANS: GENERAL APPROACHES TO RESPIRATORY DISORDERS
Impaired spontaneous ventilation with or without impaired gas exchange

---

GOALS/OUTCOMES Within 12 to 24 hours of treatment, patient has adequate gas exchange, reflected by PaO_2 greater than 80 mm Hg, $PaCO_2$ 35 to 45 mm Hg, pH 7.35 to 7.45, presence of normal breath sounds, and absence of adventitious breath sounds. RR is 12 to 20 breaths/min with normal pattern and depth or back to normal baseline.
NOC Respiratory Status: Ventilation, Vital Signs Status, Respiratory Status: Gas Exchange, Symptom Control Behavior, Comfort Level, Endurance

Ventilation Assistance
1. Assess for patent airway; if snoring, crowing, stridor, or strained respirations are present, indicative of partial or full airway obstruction, open airway using chin lift or jaw thrust.
2. Insert an oral airway if patient becomes unconscious and cannot maintain patent airway; use a nasopharyngeal airway if patient is conscious to avoid provoking vomiting. If severely distressed, patient may require endotracheal intubation.
3. Position patient to alleviate dyspnea and insure maximal ventilation; generally, sitting in an upright position unless severe hypotension is present.
4. Monitor changes in oxygenation following position change: SpO_2, SvO_2, $ScVO_2$, end-tidal CO_2, $A—aDO_2$ levels and arterial blood gases (ABGs).
5. Clear secretions from airway by having patient cough vigorously, or provide nasotracheal, oropharyngeale, or endotracheal tube suctioning, as needed.
6. Have patient breathe slowly or manually ventilate with manual resuscitator or bag-valve-mask device slowly and deeply between coughing or suctioning attempts.
7. Assist with use of incentive spirometer as appropriate.
8. Turn patient every 2 hours if immobile. Encourage patient to turn self, or get out of bed as much as tolerated if he or she is able.
9. Provide mucolytic and bronchodilating medications orally, intravenously, or by inhaler, aerosol, or nebulizer as ordered to assist with thinning secretions and relaxing muscles in lower airways.
10. Provide chest physical therapy as appropriate, if other methods of secretion removal are ineffective.

Oxygen Therapy
1. Ensure humidity is provided when using O_2 or bilevel positive airway pressure (BiPAP) device for more than 12 hours to help thin secretions.
2. Administer supplemental O_2 using liter flow and device as ordered.
3. Restrict patient and visitors from smoking while O_2 is in use.
4. Document pulse oximetry with O_2 liter flow in place at time of reading as ordered. Oxygen is a drug; the dose of the drug must be associated with the O_2 saturation or the reading is meaningless.
5. Obtain arterial blood gases if patient experiences behavioral changes or respiratory distress to check for hypoxia or hypercapnia.
6. Monitor for hypoventilation, especially in patients with COPD.
7. Monitor for changes indicative of O_2 toxicity in patients receiving higher concentrations of O_2 (more than FIO_2 45%) for longer than 24 hours. Changes will be apparent in chest radiograph and breath sounds. Absorption atelectasis may be present. The higher the O_2 concentration, the greater is the chance of toxicity.

8. Monitor for skin breakdown where O_2 devices are in contact with the skin, such as nares, around the ears, and around edges of mask devices.
9. Provide O_2 therapy during transportation and when patient gets out of bed.
10. If patient is unable to maintain Spo_2 reading of more than 88% off O_2, consult with the respiratory care practitioner/therapist and the physician about the need for home O_2 therapy.

Respiratory Monitoring

1. Monitor rate, rhythm, and depth of respirations.
2. Note chest movement for symmetry of chest expansion and signs of increased work of breathing such as use of accessory muscles or retraction of intercostal or supraclavicular muscles. Consider use of noninvasive positive pressure ventilation for impending respiratory failure.
3. Monitor for snoring, coughing, and possibly choking-type respirations when patients have a decreased level of consciousness to assess if airway is obstructed by tongue.
4. Monitor for new breathing patterns that impair ventilation, which may need aggressive management in a specialized, highly skilled setting.
5. Note that trachea remains midline, as deviation may indicate patient has a tension pneumothorax.
6. Auscultate breath sounds before and after administration of respiratory medications to assess for improvement.
7. Evaluate changes in O_2 saturation (Sao_2), pulse oximetry (Spo_2), end-tidal CO_2 ($ETCO_2$), $ScVO_2$, and ABGs as appropriate.
8. Monitor for dyspnea and note causative activities/events.
9. If increased restlessness or unusual somnolence occur, evaluate patient for hypoxemia and hypercapnia as appropriate.
10. Monitor chest radiograph reports as new images become available.

NIC Cough Enhancement, Acid-Base Management, Mechanical Ventilation, Artificial Airway Management, Oral Health Maintenance

ACUTE ASTHMA EXACERBATION

PATHOPHYSIOLOGY

The problem of asthma affects over 22 million people in the United States, including 6 million children, making it one of the most common childhood diseases. Asthma manifests variable, recurrent symptoms related to airflow limitation stemming from chronic airway inflammation. Bronchiolar smooth muscles manifest overactive bronchoconstriction and are hyperresponsive to internal and environmental stimuli. Airflow obstruction is fully or partially reversible, but as the disease progresses, the chronic airway inflammation creates edema, mucus, and eventually mucus plugging, which further decreases airflow. Eventually, irreversible changes in airway structure occur, including fibrosis, smooth muscle hypertrophy, mucus hypersecretion, injury to epithelial cells, and angiogenesis. Asthmatic persons eventually develop air trapping, increased functional residual capacity, and decreased forced vital capacity. Several types of cells and cellular elements are affected, including mast cells, epithelial cells, T lymphocytes, macrophages, eosinophils, and neutrophils, which when triggered can prompt sometimes sudden, fatal exacerbations of coughing, wheezing, chest tightness, and breathlessness.

Life-threatening asthma exacerbation results from bronchial smooth muscle contraction (bronchospasm), bronchial inflammation leading to airway edema, and mucus plugging. When an episode of bronchospasm (critical airway narrowing) is not reversed after 24 hours of maximal doses of traditional inhaled short-acting beta$_2$-adrenergic agonists (SABAs) such as albuterol or levalbuterol, injected systemic beta$_2$-agonists such as epinephrine, inhaled anticholinergics such as ipratropium, and systemic steroid therapy with prednisone, prednisolone, or methylprednisolone, the refractory patient may be diagnosed with status asthmaticus (SA). Common triggers for asthma exacerbations include respiratory tract infections, allergens (airborne or ingested), air pollutants, smoke, and physical irritants (e.g., cold air, exercise). Anxiety or "panic" attacks and use of beta-adrenergic blocking agents and nonsteroidal anti-inflammatory drugs (NSAIDs) may predispose patients to development or exacerbation of severe asthma.

Several clinical patterns for development of an asthma exacerbation are recognized. An "attack" can happen suddenly (over several hours), or it may take several days to reach a critical airway obstruction. The more common gradual presentation manifests with increasing symptoms of sputum production, coughing, wheezing, and dyspnea. As air trapping increases, lung hyperinflation prompts increased work of breathing. Rapid exhalations increase insensible water loss through exhaled water vapor and diaphoresis. Oral intake may be decreased, contributing to hypovolemia. Without adequate oral intake to promote hydration, mucus becomes thick and begins to plug the airways. Terminal bronchioles can become occluded completely from mucosal edema and tenacious secretions. Ventilation-perfusion mismatch or shunting occurs as poorly ventilated alveoli continue to be perfused, which leads to hypoxemia. Tachycardia is an early compensatory mechanism to increase O_2 delivery to the body cells, but it increases myocardial O_2 demand. Oxygen requirements and work of breathing increase, leading to respiratory failure, hypercapnia, and respiratory arrest if not managed promptly and appropriately.

ASSESSMENT
Goal of System Assessment
- Evaluate for ineffective breathing patterns, impaired gas exchange, and airway obstruction.
- Determine patient's prior treatment regimen; classify which "step" of treatment has been needed to control symptoms; patient may need to move to the next step of treatment to maintain control.
- Classify severity of exacerbation: should be determined following initial assessment and diagnostic testing.

History and Risk Factors
For Asthma
- *Asthma symptoms*: Cough (especially if worse at night), wheezing, recurrent difficulty breathing, recurrent chest tightness
- *Family history*: Patients with either family history or atopic disease are at higher risk of asthma.
- *Common triggers*: Symptoms worsen with viral respiratory infections, environmental airborne allergens, irritants in the home (mold, mildew, wood-burning stove, cockroaches, dust mites, animal dander, carpeting laid over concrete), recent emotional upset, aggressive exercise, fear, frustration, food, new medications, changes in weather (especially exposure to cold air), occupational chemicals or allergens, and hormonal changes (menstrual cycle).
- *Comorbid conditions*: Sinusitis, rhinitis, gastroesophageal reflux disease (GERD), obstructive sleep apnea (OSA), allergic bronchopulmonary aspergillosis (ABPA)

For Asthma Exacerbation
1. *Classify asthma severity*: **Intermittent** (step 1 treatment) or **persistent**: mild, moderate, severe (steps 2, 3, 4, 5, and 6 treatments); steps differ for children under age 5, children between 5 and 12 years old, and adults.
2. *Classify severity of exacerbation:* Mild to severe or life threatening
3. *Assess control*: Determine if pattern of previous exacerbations is inherent to the current episode.
4. *Compliance/ability to control*: Assess the patient's knowledge and skills for self-management.
5. *Identify precipitating factors*: **Situation**: exposure at home, work, daycare, or school to inhalant allergens or irritants; time of day, season or time of year, relationship of symptoms to meals, deterioration in other health conditions or menses
6. *Identify comorbid conditions* that may impair asthma management (e.g., sinusitis, rhinitis, GERD, OSA, obesity, stress, or depression).
7. *Surgery*: Asthmatic patients are at high risk for exacerbations following endotracheal intubation, general anesthesia, and ventilation provided during surgical or other invasive procedures. Impaired cough, hypoxemia, and hypercapnia may trigger exacerbation.

Spirometry or Peak Expiratory Flow

- *Peak expiratory flow (PEF)*: Measurement of rate or force of exhalation; those with easier breathing will have higher values than those in distress. A peak flowmeter is used by patients at home to assess asthma control. Those with more severe asthma may have difficulty discerning worsening of symptoms and may use PEF several times daily to assess for declining rate of exhalation.
- Assesses degree of obstruction and reversibility in patients older than 5 years
- Spirometry is essential for establishing the diagnosis of asthma. Patients' perceptions of airflow obstruction are highly variable. Spirometry or PEF provides an objective measurement to help classify severity of exacerbation.
- Decreased to less than 40% of predicted value indicates severe exacerbation; less than 25% of predicted value for life threatening

Vital Signs (Severe to Life-Threatening Asthma Exacerbation)

- *Presence of fever*: Temperature elevation helps discern whether patient's condition is related to a microbe (fever) versus an allergen (afebrile).
- *Pulse oximetry*: Oxygen saturation is decreased from patient's baseline value.
- Tachycardia (HR greater than 140 bpm) and tachypnea (RR greater than 40 breaths/min)
- Hypotension may be present; hypotension is exacerbated by underlying dehydration often present with patients with severe asthma.

Observation

- Severe attacks render patients unable to speak due to breathlessness.
- Use of accessory muscles; fatigued, with or without diaphoresis
- Ashen, pale, or gray/blue facial color, lip color, or nail beds
- Chest expansion may be decreased or restricted.
- Altered level of consciousness (confusion, disorientation, agitation)
- Agitation is more commonly associated with hypoxemia while somnolence is associated with hypercapnia (elevated CO_2 level).
- Frequent coughing
- Increased nasal secretions, mucosal swelling, nasal polyps
- Prolonged phase of forced expiration

Auscultation

- Wheezing bronchial breath sounds; wheezing on inspiration is more indicative of acute airway narrowing, versus wheezing on expiration, which is more common.
- Wheezing during normal breathing is common.
- Chest may be nearly silent if airflow is severely obstructed.

Palpation

- Palpate to assess for chest expansion; chest may be hyperinflated or may be asymmetrical; chest expansion during inspiration may be decreased.
- Decreased tactile fremitus may be present.

Percussion

- May reveal hyperresonance (pneumothorax), a complication of asthma

Screening Labwork

- *Complete blood count (CBC with WBC differential)*: Evaluates for elevated white blood cells indicative of chronic inflammation due to allergic response and infection including presence of eosinophils, neutrophils, and mononuclear cells
- *ABG Analysis*: Evaluates for hypoxemia and hypercapnia

RESEARCH BRIEF 4-1

A series of studies with conflicting results has identified the possibility of increased risk of asthma associated with acetaminophen use. The researchers searched all major medical databases, to identify all clinical trials and observational studies related to this correlation since 1966. Results revealed thirteen cross-sectional studies, four cohort studies, and two case-control studies of a total of 425,140 subjects. The pooled odds ratio (OR) for asthma among subjects using acetaminophen was 1.63. The risk of childhood asthma among acetaminophen users during the year preceding the diagnosis of asthma and within the first year of life was elevated (OR: 1.60 and 1.47, respectively). Only one study reported the association between high acetaminophen dose and asthma in children. Risk of asthma and wheezing was increased with prenatal use of acetaminophen (OR: 1.28 and 1.50, respectively). Results were consistent with an increased risk of asthma and wheezing in both children and adults exposed to acetaminophen. Future studies are needed to confirm the correlation.

From Etminan M, Sadatsafavi M, Jafari S, et al: Acetaminophen use and the risk of asthma in children and adults. *Chest* 136(5):1316–1323, 2009.

 Safety Alert *Patients with severe wheezing who have not been diagnosed with asthma should be evaluated for other causes of upper airway obstruction and "cardiac asthma." Patients with left ventricular failure may wheeze if interstitial fluid increases to the point where bronchioles are compressed or if the pulmonary interstitial edema is severe enough to cause bronchospasm. Asymmetric breath sounds or chest pain may signal that the patient has a pneumothorax. Stridor may indicate the patient has an impending respiratory emergency, versus wheezing that may be present regardless of situation in poorly controlled asthmatics. Stridor is commonly seen with acute airway narrowing related to acute allergic reaction or anaphylaxis.*

Diagnostic Tests for Acute Asthma Exacerbation

Test	Purpose	Abnormal Findings
Arterial blood gas analysis (ABG)	Assess for abnormal gas exchange or compensation for metabolic derangements. Initially Pao_2 is normal and then decreases as the ventilation-perfusion mismatch becomes more severe. A normal Pco_2 in a distressed asthma patient receiving aggressive treatment may indicate respiratory fatigue, which causes a progressively ineffective breathing pattern, which can also lead to respiratory arrest. Oxygenation assessment differs from acid base balance assessment, wherein the Pco_2 value is used as the hallmark sign for respiratory failure induced acidosis.	*pH changes*: Acidosis may reflect respiratory failure; alkalosis may reflect tachypnea. *Carbon dioxide*: Elevated CO_2 reflects respiratory failure; decreased CO_2 reflects tachypnea; rising Pco_2 is an ominous, since it signals severe hypoventilation, which can lead to respiratory arrest. *Hypoxemia*: Pao_2 less than 80 mm Hg) *Oxygen saturation*: SaO_2 less than 92% *Bicarbonate*: HCO_3 less than 22 meq/L *Base Deficit*: less than -2
Complete blood count (CBC) with WBC differential	WBC differential evaluates the strength of the immune system's response to the trigger of exacerbation and for presence of infection.	*Eosinophils*: increased in patients not receiving corticosteroids; indicative of magnitude of inflammatory response. *Increased WBC count*: More than 11,000/mm^3 is seen with bacterial pneumonias. WBCs may be increased by asthma in the absence of infection. The *Hematocrit (Hct)*: may be increased from hypovolemia and hemoconcentration.

Continued

Diagnostic Tests for Acute Asthma Exacerbation—cont'd

Test	Purpose	Abnormal Findings
Pulmonary function tests (PFTs)/ spirometry	The hallmark sign of asthma is a decreased FEV_1 (forced expiratory volume in the first second)/FVC (forced vital capacity.) If PEF rate does not improve with initial aggressive inhaled bronchodilator treatments, morbidity increases.	*Forced expiratory volume (FEV):* decreased during acute episodes; if less than 0.7, narrowed airways prevent forceful exhalation of inspired volume (Table 4-1). *Peak expiratory flow rate (PEF):* less than 100–125 L/min in a normal-sized adult indicates severe obstruction to air flow.
Pulse oximetry (SpO_2)	Noninvasive technology that measures the oxygen saturation of arterial blood intermittently or continuously using a probe placed on the patient's finger or ear. When using pulse oximetry, it is helpful to obtain ABG values to compare the oxygen saturation and evaluate the PaO_2, $PaCO_2$, and pH.	Normal SpO_2: more than 95%. Correlation of SpO_2 with SaO_2 (arterial saturation) is within 2% when SaO_2 is more than 50%. Temperature, pH, $PaCO_2$, anemia, and hemodynamic status may reduce the accuracy of pulse oximetry measurements. Presence of other forms of Hgb in the blood (carboxyhemoglobin or methemoglobin) can produce falsely high readings.
Serologic studies	Acute and convalescent titers are drawn to diagnose a viral infection.	*Increased antibody titers:* a positive sign for viral infection.
Chest radiograph	Evaluates the severity of air trapping; also useful in ruling out other causes of respiratory failure (e.g., foreign body aspiration, pulmonary edema, pulmonary embolism, pneumonia).	The x-ray usually shows lung hyperinflation caused by air trapping and a flat diaphragm related to increased intrathoracic volume.
12-Lead ECG (electrocardiogram)	Evaluates for dysrhythmias associated with stress response and asthma medications.	*Sinus tachycardia:* important baseline indicator; use of some bronchodilators (e.g., metaproterenol) may produce cardiac stimulant effects and dysrhythmias.
Sputum gram stain, culture and sensitivity	Culture and sensitivity may show microorganisms if infection is the precipitating event. The most reliable specimens are obtained via bronchoalveolar lavage (BAL) during bronchoscopy, or using a protected telescoping catheter (mini or using BAL) to decrease risk of contamination from oral flora.	Gross examination may show increased viscosity or actual mucous plugs. *Gram stain positive:* Indicates organism is present. *Culture:* Identifies organism. *Sensitivity:* Reflects effectiveness of drugs on identified organism.
Diagnostic fiberoptic bronchoscopy using PSB (protected specimen brush) and BAL	Obtains specimens during simple bronchoscopy without contaminating the aspirate; modified technique (mini-BAL) is also effective without the need of full bronchoscopy.	*Gram stain positive:* Indicates organism is present. *Culture:* Identifies organism. *Sensitivity:* Reflects effectiveness of drugs on identified organism.
Serum theophylline level	Important baseline indicator for patients who take theophylline regularly; therapeutic level is close to the toxic level. If additional theophylline is given, serial levels should be measured within the first 12–24 hr of treatment and daily thereafter. Patients are monitored for side effects (e.g., nausea, nervousness, dysrhythmias).	Acceptable therapeutic range is 10–20 mcg/ml. There is little evidence to support clinical benefit for adding theophylline to inhaled β-adrenergic blocking agents and steroids for patients with acute, severe asthma who were not already using theophylline regularly.

COLLABORATIVE MANAGEMENT
Care Priorities
The goal of asthma management is to control the disease using a stepped approach to therapies. Ideal control is attained when patients are free of daytime symptoms, do not awaken breathless or coughing at night, have few or no limitations on activities, do not regularly use rescue medications, have no exacerbations, and maintain a forced expiratory volume in 1 second (FEV_1) and/or peak expiratory flow rate (PEFR) greater than 80% of the predicted value. When prevention fails, the potential for life-threatening respiratory failure is high during exacerbations unresponsive to treatment within the first hour. Management is directed toward decreasing bronchospasm and increasing ventilation. Other interventions are directed toward treatment of complications (Table 4-1).

1. **Determine severity of asthma exacerbation:**
   a. *Acute severe:* PEFR is less than 40% of predicted or personal best in a patient who is unable to speak a complete sentence in one breath, with RR greater than 25 breaths/min and HR greater than 110 bpm.
   b. *Life threatening:* In a patient with severe asthma, the PEFR is less than 25% of predicted or personal best, SpO_2 less than 92%, PaO_2 less than 80 mm Hg; PcO_2 35 to 35 mm Hg, silent chest, weak respiratory effort, exhaustion, cyanosis, bradycardia, hypotension, dysrhythmias, confusion, coma.
   c. *Near fatal:* PcO_2 greater than 45 mm Hg and/or requiring mechanical ventilation using increased positive pressure to overcome inspiratory pressures; patient also has other findings of life-threatening exacerbation.

2. **Oxygen therapy:** Patients have profound hypoxia and can tolerate high doses of O_2 (FIO_2) unless they retain CO_2 and breathe by hypoxic drive. Most asthmatics are able to tolerate high flow O_2, versus those with other obstructive lung disease who cannot. Oxygen dosage must be limited in nonintubated, mechanically ventilated patients who breathe via hypoxic drive to avoid hypoventilation and respiratory arrest. Humidified O_2 therapy is begun immediately to correct hypoxemia and thin secretions. PaO_2 is kept slightly above normal unless the patient retains CO_2, to compensate for the increased O_2

Table 4-1	PULMONARY FUNCTION TESTS IN ASTHMA EXACERBATION		
Test	**Description**	**Normal Values**	**Exacerbation Values**
FEV_1 Forced expiratory volume (1 second)	Volume of gas exhaled over first second of full exhalation measured by FVC	≥75% of predicted normal	*Severe:* less than 40% of predicted or personal best *Life threatening:* less than 25% of predicted or personal best Decreased due to narrowed airways, which are resistant to airflow during exhalation
FVC Forced vital capacity	Total amount of gas exhaled as forcefully and rapidly as possible after maximal inspiration	≥80% of predicted normal	With severe or life-threatening exacerbation: decreased because of air trapping
FEF Forced expiratory flow	Average rate of flow during middle half of FEV; an accurate estimate of airway resistance	≥80% of predicted normal	Decreased because of small airways obstruction; may return to normal after inhalation of aerosolized bronchodilator
PEFR or *PEF* Peak expiratory flow rate	Maximal rate of air flow throughout FVC	<100–125 L/min in a normal-sized adult indicates severe obstruction to air flow.	Decreased because of small airways obstruction; may return to normal after inhalation of aerosolized bronchodilator

demands imposed by the increased work of breathing. The degree of hypoxemia and patient response determine the method of O_2 delivery. A high-flow device (e.g., 100% nonrebreather mask) delivers more precise and higher FIO_2. Management of anxiety must be considered, especially if the patient will not wear a mask because of feelings of suffocation.

3. **Heliox therapy:** A blended mixture of helium and O_2, available in mixtures of 60:40, 70:30, and 80:20, which is delivered either through a tight-fitting face mask or through a mechanical ventilator circuit. Use results in decreased inspiratory and expiratory airway resistance, may increase removal of CO_2, and may improve oxygenation.

4. **Intubation and mechanical ventilation:** Strongly considered when the patient has severe hypoxemia or hypercapnia indicative of impending respiratory failure: confusion, somnolence, agitation, or central cyanosis; or if patient experiences intolerable respiratory distress. Mechanical ventilation ensures adequate alveolar ventilation, and the endotracheal (ET) tube provides a pathway for clearing airway secretions by means of suctioning. Initial ventilator settings may include a tidal volume of 5 to 8 ml/kg and a rate of 12 to 15 breaths/min. Controlled mandatory ventilation may be required, along with heavy sedation, analgesia. In exceptionally severe cases, neuromuscular blockade may be warranted in addition to sedation and analgesia.

5. **Pharmacotherapy to manage acute asthma exacerbation:** Vigorous therapy is initiated to decrease bronchospasms, help reduce airway inflammation, and help remove secretions. Treatment is continued until wheezing is eliminated and pulmonary function tests return to baseline (Table 4-1).

   - *Bronchodilators*: Dilate smooth muscles of the airways to help relieve bronchospasms, resulting in increased diameter of functional airways. SABAs are the mainstay of asthma exacerbation management, while long-acting beta-adrenergic agonists (LABAs) are used for long-term control of asthma. Theophylline and aminophylline are no longer recommended for management of acute bronchospasms.
   - *Corticosteroids*: Given intravenously during the acute phase of the exacerbation to decrease the inflammatory response, which causes edema in upper airways. Administration should decrease reactivity and swelling of the airways. Dosage varies according to severity of episode and whether patient currently is taking steroids. The patient may be converted to inhaled corticosteroids once the acute phase has been resolved. Acute adrenal insufficiency can develop in patients who take steroids routinely at home, if these drugs are not given to the patient during hospitalization.
   - *Anticholinergics*: Inhaled medications used to reduce vagal tone of the airways, thus helping to reduce bronchospasms. Ipratropium (Atrovent) is used in combination with inhaled SABAs for severe, acute asthma.
   - *Magnesium sulfate*: American Thoracic Society asthma management guidelines (2008) recommend consideration of a single dose of magnesium sulfate 1.2 to 2 g over 20 minutes for patients with severe, life-threatening, or fatal exacerbation who have an inadequate or ineffective response to inhaled bronchodilators.
   - *Sedatives and analgesics*: Used in more limited doses in patients who are not intubated or mechanically ventilated, unless the person is extremely agitated and unable to cooperate with therapy. These agents depress the central nervous system (CNS) response to hypoxia and hypercapnia. Once mechanical ventilation is in place, the dosage is titrated until the patient is comfortable and/or hypoxemia or hypercapnia begins to resolve.
   - *Buffers*: Sodium bicarbonate may be given to correct severe acidosis not corrected by intubation and mechanical ventilation. Generally, this is only a temporizing measure to help relieve lactic acidosis. The physiologic response to bronchodilators improves with correction of metabolic acidosis.
   - *Antibiotics*: Given if a respiratory infection is suspected, as evidenced by fever, purulent sputum, or leukocytosis.

6. **Fluid replacement:** To liquefy secretions and replace insensible losses. Generally, crystalloid fluids (e.g., D_5W, D_5NS) are used.

7. **Chest physiotherapy:** Generally contraindicated in acute phases of exacerbation because of acute respiratory decompensation and hyperreactive airways. Once the crisis is over, the patient may benefit from percussion and postural drainage every 2 to 4 hours to help mobilize secretions.

Table 4-2	MEDICATIONS USED FOR ASTHMA EXACERBATION		
Drug Type	**Medication and Dosage**	**Action**	**Side Effects**
Short-acting inhaled β_2^- adrenergic agonist (SABA)	*Albuterol:* Nebulized 2.5–5 mg every 20 minutes for 3 doses, then 2.5–10 mg every 1–4 hours as needed, or 10–15 mg/hr continuously *Levalbuterol [(R)-albuterol]:* Nebulizer solution (0.63 mg/3 ml, 1.25 mg/0.5 ml, 1.25 mg/3 ml) given 1.25–2.5 mg every 20 minutes for 3 doses, then 1.25–5 mg every 1–4 hours as needed	Immediate adrenergic stimulant effects; activates β_2 adrenergic receptors; relaxes smooth muscle to relieve bronchospasm	Slightly increased heart rate, possible anxiety, nervousness, tremors, palpitations
Nonselective β-agonist therapy	*Epinephrine:* 0.3–0.5 mg every 20 minutes for 3 doses subcutaneously (SC) *Terbutaline:* 0.25 mg every 20 minutes for 3 doses SC; also available orally as 5 mg PO TID (maximum dose 15 mg daily) *There is no proven advantage of systemic therapy over aerosolized therapy.	Stimulates both α- and β-adrenergic receptors; relaxes bronchial smooth muscle; epinephrine may cause peripheral vasoconstriction; terbutaline is the drug of choice in pregnant women.	Increased HR (>120 bpm), nervousness, tremor, palpitations, nausea, vomiting, headache, paradoxical bronchospasm
Corticosteroids	*Prednisone, methylprednisolone, or prednisolone:* 40–80 mg/day in 1 or 2 divided doses until PEF rate reaches 70% of predicted or personal best	Anti-inflammatory effects help to decrease both swelling and reactivity of airways	Mood swings, insomnia, agitation, osteoporosis, gastrointestinal upset: nausea, heartburn; if tapered improperly, patient may experience adrenal insufficiency
Anticholinergics	*Ipratropium bromide nebulizer solution 0.25mg/ml (Atrovent):* 0.5 mg every 20 minutes for 3 doses, then as needed; generally used in conjunction with β-agonist therapy. May mix in same nebulizer with albuterol. Should not be used as first-line therapy; should be added to SABA therapy for severe exacerbations. The addition of ipratropium has not been shown to provide further benefit once the patient is hospitalized. *Ipratropium with albuterol nebulizer solution* (each 3 ml vial contains 0.5 mg ipratropium bromide and 2.5 mg albuterol): 3 ml every 20 minutes for 3 doses, then as needed. May be used for up to 3 hours in the initial management of severe exacerbations.	Blocks action of acetylcholine at parasympathetic sites of bronchial smooth muscle to cause inhibition of nasal secretions and bronchodilation	Dry mouth, dizziness, transient increased bronchospasm; may cause narrow-angle glaucoma if eyes are contaminated in susceptible patients. Use of mouthpiece nebulizer is safer than face mask.

Note: Recommendations originate from the National Institutes of Health (NIH) expert panel on the diagnosis and management of asthma (2007). *IV theophylline and magnesium are not recommended for general use* in a hospitalized patient with acute asthma by the NIH guidelines. A 20-minute IV magnesium sulfate infusion for poorly responding patients is recommended by the British Thoracic Society guidelines. All patients receiving theophylline prior to hospitalization should have a theophylline level determined before a loading dose is given.

BP, blood pressure; *GI*, gastrointestinal; *HR*, heart rate; *IV*, intravenous; *SC*, subcutaneous; *SABA*, inhaled short-acting β_2-agonist; *PEF*, peak expiratory flow.

CARE PLANS: ACUTE ASTHMA EXACERBATION

Impaired gas exchange *related to ineffective breathing patterns secondary to narrowed airways*

GOALS/OUTCOMES Within 2 to 4 hours of initiation of treatment, patient has adequate gas exchange reflected by Pao_2 greater than 80 mm Hg, $Paco_2$ 35 to 45 mm Hg, and pH 7.35 to 7.45 (or ABG values within 10% of patient's baseline), with mechanical ventilation, if necessary. Within 24 to 48 hours of initiation of treatment, patient is weaning or weaned from mechanical ventilation, and RR is 12 to 20 breaths/min with normal baseline depth and pattern.

NOC Respiratory Status: Ventilation, Vital Signs Status, Respiratory Status: Gas Exchange, Symptom Control Behavior, Comfort Level, Endurance.

Ventilation Assistance

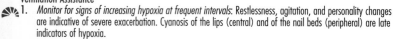

1. *Monitor for signs of increasing hypoxia at frequent intervals:* Restlessness, agitation, and personality changes are indicative of severe exacerbation. Cyanosis of the lips (central) and of the nail beds (peripheral) are late indicators of hypoxia.
2. *Monitor for signs of hypercapnia at frequent intervals:* Confusion, listlessness, and somnolence are indicative of respiratory failure and near-fatal asthma exacerbation.
3. *Monitor ABGs when continuous pulse oximetry values or patient assessment reflects progressive hypoxemia or development of hypercapnia.* Be alert to decreasing Pao_2 and increasing $Paco_2$ or decreasing O_2 saturation levels, indicative of impending respiratory failure.
4. *Monitor for decreased breath sounds or changes in wheezing at frequent intervals.* Absent breath sounds in a distressed asthma patient may indicate impending respiratory arrest.
5. *Position patient for comfort and to promote optimal gas exchange.* High-Fowler's position, with the patient leaning forward and elbows propped on the over-the-bed table to promote maximal chest excursion, may reduce use of accessory muscles and diaphoresis due to work of breathing.
6. *Monitor Fio_2 to ensure that O_2 is within prescribed concentrations.* If patient does not retain CO_2, 100% nonrebreather mask may be used to provide maximal O_2 support. If the patient retains CO_2 and is unrelieved by positioning, lower-dose O_2, bronchodilators, and steroids, intubation and mechanical ventilation may be necessary sooner than in patients who are able to receive higher doses of O_2 by mask.

Mechanical Ventilation

1. Monitor intubated and mechanically ventilated patients for increased intrathoracic pressure (auto-PEEP) due to "breath stacking," wherein the next breath is delivered prior to complete emptying of the first breath. Each subsequent breath failing to completely empty increases lung volume and predisposes the patient to volutrauma, pneumothorax, and decreased cardiac output (CO) resulting from the hyperinflated lungs causing pressure increases inside the thorax which impede venous return to the heart.
2. Monitor for hypotension. Decreased venous return can lead to hypotension. Auto-PEEP should be suspected in an intubated asthmatic patient who is hypotensive following intubation and initiation of mechanical ventilation, when there is no other obvious cause (e.g., tension pneumothorax). If auto-PEEP is suspected, consult with the respiratory therapist and the physician to modify ventilator settings.

Ineffective airway clearance *related to increased tracheobronchial secretions and bronchoconstriction; decreased ability to expectorate secretions secondary to fatigue*

GOALS/OUTCOMES Within 24 hours of initiating treatment, patient's airway has reduced secretions as evidenced by return to baseline RR (12 to 20 breaths/min) and absence of excessive coughing. Within 24 to 48 hours of resolution of severe, refractory asthma, patient reports an increased energy level with decreased fatigue and associated symptoms

NOC Respiratory Status: Airway Patency

Cough Enhancement

1. Monitor patient's ability to clear tracheobronchial secretions frequently. Set up suction equipment at the bedside.
2. Encourage oral fluid intake or administer intravenous (IV) fluids within patient's prescribed limits to help decrease viscosity of the secretions.
3. Encourage coughing to clear secretions and deep breathing unless patient is already coughing uncontrollably or going into respiratory failure. If the patient can manage to take deep breaths, respiratory failure is manageable.
4. Provide humidified O_2 to help liquefy tracheobronchial secretions.
5. Evaluate whether patient may benefit from chest physiotherapy, after crisis phase of exacerbation has been resolved. Discuss with physician. If appropriate, teach significant others to perform chest physiotherapy.

6. Teach patient proper coughing technique for effective management of secretions.
7. Instruct patient to take several deep breaths. Instruct significant others in coaching this technique.
8. After the last inhalation, teach patient to perform a succession of coughs (usually three or four) on the same exhalation until most of the air has been expelled.
9. Explain that patient may need to repeat this technique several times before the cough becomes productive.

Asthma Management
1. *Determine patient's previous asthma control status,* including which "step" of therapy was implemented (Table 4-3).
2. *Compare current status to past exacerbation responses* to determine respiratory status.
3. *Ensure spirometry measurements (FEV₁, FVC, FEV₁/FVC ratio) or PEFR readings are obtained* before and after use of a short-acting bronchodilator.
4. *Educate patient about use of a PEFR meter at home.*
5. *Determine patient's compliance* with treatments.
6. *Note onset, frequency, and duration of coughing* and advise patient to avoid triggers of coughing if identified.
7. *Coach in breathing or relaxation exercises.*
8. *Encourage patient to breathe slowly and deeply.* Teach pursed-lip breathing technique to assist patient with controlling respirations as appropriate:

Table 4-3	STEPPED MEDICATION MANAGEMENT FOR ASTHMA CONTROL				
Intermittent Asthma	**Persistent Asthma***				
Step 1	**Step 2**	**Step 3**	**Step 4**	**Step 5**	**Step 6**
SABA as needed	*Preferred* Low-dose ICS	*Preferred* Low-dose ICS + LABA Or Medium-dose ICS	*Preferred* Medium-dose ICS + LABA	*Preferred* High-dose ICS + LABA	*Preferred* High-dose ICS + LABA + oral corticosteroid
	Alternative Cromolyn, LTRA, nedocromil, theophylline	*Alternative* Low-dose ICS + either LTRA, nedocromil, theophylline, or zileuton	*Alternative* Medium-dose ICS + either LTRA, nedocromil, theophylline, or zileuton	*Alternative* Consider omalizumab for patients with allergies	*Alternative* Consider omalizumab for patients with allergies
			Asthma Specialist should manage patient		
	Consider subcutaneous allergen immunotherapy for patients with allergic asthma.				
Long-term Asthma Control Medications: Adults					
Medications	**Dosage**		**Side Effects**		
Inhaled Corticosteroids (ICS)					
Beclomethasone HFA	80–480+ mcg daily		Cough, dysphonia, oral thrush. *Cytochrome P-450 metabolism.* Drugs that inhibit isoenzyme CYP3A4 may increase systemic concentration of ICS. Systemic adverse effects may be seen. Should be used following bronchodilators after washing out the mouth.		
Budesonide DPI	160–1200+ mcg daily				
Flunisolide	500–2000+ mcg daily				
Flunisolide HFA	320–640+ mcg daily				
Fluticasone HFA/MDI	88–440+ mcg daily				
Fluticasone DPI	100–500+ mcg daily				
Mometasone DPI	200–400+ mcg daily				
Triamcinolone acetonide	300–1500+ mcg daily				

Continued

Table 4-3	STEPPED MEDICATION MANAGEMENT FOR ASTHMA CONTROL—cont'd

Long-term Asthma Control Medications: Adults

Medications	Dosage	Side Effects
Systemic Oral Corticosteroids		
Methylprednisolone Prednisolone Prednisone	7.5–60 mg daily; Short course "burst" 40–60 mg daily as single or divided doses for 3–10 days to gain control	Hyperglycemia, increased appetite, fluid retention, weight gain, peptic ulcer, aseptic necrosis *Long term*: Cushing syndrome, adrenal axis suppression, growth suppression, muscle weakness, cataracts, rarely immunosuppression
Inhaled LABAs		
Salmeterol DPI Formoterol DPI	One blister every 12 hrs One capsule every 12 hrs	Tachycardia, tremors, hypokalemia, QTc interval prolongation. Not used as a rescue inhaler for acute distress.
Combined Medications		
Fluticasone/Salmeterol Budesonide/Formoterol	One inhalation BID 2 puffs BID	See LABA and ICS; dose depends on level of control
Cromolyn/Nedocromil		
Cromolyn MDI Cromolyn Nebulizer Nedocromil MDI	2 puffs QID One ampule QID 2 puffs QID	Cough and irritation; 15–20% of patients have bad taste from nedocromil
Immunomodulators		
Omalizumab (Anti-IgE)	150–375 mg SC every 2–4 weeks	Pain, burning at injection site; possible anaphylaxis
Leukotriene Modulators		
Leukotriene Receptor Antagonists (LTRAs)		
Montelukast Zafirlukast	10 mg qhs 40 mg daily	No specific adverse effects
5-Lipoxygenase Inhibitor		
Zileuton	2400 mg daily	Liver enzyme elevation
Methylxanthines		
Theophylline	Starting dose 10 mg/kg daily up to 300mg; maximum dose 800mg daily	Tachycardia, nausea, vomiting, SVT, CNS stimulation, headache, seizures, hyperglycemia, hypokalemia, insomnia, gastric upset, increased reflux and PUD, difficulty voiding in elderly males, increased hyperactivity in children

CNS, central nervous system; *DPI*, dry powder inhaler; *MDI*, metered dose inhaler; *HFA*, hydrofluoroalkanes (ozone-benign propellant for inhalation); *ICS*, inhaled corticosteroid; *LABA*, long-acting β₂-agonist; *LTRA*, leukotriene receptor antagonist; *PUD*, peptic ulcer disease; *SABA*, short-acting β₂-agonist; *SVT*, supraventricular tachycardia.
*Information based on National Institutes of Health Asthma Management Guidelines (2007).

- Inhale through the nose.
- Form lips in an O shape as if whistling.
- Exhale slowly through pursed lips.
- Record patient's response to breathing technique. Educate significant others in coaching.

9. *Teach patient and family how to decrease metabolic demands for O_2* by limiting or pacing patient's activities and procedures.
10. *Schedule rest times after meals* to avoid competition for O_2 supply during digestion.
11. *Monitor Spo_2 by pulse oximetry during activity* to evaluate limits of activity, set future activity goals, and recommend optimal positions for oxygenation.
12. *Assess for fever 2 to 4 hours.* Consult physician and provide treatment as prescribed to decrease temperature and thus O_2 demands.

Anxiety Reduction

1. *Ascertain and alleviate the cause of restlessness to decrease metabolic demands* (e.g., if restlessness is related to anxiety, help reduce anxiety by providing reassurance, enabling family members to stay with patient, and offering distractions such as soft music or television).
2. *Be aware that restlessness may be an early sign of hypoxemia.*
3. *Explain all procedures and offer support to minimize fear and anxiety,* which can increase O_2 demands.

NIC Acid-Base Management; Acid-Base Monitoring; Airway Management; Bedside Laboratory Testing; Cough Enhancement; Emotional Support; Energy Management; Fluid Management; Fluid Monitoring; Laboratory Data Interpretation; Mechanical Ventilation; Oxygen Therapy; Positioning; Respiratory Monitoring; Vital Signs Monitoring

ADDITIONAL NURSING DIAGNOSES

Also see *Acute Respiratory Failure,* p. 383, for information about support of breathing. For other nursing diagnoses and interventions, see *Emotional and Spiritual Support of the Patient and Significant Others,* p. 200.

ACUTE LUNG INJURY AND ACUTE RESPIRATORY DISTRESS SYNDROME

PATHOPHYSIOLOGY

The terms *acute lung injury* (ALI) and *acute respiratory distress syndrome* (ARDS) are used to describe a continuum of lung dysfunction. There may be a primary (intrapulmonary) or secondary (extrapulmonary) insult to both the lung endothelium and the epithelium. The associated release of mediators, increasing vascular and alveolar permeability (leak), eventually perpetuates alveolar collapse and supports the accumulation of fluids in the pulmonary interstitium. As the capillary permeability and alveolar epithelial damage continue to worsen, surfactant activity is reduced, protein production increases, and therefore gas exchange decreases due to widened diffusion distance and intrapulmonary shunting . The alveoli tend to collapse, communicating the loss of opening pressure to other alveoli in the sac. All resist re-expansion in the absence of surfactant and the presence of significant infiltration and collapsing fluid pressure. Initially, acute hypoxemia develops, worsens, and ultimately progresses into hypercapnic respiratory failure. The shunt fraction (blood flow past de-recruited alveoli rejoins in the pulmonary venous circulation without adequate O_2 exposure) as well as alveolar (physiologic) dead space (overventilation of the unaffected alveolar sacs) increases, ultimately progressing to a profoundly noncompliant, de-recruited, and gas dysfunctional state. Current evidence supports that the over distension and force of opening-closing also profoundly affect the healthy lung. ALI and the more severe and exacerbated process, ARDS, are primarily defined once the evolution of damage has required intubation and mechanical ventilation. The progression is measured by a worsening of the patient's oxygen exchange (Table 4-4). The presence of refractory hypoxemic respiratory failure in conjunction with diffuse pulmonary infiltrates in the absence of left atrial hypertension is considered the primary indicator of the continuum of acute respiratory failure. Despite advances in the treatment of the primary inflammatory process and progress in the method of ventilatory support, the continuum of ALI/ARDS continues to be associated with high

Table 4-4	CRITERIA FOR CLASSIFICATION OF ACUTE LUNG INJURY (ALI)/ ACUTE RESPIRATORY DISTRESS CRITERIA SYNDROME (ARDS)
Criteria	**Indicators**
ALI	Acute onset
	$PaO_2/FIO_2 < 250$ mm Hg with 0.40 FIO_2 Regardless of PEEP
	Bilateral infiltrates on frontal chest radiograph
	No clinical evidence of left atrial hypertension or left ventricular dysfunction
ARDS	Same as for ALI with the exception of oxygenation issues
	$PaO_2/FIO_2 < 200$ mm Hg with 0.40 FIO_2 Regardless of PEEP

morbidity and mortality, reaching greater than 60%. Since 1964, when the continuum was first described, the understanding of etiology, pathophysiology, and epidemiology, as well as the relationship of genetic prodrome and ventilator induced lung injury process, has significantly increased (Table 4-5).

ASSESSMENT
Goal of System Assessment
Evaluate for decreasing PaO_2/FIO_2 and increasing requirements for pressure control and PEEP. (See *Acid-Base Imbalances*, p. 1)

History and Risk Factors
Shock: Trauma, hemorrhagic shock, sepsis, massive blood transfusion, and multiple liters of intravascular volume replacement
Respiratory: Inhalation of toxic substances, pneumonia, severe pneumonitis, aspiration of gastric contents, drowning, air or fat embolus, O_2 toxicity, ventilator-induced lung injury (VILI)
Other: Acute pancreatitis, post perfusion cardiopulmonary bypass, drug overdose, neurologic injury, immunosuppression, malaria

Vital Signs
- If breathing spontaneously (with or without ventilation support), respiratory rate will be rapid.
- Rapid HR if not receiving beta-antagonist therapy
- SpO_2 is lower than expected when reviewing the ventilation or O_2 support.

Observation: Oxygenation Failure
- Nasal flaring and expiratory grunt may be present.
- Use of accessory muscles indicates respiratory distress.
- May appear fatigued, with or without diaphoresis

Table 4-5	RISK FACTORS FOR ACUTE LUNG INJURY/ACUTE RESPIRATORY DISTRESS SYNDROME	
Direct Injury		**Indirect Injury**
Pneumonia		Severe sepsis
Aspiration		Trauma
Lung contusions		Pancreatitis
Inhalation/burn injury		Transfusion-related lung injury (TRALI)
Severe acute respiratory syndrome (SARS)		Ventilation-associated lung injury (VALI)

- May present with ashen, pale, or gray/blue facial color, lip color, or nail beds
- Chest expansion may be decreased, restricted, or asymmetrical with severe changes in one lung manifesting severe atelectasis or pleuritic pain.
- Altered level of consciousness (confusion, disorientation, agitation) is more common with older adults but is a very significant sign in any age group.
- Agitation is more commonly associated with hypoxemia, while somnolence is associated with hypercarbia (elevated CO_2 level).

Hypoxemic Hypoxia in Acute Lung Injury

- *Initially*: Dyspnea, restlessness, hyperventilation, cough, increased work of breathing; chest may appear to be clear on auscultation or there may be late inspiratory crackles. Patient may be significantly agitated and if intubated may appear combative.
- *Ventilator pressures*: As most of these patients will already be ventilated, increasing peak airway pressure (PawP or PIP) and a validation of increased pressure measured during inspiratory hold ($P_{plateau}$) when administering a volume-controlled breath should be evaluated and documented. The rising pressure ($P_{plateau}$) indicates a loss of functional alveolar surface, and as the compliance of the lung decreases, the pressure measured when a volume breath is delivered will rise.
- The patient's proportionate O_2 ratio will decrease (P/F). Initially there may be a shift from volume control ventilation to pressure control as well as an increase in PEEP (see Table 4-1).

Hypoxemic Hypoxia in Acute Respiratory Distress Syndrome

- *Initially*: Respiratory failure including cyanosis, pallor, grunting respirations, mid to late inspiratory rales, rapid and shallow breathing, intercostal-suprasternal retractions, tachypnea, tachycardia, diaphoresis, mental obtundation
- *Ventilator pressures*: The increasing peak and plateau pressures will be measured when the patient is given a volume control breath (cannot be measured during a pressure controlled breath).
- The O_2 (P/F) ratio will decline further and generally requires a change in ventilation support to a mean airway pressure strategy.

Auscultation

- Decreased or bronchial breath sounds
- High-pitched inspiratory crackles heard best after patient coughs
- Low-pitched inspiratory crackles caused by airway secretions

Palpation

- Palpate chest wall for tenderness indicative of inflammation.
- Palpate to assess for symmetry of chest expansion.

Percussion

- May reveal presence of consolidation or fluid (dullness) or hyperresonance (pneumothorax)

Screening Labwork

- *CBC*: Evaluates for elevated white blood cells indicative of infection. Bandemia (immature neutrophils) of greater than 10% is especially concerning.
- *Sputum gram stain, culture and sensitivity*: Identifies infecting organism
- *Blood culture and sensitivity*: If positive, may indicate organism has migrated into the bloodstream to cause a systemic infection
- *ABG analysis*: Evaluates for hypoxemia and eventually hypercapnia

A—a Gradient/A—aDo_2/P(A—a)o_2

- The A—a gradient or Alveolar—arterial O_2 tension difference is a clinically useful calculation. The calculation is based on a model as though the lung were one large alveolus and the entire blood flow of the right heart passed around it. Utilizing the rules of partial pressure as well as the laws of CO_2 production at the cell and the content of CO_2 exerting alveolar pressure, the theoretical alveolar Po_2 (PAo_2) is calculated. Once the theoretical

PAo$_2$ has been calculated, the gradient is achieved by subtracting the measured arterial Pao$_2$. The calculated "gradient" represents the difference between the calculated Alveolar oxygen (PAO$_2$) and the measured arterial oxygen (Pao$_2$).

- When the F$_{IO_2}$ is above 0.21, the A−a gradient becomes less accurate in the measurement of proportional gas exchange, although the difference should always be less than 150 mm Hg.

- *Extrapulmonary failure*: The A−a gradient generally remains normal or narrow. With shunt or V̇/Q̇ mismatch, the gradient is usually wider than normal. The A−a gradient also measures the severity of gas exchange impairment. At any age, an A−a gradient exceeding 20 mm Hg on room air or greater than 100 on increased F$_{IO_2}$ should be considered abnormal and indicative of pulmonary dysfunction.

- *P/F ratio*: The Pao$_2$ divided by the F$_{IO_2}$ (Pao$_2$/F$_{IO_2}$ ratio or, more simply, P/F) can be used to more simply assess the severity of the gas exchange defect. The normal value for the ratio of the partial pressure of arterial blood O$_2$ to F$_{IO_2}$ ({Pao$_2$/F$_{IO_2}$} F$_{IO_2}$ is expressed as a decimal ranging from 0.21 to 1.00) is 300 to 500. A value of less than 300 indicates gas exchange derangement, and a value below 200 on greater than 40% F$_{IO_2}$ is indicative of severe impairment and is a major component of the diagnostic criteria for ALI and ARDS. The inverse relationships of these measures are important to consider when discussing the level of gas exchange failure.

- Q_S/Q_T: The shunt fraction compares the nonoxygenated (shunted: Q_S) blood exiting the pulmonary bed to the total blood flow (cardiac output: Q_T). This mathematical calculation, which requires mixed venous blood gas and pulmonary blood gas, evaluates total intrapulmonary shunting. Normal physiologic shunt is 3% to 4% and may increase to 15% to 20% or more in ARDS. The routine measurements of ABGs, chest radiograph, A−a gradient, and P/F ratio as well as the presence of refractory hypoxemia are much more routinely used to diagnose intrapulmonary shunting, a core feature of ARDS.

DIAGNOSTIC TESTS

Diagnostic Tests for ALI/ARDS		
Test	**Purpose**	**Abnormal Findings**
Noninvasive Pulmonary Volumes and Pressures		
Pulmonary function studies	Evaluates inspiratory volumes and exhalation volumes as well as capacities of the lung	Persons with ALI/ARDS have decreased inspiratory volume (tidal volume and inspiratory reserve) as well as exhalation volumes (tidal volume and expiratory reserve) because the functional lung surface is significantly reduced. The amount of volume that stays in the lung at the end of a normal exhalation is significantly ↓↓ and promotes continuous alveolar collapse.
Pulmonary pressures measured during volume control breath	Measures the relationship of volume delivered and the compliance of the surface, which contains it Normal PawP or PIP when receiving a 10 ml/kg/IDW breath is <35 cm H$_2$O. Normal P$_{plateau}$ when holding a 10 ml/kg/IDW breath at the end of inspiration is <25 cm H$_2$O.	Patients presenting with lung injury and distress will have significant increases in P$_{plateau}$ pressures to more than 25 cm H$_2$O. This increase may or may not manifest as a proportional increase in PIP. For example, with a 350 ml breath, the patient with ARDS may have a PIP of 48 and a P$_{plateau}$ of 43.

Diagnostic Tests for ALI/ARDS — cont'd

Test	Purpose	Abnormal Findings
Blood Studies		
Arterial blood gas analysis	Evaluates the oxygenation of the arterial blood as well as the presence or absence of acid and the effect on the pH (environment of the cells). See *Acid-Base Imbalances*, p. 1.	Although not always predictable when in the disease process changes will occur, generally patients will develop hypoxemia, which may initially be resolved with increasing the FIO_2, but eventually will require great increases in FIO_2 and ultimately will no longer respond to oxygen therapy.
Complete blood count (CBC) Hemoglobin (Hgb) Hematocrit (Hct) RBC count (RBCs) WBC count (WBCs)	Assesses for anemia, inflammation, and infection	Decreased RBCs, Hgb, or Hct reflects anemia; WBCs and shift to the left may indicate ongoing inflammation.
Coagulation profile Prothrombin time (PT) with international normalized ratio (INR) Partial thromboplastin time (PTT) Fibrinogen D-dimer	Assesses for causes of bleeding, clotting, and disseminated intravascular coagulation (DIC) indicative of the abnormal clotting present in shock or ensuing shock	Decreased PT with low INR promotes clotting; elevation promotes bleeding. In severe sepsis, PT and INR may increase, but in the presence of ALI/ARDS, these measures along with elevated fibrinogen and D-dimer reflect a microcoagulopathy.
Radiology		
Chest radiograph (CXR)	Assesses size of lungs, presence of fluids, abnormal gas or fluids in the pleural sac, diaphragmatic margins, the pulmonary hilum, as well as integrity of the rib cage	Presence of fluids in the lung parenchyma initially presents as pulmonary edema. The continuous accumulation differentiates this edema formation to one that is not cardiac.
Computed tomography		
Cardiac CT scan	Assesses the three-dimensional lung capacities, fluid load, and primary displacement of the fluid	Normally a large gas-filled surface, the ALI/ARDS lung when seen on CT is frequently whited out, filled ¼ to ¾ with fluid that has extravagated through the endothelial deficits (capillary leak).
Invasive Measures		
Tracheal-protein/ plasma-protein ratio	A relatively new diagnostic tool used to differentiate between cardiogenic and noncardiogenic pulmonary edema (ARDS). It compares total protein in tracheal aspirate with total protein in plasma.	Ratio in cardiogenic pulmonary edema is <0.5, whereas the ratio in ARDS generally is >0.7.

COLLABORATIVE MANAGEMENT

Maintaining adequate arterial oxygenation while protecting the functional lung is the highest priority in both traditional and more recent approaches to ventilator management for ARDS. In addition, the primary goal is to determine and treat the underlying pathophysiologic condition.

Care Priorities

1. **Augment oxygen content with oxygen therapy:** The goal is to provide acceptable Pao_2 levels (greater than 60 mm Hg) with Fio_2 less than 0.50, but Fio_2 up to 1.00 may be necessary for a short time as other adjustments are made. If an increase in Fio_2 exceeds 50%, clinicians should consider increasing PEEP (by increments of 2 to 5 cm H_2O every 1 to 2 hours, until 15 or 20 cm H_2O of PEEP is reached) to reduce the right-to-left shunt and promote oxygenation. PEEP improves arterial oxygenation, primarily by recruiting collapsed and partially fluid-filled alveoli, therefore increasing the functional residual capacity (FRC) at end-expiration, which decreases the effort and sheer stress (which may damage the alveoli) of opening the alveoli again during the next inspiration. This strategy is referred to as a mean airway pressure or open lung strategy, that is, by increasing the mean airway pressure, the lung will be constantly maintained in an open state.

2. **Facilitate ventilation and gas exchange:**

   Mechanical ventilation: Provide mechanical ventilation with moderate to high levels of PEEP (to prevent tidal collapse) and low tidal volumes of about 6 ml/kg ideal body weight, to protect the functional lung from overdistention. This lung-protective ventilatory strategy has been shown to ensure adequate gas exchange, decrease the levels of intra-alveolar and systemic mediators, and improve outcomes in patients with ALI and ARDS. Many clinicians have successfully used strategies to treat ARDS by reducing the delivered tidal volume (from 8 to 10 ml/kg ideal body weight [IBW] to 4 to 6 ml/kg IBW) balanced with a RR (12–40) necessary to maintain adequate minute ventilation. This decrease of volume in the noncompliant lung reduces both peak inspiratory and plateau pressures. At the same time, the use of a lower tidal volume protects the functional lung surface from volutrauma and pressure trauma, both of which cause overdistention and stimulation of inflammation. If PEEP trials fail, other strategies designed to open and maintain opening of the alveoli may be considered. These methods such as airway pressure release ventilation (APRV), inverse ratio (I greater than E), and high-frequency oscillation (HFOV) are also mean airway pressure strategies, but the discussion of this type of advanced ventilation is beyond the scope of this book.

   Patient positioning: Primary lung edema occurs most aggressively in the dependent areas of the lung. Repositioning the patient at least every 2 hours is indicated in patients with hypoxemia; however, if staffing allows and the patient can tolerate it, more frequent (every 30 minutes) turning could be beneficial. Continuous lateral motion therapy beds may also be used to continuously turn the patient. Motion therapy assists in the redistribution of interstitial edema and may improve oxygenation.

   Prone patient positioning: Prone positioning of the patient improves the oxygenation of many patients with ARDS. There are various methods to turn the patient prone: staff generated with pillows, foam wedges, Vollman prone positioned, or mechanically with the Roto-Prone bed.

3. **Maintain adequate cardiac output with fluid therapy:** Usually, the patient's fluid volume is kept slightly depleted to minimize leakage of excess fluids into the interstitium through damaged capillary membrane. The balance between dehydration and euvolemia is a difficult one to achieve. New measures of total blood volume and arterial stroke volume may assist the provider in achieving adequate fluid without causing volume overload. The use of crystalloid versus colloid fluids has been and remains controversial, but the SAFE Study Investigators (2004) validated that the use of colloids in the general population of patients did not improve outcomes but significantly increased cost.

4. **Reduce anxiety:** Before any medication is administered, the provider must ascertain that the ventilation is tailored to the patient. This can best be evaluated by analyzing the volume-pressure loop and the flow/time graph. The respiratory therapist is an invaluable resource for this method of evaluation. After insuring adequate ventilation, many patients will require anxiety reduction with medication such as fentanyl, and anxiolytics. Those patients who cannot be adequately oxygenated and ventilated with mechanical ventilation may be given anxiety-reducing agents such as midazolam or lorazepam. A sedation scale and protocol should be used to standardize this practice. In addition, the bedside nurse must ascertain if the patient is in pain and administer analgesics appropriately. A wide variety of pain scales can be effectively utilized.

   Patients who are unable to achieve appropriate ventilation due to agitation and dyssynchrony or are hemodynamically unstable may require heavy sedation with agents such as propofol (Diprivan) or, in extreme cases, the diaphragm may need to be paralyzed with a neuromuscular blocking agent such as vecuronium bromide (Norcuron) or cisatracurium (Nimbex). Although very user dependent, train of four should be performed when evaluating level of pharmacologic paralysis. The caregiver must recognize that, although pharmacologically paralyzed patient may appear to be resting quietly or may even be comatose, he or she may be alert and extremely anxious because of the total lack of muscle control. These patients must receive appropriate sedation (e.g., lorazepam [Ativan]) and analgesia (e.g., morphine), and they will require expert psychosocial nursing interventions. See *Sedating and Neuromuscular Blockade*, p. 158. When patients appear agitated, ventilation should be evaluated first (as long as the patient is not in danger of extubation or self-harm) followed by pain evaluation and analgesia, followed by anxiety-relieving medications. Neuromuscular paralysis should be performed as a last resort and only when necessary to control ventilation.

 5. **Provide nutritional support:** Energy outlay with respiratory failure is high, in part because of the increased work of breathing. If the patient is unable to consume adequate calories with enteral feedings, total parenteral nutrition (TPN) is added. It is important to perform an occasional evaluation of the patient's caloric and metabolic needs to make certain that the patient is being adequately nourished but not overfed. All efforts should be made to feed enterally so the gut is used. Newer elemental feedings require no digestion and can be used in the stomach, duodenum, or jejunum. (See *Nutritional Support*, p. 117.)

RESEARCH BRIEF **4-2**

This multicenter, randomized, crossover trial studied the effects of alveolar recruitment maneuvers in ALI/ARDS patients receiving lung protective mechanical ventilation using both smaller tidal volumes and higher levels of PEEP than traditionally used. Patients receiving recruitment maneuvers (RMs) experienced greater decreases in systolic BP and SpO_2 during the first 10 minutes. RMs was terminated in three instances. RMs did not cause greater and sustained improvements in SpO_2 and FiO_2/PEEP. Most patients in this study had ALI/ARDS from pneumonia or aspiration. There may be greater potential for lung recruitment in sepsis or trauma-induced ALI/ARDS.

From The ARDS Clinical Trials Network; National Heart, Lung, and Blood Institute; National Institutes of Health: Effects of recruitment maneuvers in patients with acute lung injury and acute respiratory distress syndrome ventilated with high positive end-expiratory pressure. *Crit Care Med* 31(11):2592–2597, 2003.

RESEARCH BRIEF **4-3**

Goldhill DR, Imhoff M, McLean B, et al. performed a meta analysis of the published studies regarding use of rotational turning beds. Twenty prospective randomized controlled trials on rotational therapy were published between 1987 and 2004. Various types of beds were studied, but few details on the rotational parameters were reported. The usual control was manual turning of patients by nurses every 2 hours. One animal investigation and 12 clinical trials addressed the effectiveness of rotational therapy in preventing respiratory complications. Significant benefits to patients were reported in the animal study and 4 of the trials. Significant benefits to patients were reported in two of another four studies focused on treatment of established complications. Little convincing evidence is available regarding the most effective rotation parameters (e.g., degree, pause time, and amount of time per day). Meta-analysis suggests that rotational therapy decreases the incidence of pneumonia but has no effect on duration of mechanical ventilation, number of days in intensive care, or hospital mortality.

From Rotational bed therapy to prevent and treat respiratory complications: a review and meta-analysis. *Am J Clin Cardiol* 16(1), 2007.

CARE PLANS FOR ALI AND ARDS

Impaired gas exchange *related to alveolar-capillary membrane changes secondary to increased permeability with alveolar injury and collapse*

GOALS/OUTCOMES On initiation of therapy, and the titration of ventilatory support, the patient has adequate gas exchange as evidenced by the following ABG values: Pao_2 greater than 60 mm Hg, $Paco_2$ less than 45 mm Hg, pH 7.35 to 7.45. Success is achieved when the patient can maintain his or her Pao_2 even with Fio_2 decreases.
NOC Respiratory Status: Ventilation, Vital Signs Status, Respiratory Status: Gas Exchange, Symptom Control Behavior, Comfort Level, Endurance

Respiratory Monitoring
1. Assess and document character of respiratory effort: rate, depth, rhythm, and use of accessory muscles of respiration.
2. Assess patient for signs and symptoms of respiratory distress: restlessness, anxiety, confusion, tachypnea (RR greater than 20 breaths/min), and use of accessory muscles.
3. Assess breath sounds with each vital signs check. Adventitious sounds, which usually are present in the later stages of ARDS, are not as likely to occur during the early stage.
4. Monitor serial ABG values, and consult physician for significant changes. Explain need for frequent analysis to patient and significant others.
5. Compare ABG saturation with pulse oximetry saturation for accuracy. Consult physician or mid level practitioner for pulse oximetry values less than 90%.
6. Administer O_2 and monitor Fio_2 as prescribed.
7. Monitor and record pulmonary function tests as prescribed, especially tidal volume and minute ventilation. Expect decreased tidal volume and increased minute ventilation with respiratory distress.
8. Position patient for comfort and to promote adequate gas exchange. Usually, semi-Fowler's to high Fowler's position is therapeutic.
9. Keep oral airway and self-inflating manual ventilating bag at the bedside for emergency use. Keep emergency intubation equipment at the bedside for use should patient's condition deteriorate.

Risk for injury *related to dislodging of life-sustaining equipment during positioning or repositioning*

GOALS/OUTCOMES Patient can be turned, placed prone, or repositioned without dislodging life-sustaining equipment or devices. When Pao_2 and Spo_2 return to an acceptable level, or the chest radiograph shows improvement, the bed may be discontinued.
NOC Personal Safety Behavior; Risk Control

Environmental Management: Safety
1. Secure the ET tube/other devices to prevent accidental movement or dislodging.
2. Provide the appropriate length ventilator tubing to facilitate positioning of the patient without risk of pulling on the ET tube.
3. Facilitate tolerance of rotational therapy by managing anxiety and promoting sleep with medications.
4. Assess oxygenation once patient is prone. Typical responders will demonstrate at least 10 mm Hg increase in Pao_2 within 10 minutes of being placed prone.
5. Collaborate with the respiratory care practitioner to decrease the delivered O_2 as the patient's oxygenation status improves.

NIC Acid-Base Management; Airway Management; Bedside Laboratory Testing; Laboratory Data Interpretation; Mechanical Ventilation; Oxygen Therapy; Positioning; Respiratory Monitoring; Ventilation Assistance; Vital Signs Monitoring

ADDITIONAL NURSING DIAGNOSES

Also see nursing diagnoses and interventions in Nutritional Support (p. 117), Mechanical Ventilation (p. 99), Prolonged Immobility (p. 149), Acid-Base Imbalances (p. 1), and Emotional and Spiritual Support of the Patient and Significant Others (p. 200).

ACUTE PNEUMONIA

PATHOPHYSIOLOGY

Pneumonia is the sixth leading cause of death in the United States and the leading cause of death due to infectious disease. Pneumonia is an acute infection that causes inflammation of the lung parenchyma (alveolar spaces and interstitial tissue), resulting in the alveoli filling with liquid. Pneumonias can be classified into two groups: community-acquired (CAP) and hospital-associated/nosocomial (HAP). (See Table 4-6 for a detailed discussion by pneumonia type.)

Immunosuppression and neutropenia are predisposing factors in the development of all pneumonias. Severely immunocompromised patients are affected by bacteria, fungi (*Candida, Aspergillus*), viruses (cytomegalovirus), and protozoa (*Pneumocystis carinii*). *P. carinii* is seen most often in patients who are positive for HIV or who have received organ transplants.

Patients generally require critical care when an underlying medical condition increases morbidity. Common conditions include COPD, cardiac disease, diabetes mellitus, liver, renal, or cerebrovascular disease, malignancy, or an immunocompromised state. Pneumonias sometimes lead to sepsis, septic shock, and respiratory failure. Patients with underlying, chronic illnesses are more likely to experience sepsis.

Community-Acquired Pneumonia

A pneumonia that is acquired outside the hospital or nursing home, which varies from a mild to severe illness. Approximately 4 million patients develop CAP annually, resulting in 600,000 hospitalizations at a cost of approximately $23 billion. Mortality rates range from 5.1% for hospitalized and ambulatory patients to 36.5% for patients requiring critical care. The disease occurs in all age groups but is most common in those from the mid-50s to the late 60s.

Nosocomial/Hospital Associated Pneumonia (HAP)

The hospital-acquired infection is most likely to be lethal to patients. Critically ill patients are at high risk for HAP. The Centers for Disease Control and Prevention (CDC) defines *nosocomial pneumonia* as a condition occurring at least 72 hours after hospital admission, reflecting an infiltrate on chest radiograph studies, lung crackles on auscultation, or dullness with chest percussion. Either purulent sputum, a pathogenic organism in the sputum or blood, a virus from the lower respiratory tract, or serologic/pathologic evidence must be present to confirm HAP. In addition to enhanced risk by comorbidities, hospitalized patients may acquire pneumonia due to therapeutic interventions. Use of antibiotics, corticosteroids, sedatives, agents to neutralize gastric pH, artificial airway in the trachea, and respiratory therapy equipment (e.g., mechanical ventilation where bacteria can be inhaled from aerosols) are associated with HAP. Pneumonia, along with all hospital-acquired infections, may be acquired from the caregiver's hands.

Aspiration Pneumonia

Occurs after aspiration of oropharyngeal flora in an individual whose resistance is altered or whose coughing mechanisms are impaired. Aspiration pneumonia can lead to acute lung injury (ALI) or respiratory distress syndrome (ARDS). Gram negative pneumonias are more commonly seen in patients given gastric pH altering medications.

Ventilator-Associated Pneumonia

A patient who acquires pneumonia more than 48 hours following endotracheal intubation and initiation of mechanical ventilation may be classified as having ventilator-associated pneumonia (VAP), a subgroup of HAP. VAP is the leading cause of death compared with all hospital-acquired infections. Hospital mortality of ventilated patients who develop VAP is 46% compared to 32% for mechanically ventilated patients without VAP. VAP prolongs time on the ventilator and increases length of ICU stay and length of hospital stay following discharge from the ICU, adding an estimated cost of $40,000 to an average hospital admission. The Centers for Medicare and Medicaid (CMS) have recognized VAP as a preventable illness when appropriate patient care is provided. Studies have identified a series of interventions that comprise the "VAP Bundle," which is considered the standard of care for prevention of VAP (see *Collaborative Management*, p. 379).

Table 4-6	ASSESSMENT GUIDELINES BY PNEUMONIA TYPE			
Type/Pathogen	Risk Groups	Onset	Defining Characteristics	Complication/Comments
Community Acquired				
Pneumococcal (*Pneumococcus pneumoniae, Streptococcus pneumoniae*)	Persons >40 yr, especially males. Risk increases with alcoholism and debilitating diseases (e.g., COPD, heart failure, multiple myeloma, sickle cell disease). Viral upper respiratory tract infections, including influenza, often precede this pneumonia.	Abrupt	Single shaking chill, fever, pleuritic chest pain, severe cough, SOB, rust-colored sputum, and diaphoresis. Many patients also have herpes labialis, abdominal pain and distention, and paralytic ileus.	Pleural effusions, empyema, impaired liver function, bacteremia, and meningitis. Incidence of pneumococcal pneumonia peaks in winter and early spring. Mortality rate increases if more than one lobe is involved.
Mycoplasma (*Mycoplasma pneumoniae*)	School-age children to young adult (5–30 yr). Intrafamilial spread is common.	Gradual	Cough, sore throat, fever, headache, chills, malaise, anorexia, nausea, vomiting, diarrhea. In children, arthralgia involving the large joints is common.	Rare. Persistent cough and sinusitis are possible. Pulse-temperature dissociation is common.
Legionnaires (*Legionella pneumophila*)	Middle-age, older adult (males at increased risk) populations; smokers; individuals with malignancy, immunosuppression, or chronic renal failure; exposure to contaminated construction site. Hgb not elevated.	Abrupt	Malaise, headache within 24 hr, fever with normal HR, shaking chills, progressive dyspnea, cough that may become productive; GI symptoms, including anorexia, vomiting, diarrhea; arthralgia, myalgia	Respiratory failure, hypotension, shock, acute renal failure
Viral influenza A	Elderly persons with chronic diseases (e.g., COPD, diabetes mellitus, heart failure); pregnancy	1 wk after onset of influenza symptoms	Severe dyspnea, cyanosis, scant sputum occasionally with blood, fever, persistent and dry cough	Rapid course leading frequently to acute respiratory failure; secondary bacterial pneumonia
Haemophilus influenzae	Adults (especially ≥50 yr of age) with chronic diseases (e.g., diabetes mellitus, COPD, chronic alcohol ingestion)	2–6 wk after URI	Fever, chills, dyspnea, cough, nausea, vomiting, pain	Fever may be minimal or absent; HR and RR may be normal

Type/Pathogen	Risk Groups	Onset	Defining Characteristics	Complication/Comments
Nosocomial				
Klebsiella (*Klebsiella pneumoniae*) (also may be acquired in the community), *Enterobacter, Serratia*	Males >40 yr of age, chronic disease (e.g., diabetes mellitus, COPD, chronic alcohol ingestion, heart disease); those previously treated with antibiotics or ET intubation	Abrupt	Chills, fever, productive cough (copious), purulent, green, or "currant jelly" sputum) Severe pleuritic chest pain, dyspnea, cyanosis, jaundice, vomiting, and diarrhea	Lung abscess and empyema, necrotizing pneumonitis with cavitation, acute respiratory failure. High mortality rate (≤50%). Aspiration of oropharyngeal flora believed responsible for many nosocomial and community-acquired cases.
Pseudomonas (also may be acquired in the community)	Patients who are neutropenic as a result of chemotherapy or are immunosuppressed secondary to cortisone therapy or other illnesses	Gradual	Fever, chills, confusion, delirium, bradycardia, purulent sputum (green, foul smelling)	Rarely occurs in previously healthy adults; high mortality rate
Proteus	Older adults with debilitating underlying diseases	Abrupt	High fever, chills, pleuritic chest pain	Rare. Localizes to areas that already are damaged. Occurs as a mixed infection; has four pathogenic species with differing antibiotic susceptibilities.
Staphylococcus aureus, methicillin-resistant *S. aureus* (MRSA)	Patients with debilitating diseases (e.g., diabetes mellitus, renal failure, liver disease, COPD); prior viral influenza infection; IV drug abusers	Abrupt with community acquired; insidious with hospital association	Cough, chills, high fever, pleuritic pain, progressive dyspnea, cyanosis, bloody sputum	Pulmonary abscesses, empyema, pleural effusions; slow response to antibiotics
Aspiration of gastric contents	Patients with impaired gag/cough reflexes; general anesthesia; presence of NG/ET tube	Gradual: latent period between aspiration and onset of symptoms	Fever, wheezes, crackles (rales), rhonchi, dyspnea, cyanosis	Physiologic response depends on pH of material aspirated; ≥2.5, little necrosis occurs; <2.5, atelectasis, pulmonary edema, hemorrhage, and necrosis can occur.

Continued

Table 4-6	ASSESSMENT GUIDELINES BY PNEUMONIA TYPE—cont'd			
Type/Pathogen	Risk Groups	Onset	Defining Characteristics	Complication/Comments
Immunocompromised patient				
Pneumocystis (*Pneumocystis carinii*)	Patients with AIDS or organ transplants	Insidious	Several weeks of fever, nonproductive cough, night sweats, dyspnea; hypoxemia with few auscultatory signs	Bronchoscopy with transbronchial biopsy usually required for diagnosis.
Aspergillosis (*Aspergillus*)	Patients with AIDS, COPD, and transplants (especially autologous bone marrow transplant); also those receiving cytotoxic agents or steroids	Abrupt with immunosuppression; insidious with COPD	High fever; fungal ball within lung cyst or cavity; nonproductive cough; pleuritic chest pain	Cavitation frequently occurs; hematogenous spread common in immunocompromised patients.

AIDS, acquired immunodeficiency syndrome; *COPD*, chronic obstructive pulmonary disease; *ET*, endotracheal; *GI*, gastrointestinal; *HR*, heart rate; *IV*, intravenous; *NG*, nasogastric; *RR*, respiratory rate; *SOB*, shortness of breath; *URI*, upper respiratory infection.

ASSESSMENT
Goal of System Assessment

Evaluate for ineffective breathing patterns, impaired gas exchange, and airway obstruction. Findings are influenced by patient's age, extent of the disease process, underlying medical condition, and pathogen involved. Severity of pneumonia should be determined following initial assessment and diagnostic testing.

History and Risk Factors

In addition to the risk factors listed in Table 4-6, any factor that alters the integrity of the lower airways, thereby inhibiting ciliary activity, increases the likelihood of pneumonia. Impairment of the "mucociliary elevator" system impairs the ability of the patient to move secretions from the airways to the oral cavity for expectoration. These factors include hypoventilation, hyperoxia (increased FIO_2), hypoxia, airway irritants such as smoke, and the presence of an artificial airway.

Cough

- Can be unrelenting and severe; may induce vomiting in some patients
- May be productive, weak, strong, or dry (nonproductive)
- Sputum varies in color depending on pathogen and degree of inflammation (yellow, green, rust, brown; blood-tinged with severe inflammation)
- May be associated with pleuritic chest pain

Chest Radiograph

- Determines presence of pneumonia, but initial radiograph is often negative if the patient is dehydrated
- Reflects infiltrates (abnormal "white" areas) in various patterns, reflective of abnormal fluid distribution in lungs; can be mistaken for heart failure

Vital Signs

- Fever occurs in response to infection; some patients are not febrile.
- Pulse oximetry: Oxygen saturation is decreased from patient's normal baseline value.
- P/F ratio (ratio of arterial O_2 tension to fractional inspired O_2) is decreased when O_2 therapy is applied.
- Tachycardia and tachypnea are present if pneumonia is moderate to severe.
- Hypotension may be present if sepsis is ensuing; hypotension is exacerbated by underlying dehydration often present with pneumonia patients.
- Hypovolemia alone may prompt tachycardia.

Observation

- Nasal flaring and expiratory grunt may be present.
- Use of accessory muscles indicates respiratory distress.
- May appear fatigued, with or without diaphoresis if coughing has been relentless
- Ashen, pale, or gray/blue facial color, lip color, or nail beds
- Chest expansion may be decreased, restricted, or asymmetrical with severe pneumonia in one lung manifesting severe atelectasis or pleuritic pain.
- Altered level of consciousness (confusion, disorientation, agitation) is more common with older adults.
- Agitation is more commonly associated with hypoxemia, while somnolence is associated with hypercarbia (elevated CO_2 level).

Auscultation

- Decreased or bronchial breath sounds
- High-pitched inspiratory crackles heard best after patient coughs
- Low-pitched inspiratory crackles caused by airway secretions

Palpation

- Palpate chest wall for tenderness indicative of inflammation.
- Palpate to assess for symmetry of chest expansion.

Percussion
- May reveal presence of consolidation or fluid (dullness) or hyperresonance (pneumothorax)

Screening Labwork
- *CBC*: Evaluates for elevated white blood cells indicative of infection
- *Sputum gram stain, culture and sensitivity*: Identifies infecting organism
- *Blood culture and sensitivity*: If positive, indicates pneumonia organism has migrated into the bloodstream to cause a systemic infection
- *ABG analysis*: Evaluates for hypoxemia and hypercapnia

Diagnostic Tests for Acute Pneumonia

Test	Purpose	Abnormal Findings
Arterial blood gas analysis (ABG)	Oxygenation status and acid/base balance are evaluated with ABGs.	*pH changes*: Acidosis may reflect respiratory failure; alkalosis may reflect tachypnea. *Carbon dioxide*: Elevated CO_2 reflects respiratory failure; decreased CO_2 reflects tachypnea. *Hypoxemia*: Pao_2 <80 mm Hg *Oxygen saturation*: Sao_2 < 92% *Bicarbonate*: HCO_3 <22 mEq/L *Base deficit*: < −2
Complete blood count (CBC)	Evaluates for presence of infection	*Increased WBC count*: >11,000/mm^3 is seen with bacterial pneumonias. *Normal or low WBC count*: Seen with viral or mycoplasma pneumonias
Sputum gram stain, culture and sensitivity	Identifies infecting organism; A sputum culture should be obtained from the lower respiratory tract before initiation of antimicrobial therapy. The most reliable specimens are obtained via bronchoalveolar lavage (BAL) during bronchoscopy, suctioning with a protected telescoping catheter (mini-BAL), or open-lung biopsy (used occasionally to reduce contamination of specimen with oral flora).	*Gram stain positive*: Indicates organism is present *Culture*: Identifies organism *Sensitivity*: Reflects effectiveness of drugs on identified organism
Blood culture and sensitivity	Identifies whether pneumonia organism has become systemic; blood cultures help to identify the causative organism.	*Secondary bacteremia*: A frequent finding; patients with bacteremia are at higher risk for developing respiratory failure.
Serologic studies	Acute and convalescent titers are drawn to diagnose viral pneumonia. Both serologic and urine tests are available for Legionnaires pneumonia.	*Increased antibody titers*: A positive sign for viral infection
Acid-fast stain	To rule out mycobacterial infection (e.g., tuberculosis)	*Positive*: Mycobacterial infection is present.

Continued

Diagnostic Tests for Acute Pneumonia—cont'd

Test	Purpose	Abnormal Findings
Chest radiograph	Identifies anatomic involvement, extent of disease, presence of consolidation, pleural effusions, or cavitation	*Lobar:* Entire lobe involved *Segmental (lobular):* Only parts of a lobe involved *Bronchopneumonia:* Affects alveoli contiguous to the involved bronchi
Diagnostic fiberoptic bronchoscopy using PSB (protected specimen brush) and BAL	Obtains specimens during simple bronchoscopy without contaminating the aspirate; modified technique (mini-BAL) is also effective without the need of full bronchoscopy.	*Gram stain positive:* Indicates organism is present *Culture:* Identifies organism *Sensitivity:* Reflects effectiveness of drugs on identified organism
Thoracentesis	Removal of pleural effusion fluid from the pleural space using a needle to drain the chest cavity. Pleural effusion fluid may be cultured following thoracentesis to identify the causative organism.	*Gram stain positive:* Indicates organism is present *Culture:* Identifies organism *Sensitivity:* Reflects effectiveness of drugs on identified organism

COLLABORATIVE MANAGEMENT

COMMUNITY-ACQUIRED PNEUMONIA (CAP) HOSPITAL QUALITY ALLIANCE (HQA) INDICATORS

In December 2002, the American Hospital Association (AHA), Federation of American Hospitals (FAH), and Association of American Medical Colleges (AAMC) launched the Hospital Quality Alliance (HQA), an initiative to provide the public with specific reported information about hospital performance. This national public-private collaboration encourages hospitals to voluntarily collect and report quality performance information. The Centers for Medicare and Medicaid Services and The Joint Commission participate in HQA. Hospitals are expected to track and analyze their performance ratings and use the information to improve quality. The table below reflects HQA measures considered essential when caring for patients with community-acquired pneumonia (CAP). All indicators are evidence-based actions that should be included in the plan of care. The measurement describes the details of each indicator. Evidence of performance is derived from review of each patient's medical record following hospital discharge.

Indicators	Measure
Initial antibiotic timing	Initial antibiotic is received within 4 hours of hospital arrival.
Appropriate antibiotic selection	Initial antibiotic is appropriate for CAP in immunocompetent patients.
Blood cultures drawn	Cultures are performed within 24 hours prior to or after hospital arrival.
Blood cultures prior to antibiotics	Blood culture is performed before the first antibiotic is received in the hospital.
Oxygenation assessment	Assessed after arriving at the hospital
Pneumococcal vaccination	Administered during hospitalization
Influenza vaccination	Administered during hospitalization
Smoking cessation counseling	Counseling is provided for patients with history of smoking.

Care Priorities

1. **Relieve hypoxemia:**
   - *Oxygen therapy:* Administered when patient has an SpO_2 less than 92% or becomes symptomatic for air hunger. Special care must be taken not to abolish the hypoxic drive needed for effective breathing if patient has COPD and is known to retain CO_2.

For patients with chronic CO_2 retention, O_2 is delivered in low concentrations while O_2 saturation (SpO_2) is closely monitored. The physician should be consulted for parameters of "acceptable" O_2 saturation values in any patient with CO_2 retention. Patients in need of higher-level O_2 may be considered for noninvasive, positive pressure ventilation to help reduce work of breathing.

- *Intubation and mechanical ventilation*: Intubation may be necessary if a patient experiences progressive respiratory distress despite treatments. Mechanical ventilation is required if patient is unable to maintain adequate ABG values (PaO_2 greater than 60 mm Hg) with supplemental O_2. High concentrations of O_2 and positive end-expiratory pressure (PEEP) may be necessary in severe cases of pneumonia that lead to acute respiratory failure. (See *Acute Respiratory Failure*, p. 383.)

2. **Determine severity of pneumonia:** Mortality rates for severe pneumonia range from 20% to 53%. When pneumonia is confirmed, presence of any single parameter below is indicative pneumonia is severe:
   - RR greater than 30 breaths/min
   - Systolic blood pressure (BP) less than 90 mm Hg
   - Diastolic BP less than 60 mm Hg
   - Bilateral or multilobar involvement on chest radiograph
   - P/F ratio (ratio of PaO_2 to FIO_2) less than 250
   - Urine output less than 20 ml/hr or a total output of less than 80 ml/hr over 4 hours
   - Acute renal failure
   - A 50% increase in size of the pulmonary infiltrate during the first 48 hours following diagnosis
   - Patient requires endotracheal intubation and mechanical ventilation.
   - Initiate Early Goal Directed Therapy and Surviving Sepsis Guidelines if patient is septic (http://www.survivingsepsis.com/aboutcampaign).

3. **Control infection:**
   - *Antibiotics or anti-infectives*: Prescribed empirically on the basis of presenting signs and symptoms, clinical findings, and chest radiograph results until sputum or blood culture results are available. *Pneumococcus* is the most common pathogen associated with CAP, whereas enteric gram-negative bacteria are the most common pathogens identified with HAP. *Pseudomonas aeruginosa* and methicillin-resistant *Staphylococcus aureus* are the most common organisms seen in patients on long-term mechanical ventilation. Antimicrobial therapy in critically ill patients usually is parenteral and guided by sensitivity of the causative organism. Many of the organisms responsible for nosocomial pneumonias are resistant to multiple antibiotics or antimicrobials. Proper identification of the organism, determination of sensitivity to the medication, and attainment of therapeutic drug levels are critical for effective therapy.
   - *Isolation*: Some patients with pneumonia may require isolation and transmission-based precautions.

4. **Control cough:** *Antitussives are used to relieve coughing.* Occasionally narcotics such as codeine are required if coughing is unrelieved by other agents. If cough is productive, adding an expectorant to help manage thicker secretions may assist patient. Coughing should be controlled to a reasonable level, but not at the expense of expectorating sputum.

5. **Provide hydration:** IV fluids may be necessary to replace fluids lost from insensible sources (e.g., tachypnea, diaphoresis with fever). Dehydration causes secretions to become thick, tenacious, and difficult to expectorate. Hydration thins secretions for easier removal or expectoration.

6. **Reduce fever:** Analgesic antipyretics such as acetaminophen are used to reduce body temperature. Aspirin is generally not used for temperature control.

7. **Provide pain relief:** *Analgesics are used to relieve pleuritic pain.* Patients with pneumonia may have significant pleuritic pain that requires administration of opioid analgesics for relief. When opiates (e.g., codeine, morphine sulfate, meperidine) are given, varying degrees of respiratory depression occur, but these agents are often effective in controlling severe coughing. Careful and frequent monitoring of the patient's RR and depth, as well as O_2 saturation via pulse oximetry, is necessary.

8. **Support nutritional status:** Malnutrition is a causative factor in development of infections. In severely ill patients, enteral nutrition may provide the best protection against development of sepsis, owing to probable prevention of bacterial translocation

from the gut. A nutritional therapy consultation is warranted for all patients who have developed an infection and those at high risk of infection.

9. **Relieve congestion:** Percussion and postural drainage are indicated if deep breathing, coughing, and moving about in bed or ambulation are ineffective in raising and expectorating sputum. Consult with respiratory therapy as indicated.

INSTITUTE FOR HEALTHCARE IMPROVEMENT (IHI) VENTILATOR-ASSOCIATED PNEUMONIA (VAP) BUNDLE

The IHI has composed a group of interventions for all patients on mechanical ventilation that when implemented together, result in better outcomes than when implemented individually. Reducing mortality due to VAP requires an organized approach to early recognition and consistent use of evidence-based practices.

Indicator	Measure
Elevation of head of the bed	Head of the bed is elevated ≥30 degrees for the majority of the day (unless medically contraindicated).
Daily "sedation vacation" with assessment for readiness to extubate	Sedation is interrupted until the patient is able to follow commands and can be assessed for discontinuation of mechanical ventilation.
Peptic ulcer disease (PUD) prophylaxis	Gastric acid–controlling medications are administered to increase gastric pH. H_2 blockers are preferred over sucralfate. Proton pump inhibitors have not been fully studied.
Deep vein thrombosis (DVT) prophylaxis	Thrombin-inhibiting medications or mechanical devices are used to reduce the risk of clot development in lower extremities.

CARE PLANS FOR ACUTE PNEUMONIA

Risk for injury *related to respiratory compromise present with pneumonia*

GOALS/OUTCOMES Patient is free of infection reflected by normothermia and negative cultures; WBC count is within normal limits for patient; and sputum is clear to white in color.

NOC Infection Severity, Infection Protection

Infection Control
1. Implement standard precautions for infection prevention.
2. Provide additional infection control measures if infecting organism requires isolation.
3. Maintain a closed or inline suction system or an aseptic environment when suctioning the patient.
4. Inform visitors of effective precautions or pertinent isolation procedures.
5. Encourage and help provide turning, coughing, deep breathing, and use of incentive spirometer. Educate significant others to assist with these activities.
6. Encourage and assist with ambulation as soon as possible.

Infection Risk
1. Identify presurgical candidates at increased risk for nosocomial pneumonia (see Table 4-6).
2. Provide presurgical patients and significant others with verbal and written instructions and demonstrations of turning, coughing, and deep-breathing exercises performed after surgery to prevent atelectasis, which may lead to pneumonia.
3. Postoperatively encourage lung expansion: turning and repositioning in bed, deep breathing, coughing at frequent intervals. Mobilization of secretions is facilitated by movement.
4. Encourage and assist with ambulation as soon as possible.
5. Recognize the following ways in which nebulizer reservoirs can contaminate patient: introduction of nonsterile fluids or air; manipulation of nebulizer cup; or backflow of condensation into reservoir or into patient when delivery tubing is manipulated.
6. Use only sterile fluids, and dispense them aseptically.

7. Recognize and manage risk factors for patients with tracheostomy or ET tubes and mechanically ventilated patients:
   - Presence of underlying lung disease or other serious illness
   - Colonization of oropharynx or trachea by aerobic gram-negative bacteria
   - Greater access of bacteria to lower respiratory tract
   - Cross contamination is more likely with manipulation of these tubes.
   - Change breathing circuits according to CDC guidelines.
   - Discard any fluid that has condensed in tubing; do not allow it to drain back into reservoir or into patient.
   - Use "no-touch" technique, or use sterile gloves on both hands until a new tracheostomy wound has healed or formed granulation tissue around the tube.
   - Suction on an "as needed" rather than a routine basis. Frequent suctioning increases the risk of trauma and cross-contamination.

8. For patients who cannot remove secretions effectively by coughing, perform procedures that stimulate coughing such as chest physiotherapy, which includes breathing exercises, postural drainage, and percussion.

9. If pain interferes with lung expansion, control it by administering as-needed analgesics 0.5 hour before deep-breathing exercises, and provide splint support of wound areas with hands or pillows placed firmly across site of incision.

10. Identify patients at risk for aspiration, such as those with a decreased level of consciousness or dysphagia or who have a nasogastric or gastric tube in place.

11. For patients with decreased level of consciousness (LOC) who are unable to eat normally, consult physician regarding need for a method of feeding in which risk of aspiration is minimal such as postpyloric feeding (e.g., weighted small bore feeding tube that imports enteral feeding to the duodenum or percutaneous endoscopic gastrostomy [PEG tube]).

12. Elevate head of bed (HOB) to at least 30 degrees during feedings and for 1 hour after any feeding or medication to reduce the risk of aspiration.

Deficient fluid volume *related to insensible fluid losses associated with pneumonia*

GOALS/OUTCOMES Patient is normovolemic reflected by no clinical evidence of hypovolemia (e.g., furrowed tongue), stable weight, BP within patient's normal range, central venous pressure (CVP) 2 to 6 mm Hg, pulmonary artery pressure (PAP) 20 to 30/8 to 15 mm Hg, cardiac output (CO) 4 to 7 L/min, mean arterial pressure (MAP) 70 to 105 mm Hg, HR 60 to 100 beats/min (BPM), and systemic vascular resistance (SVR) 900 to 1200 dynes/sec/cm^{-5}.
NOC Fluid Balance, Electrolyte and Acid-Base Balance

Fluid Management
1. Identify patients at risk for dehydration, including those with poor nutritional status, reduced fluid intake, history of severe coughing (may be associated with inability to eat and/or vomiting), increased insensible loss secondary to hyperventilation, fever, and use of supplemental O_2.
2. Monitor input and output (I&O) hourly. Initially, intake should exceed output during volume replacement therapy. Consult physician for urine output less than 0.5 ml/kg/hr for 2 consecutive hours.
3. Monitor vital signs and hemodynamic pressures for signs of continued hypovolemia. Be alert to decreased values in BP, CVP, PAP, CO, and MAP, as well as increased HR and SVR.
4. Weigh patient daily, at the same time of day (preferably before breakfast), on a balanced scale, with the patient wearing the same type of clothing.
5. Administer fluids by mouth (PO) and IV as prescribed. Document patient's response to replacement therapy.
6. Monitor for signs and symptoms of fluid overload or too-rapid fluid administration: crackles (rales), shortness of breath (SOB), tachypnea, tachycardia, increased CVP, increased PAPs, jugular vein distention, and edema.

NIC Aspiration Precautions; Chest Physiotherapy; Cough Enhancement; Environmental Management; Fluid/Electrolyte Management; Fluid Monitoring; Hypovolemia Management; Infection Control; Intravenous Therapy; Mechanical Ventilation; Nutrition Management; Positioning; Surveillance; Respiratory Monitoring; Vital Signs Monitoring

ADDITIONAL NURSING DIAGNOSES

Also see *Drowning* (p. 307), and *Acute Asthma Exacerbation* (p. 354). As appropriate, see nursing diagnoses and interventions in *Nutritional Support* (p. 117), *Acute Respiratory Failure* (p. 383), *Mechanical Ventilation* (p. 99), *Prolonged Immobility* (p. 149), and *Emotional and Spiritual Support of the Patient and Significant Others* (p. 200).

RESEARCH BRIEF 4-4

Oral care practices in ICUs are not consistent or standardized. A recent survey of oral care practices in 59 European ICUs documented that oral care practices were carried out once daily in 20%, twice daily in 31%, and three times daily in 37% of patients. Oral care consisted primarily of mouth washes (55%) performed with chlorhexidine (61%). In contrast, only 41% used manual toothbrushes for oral care, and electric toothbrushes were never used. A study of critical care units in the United States had similar findings.

From Rello J, Koulenti D, Blot S, et al: Oral care practices in intensive care units: a survey of 59 European ICUs. *Intensive Care Med* 33(6):1066-1070, 2007; and Binkley C, Furr LA, Carrico R, et al: Survey of oral care practices in US intensive care units. *Am J Infect Control* 32(3):161-169, 2004.

ACUTE RESPIRATORY FAILURE

PATHOPHYSIOLOGY

The primary goal of the pulmonary system is to promote an appropriate and reasonable gas exchange at the alveolar-capillary surface, generally measured by pulse oximetry and arterial blood gases. *Acute respiratory failure* is a general term that identifies a primary lung dysfunction. That dysfunction results in failure to remove CO_2 (known as hypoventilation), and/or failure to promote appropriate and proportionate O_2 uptake at the alveolar-capillary interface. Type I (*hypoxemic*) is oxygenation failure, whereas type II (*hypercapnic*) is ventilation failure. Many patients manifest respiratory failure of types I and II simultaneously. Clinically, type I failure exists when Pao_2 is less than 50 mm Hg with the patient at rest and breathing room air ($Fio_2 = 0.21$ or 21% of the atmospheric pressure, which is 760 mm Hg at sea level). $Paco_2$ greater than 50 mm Hg is significant for acute ventilation failure or hypercapnia. A wide variety of disease states create a single or mixed respiratory failure. One of the simplest methods of evaluating patients relates to the understanding of basic gas exchange. Oxygenation occurs primarily during inspiration and the removal of CO_2 occurs during exhalation. The basic concepts applied here include compliance and recoil. Lung compliance is the measure of expansion of the alveoli (the gas-exchanging surface), which occurs on inspiration, whereas elasticity refers to the ability of the alveoli to recoil, as they do on exhalation. Restrictive airway diseases general present with significant hypoxemia, whereas obstructive disorders are more likely to develop a persistent and chronic hypercapnia. See Box 4-1 for a description of some of the disease processes that can lead to acute respiratory failure. Careful consideration should be given to evaluate neurologic conditions and OSA as these are commonly overlooked causes of respiratory failure. The evaluation of respiratory failure includes the understanding of the following:

$\dot{V}/\dot{Q}$ Match

This general term refers to the relationship of gas distribution ($\dot{V}$) to the amount of blood ($\dot{Q}$), which passes the total alveolar surface in 1 minute of time. Normal alveolar ventilation occurs at a rate of 4 L/min, and normal pulmonary vascular blood flow occurs at a rate of 5 L/min. The normal $\dot{V}/Q$ ratio is therefore 4 L/min divided by 5 L/min, or a ratio of 0.8, almost in a 1:1 ratio. Any disease process that interferes with either side of the equation upsets the physiologic balance, causing a $\dot{V}/Q$ mismatch.

Components of an abnormal $\dot{V}/Q$ ratio include:

Alveolar dead space ventilation: This is a primary problem with pulmonary perfusion. Alveoli may be compliant and elastic, but in a condition where the alveoli are normal or hyperventilated, and the perfusion is proportionately lower than the ventilation, there is a primary gas exchange problem. This is measured or evaluated as a high $\dot{V}/Q$ mismatch, wherein ventilation is proportionately greater than perfusion. This is frequently seen with low cardiac output states, or pulmonary embolus, and in overventilation of the independent lung surface.

| Box 4-1 | DISEASE PROCESSES LEADING TO THE DEVELOPMENT OF RESPIRATORY FAILURE |

Obstructive disease states, impaired exhalation, impaired minute ventilation, CO_2 retention
- COPD (emphysema, bronchitis, asthma, cystic fibrosis)
- Neuromuscular defects (Guillain-Barré syndrome, myasthenia gravis, multiple sclerosis, muscular dystrophy, polio, brain/spinal injury)
- Depression of respiratory control centers (drug-induced cerebral infarction, inappropriate use of high-dose oxygen therapy, drug/toxic agents)

Restrictive disease states, impaired inspiration, impaired alveolar recruitment: hypoxemia, refractory hypoxemia
- Restrictive pulmonary disease (interstitial fibrosis, pleural effusion, pneumothorax, kyphoscoliosis, obesity, diaphragmatic paralysis)
- Pulmonary emboli
- Atelectasis
- Pneumonia
- Bronchiolitis
- ARDS
- Chest trauma (rib fractures)
- Chest wall issues

Diffusion disturbances
- Pulmonary/interstitial fibrosis
- Pulmonary edema
- ARDS
- Anatomic loss of functioning lung tissue (pneumonectomy)

ARDS, acute respiratory distress syndrome; *COPD*, chronic obstructive pulmonary disease.

Diffusion distance: O_2 and CO_2 must cross the barrier created by the alveolar epithelium, the interstitial space, and the capillary endothelium. That space between is typically fluid and product free, allowing gas to move rapidly across. Diffusion is affected when an increase in anatomic distance and/or product (fluid, proteins, neutrophils) alters the ability of gas exchange between alveoli and capillary bed. Pulmonary edema is a major problem which interferes with diffusion.

Intrapulmonary Right to left shunt: Large amounts of blood pass from the right side of the heart to the left and out into the general circulation without adequate oxygenation. This process occurs when alveoli are not recruited on inspiration due to atelectasis or the alveoli are flooded. Primary causes of intrapulmonary shunt are atelectasis and ARDS.

ASSESSMENT
Goal of System Assessment
To evaluate for poor gas exchange and increased ventilatory support requirements (see *Acid-Base Balance*, p. 1, and *Mechanical Ventilation*, p. 99).

History and Risk Factors
Indicators of acute respiratory failure vary according to the underlying disease process and severity of the failure. Acute respiratory failure is one of the most common causes of impaired LOC and agitation. Respiratory failure is often associated with heart failure, pneumonia, or stroke. Sometimes the onset of acute respiratory failure is so insidious it is missed or misinterpreted. A patient may be somnolent due to hypercapnia (CO_2 retention causing elevated CO_2) from ventilatory failure or agitated and combative due to hypoxia. Patients with COPD have reduced airway diameter as well as chronic inflammation and airway remodeling, and when the underlying chronic condition is exacerbated, mucus hypersecretion and airway edema compound the initial condition. Increased effort is needed to mobilize gas in and out of the lungs, particularly during exhalation. The failure to exhale leads to

air trapping and hyperinflation, which further compromise inspiratory effort and contribute to increasing hypoxia and hypercapnia.

Vital Signs

- *Early indicators*: Dyspnea, restlessness, anxiety, headache, fatigue, cool and dry skin, increased BP, tachycardia, and persistent rapid respiratory rate, which indicate hypoxia. Hypercapnia results in slurred speech and headache.
- *Intermediate indicators*: Confusion, profound lethargy, tachypnea, hypotension and somnolence (if pH is less than 7.25), and cardiac dysrhythmias
- *Late indicators*: Cyanosis, diaphoresis, coma, and respiratory arrest

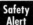 **Safety Alert** *A patient with a history of COPD may increasingly or excessively use inhaled beta$_2$-agonists. If this is the case, evaluation of tachycardia may be indicative of recent medication use.*

Observation

Skin: Facial and lip pallor, ashen or diaphoretic appearance
Nail beds: Ashen or cyanotic nail beds
Respiratory: Use of accessory muscles for breathing, work of breathing, synchronous or asynchronous lung expansion and edema (especially dependent areas)

Auscultation

Evaluate the presence of normal breath sounds and synchronous lung expansion. Auscultate for the presence of:

1. *Late inspiratory rales* (crackles): Anterior, lateral, and posterior: alveolar fluid or late opening
2. *Mid inspiratory rales* (crackles): Anterior, lateral, and posterior alveolar consolidation
3. *Early loud, coarse rales* (bubbles or rhonchi): Anterior, lateral, and posterior: conducting airway inflammation and mucus secretion
4. *Inspiratory wheezes*: Anterior, lateral, and posterior: early airway narrowing
5. *Expiratory wheezes*: Anterior, lateral, and posterior: late airway narrowing

Screening Labwork

Blood gas evaluation can determine primary and secondary problems, or primary problems with compensation (see *Acid-Base Balance*, p. 1).
Pulse oximetry is used for continuous monitoring of O_2 saturation.

Diagnostic Tests for Acute Respiratory Failure

Test	Purpose	Abnormal Findings
Blood Studies		
Arterial blood gas analysis	Assesses adequacy of oxygenation and effectiveness of ventilation. Evaluates the oxygenation of the arterial blood as well as the presence or absence of acid and the effect on the pH (environment of the cells).	Typical results predicting respiratory failure are Pao$_2$ <60 mm Hg, Paco$_2$ >45 mm Hg, with a pH that may be within normal range consistent with compensation via an increase in HCO$_3$ (bicarbonate), or the pH may be less than 7.35 consistent with acute (uncompensated) respiratory acidosis. Although changes are not always predictable in the disease process, generally patients will develop hypoxemia, which may initially be resolved with increasing the Fio$_2$ but eventually will require great increases in Fio$_2$ and ultimately will no longer respond to oxygen therapy.

Continued

Diagnostic Tests for Acute Respiratory Failure — cont'd

Test	Purpose	Abnormal Findings
Pa_{O_2}/F_{IO_2} ratio	The Pa_{O_2} divided by the F_{IO_2} (Pa_{O_2}/F_{IO_2} ratio, or more simply P/F) can be used to more simply assess the severity of the gas exchange defect. The normal value for the ratio of the partial pressure of oxygen in arterial blood to F_{IO_2} (Pa_{O_2}/F_{IO_2}) (F_{IO_2} is expressed as a decimal ranging from 0.21 to 1.00) is 300–500.	A value of less than 300 indicates gas exchange derangement, and a value below 250 is indicative of severe impairment, and compliance calculations should be performed to encourage alveolar recruitment strategies.

Radiology

Test	Purpose	Abnormal Findings
Chest radiograph (CXR)	Assesses the size of lungs, presence of fluids, abnormal gas or fluids in the pleural sac, diaphragmatic margins, the pulmonary hilum, and the integrity of the rib cage	Presence of fluids in the lung parenchyma initially presents as pulmonary edema. The continuous accumulation differentiates this edema formation to one that is not cardiac.
Computed tomography (CT) lung scan	Assesses the three-dimensional lung capacities, fluid load, and primary displacement of the fluid	Normally a large gas-filled surface, the ALI/ARDS lung when seen on CT is frequently fluffy and white due to fluid that has extravagated through the endothelial deficits (capillary leak).

COLLABORATIVE MANAGEMENT
Care Priorities

1. **Correction of hypoxemia: First treatment priority:** Pa_{O_2} levels less than 30 mm Hg for longer than 5 minutes may cause permanent brain damage or death. High-concentration O_2 therapy, in conjunction with pharmacotherapy (e.g., bronchodilators, steroids, antibiotics), often improves ABG levels sufficiently to remove the patient from danger, but increasing F_{IO_2} is a temporary solution and does not actually treat the problem.

   Patients with COPD who chronically retain CO_2 (chronic hypercapnia) are unable to receive high concentrations of O_2 unless ventilation is highly supported with an underlying rate control strategy such as noninvasive positive pressure ventilation (NPPV or NiPPV), continuous positive airway pressure (CPAP) or bilevel positive airway pressure (BiPAP), or invasive mechanical ventilation.

2. **Correction of respiratory acidosis (hypercapnia):** May be corrected using NPPV such as BiPAP, or invasive mechanical ventilation following ET intubation. Exhalation time should be increased and particular attention to that time must be applied when altering tidal volume or respiratory rate. Because CO_2 is removed during exhalation time in the respiratory cycle, any patient with CO_2 retention must be provided with a longer E time.
   - Noninvasive (NPPV): Ventilator support that is given without endotracheal intubation or tracheotomy. Administered via a face or nasal mask. Requires skilled management but not necessarily intensive care admission. NPPV or invasive mechanical support is used as a continuous replacement for normal lung function until the underlying cause of the failure can be corrected and the patient can resume ventilatory efforts independently.
   - Invasive: Ventilator support that is given through endotracheal intubation or tracheotomy; requires intensive or high-acuity care. The purposes of intubation and mechanical ventilation are to restore alveolar ventilation and systemic oxygenation, provide compensation in metabolic acidosis/alkalosis, and decrease work of breathing. Early intubation can prevent further airway collapse and tissue injury. In most cases of respiratory failure, the patient will require intubation and mechanical ventilation to support adequate respiratory function and stabilize ABG levels. (See *Mechanical Ventilation*, p. 99.)

3. **Correction of acidotic pH due to hypercapnia (hypoventilation):** Adequate cellular and metabolic functioning are hindered when pH level remains outside the normal range

of 7.35 to 7.45. When the pH is less than 7.20, evaluate for signs of systemic compromise such as failure to maintain vascular tone and therefore BP. After efforts to correct ventilation have failed or if the patient presents with clinical symptoms such as hypotension refractory to volume and vasopressors, IV sodium bicarbonate may be used conservatively to return the pH to a level higher than 7.25. The use of sodium bicarbonate is a short-term solution for most acid-base disturbances and its use may actually make the overall situation worse.

4. **Correction of alkalotic pH due to hypocapnia (hyperventilation):** A pH greater than 7.45 may indicate primary hyperventilation with a high minute ventilation (F or V_T). If possible, assess the patient for anxiety and rapid respiratory rate. If the patient is intubated, assess the settings on the ventilator to assure an appropriate method is being utilized.

If the minute ventilation is not the causative problem or cannot be adjusted, evaluate for a primary metabolic alkalosis. Causative factors of primary metabolic alkalosis may be over diuresis, diarrhea, or aggressive nasogastric (NG) drainage. The pH may be managed by compensation with CO_2 retention via a rebreathing mask, decreasing minute ventilation, or by increasing dead space on mechanical ventilator circuitry.

RESEARCH BRIEF 4-5

A severely altered level of consciousness (ALC) has been considered a contraindication to non invasive positive pressure ventilation (NiPPV). This 5-year, prospective, case-controlled study of eighty patients (total 153 patients evaluated and consecutively collected) compared the clinical outcome of patients with acute respiratory failure (ARF) due to COPD exacerbations and their different degrees of altered levels of consciousness as they related to NiPPV. The study confirmed the lower the ALC, the better the response to NiPPV, although all patients responded better than expected. The cut point was related to a Kelly score of greater than 3 as well as to the baseline pH, but not the patient's CO_2 level. A Kelly score of 1 is considered a normal level of consciousness, while a 6 is considered severely impaired consciousness.

From Scala R, Naldi M, et al: Noninvasive positive pressure ventilation in patients with acute exacerbations of COPD and varying levels of consciousness. *Chest* 128(3):1657–1666, 2005.

CARE PLANS FOR ACUTE RESPIRATORY FAILURE
Impaired gas exchange *related to disease process underlying impending respiratory failure*

GOALS/OUTCOMES Within 2 to 4 hours of initiation of treatment, patient has adequate gas exchange reflected by PaO_2 greater than 80 mm Hg, $PaCO_2$ 35 to 45 mm Hg, and pH 7.35 to 7.45 (or ABG values within 10% of patient's baseline), with mechanical ventilation, if necessary. Within 24 to 48 hours of initiation of treatment, patient is weaning or weaned from mechanical ventilation, and RR is 12 to 20 breaths/min with normal baseline depth and pattern.

NOC Respiratory Status: Ventilation, Vital Signs Status, Respiratory Status: Gas Exchange, Symptom Control Behavior, Comfort Level, Endurance

Respiratory Monitoring
1. Monitor for signs of increasing hypoxia at frequent intervals: restlessness, agitation, and personality changes are indicative of severe exacerbation. Cyanosis of the nail beds (peripheral) and/or lips (central) are early and late indicators of hypoxia, respectively.
2. Monitor for signs of hypercapnia at frequent intervals: confusion, listlessness, and somnolence may indicate respiratory failure or near-fatal asthma exacerbation.
3. Monitor ABGs when continuous pulse oximetry values or patient assessment reflects progressive hypoxemia or development of hypercapnia. Be alert to decreasing PaO_2 and increasing $PaCO_2$ or decreasing O_2 saturation levels, indicative of impending respiratory collapse.
4. Monitor for synchronous, bilateral lung expansion, decreased breath sounds, or changes in wheezing at frequent intervals. Absent breath sounds in a distressed asthma patient may indicate impending respiratory arrest.

Anxiety Reduction
1. Ascertain and alleviate the cause of restlessness to decrease metabolic demands (e.g., if restlessness is related to anxiety, help reduce anxiety by providing reassurance, enabling family members to stay with patient, and offering distractions such as soft music or television).
2. Be aware that restlessness may be an early sign of hypoxemia.
3. Explain all procedures and offer support to minimize fear and anxiety, which can increase O_2 demands.

Oxygen Therapy
1. Provide humidity in O_2 if used for more than 12 hours to help thin secretions.
2. Administer supplemental O_2 using liter flow device as ordered.
3. Document pulse oximetry with O_2 liter flow in place at time of reading as ordered. Oxygen is a drug; the dose of the drug must be associated with the O_2 saturation or the reading is meaningless.
4. Monitor for skin breakdown where O_2 devices are in contact with the skin, such as nares, and around edges of mask devices.
5. Monitor F_{IO_2} to ensure that O_2 is within prescribed concentrations. If patient does not retain CO_2, 100% nonrebreather mask may be used to provide maximal O_2 support. If the patient retains CO_2 and is unrelieved by positioning, lower-dose O_2, bronchodilators, and steroids, intubation, and mechanical ventilation may be necessary sooner than in patients who are able to receive higher doses of O_2 by mask.

Ventilation Assistance
1. Obtain arterial blood gases if patient experiences behavioral changes or respiratory distress to check for hypoxia or hypercapnia.
2. Monitor for induced hypoventilation, especially in patients with COPD.
3. Monitor for changes in chest radiograph and breath sounds indicative of O_2 toxicity and absorption atelectasis in patients receiving higher concentrations of O_2 (more than F_{IO_2} 45%) for longer than 24 hours. The higher the O_2 concentration, the greater is the chance of toxicity.
4. Position patient for comfort and to promote optimal gas exchange. High-Fowler's position, with the patient leaning forward and elbows propped on the over-the-bed table to promote maximal chest excursion, may reduce use of accessory muscles and diaphoresis due to work of breathing.
5. Consider use of NPPV prior to endotracheal intubation and mechanical ventilation.

NIC Acid-base Management; Acid-base Monitoring; Airway Management; Bedside Laboratory Testing; Cough Enhancement; Emotional Support; Energy Management; Fluid Management; Fluid Monitoring; Laboratory Data Interpretation; Mechanical Ventilation; Oxygen Therapy; Positioning; Respiratory Monitoring; Vital Signs Monitoring

ADDITIONAL NURSING DIAGNOSIS
See sections relating to patient's underlying pathologic condition. Refer to *Mechanical Ventilation*, p. 99, for further information.

PNEUMOTHORAX

PATHOPHYSIOLOGY
Pneumothorax is an accumulation of air between the parietal and visceral pleura with secondary lung collapse. There are three types of pneumothorax.

Spontaneous
A type of closed pneumothorax in which the chest wall remains intact with no leak to the atmosphere. Both primary and secondary pneumothoraces result from the rupture of a bleb or bulla on the visceral pleural surface, usually near the apex. A *primary* spontaneous pneumothorax is rarely life-threatening and generally occurs in healthy, 20- to 40-year-old men who smoke. The cause of the rupture is unknown, although it may result from a weakness related to a respiratory infection. Symptoms generally occur at rest rather than with vigorous exercise or coughing. The potential for recurrence is great, with the second pneumothorax occurring an average of 2 to 3 years after the first. A *secondary* spontaneous pneumothorax may occur in all age groups resulting from an underlying lung disease (COPD, cystic fibrosis, tuberculosis, malignant neoplasm). Symptoms are more likely to be life-threatening than with a primary spontaneous pneumothorax, and recurrence rates

are high in this population. The rate of reabsorption of spontaneous pneumothoraces is 1.25% to 1.8% of the volume of the hemithorax every 24 hours. A 15% pneumothorax would require 8 to 12 days to fully resolve without treatment.

Traumatic

The integrity of the chest wall may or may not be disrupted prior to lung collapse. An *open* pneumothorax occurs when air enters the pleural space from the atmosphere through an opening in the chest wall, such as with a penetrating injury or an invasive medical procedure (e.g., lung biopsy, thoracentesis, placement of a central line into a subclavian vein). A *closed* pneumothorax occurs when the visceral pleura is penetrated but the chest wall remains intact, with no atmospheric leak. Closed chest wall lung collapse occurs with blunt trauma, including cardiopulmonary resuscitation, when an external impact on the chest fractures and dislocates the ribs. It also may occur from the use of high-level PEEP therapy. For more information about blunt chest injuries, see *Chest Trauma*, p. 238.

Tension

Tension pneumothorax is a life-threatening medical emergency most often associated with trauma or infection. Tension can ensue with a spontaneous pneumothorax or during positive pressure mechanical ventilation. The integrity of the chest wall may or may not be disrupted prior to lung collapse. Air enters the pleural space during inspiration through a pleural tear and continues to accumulate inside the pleural cavity. The air cannot escape during expiration because the intrapleural pressure is greater than alveolar pressure, which creates a one-way or flap-valve effect. The increasing intrathoracic pressure is transmitted to the mediastinum, resulting in a mediastinal shift toward the unaffected side. The encroachment of the enlarging affected side makes it impossible for the unaffected side to fully expand. The increased pressure also compresses the vena cava, which impedes venous return, and reduces preload/end-diastolic volume. Cardiac output is progressively reduced as the intrathoracic pressure and vena caval compression increases, leading to circulatory collapse if not promptly diagnosed and managed. Bilateral tension pneumothoraces may occur, and generally result in cardiac arrest shortly after the lungs collapse.

ASSESSMENT
Goal of System Assessment

Evaluate for ineffective breathing patterns and impaired gas exchange. The clinical presentation will vary in degree, depending on the type and size of the pneumothorax. With tension pneumothorax, evaluate for decreased cardiac output and decreased tissue perfusion. See *Respiratory Assessment: General*, p. 352, and *Cardiac Assessment: General*, p. 418.

History and Risk Factors:

Trauma, pulmonary infection, high-level positive pressure mechanical ventilation: Many patients with primary pneumothoraces do not seek medical advice for several days. Nearly 46% delay seeking help with managing symptoms for more than 2 days. Assessing for delay is important because the occurrence of reexpansion pulmonary edema (RPO) after reinflation may be related to the length of time the lung has been collapsed.

Chest Radiograph
- Determines presence of pneumothorax
- Reflects absence of lung markers; includes absence of "white" blood vessels
- No circulation is present in collapsed area filled with air (black).

Vital Signs
- Tachycardia, tachypnea
- Possible fever
- BP may increase or decrease, depending on response to any changes in cardiac output, which are profound with tension pneumothorax.
- Small pneumothoraces may not affect vital signs at all.

Observation/Inspection

Spontaneous or traumatic pneumothorax
- Sudden onset of sharp, stabbing chest pain on the affected side, radiating to the shoulder if pneumothorax is large enough (greater than 20% collapse)
- British Thoracic Society guidelines define "small" as a pneumothorax of less than 2 cm and "large" as a pneumothorax of greater than 2 cm. Percentages of lung that have collapsed are also used to quantify the extent of lung collapse in clinical practice.
- Moderate to severe dyspnea and anxiety may be present if pneumothorax is large enough (greater than 30% collapse)
- Decreased chest wall movement on the affected side if the pneumothorax is large enough (greater than 40% collapse)
- Pale appearance is likely with a larger pneumothorax (greater than 50% collapse).
- With a small pneumothorax (10% to 20% collapse), the patient may have no pain and no abnormality in chest wall movement and be unaware lung collapse has occurred.

Tension pneumothorax
- Severe dyspnea
- Chest pain on affected side
- Pale progressing to gray/blue, cool, clammy, mottled skin
- Anxiety and restlessness resulting from progressive hypoxemia
- Decreased chest wall movement on affected side
- Expansion of affected side throughout respiratory cycle, rather than expansion and relaxation
- Progressively increasing jugular vein distention as vena cava is compressed
- Cardiac arrest is possible with bilateral tension pneumothoraces.

Palpation

Spontaneous or traumatic pneumothorax
- Subcutaneous emphysema (crepitus)
- Tactile and vocal fremitus decreased or absent on affected side

Tension pneumothorax
- Tracheal shift toward unaffected side
- Subcutaneous emphysema in neck and chest

Percussion

Spontaneous or traumatic pneumothorax
- Hyperresonance on affected side

Tension pneumothorax
- Hyperresonance on affected side

Auscultation

Spontaneous or traumatic pneumothorax
- Absent or decreased breath sounds on affected side
- Increased RR
- Moderate tachycardia (HR greater than 140 bpm) may be present.

Tension pneumothorax
- Absent or decreased breath sounds on affected side
- Distant heart sounds
- Tachypnea/increased RR (greater than 30 breaths/min)
- Hypotension/decreased BP (more than a 20% drop from previous BP)
- Tachycardia/increased HR (greater than 140 bpm)

 Safety Alert   *Tension pneumothorax is life-threatening. Immediate medical intervention is critical.*

Diagnostic Tests for Pneumothorax

Test	Purpose	Abnormal Findings
Chest radiograph A lateral chest or lateral decubitus radiograph should be done if the clinical suspicion of pneumothorax is high, but a PA radiograph is normal. Expiratory chest radiographs are not recommended for the routine diagnosis of pneumothorax.	Reveals the size of the pneumothorax and presence of tracheal shift	*Affected side*: Air is present in the pleural space (black); lung markings are absent in area of collapse (black); abnormal expansion of the chest wall with tension pneumothorax with lowering/flattening of the diaphragm.
Chest CT scan	CT scanning is recommended when differentiating a pneumothorax from bullous lung disease, when incorrect tube placement is suspected, and when the chest radiograph is obscured by surgical emphysema.	Presence of blackened areas indicative of air, with absence of white areas indicative of blood circulating in tissues, which may have been obliterated or unclear on the chest radiograph
Arterial blood gas (ABG) analysis	Assess for hypoxemia and acidosis.	Hypoxemia (Pao_2 <80 mm Hg on room air) is generally present with a 20% or greater lung collapse. Mild hypoxemia is present with smaller pneumothoraces. Tension pneumothoraces may cause both respiratory and lactic acidosis (pH <7.35) from impending respiratory failure and circulatory collapse. Elevated carbon dioxide and lactate lower the blood pH.
12-Lead ECG	Rule out acute coronary syndrome as a cause for chest pain with vital sign changes indicative of deterioration.	Vena cava compression from tension pneumothorax affects perfusion of the coronary arteries if pneumothorax is not diagnosed and managed promptly. ST-segment depression, indicative of myocardial ischemia, may be present, along with decreased QRS amplitude/decreased R waves, rightward axis deviation.
Pulmonary function tests	Pulmonary function tests provide minimally sensitive data to validate presence or size of pneumothorax.	Not recommended.

COLLABORATIVE MANAGEMENT
Care Priorities

Patients with shortness of breath should not be left without intervention regardless of the size of the pneumothorax seen on the chest radiograph.

1. **Relieve hypoxemia:**
   - *Oxygen therapy/Adjustment in mechanical ventilation:* Oxygen is administered when ABG values demonstrate the presence of hypoxemia. If patient is already receiving mechanical ventilation, Fio_2 is increased while evaluation is done regarding amount of positive pressure used during inspiratory and expiratory phases of ventilation. If positive pressure is a suspected cause of the pneumothorax, positive pressure is reduced if possible.

- *High-flow O_2:* If a patient with a pneumothorax is admitted for observation, high-flow (10 L/min) O_2 should be administered, with appropriate caution in COPD patients with sensitivity to high concentrations of O_2. Use of high-flow O_2 has resulted in a fourfold increase in the rate of pneumothorax reabsorption while the therapy is in progress.

2. Reexpand the collapsed lung:
    - *Observation:* No treatment may be required for small, closed pneumothoraces without significant dyspnea or breathlessness.
    - *Simple aspiration:* Recommended as first line of treatment for all primary pneumothoraces in need of intervention. Performed immediately in tension pneumothorax to remove air from the chest cavity. A large-bore needle is inserted into the second intercostal space, midclavicular line, which correlates to the superior portion of the anterior axillary lobe. A sudden rushing out of air confirms the diagnosis of tension pneumothorax. To decrease the risk of further pleural laceration as the chest reexpands, a stylet introducer needle with a plastic sheath may be used. The needle is removed after penetration, and the plastic catheter sheath is left in place to allow decompression of the chest cavity. Simple aspiration is less likely to succeed in secondary pneumothoraces and is recommended as an initial treatment in small (less than 2 cm) pneumothoraces in patients under 50 years of age with mild SOB. Large secondary pneumothoraces (larger than 2 cm), especially in patients over the age of 50, are generally not successfully managed using simple aspiration and are at high risk for recurrence. Intercostal/chest tube drainage is recommended as appropriate initial treatment. Once air is removed from the pleural space, the lung is able to reexpand.
    - *Catheter aspiration:* Catheter aspiration of simple pneumothorax (CASP) is done by passing a small ($\sim$8 Fr) catheter over a guidewire into the pleural space. A three-way stopcock is attached and air may be aspirated via a 50-ml syringe. Addition of a Heimlich valve and suction may improve success rates to over 60%. If simple aspiration or catheter aspiration drainage are unsuccessful, a chest/intercostal tube should be inserted.
    - *Chest tube placement/tube thoracostomy:* Recommended in secondary pneumothorax except in symptomatic patients with a very small (less than 1 cm or apical) pneumothorax. Chest tubes cause inflammation, ultimately scarring the pleura to help prevent recurrent spontaneous pneumothoraces. Patients with recurrent lung collapse or extensive lung disease generally require chest tubes rather than needle decompression because their visceral pleura does not seal promptly. Chest tubes are inserted in the second or third lateral intercostal space, midclavicular line, or in the fourth intercostal space at mid-thoracic line for a posterior pneumothorax. During insertion, the patient should be in an upright position so that the lung falls away from the chest wall. A small (1 to 2 cm) incision is made, and the chest tube is placed, sutured in place, and connected to an underwater-seal drainage system. Usually simple underwater-seal drainage is all that is necessary for 6 to 24 hours. A one-way flutter valve may be placed on the chest tube instead of the underwater-seal drainage system, to allow air to escape while preventing reentry. After chest tube insertion and removal of air from the pleural space, the lung begins to reexpand. There is no evidence large tubes (20 to 24 Fr) are more effective than small tubes (10 to 14 Fr). The initial use of large (20 to 24 Fr) intercostal tubes is not recommended. If a persistent air leak is present, it may be necessary to replace a small chest tube with a larger one. Suction may be used, depending on the size of the pneumothorax, the patient's condition, and the amount of drainage. Suction can be applied with a flutter valve in place.
    - *Chest tube suction:* Suction should not be applied directly after tube insertion, but rather, added after 48 hours if persistent air leak is present or the pneumothorax fails to reexpand. High-volume, low-pressure (-10 to -20 cm H_2O) suction systems are recommended. Patients requiring suction should be managed by physicians and nurses who have experience managing complex pneumothoraces. There is no evidence to support routine use of immediate suction with chest drain systems in the treatment of spontaneous pneumothorax.
    - Chemical pleurodesis: The instillation of caustic substances into the pleural space, resulting in aseptic inflammation with formation of dense adhesions, which can seal persistent air leaks. Pleurodesis is associated with a high recurrence rate of primary and secondary pneumothoraces, despite use of various sclerosants to reduce these rates. The chemicals are instilled either through chest tubes or during surgery.

Doxycycline and talc slurry are the preferred sclerosing agents. Few usage guidelines are available for physicians. Prevention of additional recurrent pneumothoraces should be managed surgically in most cases.

3. **Relieve pain:**
   - *Analgesic:* Provides relief of pain of pneumothorax or its treatment. A chest tube may cause pleuritic pain, slight temperature elevation, and pleuritic friction rub. The nurse should administer analgesics and monitor the patient's response to the analgesics administered during the procedure.

4. **Remove chest drainage device:**
   - *Stepped/staged approach:* Remove chest tube using a stepped/stage approach to ensure the air leak has resolved. A chest radiograph demonstrating complete resolution of the pneumothorax with no clinical evidence of air leak should be done first. Secondly, chest tube suction is discontinued. Clamping prior to discontinuation of the chest tube is controversial and performed by only half of trained practitioners.
   - *Chest radiograph before tube removal:* Chest radiographs are obtained following the last evidence of air leak but before chest tube removal at intervals ranging from less than 4 to 24 hours after the last air leak assessment. Nearly two-thirds of practitioners wait 5 to 12 hours after last evidence of air leak before obtaining the preremoval radiograph. Practices range from less than 4 to 24 hours.

5. **Manage persistent air leak:**
   - *Continued observation:* Patients should be observed for 4 days to assess for spontaneous closure of a pneumothorax caused by bronchopleural fistula. If the air leak persists longer than 4 days, patients should be evaluated for surgery to close the air leak with additional pleurodesis procedure to prevent recurrence. Thoracoscopy is the preferred management procedure.
   - *Additional closure techniques:* Use of an additional chest tube or bronchoscopy in an attempt to seal endobronchial sites of air leakage is not indicated. Except in special circumstances where surgery is contraindicated or a patient refuses surgery, chemical pleurodesis should not be used in the management of most patients.

6. **Provide surgical intervention for recurrent pneumothoraces:**
   - *Thoracoscopy:* Thoracoscopy can be performed with or without video assistance. Intraoperative bullectomy should be performed by staple bullectomy in patients with apical bullae visualized at surgery.
   - *Thoracotomy:* May be indicated when a patient is at high risk for repeated recurrence and is not successfully managed by thoracoscopy. High-risk status is present when at least two spontaneous pneumothoraces occurred in the same lung or if resolution of the pneumothorax has not occurred within 7 days. Thoracotomy may involve mechanical abrasion or decortication of the pleural surfaces with a dry, sterile sponge or chemical abrasion via an agent such as tetracycline (e.g., doxycycline) solution or talc, both of which result in pleural adhesions to prevent recurrence. A partial pleurectomy may be performed instead of mechanical or chemical abrasion.

CARE PLANS FOR PNEUMOTHORAX

Impaired spontaneous ventilation and impaired gas exchange *related to collapsed lung*

GOALS/OUTCOMES Within 2 to 6 hours of initiation of treatment, patient exhibits adequate gas exchange as evidenced by $Pao_2 \geq 60$ mm Hg and $Paco_2 \leq 45$ mm Hg (or values within 10% of patient's baseline values, which depend on underlying pathophysiology), RR less than 20 breaths/min with normal depth and pattern), and orientation to time, place, and person.

NOC Respiratory Status: Ventilation, Vital Signs Status, Respiratory Status: Gas Exchange, Symptom Control Behavior, Comfort Level, Endurance

Ventilation Assistance

1. Position patient to allow for full expansion of unaffected lung. Semi-Fowler's position usually provides comfort and allows adequate expansion of chest wall. The patient also can be turned unaffected side-down with the HOB elevated to ensure a better $\dot{V}/\dot{Q}$ match.
2. Change patient's position every 2 hours to promote drainage and lung reexpansion and to facilitate alveolar perfusion.
3. Encourage patient to take deep breaths, providing necessary analgesia to decrease discomfort during deep-breathing exercises. Deep breathing will promote full lung expansion and may decrease the risk of atelectasis.
4. Ensure delivery of prescribed concentrations of O_2.

Environmental Management: Safety

1. Assist physician or midlevel practitioner with chest tube insertion according to institutional guidelines.
2. Assess and maintain closed chestdrainage system:

 Closed chest drainage systems include Heimlich/flutter valve devices with/without collection chamber, disposable "wet" suction, disposable "dry" suction, Emerson disposable suction, or a manually assembled 1-4 bottle water seal drainage system. Tape all connections, and secure chest tube to thorax with tape.

- Avoid all kinks in the tubing, and ensure that the bed and equipment are not compressing any component of the system.
- Closed systems must remain intact/airtight to maintain negative pressure and avoid air entrapment in the pleural space.
- Stabilize chest drainage system with appropriate device/holder on the floor to prevent tipping or other disruption, which may open the system to air.
- Ensure system is appropriately vented at all times to help prevent possibility of tension pneumothorax should the system be disrupted. Air should be released if the system is vented.
- Drainage system should be kept below the level of the chest to maintain appropriate pressure dynamics.
- Maintain fluid in underwater-seal chamber, and suction chamber at appropriate levels. Check the water level in "wet" suction controlled units at least every shift, as the water evaporates.
- Be aware that the suction apparatus does not regulate the amount of suction applied to the closed drainage system. The amount of suction is determined by the water level in the suction control chamber. Minimal bubbling is optimal. Excessive bubbling causes rapid evaporative loss.
- Suction aids in the reexpansion of the lung. Removing suction for short periods of time will not be detrimental to the patient as long as the system is appropriately vented to allow for the escape of the air.
- Fluctuations in the underwater-seal chamber indicate the tube is patent. Fluctuations stop when either the lung has reexpanded or there is a kink or obstruction in the chest tube.
- Bubbling in the underwater-seal chamber occurs only during expiration and reflects air is leaving the pleural space through the drainage system.
- Continuous bubbling *on both inspiration and expiration* in the underwater-seal chamber is a signal that air is leaking into the drainage system. Locate and seal the system's air leak, if possible.

Safety Alert *A bubbling chest tube should never be clamped. Chest tubes should generally remain unclamped. Clamping a chest tube inserted for pneumothorax should be done under the supervision of a respiratory physician or thoracic surgeon if required. If a patient with a clamped drain experiences shortness of breath or develops subcutaneous emphysema, the tube must be unclamped immediately.*

---

3. Keep necessary emergency supplies at the bedside: (1) petroleum gauze pad to apply over insertion site if the chest tube becomes dislodged and (2) sterile water in which to submerge the chest tube if it becomes disconnected from the underwater-seal system. Never clamp a chest tube without a specific directive from the physician: clamping may lead to tension pneumothorax because the air can no longer escape.
4. Assist with chest tube removal in accordance with institutional guidelines.

Oxygen Therapy
1. Provide humidity in O_2 if used for more than 12 hours to help thin secretions.
2. Administer supplemental O_2 using liter flow device as ordered.
3. Document pulse oximetry with O_2 liter flow in place at time of reading as ordered. Oxygen is a drug; the dose of the drug must be associated with the O_2 saturation or the reading is meaningless.
4. Monitor for skin breakdown where O_2 devices are in contact with the skin, such as nares, and around edges of mask devices.

NIC Cough Enhancement, Oral Health Maintenance

Respiratory Monitoring
1. Obtain arterial blood gases if patient experiences behavioral changes or respiratory distress to check for hypoxia or hypercapnia.
2. Monitor for induced hypoventilation, especially in patients with COPD.
3. Monitor for changes in chest radiograph and breath sounds indicative of O_2 toxicity and absorption atelectasis in patients receiving higher concentrations of O_2 (more than FIO_2 of 45%) for longer than 24 hours. The higher the O_2 concentration, the greater the chance of toxicity.

NIC Acid-Base Management

Acute pain *related to chest tube placement and pleural irritation*

GOALS/OUTCOMES Within 1 to 2 hours of initiating analgesic therapy, patient's subjective evaluation of discomfort improves as documented by a pain scale. Nonverbal indicators of discomfort, such as grimacing and splinting on inspiration, are absent.
NOC Comfort Level, Pain Control Behavior, Pain Level

Pain Management
1. At frequent intervals, assess patient's degree of discomfort, using patient's verbal and nonverbal cues. Devise a pain scale with patient, rating discomfort on a scale of 0 (no pain) to 10 (worst pain). Medicate with analgesics as prescribed, evaluating and documenting the effectiveness of the medication on the basis of the pain scale.
2. Position patient on unaffected side to minimize discomfort from chest tube insertion site. Administer medication 30 minutes before initiating movement.
3. Teach patient to splint affected side during coughing, moving, or repositioning. Move patient as a unit to enhance stability and comfort.
4. Schedule activities to provide for periods of rest, because fatigue may lower patient's pain threshold.
5. Stabilize chest tube to reduce pull or drag on latex connector tubing. Tape chest tube securely to thorax, and loop latex tubing on bed beside patient.

Self-Responsibility Facilitation
1. Teach patient to maintain active range of motion (ROM) on the involved side to prevent development of a stiff shoulder from the immobility.
2. Give patient and significant others appropriate information regarding chest tube placement and maintenance.

NIC Acid-Base Management; Acid-Base Monitoring; Analgesic Administration; Environmental Management: Comfort; Exercise Promotion; Laboratory Data Interpretation; Medication Administration; Medication Management; Oxygen Therapy; Pain Management; Positioning; Respiratory Monitoring; Vital Signs Monitoring

ADDITIONAL NURSING DIAGNOSES

Also see *Activity Intolerance* in *Acute Asthma Exacerbation* (p. 354). See appropriate nursing diagnoses and interventions in *Emotional and Spiritual Support of the Patient and Significant Others* (p. 200).

RESEARCH BRIEF 4-6

Emergency management of primary spontaneous pneumothorax remains controversial. The researchers searched MEDLINE, EMBASE, the Cochrane Library, and other databases to locate studies for inclusion. Only 3 studies met the inclusion criteria defined as treating hemodynamically stable patients with no underlying lung disease receive either needle aspiration or tube thoracostomy. Outcome measures included admission rate, length of hospital stay, recurrence rate, failure rate of the procedure, dyspnea score during or after the procedure, pain score during or after the procedure, and complications. Results revealed there was no significant difference between needle aspiration and tube thoracostomy for the outcomes of immediate failure, 1-week failure, risk of complication, and 1-year recurrence rate. Needle aspiration required less analgesia in one trial and was associated with lower pain scores in another. Evidence indicates needle aspiration is as safe and effective as tube thoracostomy for management of primary spontaneous pneumothorax. Also, needle aspiration patients required fewer hospital admissions and had a shorter length of hospital stay.

From *Ann Emerg Med* 51:91–100, 2008.

PULMONARY EMBOLUS

PATHOPHYSIOLOGY

Pulmonary embolism (PE) is a blockage in the pulmonary circulation created by a lodged blood clot, vasculitis from fatty acids, or presence of air or other endogenous substances. Pulmonary emboli resulting from deep vein thrombosis (DVT) affect 600,000 patients annually in the United States. PE has occurred in nearly 70% of patients with venous thrombosis in veins proximal to the knee and is less common with more distal thrombosis. PE is associated with recurrent embolic events in over 50% of undiagnosed and untreated patients. Prevention of venous thromboembolism (VTE) has received recent attention from both researchers and quality improvement organizations as a leading strategy to help reduce morbidity and mortality in hospitalized patients. Acute right ventricular failure with resultant low cardiac output is the leading cause of death related to PE. Despite strong evidence, recommended evidence-based practices are inconsistently implemented. VTE rates are increasing as the U.S. population ages, is progressively obese, and is living longer with chronic diseases, which may promote thrombus formation. Venous thrombosis is the most common cause of PE, followed by fat emboli. Emboli related to venous air, foreign bodies, and other sources (amniotic fluid, sepsis/infection, and tumors) occur more rarely.

Venous Thrombotic Emboli

A formed blood clot from a large vein dislodges and travels to the pulmonary circulation, where it may obstruct one (massive PE) or both branches (saddle embolus) of the pulmonary artery or a smaller, distal vessel. Blood clots typically originate in the deep veins of the legs, the iliofemoral system, or pelvis. Many patients with VTEs have no symptoms of DVT. Thrombus formation can result from blood stasis, alterations in clotting factors, and injury to vessel walls. Emboli are classified by size and location and include submassive, massive, and saddle emboli. Total obstruction of blood flow leading to pulmonary infarction is rare. Prevention, early diagnosis, and appropriate treatment may reduce development of DVT and PE by 68% and mortality to less than 10%. Although most thrombotic emboli resolve completely, leaving no residual deficits, some patients may be left with chronic pulmonary hypertension (Table 4-7).

Fat Emboli

The most common nonthrombotic cause of PEs, which occurs in less than 1% of patients. The event and subsequent syndrome most often occurs within 12 to 36 hours after skeletal trauma or major orthopedic surgery but may be fulminant, with rapid embolization of fat into the

Table 4-7	INCIDENCE OF VTE IN HOSPITALIZED PATIENTS
Incidence	**Patient Type**
10–26%	Medical/nonsurgical
11–75%	Stroke
15–40%	Major surgery: general, gynecologic, urologic
15–40%	Neurosurgery
15–80%	Critically ill patients admitted to intensive care units
40–60%	Hip or knee surgery/orthopaedic surgical patients
40–60%	Major trauma
60–80%	Spinal cord injury

Composite of statistics from British Thoracic Society (2003), American College of Chest Physicians (2008), European Society of Cardiology (2008), and IMPROVE (2007) registry data on prevention of venous thromboembolism.

pulmonary and systemic circulation, followed by right ventricular failure and cardiovascular collapse. Fat emboli most often result from the release of free fatty acids during the surgical procedure, prompting toxic vasculitis followed by thrombosis and obstruction of small pulmonary arteries by fat. More recently, fat embolism has been reported following liposuction, with lipid and propofol infusions, fatty liver, and hepatic necrosis.

Venous Air Emboli

Almost always an iatrogenic complication caused by a large volume of air that enters the venous circulation and travels to the pulmonary circulation. Smaller amounts of air may be completely unproductive of symptoms, since air can be rapidly resorbed. Surgical procedures, insertion of pulmonary artery catheters, central venous catheters, hemodialysis, endoscopy, and use of automatic injectors such as those used for contrast media can prompt symptomatic air emboli. A larger bolus of air into the right ventricle may completely obstruct pulmonary blood flow, leading to cardiac arrest. In severe cases, venous air embolus has a mortality rate greater than 50%. Rapid diagnosis and treatment are essential. Case reports describe the adult lethal volume of air as approximately 200 to 300 ml delivered rapidly. Air occludes the right ventricular pulmonary outflow tract, or the smaller pulmonary arteriole with a mixture of air and fibrin clots, which results in right ventricular failure and cardiogenic shock.

Intravascular Foreign Bodies

Most foreign bodies in the central circulation are parts of intravascular catheters, a guidewire, or an inferior vena cava filter that has accumulated clot and migrated. More recently, coils for embolization and endovascular stenting have also migrated from their desired position. Most foreign bodies travel to the pulmonary arteries, with the right heart and vena cava being the secondary locations.

Other Pulmonary Emboli

Amniotic fluid embolism occurs in less than 1:8,000 to 80,000 women due to amniotic fluid being forced into the central circulation through tears in the uterine veins that may occur during normal labor. Death of both the mother and fetus may result during the delivery. Septic pulmonary emboli are infected clots dislodged from either peripheral or abdominal vein, septic thrombophlebitis, or right heart endocarditis. Prognosis is dependent on the overall patient condition and severity of the sepsis. Tumor embolism occurs with many types or carcinoma and sarcoma but causes significant respiratory symptoms in less than 3% of affected patients. Talc embolism results from drug users grinding up and injecting oral medications that are made with talc particles, which lodge in the small vessels of the pulmonary system.

ASSESSMENT
Goal of System Assessment
Evaluate for ineffective breathing patterns and impaired gas exchange. The clinical presentation will vary in degree, depending on the type and size of the embolus. With a submassive or massive embolism, evaluate for decreased cardiac output and decreased tissue perfusion. Massive embolism may prompt cardiogenic shock. For saddle embolus, identifying pulmonary embolus as the cause for acute cardiopulmonary decompensation is of paramount importance so life-saving treatments can be provided. (See *Respiratory Assessment: General*, p. 352, and *Cardiac Assessment: General*, p. 418.)

History and Risk Factors for VTE
The American College of Chest Physicians, American Thoracic Society, American College of Physicians, American Academy of Family Physicians, European Society of Cardiology, British Thoracic Society, and an array of medical and surgical specialty organizations have created guidelines for VTE prophylaxis and management. VTE prophylaxis protocols should be initiated when patients are admitted to the hospital, to help prevent development of DVT (Tables 4-8 and 4-9).

Determine Probability Based on Risk Factors
- Helps determine presence of pulmonary embolus: More than six factors is considered high, two to six is moderate, and less than two is considered low probability.
- Diagnostic tests chosen are dependent on the probability a DVT or VTE is present; a scoring system may be developed based on number of risks present. Reveals the presence of the infiltrates.

Table 4-8	RISK FACTORS FOR VENOUS THROMBOEMBOLISM IN HOSPITALIZED PATIENTS	
Age >50 years	Prior history of VTE	Myocardial infarction
Myeloproliferative disease	Impaired mobility, paresis, or paralysis	Acute or chronic lung disease
Dehydration	Recently bedridden >3 days	Obesity
Congestive heart failure	Inflammatory bowel disease	Known thrombophilic stroke
Active malignancy/cancer	Active rheumatic disease	Varicose veins or chronic venous stasis
Moderate to major surgery	Nephrotic syndrome	Pregnancy
Hormone replacement therapy	Sickle cell disease	Recently postpartum with immobility
Central venous catheter in place		Estrogen therapy or estrogen contraceptives

Note: Patients who have more than a single condition are at increased risk of developing VTE. The more conditions present, the higher the risk.

Table 4-9	RISK STRATIFICATION FOR VENOUS THROMBOEMBOLISM	
Low Risk	**Intermediate Risk**	**High Risk**
Minor surgery in mobile patients	General, open gynecologic or urologic surgery	Hip or knee arthroplasty, hip fracture surgery
Fully mobile medical patients	Medical patients, acutely ill or on bed rest	Major trauma, spinal cord injury
	Moderate VTE risk plus high bleeding risk	High VTE risk plus high bleeding risk

Vital Signs
- Severity of all findings varies with size of the embolus; patients with small emboli may be asymptomatic.
- Tachycardia (HR greater than 100 bpm), tachypnea (RR greater than 20 breaths/min), fever (greater than 99.5°F)
- *Massive embolus:* Hypotension (BP decreases by greater than 20%)
- *Saddle embolus:* May result in immediate cardiopulmonary arrest

Observation/Inspection
- Dyspnea, nonproductive cough, nausea
- Syncope, pallor, and palpitations
- Restlessness and anxiety
- Diaphoresis, cool and clammy skin
- Pleuritic chest pain, hemoptysis
- Signs of lower limb DVT: leg/calf tenderness, swelling, and/or edema
- *Submassive embolus:* any combination of the symptoms listed above
- *Massive embolus:* severe chest pain, cyanosis, acute respiratory distress
- *Saddle embolus:* sudden-onset acute respiratory distress with cyanosis, which may progress to cardiopulmonary arrest

Palpation
- Possible reduced chest excursion on affected side due to splinting for pain

Percussion
- Unchanged

Auscultation
- Crackles
- S_3 and S_4 gallop rhythms
- Transient pleural friction rub may be present.

HIGH ALERT!   Saddle pulmonary embolus is life-threatening. Immediate medical or surgical intervention is critical. Thrombolysis directed at the pulmonary embolus will also prompt lysis of other clots, and may lead to other bleeding complications. If thrombolysis is contraindicated, surgical or percutaneous catheter-mediated embolectomy is performed immediately.

Fat Emboli
History and Risk Factors
- Multiple long bone fractures; particularly the femur and pelvis
- Lower limb amputation
- Trauma to adipose tissue or liver
- Burns: See p. 279
- Hemolytic crisis: See Chapter 10
- Osteomyelitis

Observation/Inspection
Patients are often asymptomatic for 12 to 24 hours after the embolization occurs. This period ends with a sudden deterioration in cardiopulmonary and neurologic status.
- Dyspnea, acute respiratory distress
- Restlessness, confusion, delirium, and coma
- Petechial rash may appear especially over the upper torso and axillae, secondary to thrombocytopenia. The platelets aggregate in the presence of circulating fats.

Vital Signs
- RR greater than 20 breaths/min, HR greater than 100 bpm
- Increased BP, elevated temperature

Auscultation
- Inspiratory crowing, expiratory wheezes

Venous Air Emboli
History and Risk Factors
- Recent surgical procedure
- Pulmonary artery/central venous catheter insertion
- Misuse of closed-wound suction unit
- Cardiopulmonary bypass
- Hemodialysis
- Endoscopy

Clinical Presentation
Depends on severity of the bolus

Observation/Inspection
Agitation, confusion, cough, dyspnea, and chest pain

Vital Signs
RR greater than 20 breaths/min, HR greater than 100 bpm, hypotension

Auscultation
Wheezing, "mill wheel" hypotension, heart murmur

Foreign Bodies
History and Risk Factors
- Physician or midlevel practitioner accidentally lets go of the guidewire during central line insertion.
- Vena cava filter has not been retrieved within recommended time frame.
- Intravascular catheter breaks during insertion.
- Coils or stent components are accidentally released or not properly secured during insertion.

Diagnostic Tests for Venous Thrombotic Pulmonary Embolism		
Test	**Purpose**	**Abnormal Findings**
D-dimer Several assays are available with variable levels of sensitivity and specificity. Test may not be needed in high-risk or high-probability patients. Hospitals should provide information on specificity and sensitivity of test used.	Predicts likelihood a thrombus is present in low- or intermediate-risk patients. When value exceeds the cutoff, the test is positive. A negative D-dimer test reliably excludes PE in patients with low or intermediate clinical probability.	*Positive:* A thrombus is present. Scales range from 250 to 1000 ng/ml; the most common cutoff value is 500 ng/ml. Low and intermediate risk patients do not require imaging for VTE if the D-dimer is negative.
Lower extremity duplex ultrasound imaging A single normal test cannot be used to rule to subclinical DVT.	Reveals slow or obstructed flow in the venous system. Test is done on patients at high or moderate risk of DVT.	*Positive:* Reduced or obstructed blood flow is detected.
Chest radiograph: PA and lateral chest radiograph (CXR) Cannot be used alone to diagnose pulmonary embolus	Reveals abnormal lung markings and fluid shifts which occur during flow obstruction and pulmonary infarction. A baseline CXR is helpful for comparison with subsequent films to identify changes.	*Affected side:* Initially the CXR shows normal findings or an elevated hemidiaphragm. After 24 hr, small infiltrates secondary to atelectasis from decrease in surfactant may develop. If pulmonary infarction is present, infiltrates and pleural effusions may be seen within 12–36 hr.

Diagnostic Tests For Venous Thrombotic Pulmonary Embolism—cont'd

Test	Purpose	Abnormal Findings
Spiral CT angiography with contrast Older technology may be insufficient to rule out PE. Current technology is nearly 100% accurate.	Reveals flow obstruction in pulmonary circulation. Recommended for patients with intermediate-to-high probability of lower extremity DVT.	Generally reveals right ventricular dilatation. Patients with intermediate or high pretest probability of PE require diagnostic imaging studies.
Ventilation-perfusion lung scan The patient inhales radioactive-tagged gases, and radioactive particles are injected peripherally.	Assesses for $\dot{V}/\dot{Q}$ or ventilation/perfusion mismatching; a good alternative for patients who cannot receive contrast needed for spiral CT angiography.	If there is a mismatch of ventilation and perfusion (e.g., normal ventilation with decreased perfusion), vascular obstruction is likely. Results may not be definitive. False positives are more common than false negative results.
Arterial blood gas (ABG) analysis Pulse oximetry may be used to monitor O_2 saturation changes. CO_2 increases and pH changes require ABG analysis.	Assesses for hypoxemia and acidosis. Saddle embolus may cause both respiratory and lactic acidosis (pH <7.35) from impending respiratory failure and circulatory collapse.	Initially, hypoxemia (Pao_2 <80 mm Hg), hypocapnia ($Paco_2$ <35 mm Hg), and respiratory alkalosis (pH >7.45). A normal Pao_2 does not rule out the presence of TE. Mild hypoxemia may be present with smaller emboli.
12-Lead ECG Vitally important since chest pain can mimic severe angina or acute myocardial infarction	Rule out acute coronary syndrome as a cause for chest pain with vital sign changes indicative of deterioration.	If VTEs are extensive, signs of acute pulmonary hypertension may be present: right-shift QRS axes, tall and peaked P waves, ST segment changes, and T wave inversion in leads V_1–V_4.
Echocardiogram	Diagnose presence of right ventricular impairment or failure as part of risk stratification.	May reveal RV hypokinesis, dilatation or elevated pressures. RV dilatation is found in >25% of patients with PE.
Pulmonary angiography The Miller (European) and Walsh (United States) scores were used to define the amount of luminal obstruction. Improved accuracy with current CT angiography has markedly reduced the need for this invasive procedure.	A definitive study for VTEs. The right ventricle is catheterized and dye is injected into the pulmonary artery (PA) to visualize pulmonary vessels. Formerly, the gold standard for definitive diagnosis.	An abrupt vessel "cutoff" may be seen at the site of embolization. Usually, filling defects are seen. Used when other tests are inconclusive, since the procedure has a 0.2% mortality rate.
Hemodynamic studies	To determine if obstruction of blood flow is significant enough to cause pulmonary hypertension or right heart failure	PA pressures increase (>20 mm Hg) if 30% to 50% of the pulmonary arterial tree is affected. Massive VTEs cause pressure increases to >40 mm Hg, resulting in right ventricular failure, decreased CO, and hypotension.

Fat Emboli

- *ABG values:* Hypoxemia (Pao_2 less than 80 mm Hg) and hypercapnia ($Paco_2$ more than 45 mm Hg) will be present with a respiratory acidosis (pH less than 7.35).
- *Chest radiograph:* A pattern similar to ARDS is seen: diffuse, extensive, bilateral interstitial and alveolar infiltrates.
- *CBC with WBC differential:* May reveal decreased hemoglobin (Hgb) and Hct secondary to hemorrhage into the lung, thrombocytopenia, and possibly mild leukocytosis.

Venous Air Emboli

- *ABG values:* Hypoxemia (Pao_2 less than 80 mm Hg), hypercapnia ($Paco_2$ more than 45 mm Hg), and respiratory acidosis (pH less than 7.35) generally are present in severe cases.
- *Chest radiograph:* Reveals changes consistent with pulmonary edema or air-fluid levels in the main pulmonary artery system.
- *Pulmonary artery pressure:* Systolic, diastolic, and mean pressures are acutely elevated, but slight elevation of PAWP remains within normal limits (WNL).

Foreign Bodies

- *Chest radiograph:* All devices are radiopaque for easy identification using radiographs. The "lost" device should be easily visible using a chest radiograph.

COLLABORATIVE MANAGEMENT
Care Priorities: Venous Thrombotic Emboli

Patients with shortness of breath should not be left without intervention regardless of the probability VTE is present.

1. **Relieve hypoxemia:** Patent foramen ovale (or atrial septal defect) may augment hypoxemia if right atrial pressure exceeds left atrial pressure, causing deoxygenated blood to shunt from the right to the left atrium.
   - *Oxygen therapy/adjustment in mechanical ventilation*: Oxygen is administered when ABG values demonstrate the presence of hypoxemia. If patient is already receiving mechanical ventilation, Fio_2 is increased while evaluation is done regarding amount of positive pressure needed during inspiratory and expiratory phases of ventilation.
2. **Manage right ventricular failure in patients with hypotension or shock:**
   - Hemodynamic stabilization is achieved using a combination of fluid therapy to increase the end-diastolic volume in the right ventricle and positive inotropic agents to increase the force of right ventricular contraction. Management of right heart failure is complex. Efforts should be directed at restoring patency of pulmonary circulation in VTE patients. When the obstruction is relieved, the patient generally improves rapidly. See *Heart Failure*, p. 421 and *Cardiogenic Shock*, p. 472.
   - Initiate cardiopulmonary resuscitation if patient arrests with saddle embolus. Generally, these patients require pulmonary embolectomy since VTE has resulted in lethal cardiogenic shock. Sophisticated centers can use extracorporeal devices as a bridge to clot removal.
3. **In less severely ill patients, or those in need of VTE prophylaxis, prevent clot development or clot extension:**
   - *Pharmacologic therapy*: All patients at risk of developing VTE should be screened for bleeding risk prior to implementing prophylaxis using medications, since all agents have the potential to cause bleeding. Thromboprophylaxis medications include low-molecular-weight heparin (LMWH) (enoxaparin [Lovenox], dalteparin [Fragmin]), low-dose unfractionated heparin (UFH), fondaparinux (Arixtra), direct thrombin inhibitors (argatroban, lepirudin, bivalirudin), and warfarin (Coumadin). Warfarin requires 3 and 5 days of oral therapy to attain therapeutic effect, during which time the patient requires an injectable medication as a "bridge" to warfarin. Ongoing therapy may include low- or regular-dose aspirin.

VTE PROPHYLAXIS: CONSIDERATIONS FOR CONTRAINDICATION/ COMPLICATIONS

Absolute Contraindications	Relative Contraindications	Other Conditions That May Complicate Therapy
Active hemorrhage	Intracranial hemorrhage within the last year	Immune-mediated heparin-induced thrombocytopenia (HIT)
Allergy		
Severe head or spinal cord trauma within 4 weeks	Craniotomy within 2 weeks	Epidural analgesia; catheter present, or will be present in the spine

VTE PROPHYLAXIS: CONSIDERATIONS FOR CONTRAINDICATION/ COMPLICATIONS — cont'd

Absolute Contraindications	Relative Contraindications	Other Conditions That May Complicate Therapy
Note: *Absolute contraindication means therapy should not be administered to the affected patients under any circumstances, as the risk of bleeding outweighs the benefits of clot prevention.*	Intraocular surgery within 2 weeks Active intracranial lesions or neoplasms Thrombocytopenia (platelets <50,000) Coagulopathy (PT >18 sec) End-stage liver disease GI, GU hemorrhage within 1 month Current hypertensive urgency or emergency Current postoperative bleeding	Note: *Unfractioned heparin (UFH) and low-molecular-weight heparins (LMWH) can stimulate HIT (heparin-induced thrombocytopenia), an immune response which destroys platelets.* ***Nonheparin anticoagulants:*** *Argatroban (Argatroban)* *Bivalirudin (Angiomax)* *Fondaparinux (Arixtra)* *Lepirudin (Refludan)* **Danaparoid (Orgaron) (unavailable in the USA)*

- *Risk stratification:* Provide appropriate therapy based on evaluation for level of risk of development of VTE and risk of bleeding:

VTE PROPHYLAXIS BASED ON LEVEL OF RISK (SELECT ONE DRUG/ONE DOSAGE REGIMEN)

Low Risk	Intermediate Risk	High Risk
Early aggressive ambulation Short-term mechanical thromboprophylaxis may be recommended for "borderline" risk patients	Heparin 5000 units SC every 8 hr Heparin 7500 units SC every 12 hr Heparin 5000 units SC every 12 hr (if <50 kg or >75 years old) Enoxaparin 40 mg SC daily Dalteparin 2500 units daily for low or intermediate risk Consider adding SCDs	Enoxaparin 30 mg SC every 12 hr Enoxaparin 40 mg SC daily Dalteparin 5000 units SC daily Fondaparinux 2.5 mg SC daily Warfarin until INR is 2–3 Add SCDs

- *Mechanical prophylaxis:* Sequential compression devices (SCDs) may be used as the sole preventive strategy in low-risk patients, and in moderate-to high-risk patients who are not able to receive thromboprophylaxis drugs due to risk for bleeding. Plexi-pulse and elastic compression stockings are not considered sufficient as a sole VTE prophylaxis strategy for hospitalized patients. Compression stockings with a pressure of 30 to 40 mm Hg at the ankle may be implemented prior to discharge and used post-hospitalization.

4. **Prevent clot extension or migration in patients with DVT or VTE:**
Pharmacologic therapy: To inhibit thrombus growth, promote resolution of the formed thrombus, and prevent further embolus formation. The goals are achieved by keeping the aPTT at 1.5 to 2.5 times the normal. Platelet counts should be obtained every 3 days, to monitor for thrombocytopenia and paradoxic arterial thrombosis associated with heparin therapy in predisposed patients. (See *Bleeding and Thrombotic Disorders*, p. 837.)

- *Weight-based IV heparin (unfractionated) therapy:* Treatment of choice; started immediately in patients without bleeding or clotting disorders and in whom VTE is strongly suspected. Initial dose: 80 units/kg IV bolus. Dosage should be given based on the patient's weight.
- *Maintenance dose:* Following initial dose, a continuous IV infusion is usually begun at 18 units/kg/hr and titrated by serial activated partial thromboplastin time (aPTT)

Table 4-10	UNFRACTIONATED HEPARIN IV INFUSION DOSAGE TITRATION
Activated Partial Thromboplastin Time (aPTT; in seconds)	**Dosage Titration**
Less than 35 (<1.2 times the control)	80 units/kg bolus; begin infusion at 18 units/kg/hr; increase infusion rate by 4 unit/kg/hr
35–45 (1.2–1.5 times the control)	40 units/kg bolus; increase infusion rate by 2 units/kg/hr
46–70 (1.6–2.3 times the control)	No change; this is the desirable range
71–90 (2.4–3 times the control)	Decrease infusion rate by 2 units/kg/hr
>90 (>3 times the control)	Hold/stop infusion for 1 hour; then restart at 3 units/kg/hr less than when stopped
Active hemorrhage	Vitamin K, fresh-frozen plasma, and protamine sulfate may be used to help reverse heparin effects.

values to determine level of anticoagulation. Titration is done according to institutional protocol (see Table 4-10).

- Heparin requirements are the largest in the initial 72 hours of therapy. Maintenance continues for 7 to 14 days, during which time the patient is placed on bed rest to ensure the thrombus is firmly attached to the vessel wall before ambulation. Platelets should be monitored, as patients sometimes experience heparin-induced thrombocytopenia (HIT), or low platelets. Protamine sulfate is a: heparin antidote, which should be readily available during heparin therapy. Fatal hemorrhage occurs in 1% to 2% of patients undergoing heparin therapy. Risk of bleeding is greatest in women greater than 60 yr of age.
- *Subcutaneous (SC) low-molecular-weight heparin (dalteparin, enoxaparin):* An alternative to unfractionated heparin with longer half-life, greater bioavailability, and more predictable anticoagulant activity. Enoxaparin is given 1 mg/kg subcutaneously (SC) every 12 hours or 1.5 mg/kg SC daily. Dalteparin is given 200 units (IU)/kg SC daily to a maximum daily dose of 18,000 IU, while patient is being bridged to warfarin.
  - *SC Tinzaparin:* A heparin alternative given 175 units SC daily.
  - *SC Fondaparinux:* Dose is given based on three body sizes.
  - 5 mg SC daily: weight less than 50 kg
  - 7.5 mg SC daily: weight 50 to 100 kg
  - 10 mg SC daily: weight greater than 100 kg

Inferior vena cava (IVC) filter: Also known as a "Greenfield filter," the devices are designed to trap emboli before they enter the heart and pulmonary arteries. Various types of IVC filters are available, with different recommendations governing the removal/retrieval of each device. The filter is inserted through an introducer sheath into the femoral vein, threaded through the venous system, and deployed below the level of the renal veins in the IVC. The American College of Chest Physicians recommends most retrievable devices are removed approximately 2 weeks following insertion. Many devices are left in place for longer periods, with associated complications of device thrombosis and migration in 10% of patients. Permanent IVC filters are associated with recurrent DVT (in 20% of patients) and post-thrombotic syndrome (in 40% of patients). Routine use is not recommended for management of VTE.

5. **Dissolve clot using thrombolytic drugs in patients with massive or saddle embolus:** These "clot buster" drugs lyse clots via conversion of plasminogen to plasma and may be given within 72 hours of VTE to speed the process of clot lysis. These medications are not often used but can be used immediately when severe cardiopulmonary compromise or arrest has occurred. Heparin therapy is used following thrombolytic infusion. As many as 33% of patients who receive thrombolytic therapy have hemorrhagic complications. The drug should be discontinued, and fresh-frozen plasma infusion may be initiated for severe bleeding complications.

- *Streptokinase:* Loading dose of 250,000 IU in normal saline or D_5W given IV over a 30-minute period. Maintenance dose is 100,000 IU/hours given IV for 12 to 24 hours.
- *Tissue plasminogen activator (Alteplase, rTPA):* 100 mg IV infusion over 2 hours, or 0.6 mg/kg over 15 minutes (maximum dose 50 mg).
- *Urokinase:* 4400 IU/kg as a loading dose over 10 minutes, followed by an infusion of 4400 IU/kg/hr for 12 to 14 hours.

6. **Remove thrombus with an invasive procedure:**
   - *Surgical pulmonary embolectomy:* Often reserved for patients in cardiopulmonary arrest; can also be used for patients with contraindications to thrombolytic therapy, those with patent foramen ovale, and those with intracardiac thrombi. Anesthesia is rapidly induced, a median sternotomy performed, and the pulmonary artery incised to remove the clot. Cardiopulmonary bypass should be avoided in patients with patent foramen ovale or intracardiac thrombi.
   - *Percutaneous catheter embolectomy with fragmentation:* A possibly life-saving measure wherein a Greenfield suction embolectomy catheter (or other rotoblade cardiac catheter) is inserted through an introducer sheath, threaded through the pulmonary valve into the pulmonary artery, wherein the clot is macerated and fragmented, with the fragments immediately suctioned from the vessel to avoid distal embolization.

7. **Long-term anticoagulation to prevent recurrence of VTE:** Active cancer places a patient at high risk of recurrence of PE, with 20% of patients having another VTE within the first year. Other patient populations have lower, variable rates of recurrence based on whether the precipitating event was due to a modifiable risk factor or isolated event such as trauma or surgery. Patients with idiopathic PE are more difficult to stratify for risk of recurrence. Risk of bleeding must be considered when prescribing the duration of therapy.
   - *Low-molecular-weight heparin:* Subcutaneous injections may be indicated for a period of 6 months following hospitalization when a patient is at high risk for repeated recurrence.
   - *Vitamin K antagonists (VKAs):* Oral warfarin (Coumadin) is prescribed at doses to keep International Normalized Ratio (INR) 2 to 3. It is started within 24 hours of initiation of heparin therapy. An average initial dose is 5 to 10 mg. Both agents are given simultaneously for 4 to 6 days to allow time for warfarin to inhibit vitamin K–dependent clotting factors before heparin is discontinued. Daily warfarin dose is adjusted according to INR, and correct dosage is individualized per patient based on frequent INR determinations.
   - *Prothrombin time (PT):* Monitored daily, with a goal of 1 to 1.5 times normal. Once the patient's condition has stabilized and the heparin is discontinued, weekly monitoring of INR is acceptable. After hospital discharge the PT should be monitored every 2 weeks for as long as the patient continues to take warfarin.
   - *Maintenance:* May be approximately 10 mg/day, but dosage varies greatly depending on patient's age, weight, other medications taken, diet, and other factors. Warfarin is continued for 3 to 6 months and based on the continued presence of risk factors.
   - *Vitamin K administration:* For bleeding emergencies, reverses the effects of warfarin in 24 to 36 hours. Fresh-frozen plasma may be required in cases of serious bleeding.
   - *Caution:* Warfarin crosses the placental barrier and can cause spontaneous abortion and birth defects.

8. **Special considerations during pregnancy:** Getting an accurate diagnosis is of paramount importance, since a prolonged course of heparin or low-molecular-weight heparin therapy is needed to resolve the emboli. Neither drug crosses the placental barrier or is found in breast milk in significant amounts. All diagnostic modalities, including CT scanning, may be used without putting the fetus at significant risk for harm. Use of subcutaneous low-molecular-weight heparin has been increasingly recommended as evidence evolves. Warfarin or another VKA is not recommended during the first and third trimesters and is used with caution during the second trimester. Anticoagulant therapy should be continued for 3 months postpartum.

RESEARCH BRIEF 4-7

In patients with pulmonary embolism, it is not uncommon to see patients with right heart thrombi admitted to the intensive care unit. These patients have lower systolic blood pressure, a higher prevalence of overall hypotension, higher heart rate, and have an increased incidence of right ventricular dysfunction or hypokinesis than patients without right heart thrombi. Right heart thrombi are revealed by echocardiographic studies, but given a 4% overall prevalence, routine screening echocardiography is not recommended for all patients suspected of VTE. These thrombi may not be fully resolved following use of thrombolytic therapy for PE.

From Ferrari E, Benhamou M, Berthier F, et al: Mobile thrombi of the right heart in pulmonary embolism: delayed disappearance after thrombolytic treatment. *Chest* 127:1051–1053, 2005.

Care Priorities: Fat Emboli

1. **Manage hypoxemia:** Concentration of O_2 is based on clinical presentation, ABG results, and the patient's prior respiratory status. Intubation and mechanical ventilation may be required.
2. **Control toxic vasculitis:** Corticosteroids including cortisone and methylprednisolone have been used to decrease local injury to pulmonary tissue and pulmonary edema.
3. **Manage pulmonary edema:** Pulmonary edema develops in approximately 30% of patients with fat emboli, necessitating use of diuretics to remove fluid from the vascular system.
4. **Manage right heart failure and cardiogenic shock:** Although rare, fulminant, sudden onset cases of cardiovascular collapse have been reported. See *Heart Failure*, p. 421, and *Cardiogenic Shock*, p. 472.

Care Priorities: Venous Air Emboli

 Emphasis is on prevention. Ensure that central venous catheter is inserted with the patient in Trendelenburg position. Use Luer-Lok connectors on all IV tubing to prevent a disconnection. Should venous air embolus occur despite precautions, the following measures are anticipated.

Prevent further air entry:
If central line is being inserted, catheter hub should be occluded using a clamp, or the inserter's gloved finger.

Manage hypoxemia:
Oxygen using 100% FIO_2 is initiated immediately.

Minimize dispersion of air bolus into central circulation:
Place the patient in Trendelenburg position with a left decubitus tilt (turned to left side, bed in "head down" position) to minimize further movement of air bolus through the heart and into the pulmonary vasculature and beyond.

Remove air, if possible:
If a central venous catheter is in place near the right atrium, an attempt is made to aspirate the air using a syringe.

Hyperbaric oxygen therapy:
Case reports reveal the therapy to be beneficial with all types of air embolization. Impressive results have been gleaned with cerebral air embolization.

Care Priorities: Intravascular Foreign Bodies

1. **Remove the foreign body:** Physician or midlevel practitioner retrieves the migrated device or part of a device using a snare.

CARE PLANS FOR PULMONARY EMBOLISM

Risk for ineffective cardiopulmonary tissue perfusion *related to partial to complete obstruction of the lumen of one/both pulmonary arteries or smaller pulmonary vessels: The nurse will identify and provide preventive measures and appropriate treatments for patients at risk of DVT and/or VTE and other pulmonary emboli.*

- -

GOALS/OUTCOMES Patient is free of hemodynamic instability and shortness of breath reflected by normal (return to patient's stable baseline) vital signs and normal work of breathing. Within 12 hours of initiation of therapy, patient has adequate gas exchange reflected by the following ABG values: PaO_2 greater than 60 mm Hg, $PaCO_2$ 35 to 45 mm Hg, and pH 7.35 to 7.45. Within 2 to 4 days of initiating anticoagulant therapy, patient's RR is 12 to 20 breaths/min with normal depth and pattern. Unobstructed, unidirectional blood flow at an appropriate pressure is restored through large vessels of the pulmonary and systemic circuits.

NOC Circulation Status, Cardiac Pump Effectiveness, Respiratory Status: Gas Exchange

Embolus Precautions

1. Assess patient for risk factors associated with VTE (see Table 4-8).
2. Implement VTE precautions appropriate for patient's risk level.
3. Instruct patient not to cross legs, either when in bed or sitting in chair.
4. Apply sequential compression hose for bedridden patients. If patient is aggressively ambulating, use of sequential compression hose is not necessary.
5. Aggressively ambulate all appropriate patients following surgical procedures.
6. Administer subcutaneous anticoagulants as ordered or according to VTE prophylaxis protocol/guidelines.

Embolus Care: Pulmonary

1. Evaluate chest pain for intensity, location, and precipitating and relieving factors.
2. Auscultate breath sounds to assess for presence of crackles or other changes that may account for shortness of breath.
3. Monitor respiratory pattern for increased work of breathing.
4. Monitor the determinants of tissue O_2 delivery as possible (cardiac output, hemoglobin level, O_2 saturation/pulse oximetry/ABGs).
5. Evaluate arterial blood gas for decreased PaO_2 (hypoxemia), increased level of CO_2 (hypercapnia), and decreased pH (acidosis).
6. Assess for symptoms of respiratory failure and inadequate tissue oxygenation including altered mental status, anxiety, restlessness, increased work of breathing, pallor, cyanosis, and inability to maintain O_2 saturation without repeated increases in amount of supplemental O_2.
7. Instruct the patient/family/support system regarding diagnostic tests needed as part of differential diagnosis.
8. Screen patient for risk of bleeding (see VTE prophylaxis chart, p. 402) in preparation for anticoagulant and possibly thrombolytic drug administration.
9. Administer anticoagulants as ordered and monitor for bleeding complications. If unfractionated or low-molecular-weight heparin is used, monitor for decreased platelet count, which may signal development of heparin-induced thrombocytopenia.
10. Administer thrombolytic agents as ordered, and monitor for bleeding complications.
11. Consult with dietician to ensure patient maintains a diet with consistent intake of vitamin K if VKAs, such as warfarin (Coumadin), are initiated. Varying vitamin K intake may have a marked effect on the ability to regulate the appropriate dose of medication to avoid bleeding and clotting complications.
12. Consult with pharmacist about use of IV protamine sulfate, if patient has the need for heparin reversal due to severe bleeding.
13. To avoid negative interactions with anticoagulants or thrombolytic therapy, establish compatibility of all drugs before administering them:
    - *Heparin:* Digitalis, tetracyclines, nicotine, and antihistamines decrease the effect of heparin therapy. Establish compatibility before infusing other IV drugs through heparin IV line.
    - *Warfarin sodium:* Numerous drugs result in a decrease or an increase in response to treatment with warfarin. Consult with pharmacist to obtain specific information about patient's medication profile.
    - *Thrombolytic therapy:* Do not infuse other medications through the same IV line.
14. Monitor PT (prothrombin time) with INR when using warfarin and aPTT when using heparin. Adhere carefully to drug titration and/or dosage guidelines.
15. Monitor neurologic status for deterioration since recurrent embolism, shock due to bleeding, cardiogenic shock, and intracranial bleeding are possible. Neurologic changes are the first subtle sign shock may be ensuing.
16. Medicate for pain as needed.

Hemodynamic Regulation

1. Recognize presence of blood pressure alterations.
2. Auscultate heart and breath sounds.
3. Monitor SVR and PVR. PVR will be elevated with massive or saddle embolus, and can prompt right heart failure. SVR changes with the stages of shock. Initially, SVR is high as the body attempts to raise blood pressure in the presence of cardiogenic shock if right heart failure has ensued.
4. Implement recommendations for managing right heart failure as ordered.
   - Systemic hypotension should be managed to avoid progression of right heart failure.
   - Regulate vasoactive drugs. Vasopressor drugs such as dopamine or Levophed will increase afterload and may worsen heart failure. Inodilating drugs such as milrinone, amrinone, and, to a lesser extent, dobutamine may not work well, since all decrease venous return, which may also worsen right heart failure.
   - Aggressive fluid challenge is not recommended, despite some evidence of efficacy in right heart failure. Hemodynamics of right heart failure differs in the scenario of acute PE, since heart disease is not the root cause of the problem.
5. Monitor for hypovolemic shock due to excessive bleeding when using thrombolytics or anticoagulants. Patients may develop either hypovolemic or cardiogenic shock in the setting of PE. Differential diagnosis of shock states may be assisted by examining the pulmonary artery pressures and cardiac output.
   - Cardiogenic shock/right heart failure related to PE: elevated CVP, elevated PVR, decreased CO
   - Hypovolemic shock related to hemorrhage: decreased CVP, decreased PVR, decreased CO
   - Combined right heart failure and bleeding: Since CVP and PVR effects are opposites, hemodynamic readings may be difficult to interpret.

Bleeding Precautions

1. Maintain bed rest during active bleeding.
2. Administer blood products (fresh-frozen plasma, platelets, cryoprecipitate) as ordered.
3. Protect the patient from trauma, which may cause bleeding.
4. Avoid taking rectal temperatures.
5. Avoid puncturing the skin for injections, blood samples, and starting IV lines as much as possible.
6. Patient should wear shoes when ambulating, to avoid injuring the feet.
7. Patient should use a soft toothbrush for oral care.
8. Patient should use an electric razor for shaving.
9. Coordinate timing of invasive procedures with administration of fresh-frozen plasma and platelets as much possible to lessen the chance of bleeding.
10. Refrain from inserting devices into bleeding orifices.

Bleeding Reduction

1. Identify the cause of the bleeding.
2. Note hemoglobin/hematocrit levels before and after blood loss.
3. Maintain patent IV access so transfusions can occur quickly if needed.
4. Arrange for the availability of blood products, possibly using blood typing, screening, and holding the sample until products are needed.
5. Administer blood products if needed, and monitor for transfusion reaction.
6. Instruct the patient and family regarding signs of bleeding (bruising, nosebleeds, bleeding gums) and to notify the nurse if bleeding ensues.
7. Instruct the patient on activity restrictions and how to apply direct pressure if bleeding ensues prior to when nurse arrives.
8. Discuss severity of bleeding and measures being provided to manage the situation.
9. Avoid use of drugs containing aspirin and NSAIDs (e.g., ibuprofen), which are platelet-aggregation inhibitors that prolong episodes of bleeding.
10. Monitor serial coagulation or thrombin times. Report values outside the desired therapeutic ranges. Optimal range for aPTT is 1.5 to 2.5 times control value. A therapeutic INR is 2 to 3. Optimal range for thrombin time is 2 to 5 times normal.
11. Ensure easy access to antidotes for prescribed treatment:
    - *Protamine sulfate:* 1 mg counteracts 100 units of heparin. Usually, the initial dose is 50 mg.
    - *Vitamin K:* 20 mg given subcutaneously
    - *Epsilon-aminocaproic acid* (e.g., Amicar): Reverses the fibrinolytic condition related to thrombolytic therapy

Teaching: Oral Anticoagulant Therapy

1. Determine patient's knowledge of oral anticoagulant therapy.
2. Discuss the drug name, purpose, dosage, schedule, potential side effects, and complications of therapy.
3. Inform patient of the potential side effects and complications of anticoagulant therapy: easy bruising, prolonged bleeding from cuts, spontaneous nosebleeds, black and tarry stools, blood in urine and sputum.
4. Teach the rationale and application procedure for antiembolism stockings. Explain that patient should put them on in the morning before getting out of bed.
5. Stress the importance of preventing impairment of venous return from the lower extremities by avoiding prolonged sitting, crossing the legs, and wearing constrictive clothing.
6. Teach patient about foods high in vitamin K (e.g., fish, bananas, dark-green vegetables, tomatoes, cauliflower), which can interfere with anticoagulation. Patient must understand the importance of a consistent intake of foods high in vitamin K to avoid bleeding or clotting complications.
7. Caution patient that a soft-bristle toothbrush, rather than a hard-bristle one, and an electric razor, rather than a safety razor, should be used during anticoagulation therapy while at home.
8. Instruct patient to consult with physician before taking any new over-the-counter (OTC) or prescribed drugs. The following are among many drugs that enhance the response to warfarin: aspirin, ibuprofen, cimetidine, and trimethoprim. Drugs that decrease the response include antacids, diuretics, oral contraceptives, and barbiturates, among others.

NIC Acid-Base Management; Acid-Base Monitoring; Bedside Laboratory Testing; Health Education; Oxygen Therapy; Respiratory Monitoring; Surveillance; Teaching: Individual; Teaching: Prescribed Medication; Respiratory Monitoring, Vital Signs Monitoring

PULMONARY HYPERTENSION

PATHOPHYSIOLOGY

Pulmonary hypertension and pulmonary arterial hypertension (PAH) are complex, progressive, often fatal diseases caused by elevated PAPs, defined as a mean pulmonary artery pressure (MPAP) greater than 30 mm Hg, pulmonary capillary wedge pressure (PCWP) or left atrial pressure or left ventricular end-diastolic pressure less than 15 mm Hg, and PVR greater than 3 Wood units. The pulmonary vasculature is normally a highly distensible, low-resistance system. All types of pulmonary hypertension or PAH may result in right heart failure, since the right ventricle is under constant strain to pump into the highly resistant pulmonary vasculature. (See Table 4-11 for WHO classifications.)

Primary pulmonary hypertension (PPH) is rare, has a poor prognosis, and affects primarily middle-aged and young women. Causes of PAH are unclear. One type of heritable PAH is thought to be familial with a link to the bone morphogenic receptor 2 (*BMPR2*). *Secondary pulmonary hypertension* is more common, with management directed at treating the underlying cause and lowering PAPs using vasodilating drugs. PPH is often unresponsive to conventional treatments.

Rising MPAP increases PVR, which in turn causes two responses in the vasculature: "standby vessels" open to increase the surface area available for perfusion and the capillaries distend to accommodate the increased blood flow. Although these responses reduce PVR initially, the system eventually fails. Although most of the vascular system responds to hypoxia by dilating in an effort to increase blood flow to vital organs, the pulmonary vasculature responds to alveolar hypoxia by vasoconstriction, a beneficial mechanism that shunts blood away from underventilated areas to better ventilated areas in the lungs, thereby improving oxygenation. This regional mechanism is not strong enough to correct the V/Q imbalance, however. Generally, Pao_2 decreases to less than 60 mm Hg before vasoconstriction occurs; the lower the Pao_2, the more severe is the vasoconstriction.

The rise in PAP and the resulting increase in PVR from acute hypoxia are completely reversible once the hypoxia has been resolved. However, in the presence of chronic hypoxia, the pulmonary vasculature undergoes permanent changes (i.e., hypertrophy, hyperplasia), causing thickening of the vessel and narrowing of the lumen, a process known as vascular remodeling. Unfortunately, remodeling reduces vascular flexibility and causes further elevation of pressures. In addition, polycythemia develops as a compensatory mechanism to increase O_2 transport; this condition increases blood viscosity, which in turn increases PVR.

Table 4-11	WORLD HEALTH ORGANIZATION (WHO) CLASSIFICATION OF PULMONARY HYPERTENSION
WHO Class/Group	**Subsets/Examples of Causes**
Pulmonary arterial hypertension (PAH)	*Idiopathic PAH (IPAH):* Occurs at random. Also known as primary pulmonary hypertension *Heritable:* Formerly familial PAH; includes 2 types of PAH *Drug and toxin induced:* Includes antiobesity drugs like Fen-Phen (fenfluramine + phentermine), methamphetamine, and cocaine *Associated with other disorders:* Diseases include connective tissue disorders (e.g., scleroderma [SSC], CREST syndrome lupus [CSL]), HIV, portal hypertension, congenital left-to-right shunts, and hemoglobinopathies such as sickle-cell disease.
Pulmonary hypertension (PH) with left heart disease	Left-sided atrial or ventricular dysfunction, left-sided valvular heart disease
PH associated with lung diseases and/or hypoxemia	COPD, interstitial lung disease, sleep apnea, alveolar hypoventilation disorders, chronic exposure to high altitude, developmental abnormalities
PH due to chronic thrombolytic and/or embolic disease (CTEPH)	Pulmonary thromboembolism or embolism due to fat, tumor, parasites, foreign material
Miscellaneous	Sarcoidosis, histiocytosis X, lymphangiomatosis, compression of pulmonary vessels (adenopathy, tumor, fibrosing mediastinitis)

COPD, chronic obstructive pulmonary disease.
From McLaughlin W, et al. ACCF/AHA 2009 Expert consensus document on pulmonary hypertension. *Circulation* 119(16):2250–2294, 2009.

The functions of the heart and lungs are interdependent. Increased PVR stimulates the right ventricle to increase the pumping force to maintain adequate cardiac output. The right ventricle dilates and hypertrophies under the constant strain and workload. Eventually, the right side of the heart weakens and is unable to accommodate venous blood returning to the heart. As a result, pressure in the systemic venous circulation increases, causing cor pulmonale, or right-sided heart failure. See *Heart Failure* (p. 421) for further discussion of right-sided heart failure.

ASSESSMENT
Goal of Assessment
Because the low-resistance pulmonary vascular bed is clinically silent until late in the disease process, onset is insidious. Assessment prior to late stages of the disease should focus on discerning the cause of early indicators and classifying functional status (Box 4-2) so an appropriate plan of care is created.

History and Risk Factors
Factors associated with secondary pulmonary hypertension include congenital anomalies (patent foramen ovale [PFO] or ventricular septal defect [VSD]) by which additional blood is shunted from the left heart to the right heart, left ventricular failure, acidemia, COPD, sleep apnea, interstitial lung disease or pulmonary fibrosis, massive pulmonary embolism, sepsis, acute respiratory distress syndrome (ARDS) resulting in noncardiogenic pulmonary edema and an array of other causes. See Table 4-11 for etiologic factors.

Clinical Presentation
Early indicators Hyperventilation, vague chest discomfort
Late indicators Tachypnea, dyspnea, orthopnea, chest congestion

Vital Signs
- Tachycardia, tachypnea
- Blood pressure may increase or decrease, depending on response to any changes in cardiac output, which may be significant with markedly elevated pulmonary artery pressures.

Box 4-2	WHO CLASSIFICATION: FUNCTIONAL STATUS OF PATIENTS WITH PULMONARY HYPERTENSION

Class I No limitation of usual physical activity; ordinary physical activity does not cause dyspnea, fatigue, chest pain, or syncope

Class II Mild limitation of physical activity; no discomfort at rest, but normal activity causes increased dyspnea, fatigue, chest pain, or presyncope

Class III Marked limitation of activity; no discomfort at rest, but less than normal physical activity causes increased dyspnea, fatigue, chest pain, or presyncope

Class IV Unable to perform physical activity at rest; may have signs of RV failure; symptoms increased by almost any physical activity

From Gladwin and Ghofrani. Update on Pulmonary Hypertension 2009. *Am. J. Respir. Crit. Care Med.* 181: 1020–1026, 2010.

Observation/Inspection
- Cyanosis of the lips and nail beds
- Edema of the hands and feet
- Increasing abdominal girth
- Anasarca (generalized, massive edema)
- Distended jugular veins

Palpation
- Right ventricular heave (visible left parasternal systolic lift)

Auscultation
- Accentuated pulmonary component of the second heart sound
- Right ventricular diastolic gallop, pulmonary ejection click
- Distant breath sounds
- Basilar crackles in lung fields

Screening Diagnostic Tests
- *Chest radiograph:* Validates presence of underlying pathology which may have prompted development of pulmonary hypertension
- *12-Lead ECG:* Assess if patient has an acute myocardial infarction associated with heart failure. May show right ventricular hypertrophy, right-axis deviation, right bundle-branch block, and enlarged P waves.

Diagnostic Tests for Pulmonary Hypertension		
Test	**Purpose**	**Abnormal Findings**
Arterial blood gas (ABG) values	Important to the differential diagnosis of the cause of pulmonary hypertension	Values vary: Generally Pao_2 will be less than 60 mm Hg. $Paco_2$ will be within normal limits (35–45 mm Hg) unless COPD is the cause of the pulmonary hypertension, in which case $Paco_2$ is usually elevated.
Chest radiograph (CXR)	Will confirm anatomic abnormalities associated with chronic right ventricular failure	Right ventricular dilation or hypertrophy, enlarged pulmonary artery secondary to increased pressure, and diminished diaphragmatic excursion
CT scan	Helps to identify specific pathology	Will confirm the presence of interstitial lung disease

Continued

Diagnostic Tests for Pulmonary Hypertension — cont'd

Test	Purpose	Abnormal Findings
Hemodynamic measurements	Helps to confirm presence of elevated pulmonary artery pressures and monitor treatment effectiveness. Pressures in the pulmonary vasculature are measured by a pulmonary artery (e.g., Swan-Ganz) catheter.	Cardiac output can be a better measure of disease severity than the pulmonary artery pressures. Used for definitive diagnosis of pulmonary hypertension.
Right heart catheterization (RHC)	May be required to make a definitive diagnosis	Data will differentiate or quantify the contribution of the left or right ventricular failure and measure the response to pharmacotherapy.
Echocardiography	Assesses for elevated pulmonary artery systolic pressure, but not the MPAP. Hemodynamic monitoring is used for definitive diagnosis.	May reveal enlarged right atrium and right ventricle, diminished wall motion, and pulmonic valve malfunction (midsystolic closure or delayed opening). Unfortunately, false positives are common with echocardiography.
Pulmonary function tests	Important for differential diagnosis of the underlying pathologic condition	Will vary according to cause
Pulmonary angiography and perfusion scans	To rule out an embolic event as the underlying cause	Will NOT be positive if the cause is pulmonary hypertension
Red blood cell (RBC)/ hematocrit values	Screens for polycythemia associated with chronic hypoxia	May be increased above normal
Type B naturetic peptide (BNP) level	Monitors the progress of any associated heart failure	Will be progressively elevated as heart failure worsens
Other blood tests	Used to rule out other possible diagnoses, such as liver disease, HIV, and autoimmune disease	Various values will be positive for specific pathologies.

COLLABORATIVE MANAGEMENT

The goal of interdisciplinary management is to diagnose and treat the underlying disorder or process causing the pulmonary hypertension and improve the patient's symptoms, quality of life, and survival. Treatment is directed primarily toward increasing myocardial contractility, reducing right ventricular afterload caused by the high PVR, and reversal of vascular remodeling.

Care Priorities

1. **Relieve hypoxemia and improve gas exchange:**
   - *Oxygen therapy:* To eliminate hypoxia, a cause of pulmonary vascular vasoconstriction, and the resulting right ventricular afterload
   - *Bronchodilators (e.g., aminophylline, isoproterenol, terbutaline):* Act as afterload reducers by decreasing pulmonary vascular resistance and increasing right ventricular ejection fraction. By improving gas exchange, bronchodilators may decrease hypoxic vasoconstriction of the pulmonary vascular bed.
2. **Promote dilation of the pulmonary vasculature to promote blood flow and better gas exchange:**
   - *Nitric oxide therapy:* Nitric oxide gas is administered through either a face mask, a tracheostomy, or an ET tube to promote pulmonary vasodilation. The vasodilation reduces blood pressure in the pulmonary circulation. Available in a limited number of centers. Use is increasing across the United States, especially in pediatric patients.
   - *Vasodilators (e.g., nitrates, hydralazine, calcium channel blockers):* Reverse pulmonary vasoconstriction, to reduce right ventricular afterload and enhance pulmonary blood flow.

- *Endothelin blockers:* Medications such as bosentan (Tracleer) block endothelin, which contributes to vasoconstriction and vascular remodeling. Liver function tests must be performed monthly.
- *Prostacyclin (PGI₂) analogues:* Produced in endothelial cells from prostaglandin H₂, PGI₂ vasodilates the pulmonary vessels. Prostacyclin also prevents formation of platelet plugs. Synthetic prostacyclin analogues (epoprostenol [Flolan], iloprost [Ventavis], treprostinil [Remodulin, Tyvaso]) are given IV, SC, or by inhalation. Continuous IV infusion of epoprostenol is the preferred treatment option for the most critically ill patients. *NOTE: Prostacyclin is inhibited by NSAIDs, so the patient must be educated to avoid them.*
- *Phosphodiesterase-5 (PDE-5) inhibitors:* Vasodilate the pulmonary vessels. Sildenafil, the active ingredient in Viagra, is a drug in this class that has been U.S. Food and Drug Administration (FDA) approved for use in pulmonary hypertension under the trade name Revatio.

3. **Reduce circulating blood volume to reduce strain on the right heart:**
   - *Diuretics:* Reduce circulating volume via loss of sodium and water, which may decrease PAP and right ventricular workload. In turn, this reduces leftward septal bulging seen with right ventricular overload. Carefully evaluate response; if patient's condition declines, a volume infusion may be needed if patient is in right heart failure. Higher RV pressure may be needed to overcome the elevated PAP to promote RV ejection.

4. **Enhance myocardial contractility to improve blood flow through the pulmonary and systemic circulation:**
   - *Digitalis:* Generally used only with biventricular failure when other therapies have not been sufficient. The inotropic effects of digitalis can increase CO and pulmonary resistance, which are deleterious in the presence of right ventricular failure.

5. **Prevent pulmonary thromboembolism:**
   - *Anticoagulants:* Heparin is used for acute management, if the patient is actively thrombosing/embolizing. Warfarin is used for ongoing prevention of pulmonary emboli (blood clots in the lungs).

CARE PLANS FOR PULMONARY HYPERTENSION

Risk for ineffective cardiopulmonary tissue perfusion *related to blood flow anomalies stemming from pulmonary hypertension and right ventricular strain*

GOALS/OUTCOMES Within 24 hours of initiating vasodilating medications, diuretics, and inotropic agents, PAPs are reduced by at least 10%, CVP or RAP is maintained at a level that facilitates forward flow of blood if patient has right heart failure, PVR is reduced below 300 dynes/sec/cm⁻⁵, and cardiac index is at least 2 L/min/m². Systemic blood pressure is maintained at no less than 90 mm Hg systolic, with diastolic pressure at least 50 mm Hg.

NOC Tissue Perfusion: Pulmonary; Tissue Perfusion: Cardiac; Cardiac Pump Effectiveness; Respiratory Status: Gas Exchange; Circulation Status

Hemodynamic Regulation
1. Monitor PAPs and cardiac output in response to vasodilating medications, diuretics, and inotropic medications.
2. Monitor arterial BP hourly for improvement. Patient may be hypotensive if heart failure has ensued. Medications and intravascular volume regulation may help improve cardiac output and systemic circulation. Those with right heart failure require a delicate balance between medication administration and volume regulation.
3. Auscultate breath sounds to assess for crackles at least every 2 hours.
4. Monitor for decreased urine output every 2 hours. Improvement in urine output is reflective of improved systemic circulation, resulting in improved renal blood flow.
5. Judiciously monitor CVP or RAP if patient has right heart failure. Preload must be maintained at a sufficient level to be able to overcome the increased resistance to ejection (RV afterload) created by pulmonary hypertension. Patient may require a CVP that is considerably higher than normal to facilitate forward flow of blood. If diuretics worsen hemodynamics, a volume infusion may be attempted to see if the cardiac output improves.

Impaired gas exchange *related to altered blood flow secondary to pulmonary capillary constriction and fluid which may be present in the alveoli secondary to heart failure*

GOALS/OUTCOMES Gas exchange improves within 12 hours of initiating therapies, toward a goal of at least 90%. Those who are O_2 dependent must be assessed using their baseline value coupled with their activity tolerance, since both are lower than expected for the general population.

NOC Respiratory Status: Gas Exchange

Oxygen Therapy
1. Administer O_2 as prescribed. Advance O_2 delivery devices as needed. If patient requires consistent increases in FiO_2 to maintain the same O_2 saturation, notify physician or midlevel practitioner, as this is a sign of deteriorating gas exchange.
2. Assess respiratory pattern, rate, and depth; chest excursion and use of accessory muscles.
3. Monitor ABG results for hypoventilation, a sign of impending respiratory failure. (See *Acute Respiratory Failure*, P. 383.)

Ventilation Assistance
1. Monitor for changes in O_2 saturation and work of breathing in response to pulmonary vasodilating medications. If patient fails to improve and respiratory distress increases, patient must be intubated and placed on mechanical ventilation. (See *Mechanical Ventilation* for detailed information.)
2. Provide emotional and spiritual support for the patient and his or her support system. (See *Emotional and Spiritual Support of the Patient and Significant Others*, P. 200.)
3. Once patient is on mechanical ventilation, more aggressive strategies such as nitric oxide therapy can be initiated for severely ill patients unresponsive to other vasodilating medications. Patients receiving nitric oxide should improve their O_2 saturation within 24 hours of initiating treatment.
4. If patient is unable to sustain an improved O_2 saturation on nitric oxide, the physician or midlevel practitioner may need to approach the patient (if aware and oriented) and support system about ECMO (extracorporeal membrane oxygenation) if they are a candidate for heart-lung transplantation. If there are no further options available, discontinuation of life support may need to be addressed (see *Ethical Considerations in critical Care*, p 215).

Deficient knowledge *related to disease process and treatment of pulmonary hypertension and associated underlying diseases if present*

GOALS/OUTCOMES Throughout the hospitalization, patient and support system voice understanding of the plan of care; within 24 hours of hospital discharge, the patient and support system verbalize sufficient knowledge of management of the disease process(es) and treatments to sustain the patient outside the hospital.

NOC Knowledge: Disease Process; Knowledge: Treatment and Procedure(s)

Teaching: Treatments and Procedures
1. Explain all steps in the process of providing various O_2 delivery and ventilatory support strategies.
2. Discuss the selection of various modalities of vasodilator therapies. Inhaled medications and subcutaneous and intravenous infusions that will be continued outside the hospital require more extensive education than oral medications.
3. Involve case manager and discharge planner in discussions of medications, so all resource options are clarified. Many of the medications used are quite expensive to sustain if the patient is underinsured.
4. If patient requires mechanical ventilation, ensure the patient understands how to communicate with care providers (see *Mechanical Ventilation* care plans for further details , p. 99).
5. When preparing for discharge home, discuss the purpose of medications designed to reduce the workload on the heart (vasodilators), relax the heart (calcium channel blocking agents), and prevent fluid accumulation (diuretics).
6. Ensure patient is familiar with the home health providers who will provide O_2 therapy and other ventilation strategies, such as a nebulizer or aerosol, if needed.

Teaching: Disease Process
1. Assess patient's level and key support system members' level of understanding of the disease process.
2. If the cause of pulmonary hypertension has been identified, discuss appropriate management strategies of the associated disease process.
3. Discuss lifestyle changes that could prevent further complications.
4. Explain the value of learning relaxation therapy, including various breathing and visualization exercises, listening to music, meditation, and biofeedback.
5. Explain how smoking and second-hand smoke increase the workload of the heart by causing vasoconstriction. The patient should be encouraged to live in a smoke-free environment. Support system members who smoke should be given the opportunity to understand this vital information. Smoking cessation information should be provided.

6. If activity has been progressively impaired, consult with a physical therapist and respiratory therapist regarding an appropriate exercise program.
7. Have a dietician visit the patient to offer assistance with meal planning.

NIC Activity Therapy; Airway Management; Acid-Base Monitoring; Anxiety Reduction; Cardiac Care: Acute; Coping Enhancement; Invasive Hemodynamic Monitoring; Medication Administration: Intravenous; Medication Administration: Inhalation; Medication Administration: Oral; Self-Care Assistance; Sleep Enhancement; Support Group

SELECTED REFERENCES

American Association of Critical Care Nurses: AACN Practice Alert: Ventilator associated pneumonia. Retrieved April 25, 2009, from http://www.aacn.org/WD/Practice/Docs/Ventilator_Associated_Pneumonia_1-2008.pdf

American College of Chest Physicians: Consensus Panel on the Management of Spontaneous Pneumothorax: Primary pneumothorax. 2008. Retrieved April 30, 2009, from http://www.chestnet.org/education/cs/pneumothorax/qrg/page02.php

American College of Chest Physicians: Consensus Panel on the Management of Spontaneous Pneumothorax: Secondary pneumothorax. 2008. Retrieved April 30, 2009, from http://www.chestnet.org/education/cs/pneumothorax/qrg/page03.php

American Thoracic Society and Infectious Diseases Society of America: Guidelines for the management of adults with hospital-acquired, ventilator-associated, and healthcare-associated pneumonia. *Am J Respir Care* 171:388–416, 2005.

Baumann ME: Management of spontaneous pneumothorax. *Clin Chest Med* 27(2):369–381, 2006.

Berry AM, Davidson PM: Beyond comfort: oral hygiene as a critical nursing activity in the intensive care unit. *Intensive Crit Care Nur* 22(6):318–328, 2006.

Bonatti HJR, Sawyer RG, Pruett TL: Infection control in immunosuppressed patients. *Crit Connections Newsletter*, February 2009. Society of Critical Care Medicine. Retrieved April 21, 2009, from http://www.sccm.org/Publications/Critical_Connections/Archives/February2009/Pages/Infection%20Control.aspx

British Thoracic Society Standards of Care Committee and Pulmonary Embolism Guideline Development Group: British Thoracic Society Guidelines for the management of suspected acute pulmonary embolism. *Thorax* 58:470–484, 2003.

British Thoracic Society, Scottish Intercollegiate Guidelines Network. British guideline on the management of asthma. Quick Reference Guide, May 2008. Retrieved April 23, 2009, from http://www.brit-thoracic.org.uk/ClinicalInformation/Asthma/AsthmaGuidelines

Brun-Bruisson C, Minelli C, Bertolini G, et al: Epidemiology and outcome of acute lung injury in European intensive care units. Results from the ALIVE study. *Intensive Care Med* 30:51–61, 2004.

Carlson KK: Thoracentesis (assist). In Weigand DJLM, Carlson KK, editors: *AACN procedure manual for critical care*, ed 5. Philadelphia, 2005, Elsevier Saunders, pp. 181–185.

Carlson KK: Thoracentesis (perform). In Weigand DJLM, Carlson KK, editors: *AACN procedure manual for critical care*, ed 5. Philadelphia, 2005, Elsevier Saunders, pp. 174–180.

Cepkova M, Matthay MA: Pharmacotherapy of acute lung injury and the acute respiratory distress syndrome. *J Intensive Care Med* 21(3):119–143, 2006.

Dickinson S, Zalewski CA: Oral care during mechanical ventilation: critical for VAP prevention. *Critical Connections Newsletter*, February 2008. Society of Critical Care Medicine. Retrieved April 22, 2009, from http://www.sccm.org/Publications/Critical_Connections/Archives/February_2008/Pages/OralCaretoPreventVAP.aspx

Fedullo PF, Tapson VF: The evaluation of suspected pulmonary embolism. *N Engl J Med* 49:1247–1256, 2003.

Geerts WH, Bergqvist D, Pineo GF, et al: Prevention of venous thromboembolism: American College of Chest Physicians evidence-based clinical practice guidelines, ed 8. *Chest* 133(suppl 6):S381–S453, 2008.

Ghofrani HA, et al: Uncertainties in the diagnosis and treatment of pulmonary arterial hypertension. *Circulation* 118:1195–1201, 2008.

Goldhill DR, Imhoff M, McLean B, et al: Rotational bed therapy to prevent and treat respiratory complications: a review and meta-analysis. *Am J Clin Cardiol* 16(1), 2007.

Goodrich C: Needle thoracostomy (perform). In Weigand DJLM, Carlson KK, editors: *AACN procedure manual for critical care*, ed 5. Philadelphia, 2005, Elsevier Saunders, pp. 170–173.

Guerin C, Gaillard S, Lemasson S: Effects of systematic prone positioning in hypoxemic acute respiratory failure: a randomized controlled trial. *JAMA* 292(19):2379–2387, 2004.

Henry M, Arnold T, Harvey J, on behalf of the BTS Pleural Disease Group, a subgroup of the BTS Standards of Care Committee: BTS guidelines for the management of spontaneous pneumothorax. *Thorax* 58(suppl II):39–52, 2003. Retrieved April 26, 2009, from http://www.brit-thoracic.org.uk/Portals/0/ClinicalInformation/PleuralDisease/Guidelines/PleuralDiseaseSpontaneous.pdf

Hill N: Non-invasive ventilation in critical care. *Critical Connections Newsletter,* February 2008. Society of Critical Care Medicine. Retrieved April 22, 2009, from http://www.sccm.org/Publications/Critical_Connections/Archives/February_2008/Pages/Noninvasive Ventilation.aspx

Kesslert R, Ståhi E, et al: Patient understanding, detection, and experience of COPD exacerbations. *Chest* 130:133–142, 2006.

Kirkwood P: Chest tube removal (perform). In Weigand DJLM, Carlson KK, editors: *AACN procedure manual for critical care,* ed 5. Philadelphia, 2005, Elsevier Saunders, pp. 140–145.

Lawrence DM, Carlson KK: Chest tube placement (assist). In Weigand DJLM, Carlson KK, editors: *AACN procedure manual for critical care,* ed 5. Philadelphia, 2005, Elsevier Saunders, pp. 134–139.

Lawrence DM: Chest tube placement (perform) In Weigand DJLM, Carlson KK, editors: *AACN procedure manual for critical care,* ed 5. Philadelphia, 2005, Elsevier Saunders, pp. 125–133.

Mandel LA, Wunderlink RG, Anzueto A, et al: Infectious Diseases Society of America/American Thoracic Society Consensus Guidelines on Management of Community Acquired Pneumonia in Adults. *Clin Infect Dis* 44(suppl 2):S27–S72, 2007.

Marik PE, Pastores S, Annane D, et al: Clinical practice guidelines for the diagnosis and management of corticosteroid insufficiency in critical illness: recommendations of an international task force. *Crit Care Med* 36:1937–1949, 2008.

McLaughlin V, McGoon M: Pulmonary arterial hypertension. *Circulation* 114:1417–1431, 2006.

McLaughlin W, et al: ACCF/AHA 2009 Expert consensus document on pulmonary hypertension. *Circulation* 119(16):2250–2294, 2009.

Pickett JD: Closed chest drainage system. In Weigand DJLM, Carlson KK, editors: *AACN procedure manual for critical care,* ed 5. Philadelphia, 2005, Elsevier Saunders, pp. 151–169.

Reddel HK, Taylor DR, Bateman ED, et al: An Official American Thoracic Society/European Respiratory Society Statement: Asthma Control and Exacerbations. *Am J Respir Crit Care Med* 180:59–99, 2009. Retrieved November 22, 2009, from http://www.thoracic.org/sections/publications/statements/resources/asthma-control.pdf

Rubenfeld GD, Caldwell E, Peabody E, et al: Incidence and outcomes of acute lung injury. *N Engl J Med* 353:1685–1693, 2005.

Scala R, Naldi M, et al: Noninvasive positive pressure ventilation in patients with acute exacerbations of COPD and varying levels of consciousness. *Chest* 128(3):1657–1666, 2005.

Sona C, Schallom L: Nursing practice excellence: a key to infection prevention. *Critical Connections Newsletter,* February 2009. Society of Critical Care Medicine. Retrieved April 21, 2009, from http://www.sccm.org/Publications/Critical_Connections/Archives/February2009/Pages/NursingPracticeExcellence.aspx

Souza R, Jardim C: Trends in pulmonary arterial hypertension. *Eur Respir Rev* 18(111):7–12, 2009.

Sweet DD, Naismith A, Keenan SP, et al: Missed opportunities for noninvasive positive pressure ventilation: a utilization review. *J Crit Care* 23:111, 2008.

Tang B, Craig J, Eslick G, et al: Use of corticosteroids in acute lung injury and acute respiratory distress syndrome: a systematic review and meta-analysis. *Crit Care Med* 37:1594–1603, 2009.

Tapson VF, Decousus H, Pini M, et al: Venous thromboembolism prophylaxis in acutely ill, hospitalized medical patients: findings from the International Medical Prevention Registry on Venous Thromboembolism. *Chest* 132 (3): 936–945, 2007

Taylor DR, Bateman ED, Boulet L-P, et al: A new perspective on concepts of asthma severity and control. *Eur Respir J* 32:545–554, 2008.

The ARDS Clinical Trials Network, National Heart, Lung, and Blood Institute; National Institutes of Health: Effects of recruitment maneuvers in patients with acute lung injury and acute respiratory distress syndrome ventilated with high positive end-expiratory pressure. *Crit Care Med* 31(11): 2592–2597, 2003.

The NHLBI ARDS Clinical Trials Network: Comparison of two fluid-management strategies in acute lung injury. *N Engl J Med* 354(24):2564–2575, 2006.

The NHLBI ARDS Clinical Trials Network: Pulmonary-artery versus central venous catheter to guide treatment of acute lung injury. *N Engl J Med* 354(21):2213–2224, 2006.

Torbicki A, Perrier A, Konstantinides S, et al: The Task Force for the Diagnosis and Management of Acute Pulmonary Embolism of the European Society of Cardiology. Guidelines on the diagnosis and management of pulmonary embolism. *Eur Heart J* 29:2276–2315, 2008.

US Dept of Health and Human Services, National Institutes of Health: National Asthma Education and Prevention Program Expert Panel Report 3. Guidelines for the Diagnosis and Management of Asthma (Summary Report 2007). Retrieved April 1, 2009, from http://www.nhlbi.nih.gov/guidelines/asthma/index.htm

Ware LB: Prognostic determinants of acute respiratory distress syndrome in adults: impact on clinical trial design. *Crit Care Med* 33(3 suppl):S217–S222, 2005.

Weigand DJLM, Carlson KK, editors: *AACN procedure manual for critical care*, ed 5. Philadelphia, 2005, Elsevier Saunders.

Zehtabshi S, Rios CL: Management of emergency department patients with spontaneous pneumothorax: needle aspiration or tube thoracostomy? *Ann Emerg Med* 51(1):91–100, 2008.

Cardiac and Vascular Disorders

CARDIOVASCULAR ASSESSMENT: GENERAL

Goal of System Assessment

Evaluate for decreased cardiac output and decreased tissue perfusion.

Vital Sign Assessment

Measure heart rate (HR), heart rhythm, and blood pressure (BP) to evaluate cardiac output and perfusion.

- Measure BP on both arms.
- Compare cuff BP to arterial line BP if arterial line is in place; decide which pressure is deemed the most accurate; treat BP using that value.
- Note pulse pressure.

12-Lead Electrocardiogram

Evaluate for changes from last electrocardiogram (ECG) to assess for worsened heart disease (myocardial damage) or for electrolyte imbalances, which may decrease cardiac output; this should be done on every patient to use for comparison.

- Heart rate: diagnose type of tachycardia, bradycardia, or irregular rhythm
- PR, QRS, and QT intervals
- ST-segment and T-wave changes such as depression or elevation
- Pacing and conduction: regular, normal rate and velocity

Observation

- Evaluate for facial and lip color, appearance of skin and nails, and patterns of edema (especially dependent areas) to evaluate for decreased tissue perfusion.
- Inquire about the presence of chest, arm, and jaw discomfort.
- Inquire about compliance with taking cardiac medications as prescribed.

Palpation

Pulse assessment to evaluate for decreased tissue perfusion:

- Pulse quality and regularity bilaterally (scale 0 to 4+)
- Edema (scale 0 to 4+): extremities, back, and sacrum
- Capillary refill
- Evaluate all peripheral pulses to assess for vascular disease.
- Auscultation
- Heart sounds to evaluate for contributors to decreased cardiac output (note changes with body positioning and respirations):
  - Aortic, pulmonic, Erb's point, tricuspid, mitral

- S_1 (lub) and S_2 (dub): quality, intensity, pitch
- Extra sounds: S_3 (after S_2), S_4 (before S_1) indicative of heart failure (HF)
- Extra sounds: Murmurs, clicks (may indicate valve disease)
- Extra sounds: Friction rub indicative of pericarditis

Labwork

Blood studies can reveal causes of dysrhythmias or changes in pacing/conduction or HR changes:
- Electrolyte levels: ↑ or ↓ potassium or magnesium
- Complete blood counts: anemia, ↑ white blood cells (WBCs)
- Coagulation studies
- Lipid profile
- Cardiac enzymes/isoenzymes
- B-type natriuretic peptide (BNP)
- Levels of cardiac medications

CARE PLANS FOR GENERALIZED CARDIOVASCULAR DYSFUNCTIONS

Activity intolerance *related to decreased cardiac output*

GOALS/OUTCOMES Within the 12- to 24-hour period before discharge from the critical care unit (CCU), patient exhibits cardiac tolerance to increasing levels of activity as evidenced by respiratory rate (RR) less than 24 breaths per minute (breaths/min), normal sinus rhythm (NSR) on ECG, BP within 20 mm Hg of patient's normal range, HR less than 120 beats per minute (bpm) (or within 20 bpm of resting HR for patients on beta blocker therapy), and absence of chest pain.
NOC Endurance

Energy Management
1. Determine patient's physical limitations.
2. Determine causes of fatigue and perceived causes of fatigue.
3. Monitor cardiorespiratory response to activity (tachycardia, other dysrhythmias, tachypnea, dyspnea, diaphoresis, pallor) and hemodynamic response (elevated pulmonary artery pressures [PAPs], central venous pressure [CVP], or no change/little increase in cardiac output) if a pulmonary artery catheter or bioimpedance device is in place.
4. Monitor for chest discomfort during activity.
5. Reduce all causes of discomfort, including those induced by the patient's environment, such as uncomfortable room temperature or position, thirst/dry mouth, and wrinkled or damp bedding.
6. Provide alternating periods of rest and activity.

Self-Care Assistance: Instrumental Activities of Daily Living (IADLs)
1. Determine need for assistance with IADLs including walking, cooking, shopping, housekeeping, transportation, and money management.
2. Provide for methods of contacting support of assistance people (such as lifeline services, emergency response services including readily accessible telephone numbers if patient's area is not 911 accessible).
3. Determine financial resources and personal preferences for modifying their home to accommodate any disabilities.

Decreased cardiac output *related to altered cardiac pump function*

GOALS/OUTCOMES Within 24 hours of this diagnosis, patient exhibits adequate cardiac output, as evidenced by BP within normal limits for patient, HR 60 to 100 bpm, NSR on ECG, peripheral pulses greater than 2+ on a 0 to 4+ scale, warm and dry skin, hourly urine output greater than 0.5 ml/kg, measured cardiac output (CO) 4 to 7 L/min, CVP 4 to 6 mm Hg, PAP 20 to 30/8 to 15 mm Hg, pulmonary artery wedge pressure (PAWP) 6 to 12 mm Hg, and patient awake, alert, oriented, and free from anginal pain.
NOC Circulation Status

Cardiac Care: Acute
1. Palpate and evaluate quality of peripheral pulses, for presence of edema, capillary refill, and skin color and temperature of extremities.
2. Monitor ECG continuously, noting HR and rhythm. Select the most diagnostic lead(s) for monitoring patient. Consider use of ST-segment monitoring if available.

3. Compare current ECG readings with past readings and report abnormal findings that create instability or have the potential to create instability.
4. Use a 12- or 15-lead ECG to diagnose heart rhythm changes, because one or two leads are often insufficient to fully diagnose ECG changes.
5. Provide antidysrhythmic medications as appropriate to abate heart rhythms that prompt hypotension.
6. Provide positive inotropic drugs as appropriate to help increase cardiac output to maintain stable BP.
7. Monitor effects of negative inotropic medications (e.g., beta blockers) carefully, as the decreased myocardial workload may prompt hypotension.
8. Evaluate chest pain for location, radiation, intensity, duration, and precipitating factors. Emphasize to patient the importance of reporting all instances of chest pain and pressure and arm, neck, and jaw pain.
9. Apply oxygen when chest pain is present, according to Advanced Cardiac Life Support (ACLS) guidelines.
10. Monitor pacemaker function as appropriate to insure device is sensing, pacing and capturing appropriately.
11. Auscultate heart tones; be alert for development of new S_3 and S_4, new "split" sounds, or pericardial friction rubs.
12. Auscultate lungs for rales, crackles, wheezes, rhonchi, pleural friction rubs, or other adventitious sounds indicative of fluid retention.
13. Monitor for diminished level of consciousness, which may signal cerebral perfusion is compromised secondary to decreased cardiac output.
14. Auscultate abdomen and monitor for decreased bowel sounds and/or abdominal distention, which may indicate abdominal perfusion is compromised.
15. Record intake and output, urine output, and daily weight and evaluate for fluid retention, which may indicate renal perfusion is compromised.
16. Note electrolyte values at least daily, monitoring closely for changes in potassium and magnesium, which may prompt dysrhythmias; increased blood urea nitrogen (BUN) or increased creatinine, which may indicate low CO is causing renal insufficiency; and hyperglycemia, which may indicate patient has underlying diabetes.
17. Monitor for increasing activity intolerance, dyspnea, excessive fatigue, and orthopnea, which may all indicate CO is lessening.
18. Keep head of the bed (HOB) elevated if patient is unable to breathe comfortably when flat in bed.
19. Insert urinary catheter if patient is unable to void without markedly increasing activity level, or anuria is noted, as appropriate.

Hemodynamic Regulation
1. Monitor values generated by pulmonary artery catheter to directly assess CO.
2. Assess for further decreases in CO reflected by elevated pulmonary artery occlusive/wedge pressure, elevated CVP, and elevated pulmonary vascular resistance (PVR).
3. Monitor for fluid overload by assessing for elevated systemic vascular resistance (SVR).
4. Monitor the effects of all medications on hemodynamic readings, including effects of positive or negative inotropic agents, antidysrhythmics, and vasodilating or vasoconstricting medications.

Impaired gas exchange *related to decreased perfusion to the lungs*

GOALS/OUTCOMES Within 12 to 24 hours of treatment, patient has adequate gas exchange as evidenced by Pao_2 greater than 80 mm Hg, $Paco_2$ 35 to 45 mm Hg, pH 7.35 to 7.45, presence of normal breath sounds, and absence of adventitious breath sounds. RR is 12 to 20 breaths/min with normal pattern and depth.
NOC Respiratory Status: Ventilation

Airway Management
1. Assess for patent airway; if snoring, crowing, or strained respirations are present, indicative of partial or full airway obstruction, open airway using chin-lift or jaw-thrust.
2. Insert oral or nasopharyngeal airway if patient cannot maintain patent airway; if severely distressed, patient may require endotracheal intubation.
3. Position patient to alleviate dyspnea and ensure maximal ventilation — generally in a sitting upright position unless severe hypotension is present.
4. Clear secretions from airway by having patient cough vigorously, or provide nasotracheal, oropharyngeal, or endotracheal tube suctioning as needed.
5. Have patient breathe slowly or manually ventilate with Ambu bag slowly and deeply between coughing or suctioning attempts.
6. Assist with use of incentive spirometer as appropriate.
7. Turn patient every 2 hours if immobile. Encourage patient to turn self, or get out of bed as much as tolerated if able.

8. Provide mucolytic and bronchodilating medications orally, intravenously (IV), or by inhaler, aerosol, or nebulizer as ordered to assist with thinning secretions and relaxing muscles in lower airways.
9. Provide chest physical therapy as appropriate, if other methods of secretion removal are ineffective.

Oxygen Therapy
1. Provide humidity in oxygen or bilevel positive airway pressure (BiPAP) device if used for longer than 12 hours to help thin secretions.
2. Administer supplemental oxygen using liter flow and device as ordered.
3. Restrict patient and visitors from smoking while oxygen is in use.
4. Document pulse oximetry with oxygen liter flow in place at time of reading as ordered. Oxygen is a drug; the dose of the drug must be associated with the oxygen saturation reading or the reading is meaningless.
5. Obtain arterial blood gases (ABGs) if patient experiences behavioral changes or respiratory distress to check for hypoxemia or hypercapnia.
6. Monitor for oxygen-induced hypoventilation, especially in patients with chronic obstructive pulmonary disease (COPD).
7. Monitor for changes in chest radiograph and breath sounds indicative of oxygen toxicity and absorption atelectasis in patients receiving higher concentrations of oxygen (greater than FiO_2 45%) for longer than 24 hours. The higher the oxygen concentration, the greater is the chance of toxicity.
8. Monitor for skin breakdown where oxygen devices are in contact with skin, such as nares and around edges of mask devices.
9. Provide oxygen therapy during transportation and when patient gets out of bed.
10. If patient is unable to maintain SpO_2 reading of greater than 88% off oxygen, consult with respiratory care practitioner and physician about the need for home oxygen therapy.

Respiratory Monitoring
1. Monitor rate, rhythm, and depth of respirations.
2. Note chest movement for symmetry of chest expansion and signs of increased work of breathing such as use of accessory muscles or retraction of intercostal or supraclavicular muscles. Consider use of BiPAP for impending respiratory failure.
3. Ensure airway is not obstructed by tongue (snoring or choking-type respirations) and monitor breathing patterns. New patterns that impair ventilation should be managed as appropriate for setting.
4. Note that trachea remains midline, as deviation may indicate patient has a tension pneumothorax.
5. Auscultate breath sounds following administration of respiratory medications to assess for improvement.
6. Note changes in oxygen saturation (SaO_2), pulse oximetry (SpO_2), and end-tidal CO_2 ($ETCO_2$) and ABGs as appropriate.
7. Monitor for dyspnea and note causative activities or events.
8. If increased restlessness or unusual somnolence occur, evaluate patient for hypoxemia and hypercapnia as appropriate.
9. Monitor chest radiograph reports as new films become available.

HEART FAILURE

PATHOPHYSIOLOGY

HF is a syndrome stemming from impaired cardiac pump function, resulting in systemic perfusion that is inadequate to meet the body's metabolic demands for energy production. The condition may be divided into systolic or diastolic HF. In systolic HF, there is reduced cardiac contractility, while in diastolic HF, there is impaired cardiac relaxation and abnormal ventricular filling. HF is the leading cause of death in the United States, affecting approximately 5 million patients. One in five patients dies within 1 year of diagnosis. The annual medical cost is over $30 billion. Although much progress has been made in the treatment, the annual mortality rate remains high (5% to 20%). The greatest number of patients die from New York Heart Association (NYHA) Class IV symptoms, including progressive pump failure and congestion. Over half die from sudden cardiac death. Many die from end-organ failure resulting from inadequate perfusion. The kidneys are especially vulnerable. Those with a poor cardiac prognosis typically manifest a higher NYHA HF class, high catecholamine and BNP levels, renal dysfunction, cachexia, valvular regurgitation, ventricular dysrhythmias, lower ejection fraction, hyponatremia, and left ventricular (LV) dilation. Patients with both systolic and diastolic LV dysfunction have a worse prognosis than do patients with either condition alone.

HF is a degenerative process manifested by progressive pathologic changes in the cardiac structure and function resulting from increased pressure (e.g., hypertension, aortic stenosis), excessive intracardiac volume (e.g., mitral regurgitation), or cardiac injury (e.g., myocardial infarction [MI], myocarditis, or cardiomyopathy) associated with neurohormonal changes. The affected chamber wall dilates, hypertrophies, and becomes more spherical—a process known as *remodeling*. The remodeling process itself increases the wall stress, causing further remodeling. Therefore, reduction of remodeling is an important goal of therapy. There are several strategies used to reduce remodeling, including medications (e.g., angiotensin-converting enzyme [ACE] inhibitors [ACEIs], angiotensin receptor blockers [ARBs], beta adrenergic blockers, neurohormonal agents, and diuretics), devices, and surgery.

Effective pumping of the heart depends on the elements of the cardiac cycle (systole and diastole) that determine CO: preload (end-diastolic volume in the ventricles), which stretches the myocardial fibers; afterload (resistance to ejection); and contractility of the myocardium. Myocardial contractility depends heavily on the delivery of oxygen and nutrients to the heart. Patients with cardiomyopathy, valvular disease, hypertension, or coronary artery disease (CAD) may have oxygen deprivation to a portion of the myocardium (local) or across the entire ventricle (global), resulting in alterations in both ventricular wall motion and contractility. Deprived areas can become hypokinetic (weakly contractile), akinetic (noncontractile), or dyskinetic (moving opposite from the normal tissues). Compromised patients may also have dysrhythmias that disturb depolarization and repolarization, resulting from damage to the conduction pathways. Less frequently, the heart cannot compensate for greatly increased metabolic demands caused by disease states such as thyroid storm. These metabolically deranged patients manifest symptoms of HF as a result of oxygen delivery that is insufficient to compensate for an elevated metabolic rate.

One ventricle typically fails before the other, so pump failure may be described as either left-sided, right-sided, or both (biventricular).

Left-Sided Heart Failure

Patients may have left-sided HF resulting from problems with either ventricular systole or diastole. CAD is the cause of left-sided HF in about two-thirds of patients with LV systolic dysfunction (LVSD). With inadequate contraction of the heart during systole, blood cannot move forward effectively through the arterial system to deliver oxygen and nutrients to the rest of the body systems. Problems with diastole are related to failure of the ventricle to effectively "relax" during diastole, resulting in inadequate filling. Either cause of HF can result in pulmonary vascular congestion and edema.

Right-Sided Heart Failure

Failure of the right side of the heart results from increased resistance to right ventricular (RV) ejection, most often due to left-sided HF, pulmonary hypertension, or lung disease. RV MI, cardiomyopathy, or trauma often results in ineffective, abnormal RV wall motion, resulting in reduced ejection into the pulmonary circulation with subsequent congestion in the venous system (inferior and superior vena cava and branching vessels). Perfusion to the left ventricle is also compromised because blood does not flow at the normal rate from the right ventricle through the pulmonary vasculature into the left side of the heart.

Biventricular Failure

Patients who experience both LV and RV MI (a combination often seen with inferior wall MI) experience hemodynamics that are extremely complex to manage. The impaired right ventricle needs volume infusion to promote better expansion, or "more stretch," of the ventricle, whereas the left ventricle may be unable to accommodate a normal or pre-MI volume and requires volume reduction. Deviation of the intraventricular septum associated with right-sided HF caused by distention of the ventricle can significantly reduce the size of the left ventricle. Ultimately, failure in either side of the heart will affect both sides, because the ventricles are interdependent.

CARDIOVASCULAR ASSESSMENT: HEART FAILURE

Goal of System Assessment

Evaluate for decreased CO and decreased tissue perfusion initially with General Assessment, p. 418. If patient has developed HF secondary to acute coronary syndrome, see *Assessment in Acute Coronary Syndromes*, p. 434.

History and Risk Factors

History of HF, CAD, and MI; familial history of CAD; age greater than 65 years; cigarette smoking; alcohol use; hypercholesterolemia; hypertension; diabetes; obesity; dysrhythmias; weight gain; and decreasing activity tolerance. Fatigue may be the only presenting symptom. Other important data include understanding of and compliance with low-sodium diet, fluid restriction or medications, and a decreased exercise tolerance.

Heart Failure Assessment

Left-Sided Heart Failure Pulmonary Edema and Congestion	Right-Sided Heart Failure Cor Pulmonale and Systemic Congestion	Biventricular Failure Pulmonary and Systemic Congestion
Clinical Presentation		
Anxiety, air hunger, tachypnea, nocturnal dyspnea, dyspnea on exertion (DOE), orthopnea, moist cough with frothy sputum, tachycardia, diaphoresis, cyanosis or pallor, insomnia, palpitations, weakness, fatigue, anorexia, and changes in mentation	Fluid retention, peripheral edema, weight gain, decreased urinary output, abdominal tenderness, nausea, vomiting, constipation, and anorexia. Because the edema of heart failure is dependent, patients on bed rest may have edema of the feet, ankles, legs, hands, and/or sacrum.	All signs of both right- and left-sided heart failure, as stated, along with possible signs of cardiogenic shock in acutely ill patients: peripheral cyanosis, fatigue, decreased tissue perfusion, decrease in metabolism, and low urinary output
Physical Assessment		
Decreased BP, orthostasis (drop in BP with sitting or standing), tachycardia, dysrhythmias, tachypnea, crackles or bibasilar (or dependent) rales, S_3, or summation gallop	Hepatomegaly, splenomegaly, dependent pitting edema, jugular venous distention, positive hepatojugular reflex, and ascites	Hypotension, tachycardia, tachypnea, pulmonary edema, dependent pitting edema, hepatosplenomegaly, distended neck veins, pallor, and cyanosis
Monitoring		
Decreased CO/CI, Spo_2 and Svo_2; elevated PAP, PAWP, SVR; dysrhythmias	Dysrhythmias, elevated RAP and CVP, precipitous drop in Svo_2 with minimal activity, and possibly decreased CO/CI, caused by failure of right ventricle to pump adequate blood through the pulmonary vasculature to maintain adequate left ventricular filling volumes for normal cardiac output	Elevated PAP, PAWP, SVR, pulmonary vascular resistance (PVR), RAP, and CVP, decreased CO/CI, dysrhythmias, and decreasing Spo_2 and Svo_2, despite increasing administered oxygen

Heart Failure

Diagnostic Tests for Acute Heart Failure

Test	Purpose	Abnormal Findings
Noninvasive Cardiology		
Electrocardiogram 12-, 15-, or 18-lead ECG	Assess for ischemic heart disease and acute or older myocardial infarction (MI); may reveal atrial and/or ventricular hypertrophy, dysrhythmias such as atrial fibrillation, which may precipitate heart failure by decreasing cardiac output, and dysrhythmias associated with electrolyte imbalance.	Presence of ST-segment depression or T wave inversion (myocardial ischemia), or pathologic Q waves (resolved MI) in 2 contiguous or related leads *Contiguous leads indicative of location of ischemia or old MI:* *V1 and V2:* Intraventricular septum *V3 and V4:* Anterior wall of left ventricle *V5 and V6:* Lateral wall of left ventricle *V7–V9:* Posterior wall of left ventricle *II, III, AVF:* Inferior wall of left ventricle *V1, V1R–V6R:* Right ventricle
Blood Studies		
Digitalis levels	Digitalis levels are often difficult to manage in heart failure patients, so levels should be done daily if the dosage is being altered.	Chronic heart failure predisposes the patient to digitalis toxicity because of the low cardiac output state, which also causes decreased renal excretion of the drug.
Complete blood count (CBC) Hemoglobin (Hgb) Hematocrit (Hct) RBC count (RBCs) WBC count (WBCs)	Assess for anemia, inflammation, and infection; assists with differential diagnosis of chest discomfort and fluid balance.	May reveal decreased Hgb and Hct levels in the presence of anemia or dilution.
Electrolytes Potassium (K^+) Magnesium (Mg^{2+}) Calcium (Ca^{2+}) Sodium (Na^+)	Assess for possible causes of dysrhythmias and/or heart failure.	Abnormal levels of K^+, Mg^{2+}, or Ca^{2+} may cause dysrhythmias; elevation of Na^+ may indicate dehydration (blood is more coagulable); may reveal hyponatremia (dilutional); and may reveal hypokalemia, which can result from use of diuretics, or hyperkalemia, if glomerular filtration is decreased. Hyperkalemia can also be a side effect of angiotensin-converting enzyme inhibitors (ACEIs) and potassium-sparing diuretics.
Coagulation profile Prothrombin time (PT) with international normalized ratio (INR) Partial thromboplastin time (PTT) Fibrinogen D-dimer	Assess for efficacy of anticoagulation in heart failure patients receiving warfarin therapy; also helps to evaluate for the presence of cardiogenic shock or hypoperfusion.	Decreased PT with low INR promotes clotting and reflects inadequate anticoagulation; elevation promotes bleeding; elevated fibrinogen and D-dimer reflects abnormal clotting is present.

Diagnostic Tests for Acute Heart Failure—cont'd

Test	Purpose	Abnormal Findings
B-type natriuretic peptide (BNP)	BNP, a hormone secreted by the ventricles, can be useful in distinguishing dyspnea due to heart failure from dyspnea due to pulmonary causes and in monitoring response to therapy.	Levels >100 pg/ml support the diagnosis of heart failure. However, though the BNP level decreases with effective therapy, it may remain chronically >100, even when the patient is no longer symptomatic.
Arterial blood gas (ABG) analysis	Assesses for changes in pH and problems with oxygenation	May reveal hypoxemia caused by the decreased oxygen available from fluid-filled alveoli. Decreased pH may be present reflecting hypoperfusion at the cellular level resulting in lactic acidosis. Lactate level may be done in addition to the ABG to assess if shock is ensuing. If the lactate level is more than 4, the patient may be in cardiogenic shock.
Hepatic enzymes and serum bilirubin levels	Serum glutamate oxaloacetate transaminase/aspartate aminotransferase (SGOT/AST), serum glutamate pyruvate transaminase/alanine aminotransferase (SGPT/ALT), and serum bilirubin levels may be elevated because of hepatic venous congestion.	Elevation reflects vascular congestion resulting from heart failure that has caused decreased forward blood flow from the liver to the heart. The liver becomes engorged with blood, which results in increased hepatic enzymes and bilirubin.
Blood urea nitrogen (BUN) and creatinine levels	Rising BUN and creatinine indicate undesirable renal response to diuretic therapy.	Elevation places patients at higher risk for renal failure secondary to heart disease.
Radiology		
Chest radiograph (CXR)	Assesses size of heart, thoracic cage (for fractures), thoracic aorta (for aneurysm) and lungs (pneumonia, pneumothorax); assists with differential diagnosis of chest discomfort and activity intolerance	May reveal pulmonary edema, increased interstitial density, infiltrates, engorged pulmonary vasculature, and cardiomegaly *Note:* Portable CXR should be done with patient centered on the plate and with head of bed elevated whenever possible.
Cardiac magnetic resonance imaging (MRI)	Assesses ventricular size, morphology, function, status of cardiac valves, and circulation	Enlarged heart, remodeled heart, incompetent of stenotic heart valves, narrowed or occluded coronary arteries, which may be the cause of heart failure.
Cardiac computed tomography (CT scan)	Assesses ventricular size, morphology, function, status of cardiac valves, and circulation	Enlarged heart, remodeled heart, incompetent of stenotic heart valves, narrowed or occluded coronary arteries; technology is improving in accuracy; may eventually reduce the need for cardiac catheterization.
Cardiac ultrasound echocardiography (echo)	Assess for mechanical and structural abnormalities related to effective pumping of blood from both sides of the heart.	May reveal a reduced ejection fraction (ejection fraction <40%), ventricular wall motion disorders, valvular dysfunction, cardiac chamber enlargement, pulmonary hypertension, or other cardiac dysfunction

Heart Failure

Continued

Diagnostic Tests for Acute Heart Failure—cont'd

Test	Purpose	Abnormal Findings
Transesophageal echo	Assess for mechanical and structural abnormalities related to effective pumping of blood from both sides of the heart using a transducer attached to an endoscope.	Same as for echo but can provide enhanced views, particularly of the posterior wall of the heart
Cardiac positron emission tomography (PET scan)	Isotopes are used to assess if viable cardiac tissue is present.	Viable tissue has increased uptake of the glucose tracer and decreased uptake of the blood flow tracer (ammonia).
Invasive Cardiology		
Coronary angiography/ cardiac catheterization	Assesses for presence and extent of CAD, left ventricular function, and valvular disease using a radiopaque catheter inserted through a peripheral vessel and advanced into the heart and coronary arteries	Treatable coronary artery blockages are a major cause of new-onset HF. Low ejection fraction indicates heart failure, stenotic or incompetent heart valves can decrease CO, narrowed or occluded coronary arteries cause chest pain, abnormal pressures in the main coronary arteries indicate impaired circulation, elevated pressures inside the chambers of the heart indicate heart failure, abnormal ventricular wall motion decreases CO, and elevated pulmonary artery pressures indicate heart failure.

See diagnostic tests in *Acute Coronary Syndromes*, p. 434.

COLLABORATIVE MANAGEMENT

Care Priorities

1. **Treat the underlying cause and precipitating factors.**
Initial therapy focuses on stabilizing the hemodynamic and respiratory status and searching for reversible causes of HF. The goals of long-term therapy focus on improvement of the quality of the patient's life and management of the compensatory mechanisms causing the patient's symptoms. ACEIs and beta blockers have been shown to improve mortality and morbidity and are now the standard of care.

- *Diseases/conditions causing left-sided HF:* Atherosclerotic heart disease, acute MI (AMI), dysrhythmias, cardiomyopathy, increased circulating volume, systemic hypertension, aortic stenosis, aortic regurgitation, mitral regurgitation, coarctation of the aorta, atrial septal defect, ventricular septal defect, cardiac tamponade, and constrictive pericarditis
- *Diseases/conditions causing right-sided HF:* Left-sided HF, pulmonary hypertension, atherosclerotic heart disease, AMI, dysrhythmias, pulmonary embolism, fluid overload or excess sodium intake, COPD, mitral stenosis, pulmonary stenosis, and myocardial contusion
- *Diseases/conditions causing biventricular failure:* Any combination of the diseases that cause either right- or left-sided HF

2. **Provide oxygen therapy and support ventilation.**
Supplemental oxygen is required to optimize the patient's oxygen saturation.

Safety Alert	*Pulse oximetry is done in combination with respiratory assessment, as use of pulse oximetry alone is an inaccurate reflection of efficacy of oxygenation at the cellular level. If patient is tachypneic with increased work of breathing, noninvasive positive pressure ventilation (NiPPV, NPPV, BiPAP) may be used to reduce the work of breathing, and thus relieve additional stress associated with HF (see Acute Respiratory Failure, p. 383, for additional information regarding NiPPV, mechanical ventilation, and oxygen therapy).*

- *Pulse oximetry:* Device placed on the patient's finger or ear to determine efficacy of ventilation through measurement of oxygen saturation

3. **Provide goal-directed pharmacotherapy to help relieve symptoms and promote stabilization during acute episodes.**

Medications help reduce intravascular volume, promote vasodilation to reduce resistance to ventricular ejection, and promote enhanced myocardial contractility.

- *Diuretics:* Reduce blood volume and decrease preload. Should be used in conjunction with an ACEI or ARB. A loop diuretic is generally used initially, while a thiazide diuretic is added for patients refractory to the loop diuretic (diuretic resistance or possibly, cardiorenal syndrome) (Table 5-1). Diuretics effectively manage respiratory distress but have not been shown to improve survival. Diuretics may cause azotemia, hypokalemia, metabolic alkalosis, and elevation of neurohormone (e.g., BNP) levels.
- *Morphine:* Induce vasodilation and decrease venous return, preload, sympathetic tone, anxiety, myocardial oxygen consumption, and pain.
- *Inodilators (milrinone and inamrinone):* Phosphodiesterase-inhibiting drugs increase contractility of the heart and lower SVR through vasodilation. This allows the failing heart to pump against less pressure (reduced afterload), resulting in increased CO. Milrinone is used for hypotensive patients with low-CO HF and pulmonary hypertension. It is a more potent pulmonary vasodilator than dobutamine. Milrinone is superior to dobutamine for patients on chronic oral beta blocker therapy who develop acute hypotensive HF.
- *Inotropic agents:* Administer digitalis to slow HR, giving the ventricles more time to fill, and to strengthen contractions; administer dopamine or dobutamine to support BP and enhance contractility (see Appendix 6). Digoxin is excreted by the kidneys, so the dose is reduced for those with renal failure. Digoxin may be prescribed for patients with LVSD who remain symptomatic on standard therapy, especially if they develop atrial fibrillation. Dobutamine enhances contractility by directly stimulating cardiac beta$_1$ receptors. IV dobutamine infusions are sometimes used for patients with acute

Table 5-1	**DIURETICS**	
Type of Diuretic	**Generic Name and Initial Dose**	**Usage Information**
Loop	Furosemide (Lasix) 20 mg	Given PO or IV; PO dosage is doubled for the equivalent effect of IV dosing.
	Bumetanide (Bumex) 0.5 mg	PO and IV dosing result in the same effects from the same dosage.
	Torsemide (Demadex) 10–20 mg	Given PO or IV. Has strongest PO effects of all loop diuretics.
	Ethacrynic Acid (Edecrin) 50 mg	Given IV to patients who are allergic to furosemide, or other loop diuretics
Thiazide	Hydrochlorothiazide (HCTZ) 12.5 mg	Given PO mainly to manage hypertension; can easily lead to hypokalemia, hyponatremia, and dehydration
	Metolazone (Zaroxolyn) 2.5 mg	Given PO; should be given 30 minutes before furosemide if used together; has high incidence of hypokalemia

Heart Failure

hypotensive HF or shock. The dose of dobutamine should always be titrated to the lowest dose that maintains hemodynamic stability, to minimize adverse events. As with many inotropes, long-term infusions of dobutamine may increase mortality due to lethal dysrhythmias. Chronic dobutamine infusions should be reserved as part of palliative symptom relief and for those who have an implantable cardioverter-defibrillator (ICD) while awaiting heart transplantation. Intermittent outpatient infusions of dobutamine are no longer recommended for routine management of HF. Dopamine and dobutamine are both associated with tachycardia, which can reduce ventricular filling time.

- *Aldosterone antagonists:* Spironolactone and eplerenone have been approved for patients with HF. Aldosterone inhibition reduces sodium and water retention, endothelial dysfunction, and myocardial fibrosis but may cause hyperkalemia. Serum potassium levels must be closely monitored. These drugs should not be used in patients with a creatinine level higher than 2.5 mg/dl. Data are inconclusive for patients with mild HF. Adding an aldosterone antagonist is reasonable for those with moderately severe to severe symptoms of HF and reduced CO who agree to have both renal function and potassium concentration closely monitored. The RALES trial reported a 30% reduction in mortality and hospitalizations when spironolactone was added to standard therapy for patients with advanced HF. The EPHESUS trial reported a 15% reduction in the risk of death and hospitalization in patients receiving eplerenone with low CO HF with an ejection fraction less than 40% after an MI.

- *Vasodilators:* Nitrates (oral, topical, or IV) to dilate venous or capacitance vessels, thereby reducing preload and cardiac and pulmonary congestion. Hydralazine will dilate the resistant vessels and reduce afterload, thus increasing forward flow. The combination of hydralazine and nitrate is inferior to an ACEI in improving survival but better than the ACEI in improving hemodynamics. Nitroprusside is used when oral agents, hydralazine, or nitrates are ineffective. Prior to discontinuing nitroprusside infusions, patients should be converted to oral vasodilators (e.g., ACEIs, ARBs, or hydralazine and a nitrate.) Nitroprusside is ideally used only for a short time in patients with advanced renal disease to avoid thiocyanate toxicity, an accumulation of this byproduct of the hepatic metabolism of nitroprusside. Thiocyanate is renally excreted and may not be excreted well in those with severe azotemia or kidney failure. Nitroprusside should also be avoided in patients with acute coronary syndrome because it may cause coronary steal syndrome, which shunts blood away from the ischemic myocardium to better-perfused muscle.

- *Cardiac neurohormones:* Infusion of BNP/nesiritide is used for patients with cardiorenal syndrome, which is renal insufficiency resulting from reduced renal perfusion due to HF. Nesiritide increases CO by inducing vasodilation without increasing HR or oxygen consumption. The drug helps to regulate vasoconstrictive and sodium-retaining effects of other neurohormones. Nesiritide is administered to patients with acutely decompensated HF as a weight-based bolus followed by continuous IV infusion. It may be initiated in the emergency department and does not require hemodynamic monitoring or frequent titration. Drug tolerance and dysrhythmias are unlikely.

 - *ACEIs (benazepril, captopril, enalapril, fosinopril, lisinopril, moexipril, perindopril, quinapril, ramipril, trandolapril):* ACEIs affect the renin-angiotensin system by inhibiting the conversion of circulating angiotensin I into angiotensin II. They reduce remodeling, and both preload and afterload, to decrease the work of the ventricles while resulting in increased CO and systemic perfusion/oxygenation. Vasodilation and neurohormonal modulation with ACEIs reduce mortality and HF symptoms while improving exercise tolerance and LV ejection fraction. Emergency department visits and hospitalizations are also decreased. All patients with LVSD should be treated with an ACEI unless they have a contraindication or intolerance. ACEIs should be used in combination with beta blockers in most HF patients, particularly those with a prior MI, regardless of CO or ejection fraction. These drugs help prevent HF in patients at high risk with atherosclerosis, diabetes mellitus, or hypertension with other cardiovascular risk factors. ACEI dose should be titrated to the maximum tolerated; however, 10% to 20% of patients are ACEI intolerant. The most troubling side effect from ACEIs is cough, which may prompt a change to an angiotensin II receptor blocker (ARB) or a combination of hydralazine and a nitrate.

> **Safety Alert** *The majority of patients who cough on ACEIs are doing so because of HF rather than intolerance to the ACEI. Cough may disappear with increased diuresis. Development of either angioedema or acute renal failure requires that the drug be stopped immediately.*

- *AT$_1$ receptor antagonist (candesartan, eprosartan, irbesartan, olmesartan, losartan, telmisartan):* Have effects similar to ACEIs but have not proved to reduce mortality. AT$_1$ receptor-blocking agents are used in patients who are ACEI intolerant. These drugs were not found to be superior to ACEIs in improving mortality, but they generally have fewer side effects. ARBs are recommended as second-line therapy in patients who are intolerant to ACEIs because of cough or angioedema. ARBs help to prevent HF in high-risk patients with atherosclerosis, diabetes mellitus, and hypertension. ARBs should not be substituted for ACEIs in patients with hyperkalemia or renal dysfunction, as they are associated with similar complications.
- *Beta adrenergic blocking agents (acebutolol, atenolol, betaxolol, bisoprolol, carteolol, carvedilol, esmolol, labetalol, metoprolol, nadolol, oxprenolol, propanolol, penbutolol, sotalol, pindolol, timolol):* Not all beta adrenergic blockers are approved for use in managing HF. Only three (carvedilol, metoprolol succinate [Toprol XL], and bisoprolol) have improved survival. All stable patients with current or prior symptoms of HF and reduced ejection fraction should receive a beta blocker unless contraindicated. These drugs block the effects of circulating catecholamines released during HF. Catecholamines cause peripheral vasoconstriction, increased resistance to ventricular ejection, increased HR, and increased myocardial oxygen consumption and may precipitate myocardial ischemia and ventricular dysrhythmias. Beta blockers reduce contractility, resulting in decreased myocardial oxygen consumption and demand. Historically, reduction in contractility was the main reason many physicians hesitated to prescribe beta blockers to HF patients. Diabetes mellitus, COPD, and peripheral arterial disease do not contraindicate the use of beta blockers; however, patients with severe bronchospasm and hypotension may not tolerate these drugs. The combination of ACEI, diuretics, and beta blockers administered together may cause hypotension. Spacing the drug administration times by at least 2 hours usually relieves this effect.

4. **Manage acute pulmonary edema; include the following immediate interventions.**
   - Monitoring for signs and symptoms of *acute respiratory failure*
   - Titrating *supplemental oxygen* to maintain adequate oxygenation
   - Providing *NiPPV* for patients with increased work of breathing
   - *Elevating HOB* as needed to promote oxygenation
   - If NiPPV is unsuccessful, consider *endotracheal (ET) intubation with mechanical ventilation* (see *Acute Respiratory Failure*, p. 383).
   - *Diuretic therapy:* In severely ill patients, furosemide or bumetanide may be used as continuous IV infusion to assist with constant fluid removal. Patients with renal impairment/failure may require infusions of appropriate diuretics or ultrafiltration if other efforts to remove fluid fail.
   - *Pharmacologic therapy,* including continuous IV infusions of inotropic agents, vasodilators, beta blockers, and IV morphine. If cardiogenic shock ensues, vasopressors and intra-aortic balloon pumping (IABP) may also be necessary. If the person has evidence of renal insufficiency or failure, ACEI dosage may be reduced or the drug discontinued.

5. **Initiate a low-calorie (if weight control is necessary) and low-sodium diet.**
   - Extra salt and water are held in the circulatory system, causing increased strain on the heart. Limiting sodium (Table 5-2) will reduce the amount of fluid retained by the body. In addition, fluids may be limited to 1500 to 2000 ml/day.

6. **Initiate device or electronic therapy.**
   - *Cardiac resynchronization therapy:* Consider biventricular pacing, wherein a third electrode is implanted in a left cardiac vein via the coronary sinus so that the right and left ventricles are activated simultaneously. Relief of symptoms is achieved in approximately 70% of patients because of improved ventricular contraction and reduction of mitral regurgitation. Multiple clinical trials have shown the benefit of cardiac resynchronization therapy (CRT) for those with severe symptomatic HF with a wide QRS complex.
   - *ICD:* Approximately 50% of patients with HF die of sudden death. Implanting an ICD may improve survival in some of these patients. ICD therapy has been superior

Heart Failure

Table 5-2	**LOW-SODIUM DIETARY GUIDELINES**
Foods High in Sodium*	**Foods Low in Sodium**
Beans and frankfurters	Bread
Bouillon cubes	Cereal (dry or hot); *read labels*
Canned or packaged soups	Fresh fish, chicken, turkey, veal, beef, and lamb
Canned, smoked, or salted meats; salted fish	
Dill pickles	Fresh fruits and vegetables
Fried chicken dinners and other fast foods	Fresh or dried herbs
Monosodium glutamate (e.g., Accent)	Gelatin desserts
Olives	Oil, salt-free margarine
Packaged snack foods	Peanut butter
Pancake or waffle mix	Tabasco sauce
Processed cheese	Low-salt tuna packed in water
Seasoned salts (e.g., celery, onion, garlic)	
Sauerkraut	
Soy sauce	
Vegetables in brine or cans	
Additional suggestions	
Do not add table salt to foods.	Do not buy convenience foods; remember that fresh is best.
Season with fresh or dried herbs.	Read all labels for salt, sodium, or sodium chloride content.
Avoid salts or powders that contain salt.	

*Many of these foods now are available in low-salt or salt-free versions.

to antiarrhythmic drug therapy in preventing sudden death. Cardiac resynchronization therapy can be combined with an ICD as a single device if the patient meets the requirements for both therapies.

- *LV assist devices (LVADs):* Some patients with cardiogenic shock unresponsive to intra-aortic balloon counterpulsation and IV inotrope therapy may be referred for mechanical circulatory support. At present, LVADs are most often used as a bridge to cardiac transplantation in patients who are appropriate candidates. The inflow cannula of an LVAD is connected to the apex of the left ventricle. Blood is pumped by the device via the outflow cannula to the aorta. Complications include stroke, infection, coagulopathy with bleeding, multiple organ dysfunction syndrome (MODS), and prosthetic valve insufficiency. LVADs have been used as permanent implants (destination therapy), and advances in technology have allowed for more widespread implementation.
- *Ventricular reconstruction surgery:* Ventricular remodeling surgery, or a Dor procedure, is used to manage HF secondary to ischemic cardiomyopathy. There are several components to the procedure including coronary artery bypass grafting (CABG), mitral and tricuspid valve repair, resection of LV scar or aneurysm, reshaping the left ventricle from the remodeled spherical shape back to an elliptical shape, and epicardial LV pacing lead placement. Candidates for this procedure have CAD, severe ischemia or hibernating myocardium, LV dysfunction with akinetic or dyskinetic ventricular segments, and mitral or tricuspid regurgitation.

- *Cardiac transplantation:* Replacing the heart is a procedure of limited availability done on patients with little disease outside of end-stage HF with severely functional impairment despite optimal medical management. Patients are not transplant candidates if they have significant comorbidities, pulmonary hypertension, active infection, significant psychosocial issues, or history of medical noncompliance. Survival following a heart transplant is about 85% at 1 year. Survival declines by an additional 4% annually. Complications include rejection of the transplanted heart, infection, transplant-related CAD, and malignancy. Following cardiac transplantation, patients must maintain lifelong immunosuppression to prevent rejection, which places them at high risk for opportunistic infections and malignancies.

CARE PLANS FOR HEART FAILURE

Excess fluid volume *related to compromised regulatory mechanism secondary to decreased cardiac output*

GOALS/OUTCOMES Within 24 hours of treatment, patient becomes normovolemic as evidenced by absence of adventitious lung sounds, decreased peripheral edema, increased urine output, weight loss, PAWP less than 18 mm Hg (reasonable outcome for these patients), SVR less than 1200 dynes/sec/cm^{-5}, and CO greater than 4 L/min.
NOC Fluid Overload Severity; Fluid Balance; Electrolyte and Acid-Base Balance

Fluid/Electrolyte Management
1. Auscultate lung fields for presence of crackles and rhonchi or other adventitious sounds.
2. Monitor input and output (I&O) closely. Report positive fluid state or decrease in urine output to less than 0.5 ml/kg/hr.
3. Weigh patient daily; report increases in weight. An acute gain in weight of 1 kg can signal a 1-L gain in fluid.
4. Note changes from baseline assessment to detect worsening of HF, such as increased pedal edema, increased jugular venous distention, development of S_3 heart sound or new murmur, and dysrhythmias.
5. Monitor hemodynamic status every 1 to 2 hours and on an as-needed basis. Note response to drug therapy as well as indicators of the need for more aggressive therapy, including increasing PAWP and SVR and decreasing CO.
6. Administer diuretics, positive inotropes, inodilators, beta blockers, and vasodilators as prescribed. (See Appendix 6 for more information about inotropic and vasoactive drugs.)
7. Watch for signs and symptoms of renal insufficiency.
8. Limit oral fluids as prescribed, and offer patient ice chips or frozen juice pops to decrease thirst and relieve discomfort of dry mouth.

NIC Invasive Hemodynamic Monitoring; Medication Management; Nutrition Counseling; Surveillance; Teaching: Disease Process; Hemodialysis Therapy

Decreased CO *related to disease process that has resulted in decreased ability of the heart to provide adequate pumping to maintain effective oxygenation and nutrition of body systems*

GOALS/OUTCOMES Within 24 hours of initiating treatment, the patient has attained a cardiac index (CI) of at least 2.0, PAP is reduced to within 10% of patient's normal baseline, BP has stabilized to within 10% of baseline, and HR is controlled to within 10% of normal baseline.
NOC Cardiac Pump Effectiveness; Circulation Status

Cardiac Care: Acute Hemodynamic Regulation
1. Monitor cardiac rhythm and rate continuously.
2. Monitor CO, CI, pulmonary and systemic vascular pressures, and other hemodynamic values at least hourly, as appropriate. Implement continuous CO and Svo$_2$ monitoring if available.
3. Monitor neurologic status to assess for adequate cerebral perfusion.
4. Monitor renal function (BUN and creatinine) daily, as appropriate.
5. Monitor liver studies (SGOT/AST, SGPT/ALT, and/or bilirubin), as appropriate.
6. Monitor the other determinants of oxygen delivery, including level of Hgb and oxygen saturation.
7. Refrain from taking rectal temperatures, to prevent bradycardias.

8. Control tachycardia as soon as possible with beta blockers or other appropriate measures as determined by the physician and ACLS guidelines.
9. Obtain 12/15/18-lead ECG to assess new dysrhythmias or profound instability.
10. IABP may be necessary; prepare needed equipment for insertion of the balloon catheter and implementation of pumping.
11. If patient has atrial fibrillation, ensure that patient has been receiving appropriate anticoagulants or antiplatelet agents to prevent thrombus formation.

NIC Cardiac Care: Acute; Circulatory Care: Mechanical Assist Device; Hemodynamic Regulation; Shock Management: Cardiac; Neurologic Monitoring; Medication Management; Dysrhythmia Management

Impaired gas exchange *related to alveolar-capillary membrane changes secondary to fluid collection in the alveoli and interstitial spaces*
- -

GOALS/OUTCOMES Within 24 hours of initiation of treatment, patient has improved gas exchange as evidenced by Pao_2 at least 80 mm Hg, RR 12 to 20 breaths/min with normal pattern and depth and absence of adventitious breath sounds.
NOC Respiratory Status: Gas Exchange; Mechanical Ventilation Response: Adult

Respiratory Monitoring
1. Monitor respiratory rate, rhythm, and character every 1 to 2 hours. Be alert to RR greater than 20 breaths/min, irregular rhythm, use of accessory muscles of respiration, or cough.
2. Auscultate breath sounds, noting presence of crackles, wheezes, and other adventitious sounds.
3. Provide supplemental oxygen as prescribed and titrate to Spo_2.
4. Monitor Spo_2 for decreases to less than 92%.
5. Assess ABG findings; note changes in response to oxygen supplementation or treatment of altered hemodynamics.
6. Suction patient's secretions as needed.
7. Establish a protocol for deep breathing, coughing, and turning every 2 hours.
8. Place patient in semi-Fowler's or high Fowler's position to maximize chest excursion.
9. If mechanical ventilation is necessary, monitor ventilator settings, ET tube function and position, and respiratory status.

NIC Airway Management; Anxiety Reduction; Cardiac Care: Acute; Medication Management; Oxygen Therapy; Respiratory Monitoring

Activity intolerance *related to imbalance between oxygen supply and demand secondary to decreased functioning of the myocardium*
- -

GOALS/OUTCOMES Within the 12- to 24-hour period before discharge from the critical care unit, patient exhibits cardiac tolerance to increasing levels of activity as evidenced by RR less than 24 breaths/min, NSR on ECG, and HR 120 bpm or less (or within 20 bpm of resting HR).
NOC Activity Tolerance; Energy Conservation

Energy Management
1. Maintain prescribed activity level, and teach patient the rationale for activity limitation.
2. Organize nursing care so that periods of activity are interspersed with extended periods of uninterrupted rest.
3. To help prevent complications of immobility, assist patient with active/passive range-of-motion (ROM) exercises, as appropriate. Encourage patient to do as much as possible within prescribed activity allowances.
4. Note patient's physiologic response to activity, including BP, HR, RR, and heart rhythm. Signs of activity intolerance include chest pain, increasing SOB, excessive fatigue, increased dysrhythmias, palpitations, HR response greater than 120 bpm, SBP greater than 20 mm Hg from baseline or greater than 160 mm Hg, and ST-segment changes. If activity intolerance is noted, instruct patient to stop the activity and rest.
5. Administer medications as prescribed, and note their effect on patient's activity tolerance.
6. As needed to help prevent muscle loss and wasting, refer patient to physical therapy department.

NIC Activity Therapy; Energy Management; Teaching: Prescribed Activity/Exercise; Dysrhythmia Management; Pain Management; Medication Management

Deficient knowledge *related to disease process with HF; need to stop smoking, if applicable; activity requirements and limitations; need for daily weight log; symptoms to report; prescribed diet and fluid restriction and medications*

GOALS/OUTCOMES Within the 24-hour period before discharge from CCU, patient and significant others verbalize understanding of patient's disease, as well as the prescribed diet and medication regimens.

NOC Knowledge: Cardiac Disease Management

Teaching: Disease Process

1. Teach patient the physiologic process of HF, discussing in terms appropriate to the patient how fluid volume increases because of poor heart function.
2. Teach the patient about the adverse effects of smoking and how smoking cessation may benefit him or her. Provide information about smoking cessation classes and nicotine patches and medications prescribed to help people stop smoking, such as varenicline and bupropion.
3. Teach patient about the importance of a low-sodium diet to help reduce volume overload. Provide patient with a list of foods that are high and low in sodium. Teach patient how to read and evaluate food labels.
4. Teach patient the signs and symptoms of fluid volume excess that necessitate medical attention: irregular or slow pulse, increased SOB, orthopnea, decreased exercise tolerance, and steady weight gain ($\geq$1 kg/day for 2 successive days).
5. Advise patient about the need to keep a journal of daily weight. Explain that an increase of $\geq$1 kg/day on 2 successive days of normal eating necessitates notification of physician.
6. If patient is taking digitalis, teach the technique for measuring pulse rate. Provide parameters for withholding digitalis (usually for pulse rate less than 60/min) and notifying the physician.
7. Teach patient how to manage any advanced therapy that is used, biventricular pacemaker or internal cardiac defibrillator used for CRT, ventricular assist device (VAD), or heart transplant.
8. Instruct patient regarding the prescribed activity progression after hospital discharge, signs of activity intolerance that signal the need for rest, and use of prophylactic nitroglycerin (NTG) to reduce congestion of the heart and lungs. General activity guidelines are as follows:
   - Get up and get dressed every morning.
   - Weigh before breakfast.
   - Space your meals and activities to allow time for rest and relaxation.
   - Perform activities at a comfortable, moderate pace. If you get tired during any activity, stop to rest for 15 minutes before resuming.
   - Avoid activities that require straining or lifting.
   - Plan at least two periods a day of walking, following the guidelines in Table 5-3.
   - Warning signals to stop your activity and rest: chest pain, shortness of breath (SOB), dizziness or faintness, unusual weakness.

NIC Cardiac Care: Rehabilitation; Exercise Promotion; Smoking Cessation Assistance; Teaching: Prescribed Activity/ Exercise; Emotional Support; Progressive Muscle Relaxation; Weight Management; Mutual Goal Setting; Teaching: Prescribed Diet; Teaching: Prescribed Medication

ADDITIONAL NURSING DIAGNOSES

Also see nursing diagnoses and interventions in *Hemodynamic Monitoring* (p. 75), *Prolonged Immobility* (p. 149), and *Emotional and Spiritual Support of the Patient and Significant Others* (p. 200).

Table 5-3	ACTIVITY PROGRESSION AFTER HOSPITAL DISCHARGE	
Week	**Distance Walked**	**Time**
1–2	¼ mi	Leisurely; twice daily
2–3	½ mi	15 min
3–4	1 mi	30 min
4–5	1½ mi	30 min
5–6	2 mi	40 min

Heart Failure

ACUTE CORONARY SYNDROMES

PATHOPHYSIOLOGY

Acute or unstable coronary syndromes include chest discomfort caused by either myocardial ischemia or pain associated with MI. *Angina pectoris* is chest discomfort or pain associated with myocardial ischemia, caused by insufficient coronary blood flow to meet myocardial oxygen demands (e.g., during exercise). If the pain has a predictable pattern, it is considered stable. Those with ischemic pain that occurs at rest or with normal activity have unstable angina. Angina may occur when the coronary blood flow is reduced as a result of vessel lumen narrowing by plaque or when perfusion pressure is low, as in sudden hypotension. Angina may also be due to increased myocardial workload as in aortic stenosis, when oxygen demands are greatly elevated. The heart's workload is significantly increased by pumping against the tremendous resistance to ejection created by the narrowed aortic valve. Dysrhythmias may also cause chest discomfort caused by either increased workload (e.g., with tachycardias) or coronary perfusion deficit (e.g., with bradycardias).

AMI is necrosis of myocardial tissue resulting from relative or absolute lack of blood supply to the myocardium. Most AMIs are caused by atherosclerosis, which results in plaque formation within the coronary arteries. Plaque deposition results in endothelial changes, which over time cause narrowing of the lumen of the coronary artery. If an unstable plaque ruptures, the immune system responds with localized inflammation, platelets aggregate at the site of the injured plaque, and a thrombus forms; and if the lesion is large enough to fill the vessel lumen, this process results in total occlusion of blood flow. Occlusion can also be caused by coronary artery spasm. The site and size of MI are determined by the location of the arterial occlusion. Research has revealed that the presence of specific inflammatory substrates may be an effective tool to help diagnose progressive coronary vascular disease.

American Heart Association (AHA)/American College of Cardiology (ACC) standards recommend treatment protocols for three types of acute coronary syndromes: unstable angina, MI with ST-segment elevation (STEMI), and MI without ST-segment elevation (NSTEMI or non-STEMI). Patients with STEMI and NSTEMI evolve to an ECG with or without Q waves. The type of clot present in the coronary artery determines the appropriate treatment. Platelet-rich clots often result in unstable angina or NSTEMI, whereas fibrin-rich clots result in STEMI.

The cause of acute chest pain may not be related to myocardial ischemia. Differential diagnosis of cardiac pain versus other origins is critical and can challenge the most experienced clinician. Extracardiac causes of chest pain include pulmonary embolus, pneumonia, bronchitis, pneumothorax, aortic arch or high thoracic aortic aneurysm, esophagitis, hiatal hernia, cholecystitis, cholelithiasis, gastroesophageal reflux disease (GERD), costochondritis, musculoskeletal strain, anemia, hypoglycemia, fractured ribs or sternum, hyperthyroidism, hypothyroidism, obstipation, and bowel obstruction. Cardiac causes of chest pain not directly related to ischemia include valvular disease, cardiac trauma, cardiac tamponade, pericarditis, and endocarditis.

The diagnostic process should initially focus on ruling out MI. It is the most common cause of severe, unrelieved chest pain and requires immediate reperfusion therapy to minimize loss of myocardium. Left unchecked, patients with large areas of necrosis can progress to cardiogenic shock quickly. The patient's history and physical examination provide the initial framework for treatment decisions, coupled with the initial diagnostic ECG and assessment of serum enzyme levels and, more recently, of the presence of inflammatory substrates to evaluate for acute or impending MI. If MI does not appear likely from these findings, differential diagnosis of chest pain should then focus on identification of other life-threatening events such as dissecting thoracic or aortic arch aneurysms, large pulmonary embolism, or cardiac tamponade.

CARDIOVASCULAR ASSESSMENT: ACUTE CORONARY SYNDROME

Goal of System Assessment

- Evaluate for decreased CO and decreased tissue perfusion initially with General Assessment, p. 418.

History and Risk Factors

- Family history of CAD, age greater than 70 years, male sex, postmenopausal females, cigarette smoking, hypercholesterolemia, hyperlipidemia, hypertension, hyperglycemia, increased waist circumference, diabetes, obesity, increased stress, sedentary lifestyle, noncompliance with medication management (beta adrenergic blockers, diuretics, ACEIs, ARBs, nitrates, aspirin or other platelet inhibitors)

Chest Pain: Angina

- May result from exertion or emotional stress
- Onset can be abrupt or gradual
- *Stable angina:* Gradually increases in severity during episodes over several months; does not occur with rest; subsides gradually with rest
  - Lasts for 1 to 4 minutes; can last up to 30 minutes
  - Should be relieved by NTG in 45 to 90 seconds
- *Unstable angina:* Pain that has changed significantly from past patterns and can occur at rest; includes Wellens syndrome (left anterior descending coronary artery lesion), rest angina, preinfarction (crescendo) angina (may cause slight ST elevation and increased troponin level), Prinzmetal's angina (from coronary artery vasospasms at rest), and new-onset angina
- *Most common feelings:* Substernal pressure, chest tightness, heaviness or squeezing in the chest
- *Extreme pain:* Crushing substernal chest pain radiating down the left arm, or up to the jaw with shortness of breath
- *Variations:* Jaw or arm pain only, right- or left-sided chest discomfort, pain in the teeth, nausea, heartburn, syncope
- *No pain:* Does not rule out ischemia; common in elders, women, and diabetics, who may feel extreme, sudden onset fatigue rather than pain

Chest Pain: Acute Myocardial Infarction

- Onset can be abrupt or gradual.
- Does not subside with rest
- Lasts for longer than 30 minutes
- NOT relieved by NTG
- *Most common feelings:* Continuous substernal pressure, chest tightness, heaviness or squeezing in the chest
- *Extreme pain:* Continuous crushing substernal chest pain radiating down the left arm or up to the jaw, nausea, vomiting, SOB, orthopnea, anxiety, apprehension, diaphoresis, cyanosis, syncope, strokelike symptoms
- *Variations:* Jaw or arm pain only, right- or left-sided chest discomfort, pain in the teeth, heartburn
- *No pain:* Does not rule out infarction; 25% of MIs are "silent" or without pain; common in older adults, women, and diabetic persons, who may feel extreme, sudden-onset fatigue rather than pain

12-Lead Electrocardiogram: Angina and Acute Myocardial Infarction

- Compare current ECG with past ECG.
- *Angina:* Review for ST-segment depression in at least two contiguous leads, which indicates myocardial ischemia.
- *Acute MI:* Review for ST-segment elevation in at least two contiguous leads, which indicates active myocardial damage (acute infarction); may or may not form Q waves.
- *Evaluate pacing and conduction:* Rhythm regularity, rather, and conduction velocity (PR, QRS, QT intervals)
- *Dysrhythmias:* New bundle branch block (especially left) is diagnostic for MI; sinus bradycardia, atrioventricular (AV) heart blocks, and ventricular ectopy may also be present.

Vital Signs

- Possible fever in patients with AMI
- BP may increase or decrease, depending on sympathetic nervous system (SNS) response to change in CO.

- HR may increase or decrease depending on SNS response and ensuing damage to the conduction pathway, hypoxia; SNS response is blunted by beta adrenergic blocking agents.

Observation

Evaluate for facial and lip pallor, ashen or diaphoretic appearance of skin, ashen or cyanotic nail beds, and edema (especially dependent areas) to determine decreased tissue perfusion.

- Instruct patient to report any discomfort immediately.
- Inquire about compliance with taking cardiac medications as prescribed.

Palpation

Pulse amplitude may be increased or decreased, depending on SNS response; evaluate for:

- Pulse quality and regularity bilaterally (scale 0 to 4+)
- Edema (scale 0 to 4+): extremities and sacrum
- Slow capillary refill (longer than 2 seconds)

Auscultation

Heart sounds to evaluate for contributors to decreased CO (note changes with body positioning and respirations):

- S_1 and/or S_2 split indicative of altered conduction
- S_3 indicative of HF
- S_4 indicative of HF
- Murmurs, clicks indicative of valve disease
- Friction rub indicative of pericarditis

Labwork

Blood studies can reveal causes of dysrhythmias or changes in pacing/conduction or HR changes:

- Electrolyte levels: ↑ or ↓ potassium or magnesium
- Complete blood counts: Possible anemia, ↑ WBCs
- Cardiac enzymes/isoenzymes: Elevated if MI has occurred
- BNP: Elevated if HF is present
- Levels of cardiac medications: Low levels may reveal noncompliance with ordered medications.

Diagnostic Tests for Acute Coronary Syndrome

Test	Purpose	Abnormal Findings
Noninvasive Cardiology		
Electrocardiogram (ECG) 12-, 15-, and 18-lead ECG: must be obtained during an episode of chest pain for full benefit of help with diagnosis; should be done in a series to view evolving changes; may not reveal changes if not during an episode of chest pain	Assess for ischemic heart disease and acute or older myocardial infarction (MI); helps identify ST-segment elevation MI (STEMI) versus non–ST-segment elevation MI (NSTEMI); frames need for antiplatelet drugs versus thrombin inhibitors versus thrombolytic drugs or angioplasty (for STEMI).	Presence of ST segment depression or T wave inversion (myocardial ischemia), ST elevation (acute MI), new bundle branch block (especially left BBB) or pathologic Q waves (resolving/resolved MI) in 2 contiguous or related leads Contiguous leads indicative of location of ischemia or infarction: *V1 and V2:* Intraventricular septum *V3 and V4:* Anterior wall of left ventricle *V5 and V6:* Lateral wall of left ventricle *V7–V9:* Posterior wall of left ventricle *II, III, AVF:* Inferior wall of left ventricle *V1, V1R–V6R:* Right ventricle

Diagnostic Tests for Acute Coronary Syndrome—cont'd

Test	Purpose	Abnormal Findings
Stress tests Stress test on a treadmill with or without thallium Thallium stress test using medications	Assess for cardiac ischemia by monitoring ECG changes and chest pain during exercise on a treadmill. Thallium scan is done following the exercise to further assess for ischemic areas. Stress can also be induced using drugs that increase cardiac workload instead of treadmill exercise.	ST depression on ECG, chest pain during exercise; thallium does not accumulate normally in ischemic areas (cold spots) of the heart; for MI patients, generally used after the acute phase of MI
Cardiac radionuclide imaging Technetium-99m with pyrophosphate Technetium-99m with sestamibi	Assess myocardial perfusion to determine areas of infarction and ischemia.	Infarcted areas of myocardium appear as "hot spots" on the scan up to 10 days after MI.
Blood Studies		
Serial cardiac enzymes Myoglobin CK-MB isoform CK-MB Troponin I Troponin T	Assess for enzyme changes indicative of myocardial tissue damage; diagnostic for MI; should be done at least every 8 hours during the first 24 hours following severe chest pain.	Elevated enzymes reflect muscle damage; if CK-MB and troponins are elevated, MI has occurred. *Myoglobin:* Elevation begins in 1–3 hours, peaks 6–7 hours, subsides 24 hours *CK-MB isoform:* Elevation begins in 2–6 hours, peaks 18 hours, subsides (varies) *CK-MB:* Elevation begins in 3–12 hours, peaks 24 hours, subsides in 48–72 hours *Troponin I:* Elevation begins in 3–12 hours, peaks 24 hours, subsides 5–10 days *Troponin T:* Elevation begins in 3–12 hours, peaks 12–48 hours, subsides 5–10 days Ratio of the MB2 (cardiac) to MB1 (all muscle) types of CK-MB is also diagnostic for MI if the ratio becomes >2.5. Normal levels may vary from one institution or laboratory instrument to another. If MI is strongly suspected and CK total and MB are within normal limits (WNL), testing for troponin will provide the best diagnostic information.
Complete blood count (CBC) Hemoglobin (Hgb) Hematocrit (Hct) RBC count (RBCs) WBC count (WBCs)	Assess for anemia, inflammation and infection; assists with differential diagnosis of chest pain.	Decreased RBCs, Hgb, or Hct reflects anemia, which exacerbates chest pain; MI may increase WBCs.
Electrolytes Potassium (K^+) Magnesium (Mg^{2+}) Calcium (Ca^{2+}) Sodium (Na^+)	Assess for possible causes of dysrhythmias and/or heart failure.	Decrease in K^+, Mg^{2+}, or Ca^{2+} may cause dysrhythmias; elevation of Na^+ may indicate dehydration (blood is more coagulable); low Na^+ may indicate fluid retention and/or heart failure.

Acute Coronary Syndromes

Continued

Diagnostic Tests for Acute Coronary Syndrome—cont'd

Test	Purpose	Abnormal Findings
Coagulation profile Prothrombin time (PT) with international normalized ratio (INR) Partial thromboplastin time (PTT) Fibrinogen D-dimer	Assess for causes of bleeding, clotting, and disseminated intravascular coagulation (DIC) indicative of abnormal clotting present in shock or ensuing shock.	Decreased PT with low INR promotes clotting; elevation promotes bleeding; elevated fibrinogen and D-dimer reflect abnormal clotting is present.
B-type natriuretic peptide (BNP)	Assess for heart failure.	Elevation indicates heart failure is present.
Lipid profile and lipoprotein-cholesterol fractionation Total cholesterol High-density lipoprotein (HDL) cholesterol Low-density lipoprotein (LDL) cholesterol Very-low-density lipoprotein (VLDL) cholesterol Triglycerides	Assess for causes of arterial plaque formation contributing to coronary artery disease (CAD). Total cholesterol measures circulating levels of free cholesterol and cholesterol esters. Triglycerides assesses storage form of lipids.	Elevation of total cholesterol, LDL, VLDL, and triglycerides indicates a greater potential for developing CAD; elevated HDL lowers probability of CAD. Concentrations vary with age. *Total cholesterol:* Many physicians prefer patients to have a total cholesterol level of <200 mg/dl, but if fractionation is used, other risk factors are considered prior to recommending patients lower their cholesterol level if >200 mg/dl.
C-reactive protein (CRP)	Assess for inflammation of coronary plaque.	Elevation places patients at higher risk for acute MI.
Homocysteine	Assess for potential of accelerated plaque formation.	Elevation places patients at higher risk for acute MI.
Radiology		
Chest radiograph (CXR)	Assess size of heart, thoracic cage (for fractures), thoracic aorta (for aneurysm) and lungs (pneumonia, pneumothorax); assists with differential diagnosis of chest pain.	Cardiac enlargement, increased vascular markings and bilateral infiltrates reflect heart failure (pulmonary edema). *Note:* Portable CXR should be done with patient centered on the plate and with head of bed elevated whenever.
Magnetic resonance imaging (MRI) Cardiac MRI	Assesses ventricular size, morphology, function, status of cardiac valves and circulation	Enlarged heart, remodeled heart, incompetent of stenotic heart valves, narrowed or occluded coronary arteries
Computed tomography (CT) Cardiac CT scan	Assesses ventricular size, morphology, function, status of cardiac valves and circulation	Enlarged heart, remodeled heart, incompetent of stenotic heart valves, narrowed or occluded coronary arteries; technology is improving in accuracy; may eventually reduce the need for cardiac catheterization
Ultrasound echocardiography (echo)	Assess for mechanical and structural abnormalities related to effective pumping of blood from both sides of the heart.	Abnormal ventricular wall movement or motion, low ejection fraction, incompetent or stenosed heart valves, abnormal intracardiac chamber pressures

Diagnostic Tests for Acute Coronary Syndrome—cont'd

Test	Purpose	Abnormal Findings
Transesophageal echo	Assess for mechanical and structural abnormalities related to effective pumping of blood from both sides of the heart using a transducer attached to an endoscope.	Same as above but can provide enhanced views, particularly of the posterior wall of the heart
Positron emission tomography (PET) PET scan: cardiac	Isotopes are used to assess if viable cardiac tissue is present.	Viable tissue has increased uptake of the glucose tracer and decreased uptake of the blood flow tracer (ammonia).
Indium-111 anti-myosin imaging Indium scan: cardiac	Anti-myosin antibodies are injected along with radioactive indium-111 to visualize damaged areas	Antibodies are taken up by damaged myocardial cells as white blood cells rush to the area as part of the inflammatory process.
Invasive Cardiology		
Coronary angiography cardiac catheterization	Assesses for presence and extent of CAD, left ventricular function, and valvular disease using a radiopaque catheter inserted through a peripheral vessel and advanced into the heart and coronary arteries; allows direct injection of thrombolytic drugs	Low ejection fraction indicates heart failure, stenotic or incompetent heart valves can decrease CO, narrowed or occluded coronary arteries cause chest pain, abnormal pressures in the main coronary arteries indicate impaired circulation, elevated pressures inside the chambers of the heart indicate heart failure, abnormal ventricular wall motion decreases CO, and elevated pulmonary artery pressures indicate heart failure. Test is used to prescribe the most appropriate treatment: percutaneous coronary intervention (PCI) or cardiac surgery.

ECG Monitoring and Interpretation

First ECG: The first ECG is done immediately and is used as part of the process to differentiate AMI from angina pectoris or other causes of chest pain and to help determine suitability for antiplatelet medications (often given to patients with unstable angina and NSTEMI) versus thrombolytic therapy or other reperfusion strategy (e.g., coronary angioplasty) for MI. Reperfusion strategies should be implemented immediately for STEMI patients.

Standard 12-lead ECG: The standard 12-lead ECG is designed for evaluation of the anterior, inferior, and lateral walls of the left ventricle. Infarcts that extend to the right ventricle and/or the posterior wall of the left ventricle cannot be clearly detected by the 12-lead ECG.

15- to 18-lead ECG: Indications for performing additional ECG evaluation with 15 or 18 leads include ST-segment elevation suggestive of an inferior wall MI (II, III, AVF); isolated ST-segment elevation in V_1 or ST-segment elevation in V_1 greater than in V_2; borderline ST-segment elevation in V_5 and V_6 or in V_1 through V_3; and ST-segment depression or suspicious isoelectric ST segments in V_1 through V_3.

Serial ECGs: ECGs are then done in a series (initially and then every 30 minutes for the first 2 hours). Characteristic changes in certain lead groups identify the area and evolution of infarct. After the initial evaluation phase, ECGs may be done every 8 to 24 hours and with chest pain.

Significant Electrocardiogram Changes

ST-segment changes and new bundle branch block: The presence or absence of ST-segment elevation is used to risk stratify patients and determine the best treatment plan. ST segments are elevated in the leads "over" or facing the infarcted area. Reciprocal changes

(ST-segment depressions) will be found in leads 180 degrees from the area of infarction. New bundle branch block, especially left bundle branch block, coupled with other findings, may also indicate MI is present. Patients with STEMI are candidates for emergency reperfusion strategy: either thrombolytics within 30 minutes of arrival or percutaneous coronary intervention (PCI) within 90 minutes of arrival.

Not all patients experience STEMI. The 2007 ACC/AHA guidelines have expanded the treatment options for NSTEMI patients, who do not have ST-segment elevation, and revised treatment guidelines for patients with coronary stents in place.

Q waves: Are a later ECG change and may or may not be present with patients presenting with an MI. Are indicative of MI or are "pathologic" if they meet one of two criteria: wide (longer than 0.04 seconds) and/or deep (greater than 25% of the total voltage of the QRS). Q waves have been used as one of the diagnostic criteria for AMI to determine if a reperfusion strategy is appropriate for the patient. Patients who initially are without Q waves may develop them later, or the tissue necrosis may extend itself if a reperfusion strategy is withheld.

Safety Alert *Fewer than 42% of patients with AMI have diagnostic ST-segment elevation on their emergency department admission 12-lead ECG. Also, left bundle branch blocks (and, to a lesser extent, right bundle branch blocks) can distort the 12-lead ECG, making recognition of ST-segment elevation difficult to impossible. Mild ST-segment elevation is seen in some patients before MI, related to microemboli breaking off the ruptured plaque where the clot is evolving in the damaged coronary vessel.*

Twelve-lead ECG diagnosis of posterior wall MI can only be made by noting the reciprocal change is the anterior leads (V_1–V_3). Lead V_1 is the only lead that may indicate an isolated RV MI. Use of 15- or 18-lead ECGs that provide a more direct view of the posterior and RV walls of the heart is recommended for more accurate diagnosis of both posterior wall and RV MI.

T-wave changes: Within the initial hour of infarction, tall, peaked, "hyperacute" upright T waves may be seen in leads over the infarct. Within several hours to days, the T wave becomes inverted. Gradually over time, the ST segment becomes isoelectric and the T wave may remain inverted. T-wave changes may last for weeks and return to normal or remain inverted for the rest of the patient's life. T-wave changes reflective of posterior and RV MI are not clearly seen in the 12-lead ECG. Use of 15- or 18-lead ECGs should provide clearer information about these areas (Table 5-4).

Table 5-4	12- TO 18-LEAD ECG LOCATION OF MYOCARDIAL INFARCTION (MI)		
MI Location	**Leads Reflecting MI**	**Reciprocal Leads**	**Affected Artery(ies)**
Intraventricular septum	V_1, V_2	Not seen	Left coronary, LAD septal branch
Anterior LV	V_3, V_4	II, III, AVF	Left coronary, LAD diagonal branch
Lateral LV	V_5, V_6	V_1–V_3	Left coronary circumflex branch
Posterior LV	V_7–V_9 *	V_1–V_4	Right coronary or circumflex branch
Right ventricle (RV)	V_{1R}–V_{6R} *	Not seen	Right coronary with proximal branches
Inferior LV	II, III, AVF	I, AVL	Right coronary posterior descending branch

*Leads must be added to normal 12-lead ECG.
LAD, left anterior descending artery; LV, left ventricle.

COLLABORATIVE MANAGEMENT

ACUTE MYOCARDIAL INFARCTION HOSPITAL QUALITY ALLIANCE INDICATORS

In December 2002, the American Hospital Association (AHA), Federation of American Hospitals (FAH), and Association of American Medical Colleges (AAMC) launched the Hospital Quality Alliance (HQA), an initiative to provide the public with specific reported information about hospital performance. This national public-private collaboration encourages hospitals to voluntarily collect and report quality performance information. The Centers for Medicare and Medicaid Services (CMS) along with The Joint Commission participate in the HQA. Hospitals are expected to track and analyze their performance ratings and use the information to improve quality. The table reflects HQA measures considered essential when caring for patients following an acute MI. All indicators are evidence-based actions that should be included in the plan of care. The measurement describes the details of each indicator. Evidence of performance is derived from review of each patient's medical record following hospital discharge.

Indicators	Measure
Aspirin at arrival	Acute myocardial infarction (AMI) patients without aspirin contraindications who received aspirin within 24 hours before or after hospital arrival
Aspirin at discharge	AMI patients without aspirin contraindications who were prescribed aspirin at hospital discharge
Angiotensin-converting enzyme (ACE) inhibitor or ARB for left ventricular systolic dysfunction	AMI patients with left ventricular systolic dysfunction (LVSD) and without both ACE inhibitor and angiotensin receptor blocker (ARB) contraindications who were prescribed an ACE inhibitor or an ARB at hospital discharge
Beta-blocker at discharge	AMI patients without beta-blocker contraindications who were prescribed a beta-blocker at hospital discharge
Fibrinolytic agent received within 30 minutes of hospital arrival	AMI patients receiving thrombolytic therapy during hospital stay with a time from hospital arrival to thrombolysis of 30 minutes or less
Percutaneous coronary intervention (PCI) received within 90 minutes of hospital arrival	AMI patients receiving a PCI during the hospital stay with a time from hospital arrival to PCI of 120 minutes or less
Smoking cessation advice/counseling	AMI patients with a history of smoking cigarettes, who are given smoking cessation counseling during a hospital stay
30-day risk adjusted heart attack mortality	The measures comply with standards for publicly reported outcomes models that have been endorsed by the American Heart Association and the American College of Cardiology. These measures have been published in peer review literature and approved by the rigorous process of the National Quality Forum.

Care Priorities for All Acute Coronary Syndromes

Prevention of initial or further coronary thrombus formation may include administration of anticoagulant/antithrombin medications (i.e., unfractionated or low-molecular-weight heparin) and antiplatelet drugs (e.g., aspirin, clopidogrel, or glycoprotein [GP] IIb/IIIa inhibitors such as abciximab, eptifibatide, or tirofiban). In patients evolving toward AMI, these agents are thought to abate complete closure of the coronary arteries or to prevent more extensive clot formation. Cardiac catheterization is often performed to assess the size and location of coronary lesions. If significant lesions are found, PCI can immediately follow the cardiac catheterization in facilities that offer PCI.

1. **Relief of acute ischemic pain:**

Drugs are administered and titrated to reduce or eliminate chest pain. Morphine, oxygen, nitrates, and aspirin (MONA) are considered primary treatment modalities. The preferred order of these basic interventions is oxygen, aspirin (if not already given), nitrates, and morphine.

- *Oxygen:* Usually 2 to 4 L/min by nasal cannula, or mode and rate as directed by ABG values, to promote both myocardial and generalized increases in oxygenation. As oxygen delivery to the heart is enhanced, pain can be relieved. If the patient deteriorates, other methods of oxygen delivery may be implemented (e.g., nonrebreather mask with reservoir and mechanical ventilation for those who deteriorate markedly).

- *Aspirin:* 160 to 320 mg ideally chewed should be given immediately if the patient has not been given aspirin prior to arrival at the hospital.
- *Oral, sublingual, and other forms of nitrates/NTG:* Can be used for short-term therapy or longer-lasting prophylactic effects. These non-IV medications are used for management of myocardial ischemia or angina pectoris rather than for MI.
- IV *nitrates/NTG:* For unstable angina or evolving MI, it is titrated until relief is obtained, generally up to 200 mcg/min as long as the patient maintains a systolic BP (SBP) of at least 80 mm Hg.

 Safety Alert *Patients with chest discomfort that is unrelieved by oxygen and nitrates are in all probability having an AMI and should be evaluated immediately for a reperfusion strategy.*

- *IV or oral immediate-release morphine sulfate:* Given in small increments (e.g., 2 mg) until relief is obtained. This medication is usually not necessary unless an MI is occurring. Low BP may contraindicate administration.
2. Prevention of coronary artery clot formation:
   - *Antithrombin therapy:* Heparin (unfractionated) or low-molecular-weight heparin (fractionated) infusion is sometimes implemented to prevent clot extension and/or formation, particularly if significant ST depression (greater than 1 mm) is noted or troponins are slightly positive. Dosage should be weight based and follow a titration protocol based on ongoing studies of PTT/aPTT (partial thromboplastin time/activated partial thromboplastin time). If patients experience a drop in platelets with heparins, a direct thrombin inhibitor (i.e., Argatroban) may be used.
   - *Antiplatelet therapy:* Infusion of GP IIb/IIIa inhibitors (e.g., abciximab, eptifibatide, tirofiban) is implemented more regularly since receiving support in the AHA/ACC 2000 ACLS standards of emergency cardiac care. In patients with marked ST-segment depression (greater than 1 mm) or progressively unstable angina, antiplatelet therapy may halt the vessel occlusion process by interrupting platelet aggregation. Clots are unable to form without the "white clot scaffolding" provided by platelet aggregation. Aspirin is an antiplatelet drug.
   - *Direct thrombin inhibitors:* A new class of anticoagulants that bind directly to thrombin and block its interaction with its substrates, DTIs act independently of antithrombin, so they can inhibit thrombin bound to fibrin or fibrin degradation products. Bivalirudin is commonly used during PCI because its duration of action is short. Coagulation times return to baseline approximately 1 hour following cessation of administration.
3. Reduction of myocardial workload and myocardial oxygen consumption:
   - *Limit activities:* Restrictions based on patient's activity tolerance. Bed rest with bedside commode privileges generally is recommended for patients with AMI for up to 12 hours after symptom onset. Longer periods of bedrest can promote development of orthostatic intolerance, which is prevented by elevation of the HOB, dangling the lower extremities, and other low-exertion activities. Patients should be instructed to avoid the Valsalva maneuver when toileting, because it may predispose them to ventricular dysrhythmias.
   - *Administer medications:*
     - *Beta adrenergic blocking agents* (e.g., metoprolol, carvedilol, propranolol): To decrease HR, BP, and myocardial contractility. Strongly recommended as part of primary pharmacologic therapy for AMI patients.
     - *ACEIs* (e.g., enalapril, ramipril, quinapril): To decrease BP and thus reduce the resistance to ventricular ejection. Used for patients with myocardial ischemia and after MI if patients need long-term BP control. Effective in prevention and treatment of HF.
     - AT_1 *receptor antagonists (ARBs)* (candesartan, eposartan, irbesartan, olmesartan, losartan, telmisartan): Have similar effects to ACEIs but have not been proved to reduce mortality. ARBs are used in patients who are ACEI intolerant.
     - *Calcium channel blockers* (e.g., nifedipine, diltiazem): No longer recommended for management of patients with acute coronary syndromes unless coronary artery spasms are strongly suspected.
4. Prevention, recognition, and treatment of dysrhythmias:
ACLS algorithms or agency protocol is used.

HIGH ALERT! Caution should be exercised in the use of antidysrhythmic agents in AMI patients, especially with the management of reperfusion dysrhythmias, because instability of the conduction system with AMI is sometimes aggravated by use of antidysrhythmic agents. Electrical therapies such as synchronized cardioversion, defibrillation, external/transthoracic pacing, or transvenous pacing may provide a safer management strategy for these patients.

5. **Prevention of contrast-induced nephropathy related to use of contrast during coronary angiography/PCI:**
   - Hydration using IV and oral fluids is paramount. Mucomyst may be used to help prevent contrast-induced nephropathy.

Additional Treatments

1. **Management of unstable AMI with ST-segment elevation (STEMI):**
   - *Hemodynamic monitoring:* Used in a patient with a complicated MI resulting in ventricular failure with threat of cardiogenic shock. Pulmonary artery (PA) and capillary pressures are measured, along with CO and SVR. Unstable patients may manifest increased PAP, increased PAWP, decreased CO, and increased SVR.
2. **Acute STEMI: PCI procedures:**
   - *Percutaneous transluminal coronary angioplasty (PTCA):* The original PCI performed for improving blood flow through stenotic coronary arteries. A balloon-tipped catheter is inserted into the coronary arterial lesion, and the balloon is inflated to compress the plaque material against the vessel wall, thereby opening the narrowed lumen. PTCA is performed on individuals with AMI, postinfarction angina, postbypass angina, and chronic stable angina. The ideal candidate has single-vessel disease with a discrete, proximal, noncalcified lesion. As technology has improved, patients with more complex conditions have become routine candidates for the procedure if performed by an experienced invasive cardiologist. During the procedure, the patient is sedated lightly and is given a local anesthetic at the insertion site—usually the femoral artery. ECG electrodes are placed on the chest. An introducer sheath is inserted into the femoral artery, a guide wire is passed into the aorta and coronary artery, and the balloon catheter is passed over the guide wire to the stenotic site. The patient may be asked to take deep breaths and cough to facilitate passage of the catheter. Heparin, GP IIb/IIIa inhibitor, and/or a direct thrombin inhibitor, such as bivalirudin, is administered to prevent clot formation. The balloon is inflated repeatedly for 60 to 90 seconds at a pressure of 4 to 15 atmosphere (atm). Subsequently, radiopaque dye is injected to determine whether the stenosis has been reduced to less than 50% of the vessel diameter, which is the goal of the procedure. The femoral artery site may be closed using a device or the introducer sheath left in the femoral artery until the effect of anticoagulant medications has diminished.
   - *Complications after PTCA:* These include acute coronary artery occlusion, coronary artery dissection, reocclusion in AMI patients, AMI, coronary artery spasm, bleeding, circulatory insufficiency, renal hypersensitivity to contrast material, hypokalemia, vasovagal reaction, dysrhythmias, and hypotension. Restenosis can occur 6 weeks to 6 months after PCI, although the patient may not experience angina.
   - *Coronary artery atherectomy:* A PCI that removes atherosclerotic plaque from coronary arteries using a special catheter equipped with a cutting device that shaves the lesion. Fragments from the technique are collected into the "nose cone" of the device (directional atherectomy); pulverized and dispersed into the circulation (rotational or "rotoblade" atherectomy); or aspirated (transluminal extraction catheterization [TEC]). May be used for patients with myocardial ischemia and during or after an AMI.
   - *Intracoronary stent procedure:* A PCI wherein endovascular stents (metal-mesh tubes) are used to keep arteries open. A variety of designs, materials, and deployment procedures are available. Newer "drug-eluting" stents are coated with drugs to help prevent restenosis of the affected artery. Balloon-expanded stents are most commonly used in the United States and are inserted during PCI. May be used for stenosed coronary arteries or to reopen stenotic CABG replacement vessels (grafts).
   - *Laser coronary angioplasty:* A PCI that enables debulking of distal coronary lesions in tortuous arteries to allow for reperfusion. The laser is a part of the coronary artery catheter (similar to the device used in PTCA) and ablates only the tissue it contacts.

3. **Surgical revascularization:**
   - Surgical revascularization procedures are seldom used as the primary management strategy for AMI. Several approaches are available for myocardial revascularization, including CABG via median sternotomy or minimally invasive technique. Patients with multivessel or diffuse CAD are the most appropriate candidates for these procedures. Surgical indications include (1) stable angina with 50% stenosis of the left main coronary artery, (2) stable angina with three-vessel CAD, (3) unstable angina with three-vessel disease or severe two-vessel disease, (4) recent MI, (5) ischemic HF with cardiogenic shock, and (6) signs of ischemia or impending MI after angiography procedure. Robotics have been used recently to assist the surgeon with the procedure. Cardiac surgery should be readily available for patients who experience complications undergoing any diagnostic or treatment procedures in the cardiac catheterization laboratory.

4. **Acute STEMI: Thrombolytic therapy:**
   - *Thrombolytic therapy (lysis of coronary arterial clot):* Used for reperfusion of the occluded coronary vessel(s) that causes AMI. Drugs include tenecteplase (TNK-TPA), alteplase (rtPA, Activase), reteplase (Retavase), streptokinase, urokinase, and anisoylated plasminogen streptokinase activator complex (APSAC, Eminase) (Box 5-1 and Table 5-5). Thrombolytic therapy is an AHA/ACC Class I intervention for patients with ST-segment elevation in two or more contiguous leads, bundle branch block (obscuring ST-segment analysis), and history suggestive of AMI who present within 12 hours of symptom onset and are less than 75 years of age. Patients must be carefully screened for risk of bleeding before administration of these IV medications (Box 5-2). Time from the entry of the patient into the emergency department of the hospital to treatment with thrombolytics should be within 30 minutes of arrival. Thrombolytics are also used for direct injection into the coronary arteries as part of coronary angiography during cardiac catheterization and angioplasty.

Box 5-1 | THROMBOLYTICS

First-generation thrombolytics

Streptokinase: An enzyme derived from group C beta-hemolytic streptococci. Because it is an antigen, patients who have had previous exposure to streptococcal organisms may have antibodies against streptokinase. Therefore steroids or antihistamines are administered before streptokinase therapy to prevent a hypersensitivity reaction.

Anistreplase: A plasminogen activator that induces clot lysis with fewer systemic lytic effects than does streptokinase. Allergic and anaphylactic reactions are possible.

Second-generation thrombolytics

These are fibrin-specific, they decrease systemic activation of plasminogen and the resulting degradation of circulating fibrinogen compared to first-generation thrombolytics, and they are nonantigenic.

Alteplase: A recombinant tissue plasminogen activator (rtPA) with the same amino acid sequence as endogenous tissue plasminogen activator (tPA). Has a shorter half-life than do the other agents, less than 5 minutes. Several dosage regimens are approved for coronary thrombolysis.

Reteplase: A recombinant deletion mutein of tPA. Catalyzes cleavage of endogenous plasminogen to generate plasmin. It is not clot-specific, so fibrinogen levels fall to lower levels than those seen with rtPA (alteplase), with a return to baseline value within 48 hours after infusion. The half-life is 13 to 16 minutes, and the drug is cleared by the liver and kidneys. Dosage: given as two boluses 30 minutes apart, each over 2 minutes.

Tenecteplase: A modified form of human tPA that binds to fibrin and converts plasminogen to plasmin. In the presence of fibrin, conversion of plasminogen to plasmin is increased relative to its conversion in the absence of fibrin. This fibrin-specificity decreases systemic activation of plasminogen and the resulting degradation of circulating fibrinogen compared to a molecule lacking this property. Following administration of tenecteplase, there are decreases in circulating fibrinogen and plasminogen. Tenecteplase is given as a single 5-second bolus and is dosed by weight.

Table 5-5	THROMBOLYTIC DOSAGE REGIMENS					
Name of Agent: Generic and Brand Names	Streptokinase (Streptase)	Anistreplase (APSAC, Eminase)	Reteplase (Retavase)	Alteplase (Activase)	Alteplase (Activase)	Tenecteplase (TNKase)
Regimen	Original	Original	Double bolus	Accelerated	Original	Single bolus
Total time of regimen	30–60 min	2–5 min	30 min	90 min	180 min	5 sec.
Initial IV bolus		30 units over 2–5 min	10 units over 2 min	15 mg	6–10 mg	Weight / Dose
						<60 kg / 30 mg
						≥60 to <70 kg / 35 mg
						≥80 kg / 50 mg
Second IV bolus at time: 30 min			10 units over 2 min			
Infusion from time 0 to ≥30 min	1.5 million units IV over 30–50 min			0.75 mg/kg, max dose 50 mg		
Infusion from time 0 to 60 min					50–54 mg: 1hr total 60 mg	
Infusion from 30 to 90 min				0.50 mg/kg, max dose 35 mg		
Infusion from 60 to 120 min					20 mg	
Infusion from 120 to 180 min					20 mg	
Total dose	1.5 million units	30 units	20 units	Varies by weight, max dose 100 mg	100 mg	50 mg

Acute Coronary Syndromes

| Box 5-2 | Contraindications and Warnings for Thrombolytic Therapy |

Contraindications
- Known hypersensitivity to thrombolytic agents
- Active internal bleeding
- History of stroke
- Recent intracranial or intraspinal surgery or trauma
- Known bleeding diathesis
- Severe, uncontrolled hypertension

Warnings (risks may be increased and should be weighed against anticipated benefits)
- Recent major surgery (e.g., coronary artery bypass graft, obstetric delivery, organ biopsy)
- Previous puncture of noncompressible vessels
- Cerebrovascular disease
- Recent gastrointestinal or genitourinary bleeding
- Recent trauma
- Hypertension (systolic BP ≥180 mm Hg and/or diastolic BP ≥110 mm Hg)
- High likelihood of left-sided heart thrombus (e.g., mitral stenosis with atrial fibrillation)
- Acute pericarditis
- Subacute bacterial endocarditis
- Hemostatic defects including those secondary to severe hepatic or renal disease
- Severe hepatic or renal dysfunction
- Pregnancy
- Diabetic hemorrhagic retinopathy or other hemorrhagic ophthalmic conditions
- Septic thrombophlebitis or occluded arteriovenous cannula at a seriously infected site
- Advanced age
- Currently receiving anticoagulants (e.g., warfarin sodium)
- Any other condition in which bleeding constitutes a significant hazard or would be particularly difficult to manage because of its location

CARE PLANS FOR ACUTE CORONARY SYNDROMES

Activity intolerance *related to imbalance between oxygen supply and demand secondary to decreased cardiac output associated with coronary artery disease*

GOALS/OUTCOMES Within the 12- to 24-hour period before discharge from the CCU, the patient exhibits cardiac tolerance to increasing levels of activity as evidenced by RR less than 24 breaths/min, NSR on ECG, BP within 20 mm Hg of patient's normal range, HR less than 120 bpm (or within 20 bpm of resting HR for patients on beta-blocker therapy), and absence of chest pain.

NOC Energy Conservation, Instrumental Activities of Daily Living (IADL)

Energy Management
1. Assist patient with identifying activities that precipitate chest pain, and teach patient to use NTG prophylactically before the activity.
2. Assist patient as needed in progressive activity program, beginning with level I and progressing to level IV, as tolerated (Table 5-6).
3. Assess patient's response to activity progression. Be alert to presence of chest pain, SOB, excessive fatigue, and dysrhythmias. Monitor for a decrease in BP greater than 20 mm Hg and an increase in HR to greater than 120 bpm (greater than 20 bpm above resting HR in patients receiving beta-blocker therapy).
4. Teach patient about measures that prevent complications of decreased mobility, such as active ROM exercises. (For additional details, see "Prolonged Immobility," p. 149.)

NIC Energy Management, Self-Care Assistance: IADL

Table 5-6	**ACTIVITY LEVEL PROGRESSION FOR HOSPITALIZED PATIENTS***	
Level	**Activity**	
I	Bed rest	Flexion and extension of extremities 4 times daily, 15 times each extremity; deep breathing 4 times daily, 15 breaths; position change from side to side every 2 hr
II	OOB to chair	As tolerated, 3 times daily for 20–30 min
III	Ambulate in room	As tolerated, 3 times daily for 20–30 min
IV	Ambulate in hall	Initially, 50–200 ft twice daily; progressing to 50–200 ft 4 times daily

*Signs of activity intolerance: Decrease in BP <20 mm Hg; increase in HR to >120 beats/min (or >20 beats/min above resting HR in patients receiving beta-blocker therapy).
BP, blood pressure; *HR*, heart rate; *OOB*, out of bed.

Risk for deficient fluid volume *related to increased risk of bleeding*

GOALS/OUTCOMES The patient will not experience bleeding or a decrease in hemoglobin (Hgb) or hematocrit (Hct).
NOC Fluid Balance

Bleeding Precautions
1. Monitor dosing of all drugs known to increase bleeding, including aspirin and other antiplatelet drugs, GP IIb/IIIa inhibitors, direct thrombin inhibitors, and thrombolytics.
2. Monitor Hgb and Hct closely. Report Hgb drop greater than 2 g to physician immediately.
3. Monitor vital signs closely. Drop in BP and increase in HR may indicate developing shock, which may be cardiogenic or indicate hidden bleeding.
4. After PCI via femoral sheath, keep HOB less than 30 degrees and affected leg straight as ordered.
5. After PCI, monitor vital signs, sheath site, and distal pulses every 15 minutes until sheath is removed, then every 15 minutes × 2, then every 30 minutes × 2, then every 4 hours.
6. Carefully follow physician's orders for sheath removal after PCI.
7. If bleeding occurs at the insertion site, position the patient flat and apply pressure until hemostasis is achieved and obtain stat CBC. Notify physician or midlevel practitioner for drop in Hgb.
8. Instruct the patient to report any discomfort. Groin pain may indicate pseudoaneurysm; back pain may indicate retroperitoneal bleed.

NIC Bleeding Reduction; Surveillance; Hemorrhage Control; Neurologic Monitoring

Decreased CO (or risk for same) *related to alterations in rate, rhythm, and conduction secondary to increased irritability of ischemic tissue during reperfusion (usually occurs within 1 to 2 hours after initiation of therapy); reocclusion of thrombolysed vessels; negative inotropic changes secondary to cardiac disease; hypotension secondary to blood loss*

GOALS/OUTCOMES Within 12 hours of initiation of thrombolytic therapy or PCI, patient has adequate CO as evidenced by NSR on ECG, peripheral pulses greater than 2+ on a 0 to 4+ scale, warm and dry skin, and hourly urine output ≥0.5 ml/kg/hr. Patient is awake, alert, and oriented without palpitations, chest pain, or dizziness. Within 48 hours, patient maintains stability as just described.

Safety Alert	*Reocclusion occurs in as many as 16% of patients within 24 to 48 hours after thrombolysis.*

NOC Circulation Status

Cardiac Care
1. Monitor ECG continuously for evidence of dysrhythmias. Consult physician or midlevel practitioner for significant dysrhythmias or new or worsening ST-segment elevation.
2. With any dysrhythmia, check vital signs and note accompanying signs and symptoms such as dizziness, lightheadedness, syncope, and palpitations.

3. Ensure availability of emergency drugs and equipment: atropine, isoproterenol, epinephrine, amiodarone, lidocaine (use cautiously with AMI), defibrillator-cardioverter, and external and transvenous pacemaker.
4. Evaluate patient's response to medications and emergency treatment.
5. Monitor patient for signs of reocclusion: chest pain, nausea, diaphoresis, and dysrhythmias.
6. Consult physician for any signs of reocclusion.
7. Obtain 12/15/18-lead ECG if reocclusion is suspected.
8. Anticipate and prepare patient for cardiac catheterization, PCI with stent, or repeated thrombolytic therapy.
9. Monitor for signs of bleeding and bleeding complications: bleeding at sheath site or at IV sites, back pain (may indicate retroperitoneal bleed), signs and symptoms of cerebrovascular accident (CVA)/stroke (see *Stroke: Acute Ischemic and Hemorrhagic*, p. 674).

NIC Hemodynamic Regulation; Circulatory Care; Dysrhythmia Management; Cardiac Care: Acute

Risk for injury *related to potential for allergic or anaphylactic reaction to streptokinase or anistreplase secondary to antigen/antibody response*

GOALS/OUTCOMES Patient has no symptoms of allergic response as evidenced by normothermia, RR 12 to 20 breaths/min with normal pattern and depth, HR less than 100 bpm, BP at baseline or within normal limits, natural skin color, and absence of itching, urticaria, headache, muscular and abdominal pain, and nausea.
NOC Risk Control

Risk Identification
1. Before treatment, question patient about history of previous streptokinase therapy or streptococcal infection. Consult physician or midlevel practitioner for positive findings.
2. Administer prophylactic hydrocortisone as prescribed.
3. Monitor patient during and for 48 to 72 hours after infusion for indicators of allergy: hypotension (brief or sustained), urticaria, fever, itching, flushing, nausea, headache, muscular pain, bronchospasm, abdominal pain, dyspnea, or tachycardia. These indicators can appear immediately after or as long as several days after streptokinase therapy.
4. If hypotension develops, increase rate of IV infusion/administer volume replacement as prescribed. Prepare for vasopressor administration if there is no response to volume replacement.
5. Treat allergic response with diphenhydramine or other antihistamine as prescribed.

NIC Shock Management: Vasogenic; Shock Management

Decreased cardiac output *related to cardiac dysfunction following acute coronary event*

GOALS/OUTCOMES Within 24 hours of this diagnosis, patient exhibits adequate CO, as evidenced by BP within normal limits for patient, HR 60 to 100 bpm, NSR on ECG, peripheral pulses greater than 2+ on a 0 to 4+ scale, warm and dry skin, hourly urine output greater than 0.5 ml/kg, measured CO 4 to 7 L/min, right atrial pressure (RAP) 4 to 6 mm Hg, PAP 20 to 30/8 to 15 mm Hg, PAWP 6 to 12 mm Hg, and the patient awake, alert, oriented, and free from anginal pain.
NOC Tissue Perfusion: Cardiac

Cardiac Care, Acute
1. See Care Plans for Generalized Cardiovascular Dysfunctions, p. 419.
2. Monitor for ST-segment elevation indicative of myocardial injury, ST depression indicative of myocardial ischemia, new left bundle branch block, and Q waves indicative of MI. All ECG changes must be present in at least two contiguous (related) leads.
3. Collaborate with physician if decreased CO does not respond to acute cardiac care interventions.
4. Maintain fluid balance carefully, with close assessment for need for fluids versus diuretics. Patients with right HF may require support with IV fluids, while those with left HF may respond better to diuretics.
5. Provide patient with platelet inhibiting (e.g., clopidogrel, aspirin, abciximab) and thrombin-inhibiting medications (e.g., heparin, enoxaparin, fondaparinux, bivalirudin) as appropriate, according to AHA guidelines for STEMI or NSTEMI.

Hemodynamic Regulation
1. Monitor for unstable BP and use hemodynamic readings to help assess need for titration of vasoactive, inotropic, and antidysrhythmic medications.
2. Collaborate with physician to assess if patients with severe bundle branch block might benefit from biventricular cardiac pacing to improve synchrony of ventricular contraction.
3. Assess effects of fluid challenges on CVP and pulmonary artery occlusive pressure (PAOP); especially in patients with RV infarction.
4. Elevate legs rather than placing patients in Trendelenberg position to help augment venous return to increase BP.

Circulatory Care: Mechanical Assist Device
1. Assess peripheral circulation meticulously when intra-aortic balloon catheter is in place.
2. Evaluate impact of changes in balloon counterpulsation settings on CO, CI, all hemodynamic pressures, and BP.
3. Examine all cannulas for kinking or disconnection if patient becomes suddenly unstable without other notable cause.
4. Use strict aseptic technique when changing device-related dressings.
5. Administer anticoagulants or thrombolytics as appropriate.
6. Collaborate with physician regarding need for further interventions if patient remains unstable despite mechanical assist device and vasoactive, inotropic, and antidysrhythmic medications.

Deficient knowledge: coronary artery disease process and its lifestyle implications *related to the need to help prevent further incidence of heart disease*

GOALS/OUTCOMES Within the 24-hour period before discharge from the step-down unit, patient verbalizes understanding of his or her disease, as well as the necessary lifestyle changes that may modify risk factors.
NOC Knowledge: Disease Process; Knowledge: Medication; Knowledge: Diet; Knowledge: Energy Conservation; Sexual Identity: Acceptance; Knowledge: Sexual Functioning

Teaching: Cardiac Disease Process
1. Teach patient about ischemia and its resultant chest pain, referred to as angina pectoris.
2. Discuss the pathophysiologic process underlying patient's angina, using drawings or heart models as indicated.
3. Assist patient in identifying his or her own risk factors (e.g., cigarette smoking, high-stress lifestyle, hyperglycemia, high-fat diet).
4. Teach patient about risk factor modification:
   - *Smoking cessation:* Teach patient that smoking causes the coronary arteries to constrict, thus decreasing blood flow to the heart.
   - *Stress management:* Discuss the role that stress plays in angina. Explain that stress increases sympathetic tone, which can cause the BP and HR to increase, resulting in increased oxygen demand. By using relaxation techniques such as imagery, meditation, or biofeedback, one can decrease the effects of stress on the heart. For a sample relaxation technique, see *Appendix 7.*

NIC Teaching: Individual; Teaching: Disease Process, Thrombolysis

Altered protection *related to risk of bleeding/hemorrhage secondary to nonspecific thrombolytic effects of therapy*

GOALS/OUTCOMES Symptoms of bleeding complications are absent as evidenced by BP within patient's normal range, HR less than 100 bpm, blood-free secretions and excretions, natural skin color, baseline or normal level of consciousness (LOC), and absence of back and abdominal pain, hematoma, headache, dizziness, and vomiting.
NOC Risk Control

Risk Identification
1. When patient is admitted, obtain a thorough history, assessing for the following:
   - Risk factors for intracranial hemorrhage: uncontrolled hypertension, cerebrovascular pathology, central nervous system (CNS) surgery within previous 6 months
   - Bleeding risks: recent or active gastrointestinal (GI) bleeding, recent trauma, recent surgery, bleeding diathesis, advanced liver or kidney disease
   - Risk of systemic embolization: suspected left-sided heart thrombus
   - History of streptococcal infection or previous streptokinase therapy

2. Monitor clotting studies per agency protocol. Regulate heparin drip to maintain PTT at $1\frac{1}{2}$ to 2 times control levels or according to protocol. Never discontinue heparin without consulting with a physician or midlevel practitioner.
3. Apply pressure dressing over puncture sites. If cardiac catheterization was performed, inspect site at frequent intervals for evidence of hematoma formation. Immobilize extremity for 6 to 8 hours after catheterization procedure.
4. Avoid unnecessary venipunctures, IM injections, or arterial puncture. Obtain laboratory specimens from heparin-lock device.
5. Monitor patient for indicators of internal bleeding: back pain, abdominal pain, decreased BP, pallor, and bloody stool or urine. Report significant findings to physician or midlevel practitioner.
6. Monitor patient for signs of intracranial bleeding every 2 hours: change in LOC, headache, dizziness, vomiting, and confusion.
7. Test all stools, urine, and emesis for occult blood.
8. Use care with oral hygiene and when shaving patient. For more information about safety precautions, see *Pulmonary Embolus*, p. 396.

Teaching: Diet and Prescribed Medications
1. *Diet low in cholesterol and saturated fat:* Provide sample diet plan for meals that are low in cholesterol and saturated fat. Teach patient about foods that are high and those that are low in cholesterol and saturated fat. Stress the importance of reading food labels.
2. *Blood pressure control:* If patient was found to have hypertension associated with MI, the patient should be taught the importance of taking appropriate medications to control BP and to follow recommended dietary guidelines to minimize sodium intake. Sodium promotes water retention, which can increase the BP. Higher systemic BP increases the workload of the heart, demanding that more myocardial oxygen be consumed.
   - Teach patient about the prescribed medications, including name, purpose, dosage, action, schedule, precautions, and potential side effects.
   - Teach patient the actions that should be taken if chest pain is unrelieved or increases in intensity.

Teaching: Activity/Exercise
If chest pain occurs:
1. Stop and rest.
2. Take 1 NTG; wait 5 minutes. If pain is not relieved, take a second NTG; wait 5 minutes. If pain is not relieved, take a third NTG.
3. Lie down if headache occurs. The vasodilation effect of NTG causes a decrease in BP, which may result in orthostatic hypotension and transient headache.
4. If the pain is not relieved after 3 NTGs taken over a 15-minute period, dial 911 or the local emergency number.
5. Explain to the patient that it is no more beneficial to be in the emergency department than it is to be at home during episodes of chest pain caused by angina and therefore traveling to a hospital at the first sign of chest pain usually is unnecessary.
6. Review activity limitations and prescribed progressions (see Tables 5-3 and 5-6). Provide the following information:
   - When you are discharged from the hospital, it is important that you continue your walking program. Do not overestimate your ability; rather, start off slowly and build up. Depending on how you feel, you may only be able to stay at one level or you may progress to 2 miles quickly. Remember to warm up and cool down with stretches for 5 to 7 minutes and to walk three to five times each week.
   - Avoid sudden energetic activities.
   - Plan for regular rest periods in the afternoon.
   - Let your body guide you regarding whether to increase or decrease activity.
   - Inform your physician of any changes in activity tolerance, such as the development of new symptoms with the same activity.
7. Avoid exercising outdoors in very cold, hot, or humid weather. Extreme weather places an additional stress on the heart. If you do exercise in extremes of weather, decrease the pace and monitor your response carefully.
8. Pulse monitoring: Teach patient how to take pulse, including parameters for target HRs and limits.

Teaching: Sexuality
Sexual activity guidelines: Because sexual activity is a physical activity, certain guidelines can help the patient and his or her partner enjoy a satisfying sexual relationship while minimizing the workload of the heart:
1. Rest is beneficial before engaging in intercourse.
2. Find a position that is comfortable for you and your partner. Assuming a different position that is uncomfortable to both may increase the workload of the heart.

3. Medications such as NTG may be taken prophylactically by the patient before intercourse to prevent chest pain.
4. Postpone intercourse for 1 to 2 hours after eating a heavy meal.
5. Report the following symptoms to your physician if they are experienced after sexual relations: SOB, increased HR that persists for longer than 15 minutes, unrelieved chest pain.

NIC Teaching: Disease Process; Teaching: Prescribed Activity/Exercise; Teaching: Prescribed Medication; Teaching: Sexuality

Acute pain (chest) *Related to biophysiologic injury related to decreased oxygen supply to the myocardium*

GOALS/OUTCOMES Within 30 minutes of intervention, patient's subjective evaluation of discomfort improves, as documented by a pain scale. Nonverbal indicators, such as grimacing, are absent. Vital signs return to baseline. ECG changes present during event resolve.
NOC Pain Control

Pain Management
1. Assess and document the character of the patient's chest pain, including location, duration, quality, intensity, precipitating and alleviating factors, presence or absence of radiation, and associated symptoms. Devise a pain scale with patient, rating discomfort from 0 (no pain) to 10 or any system that assists in objectively reporting pain level.
2. Measure BP and HR with each episode of chest pain. BP and HR may increase because of sympathetic stimulation as a result of pain. If the chest pain is caused by ischemia, the heart muscle may not be functioning normally and CO may decrease, resulting in a low BP. In addition, dysrhythmias such as bradycardia and ventricular ectopy may be noted with ischemia. If BP is low, it may not be advisable to administer nitrates and morphine, which can further reduce BP, adding to myocardial ischemia.
3. After each titration of IV NTG, evaluate patient's BP and the effects of therapy in relieving patient's chest pain. If slight hypotension occurs (80 to 90 mm Hg systolic), reduce the flow rate to one-half or less of the infusing dose. If severe hypotension (less than 80 mm Hg SBP) occurs, stop the infusion and contact the physician for further directions. In either situation, the physician may prescribe a normal saline infusion or low-dose positive inotropic agent (e.g., dopamine, dobutamine) to enhance cardiac contractility.

Safety Alert *Inotropic agents increase the oxygen demands of the myocardium and may increase ischemia.*

4. Monitor for side effects of NTG, including headache, hypotension, syncope, facial flushing, and nausea. If side effects occur, place patient in a supine position and consult physician for further interventions.
5. Administer heparin, GP IIb/IIIa inhibitors (abciximab, tirofiban, eptifibatide), and aspirin as prescribed. Heparin infusion usually should be administered using a weight-based protocol, which is titrated according to PTT results. These patients are predisposed to bleeding and may need to be placed on bleeding precautions.
6. Maintain a quiet environment and group patient care activities to allow for periods of uninterrupted rest. Consider healing touch therapy, relaxation exercises, or music therapy.
7. Position patient according to his or her comfort level.
8. Provide care calmly and efficiently; reassure patient during chest pain episodes.
9. Ensure that activity restrictions and bedrest are maintained; teach patient about activity limitation and its rationale — to minimize oxygen requirements and thus decrease chest pain. Reassure patient activities are allowed based on individual response. Often, patients may be afraid to engage in activities for fear of further deterioration.
10. Instruct patient to report any further episodes of chest pain.

Dysrhythmia Management
1. Obtain a 12/15/18-lead ECG during patient's episode of chest pain. During angina, ischemia usually is demonstrated on the ECG by ST-segment depression and T-wave inversion.
2. Administer nitrates as prescribed, titrating IV NTG so that chest pain is relieved yet SBP remains greater than 90 mm Hg. NTG drip is usually 50 mg NTG in 250 ml D_5W. Begin with 6 ml/hr, which is 5 mcg/min. Titrate by increments of 10 to 20 ml every 5 minutes (or 10 to 20 mcg/min every 5 minutes) up to a maximum dosage determined by agency protocol, physician, or midlevel practitioner.

3. As prescribed, administer beta-blockers and possibly calcium channel blockers, which relieve chest pain by (1) diminishing coronary artery spasm, causing coronary and peripheral vasodilation, and (2) decreasing myocardial contractility and oxygen demand. Monitor for side effects, including bradycardia and hypotension. Be alert to indicators of HF, including fatigue, SOB, weight gain, and edema, and to indicators of heart block, such as syncope and dizziness.
4. Administer oxygen per nasal cannula at 2 to 4 L/min, as prescribed.

NIC Analgesic Administration; Cardiac Care: Acute; Hemodynamic Regulation

CARE PLANS FOR PATIENTS UNDERGOING PERCUTANEOUS CORONARY INTERVENTION

Deficient knowledge *related to angioplasty procedure and postprocedure care*

GOALS/OUTCOMES Within the 24-hour period before the procedure, patient describes the rationale for the procedure, how it is performed, and postprocedure care. Patient relates discharge instructions within the 24-hour period before discharge from the CCU.

NOC Knowledge: Treatment Procedure(s); Knowledge: Medications; Knowledge: Disease Process

Teaching: Cardiac Disease Process
1. Assess patient's understanding of CAD and the purpose of angioplasty. Evaluate patient's style of coping and degree of information desired.
2. As appropriate for coping style, using a heart drawing, discuss the location of the patient's CAD with the patient and significant others.

Teaching: Procedure/Treatment
1. Use of local anesthesia and sedation during procedure
2. Insertion site of catheter: groin or arm
3. Sensations that may occur: mild chest discomfort, a feeling of heat as the dye is injected
4. Use of fluoroscopy during procedure. Determine patient's history of sensitivity to contrast material.
5. Ongoing observations made by nurse after procedure: BP, HR, ECG, leg or arm pulses, blood tests
6. Importance of lying flat in bed for 6 to 12 hours after procedure unless a vascular closure device was used. Patients are able to get out of bed sooner when a closure strategy is used.
7. Necessity for nursing assistance with eating, drinking, and toileting needs after procedure
8. Need for increased fluid intake after procedure to flush dye from system
9. If patient and significant others express or exhibit evidence of anxiety regarding the procedure, try to arrange for them to meet with another patient who has had a successful angioplasty.

Teaching: Prescribed Medication
Discharge instructions:
1. Importance of taking antiplatelet drugs to prevent restenosis
2. Importance of taking statins and other antilipid drugs to prevent progression of CAD
3. Avoidance of strenuous activity during first few weeks at home
4. Follow-up visit with cardiologist 1 week after hospital discharge
5. Signs and symptoms to report to health care professional (e.g., GI upset, repeat of angina, fainting)

NIC Teaching: Procedure/Treatment; Anxiety Reduction; Support Group

ADDITIONAL NURSING DIAGNOSES

Also see nursing diagnoses and interventions as appropriate in *Nutritional Support* (p. 117), *Mechanical Ventilation* (p. 99), *Hemodynamic Monitoring* (p. 75), *Prolonged Immobility* (p. 149), *Emotional and Spiritual Support of the Patient and Significant Others* (p. 200), *Acute Cardiac Tamponade* (p. 257), *Heart Failure* (p. 421), and *Dysrhythmias and Conduction Disturbances* (p. 492).

ACUTE INFECTIVE ENDOCARDITIS

PATHOPHYSIOLOGY

Infective endocarditis (IE) is infection of the endocardium (the innermost layer of the heart), often involving the natural or prosthetic valve; it is caused by bacteria, viruses, fungi, or rickettsiae. Forty percent of patients with IE have no underlying heart disease. Four mechanisms are known to contribute to the development of IE. The first is a congenital or acquired defect of the heart valve or the septum (i.e., septal defect, stenotic or insufficient valve), often accompanied by a jet-Venturi stream of blood flowing from a high-pressure area to a low-pressure area through a narrow opening. The low-pressure area beyond the narrowed jet-flow site provides an ideal site for colonization by any infecting organism. Rheumatic valvular disease evolves in about 40% of patients. The mitral valve is most often affected. The second mechanism is the formation of a sterile thrombus at the low-pressure site, which gives rise to vegetation. Third, a bacteremia occurs as a result of colonization in the vegetation. Fourth, a high level of agglutinating antibodies promotes growth of the vegetation, which usually develops on the low-pressure side of the valve leaflet within 1 to 2 cm of the tip of the leaflet.

Portals of entry for the infecting organism include the mouth and GI tract, upper airway, skin, and external genitourinary (GU) tract. All heart valves are at risk for infection, but the aortic and mitral valves are more commonly affected than the right-sided pulmonic and tricuspid valves. IV drug abuse increases the possibility of tricuspid IE. Once the infection process begins, valvular dysfunction, manifested by insufficiency with regurgitant blood flow, can occur, ultimately resulting in a decrease in CO. The vegetation may enlarge and obstruct the valve orifice, further reducing CO. The vegetation may break apart and embolize to vital organs. In severe cases, the affected valve may necrose, develop an aneurysm, and rupture or the infection may extend through the myocardium and epicardium to cause a pericarditis (see *Acute Pericarditis*, p. 461). If the conduction system is affected by the spreading infection, bundle branch block may occur. The chordae tendineae can become infected and rupture, resulting in severe acute mitral or tricuspid regurgitation. Complications of IE occur suddenly, with a dramatic change in the clinical picture. Mortality rates between 20% and 50% have been reported. The infection recurrence rate is 10% to 20%. The incidence of IE is higher in patients over age 50 years, is more common in men than in women, and is uncommon in children.

ASSESSMENT

Goal of Assessment

The goal is to identify the severity of symptoms. The severity of symptoms varies depending on the infective organism. (For example, *Staphylococcus aureus* infection is more severe than that with *Streptococcus viridans*.) Acute presentation is defined as onset within 1 week of infection, while subacute infections may take up to 4 weeks to present.

History and Risk Factors

Patients at higher risk for bacteremia leading to IE include those with valvular disease undergoing invasive procedures and insertion of devices including temporary pacemakers, PA catheters, and central IV catheters or ports; those undergoing endoscopy, surgery, or dental work, and immunosuppressed patients (e.g., with organ transplants, carcinoma, burns, or diabetes mellitus). Users of illicit IV drugs are at risk of tricuspid valve disease. Drug abusers with IE are commonly young males.

Vital Signs

- Fever, tachycardia, possible dysrhythmias, possible hypotension

Hemodynamic Measurements

Invasive monitoring devices are used cautiously with these patients, as they may cause further valvular dysfunction, embolization, and infection.

- PA catheters are used to assess hemodynamic function if necessary.
- Elevations of PAP and CVP, with reduced CO, are expected in most patients with IE.

Observation

- The skin is often pale.
- If right-sided HF is present, skin and sclera may be jaundiced and edematous, with neck vein distention, a positive hepatojugular reflex, and ascites.
- Late assessment findings include anemia, petechiae, and clubbing of the fingers.
- Splenomegaly occurs by 10 days due to the activation of the reticuloendothelial system. If marked, a splenic infarct may have occurred.
- *Acute infective stage:* Diaphoresis, fatigue, anorexia, joint pain, weight loss, and abdominal pain
- *Splinter hemorrhages:* Small red streaks on the distal third of the fingernails or toenails
- *Janeway lesions:* Painless, small, hemorrhagic lesions found on the fingers, toes, nose, or earlobes, probably occurring as the result of immune complex deposition with inflammation
- *Osler nodes:* Painful, red, subcutaneous nodules found on the pads of the fingers or on the feet, probably occurring as a result of emboli producing small areas of gangrene or vasculitis
- *Roth spots:* Retinal hemorrhages with pale centers seen on fundoscopic examination

---

 Safety Alert *If emboli of the vegetations occur in other areas, signs and symptoms of stroke or peripheral, myocardial, renal, or mesenteric arterial insufficiency, occlusion, or infarct will be seen.*

Auscultation

- A new or changed murmur may be heard as a result of the valvular dysfunction.
- If HF is present, fine crackles may be auscultated at the lung bases, and an S_3 or S_4 heart sound may be audible.

Screening Labwork

Blood studies can reveal presence of infection or further and progressive heart status, such as HF, conduction problems, or ischemia.

- Cardiac enzymes/isoenzymes: To rule out MI as a cause of chest discomfort or shortness of breath
- BNP: Elevated if HF is present
- Levels of cardiac medications: Low levels may reveal noncompliance with ordered medications.

12-Lead Electrocardiogram

Evaluates for changes from last ECG to assess for worsening of heart disease (myocardial damage). ECG changes resulting from electrolyte imbalances may also decrease CO. An initial 12-lead ECG should be done on every patient and used for comparison over the course of hospitalization.

- Heart rate: Diagnose type of tachycardia, bradycardia, or irregular rhythm. During acute episodes, atrial dysrhythmias such as PAT, PACs, atrial flutter, or atrial fibrillation may occur.
- PR, QRS, QT intervals: May increase, but may be regular with a normal rate and conduction velocity.
- ST-segment and T-wave changes: Depression or elevation

Diagnostic Tests for Infective Endocarditis

Test	Purpose	Abnormal Findings
Noninvasive Cardiology		
12-lead electrocardiogram (ECG)	Frequently performed to determine if ischemia or conduction system defects are present	Heart block may manifest if the AV node or bundle of His is affected by the infection. Atrial and/or ventricular enlargement may be seen from the prolonged effects of valve disease. Chambers may be enlarged or muscle walls thickened (see Table 5-7). Atrial dysrhythmias including premature atrial contractions (PACs), paroxysmal atrial tachycardia (PAT), and atrial fibrillation (AF) are frequently seen as chambers enlarge from volume overload (see Table 5-8).
Blood Studies		
Serial cardiac enzymes Myoglobin CK-MB isoform CK-MB Troponin I Troponin T	Assess for enzyme changes indicative of myocardial tissue damage; diagnostic for MI; rule out MI.	Elevated if MI occurs from embolization of vegetations into the coronary arteries
Complete blood count (CBC) RBC count (RBCs) WBC count (WBCs)	Assess for signs of infection.	Increased WBCs and eosinophils, with reduced RBCs/possible anemia
Electrolytes Potassium (K^+) Magnesium (Mg^{2+}) Calcium (Ca^{2+}) Sodium (Na^+)	Assess for electrolyte imbalance, which helps with differential diagnosis.	May be normal. Potassium or magnesium is sometimes increased or decreased.
ABGs	Determine effectiveness of oxygenation.	Indicative of cardiac and pulmonary status (see *Acid-Base Imbalances*, p. 1)
Coagulation profile Prothrombin time (PT) with international normalized ratio (INR) Partial thromboplastin time (PTT) Fibrinogen D-dimer	Assess for causes of bleeding, clotting, and disseminated intravascular coagulation (DIC) indicative of abnormal clotting present in shock or ensuing shock.	Decreased PT with low INR promotes clotting; elevation promotes bleeding; elevated fibrinogen and D-dimer reflects abnormal clotting is present. In the presence of effusions, anticoagulants are contraindicated because of the high risk of cardiac tamponade, which can result from bleeding into the pericardium.
Blood cultures For low suspicion of IE: 3–6 sets of aerobic and anaerobic blood cultures should be drawn from different venipuncture sites over 24 hours.	Provides definitive diagnosis of the infecting organism. Antibiotics are prescribed based on organism sensitivity. Drawn 1 hour apart over 3 hours. *If suspicion is high*, cultures should be drawn within 1–2 hours and empiric antibiotic treatment begun. Cultures can be negative when IE is present as a result of slow-growing organisms, prior antibiotic use, failure to obtain adequate number of specimens, or the organism's failure to grow in standard culture media.	The most common bacteria found in native (the patient's) valve IE are *Streptococcus viridans* (60%), *Staphylococcus aureus* (25%), and the HACEK group (*Haemophilus, Actinobacillus, Cardiobacterium, Eikenella,* and *Kingella* spp.). Manipulations of the gastrointestinal (GI) or genitourinary (GU) tract may result in IE from *Enterococcus faecalis*. Early prosthetic valve infections are caused by *Staphylococcus epidermidis* (33%), gram-negative bacteria (19%), and *S. aureus* (17%). *Candida* is the most common fungal source of IE, accounting for 8% of prosthetic valve endocarditis and 1% of native valve endocarditis.

Acute Infective Endocarditis

Continued

Diagnostic Tests for Infective Endocarditis—cont'd		
Test	**Purpose**	**Abnormal Findings**
Additional studies Rheumatoid factor Erythrocyte sedimentation rate (ESR) IE gamma globulins B-type natriuretic peptide (BNP)	To identify the causes of IE and associated diseases	Rheumatoid factor and ESR are elevated. IE gamma globulins may be present. BNP will be elevated if heart failure is present.
Radiology		
Chest radiograph (CXR)	Assess size of heart, mediastinum, thoracic cage (for fractures), thoracic aorta (for aneurysm) and lungs (pneumonia, pneumothorax); assists with differential diagnosis of chest pain.	Cardiac enlargement may reflect widening mediastinum and tamponade.
Computed tomography (CT) Cardiac CT scan	Assesses ventricular size, morphology, function, status of cardiac valves, and circulation. May be done to assess for embolization to other organs.	
Ultrasound echocardiography (echo) Transesophageal echo	Reveals valvular involvement and vegetation size and defines severity of valvular dysfunction. M-mode, two-dimensional, Doppler, and transesophageal echocardiograms (TEEs) are used. TEE is the preferred test.	Detects vegetation, especially with prosthetic valves. Obtained within 2 hours of acute presentation, the test is 90% specific and sensitive. Preexisting IE may be indistinguishable from new vegetations.
Arteriograms: renal, mesenteric, and peripheral	Assess for embolization.	If embolization is present, affected organs are compromised and may fail.

COLLABORATIVE MANAGEMENT
Care Priorities
1. **Prevent infective endocarditis in patients undergoing invasive procedures:**
The American Heart Association recommends prophylactic antibiotics for *high- or moderate-risk* patients with valvular disease, before and after selected invasive procedures (bronchoscopy, cystoscopy, biopsy of urinary tract/prostate, tonsillectomy, adenoidectomy, esophageal dilation/sclerotherapy, transurethral prostatectomy, lithotripsy, and gynecologic procedures) in the presence of infection and dental work to prevent or reduce the risk of IE. Those at *low risk* (patients who have undergone cardiac revascularization, pacemaker insertion, or atrial septal defect repair or have mitral valve prolapse with normal leaflets and no regurgitation) no longer require antibiotic prophylaxis.

- *High risk:* Includes those with bioprosthetic valve replacement, valvular repair, complex cyanotic congenital repairs, systemic or pulmonary conduits, and previous IE
- *Moderate risk:* Includes those with other noncyanotic congenital defects, valvular dysfunction, hypertrophic cardiomyopathy, and mitral valve prolapse with evidence of regurgitant blood flow or thickened valve leaflets
- *Treatment of streptococcal infected endocarditis:* Patients should be treated for at least 2 weeks in the hospital and observed for cardiac and noncardiac complications. Patients may be a candidate for outpatient and home parenteral antibiotic therapy.

Table 5-7	ASSESSMENT FINDINGS WITH VALVULAR HEART DISEASE		
Valve Dysfunction	**Murmur**	**Pathology**	**Hemodynamic Changes**
Aortic stenosis	Systolic, blowing murmur at second ICS, RSB; may radiate to the neck	Reduced flow across aortic valve with ↑ LV volume and pressure, with ↓ CO; LV hypertrophy eventually occurs	↑ LV pressure; ↑ PAEDP; ↓ CO and aortic pressure with a narrow pulse pressure reflecting the decreased stroke volume
Aortic insufficiency	Diastolic blowing murmur at second ICS, RSB, beginning immediately with S_2	Regurgitant blood flow from aorta to LV during diastole	↑ LV pressure and PAEDP; ↓ CO; ↑ systolic BP and widened pulse pressure
Mitral stenosis	Loud, long, diastolic rumbling murmur at fifth ICS, MCL; may radiate to axilla; S_1 is loud and there is an opening snap with S_2	Reduced flow across mitral valve with left atrial and pulmonary congestion	↑ Mean PAP; ↓ CO
Mitral insufficiency	Systolic murmur at fifth ICS, MCL	Regurgitant blood flow from LV to left atrium, resulting in pulmonary congestion	Giant V waves in the PA occlusive tracing; ↑ systolic PAP; ↓ CO; mean PAP may be normal
Pulmonic stenosis	Systolic blowing murmur at second ICS, LSB; may radiate to neck	Reduced flow across pulmonic valve with ↑ RV volume and pressure, with diminished LV return, resulting in ↓CO	↑ RV systolic pressure, mean RAP, PAEDP, and mean PAP
Pulmonic insufficiency	Diastolic murmur at second ICS, LSB that starts later and is lower pitched than aortic murmur	Regurgitant blood flow from pulmonary artery to RV during diastolic, resulting in RV overload	↑ systolic RV pressure with wide pulse pressure; LVEDP and CO often normal but ↓ may if disorder is severe
Tricuspid stenosis	Diastolic murmur at fourth ICS	Reduced flow across tricuspid valve with ↑ right atrial and venous congestion	CVP ↑ with accentuated A wave on the RA waveform
Tricuspid insufficiency	Pansystolic murmur at fourth ICS, LSB that increases in intensity with inspiration	Regurgitant blood flow from RV to RA; right atrial and venous congestion occurs	↑ CVP with prominent V wave on the RA tracing; normal or low PAP, LVEDP, and CO

BP, blood pressure; *CO*, cardiac output; *CVP*, central venous pressure; *ICS*, intercostal space; *LSB*, left sternal border; *LV*, left ventricle/ventricular; *LVEDP*, left ventricular end-diastolic pressure; *MCL*, midclavicular line; *PA*, pulmonary artery; *PAEDP*, pulmonary artery end-diastolic pressure; *PAP*, pulmonary artery pressure; *RA*, right atrium; *RAP*, right atrial pressure; *RSB*, right sternal border; *RV*, right ventricle/ventricular.

Acute Infective Endocarditis

- *Treatment of coagulase-negative species causing prosthetic valve endocarditis within the first year after valve replacement:* Patients are usually methicillin-resistant. They should be given. A combination of vancomycin and refampicin for at least 6 weeks with the addition of gentamicin for the initial 2 weeks.
2. **Treat infection and prevent further complications, such as emboli, HF, or cardiogenic shock:**
   - *Antibiotics:* Patients usually require 4 to 6 weeks of IV antibiotics. The first 2 weeks may be initiated during hospitalization and the remaining therapy done on outpatient status. The vegetation must be sterilized, abscesses treated, and spread of infection prevented. Initial antibiotic selection is empirical followed by therapy based on the results of the blood/tissue culture and sensitivity studies.

Table 5-8	**ECG CHANGES FREQUENTLY FOUND WITH VENTRICULAR AND ATRIAL HYPERTROPHY**
Chamber	**ECG Change**
Left ventricular enlargement	"R" voltage increases in V_{4-6}; "S" voltage increases (deeper inflection) in V_{1-2}; the sum of "S" in V_1 or V_2 and "R" in V_5 or V_6 will be more than 35 mm, or "R" in any V lead will be more than 25 mm
Left atrial enlargement	"P mitrale" in leads II, III, aV_F, and V_1; P wave is m-shaped with a duration more than 0.1 sec
Right ventricular enlargement	"R" voltage increases in V_1 or V_2; "S" voltage increases in V_5, V_6; sum of "R" in V_1 or V_2 and "S" in V_5 or V_6 will be more than 35 mm
Right atrial enlargement	"P pulmonale" in leads II, III, aV_F, and V_1; P wave is 2.5 mm voltage and 0.1 sec duration

- *Fluid and sodium restriction:* Used for optimal fluid balance with reduced heart function or HF. Specific restrictions must be individualized and based on severity of symptoms.
- *Bedrest:* May be used initially, with activity as tolerated for the remainder of treatment
- *Diet:* High in protein and calories to prevent cardiac cachexia and support the immune system
- *Watch for signs of embolization during the first 3 months of treatment:* Monitor renal status, vital signs, and oxygenation.

3. **Pharmacotherapy:**
   - *Oxygen therapy with pulse oximetry (Spo_2):* Oxygen (Fio_2) to maintain Pao_2 at 80 mm Hg or higher and pulse oximetry to monitor oxygen saturation continuously or intermittently to keep Spo_2 at 95% or higher
   - *Diuretics:* May be used to decrease symptoms of HF by reducing intravascular volume
   - *Positive inotropic agents (e.g., digoxin, dobutamine, milrinone, inamrinone):* Used to increase contractility and CO
   - *Vasodilators:* nitroprusside, nitroglycerin: Reduce cardiac work and improve coronary arterial perfusion. Both preload and afterload (end-diastolic ventricular volume and pressure) may be reduced to help relieve symptoms of HF. Aggressive vasodilation is not well tolerated by all patients
   - *Sedation:* May be necessary to allay anxiety and to reduce myocardial oxygen consumption

4. **Manage HF and/or cardiogenic shock:**
   See *Heart Failure* (p. 421) and *Cardiogenic Shock* (p. 472).

5. **Consider surgical valve replacement:**
   Required when HF worsens or if the infection fails to respond to antibiotics (see *Valvular Heart Disease*, p. 566). An abscess or infected tissue may be surgically removed if there is no response to long-term antibiotics. If the patient is hemodynamically stable, surgery may not be needed. A surgeon is usually consulted in case of an HF emergency.
   - Indications for urgent native valve replacement:
     - Heart failure due to acute aortic or mitral regurgitation
     - Persistent fever and bacteremia for longer than 8 days despite adequate antimicrobial therapy
     - Abscesses, pseudoaneurysms, abnormal communications like fistulas or rupture of one or more valves, conduction disturbances, myocarditis, or other findings indicating local spread of infection
     - Antibiotic-resistant microorganisms (e.g., fungi, *Brucella* and *Coxiella* spp.) or microorganisms with a high potential for rapid destruction of cardiac structures (e.g., *S. lugdunensis*)
   - Indications for replacement of prosthetic valves: Complications that may prompt the need to replace a prosthetic valve include primary valve failure, prosthetic valve endocarditis, prosthetic valve thrombosis, thromboembolism, and mechanical hemolytic anemia.
   Prosthetic valve endocarditis (PVE): The hallmark sign of PVE in mechanical valves is ring abscesses. Ring abscess may lead to valve dehiscence, perivalvular leakage, and formation of myocardial abscesses. Extension to the conduction system may prompt a

new atrioventricular block. Valve stenosis and purulent pericarditis are seen less often. Valve stenosis is more common with bioprosthetic valves than mechanical valves. Bioprosthetic valve PVE results in leaflet tears or perforations. Ring abscesses, purulent pericarditis, and myocardial abscesses are seen less often in bioprosthetic valve PVE.

Early PVE: Occurs within 60 days of valve insertion and is usually the result of perioperative contamination

Late PVE: Occurs 60 days or later after insertion and is usually the result of transient bacteremia from dental or GU sources, GI manipulation, or IV drug abuse

---

CARE PLANS FOR ACUTE INFECTIVE ENDOCARDITIS

Decreased cardiac output *related to altered preload, afterload, or contractility secondary to valvular dysfunction*

GOALS/OUTCOMES Within 72 hours after initiation of therapy, patient has adequate hemodynamic function with NSR or controlled atrial fibrillation as evidenced by the following: HR less than 100 bpm, BP greater than 90/60 mm Hg, stable weight, intake equal to output plus insensible losses, RR less than 20 breaths/min with normal depth and pattern, and absence of S_3 or S_4 heart sounds, crackles, distended neck veins, and other clinical signs of HF. Optimally, the following normal parameters will be achieved: CO 4 to 7 L/min, CVP 4 to 12 mm Hg, and MAP 60 to 105 mm Hg.

NOC Cardiac Pump Effectiveness; Circulation Status

Cardiac Care

1. Assess heart sounds every 2 to 4 hours. A change in the characteristics of a heart murmur may signal progression of valvular dysfunction, which can occur with insufficiency, stenosis, dislodgment of vegetation, or unseating of a prosthetic valve.
2. Assess heart sounds. A new S_3 or S_4 sound may signal HF.
3. Monitor heart rhythm continuously. Report dysrhythmias, which may indicate the spread of infection to the conduction system or atrial volume overload.
4. Monitor for signs of left-sided HF: crackles, S_3 or S_4 sounds, dyspnea, tachypnea, digital clubbing, decreased BP, increased pulse pressure, increased serum BNP levels, increased LVEDP, and decreased CO.
5. Monitor for signs of right-sided HF: increased CVP, distended neck veins, positive hepatojugular reflex, edema, jaundice, increased serum BNP levels, and ascites.
6. Monitor I&O hourly, and measure weight daily. Use the same scale and amount of clothing, and weigh patient at the same time of day for accuracy. Consult physician if patient's weight increases by more than 1 kg per day.
7. If patient's CVP is high, decrease preload by limiting fluid and sodium intake and administer diuretics and venous dilators (e.g., NTG) as prescribed.
8. If patient's MAP is high, decrease afterload with prescribed arterial dilators (e.g., nitroprusside).
9. For low CVP or BP, consult with physician or midlevel practitioner. Vasopressors may be prescribed. Patient may be developing sepsis, so monitor carefully.
10. If diastolic BP is low, coronary artery perfusion may be reduced. Prevent further reductions by avoiding administration of morphine sulfate or rapid warming of hypothermic patients. Increase contractility with inotropic drugs, as prescribed.
11. Provide activities as tolerated. Intolerance indicates ineffective oxygenation.
12. Help patient reduce stress and myocardial oxygen consumption by teaching stress-reduction techniques such as imagery, meditation, or progressive muscle relaxation. For description of a relaxation technique, see *Appendix 7*
13. Provide sedation as needed.
14. Prevent orthostatic hypotension by changing patient's position slowly. See *Cardiogenic Shock*, p. 472, for a discussion of preload and afterload medications.

NIC Energy Management

Impaired gas exchange *related to alveolar-capillary membrane changes with decreased diffusion of oxygen secondary to pulmonary congestion*

GOALS/OUTCOMES Within 24 hours of initiation of oxygen therapy and during the weaning process, patient has adequate gas exchange as evidenced by RR less than 20 breaths/min with normal pattern and depth, Svo_2 60% to 80%, Pao_2 greater than 80 mm Hg, Sao_2 greater than 95%, and natural skin color.

NOC Respiratory Status: Gas Exchange; Tissue Perfusion: Pulmonary

Ventilation Assistance
1. Assess rate, effort, and depth of respirations. RR increases in response to inadequate oxygenation. Tachypnea may indicate pulmonary congestion.
2. Assess color of skin and mucous membranes. Pallor signals impaired oxygenation.
3. Auscultate lungs every 2 hours. Report crackles, rhonchi, and wheezing.
4. If hemodynamic monitoring with oximetry is used, assess Svo_2. It may fall because increased metabolic demands have increased oxygen uptake, or because the patient has increased extraction as a result of reduced perfusion/oxygen delivery. Svo_2 values may fall before the patient is symptomatic; they correlate with CO.
5. Monitor ABG values for evidence of hypoxemia (Pao_2 less than 80 mm Hg), respiratory acidosis ($Paco_2$ greater than 45 mm Hg, pH less than 7.35), or respiratory alkalosis ($Paco_2$ less than 35 mm Hg, pH greater than 7.45) from tachypnea. Either may indicate impending respiratory failure.
6. Deliver oxygen as prescribed. Observe respiratory rate of COPD patients if oxygen is increased to avoid hypoventilation and/or respiratory arrest.
7. Assess arterial oxygen saturation with pulse oximetry. Normal oxygen saturation is 95%–99%. Levels of 90%–95% necessitate frequent assessment. Levels less than 90% require aggressive interventions to increase oxygen saturation. Consider increasing Fio_2, decreasing preload, and taking measures to improve ventilation.
8. Place patient in high Fowler's position to facilitate gas exchange as tolerated.
9. Have patient cough, deep breathe, and use incentive spirometry to prevent atelectasis.

NIC Invasive Hemodynamic Monitoring; Oxygen Therapy; Respiratory Monitoring

Risk for infection (systemic) *related to presence of invasive catheters and lines; inadequate secondary defenses secondary to prolonged antibiotic use*

GOALS/OUTCOMES Patient is free of secondary infection as evidenced by clear urine with normal odor, wound healing within acceptable time frame, and absence of erythema, warmth, and purulent drainage at insertion sites for IV lines. On resolution of acute stage of IE, patient remains normothermic with WBC count less than 11,000/mm³, negative culture results, and HR less than 100 bpm. CO is less than 7 L/min, and Svo_2 is 60% to 80%. No yeast overgrowth infections are present. Patient and significant others verbalize rationale for antibiotic therapy and identify where and how to obtain guidelines.

NOC Infection Severity

Infection Protection
1. Use strict aseptic technique to care for all invasive monitoring device insertion sites and IV lines. Rotate central lines per hospital protocol. Discuss feasibility of a tunneled catheter or peripherally inserted central catheter (PICC) line with physician.
2. Change tubing, containers, and peripheral insertion sites per agency protocol. Inspect all catheter insertion sites daily for redness, drainage, or other evidence of infection. Rotate site immediately if infection is suspected.
3. Provide mouth care at least every 4 hours to minimize fungal and other infections. Women may require antifungal medications to manage vaginal yeast infections.
4. Provide perineal care with soap and water for patients with indwelling urinary catheters. Inspect urine for evidence of infection, such as casts, cloudiness, or foul odor. Be alert to patient complaints of burning with urination after catheter is removed.
5. Monitor temperature, WBC count, and HR. Increases may be signs of infection.
6. Calculate SVR with CO measurements. Symptoms of septic shock include increased CO, decreased SVR, and increased Svo_2 during the early stages.
7. Teach patient and significant others the importance of reporting signs and symptoms of recurring infections (e.g., fever, malaise, flushing, anorexia) or HF (e.g., dyspnea, tachypnea, tachycardia, weight gain, peripheral edema).
8. Stress the importance of prophylactic antibiotics before invasive procedures such as dental examinations or surgery. The AHA publishes general guidelines for prophylactic antibiotic treatment to prevent IE.

NIC Fever Treatment; Surveillance; Infection Control

Ineffective tissue perfusion (or risk for same) renal, gastrointestinal, peripheral, cardiopulmonary, and cerebral *related to interrupted arterial blood flow secondary to emboli caused by vegetations*

GOALS/OUTCOMES Patient has adequate perfusion as evidenced by urine output at least 0.5 ml/kg/hr, at least 5 bowel sounds/min, peripheral pulses at least 2+ on a 0 to 4+ scale, warm and dry skin, BP at least 90/60 mm Hg, RR 12 to 20 breaths/min with normal pattern and depth, NSR on ECG, and orientation to time, place, and person.
NOC Circulation Status

Hemodynamic Regulation

> **Safety Alert** *Unlike peripheral venous emboli, these emboli are caused by the vegetations; therefore, prevention is difficult. Interventions are aimed at early detection of embolization and supportive therapies.*

1. Monitor I&O at frequent intervals. Be alert to urinary output less than 0.5 ml/kg/hr for 2 consecutive hours. Report oliguria, as it may signal impending acute renal failure.
2. Monitor bowel sounds every 2 hours. Report hypoactive or absent bowel sounds. Patients are at risk for decreased mesenteric perfusion and mesenteric or bowel infarction.
3. Assess peripheral pulses, color, and temperature of extremities. Weak pulses (2+ or less on a 0 to 4+ scale) with pale, cool limbs/hands/feet may denote peripheral embolization.
4. Monitor patient for confusion and changes in sensorimotor capabilities or cognition, which may signal cerebral emboli.
5. Assess for chest pain, decreased BP, SOB, ischemic or injury pattern on 12-lead ECG, or elevated cardiac enzyme levels indicative of MI caused by vegetation emboli that have migrated to the coronary arteries (see *Acute Coronary Syndromes*, p. 434).
6. Assess for and report appearance of splinter hemorrhages, Osler's nodes, Janeway's lesions, and Roth's spots (see *Assessment*, p. 418).

NIC Circulatory Care; Cardiac Care: Acute

ADDITIONAL NURSING DIAGNOSES

As appropriate, also see nursing diagnoses and interventions in *Nutritional Support* (p. 117), *Hemodynamic Monitoring* (p. 75), *Prolonged Immobility* (p. 149), *Emotional and Spiritual Support of the Patient and Significant Others* (p. 200), *Acute Cardiac Tamponade* (p. 257), *Heart Failure* (p. 421), and *Cardiogenic Shock* (p. 472).

ACUTE PERICARDITIS

PATHOPHYSIOLOGY

Pericarditis is the general term for an inflammatory process involving the pericardium and the epicardial surface of the heart. Inflammation can occur as the result of an AMI, an infection, chronic renal failure, or an immunologic, chemical, or mechanical event (Box 5-3). Often, early pericarditis manifests as a dry irritation, whereas late pericarditis (after 6 weeks) involves pericardial effusions that can lead to cardiac tamponade if severe. Pericarditis is often seen in the critical care unit as a secondary finding following coronary revascularization surgery or valve replacement or associated with chronic renal failure. A thorough assessment and recognition are essential for appropriate treatment, as symptoms can be masked by the primary condition. For example, patients are sometimes transferred into a critical care unit with acute cardiac decompensation resembling acute coronary syndrome, when in reality, the condition is caused by pericardial effusions.

The initial pathophysiologic findings of pericarditis include infiltration of polymorphonuclear leukocytes, increased vascularity, and fibrin deposition. Inflammation may spread from the pericardium to the epicardium or pleura. The visceral pericardium may develop exudates or adhesions. Large effusions can lead to cardiac tamponade. The excess fluid compresses the heart within the pericardial sac, which impairs filling of the chambers and ventricular ejection.

Acute Pericarditis

Box 5-3	CAUSES OF PERICARDITIS

- Autoimmune cardiac injury
- Dressler syndrome (post AMI)
- Drug induced (e.g., hydralazine, phenytoin)
- Hypothyroidism
- Idiopathic
- Infection (bacterial or viral)
- Myocardial infarction
- Metabolic disorders
- Neoplasms
- Postpericardiotomy syndrome
- Radiation injury
- Rheumatologic disease
- Rheumatic fever
- Rheumatoid arthritis
- Systemic lupus erythematosus
- Sarcoidosis
- Trauma
- Uremia

ASSESSMENT
Goal of Assessment
The goal is to assess severity of the symptoms and to rule out acute coronary syndrome at the cause of ECG changes (ST-segment elevation and/or depression) and chest pain. Acute pericarditis is characterized by chest pain, pericardial friction rub, and serial electrocardiographic changes. Severe pericardial effusions can cause cardiac tamponade.

History and Risk Factors
AMI, recent bacterial or viral infection, chronic renal failure, autoimmune disease including rheumatoid arthritis and systemic lupus erythematosus, radiation therapy, cardiac surgery, or chest trauma. Viral infection is the more common cause (1% to 10%) of acute pericarditis, followed by bacterial infection, which can lead to purulent pericarditis (1% to 8%). Tuberculosis causes 1% to 4% of cases.

Observation
The patient presents with chest pain, but the location and quality can vary. Pain can be a knife-like, stabbing pain that may radiate to the neck or shoulder. Usually the pain is aggravated by a supine position, coughing, deep inspiration, and swallowing. Dyspnea develops because of shallow breathing to prevent pain.

Early indicators of pericarditis: Fatigue, pallor, fever, and anorexia

Late indicators and evidence of effusions: Increased dyspnea, crackles, and neck vein distention. Joint pain may be present when inflammation is generalized. Evaluate for signs of pain, distress and tamponade.

- Dyspnea level and oxygen need
- Neck vein distention assessment
- Use of pain scale to determine progress of treatment

Vital Sign Assessment
Heart rate, heart rhythm, and BP are used to evaluate CO and perfusion.

- *BP elevated on right arm:* When BP is taken on both arms, if cardiac tamponade is ensuing, blood cannot flow into and through the constricted heart.
- *Narrowing pulse pressure:* May indicate effusion is exerting pressure around the heart
- *Pulsus paradoxus:* BP should be checked for a paradoxical pressure greater than 10 mm Hg. Normally the systolic pressure is slightly higher during the expiration and lower during inspiration. When effusions are present, this difference in systolic pressure across the respiratory cycle will be greater than 10 mm Hg.
- *Tachycardia:* Heart rate is usually rapid and regular.
- *Beck's triad:* Hypotension, elevated venous pressure with jugular venous distention, and muffled heart sounds may occur in patients with cardiac tamponade, especially if sudden intrapericardial hemorrhage occurs.

Hemodynamic Measurements

If used, the PA catheter reveals elevated CVP, PAP, and PAWP.

- *As effusions increase:* CO will decrease. If adhesions are present, the filling of the chambers may be restricted, resulting in reduced end-diastolic volumes and pressures.
- *If cardiac tamponade is developing:* Pressures in all heart chambers eventually equalize and the patient has a cardiac arrest.

Auscultation

Heart sounds may reveal an intermittent pericardial friction rub with one, two, or three components: atrial systole, ventricular systole, and rapid ventricular filling. Heart sounds can be distant, and the pulmonic component of the second heart sound will be accentuated.

Pericardial friction rub: The rub is heard best with the diaphragm of the stethoscope positioned at the left lower sternal border. The rub is often positional, so auscultation should be done with the patient in several positions (i.e., supine, sitting and leaning forward, lying on the left lateral side). A friction rub may not be heard, even in the presence of pericarditis.

Screening Labwork

- Complete blood count: May reveal elevated WBCs and anemia
- Cardiac enzymes: Isoenzymes may be elevated if the epicardium is inflamed.

12-Lead Electrocardiogram

Evaluates for changes from last ECG; assesses for worsened heart disease (myocardial damage) or electrolyte imbalances that may decrease CO; should be done on every patient to use for comparison.

- *Heart rate:* Diagnose type of tachycardia, bradycardia, or irregular rhythm. During acute episodes, atrial dysrhythmias such as PAT, PACs, atrial flutter, or atrial fibrillation may occur.
- *PR, QRS, QT intervals:* May lengthen or shorten
- *ST-segment and T-wave changes:* Depression or elevation
- *Pacing and conduction:* Regular, normal rate and velocity
- *Late dysrhythmias:* Include ventricular ectopy or bundle branch blocks if the inflammatory process involves the ventricles. Pericardial effusion may decrease the voltage of the QRS complex on the ECG. Diffuse ST-segment elevation can be documented as described in Table 5-9.

Table 5-9	ECG CHANGES WITH PERICARDITIS	
Stage	**Time of Change**	**Pattern**
1	Onset of pain	ST segments have a concave elevation in all leads except AVL and V_1; T waves are upright
2	1–7 days	Return of ST segments to baseline with T wave flattening and invert
3	1–2 wk	Inversion of T waves without R or Q changes
4	Weeks to months	ECG returns to prepericarditis state

Diagnostic Tests for Acute Pericarditis		
Test	**Purpose**	**Abnormal Findings**
Noninvasive Cardiology		
Electrocardiogram (ECG) 12-, 15-, and 18-lead ECG	Differentiate between ischemia versus inflammation	Will show ST-segment or T-wave changes, which often are confused with ischemic changes. In pericarditis, they are more diffuse and follow a four-stage pattern (see Table 5-9).

Continued

Acute Pericarditis

Diagnostic Tests for Acute Pericarditis — cont'd

Test	Purpose	Abnormal Findings
Blood Studies		
Serial cardiac enzymes Myoglobin CK-MB isoform CK-MB Troponin I Troponin T	Assess for enzyme changes indicative of myocardial tissue damage; diagnostic for MI; rule out MI.	May reveal elevation of the CK and MB bands if the epicardium is inflamed
Complete blood count (CBC) Hemoglobin (Hgb) Hematocrit (Hct) RBC count (RBCs) WBC count (WBCs) Anti–streptolysin O (ASO) titer C-reactive protein Sedimentation rate	Assess for anemia, inflammation, and infection; assists with differential diagnosis of chest pain.	Decreased RBCs, Hgb, or Hct reflects anemia from blood loss. Anti–streptolysin O (ASO) titer is elevated when the cause of the pericarditis is an immunologic disorder. If the pericarditis is the result of an infection, blood cultures will identify the infecting organism. Other markers of inflammation can be seen (elevated WBCs, C-reactive protein [CRP], lactate dehydrogenase [LDH], or erythrocyte sedimentation rate [ESR]) unless the pericarditis is secondary to uremia.
Electrolytes Potassium (K^+) Magnesium (Mg^{2+}) Calcium (Ca^{2+}) Sodium (Na^+)	Assess for electrolyte status.	Use to rule out other causes.
Coagulation profile Prothrombin time (PT) with international normalized ratio (INR) Partial thromboplastin time (PTT) Fibrinogen D-dimer	Assess for causes of bleeding, clotting, and disseminated intravascular coagulation (DIC) indicative of abnormal clotting present in shock or ensuing shock.	Decreased PT with low INR promotes clotting; elevation promotes bleeding; elevated fibrinogen and D-dimer reflect abnormal clotting is present. In the presence of effusions, anticoagulants are contraindicated because of the high risk of cardiac tamponade, which can result from bleeding into the pericardium.
Radiology		
Chest radiography (CXR)	Assess size of heart, mediastinum, thoracic cage (for fractures), thoracic aorta (for aneurysm), and lungs (pneumonia, pneumothorax); assists with differential diagnosis of chest pain.	Cardiac enlargement may reflect widening mediastinum and tamponade. Cardiac enlargement not always present with tamponade.
Computed tomography (CT) Cardiac CT scan	Check for effusions, both pericardium and epicardium. Assess ventricular size, morphology, function, status of cardiac valves, and circulation.	Will differentiate restrictive pericarditis from constrictive cardiomyopathy by means of the appearance of thickened pericardium on the cross-sectional views of the thorax, which occurs with pericarditis

Diagnostic Tests for Acute Pericarditis — cont'd

Test	Purpose	Abnormal Findings
Ultrasound Echocardiography (echo) Transesophageal echo (TEE)	Assess for mechanical abnormalities related to effective pumping of blood from both sides of the heart. Assess for fluid in both the pericardial sac and pleural space.	Will show absence of echoes in the areas of effusion. This test, which is essential for quantifying and evaluating the trend of effusions, will appear normal if the pericarditis is present without effusions. TEE may be helpful in identifying some areas of effusion and provide an enhanced view of the posterior wall of the heart.
Magnetic resonance imaging (MRI)	Check for effusions, both pericardium and epicardium.	

COLLABORATIVE MANAGEMENT
Care Priorities

1. **Relieve acute pain:**

May experience retrosternal or left precordial chest pain, nonproductive cough, and SOB. Pleural effusion may be present.

- *Oxygen:* Usually 2 to 4 L/min by nasal cannula, or mode and rate as directed by arterial blood gas (ABG) values or pulse oximetry. Used to promote both myocardial and generalized increases in oxygenation. As oxygen (O_2) delivery to the heart is enhanced, pain can be relieved. If the patient deteriorates, other methods of O_2 delivery may be implemented (e.g., nonrebreather mask with reservoir and mechanical ventilation for those who deteriorate markedly).
- *Aspirin:* 160 to 320 mg ideally chewed. Should be given immediately if the patient has not been given aspirin prior to the hospital.
- *Nonsteroidal anti-inflammatory drugs (NSAIDs):* Preferred for reducing inflammation, particularly if the patient has had an MI or cardiac surgery, since these drugs do not delay healing as do corticosteroids. NSAIDs have fewer side effects than do steroids. Examples include aspirin, indomethacin, and ibuprofen. NSAIDs can increase fluid retention and may cause renal insufficiency and worsen HF, as well as pose risk for gastrointestinal bleeding.
- *Colchicine:* Reduces inflammation in the body; may be prescribed as a first-line treatment for pericarditis or as a treatment for recurrent symptoms. Colchicine can reduce the length of pericarditis symptoms and decreases the risk that the condition will recur. However, the drug is not safe for people with certain pre-existing health problems, such as liver or kidney disease. Carefully check the patient's health history before prescribing colchicine.
- *Prednisone:* Given at 20 to 80 mg daily for 5 to 7 days if there is no response to NSAIDs. Corticosteroids are contraindicated if pericarditis occurs secondary to an AMI because they can cause thinning of the scar formation and increase risk of rupture. Must be tapered gradually to avoid adrenal insufficiency.
- *Medications to manage the cause:* Antibiotics, immunoglobulin, antifungals, chemotherapy

2. **Prevent cardiac damage and manage pericardial effusions to prevent cardiac tamponade.**

- *Subxiphoid pericardiocentesis:* Performed if effusions persist and cardiac status decompensates. A needle (used in a tamponade emergency) or catheter is used to remove the fluid compressing the heart. Echocardiography is used to guide the catheter tip and assess the amount of effusion remaining. The pericardial catheter may be removed after the fluid has been withdrawn or may be left in place for several days to allow for gradual removal of fluid. Usually 100 ml or more is withdrawn every 4 to 6 hours. The catheter is flushed with saline every 4 to 6 hours after withdrawal of the effusion to prevent clotting. Strict aseptic technique is essential for preventing infection.
- *Pericardiectomy:* A surgical procedure to prevent cardiac compression or relieve the restriction. It may be necessary in chronic pericarditis for patients with recurrent effusions or adhesions. This procedure is often required in severe and recurrent pericarditis associated with uremia.

CARE PLANS FOR ACUTE PERICARDITIS

Ineffective breathing pattern *related to guarding as a result of chest pain*

GOALS/OUTCOMES Within 48 hours of this diagnosis, patient demonstrates RR 12 to 20 breaths/min with normal depth and pattern and reports that chest pain is controlled.

NOC Respiratory Status: Ventilation

Respiratory Monitoring

1. Assess rate and depth of respirations along with the character and intensity of the chest pain. Provide prescribed pain medication as needed.
2. Teach patient to avoid aggravating factors such as a supine position. Encourage patient to alter his or her position to minimize the chest pain. The following positions may be helpful: side-lying, high Fowler's, or sitting and leaning forward.
3. Assess lung sounds every 4 hours. If breath sounds are decreased, encourage patient to perform incentive spirometry exercises every 2 to 4 hours along with coughing and deep-breathing exercises.
4. To facilitate coughing and deep breathing, teach the patient to support the chest by splinting with pillows or by holding the arms around the chest.

NIC Positioning; Pain Management

 Activity intolerance *related to bedrest, weakness, and fatigue secondary to impaired cardiac function, ineffective breathing pattern, or deconditioning*

GOALS/OUTCOMES Within 72 hours of this diagnosis, patient exhibits cardiac tolerance to increasing levels of exercise as evidenced by peak HR less than 20 bpm over patient's resting HR, peak SBP less than 20 mm Hg over patient's resting SBP, Svo$_2$ at least 60%, RR less than 24 breaths/min, NSR on ECG, warm and dry skin, and absence of crackles, murmurs, and chest pain during or immediately after activity.

NOC Energy Conservation; Endurance; Activity Tolerance

Energy Management

| **Safety Alert** | *Steroid myopathy may develop in patients who receive high doses or long-term treatment with steroids. Muscle weakness occurs in the large proximal muscles. Patients experience difficulty in lifting objects and moving from a sitting position to a standing position. Steroids also increase the risk of developing osteoporosis and bone fracture; therefore, when on chronic therapy, the patient should have recommended daily intake of calcium and vitamin D.* |

1. Assess the patient for evidence of muscle weakness; assist with activities as needed.
2. Modify the activity plan for the patient with post-MI pericarditis who is receiving steroids. A lower activity level may help prevent thinning of the ventricular wall and reduce the risk of an aneurysm or rupture of the ventricle.
3. Teach patient to resume activities as tolerated, resting between activities.
4. For other interventions, see this nursing diagnosis in *Prolonged Immobility*, p. 149.

NIC Cardiac Care: Rehabilitative; Teaching: Prescribed Activity/Exercise

ADDITIONAL NURSING DIAGNOSES

Also see *Decreased Cardiac Output* in *Acute Cardiac Tamponade* (p. 263). For other nursing diagnoses and interventions, see *Prolonged Immobility* (p. 149).

AORTIC ANEURYSM/DISSECTION

PATHOPHYSIOLOGY

An aortic aneurysm is an abnormal dilation of the vessel, with an increase of at least 50% its normal diameter. Conditions that weaken the medial layer or increase stress on the vessel wall can lead to dilation, aneurysmal formation, and eventually rupture or dissection of the aorta. Pathologies related to the aorta can be life-threatening due to the potential for disruption of blood flow to a large portion of the body, including vital organs such as the brain, heart, kidneys, and GI tract. Symptoms may mimic other conditions, and survival depends largely on timely diagnosis and rapid intervention to preserve end-organ function.

Aneurysms are usually described based on their location along the aorta (thoracic, abdominal) and their morphology. A *true aneurysm* involves all three layers of the arterial wall (intima, media, adventitia). The two forms of a true aneurysm are fusiform (symmetrical dilation of the entire circumference of the aorta) and saccular (eccentric ballooning of only a portion of the aortic wall). A *false aneurysm* or *"pseudoaneurysm"* is a hematoma caused by injury to the aortic wall, resulting in blood contained by the adventitia or surrounding tissue.

Most often aneurysms develop at the site of an atherosclerotic lesion, which precipitates degeneration of the tissue and allows the arterial wall to dilate. With advancing age, the elastin in the aorta is decreased, which further weakens the vessel wall. Hypertension increases mechanical stress on the vessel, promoting further expansion of the aneurysm. The rate at which the aneurysm increases is not predictable; however, the likelihood of rupture or dissection increases dramatically when the size exceeds 6 cm. Aortic aneurysms result in approximately 15,000 deaths per year, the majority due to rupture.

An aortic dissection is a longitudinal tear in the intimal layer of the aortic wall. As blood enters the tear, pulsatile pressure creates a false channel between the intimal and medial layers. The force of pressure generated by ventricular contraction and systemic BP can cause the dissection to extend either distally or proximally—compromising flow to structures perfused by that segment of the aorta. Precipitating factors for aortic dissection include medial degeneration from inherited (e.g., connective tissue diseases, congenital defects) or acquired (e.g., hypertension, inflammation) disorders, trauma, pregnancy, and cocaine abuse (see *Hypertensive Emergencies*, p. 531).

Aortic dissection is classified by location, using two different systems. The Debakey classification defines a dissection as Type I if it involves the entire aorta, Type II if it is confined to the ascending aorta only, and Type III if the dissection originates in the descending aorta, distal to the left subclavian artery. The Stanford system classifies dissections into two groups: Type A, which involves both the ascending and descending aorta (Debakey Types I and II), and Type B, which affects only the descending aorta (Debakey Type III). Ascending dissections occur much more frequently (65%) than descending dissections and are considered more lethal.

The morbidity and mortality associated with aortic dissection are greatest near the time of the initial injury. Patients who present for medical evaluation within 2 weeks or less of symptom onset are characterized as "acute," while a dissection diagnosed after this time is considered "chronic." Approximately 2000 episodes of acute aortic dissection occur annually, with mortality approaching 80% if left untreated.

ASSESSMENT

Goal of the Assessment

Gather information that can assist in making the differential diagnosis so appropriate management can be initiated immediately.

History and Risk Factors

Hypertension, atherosclerosis and related risk factors (e.g., smoking, CAD, hyperlipidemia), connective tissue disorders (e.g., Marfan syndrome, Ehlers-Danlos syndrome), congenital defects (e.g., coarctation of the aorta, bicuspid aortic valve), family history of aneurysm or dissection, blunt chest trauma, pregnancy, cocaine use, advanced age (older than 60 years), and male sex

Vital Signs

- Hypertension may be preexisting or an SNS response to pain; more common in descending dissections.
- Hypotension secondary to hemorrhage or complications is associated with ascending dissection (aortic regurgitation, MI, tamponade).
- BP differences between extremities reflect involvement of brachial arteries; variation of 20 mm Hg considered significant.

Observation

Pain

- Intense pain of abrupt onset, often described as tearing, ripping, or sharp
- Midline, anterior pain is typical of Type A dissection, while posterior (intrascapular), back, or abdominal pain is more common in Type B dissection.
- With rupture of an abdominal aneurysm, pain will occur along the flank or lumbar back.
- Pain may radiate, following the path of the dissection.
- Vasovagal responses to intense pain: Diaphoresis, apprehension, nausea, vomiting, faintness may occur.
- Symptoms vary based on location of the dissection and resultant compromise in tissue perfusion.
- Acute LV failure (SOB, chest pain): Results from involvement of coronary arteries or the aortic valve
- Neurologic deficits: Syncope, confusion, sensorimotor changes, and lethargy result from involvement of branches of the ascending aorta.
- Paraplegia, paresthesia, or focal deficits: From involvement of spinal arteries
- Decreased urine output: If dissection extends to renal arteries, it can cause impaired perfusion and decreased kidney function.

Palpation

- Pulse deficits (difference in pulse volume or absent pulses) are considered a classic finding; occur in only 30% of patients.
- Sudden loss of pulses indicates extension of dissection.
- Slow capillary refill and cool skin reflect diminished perfusion.

Auscultation

- Diastolic murmur: With aortic regurgitation
- Muffled heart tones: With cardiac tamponade
- Hyperactive bowel sounds: With mesenteric artery ischemia

DIAGNOSTIC TESTS

HIGH ALERT! Rapid diagnostic imaging is essential, because mortality from aortic dissection increases by the hour. Transesophageal echocardiography, CT angiography, and magnetic resonance imaging are all highly accurate in identifying the presence and extent of dissection. The choice of a study is usually determined by the clinical stability of the patient and the availability of resources at a facility. While the definitive diagnosis is made by imaging studies, additional diagnostic tests may be helpful in ruling out other potential causes of chest pain (pulmonary embolism, MI, pericarditis) or evaluating the extent of end-organ involvement (see *Diagnostic Tests* later).

Diagnostic Tests for Acute Aortic Dissection		
Test	**Purpose**	**Abnormal Findings**
Blood Studies		
Cardiac enzymes	Assess for myocardial infarction.	Elevations indicate myocardial damage but cannot rule out dissection of the ascending aorta, which may involve the coronary vessels.

Diagnostic Tests for Acute Aortic Dissection — cont'd

Test	Purpose	Abnormal Findings
Complete blood count	Evaluate for infectious processes (pericarditis) and possible blood loss.	WBCs may be elevated secondary to the stress response. Decreased hemoglobin and hematocrit indicate blood loss with aortic dissection or rupture.
Blood urea nitrogen/creatinine	Evaluate renal function.	Elevations may be seen with dissection involving the renal arteries or with prerenal failure secondary to blood loss.
D-dimer	Evaluate risk for aortic dissection and pulmonary embolism (PE).	Levels >500 mg/ml in the first 24 hours of symptoms support diagnosis of acute dissection. Further studies are needed to distinguish between AD and PE.
Noninvasive Cardiology		
Electrocardiogram (ECG)	Evaluate for presence of myocardial ischemia and infarction.	Presence of ST-segment depression or T-wave inversion (myocardial ischemia), ST-elevation (acute MI), in 2 contiguous or related leads. Changes could indicate primary MI, or dissection with coronary artery involvement.
Transesophageal echocardiogram (TEE)	Assess for presence of aneurysm or dissection, location along the aorta, involvement of other structures (aortic valve, coronary arteries), and presence of complications.	Hallmark of dissection is the presence of an intimal "flap" dividing a true and false lumen. May reveal aortic regurgitation or coronary artery damage if dissection involves ascending aorta. Cardiac tamponade and pericardial effusion may also be present.
Radiology		
Chest radiograph (CXR)	Assess for abnormalities of the ascending aorta and rule out other possible causes of chest pain.	Widened mediastinum or abnormal aortic contour may increase suspicion for aortic dissection. A normal CXR may be present in up to 16% of aortic dissections.
Computed tomography angiography (CTA)	Identify dissection and define sites of origin and termination. Also useful in determining branch vessel involvement and size of the aorta.	Visualization of intimal flap and dual lumens confirm dissection. Spiral CT provides rapid imaging of entire aorta, coronary arteries, and pulmonary vessels to differentiate between MI, AD, and PE.
Magnetic resonance imaging (MRI)	Delineate presence and extent of dissection, including site of entry and presence of thrombus.	Presence of an intimal flap, along with true and false lumens, confirms diagnosis of dissection.

Aortic Aneurysm/Dissection

COLLABORATIVE MANAGEMENT

Because of the emergent nature of this disorder, limited randomized controlled trials are available to guide the treatment of patients with aortic dissection or rupture. The establishment of the International Registry of Acute Aortic Dissection (IRAD) has provided valuable information regarding presentation, management, and outcomes for this patient population. Current treatment guidelines, based on the consensus of clinical experts, are described next.

ACUTE AORTIC DISSECTION GUIDELINES

In 2001, the European Society of Cardiology developed guidelines for the management of acute aortic dissection. Because limited clinical trials exist to guide practice, these guidelines were based on consensus of practice experts. Recommendations that received a Class I recommendation (consensus of all members) are summarized below:

Initial Management of Patients with Suspected Aortic Dissection

Detailed medical history and complete physical examination (whenever possible)
Intravenous lines, blood sample (creatine kinase, troponin T or I, myoglobin, white blood cell count, D-dimer, hematocrit, lactase dehydrogenase)
ECG: documentation of ischemia
Heart rate and blood pressure monitoring
Pain relief (morphine sulfate)
Reduction of systolic blood pressure using beta-blockers (intravenous propranolol, metoprolol, esmolol, or labetalol)
Transfer to intensive care unit
In patients with severe hypertension, or: additional vasodilator (intravenous sodium nitroprusside titrated to blood pressure of 100–120 mm Hg)
Profound hemodynamic instability: intubation and ventilation

Imaging Studies in Acute Aortic Dissection

Transesophageal echocardiography
Computed tomography
Contrast angiography (*if needed* to define anatomy in visceral malperfusion and to guide percutaneous interventions)

Therapy for Acute Type A (Types I and II) Aortic Dissection

Emergency surgery to avoid tamponade/aortic rupture
Valve-preserving surgery — tubular graft *if* normal-sized aortic root and no pathologic changes of valve cusps
Replacement of aorta and aortic valve (composite graft) *if* ectatic proximal aorta and/or pathologic changes of valve/aortic wall

Therapy for Acute Type B (Type III) Aortic Dissection

Medical therapy
Surgical aortic replacement *if* signs of persistent or recurrent pain, early expansion, peripheral ischemic complications, or rupture

From Erbel R, et al. Diagnosis and management of aortic dissection: Recommendations of the Task Force on Aortic Dissection, European Society of Cardiology. *Eur Heart J* 22:1642–1681, 2001.

Care Priorities

The immediate goal of therapy for aortic dissection or rupture is to limit propagation of the dissection by reducing the shearing forces created by myocardial contractility and BP.

1. **Preserve the tissue integrity of the aorta with beta-blocker therapy (e.g., metoprolol, esmolol):** To reduce the velocity of LV ejection, slow HR and reduce BP. Usually administered intravenously, titrating to achieve an HR of 60 to 80 bpm. In patients unable to tolerate beta-blockers (because of asthma, bradycardia, or signs of HF), calcium channel blockers (diltiazem, verapamil) may be used as an alternative.
   - *Antihypertensive therapy:* Initiated if patient remains hypertensive after beta-blockers. Usually nitroprusside or nicardipine is started, as described in *Hypertensive Emergencies*, p. 531. Labetalol is another option, with the added advantage of providing beta-blockade. An SBP of 100 to 120 mm Hg is desired.

> **Safety Alert** *Initiation of a vasodilator prior to beta-blockade can cause a reflexive increase in HR and contractility. This SNS-medicated response can lead to further dissection.*

2. **Control pain:** Usually achieved with IV morphine sulfate, 2 to 10 mg, since morphine helps diminish sympathetic outflow. If additional sedation is required, midazolam may be used.

3. **Evaluate for and facilitate surgical treatment:** Urgent operation is recommended for Type A (ascending) dissection, and Type B (descending) dissection when impending rupture, significant organ ischemia, or refractory hypertension occurs. Surgery involves removal of the affected section of the aorta and replacement with a prosthetic graft. Repair or replacement of the aortic valve may also be needed.
4. **Continue medical management:** Most often patients with Type B dissections are managed medically. After control of BP is achieved with intravenous agents, oral antihypertensive therapy is initiated, along with gradual weaning from the IV infusion. The goal of chronic therapy is to maintain an SBP less than 130 mm Hg to prevent redissection. Long-term management includes beta-blockade, lipid control, smoking cessation, and serial imaging to evaluate for further changes in the aorta.
5. **Consider interventional treatment:** Over the last decade there has been an increase in endovascular management of aortic dissection. Options include fenestrated grafts (with openings), which allow blood to flow from the aorta into branching arteries, and stent placement to relieve malperfusion to vital organs and extremities.

CARE PLANS FOR AORTIC ANEURYSM/DISSECTION

Ineffective tissue perfusion: peripheral, cardiopulmonary, renal, and cerebral *related to interruption of arterial blood flow secondary to narrowed aortic lumen*

GOALS/OUTCOMES Within 48 hours of this diagnosis, patient has adequate tissue perfusion as evidenced by distal pulses bilaterally equal and greater than 2+ on a 0 to 4+ scale, brisk capillary refill (less than 2 seconds), warm skin, bilaterally equal sensations in the extremities, bilaterally equal SBP 100 to 120 mm Hg, HR 60 to 80 bpm, NSR on ECG, urine output greater than 0.5 ml/kg/hr, equal and normoreactive pupils, and orientation to time, place, and person.
NOC Circulation Status

Shock Prevention
1. Assess cardiovascular status by monitoring HR and rhythm, ECG, and cardiac enzyme levels. A dissection along the coronary arteries will result in an MI.
2. Perform bilateral assessment of BP and distal pulses (particularly radial, femoral, and dorsalis pedis) hourly during initial phase of dissection and then every 4 hours as the patient's condition stabilizes.
3. Note changes in strength or symmetry of distal pulses. Be alert to any change in color, capillary refill, and temperature of each extremity. Report significant findings.
4. If the difference in SBP between the extremities exceeds 10 mm Hg, consult physician immediately. Titrate vasodilators based on arm with highest BP.
5. Monitor hemodynamic parameters (BP, CVP, PAP) for signs of decreased intravascular volume. Establish separate intravenous lines for volume and medications.
6. Monitor for paresthesias of the extremities — a sign of diminished perfusion to the spinal arteries.
7. Assess for signs of pericardial tamponade: distended neck veins, muffled heart sounds, decreased SBP (less than 90 mm Hg or greater than 20 mm Hg drop in systolic trend), and pulsus paradoxus.
8. Assess for signs of acute aortic regurgitation: diastolic murmur, dyspnea, decreased CO.
9. Monitor urine output hourly. Consult physician or midlevel practitioner if urine output is less than 0.5 ml/kg/hr for 2 consecutive hours.
10. Assess neurologic status hourly. Report restlessness and changes in LOC, pupil size, or reaction to light.

NIC Hemodynamic Regulation; Cardiac Care: Acute; Circulatory Care; Surveillance

---

Acute pain *related to biophysical injury secondary to necrosis at the aortic media and distal tissue hypoperfusion*

GOALS/OUTCOMES Within 24 to 48 hours of this diagnosis, patient's subjective evaluation of pain improves, as documented by a pain scale. Nonverbal indicators, such as grimacing, are decreased or absent.
NOC Pain Control

Pain Management

1. Monitor patient at frequent intervals for the presence of discomfort. Devise a pain scale with patient, rating discomfort from 0 (no pain) to 10 (severe pain). Medicate with analgesics as prescribed, and rate relief obtained, using the pain scale.
2. During episodes of pain, assess for a change in peripheral pulses or altered hemodynamics (i.e., BP, PAP, PAWP, CO, SVR), because such changes often are associated with extension of the aortic dissection.
3. Control BP during episodes of pain by titrating vasodilator or use beta-blocker to maintain specified parameters.
4. Immediately consult physician for any increase in the severity of pain, because it may indicate the need for emergency surgery.

NIC Anxiety Reduction

RESEARCH BRIEF 5-1

D-dimer has been found to be elevated in patients with acute aortic dissection (AAD), but the use of this test as a means to "rule out" patients with suspected dissection has been controversial. The efficacy of using D-dimer as a diagnostic tool for acute dissection was evaluated in a prospective multicenter study, using patients enrolled in the International Registry of Acute Aortic Dissection. Two hundred twenty patients with suspected AAD were included, of whom 87 were diagnosed with actual aortic dissection and 133 with other diagnoses, such as angina, MI, and PE. D-dimer was markedly elevated in patients with aortic dissection (>500 ng/ml) throughout the first 24 hours. The authors concluded that D-dimer could be used to risk stratify patients presenting within the first 24 hours, to rule out both pulmonary embolism and aortic dissection and help decide whether to subject the patient to further diagnostic studies.

From Suzuki D, et al: Diagnosis of acute aortic dissection by D-dimer: the International Registry of Aortic Dissection substudy on biomarkers (IRADBio) experience. *Circulation* 119:2702–2707, 2009.

ADDITIONAL NURSING DIAGNOSES

For other nursing diagnoses and interventions, also see the following as appropriate: *Hemodynamic Monitoring* (p. 75), *Prolonged Immobility* (p. 149), *Emotional and Spiritual Support of the Patient and Significant Others* (p. 200), and *Chest Trauma* (p. 238).

CARDIOGENIC SHOCK

PATHOPHYSIOLOGY

Cardiogenic shock is defined as tissue hypoperfusion induced by HF after correction of preload. It is the most severe clinical expression of LV failure. The condition is associated with extensive damage to the LV myocardium in greater than 80% of STEMI patients in whom it occurs and is the leading cause of in-hospital death in patients with AMI. Cardiogenic shock is thought to occur when greater than 40% of ventricular mass is lost to infarction. Without some form of cardiac assistance, this condition is associated with 80% mortality, and even with early revascularization, 1-year survival remains less than 50% in these patients. The condition may result from ischemic heart disease, cardiomyopathy, valvular heart disease, inflammation, cardiac contusion, and cardiac surgery. In the setting of HF leading to cardiogenic shock, there are hemodynamic (increased afterload and volume) and chemical (neurohormones, peptides, growth factors, and natriuretic peptides) signals that stimulate changes in the biology of the cardiac cells. Neurohormones or peptides include norepinephrine, angiotensin II, aldosterone, and the natriuretic peptides. The activation of the renin-angiotensin-aldosterone system (RAAS) and the SNS is primarily involved in the development of HF leading to cardiogenic shock.

At autopsy, greater than two-thirds of patients with cardiogenic shock demonstrate stenosis of 75% or more of the luminal diameter of all three major coronary vessels, including the left anterior descending coronary artery. Although the prognosis of patients with cardiogenic shock has improved due to aggressive reperfusion strategies, in-hospital mortality from all causes remains at about 50%.

ASSESSMENT
Goal of Assessment
The goals are to identify the severity of symptoms and the stage of the shock and provide data to assist with differential diagnosis of the cause. Cardiac output is decreased due to cardiomyocyte dysfunction. The kidneys initially compensate by triggering the RAAS to increase BP by vasoconstriction and fluid retention. This is detrimental in setting of pump failure, as the increase in afterload augments the resistance to LV ejection (see *Heart Failure*, p. 421, for additional assessment information).

Observation
As shock progresses from the low output state, there is evidence of vital organ hypoperfusion: clouded sensorium, oliguria, and acidosis. Skin is cool to cold, and diaphoretic due to reduced peripheral perfusion.

Vital Signs
- HR greater than 90 bpm
- SBP less than 90 mm Hg or at least 30 to 35 mm Hg below normal for the patient
- Capillary refill greater than 3 seconds

Auscultation
- S_3 or S_4 heart sounds may be present resulting from an overdistended, noncompliant ventricle.
- Pulmonary congestion and tachypnea result in crackles throughout lung fields.
- Mitral regurgitation, if present, will result in a murmur that is high-pitched holosystolic and radiates to the axilla. The intensity of the murmur may not correlate with the severity of regurgitation. Electrocardiographic changes in mitral regurgitation are nonspecific and are primarily changes of LV hypertrophy and strain.

Hemodynamic Measurements
Hemodynamic monitoring: Is necessary for cardiogenic shock patients to guide initial therapy. An arterial line and a specialized pulmonary artery catheter measure mixed venous oxygen saturation in the pulmonary artery (Svo_2). Svo_2 is one indicator of how well oxygen supply meets tissue demand for energy production (see *Hemodynamic Monitoring*, p. 75).
Measuring tissue perfusion: The major focus for the treatment of shock is the improvement and preservation of tissue perfusion. Adequate tissue perfusion depends on an adequate supply of oxygen being transported to the tissues and the cells' ability to use it. Oxygen transport is influenced by pulmonary gas exchange, CO, and Hgb levels. Oxygen use is influenced by the internal metabolic environment.
Improving cellular oxygen transport: Part of the management of cardiogenic shock focuses on improving oxygen transport to the tissues. Svo_2 falls below the normal range of 60% to 80% when oxygen supply is decreased or tissue demand is increased. Svo_2 has a positive correlation with CO. Continuous monitoring of Svo_2 provides an indirect but continuous assessment of CO and perfusion. Table 5-10 outlines the common hemodynamic characteristics in cardiogenic shock.

DIAGNOSTIC TESTS
See *Diagnostic Tests for Heart Failure*, p. 424, and *Acute Coronary Syndromes*, p. 434 (for patients with ischemic heart disease).

COLLABORATIVE MANAGEMENT
Care Priorities
It is significant that patients in cardiogenic shock have an extraordinarily high early mortality. Those patients who survive for 30 days following the initial hospital stay have a mortality rate similar to that of patients with an AMI without shock. It is imperative that "shock" patients

Table 5-10	HEMODYNAMIC CHARACTERISTICS IN CARDIOGENIC SHOCK
Heart rate (bpm)	>90
Systolic blood pressure (mm Hg)	<90
Cardiac index (L/min/m^2)	<2.2
Mean arterial pressure (mm Hg)	<60
Pulmonary artery occlusion pressure (mm Hg)	>18
Coronary perfusion pressure (mm Hg)	<60
Diuresis (ml/kg/hr)	<0.5
Central venous pressure	>8
Systemic vascular resistance	>1300
Svo$_2$ (%)	<60

receive aggressive and supportive care during their early phase to avoid the refractory multiorgan dysfunction that results in death.

Treatment of cardiogenic shock is aimed at improving symptoms and stabilizing the hemodynamics. The goals are to maximize oxygen delivery at the cellular level and to reduce causes of increased stress or workload, which increase oxygen demand. Therefore, normalization of ventricular filling pressures and optimization of cardiac index are important aspects of patient stabilization. The challenge is to augment ventricular filling pressures (preload) without increasing afterload (systemic BP/SVR and PAPs) in the process. All measures strive to increase the CO, which is the root cause of the hypotension associated with severe HF/cardiogenic shock.

Pharmacologic Support of the Failing Heart

1. **Achieve adequate ventricular filling pressures (adequate preload):** Use of fluid volume infusion to help augment RV preload should be the first strategy if the CVP is less than 8 to 12 mm Hg and/or PAWP is less than 14 to 18 mm Hg. Maintaining an elevated CVP and PAOP may be necessary for an effective RV and LV preload in the setting of cardiogenic shock. Vasopressors (norepinephrine, dopamine, vasopressin) are carefully added primarily to assist in promoting venous return to the heart, rather than to induce arterial vasoconstriction. Arterial vasoconstriction increases afterload, which vasodilators are used to control. Since cardiogenic shock patients have hypotension, and vasodilators further reduce mean arterial pressure (MAP), it is necessary to add vasopressors in the early treatment of cardiogenic shock in an attempt to balance preload and afterload. Several vasopressors and vasodilators also increase myocardial contractility, which may also be helpful in augmenting CO. (See Appendix 6, *Vasoactive Drugs*.)

2. **Control resistance to RV and LV ejection using vasodilating agents:** Several vasoactive pharmacologic agents can be administered to help control afterload after adequate preload is achieved. Current guidelines recommend the use of vasodilators—nitroglycerin, nitroprusside, or nesiritide—in addition to diuretics to achieve stable hemodynamics and symptomatic improvement in patients with elevated filling pressures and a low cardiac index (see *Heart Failure, Collaborative Management*, p. 426).

   Nitroglycerin: A nitric oxide (NO) donor that is used intravenously, primarily for coronary artery vasodilation, in patients who have been effectively supported to maintain a stable arterial BP. NTG is predominantly a systemic venodilator with mild arteriolar vasodilating effects. NTG has a rapid onset of action, usually within 3 to 5 minutes, and may be titrated rapidly to achieve specific hemodynamic effects. The coronary arterial vasodilation helps to relieve myocardial ischemia and may result in increased contractility. Dosing is usually initiated at 20 mcg/min and increased by 20 mcg/min increments until the hemodynamic goals are achieved. The most common side effect of NTG is headache. In the setting of cardiogenic shock, the arterial BP is monitored continuously, since the drug is generally being used in combination with other vasoactive medications. Outside the setting of cardiogenic shock, stable patients with acute coronary syndrome are given NTG immediately for relief of chest discomfort if the SBP is at least 90 mm Hg.

Nesiritide: Nesiritide is an IV vasodilator used specifically to reduce preload and afterload in the treatment of patients with acute decompensated HF. Nesiritide is a recombinant form of the BNP that is secreted by the ventricles in response to myocardial stretch. A clinical response from nesiritide is usually rapid with significant reduction in PAOP and symptoms of dyspnea within 10 to 20 minutes of initiation of the drug.

Nesiritide potentiates the effect of diuretics and inhibits the RAAS, leading to a reduction in plasma aldosterone. Nesiritide has a renal effect and promotes sodium excretion. The recommended starting dose of nesiritide is a 2 mcg/kg bolus followed by an infusion of 0.01 mcg/kg/min until the desired hemodynamic parameters are met.

Nitroprusside: A balanced arterial and venous vasodilator that acts by production of nitrosothial in the vasculature, which in turn generates cyclic guanosine monophosphate in vascular smooth muscle and evokes relaxation. Currently, it is recommended only in patients with HF in whom afterload is severely increased (SVR greater than 1800 dynes/sec/cm^{-5}). Nitroprusside is usually started at 10 mcg/min and titrated up to 10 to 20 mcg/min at 10 to 20 minutes, with a goal of lowering the PAOP to 16 mm Hg without causing the SBP to fall below 80 mm Hg. Dosages can also be measured as mcg/kg/min ranging from 0.5 mcg/kg/min to 10 mcg/kg/min. Dosage requirements vary from patient to patient.

3. **Increase myocardial contractility using positive inotropic agents:**
Medications frequently administered as continuous infusion in patients with cardiogenic shock to improve the hemodynamic profile. These agents may be given in addition to diuretics and vasodilators (see *Heart Failure*, p. 421).

Dobutamine: A beta adrenergic–stimulating, catecholamine agent that exerts a potent inotropic effect, along with a peripheral and pulmonary vasodilating effect. The drug should be used only for short-term management to increase contractility because of the increased risk of tachydysrhythmias and ischemia. Doses usually start at 2 mcg/kg/min with titration upward to achieve the desired hemodynamic profile. Patients who are taking beta adrenergic–blocking agents may require higher doses of dobutamine. Dosage should not exceed 10 to 15 mcg/kg/min because of the possibility of inducing dysrhythmias, including increased risk of premature ventricular contractions, and episodes of nonsustained ventricular tachycardia resulting from increased ventricular irritability from the catecholamine properties of the drug. Dobutamine infusions have also been shown to increase aldosterone levels significantly, which may prompt fluid retention.

Dopamine: Dopamine stimulates alpha and beta receptors in the heart and dopaminergic receptors that cause vasodilatation in the renal and peripheral vasculature. At lower to midrange doses, dopamine increases blood flow to the renal, mesenteric, coronary, and cerebral beds; however, at high doses (greater than 5 mcg/kg/min), it causes alpha receptor stimulation and peripheral vasoconstriction. The starting dose of dopamine is 0.5 to 1 mcg/kg/min and is increased until the desired effect is achieved. Up to 3 mcg/kg/min, dopamine is predominantly vasodilatory; however, when the dose is increased to 5 mcg/kg/min, alpha receptors are stimulated and it becomes a vasoconstrictor. When dopamine is used as a vasopressor, weaning may have to be discontinued at 3 mcg/kg/min because lower doses may promote vasodilatation and lower BP. Dopamine may promote worsening ischemia and should be used with caution in cardiogenic shock patients, especially those with a history of HF.

Milrinone: Milrinone is a phosphodiesterase inhibitor that increases contractility by improving sarcolemma calcium uptake. Milrinone promotes positive inotropic effects in the myocardium and promotes peripheral and pulmonary vasodilatation through smooth muscle relaxation. The dosage range is 0.375 mcg/kg/min titrated up to achieve the desired hemodynamic effects, usually to a dosage of about 0.5 mcg/kg/min. Hypotension may result from the titration. The elimination and half life of milrinone is 2.4 hours and is increased to at least twice that time in the presence of renal failure, since the drug is primarily renally excreted. Dosage of milrinone should be reduced for renal failure patients.

Levosimendan: The inodilator levosimendan is a relatively new agent that also has positive lusitropic effects. Levosimendan may be considered in cardiogenic shock patients. Several randomized trials have demonstrated that levosimendan is superior to dobutamine in improving hemodynamic parameters and renal function in patients with cardiogenic shock.

Cardiogenic Shock

Table 5-11 provides a summary of the hemodynamic effects of drugs used in cardiogenic shock.

Mechanical Support of the Failing Heart

4. **Reduce LV afterload and increase coronary arterial perfusion using balloon counterpulsation therapy/IABP:** IABP is the most widely used mechanical support device in the world today and is an important component in the treatment of patients with cardiogenic shock who fail to respond to standard treatment. The efficacy of IABP has not been significantly evaluated in adequately powered randomized controlled trials to date. First introduced in the 1960s for treatment of cardiogenic shock, the goals of IABP therapy are to increase coronary perfusion pressure and thus coronary artery blood flow and to decrease LV workload. These goals are achieved by displacement of volume in the aorta during systole and diastole with alternating inflation and deflation of the balloon in synchrony with the ECG. The intravascular balloon device is usually threaded from a femoral artery insertion site through the great vessels and is positioned in the aortic arch/descending thoracic aorta below the arch. The balloon inflates during diastole to augment coronary artery perfusion and deflates in synchrony with systole to create a "brief space" in the aorta, which promotes lower resistance to ventricular ejection. The increased coronary artery perfusion will improve oxygen delivery to the ischemic ventricle. Better systemic perfusion helps to reverse the acidosis often seen in shock states and decreases secondary organ dysfunction related to hypoperfusion.

5. **Support CO and systemic perfusion using an LVAD:** Profound ventricular failure is defined as a MAP less than 60 mm Hg, an SBP less than 90 mm Hg, and a CI less than 2.0 L/min/m^2. In these cases, a more aggressive treatment approach may be required. The VAD is designed to support a failing natural heart with flow assistance. Diversion of varying amounts of systemic blood flow around a failing ventricle reduces cardiac workload while maintaining adequate perfusion to sustain end-organ function. VADs can be used to support a failing right ventricle or left ventricle or both. Several VADs have been approved by the Food and Drug Administration, and a number of other devices are in clinical trials. All consist of a blood pump, cannula, and some type of power supply. Some devices displace blood to create pulsatile flow, whereas others create continuous flow and are therefore pulseless. External VADS are used primarily for short-term support, and smaller implantable VADs are used for long-term therapy. The LVAD is the most commonly used. Outflow cannulas that divert blood from the heart to the LVAD are surgically placed in the left atrium or the LV apex depending on the indication for the device. Inflow back to the heart from the pump is accomplished by cannulation of the aorta or femoral artery for the LVAD and/or the pulmonary artery for the RVAD. Flow

Table 5-11	HEMODYNAMIC EFFECTS OF DRUGS USED IN CARDIOGENIC SHOCK			
	CI	PAOP	MAP	SVR
Vasodilators				
Nitroprusside	I	D	D	D
Nitroglycerin	I	D	D	D
Nesiritide	I	D	D	D
PDE Inhibitors				
Milrinone	I	D	D	D
Ca^{2+} Sensitizers				
Levosimendan	I	D	D	D
Catecholamines				
Dopamine	I	I	I	I
Dobutamine	I	D	=	D

I, increased; *D*, decreased; =, effects depend on dosage.

rates between 1 and 6 L/min are used to maintain adequate CO while decreasing ventricular workload. The LVAD is in counterpulsation with the patient's heart, which means it is in the filling phase during LV contraction and ejecting during LV relaxation. Percutaneous ventricular assist devices (PVADs) have recently become available as a bridge to surgical LVAD. Table 5-12 outlines the various types of VADs. Complications of VADs include coagulopathy, bleeding, embolization, infection, sepsis, and renal failure.

6. **Provide other treatments for cardiogenic shock after the cause of pump failure has been identified** (see *Heart Failure*, p. 421):

* Emergency CABG or surgical reperfusion (see *Acute Coronary Syndromes*, p. 434)
* Emergency PCI with stents placed in the occluded artery (see *Acute Coronary Syndromes*, p. 434) (Current trials are under way worldwide with implantable dissolvable stents.)
* Heart transplantation (see *Organ Transplantation*, p. 906)

CARE PLANS FOR CARDIOGENIC SHOCK

Decreased CO *related to increased afterload, increased preload, or decreased contractility secondary to loss of 40% or more of myocardial functional mass*

GOALS/OUTCOMES The patient's hemodynamic function is optimized as evidenced by CO at least 4 L/min, BP greater than 90/60 mm Hg, SVR less than 1200 dynes/sec/cm^{-5}, and PAOP less than 12 mm Hg, before weaning from assist device or pharmacologic agents.

NOC Tissue Perfusion: Cardiac; Tissue Perfusion: Cerebral; Tissue Perfusion: Peripheral; Tissue Perfusion: Pulmonary; Tissue Perfusion: Abdominal Organs

Shock Management: Cardiac

1. Monitor arterial vital signs and hemodynamics continously.
2. Titrate vasoactive drugs to achieve a CO between 4 and 7 L/min, arterial BP at least 90/60, and PAOP less than 14 mm Hg.
3. Assess CO and SVR every 1 to 4 hours and after every change in pharmacologic therapy. Consult physician if SVR increases (greater than 1200 dynes/sec/cm^{-5}). A vasodilating drug such as nitroprusside or similar medication may be needed to decrease excessive afterload.
4. Auscultate lung sounds every 1 to 2 hours, and monitor urinary output. Report changes, including an increase in crackles and decreased urine output. An adjustment in IV fluid therapy or additional diuretics may be necessary.
5. Keep HOB at 30 degrees unless patient is hypotensive.
6. Treat ventricular dysrhythmias with prescribed antidysrhythmic medications.
7. Temporary cardiac pacing for symptomatic bradycardia may be necessary. Second- or third-degree heart block may occur. Transcutaneous or transvenous pacing may be used.
8. If medical management does not improve the hemodynamic profile, prepare patient for insertion of IABP or LVAD.

NIC Cardiac Care: Acute; Circulatory Care: Mechanical Assist Device; Hemodynamic Regulation

Table 5-12	VENTRICULAR ASSIST DEVICES
Type	**Indications**
External	
Thoratec PVAD	Short-term ventricular or biventricular support
Impella Recover L.P 2.5	Short-term left ventricular support
Tandem Heart	Short-term left ventricular support
Abiomed BVS 5000	Short-term univentricular or biventricular support
Implantable	
Heartmate VE	Long-term left ventricular support
Heartmate II LVAS	Long-term ventricular support
Novacor LVAS	Long-term ventricular support
(Heartmate VE is approved for bridge to transplantation and destination therapy.)	

Cardiogenic Shock

Ineffective tissue perfusion: altered cardiopulmonary, cerebral, peripheral, and/or renal tissue perfusion *related to interrupted arterial blood flow to vital organs secondary to inadequate arterial pressure*

GOALS/OUTCOMES Within 96 hours of initial diagnosis of cardiogenic shock, the patient will have adequate tissue perfusion as evidenced by orientation to time, place, and person; equal and normoreactive pupils; normal deep tendon reflexes; urine output at least 0.5 ml/kg/hr; warm and dry skin; peripheral pulses at least 2+ on a 0 to 4+ scale; brisk capillary refill (less than 2 seconds); BP at least 90/60 mm Hg, and Svo$_2$ greater than 65% or within patient's normal range.
NOC Circulation Status

Cardiac Care: Acute Hemodynamic Regulation
1. Check neurologic status every 1 to 2 hours to assess cerebral perfusion. Be alert to changes in LOC, orientation, perception, motor activity, reflexes, and pupillary response to light. Consult physician for any changes.
2. Monitor I&O hourly to assess renal perfusion; report urine output less than 0.5 ml/kg/hr for 2 consecutive hours. Assess extremities every 1 to 2 hours, noting changes in skin color, temperature, capillary refill, BP, and distal pulses.
3. Titrate vasoactive drugs to maintain SBP at least 90 mm Hg.

NIC Circulatory Care: Peripheral, Cerebral, Cardiac, Gastrointestinal

Impaired gas exchange *related to alveolar-capillary membrane changes secondary to pulmonary congestion; altered oxygen-carrying capacity of the blood secondary to acidosis occurring with anaerobic metabolism*

GOALS/OUTCOMES Before weaning from supplemental oxygen or ventilatory assistance is attempted, the patient will have adequate gas exchange as evidenced by Pao$_2$ at least 80 mm Hg, RR 12 to 20 breaths/min with normal depth and pattern, oxygen saturation at least 95%, Svo$_2$ 60% to 80%, and Scvo$_2$ at least 80%.
NOC Respiratory Status: Gas Exchange; Respiratory Status: Ventilation

Ventilation Assistance
1. At least hourly, assess rate, depth, and effort of patient's respirations. Note tachypnea or labored breaths. In-spect skin and mucous membranes for pallor or cyanosis (a late sign of hypoxia). Consult physician promptly for significant findings.
2. Auscultate lung fields every 1 to 2 hours. Be alert to crackles, rhonchi, or wheezes.
3. Monitor ABG values for hypoxemia (Pao$_2$ less than 80 mm Hg) or metabolic acidosis (pH less than 7.35 and less than 22 mEq/L).
4. Deliver oxygen as prescribed.
5. Monitor transcutaneous oxygen saturation with a pulse oximeter. Consult physician if oxygen saturation falls to less than 90%.
6. Monitor and manage Svo$_2$ by supporting CO. When CO drops, perfusion decreases and oxygen extraction increases, resulting in a lower Svo$_2$.
7. If patient's condition deteriorates, prepare for intubation and mechanical ventilation.

NIC Acid-Base Management; Airway Management; Oxygen Therapy; Mechanical Ventilation

For Patients Undergoing IABP Procedure
Decreased cardiac output (or risk for same) *related to negative inotropic changes and rate, rhythm, and conduction alterations secondary to ischemia or injury*

GOALS/OUTCOMES Within 24 hours of diagnosis of cardiogenic shock, patient's CO is effectively supported as evidenced by MAP at least 60 mm Hg to support peripheral perfusion, improved ECG rhythm, HR 60 to 100 bpm, peripheral pulses audible with Doppler or palpable, hourly urinary output at least 0.5 ml/kg/hr or renal support strategy in place, measured CO 4 to 7 L/min, CI greater than 2 L/min/m^2, PAOP less than 15 mm Hg, SVR less than 1200 dynes/sec/cm^{-5}, Svo$_2$ 60% to 80%, Scvo$_2$ at least 80%, and patient awake, alert, oriented, and free from chest discomfort.
NOC Circulation Status

Circulatory Care: Mechanical Assist Device

1. Monitor BP, PAP, RAP, Svo₂, and HR and rhythm on a continuous basis. Monitor PAOP, SVR, and CO/CI hourly. Report the following to the physician: increased PAWP, decreased CO, new ST-segment elevation or depression, deterioration in heart rhythm, decreased Svo₂, or elevated SVR.

2. Monitor hourly urinary output. Report output that is less than 0.5 ml/kg/hr for 2 consecutive hours. Monitor BUN and creatinine values daily. Report increased BUN (greater than 20 mg/dl) and serum creatinine (greater than 1.5 mg/dL), indicative of acute renal failure.

3. Monitor bilateral peripheral pulses along with color and temperature of extremities every 2 hours.

4. Provide oxygen therapy or maintain ventilator settings as prescribed.

5. Regulate IV inotropic agents such as dobutamine, dopamine, and milrinone to maintain CI at least 2.5 to 4 L/min/m². Monitor for side effects, including tachyarrhythmias, ventricular ectopy, headache, and angina. (See Appendix 6 for more information.)

6. Regulate afterload-reducing agents such as nitroprusside and nitroglycerin to maintain SVR less than 1200 dynes/sec/cm⁻⁵. Monitor for drug side effects, including hypotension, headache, dizziness, nausea, vomiting, and cutaneous flushing.

7. Administer diuretic agents as prescribed for elevated PAOP (greater than 14 mm Hg). Monitor for signs and symptoms of hypokalemia (e.g., weakness, dysrhythmias), a potential side effect of diuretics.

8. Provide a quiet environment conducive to stress reduction.

9. Administer prescribed pain medications to keep patient comfortable. Stress increases workload of the heart.

10. Monitor Hgb and Hct values daily. Loss of blood reduces oxygen delivery to the cells, prompting tachycardia and tachypnea.

NIC Surveillance; Hemodynamic Regulation

Ineffective tissue perfusion (or risk for same): peripheral: involved leg *related to interrupted arterial blood flow secondary to arterial wall dissection by sheath or thrombus formation*

GOALS/OUTCOMES Throughout hospitalization, patient has adequate perfusion in the involved leg as evidenced by Doppler or palpable peripheral pulses, normal color and sensation, warmth, full motor function, and absence of bleeding, abdominal pain, and tingling in the involved leg.

NOC Circulation Status; Sensory Function: Cutaneous; Tissue Perfusion: Peripheral

Circulatory Care: Arterial Insufficiency

1. Monitor circulation in affected leg every 30 minutes for 2 hours and every 2 hours thereafter if assessment is within normal limits. Assess pulses, temperature, color, sensation, and mobility of the toes in the involved leg. Consult physician or midlevel practitioner immediately for significant changes.

2. Instruct patient to notify staff member if pain, numbness, or tingling occurs in the involved leg.

3. Provide protection to heel of involved foot, using sheepskin, occlusive opaque dressing, or heel protector. Place lamb's wool between the toes to minimize their pressure against each other.

4. To enhance perfusion in the involved leg, have patient perform passive foot exercises 4 times daily, without bending leg at the hip: foot flexion/extension, foot circles, and quadriceps setting. A pneumatic compression device may be beneficial.

5. Administer IV medications (e.g., heparin) as prescribed to prevent clots from forming on the balloon. Monitor patient for signs of bleeding, including decreased Hct (optimal values are at least 37% [female] or at least 40% [male]), abdominal pain, hematuria, oral bleeding, or blood-tinged mucus.

6. Monitor PTT if heparin is used (optimal value is 30 to 40 seconds [activated]). Therapeutic anticoagulation is usually 1½ times that of normal. Maintain adequate hydration (2 to 3 L/day) to minimize risk of clot formation.

7. Keep HOB at 30 degrees or less to prevent upward migration of the balloon catheter, which may occlude subclavian artery.

8. Assess for the following signs of balloon migration: decreased left radial pulse, sudden decrease in urine output (less than 0.5 ml/kg/hr), flank pain, and dizziness.

9. When the balloon is no longer needed, maintain regular balloon inflation timing to prevent clot formation until balloon can be removed.

NIC Positioning; Circulatory Precautions; Lower Extremity Monitoring

Impaired tissue integrity (or risk for same) *related to external factors (pressure and immobilization); internal factors (altered circulation, possible insulin resistance, and decreased nutritional intake)*

GOALS/OUTCOMES Throughout hospitalization, patient's tissue remains intact.
NOC Tissue Integrity: Skin and Mucous Membranes

Pressure Ulcer Prevention
1. Position patient on low-pressure protective bed to enhance blood flow to dependent areas and allow air circulation across the skin, promoting evaporation of moisture.
2. Reposition patient every 2 hours, especially when spontaneous movement is diminished. When turning patient, keep involved leg extended and log-roll patient onto side.
3. Provide meticulous care to keep skin clean and dry. Inspect pressure areas (e.g., coccyx, ischial tuberosity, calcaneus, malleolus) at least tid.
4. Ensure that patient's diet is high in protein and calories, with blood glucose 80 to 110 mg/dl to promote an anabolic or "building" state. If patient's oral intake is inadequate, consider nutritional support (i.e., enteral or parenteral nutrition).
5. Teach patient how to move in bed while minimizing flexion of involved hip.

NIC Bedrest Care; Positioning; Self-Care Assistance

Ineffective breathing pattern *related to fatigue and decreased energy secondary to HF; decreased lung expansion secondary to medically imposed position (HOB at 30 degrees)*

GOALS/OUTCOMES Within 4 hours of diagnosis of HF, patient has an effective breathing pattern as evidenced by Pao_2 at least 80 mm Hg, Spo_2 at least 90%, absence of adventitious breath sounds, and RR 12 to 20 breaths/min with normal pattern and depth.
NOC Respiratory Status: Ventilation; Vital Signs; Mechanical Ventilation Response: Adult

Respiratory Monitoring
1. Monitor breath sounds every 2 hours. Assess anterior and posterior lung fields for adventitious (e.g., crackles, rhonchi) or absent sounds.
2. Monitor oxygen saturation by pulse oximetry. Maintain oxygen saturation at greater than 90%.
3. Monitor RR, rhythm, and breathing pattern hourly.
4. Assess for atelectasis (e.g., dyspnea, elevated temperature, weakness, absent or decreased breath sounds) and respiratory infection (e.g., elevated temperature, SOB, increased sputum production or coughing, and altered color of sputum).
5. Monitor temperature every 4 hours and WBC count daily for signs of infection. Be alert to low-grade fever of less than 37.8°C (less than 100°F) and increased WBC count.
6. Provide supplemental oxygen and chest physiotherapy as prescribed.
7. Encourage patient to perform deep-breathing exercises or incentive spirometry with coughing every 1 to 2 hours while awake to reduce the possibility of atelectasis.
8. If coughing is ineffective; consider suctioning if indicated.
9. Reposition patient at least every 2 hours to minimize stasis of lung secretions.
10. Monitor patient's fluid volume status to ensure adequate hydration and to keep secretions thin and mobile. Fluid intake goal may be 2 to 3 L/day.
11. Elevate HOB 30 degrees as tolerated, to promote effective breathing pattern.
12. If patient has respiratory insufficiency despite other measures, prepare for endotracheal intubation and mechanical ventilation.

NIC Airway Management; Oxygen Therapy; Mechanical Ventilation

Ineffective protection *related to risk of bleeding/hemorrhage secondary to coagulopathy or IV anticoagulants needed to maintain therapeutic equipment, such as ventricular assist devices*

GOALS/OUTCOMES Throughout hospitalization, patient's bleeding is controlled as evidenced by secretions and excretions negative for blood, chest tube drainage within acceptable amounts (less than 100 ml/hr), and absence of abdominal pain or ecchymoses.
NOC Blood Coagulation

Bleeding Precautions
1. Monitor PTT, ACT, and platelet level daily. Report and manage levels not within therapeutic range. Anticoagulation and decreased platelet levels increase the risk of bleeding and hemorrhage.
2. Monitor Hct and Hgb daily. Decreased levels may signal the presence of bleeding.
3. Test GI drainage and stool daily for blood.
4. Protect patient from injury. Pad side rails, if necessary, and turn patient carefully. Use sponge-tipped applicators for oral care.
5. Test gastric pH every 4 hours. Administer gastric acid–neutralizing drugs, such as antacids or histamine H2-receptor antagonists as prescribed to maintain gastric pH at 5 or higher.

NIC Bleeding Reduction

Patients with VADs

Risk for disuse syndrome *related to imposed restrictions against movement secondary to presence of assist device or debilitated state*

GOALS/OUTCOMES Patient maintains baseline ROM without evidence of muscle atrophy or contracture formation.
NOC Immobility Consequences: Physiological

Exercise Therapy: Joint Mobility
1. Be aware that patient can be turned gently from side to side when the heart assist device is in place. Do this every 2 hours, observing assist device cannulas closely to ensure that tension is not placed on them during patient repositioning.
2. Provide passive ROM to extremities four times daily.

NIC Energy Management

Decreased cardiac output (or risk for same) *related to altered preload and negative inotropic changes secondary to reduced right ventricular contraction occurring with left-sided heart assist device*

| Safety Alert | *This is a complication of the left-sided heart assist device, particularly when the outflow cannula is located in the left ventricle. When the left ventricle is decompressed, septal wall motion is diminished, thereby reducing RV contraction. Patients who have pulmonary hypertension or impaired RV function caused by AMI or cardiopulmonary bypass are especially prone to developing this problem.* |

GOALS/OUTCOMES Within 24 hours of diagnosis of HF, patient's CO will be adequate as evidenced by measured CO 4 to 7 L/min, RAP 4 to 6 mm Hg, PVR 60 to 100 dynes/sec/cm^{-5}, and LAP at least 10 mm Hg.
NOC Cardiac Pump Effectiveness

Circulatory Care: Mechanical Assist Device
1. Monitor patient for a decrease in CO with associated increases in RAP and PVR, which are diagnostic decreased CO.
2. An adequate preload is necessary to prevent a vacuum effect from the device, thereby decreasing CO.

NIC Circulatory Care: Mechanical Assist Device; Hemodynamic Regulation

Risk for infection *related to inadequate primary defenses secondary to presence of multiple invasive lines, movement restrictions, and stasis of body fluids*

GOALS/OUTCOMES Patient is free of infection as evidenced by normothermia, WBC count 11,000/mm^3 or less, negative culture results, and absence of erythema, swelling, warmth, tenderness, and purulent drainage at incision or cannulation sites.
NOC Infection Severity; Immune Status

Infection Protection
1. On a daily basis, monitor temperature, WBC count, and all incisions and cannulation sites for evidence of infection. Be alert to low-grade fever of approximately 37.8°C (100°F), WBC count greater than 11,000/mm³, and incision that is erythematous, warm, swollen, and tender to the touch or that has purulent discharge.
2. Culture any suspicious drainage or secretions; report positive findings.
3. Change IV tubing every 72 hours (or per agency protocol), using aseptic technique.
4. Change all dressings over catheter insertion sites per agency protocol, using aseptic technique.
5. Administer prophylactic IV antibiotics as prescribed.
6. Provide nutritional support to ensure that nitrogen balance is attained.
7. Monitor breath sounds every 2 hours. Assess for the presence of crackles, rhonchi, or signs of consolidation. Following extubation, perform coughing and deep-breathing exercises.
8. If patient is incapable of expectorating secretions independently, suction as often as needed. Inspect the mucus, noting color and consistency. Be alert to secretions that are yellow, green, or thickened.
9. Provide gentle chest physiotherapy as prescribed. Percussion and vibration can be performed over the posterior and lateral lung lobes during every positioning change, or at least four times daily.

NIC Infection Control

Imbalanced nutrition: less than body requirements *related to decreased intake secondary to oral intubation; increased nutritonal needs secondary to debilitated state and impaired tissue perfusion with concomitant nitrogen malabsorption*

GOALS/OUTCOMES Within the 24- to 48-hour period before discharge from the ICU, patient has adequate nutrition as evidenced by a balanced nitrogen state, stable weight, urine nitrogen 10 to 20 g/24 hr, thyroxine-binding prealbumin 20 to 30 mg/dL, and retinol-binding protein 4 to 5 mg/dL.
NOC Nutritional Status

Nutrition Management
1. Provide nutrition via tube feedings, or total parenteral nutrition, to ensure minimum of 1 to 5 g protein/kg/day and a calorie intake of 100 kcal/kg/day, along with other essential elements. Ask dietitian to monitor daily calorie and protein intake.
2. Weigh patient daily for trend. Report continuing decreases in weight.
3. Monitor 24-hour urinary nitrogen every 3 days for increase in excretion.
4. Monitor I&O hourly. Report positive or negative fluid state of 300 ml/hr.
5. Assess patient for signs of cardiac cachexia: muscle atrophy, weakness, anorexia, and weight loss.

NIC Nutrition Therapy; Nutritional Monitoring

CARDIOMYOPATHY

PATHOPHYSIOLOGY

Cardiomyopathy (CM) refers to a heterogeneous group of myocardial diseases that are often genetic and associated with mechanical and electrical dysfunction. Most types of CM result in inappropriate ventricular hypertrophy or dilation. The AHA 2006 expert panel on Contemporary Definitions and Classification of Cardiomyopathy categorized CM into two major groups: primary and secondary CM. Primary CMs are caused by pathology confined to the heart muscle alone, whereas secondary CMs are caused by pathology from a variety of generalized systemic (multiorgan) disorders (Table 5-13). Some common disease entities involving the heart muscle have been excluded from the present contemporary CM classification. These include pathologic myocardial processes and cardiac dysfunction caused by another cardiovascular abnormality, such as valvular heart disease, systemic hypertension, congenital heart disease, and atherosclerotic coronary artery disease. Other conditions not included in this CM classification are cardiac tumors, diseases affecting the endocardium with little or no myocardial involvement, and hypertensive hypertrophic CM. Primary and secondary CMs included in the 2006 AHA definition of CM are further classified into the following categories: hypertrophic CM (HCM), dilated CM (DCM), arrhythmogenic right ventricular CM/dysplasia (ARVC/D), and left ventricular noncompaction (LVNC). Be aware that one disease, be it primary or secondary CM, may fall into more than one CM classification, causing confusion if there is an overlap between categories. For example, some genetic primary CMs are known to cause both DCM and HCM. Furthermore, a CM may evolve, as a consequence of remodeling, from one category to another as the disease progresses. CMs, whether confined to the heart (primary CM) or part of a generalized systemic disorder (secondary CM), often lead to cardiovascular death or progressive HF-related disability.

Functional Classifications of Cardiomyopathy

Hypertrophic cardiomyopathy (HCM): HCM is characterized by inappropriate hypertrophy of the ventricular muscle leading to LV stiffness and diastolic dysfunction. HCM is commonly a genetic heart disease and is less commonly caused by an infiltrative process. Approximately 60% to 70% of patients with HCM have familial HCM, an inherited autosomal dominant condition. Other cardiovascular diseases, like hypertension and aortic stenosis, are

Table 5-13	TYPES AND CAUSES OF CARDIOMYOPATHY
Primary Types of Cardiomyopathy	**Secondary Causes of Cardiomyopathy**
Genetic Type Hypertrophic cardiomyopathy (HCM) Arrhythmogenic right ventricular cardiomyopathy/dysplasia (ARVC/D) Left ventricular noncompaction (LVNC) *Mixed Type (Genetic and Nongenetic)* Dilated cardiomyopathy (DCM) Restrictive cardiomyopathy (nonhypertrophied and nondilated) (RCM) *Acquired Type* Inflammatory (myocarditis) Stress provoked ("tako-tsubo") Peripartum Tachycardia induced	*Autoimmune/Collagen* Systemic lupus erythematosus, dermatomyositis, rheumatoid arthritis, scleroderma, polyarteritis, nodosa *Storage* Hemochromatosis, Fabry disease, glycogen storage disease (type II, Pompe), Niemann-Pick disease *Neuromuscular/Neurologic* Friedreich ataxia, Duchenne-Becker muscular dystrophy, Emery-Dreifuss muscular dystrophy, myotonic dystrophy, neurofibromatosis, tuberous sclerosis *Infiltrative* Amyloidosis, Gaucher disease, Hurler disease, Hunter disease *Inflammatory (Granulomatous)* Sarcoidosis *Endocrine* Diabetes mellitus, hyperthyroidism, hypothyroidism, hyperparathyroidism, pheochromocytoma, acromegaly *Cardiofacial* Noonan syndrome, lentiginosis *Endomyocardial* Endomyocardial fibrosis, hypereosinophillic syndrome (Löeffler endocarditis) *Nutritional Deficiencies* Beriberi (thiamine), pellagra, scurvy, selenium, carnitine, kwashiorkor *Toxicity* Drugs, heavy metals, chemical agents *Electrolyte Imbalance* *Consequence of Cancer Therapy* Anthracyclines: doxorubicin (Adriamycin), daunorubicin, cyclophosphamide, radiation

Note: This table lists common diseases associated with primary and secondary CM and is not intended to represent an exhaustive and complete list of conditions associated with CM. Some disagreement exists in the scientific community regarding the classification, definition, and nomenclature of CM; therefore, discrepancies and contradictions may occur among various scientific resources.

capable of producing the same magnitude of wall thickening seen with HCM. Obstructive HCM occurs when the enlarged heart muscle, usually the ventricular septum, obstructs the ventricular outflow channel, which may result in angina, HF, and sudden death. HCM is the most common cause of sudden cardiac death in the young, especially in athletes, but may lead to HF and disability at any age.

Dilated cardiomyopathy (DCM): DCM is characterized by marked, progressive dilation of the ventricles, resulting in decreased myocardial contractility and a reduced systolic ejection fraction (less than 40%). DCM is the the most frequent cause of heart transplantation and the third most common cause of HF behind CAD and hypertension. Infectious agents (particularly viruses producing myocarditis), cocaine, chronic excessive alcohol consumption, and chemotherapeutic agents are common causes of DCM, along with other autoimmune, neurologic, metabolic, endocrine, nutritional, and other systemic disorders. About 20% to 35% of DCM cases have been reported as familial, frequently associated with skeletal muscle or neuromuscular disorders. In patients with severe dilation, the increase in total cardiac mass may lead to ventricular hypertrophy. Alternatively, DCM may occur as a late manifestation of hypertrophic heart disease. DCM may ultimately lead to a decline in LV contractile function, ventricular and supraventricular arrhythmias, conduction system abnormalities, thromboembolism, progressive HF, and sudden or HF-related death.

Restrictive cardiomyopathy (RCM): RCM is less common than HCM or DCM and is characterized by nondilated ventricles with impaired ventricular filling from rigid or fibrotic ventricular walls. LV diastolic dysfunction occurs, often associated with very high end-diastolic pressures and moderate to marked biatrial enlargement secondary to elevated atrial pressures. Hypertrophy is typically absent, although the infiltrative and storage diseases (such as amyloid and hemochromatosis) may cause an increase in LV wall thickness. Systolic function usually remains normal, at least early in the disease. Treatment is difficult and prognosis is poor. Differentiating RCM from constrictive pericarditis is important since the two clinical pictures are similar, whereas management is markedly different.

Arrhythmogenic right ventricular cardiomyopathy/dysplasia (ARVC/D): ARVC/D is an uncommon genetic disease characterized by progressive replacement of normal myocardial cells with fatty or fibrofatty tissue. Initially thought to be a disease isolated to the right ventricle, more recent evidence shows the left ventricle is also involved in as many as 75% of cases. Clinical manifestations include ventricular dysrhythmias and HF. In young adults, ARVC/D often presents with sudden death.

Left ventricular noncompaction (LVNC): LVNC is an anatomic abnormality of LV myocardial development characterized by a "spongy" and "noncompacted" morphologic appearance of the LV myocardium. Noncompaction predominantly involves the apical portion of the LV chamber with deep intertrabecular recesses, or channels, in communication with the ventricular cavity and filled with blood from the ventricular cavity. LVNC has been associated with a high incidence of HF, thromboembolism, and ventricular arrhythmias in adults.

ASSESSMENT
Goal of Assessment
The physical assessment of patients with CM attempts to characterize the etiology and severity of cardiac dysfunction, the level of functional impairment, and the optimal therapeutic approach. Furthermore, the physical assessment should identify factors that precipitated clinical decompensation, for example, exercise or exacerbation of autoimmune disease. A good physical assessment will help differentiate heart and circulatory failure from entities that cause similar complaints and findings. During the course of treatment, the physical assessment will also provide feedback about the patient's response to therapies (Table 5-14).

Observation
A patient's clinical presentation will vary according to the type and extent of the CM and whether the patient has progressed to overt HF. The clinical presentation will reflect both the hemodynamic abnormalities caused by cardiac dysfunction and the degree of secondary compensatory mechanisms. Patients' presenting symptoms may range between asymptomatic to, unfortunately, symptoms continuous with cardiogenic shock or sudden death. Most commonly, patients will present with symptoms of HF or arrhythmias (see Table 5-14).

Table 5-14	SIGNS AND SYMPTOMS OF CARDIOMYOPATHY		
Source of Initial	Dilated	Hypertrophic	Restrictive
	Systolic dysfunction	Diastolic dysfunction	Diastolic dysfunction
Clinical presentation	• S&S of CHF usually develop insidiously and are caused by LV failure, RV failure, or biventricular failure. • Common symptoms include exertional dyspnea, fatigue, weakness, dry cough, orthopnea, PND, ascites, peripheral edema. • Patients may also have changes in mentation; i.e., confusion, restlessness, lethargy.	• Wide spectrum of S&S, depending on extent and severity of dysfunction • Most patients have few symptoms, if any. • Other patients present with the following S&S of heart dysfunction: dyspnea (caused by increasing LV diastolic pressure), PND, angina (caused by hypertrophy and relative ischemia), palpitations, fatigue (caused by decreased CO), and syncope (caused by arrhythmias or obstructive HCM).	• The least common type of CM. Hallmark S&S are from ventricular stiffness caused by LVH and endocardial fibrosis, reducing ability of the ventricle to relax and fill during diastole. • Common presenting symptoms include exercise intolerance and exertional dyspnea. • If more advanced disease, HF S&S are orthopnea, PND, peripheral edema, ascites, fatigue, and weakness. • Angina if RCM due to amyloidosis
Physical assessment	• Must estimate the severity of hemodynamic dysfunction • Common exam findings associated with HF: tachycardia, JVD, PMI displaced down and to left; +S₃ and S₄ gallops, systolic murmurs of AV valves; basilar rales; ascites and hepatomegaly, especially if RV failure; extremities cool, mottled, cyanotic; peripheral pulses weak with pulsus alternans; BP normal or low • Sinus tachycardia, atrial fibrillation, and ventricular dysrhythmias are common.	• May reveal the presence of an LV outflow tract obstruction by revealing a harsh left sternal border murmur of the aortic valve • An S₄ gallop may be present. Supraventricular dysrhythmias, especially atrial fibrillation, and ventricular dysrhythmias are common. • Sudden death can be the first symptom.	• Usually a result of elevated venous pressure and include dependent peripheral edema, ascites, and an enlarged, tender, and pulsatile liver; JVD that does not fall normally or may rise with inspiration (Kussmaul sign) • Atrial fibrillation is common. • PMI is typically in normal position and of normal character. • Heart block may be evident in patients with amyloidosis or sarcoidosis. • There may also be a loud S₃ or murmur of tricuspid or mitral regurgitation.

AV, atrioventricular; CHF, congestive heart failure; CM, cardiac myopathy; CO, cardiac output; HCM, hypertrophic cardiomyopathy; HF, heart failure; JVD, jugular venous distention; LV, left ventricular; LVH, left ventricular hypertrophy; PMI, point of maximal impulse; PND, paroxysmal nocturnal dyspnea; RCM, restrictive cardiomyopathy; RV, right ventricular; S&S, signs and symptoms.

Cardiomyopathy

Diagnostic Tests for Cardiomyopathy

Test	Purpose	Abnormal Findings
Noninvasive Cardiology		
Echocardiography (two-dimensional echo) The most useful test for diagnosis in cardiomyopathy	Measures ejection fraction (EF), LV size, and dilation of the cardiac chambers; measures ventricular wall thickness, location and degree of hypertrophy, and septal contractility. Provides helpful information about valve function and the presence of a thrombus	May reveal a reduced ejection fraction (EF <40%), ventricular wall motion disorders, valvular dysfunction, cardiac chamber enlargement, pulmonary hypertension, presence of a thrombus, or other cardiac dysfunction
48-hour electrocardiogram Holter monitoring	Can help detect the presence of intermittent dysrhythmias, including dangerous ventricular dysrhythmias	May reveal undiagnosed, significant, asymptomatic, or minimally symptomatic dysrhythmias
Electrocardiogram (ECG) 12-, 15-, or 18-lead ECG	An ECG provides valuable information about the heart rate, rhythm, electrical conduction system, electrical synchrony, and presence of hypertrophy, ischemia, or infarction.	The detection of LA enlargement, repolarization abnormalities, and pathologic Q waves is often the first clue to the presence of HCM.
Cardiopulmonary exercise test (CPX)	Determines maximal myocardial oxygen consumption (MVO_2) defined as the greatest amount of oxygen a patient can utilize while performing dynamic aerobic exercise.	This test quantifies a patient's functional limitations resulting from ventricular dysfunction and helps differentiate between cardiac and pulmonary causes. MVO_2 is usually expressed as milliliters of oxygen consumed per kilogram of body weight per minute.
Blood/Laboratory Studies		
Laboratory testing is individualized based on a patient's history, examination, and imaging tests. Specialized diagnostic laboratory testing, such as gene testing, hemochromatosis panel, autoimmune tests, and infection screening, might not always be necessary or may only be ordered on initial presentation.		
Complete blood count (CBC) Hemoglobin (Hgb) Hematocrit (Hct) RBC count (RBCs) WBC count (WBCs)	Assess for anemia, inflammation and infection; assists with differential diagnosis of chest discomfort and fluid balance.	May reveal decreased Hgb and Hct levels in the presence of anemia or dilution
Electrolytes Potassium (K^+) Magnesium (Mg^{2+}) Calcium (Ca^{2+}) Sodium (Na^+)	Assess for possible causes of dysrhythmias and/or heart failure.	Abnormal levels of K^+, Mg^{2+}, or Ca^{2+} may cause dysrhythmias; Elevation of Na^+ may indicate dehydration (blood is more coagulable); May reveal hyponatremia (dilutional); hypokalemia, which can result from use of diuretics; or hyperkalemia, if glomerular filtration is decreased. Hyperkalemia can also be a side effect of angiotensin-converting enzyme inhibitors (ACEIs) and potassium-sparing diuretics.
Digitalis levels	Digitalis levels are often difficult to manage in heart failure patients, so levels should be done daily if the dosage is being altered.	Chronic heart failure predisposes the patient to digitalis toxicity because of the low cardiac output state, which also causes decreased renal excretion of the drug.
Antidysrhythmic drug levels	Screens for possible drug toxicity or low, non-therapeutic levels	Toxicity or non-therapeutic levels may prompt significant dysrhythmias.

Diagnostic Tests for Cardiomyopathy—cont'd

Test	Purpose	Abnormal Findings
Coagulation profile Prothrombin time (PT) with international normalized ratio (INR) Partial thromboplastin time (PTT) Fibrinogen D-dimer	Assess for efficacy of anticoagulation in heart failure patients receiving warfarin therapy; also helps to evaluate for the presence of cardiogenic shock or hypoperfusion.	Decreased PT with low INR promotes clotting and reflects inadequate anticoagulation; elevation promotes bleeding; elevated fibrinogen and D-dimer reflects abnormal clotting is present.
B-type natriuretic peptide (BNP)	BNP, a hormone secreted by the ventricles, can be useful in distinguishing dyspnea due to heart failure from dyspnea due to pulmonary causes and in monitoring response to therapy.	Levels >100 pg/ml support the diagnosis of heart failure. However, though the BNP level decreases with effective therapy, it may remain chronically >100, even when the patient is no longer symptomatic.
Hepatic enzymes and serum bilirubin levels	Serum glutamate oxaloacetate transaminase/aspartate aminotransferase (SGOT/AST), serum glutamate pyruvate transaminase/alanine aminotransferase (SGPT/ALT), and serum bilirubin levels may be elevated because of hepatic venous congestion.	Elevation reflects vascular congestion resulting from heart failure has caused decreased forward blood flow from the liver to the heart. The liver becomes engorged with blood, which results in increased hepatic enzymes and bilirubin.
Troponin	Assesses for damage to myocardial cells	Elevation may indicate recent damage has occurred.
Thyroid function Thyroid-stimulating hormone (TSH) Free thyroxine index (FTI) Or thyroxine (T4)	Screens for thyroid disease, which may contribute to heart failure	TSH may be elevated unless the disease is long-standing or severe. FTI and T_4 levels may be decreased (see *Myxedema Coma*, p. 725, for more information).
Urinalysis	Helps assess for renal and urologic disease, metabolic abnormalities, and infection that may be related to cardiomyopathy.	Findings will be patient specific.
Radiology		
Chest radiograph (CXR)	Can detect cardiomegaly, pulmonary venous congestion, and characteristic lines of interstitial edema (or fluid) consistent with congestive heart failure	May reveal pulmonary edema, increased interstitial density, infiltrates, engorged pulmonary vasculature, and cardiomegaly Cardiomegaly is commonly seen in DCM, while HCM may result in a normal cardiac silhouette. CXR in patients with RCM may detect mild cardiac enlargement.
Radionuclide studies	Radionuclide ventriculography is a noninvasive method for measuring global and regional LV function.	In DCM, results may reveal diffuse left ventricular hypokinesis, left ventricular ejection fraction <40%, and elevated end-diastolic and systolic volumes. In HCM, the test may reveal vigorous systolic function, hypertrophy, and a small LV volume. With RCM, the test may reveal normal systolic function and a small to normal LV.

Cardiomyopathy

Continued

Diagnostic Tests for Cardiomyopathy—cont'd

Test	Purpose	Abnormal Findings
Invasive Cardiology		
Coronary angiography/ cardiac catheterization	A left heart catheterization with coronary angiography is the gold standard for ruling out ischemic heart disease. A right heart catheterization measures intracardiac and pulmonary pressures.	Hemodynamic findings from a right heart catheterization include cardiac output (CO), cardiac index (CI), right atrial filling pressures (RAP), pulmonary artery pressure (PAP), systemic vascular resistance (SVR), and left ventricular end-diastolic pressure or pulmonary catheter wedge pressure (PCWP). (See Table 5-15.)
Endomyocardial biopsy (EMB)	EMB is used to determine the classification and/or cause of cardiomyopathy through histologic studies that may identify an infiltrative or genetic disorder.	EMB tissue can detect inflammation, metabolic abnormalities, the presence of fibrofatty infiltration, and many other abnormalities of the myocardium. EMB is performed during cardiac catheterization.

COLLABORATIVE MANAGEMENT
Care Priorities

1. Initiate hemodynamic monitoring to help evaluate intracardiac pressures during therapeutic interventions.

For monitoring parameters, see Table 5-15.

2. Reduce activity level to decrease oxygen demand during periods of activity intolerance due to instability.

When the patient stabilizes, increase activity gradually, as tolerated to prevent complications of immobility. Document activity tolerance (including position in bed) to help reflect if treatments are effective.

3. Initiate pharmacotherapy to maintain or reestablish hemodynamic stability, control symptoms, and prevent cardiac remodeling, all of which aid in halting further disease progression.

Medications commonly used in the treatment of CM and their nursing implications (also see *Heart Failure*, p. 421, and *Cardiogenic Shock*, p. 472):

ACEI/ARB: Used in DCM to decrease preload and afterload and block the compensatory response of the renin-angiotensin system to HF. If hemodynamically monitored, the desired effect is to decrease SVR, RAP, and PAWP while increasing CO/CI. Goal SBP is greater than 90 mm Hg. Monitor patients for postural hypotension, hyperkalemia, and worsening renal function.

Beta-blockers: In patients diagnosed with HCM, beta-blockers reduce myocardial oxygen demand and increase diastolic filling time by slowing the HR, relaxing cardiac muscle, and increasing CO. Also, beta-blockers help decrease cardiac outflow obstruction during exercise and reduce sympathetic cardiac stimulation in patients with HCM. For

Table 5-15   HEMODYNAMIC PRESENTATION WITH CARDIOMYOPATHY

Pressure	Effect	Normal Values
Right atrial pressure	Increased	4–6 mm Hg
Pulmonary artery pressure	Increased	20–30/8–15 mm Hg
Pulmonary wedge pressure	Increased	6–12 mm Hg
Cardiac output	Decreased	4–7 L/min
Cardiac index	Decreased	2.5–4 L/min/m^2
Pulmonary vascular resistance	Unchanged or increased	60–100 dynes/sec/cm^{-5}
Systemic vascular resistance	Increased	900–1200 dynes/sec/cm^{-5}

DCM, the goal is to block the compensatory response of the adrenergic system to HF and increase CO/CI while keeping a stable HR (at least 60 bpm) and BP (SBP at least 90 mm Hg). *Note:* These effects are not immediate and may take days to weeks to occur. Beta-blockers should be held in patients receiving IV dobutamine. Generally, beta-blockers should be started once a patient's HR and signs and symptoms have stabilized. Initiating or increasing beta-blocker doses while a patient is experiencing signs and symptoms of HF may worsen dyspnea, edema, bradycardia, and vasodilation. Not all patients with CM tolerate target doses of beta-blockers and should be titrated individually while monitoring BP, HR, and signs and symptoms of worsening HF.

Diuretics: Diuretics reduce preload and pulmonary congestion. If a patient is hemodynamically monitored, diuretics will result in a decreased PAWP and help to achieve a negative fluid balance and ultimately a euvolemic state. Use diuretics cautiously for HCM since they are contraindicated in some patients with obstructive HCM. Monitor the patient for weakness, postural hypotension, hypokalemia (see *Hypokalemia*, p. 52), hypomagnesium, and worsening renal function.

Potassium supplements: Potassium lost in the urine as a result of diuresis may necessitate replacement with potassium supplements. Maintain serum levels in the high normal range (4.2 to 5 mEq/L).

Aldosterone antagonists: Aldosterone is a neurohormone shown to contribute to the development of LV hypertrophy (LVH) and fibrosis involved in myocardial remodeling. Aldosterone antagonists are weak diuretic drugs that block the action of aldosterone. These drugs inhibit sodium reabsorption in the distal convoluted tubule of the kidney and cause retention of potassium and magnesium. Potassium levels must be closely monitored to avoid hyperkalemia or worsening renal function. With aldosterone antagonist use, other side effects include postural hypotension and, if taking spironolactone, gynecomastia.

Vasodilators (hydralazine and nitrates):   These drugs decrease preload and afterload in DCM, resulting in improved CO and enhanced nitric oxide availability. For patients with hemodynamic monitoring, pay attention to decreasing SVR. It is important to maintain a stable BP (keep MAP at 65 mm Hg or higher). Nitrates are not typically used in HCM. Side effects of vasodilators include postural hypotension, dizziness, headache, nausea, and vomiting.

Inotropic therapy (digoxin, dobutamine, milrinone):   Inotropes enhance contractility. If a patient has hemodynamic monitoring, the goal of milrinone and dobutamine is to increase CO/CI and maintain a stable BP for adequate perfusion. Monitor for rhythm disturbances. Other potential side effects include headache and angina.

Safety Alert   *Digoxin is contraindicated in the treatment of obstructive HCM, as it may be ineffective or worsen the condition. Digoxin is also contraindicated in patients with a diagnosis of amyloidosis.*

Antidysrhythmic agents: Medications used to control atrial and ventricular dysrhythmias are common for patients diagnosed with DCM and HCM.

Anticoagulants: Anticoagulants are important to prevent thrombus formation related to atrial fibrillation or decreased ventricular contraction and emptying. INRs must be monitored with extra caution for potential for medication interactions that affect the INR.

Calcium channel blockers (CCBs):   Nonhydropyridine CCBs, such as verapamil or diltiazem, may be used to treat HCM by improving diastolic filling time, heart muscle relaxation, and exercise capacity. Most CCBs are contraindicated in DCM, except for hydropyridine CCBs (such as amlodipine), which is occasionally used to treat hypertension in patients with DCM.

4. **Initiate electrical/device-based therapy to maintain or reestablish hemodynamic stability, control symptoms, and prevent cardiac remodeling.**   (For further information, also see *Heart Failure*, p. 421, and *Cardiogenic Shock*, p. 472.)

   CRT: CRT may be considered for patients with DCM and LVEF less than 35%, a QRS duration greater than 0.12 second (cardiac dyssynchrony), sinus rhythm, and with New York Heart Association (NYHA) Class III to IV HF symptoms despite optimal recommended medical therapies.

Dual-chamber pacemakers: Pacemakers treat dangerous cardiac dysrhythmias associated with symptomatic bradycardia, ventricular dysfunction, or low CO.

ICD: ICDs treat life-threatening ventricular dysrhythmias in patients with cardiac conditions associated with a high risk of sudden death. Patients at risk for sudden death requiring ICD placment are on optimal medical therapy with a reasonable expectation of survival and with good functional status for longer than 1 year.

Alcohol ablation: During a cardiac catheterization, ethanol is injected into the septal branches of the LAD. This purposeful reduction of myocardial tissue through a limited, therapeutic septal infarction will reduce outflow obstruction in HCM.

Ultrafiltration (UF): UF, used to treat acute decompensated HF with volume overload, is the mechanical removal of excess body fluid by the generation of a convective gradient across the hemofilter membrane. The electrolyte concentration of the ultrafiltrate is equal to that of the plasma and avoids the stimulation of the renin-angiotensin-aldosterone axis.

IABP: In the presence of a failing myocardium, an IABP helps to decrease afterload and increase coronary artery perfusion

Mechanical Circulatory Support/VADs: A VAD is used in the presence of a failing myocardium to increase CO (see *Cardiogenic Shock*, p. 472).

5. **Provide surgical interventions to maintain or reestablish hemodynamic stability, control symptoms, and prevent cardiac remodeling.** (For further information, also see *Heart Failure*, p. 421, and *Cardiogenic Shock*, p. 472.)

Ventricular septal myotomy-myectomy: During this procedure, the hypertrophied ventricular septum of obstructive HCM is removed.

Heart transplantation: Open heart transplantation is pursued for patients with advanced CM refractory to optimal medical therapy. Each institution has criteria that must be met before transplantation is considered a treatment option (see *Organ Transplantation*, p. 906).

CARE PLANS FOR CARDIOMYOPATHY

Nursing care must be based on the type of CM, its associated pathology, and the patient's clinical manifestations. Acute decompensated HF (ADHF) is a gradual or rapid change in HF signs and symptoms resulting in a need for urgent therapy due to elevated LV filling pressures and/or low CO. The primary aspects of care related to ADHF are outlined since this is the most common presenting problem, for this patient population, in the acute care setting.

Decreased cardiac output *related to disease process that has resulted in decreased ability of the heart to provide adequate pumping to maintain effective oxygenation and nutrition of body systems*

- -

GOALS/OUTCOMES Within the 24-hour period before discharge from the CCU, patient has adequate CO as evidenced by:

ASSESSMENT MEASURE	GOAL
SBP	At least 90 mm Hg
MAP	At least 65 mm Hg
CI	2.5 to 4 L/min/m^2
CO	4 to 7 L/min
PAWP	Less than 18 mm Hg
Right atrial pressure (RAP)/CVP	4 to 6 mm Hg
RR	12 to 20 breaths/min
HR	Less than 100 bpm
Urinary output	More than 0.5 ml/kg/hr
Skin assessment	Warm and dry
Peripheral pulses	At least 2+ on a 0 to 4+ scale
Mental status	Orientation to time, place, and person (assuming baseline orientation ×3)

NOC Cardiac Pump Effectiveness; Circulation Status

Cardiac Care: Acute Hemodynamic Regulation

1. If a pulmonary artery (PA) catheter is present, record hemodynamic readings every 1 to 2 hours and on an as-needed basis.

2. Be alert to PAWP greater than 18 mm Hg and RAP/CVP greater than 6 mm Hg. Although normal PAWP is 6 to 12 mm Hg, these patients may need increased filling pressures for adequate preload, with wedge pressure at 15 to 18 mm Hg. Those with right HF may need an RAP/CVP 8 to 12 mm Hg. Measure CO/CI every 2 to 4 hours and on an as-needed basis. Optimally, CO should be 4 to 7 L/min and CI should be 2.5 to 4 L/min/m²; for some patients, the best CO/CI will be below expected normal values.

3. Keep accurate I&O records and weigh the patient daily at the same time every day, noting trends and goal weight. Individuals with CM may be on a strict fluid-restricted (e.g., 1000 to 2000 ml/day) and sodium-restricted (e.g., less than 2000 mg/day) diet.

4. Monitor electrolytes and renal function routinely, especially if your patient is receiving high-dose diuretics. Notify the physician if urinary output is less than 30 ml/hr or less than 500 ml the first hour after receiving a loop diuretic, or if total urine output in 24 hours is less than 1000 ml.

5. Monitor cardiac rhythm continuously for dysrhythmias, such as sinus or atrial tachycardias, atrial fibrillation, or ventricular ectopy, which may further decrease CO.

6. Assist patients with activities of daily living (ADLs) when necessary and monitor activity tolerance. Be sure to document activity tolerance and report worsening exercise tolerance. *Note:* A patient's activity intolerance is often related to an imbalance between the oxygen supply and demand secondary to decreased myocardial contractility.

7. Administer medications as prescribed, staggering the HF-related medications throughout the day rather than administering them all at once. Be sure to provide ongoing patient education regarding the purpose and common side effects for each medication.

NIC Cardiac Care: Acute; Circulatory Care: Mechanical Assist Device; Hemodynamic Regulation; Shock Management: Cardiac; Neurologic Monitoring; Medication Management; Dysrhythmia Management

Activity intolerance *related to imbalance between oxygen supply and demand secondary to decreased functioning of the myocardium*

GOALS/OUTCOMES *Within the 12- to 24-hour period before discharge from the CCU, patients should exhibit cardiac tolerance to increasing levels of activity as evidenced by respiratory rate less than 24 breaths/min, BP within 20 mm Hg of patient's normal range, HR within 20 bpm of patient's normal resting HR, return to a stable baseline ECG rhythm, and activity tolerance to a level without presence of angina/chest pain or worsening dyspnea.*
NOC Activity Tolerance; Energy Conservation

Energy Management

1. Monitor the patient's physiologic response to activity, reporting any symptoms of chest pain, new or increasing SOB, increases in HR greater than 20 bpm above resting HR, and increase or decrease in SBP greater than 20 mm Hg.

2. Monitor cardiac rhythm for the occurrence of dysrhythmias at rest or during activity.

3. Observe for and report any signs of decreased CO, e.g., changes in mentation, cool-clammy skin, or tachycardia.

4. Plan nursing care so that the patient is assured of extended periods of rest (at least 90 minutes).
   - To prevent complications of immobility, perform or teach patients and significant others active, passive, and assistive ROM exercises. For a discussion of an in-bed exercise program, see Table 5-6 and interventions in *Prolonged Immobility,* p. 149.
   - Consult the physician to ensure that exercises are within the patient's prescribed limitations.

NIC Activity Therapy; Energy Management; Teaching: Prescribed Activity/Exercise; Dysrhythmia Management; Pain Management; Medication Management

ADDITIONAL NURSING DIAGNOSES

Also see nursing diagnoses and interventions in *Hemodynamic Monitoring* (p. 75), *Heart Failure* (p. 421), *Prolonged Immobility* (p. 149), *Emotional and Spiritual Support of the Patient and Significant Others* (p. 200), and *Cardiogenic Shock* (p. 472).

DYSRHYTHMIAS AND CONDUCTION DISTURBANCES

PATHOPHYSIOLOGY

Cardiac dysrhythmias reflect abnormal function of the heart's electrical system. Cardiac electrical cells closely interface with the mechanical cells, which contain the contractile muscle filaments. Dysrhythmias may originate in any part of the electrical system, from the pacing cells (sinoatrial [SA] node, atrioventricular [AV] junction) to any portion of the conduction system (atria, His-Purkinje system, bundle branches, and ventricles). Sympathetic and parasympathetic nerve fibers influence the rate of discharge of the SA node, conduction through the AV node, and force of both atrial and ventricular contraction. The main parasympathetic influence is the vagus nerve, which slows the rate of pacing by the SA node and AV junction, and decreases force of contraction. Sympathetic nerve fibers originate from T1 to T5 and, when stimulated, produce the neurotransmitter norepinephrine, which increases HR during the stress response. Sympathetic stimulation also promotes production of catecholamines by the adrenal glands, and the hormones are received by catecholamine receptors (alpha receptors, beta receptors, dopaminergic receptors), which increase HR, force of contraction, BP, and CO. Electrical dysfunction can markedly change the CO and cause prompt deterioration in the patient's hemodynamic status (Figure 5-1).

Cardiac electrophysiology involves studying the electrical impulses and their conduction across the atria and throughout the ventricles to provide power and coordination for the cardiac cycle. Electrical impulses are created by ion exchange. Exchange of ions in the mechanical or muscle cells generates electrical activity. At rest, the muscle has slightly more positive ions (Na^+ and Ca^{2+}) on the outside of the cells and more negative ions inside the cells (resting membrane potential or polarization). K^+ is the most prevalent intracellular ion. The resting cells have a threshold for activation, based on the difference in the ion concentrations (action potential). Stimulation of a cardiac muscle cell, or depolarization, is created by a rapid influx of Na^+ followed by a slower influx of Ca^{2+} into the cell. Normally, the influx is followed by muscle contraction. The cell responds to the influx by K^+ diffusing out of the cell to help rebalance the positive ions (early repolarization and plateau phase) on both sides of the cell membrane. A slower efflux is followed by a rapid efflux of K^+ (rapid repolarization). Finally, the sodium-potassium pump must activate to fully rebalance the electrical potential of the cell, restore the ions to their original position, and achieve resting membrane potential or polarization.

Normal electrical activity of the heart produces waves or deflections on the ECG (Figure 5-2). The waves and intervals that comprise the components of the ECG make up one electrical cardiac cycle (Figure 5-3).

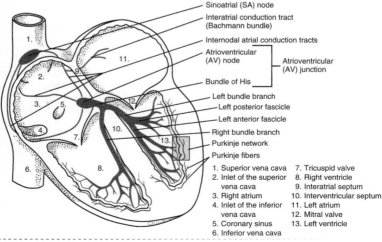

Sinoatrial (SA) node

Interatrial conduction tract (Bachmann bundle)

Internodal atrial conduction tracts

Atrioventricular (AV) node

Atrioventricular (AV) junction

Bundle of His

Left bundle branch
Left posterior fascicle
Left anterior fascicle
Right bundle branch
Purkinje network
Purkinje fibers

1. Superior vena cava
2. Inlet of the superior vena cava
3. Right atrium
4. Inlet of the inferior vena cava
5. Coronary sinus
6. Inferior vena cava
7. Tricuspid valve
8. Right ventricle
9. Interatrial septum
10. Interventricular septum
11. Left atrium
12. Mitral valve
13. Left ventricle

Figure 5-1 Electrical conduction system. (From Huszar RJ: *Basic dysrhythmias: interpretation and management,* ed 3, St Louis, MO, 2002, Mosby.)

- *P wave:* Electrical impulse originating in the SA node, the heart's primary pacemaker, which prompts atrial depolarization or the spread of the impulse across the right and left atria. It is the first positive deflection from the isoelectric baseline in most ECG leads but may be postive, negative, or biphasic in leads III, aVL, and V_1. The atria contract following the appearance of the P wave. The wave should be rounded, less than 0.11 second in duration (width), and no greater than 2.5 mm in height (voltage).
- *PR interval:* The P wave plus the isoelectric line extending to the beginning of the QRS complex, wherein the impulse spreads through the AV node, the bundle of His, the right and left bundle branches, and Purkinje fibers. The interval measures 0.12 to 0.2 second in normal adults.
- *QRS complex:* A set of three combined waves (Q, R, and S) that represents ventricular depolarization, which stimulates ventricular contraction. The wave of atrial repolarization is hidden within this larger, dominant complex. The QRS complex should be 0.06 to 0.1 second in normal adults and varies in direction depending on the ECG lead but is most recognized as positive deflection (which represents the R wave, a positive deflection from the baseline). Some normal positive complexes are "missing" a distinct Q or S wave. The complex is predominantly negative in leads aVR, V_1, and V_2 and biphasic in leads V_3, V_4, and, occasionally, lead III (which represents stronger Q- and S-wave activity, which are the negative deflections that precede and follow the R wave).
- *ST segment:* The isoelectric line between the end of the QRS complex and the T wave, which represents early ventricular repolarization. The segment changes in response to myocardial ischemia, injury, hypokalemia, pericarditis, and other ventricular tissue abnormalities. The "J" point is where the ST segment begins, where the QRS complex terminates.
- *T wave:* Represents ventricular repolarization, wherein during the first part of the wave, the tissue is refractory to further stimulation (absolute refractory period). At the peak of the T wave, the tissue becomes sensitive to stronger electrical stimuli (relative refractory period), and ventricular dysrhythmias may occur.
- *QT interval:* Represents the depolarization and repolarization of the ventricle, measured from the beginning of the QRS complex to the end of the T wave. If no Q wave is present, the interval is measured from the beginning of the R wave to the end of the T wave. As the HR increases, the QT interval should decrease proportionally. There are tables available to reflect the duration of a normal QT interval for various HRs. When the duration of the QT interval is adjusted or corrected for HR, the interval is termed the QTc interval. A QT interval that is greater than half the RR interval (distance between two R waves) is considered prolonged.
- *U wave:* A small positive waveform that sometimes follows the T wave. The significance is unknown, but it is theorized to be a wave of Purkinje fiber repolarization.

Abnormal Electrocardiogram Tracings

Myocardial ischemia, electrolyte or other chemical imbalance, and an abnormally configured electrical system are factors likely to stimulate dysrhythmias. The normal flow of impulses depends on properly nourished, well-oxygenated electrical tissues with an anatomically correct pacing and conduction system. The cardiac cycle depends on a balance of basic regulatory substances including sodium, potassium, calcium, and glucose, and appropriate amounts of catecholamines. Imbalance of these regulators can cause a disturbance in automaticity, conduction/conductivity, or myocardial contractility.

- *Automaticity:* The ability of cardiac cells to initiate an electrical impulse spontaneously, without stimulation by a nerve or other source. Hypokalemia and hypocalcemia increase automaticity. The SA node, AV junction, and Purkinje fibers possess automaticity. All cardiac muscle is electrically "irritable" or excitable due to the concentration of ions on both sides of the cell membranes, but not all cells possess automaticity. All cardiac cells are able to respond to external stimuli, including electrical and mechanical sources.
- *Conduction/conductivity:* All cardiac cells can receive electrical stimuli and transmit or conduct impulses to an adjacent cell. Intercalated disks in the cell membranes facilitate the transmission of impulses throughout the heart muscle. When impulses reach muscle cells, they stimulate muscle contraction.
- *Myocardial contractility:* Cardiac muscle cells "shorten" in response to electrical impulses, which manifests as a muscle contraction.

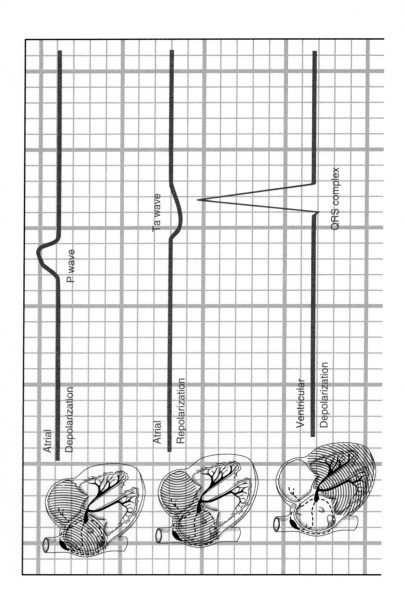

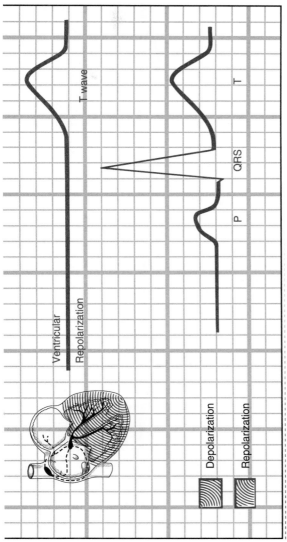

Figure 5-2 Electrical basis on the ECG. (From Huszar RJ: *Basic dysrhythmias: interpretation and management*, ed 3, St Louis, MO, 2002, Mosby.)

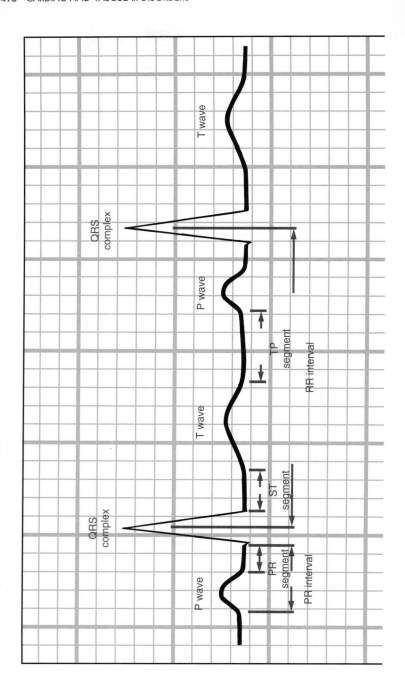

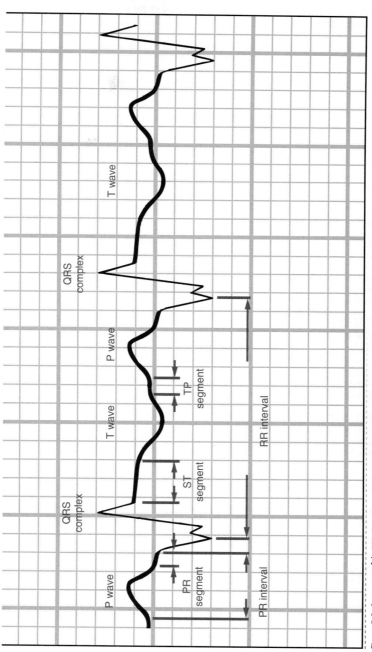

Figure 5-3 Components of the ECG. (From Huszar RJ: *Basic dysrhythmias: interpretation and management*, ed 3, St Louis, MO, 2002, Mosby.)

Dysrhythmias and Conduction Disturbances

Causes of Abnormal Rhythms

Disturbances in automaticity: May involve an acceleration or deceleration in pacing or automaticity of the SA node, such as sinus tachycardia (HR greater than 100 bpm) or sinus bradycardia (HR less than 60 bpm). Premature beats or possibly an escape or compensatory heart rhythm may arise from the atria, junction, or ventricles if the SA node is dysfunctional or arrests. Without additional catecholamines prompted by the stress response, escape rhythms generated from the AV junction or the ventricles are usually bradycardic (HR less than 60 bpm). Abnormal rhythms, such as atrial or ventricular tachycardia, may also result from excessive sympathetic stimulation or electrolyte imbalance.

Disturbances in conduction: Conduction may be too rapid, as in conditions that induce the stress response (e.g., severe/critical illness, certain endocrine diseases, profound emotional stress) or in the presence of an accessory pathway (e.g., Wolff-Parkinson-White [WPW] syndrome). Accessory pathways are extra conduction fibers that provide a direct connection between the atria and the ventricles, circumventing the AV node. Rhythms generated from these anatomically incorrect conduction systems are called AV reciprocating tachycardias and may have rates greater than 250 bpm. Reentry is a situation in which a misdirected electrical impulse reexcites a conduction pathway through which it has already passed. Once started, this impulse may circulate through the same area repeatedly, prompting an AV reentrant tachycardia. The trapped impulse becomes the pacemaker in this circumstance. Impulse conduction may be delayed or too slow (e.g., first- and second-degree AV block), or become totally blocked from continuing down the pathway by abnormal electrical tissues (e.g., third-degree or complete heart block) (Figure 5-4).

Combinations of disturbed automaticity and conduction: Several dysrhythmias may occur simultaneously (e.g., first-degree AV block [disturbance in conductivity], premature atrial complexes [PACs] [disturbance in automaticity]).

ASSESSMENT

Goal of Assessment

To diagnose the type of dysrhythmia, the cause of the rhythm (electrolyte or acid-base imbalance, structural abnormality, heart and/or renal disease, nervous system or neuroendocrine dysfunction), the impact of the dysrhythmia on the CO (BP)/coronary artery perfusion (may prompt chest discomfort), and to determine the urgency and type of treatment. Lethal dysrhythmias result in cardiac arrest.

History and Risk Factors

Acidosis or alkalosis, acute coronary syndrome (CAD, angina, MI) or other heart disease or acute conditions (pericarditis, presence of accessory conduction pathways, cardiomyopathy, HF, valvular disease, cardiac tamponade), anemia, current use of antidysrhythmic or bronchodilating drugs, recreational drug abuse, drug overdose, use of catecholamines (epinephrine, dopamine, dobutamine, norepinephrine), use of tricyclic antidepressants (TCAs), diuretics, exposure to other environmental toxins, electrolyte disturbances (especially hypokalemia, hypoglycemia, or hypomagnesemia), endocrine disease (posterior pituitary, thyroid, parathyroid, adrenal, or pancreas), hypothermia, hypoxia, hypotension, hypovolemia, hypervolemia, increased intracranial pressure, infection pneumothorax or tension pneumothorax, pulmonary disease including pulmonary embolism, peripheral vascular or peripheral arterial disease (PAD), respiratory failure, renal failure, and sepsis

Observation

The patient's appearance varies from absence of symptoms to complete cardiopulmonary arrest. Common symptoms include activity intolerance, weakness, pallor, hypotension, dizziness, SOB, dyspnea, palpitations, chest discomfort or pressure, and sensation of "racing heart" or "skipped beats." More serious symptoms include altered mental status, anxiety, respiratory insufficiency, syncope, and seizures, which may lead to HF and cardiopulmonary arrest. Pulseless ventricular tachycardia, ventricular fibrillation, asystole, and pulseless electrical activity (PEA) result in immediate cardiac arrest.

1. Prolonged PR interval (>0.20 sec)
   (first-degree AV block)

Delay of
conduction of the
electrical impulse
through the:

AV node or
bundle of His

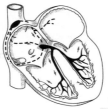

⟍ Electrical impulse
▨ Conduction delay

2. Absence of a QRS after a P wave
   (second- and third-degree AV block)

Blockage of
conduction of the
electrical impulse
through the:

AV node or
bundle of His,
or bundle branches

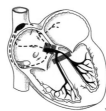

⟍ Electrical impulse
■ Conduction delay

3. Short PR interval (<0.12 sec)

a. Ectopic
pacemaker in
the atria or
AV junction

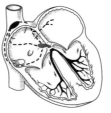

OR

b. Conduction of the
electrical impulse
through abnormal
AV conduction
pathways

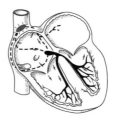

⟍ Electrical impulse

Figure 5-4 Anomalous AV conduction. (From Huszar RJ: *Basic dysrhythmias: interpretation and management*, ed 3, St Louis, MO, 2002, Mosby.)

Vital Signs

Vary with type of dysrhythmia. Vital signs may be unaffected or affected slightly. Accelerated or decelerated HR may cause hypotension, result in HF, or deteriorate into pulselessness. Symptomatic dysrhythmias most often result in a very rapid, slow, or irregular pulse, changed pulse quality, hypotension, pallor, possibly a variable HR (fast, then slow), and tachypnea. If the CO is markedly decreased, shocklike symptoms ensue including cold, clammy skin, dusky or cyanotic appearance, decreased urine output, and feeling of impending doom or imminent death.

ECG and Hemodynamic Measurements

Hemodynamic measurements will vary, depending on the effect of the dysrhythmia on the CO. If patient has HF, CO is decreased and PAP may be elevated. Right- and left-sided HF manifest differently (see *Heart Failure*, p. 421). Tachycardias usually increase CO initially, unless the rate is too fast to allow adequate ventricular filling, in which case CO decreases and may lead to HF. ECG findings seen with various dysrhythmias include abnormalities in rate such as sinus bradycardia or sinus tachycardia, irregular rhythm such as atrial fibrillation, extra beats such as PACs and premature junctional complexes (PJCs), wide and bizarre-looking beats such as premature ventricular complexes (PVCs) and ventricular tachycardia (VT), a fibrillating baseline such as ventricular fibrillation (VF), and a straight line as with asystole. Figures 5-5 through 5-30 give an overview of common rhythms, dysrhythmias, conduction disturbances, and pacemaker rhythms and their treatment. Occasionally, patients have an electrical rhythm without corresponding mechanical pumping. This condition is known as PEA. Initially, the rhythm may appear nearly normal but rapidly deteriorates as the conduction pathway becomes hypoxic.

Auscultation

If HF is present, heart sounds may include S_3 and S_4; basilar crackles or rales are audible with lung auscultation; and a wet cough with frothy sputum may be present.

Palpation

With HF, jugular veins are distended and peripheral edema is present.

Normal Sinus Rhythm

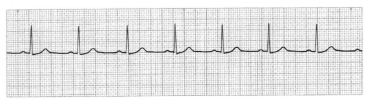

- Rhythm: regular
- Atrial rate: 60-100 beats/min
- Ventricular rate: 60-100 beats/min
- P waves: before each QRS
- QRS: normal and of normal width (less than .12 sec)
- PR interval: normal (.12-.20 sec)
- P: QRS: 1:1

Significance: Usual, normal rhythm and conduction.
Intervention: None.

Figure 5-5 Normal sinus rhythm. (From Huszar RJ: *Basic dysrhythmias: interpretation and management,* ed 3, St Louis, MO, 2002, Mosby.)

Sinus Tachycardia

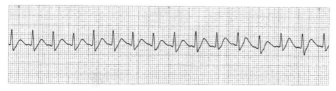

- Rhythm: regular
- Atrial rate: >100 beats/min; usually <160 beats/min
- Ventricular rate: >100 beats/min; usually <160 beats/min
- P waves: before each QRS
- QRS: normal duration
- PR interval: normal
- P: QRS: 1:1

Significance: Increased rate usually caused by sympathetic stimulation. Causes may include pain, fever, anxiety, hypovolemia, heart failure, caffeine intake, use of theophylline or sympathomimetic agents.

Intervention: Treat the cause.
Increased rate is usually caused by sympathetic stimulation. Cause may include pain, fever, anxiety, hypovolemia, heart failure, caffeine intake, use of theophylline or sympathomimetic agents.

Figure 5-6 Sinus tachycardia. (From Huszar RJ: *Basic dysrhythmias: interpretation and management*, ed 3, St Louis, MO, 2002, Mosby.)

Sinus Bradycardia

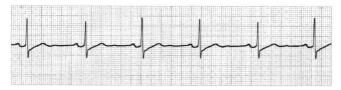

- Rhythm: regular
- Atrial rate: <60 beats/min
- Ventricular rate: <60 beats/min
- P waves: before each QRS
- QRS: normal duration
- PR interval: normal
- P: QRS: 1:1

Significance: Slow rate usually caused by increased parasympathetic stimulation. Causes may include vagal stimulation, β-adrenergic blocking agents and other drugs, AMI, increased intracranial pressure (IICP). This rhythm may be "normal" in some people.

Intervention: No treatment necessary unless patient's BP drops and/or LOC is altered or PVCs occur. Initial treatment is atropine and oxygen.
Atropine 0.5 mg may be given and repeated up to a total dose of 3 mg if bradycardia is symptomatic (hypotension, chest discomfort). Transcutaneous pacing, epinephrine (2-10 mcg/min) or dopamine (2-10 mcg/kg/min) may also be considered.

Figure 5-7 Sinus bradycardia. (From Huszar RJ: *Basic dysrhythmias: interpretation and management*, ed 3, St Louis, MO, 2002, Mosby.)

Dysrhythmias and Conduction Disturbances

Sinus Dysrhythmia

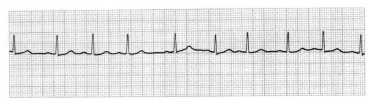

- Rhythm: regular
- Atrial rate: 60-100 beats/min
- Ventricular rate: 60-100 beats/min
- P waves: before each QRS
- QRS: normal duration
- PR interval: normal
- P: QRS: 1:1

Significance: This rhythm usually increases in rate with respiration and decreases with expiration. It can be a normal finding in children. As an abnormal finding, it may be caused by drugs, IICP, or heart disease.

Intervention: Observation; usually no treatment necessary.

Figure 5-8 Sinus dysrhythmia. (From Huszar RJ: *Basic dysrhythmias: interpretation and management,* ed 3, St Louis, MO, 2002, Mosby.)

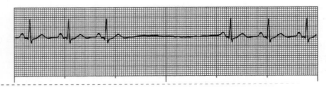

Figure 5-9 Normal sinus rhythm with sinus arrest. (From Aehlert B: *ECGs made easy: pocket reference,* ed 2, St Louis, MO, 2002, Mosby.)

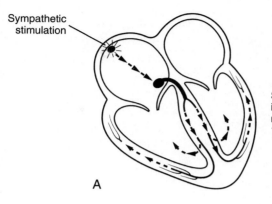

SA node originates
impulses at regular
rate of greater than
100 / minute

A

Wandering Atrial Pacemaker

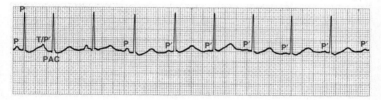

- Rhythm: irregular
- Atrial rate: usually 60-100 beats/min
- Ventricular rate: usually 60-100 beats/min
- P waves: before each QRS
- QRS: normal duration
- PR interval: usually normal; some variation
- P: QRS: 1:1

Significance: An ectopic atrial focus. Causes may include drugs, COPD, inflammatory disorders.

Intervention: Observation. If cause can be determined, treat cause. If patient is receiving digoxin, check serum level.

Figure 5-10 Sinus tachycardia with premature atrial complexes (PACs). (**Top,** from Emergency Nurses Association: *Sheehy's manual of emergency care,* ed 6, St Louis, MO, 2005, Mosby. **Bottom,** from Aehlert B: *ECGs made easy: pocket reference,* ed 2, St Louis, MO, 2002, Mosby.)

Dysrhythmias and Conduction Disturbances

Atrial Tachycardia

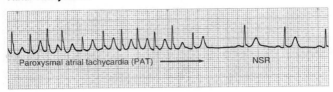

- Rhythm: mostly regular
- Atrial rate: 160-240 beats/min
- Ventricular rate: depends on AV conduction ratio
- P waves: may be difficult to identify because of fast rate
- QRS: normal; may be wide if aberrant conduction is present

Significance: Can precipitate chest pain and ischemia. Patients often experience dizziness, diaphoresis, and nausea. Many patients diagnosed with wide-complex atrial tachycardia (SVT) are found to have ventricular tachycardia when electrophysiology studies are done.

Intervention: Vagal maneuvers, diltiazem, adenosine. Other agents include digoxin, β-blockers, and procainamide. If the patient has an accessory pathway with AV reciprocating tachycardia, catheter ablation may be necessary to correct the problem.

Figure 5-11 Atrial tachycardia. (From Huszar RJ: *Basic dysrhythmias: interpretation and management,* ed 3, St Louis, MO, 2002, Mosby.)

Atrial Flutter (Type I)

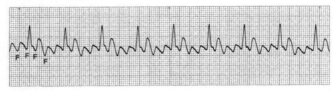

- Rhythm: regular if block is regular; may be irregular
- Atrial rate: 240-340 beats/min (type I); 340-430 beats/min (type II)
- Ventricular rate: depends on AV conduction
- P waves: saw-toothed; F waves
- QRS: normal
- PR interval: not measurable
- P: QRS: P > QRS

Significance: An atrial ectopic focus. AV conduction ratios can be variable, usually at least 2:1. The ineffective contraction can cause thrombus formation in the atria, which may subsequently embolize to the lungs, brain, and possibly other distal vessels.

Intervention: IV diltiazem, diltiazem, or β-blockers. For type I, rapid atrial pacing or cardioversion if unstable. Other agents may include IV ibutilide or amiodarone. PO flecainide, amiodarone, propafenone, or sotalol may also be used. Patients with an atrial rate of >240 may need to be anticoagulated to prevent atrial thrombus formation.

Figure 5-12 Atrial flutter (type I). (From Huszar RJ: *Basic dysrhythmias: interpretation and management,* ed 3, St Louis, MO, 2002, Mosby.)

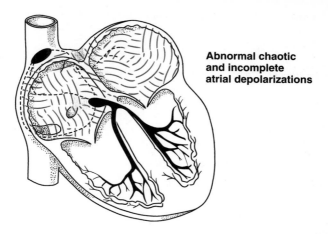

**Abnormal chaotic
and incomplete
atrial depolarizations**

Atrial Fibrillation

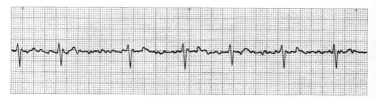

- Rhythm: irregularly irregular
- Atrial rate: >350 beats/min
- Ventricular rate: variable
- P waves: coarse or fine fibrillatory waves
- QRS: normal
- PR interval: not measurable
- P: QRS: P > QRS

Significance: Chaotic atrial firing and ineffective atrial contraction. Cardiac output usually drops because of loss of atrial "kick." Ineffective atrial contraction makes clot formation a danger.

Intervention: Patients in chronic AF with controlled ventricular response may not require intervention. For new-onset AF with a rapid ventricular response, use the same protocol as recommended for atrial flutter. Patients should be anticoagulated to prevent atrial thrombus formation, unless contraindicated because of other medical problems.

Figure 5-13 Atrial fibrillation (AF). (From Huszar RJ: *Basic dysrhythmias: interpretation and management,* ed 3, St Louis, MO, 2002, Mosby.)

AV Junctional Rhythm or Junctional Escape Rhythm

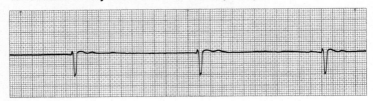

- Rhythm: regular
- Atrial rate: cannot determine
- Ventricular rate: 40-60 beats/min
- P waves: inverted before or after QRS or not present
- QRS: normal
- PR interval: <0.12 sec if P precedes QRS
- P: QRS: P ≤ QRS

Significance: AV node assumes primary pacing function from atria.
Intervention: Usually no specific therapy indicated. If patient becomes
symptomatic because of a slow rate. Atropine 0.5 mg may
be given, and repeated up to a total of 3 mg. Transcutaneous
pacing, or continuous infusions of Epinephrine (2–10 mcg/min),
or Dopamine (2–10 mcg/kg/min) may be considered.

Figure 5-14 AV junctional rhythm or junctional escape rhythm. (From Huszar RJ: *Basic dysrhythmias: interpretation and management,* ed 3, St Louis, MO, 2002, Mosby.)

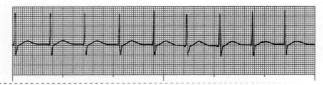

Figure 5-15 Accelerated junctional rhythm. (From Aehlert B: *ECGs made easy: pocket reference,* ed 2, St Louis, MO, 2002, Mosby.)

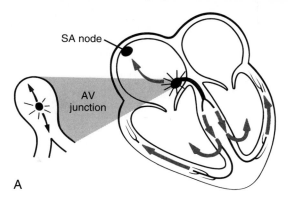

A

Premature Junctional Complexes

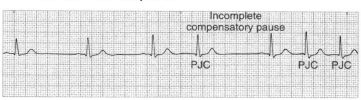

- Rhythm: irregular
- Atrial rate: cannot determine
- Ventricular rate: depends on underlying rhythm
- P waves: before, during, and after QRS
- QRS: normal
- PR interval: <0.12 sec if P precedes QRS
- P: QRS: P ≤ QRS

Significance: Less common than PACs; may precede blocks.
Intervention: Observation. Usually no treatment is necessary. If indicated, therapy is similar to that for PACs.

Figure 5-16 Premature junctional complexes. (**Top,** from Emergency Nurses Association: *Sheehy's manual of emergency care*, ed 6, St Louis, MO, 2005, Mosby. **Bottom,** from Huszar RJ: *Basic dysrhythmias: interpretation and management*, ed 3, St Louis, MO, 2002, Mosby.)

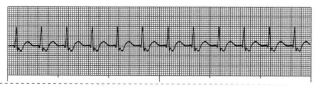

Figure 5-17 Junctional tachycardia (JT). (From Aehlert B: *ECGs made easy: pocket reference*, ed 2, St Louis, MO, 2002, Mosby.)

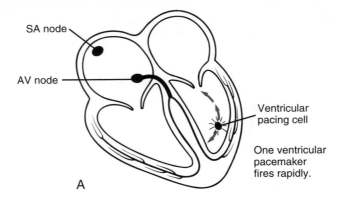

SA node

AV node

Ventricular pacing cell

One ventricular pacemaker fires rapidly.

A

Ventricular Tachycardia

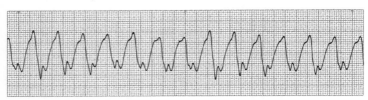

- Rhythm: slightly irregular
- Atrial rate: cannot determine
- Ventricular rate: 150-250 beats/min
- P waves: not visible
- QRS: wide (>0.12 sec)
- PR interval: cannot determine
- P: QRS: absent

Significance: Cardiac output falls significantly, cannot be tolerated for long, and will deteriorate into VF and asystole. May be monomorphic (same form repeated) or polymorphic (more than one type present).

Intervention: Current research indicates Amiodarone is useful in converting unstable VT to sinus rhythm. If pulseless, patient requires immediate defibrillation. Recent studies indicate patients who survive sudden cardiac death and those with sustained VT should be considered for an implantable cardioverter-defibrillator (ICD).

Figure 5-18 Ventricular tachycardia. (**Top,** from Emergency Nurses Association: *Sheehy's manual of emergency care*, ed 6, St Louis, MO, 2005, Mosby. **Bottom,** from Huszar RJ: *Basic dysrhythmias: interpretation and management*, ed 3, St Louis, MO, 2002, Mosby.)

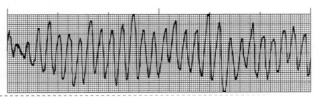

Figure 5-19 Torsade de pointes. (From Aehlert B: *ECGs made easy: pocket reference*, ed 2, St Louis, MO, 2002, Mosby.)

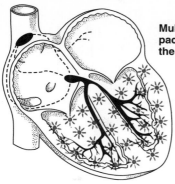

Multiple ectopic pacemaker in the ventricles

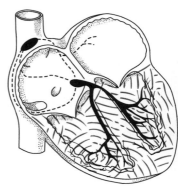

Abnormal, chaotic, and incomplete ventricular depolarizations

Ventricular Fibrillation

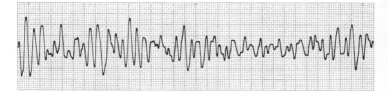

- Rhythm: irregular
- Atrial rate: cannot determine
- Ventricular rate: rapid
- P waves: not seen
- QRS: absent; fibrillatory waves
- PR interval: none
- P: QRS: none

Significance: Most common cause of sudden cardiac death. VF produces no cardiac output.

Intervention: Immediate defibrillation is required with 200 joules, or per other recommendation of the defibrillator manufacturer. Perform cardiopulmonary resuscitation until defibrillator is available. Repeat single shock defibrillation every 2 minutes while CPR continues between shocks, increasing energy to maximum of 360 joules. Patients who survive sudden cardiac death (VF) should be considered for an implantable cardioverter-defibrillator (ICD).

Figure 5-20 Ventricular fibrillation. (From Huszar RJ: *Basic dysrhythmias: interpretation and management*, ed 3, St Louis, MO, 2002, Mosby.)

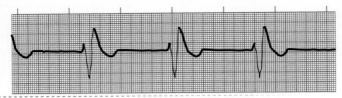

Figure 5-21 Idioventricular rhythm. (From Aehlert B: *ACLS Study Guide*, ed 3, St Louis, MO, 2007, Mosby.)

Asystole

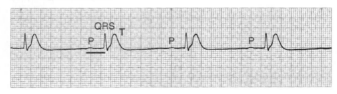

- No electrical activity
- May see a rare, wide, bizarre QRS

Significance: Mortality >95%. Always confirm asystole in 2 leads.

Intervention: Asystole means the heart is not beating or the pulse is absent. Perform cardiopulmonary resuscitation (CPR) according to current American Heart Association Basic Cardiac Life Support Guidelines, and initiate Advanced Cardiac Life Support as soon as possible. Those with symptomatic idioventricular rhythms may benefit from bradycaridia interventions if a pulse is present.

Figure 5-22 Asystole. (From Huszar RJ: *Basic dysrhythmias: interpretation and management*, ed 3, St Louis, MO, 2002, Mosby.)

First-Degree AV Block

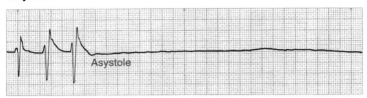

- Rhythm: regular
- Atrial rate: 60-100 beats/min
- Ventricular rate: 60-100 beats/min
- P waves: present; precede each QRS
- QRS: normal
- PR interval: prolonged (>0.2 sec)
- P: QRS: 1:1

Significance: Impulse conduction is delayed through the AV node. Causes are varied and may include heart disease, ischemia, digitalis toxicity, other drug effect, and myocarditis.

Intervention: Observation; usually no treatment needed. Atropine 0.5 mg may be given and repeated up to a total dose of 3 mg if bradycardia is symptomatic (hypotension, chest discomfort). Transcutaneous pacing, epinephrine (2-10 mcg/min), or dopamine (2-10 mcg/kg/min) may also be considered.

Figure 5-23 First-degree AV block. (From Huszar RJ: *Basic dysrhythmias: interpretation and management*, ed 3, St Louis, MO, 2002, Mosby.)

Second-Degree AV Block Type I (Wenckebach)

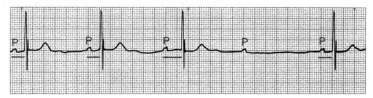

- Rhythm: irregular
- Atrial rate: exceeds ventricular rate
- Ventricular rate: less than sinus rate
- P waves: one P wave precedes each QRS except during nonconducted P waves, which occur regularly
- QRS: normal
- PR interval: lengthens progressively with each cycle until one is nonconducted

Significance: Usually a transient block that does not progress to complete heart block.

Intervention: Observation; treatment usually not necessary.
Atropine 0.5 mg may be given and repeated up to a total dose of 3 mg if bradycardia is symptomatic (hypotension, chest discomfort). Transcutaneous pacing, epinephrine (2-10 mcg/min), or dopamine (2-10 mcg/kg/min) may also be considered.

Figure 5-24 Second-degree AV block (Type I) (Wenckebach). (From Huszar RJ: *Basic dysrhythmias: interpretation and management,* ed 3, St Louis, MO, 2002, Mosby.)

Second-Degree AV Block Type II

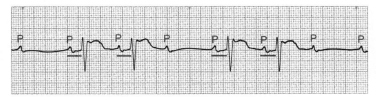

- Rhythm: irregular
- Atrial rate: exceeds ventricular rate
- Ventricular rate: depends on degree of block
- P waves: 2 or more for each QRS
- QRS: normal duration
- PR interval: normal or prolonged on the conducted complex
- P: QRS: P > QRS

Significance: This block may occur with anterior wall AMI and may progress rapidly to complete heart block.

Intervention: Observation if patient is asymptomatic. If symptoms occur, atropine 0.5 mg may be given and repeated up to a total dose of 3 mg if bradycardia is symptomatic (hypotension, chest discomfort). Transcutaneous pacing, epinephrine (2-10 mcg/min), or dopamine (2-10 mcg/kg/min) may also be considered.

Figure 5-25 Second-degree AV block (Type II). (From Huszar RJ: *Basic dysrhythmias: interpretation and management,* ed 3, St Louis, MO, 2002, Mosby.)

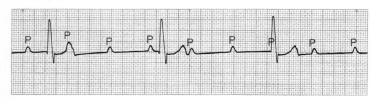

Complete Heart Block

- Rhythm: usually regular
- Atrial rate: exceeds ventricular rate
- Ventricular rate: <60 beats/min
- P waves: occur at regular intervals
- QRS: <0.12 sec if pacemaker is in the AV node; >0.12 sec if ventricular pacemaker
- PR interval: no relationship between P and QRS
- P: QRS: no relationship

Significance: No conduction of SA node impulses. The atria and ventricles beat independently of each other. The slow rate can cause myocardial ischemia.

Intervention: Pacemaker insertion necessary.
Atropine 0.5 mg may be given and repeated up to a total dose of 3 mg if bradycardia is symptomatic (hypotension, chest discomfort). Transcutaneous pacing, epinephrine (2-10 mcg/min), or dopamine (2-10 mcg/kg/min) may also be considered.

Figure 5-26 Complete (third-degree) AV block. (**Top,** from Emergency Nurses Association: *Sheehy's manual of emergency care,* ed 6, St Louis, MO, 2005, Mosby. **Bottom,** from Huszar RJ: *Basic dysrhythmias: interpretation and management,* ed 3, St Louis, MO, 2002, Mosby.)

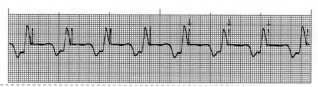

Figure 5-27 Ventricular demand pacemaker (VVI). (From Aehlert B: *ECGs made easy: pocket reference,* ed 2, St Louis, MO, 2002, Mosby.)

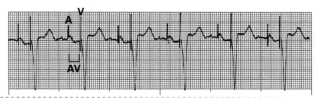

Figure 5-28 Dual-chambered pacemaker. (From Aehlert B: *ECGs made easy: pocket reference,* ed 2, St Louis, MO, 2002, Mosby.)

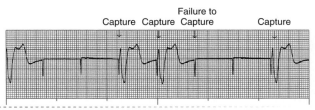

Figure 5-29 VVI pacemaker with failure to capture. (From Aehlert B: *ECGs made easy: pocket reference,* ed 2, St Louis, MO, 2002, Mosby.)

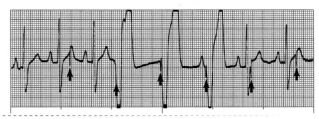

Figure 5-30 VVI pacemaker with failure to sense. (From Aehlert B: *ECGs made easy: pocket reference,* ed 2, St Louis, MO, 2002, Mosby.)

Diagnostic Tests: Cause(s) of Dysrhythmias

Test	Purpose	Abnormal Findings
Noninvasive Cardiology		
Electrocardiogram (ECG) 12-lead ECG or 15- or 18-lead ECG: Expanded method used to detect and analyze dysrhythmias, in which additional electrodes are placed on the skin of the right side of the chest and/or left posterior subscapular area to better detect problems with the perfusion to the right ventricle and posterior wall of the left ventricle (see Figure 5-32)	12-lead ECGs are the accepted standard method for detecting and analyzing dysrhythmias, including those associated with myocardial ischemia, injury, and infarction. 12 electrodes are placed on the skin of the patient's limbs and on the chest over the left ventricle (Figure 5-31).	Rapid tachycardias and profound bradycardias of all origins may prompt instability of hemodynamic status. Acute coronary syndrome manifests with presence of ST-segment depression or T-wave inversion (myocardial ischemia), ST elevation (acute MI), new bundle branch block (especially left BBB), or pathologic Q waves (resolving/resolved MI) in 2 contiguous or related leads. May be obtained during an episode of chest pain to help with establishing the relationship between the chest discomfort and the dysrhythmia.
Stress tests Stress test on a treadmill with or without thallium Thallium stress test using medications	Continuous ECG monitoring of the patient while a stressor (e.g., exercise on the treadmill; dipyradimole, dobutamine, or adenosine injection) is induced. The test continues until the patient reaches the target heart rate or becomes symptomatic (e.g., chest pain, severe fatigue, dysrhythmias).	Results determine the ability of the heart to compensate for various amounts of stress. Stress electrocardiography uses an echocardiogram immediately following the increase in heart rate to detect any regional wall motion abnormalities brought on by the tachycardia.
Ultrasound echocardiography (echo)	Assess for mechanical and structural abnormalities related to effective pumping of blood from both sides of the heart	Abnormal ventricular wall movement or motion, low ejection fraction, incompetent or stenosed heart valves, abnormal intracardiac chamber pressures
Transesophageal echocardiography (TEE)	Ultrasound technique to monitor atrial and ventricular wall motion through a high frequency two-dimensional transducer on the end of a gastroscope that the patient swallows	From this position in the esophagus, a high-resolution image of the posterior approach to the heart allows for better imaging of the aorta, valves, atria, and coronary arteries and can also detect clots that are present in the heart as a result of stasis of blood secondary to dysrhythmias (e.g., atrial fibrillation).
Ambulatory monitoring (e.g., 24-hour external Holter monitor or internal cardiac event [loop] recorder)	Continuous cardiac monitor worn externally (Holter) or for 24 hours by the patient so that ECG changes that occur during normal daily activities (including sleeping) can be determined	The loop recorder is implanted if the Holter monitor is ineffective in capturing dysrhythmias. The patient keeps a timed log of all activities/events/symptoms, which is later compared with the ECG recording to analyze the relationship of dysrhythmias to symptoms and activities. The loop recorder does not record continuously. Instead the patient activates the recorder when symptoms occur so that the cardiac "event" is recorded and then transmitted to monitoring agency via telephone

Diagnostic Tests: Cause(s) of Dysrhythmias —cont'd

Test	Purpose	Abnormal Findings
Blood Studies		
Therapeutic drug levels	Assesses for effectiveness of antidysrhythmic drugs already prescribed, as well as other medications that may cause dysrhythmias	Toxic levels of many cardiac, pulmonary, neurologic, and antidysrhythmic medications may prompt development of new, possibly more dangerous dysrhythmias. All antidysrhythmic agents are proarrhythmic, especially when certain electrolyte imbalances are present, particularly the Class I agents (e.g., quinidine, mexiletine, disopyramide).
Complete blood count (CBC) Hemoglobin (Hgb) Hematocrit (Hct) RBC count (RBCs) WBC count (WBCs)	Assess for anemia, inflammation, and infection; assists with differential diagnosis of chest pain.	Decreased RBCs, Hgb, or Hct reflects anemia, which often exacerbates dysrhythmias; MI, pericarditis, and endocarditis may increase WBCs.
Electrolytes Potassium (K^+) Magnesium (Mg^{2+}) Calcium (Ca^{2+}) Sodium (Na^+)	Both elevations and deficits of electrolytes can alter cardiac action potential, create an electrically unstable environment, and precipitate dysrhythmias.	Decrease in K^+, Mg^{2+}, or Ca^{2+} may cause dysrhythmias; elevation of Na^+ may indicate dehydration (blood is more coagulable); low Na^+ may indicate fluid retention and/or heart failure.
Toxicology screening Alterations in both automaticity and conduction can be prompted by recreational drugs.	Assesses for presence of drugs in the bloodstream and/or urine, which can alter various stages of cardiac action potential	Toxic levels of "recreational" or "street" drugs (e.g., "crack," cocaine, amphetamines, barbiturates) or mood-altering drugs (e.g., tricyclic antidepressants, sedative/hypnotics) can induce lethal dysrhythmias.
ABG values	Screens for hypoxemia or acid-based imbalance, which may prompt dysrhythmias	May reflect hypoxemia or pH abnormality that can interfere with electrolyte balance, both of which can cause dysrhythmias. Hypoxemia can also result from dysrhythmias that significantly decrease cardiac output.
B-type natriuretic peptide (BNP)	Assess for heart failure.	Elevation indicates heart failure is present.
C-reactive protein (CRP)	Assess for inflammation.	Elevation places patients at higher risk for acute MI, pericarditis, and endocarditis.
Radiology		
Chest radiograph (CXR)	Assess size of heart, thoracic cage (for fractures), thoracic aorta (for aneurysm), and lungs (for pneumonia, pneumothorax).	Cardiac enlargement, increased vascular markings, and bilateral infiltrates reflect heart failure (pulmonary edema).
Magnetic resonance imaging (MRI) Cardiac MRI	Assess ventricular size, morphology, function, status of cardiac valves, and circulation.	Enlarged heart, remodeled heart, incompetent of stenotic heart valves, narrowed or occluded coronary arteries

Continued

Diagnostic Tests: Cause(s) of Dysrhythmias—cont'd

Test	Purpose	Abnormal Findings
Computed tomography (CT) Cardiac CT scan	Assess ventricular size, morphology, function, status of cardiac valves, and circulation.	Enlarged heart, remodeled heart, incompetent of stenotic heart valves, narrowed or occluded coronary arteries; technology is improving in accuracy; may eventually reduce the need for cardiac catheterization.
Invasive Cardiology		
Electrophysiologic studies (EPS) Invasive test in which 2 or 3 catheters are placed into the heart at the sinus node and along the conduction system	This test can help to assess the SA node, AV node, and the His-Purkinje system; determine the characteristics of reentrant dysrhythmias; and "map" the location of suspected proarrhythmic sites or accessory pathways.	Rapid pacing stimuli at those sites with various voltages of electricity can induce dysrhythmias. Results help to determine the type of device and medications the patient may need to maintain cardiac electrical stability. Various medications, electrical therapies, and ablation are then implemented to terminate the induced dysrhythmias.

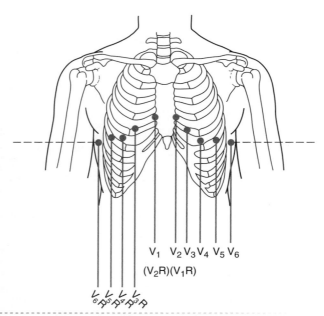

V_1 V_2 V_3 V_4 V_5 V_6

$(V_2R)(V_1R)$

V_6R V_5R V_4R V_3R

Figure 5-31 Placement of the left and right chest leads. (From Aehlert B: *ACLS Study Guide,* ed 3, St Louis, MO, 2007, Mosby.)

Posterior view

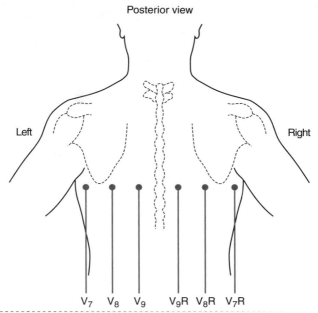

Figure 5-32 Posterior chest lead placement. (From Aehlert B: *ACLS Study Guide*, ed 3, St Louis, MO, 2007, Mosby.)

COLLABORATIVE MANAGEMENT
Care Priorities

1. **Identify the dysrhythmia and assess for symptoms:**
Diagnose the type of dysrhythmia and the effect of the rhythm on the patient's hemodynamic status. Rhythms resulting in hypotension, respiratory distress, chest discomfort, or pulseless-ness are considered unstable and require immediate management. When evaluating rhythms, the following basic assessments can be made prior to diagnosing the exact dysrhythmia:

Consciousness: Is the patient responsive or unconscious? If unconscious, is he or she breathing? If not breathing, open the airway and check the pulse. If still not breathing, and pulse is not present, patient is in cardiac arrest (regardless of rhythm) and cardiopul-monary resuscitation (CPR) must be initiated while another person obtains the cardiac monitor, defibrillator, or automated external defibrillator (AED). An ECG rhythm is sometimes present without a pulse (PEA).

HR and rhythm: Too fast or too slow? Regular or irregular? When the HR exceeds 150 or is less than 50, patients are more likely to experience adverse effects. Fast rhythms include sinus tachycardia, atrial tachycardia, atrial flutter, atrial fibrillation, junctional tachycardia, and VT with a pulse. Slow rhythms include sinus bradycardia, junctional rhythms, ventricular or idio-ventricular rhythms, and second- and third-degree heart blocks.

Appearance of QRS complexes: Wide or narrow? Tachycardias with QRS that exceed 0.10 second in duration are more likely to originate from the ventricles, unless the patient has reason to have aberrant conduction or has a history of bundle branch block.

Presence of P waves/PR interval: Is there one P wave preceding each QRS complex? Is the P wave normal in appearance? Is the PR interval short, normal, or prolonged?

Stable or unstable vital signs and assessment: Unstable patients require immediate manage-ment. Symptomatic bradycardia resulting in hypotension may be best managed with transcutaneous cardiac pacing if atropine is ineffective. Symptomatic tachycardias may be best managed using synchronized cardioversion. Pulseless patients with tachycardia are managed with unsynchronized cardioversion/defibrillation.

Cardiopulmonary arrest: All patients receive CPR and IV or intraosseous (IO) epinephrine 1 mg immediately, and every 3 to 5 minutes throughout resuscitation. Vasopressin 40 mg may be given instead of the first or second dose of epinephrine. Atropine 1 mg may be given to patients with slow-rate PEA or asystole every 3 to 5 minutes up to 3 mg total dose. Patients with pulseless VT or VF require immediate defibrillation.

2. **Determine the urgency of correcting the dysrhythmia, and whether drugs or electrical therapy is the most appropriate approach for the patient's situation.**

The more unstable the patient, the more aggressive is the treatment. There are situations wherein dysrhythmias do not readily respond to treatment, requiring further evaluation. Some lethal dysrhythmias may be resistant to correction, resulting in death. Generally, electrical therapies provide almost immediate correction of the instability associated with dysrhythmias, if the patient is able to respond to treatment. Boluses of medications such as atropine, adenosine, and ibutilide work quickly. Loading doses of medications that are followed by infusions such as amiodarone or diltiazem sometimes result in correction of rhythms but generally require the medication infusion to attain full correction and stability. Each patient's situation must be managed using a thorough evaluation of their history, and under the guidance of the AHA guidelines for ACLS. *A Handbook of Emergency Cardiac Care for Health Providers* is updated regularly to reflect current research. The resource includes information reviewed by AHA's Committee on Emergency Cardiovascular Care, and Subcommittees on Basic Life Support, Pediatric Resuscitation, and Advanced Cardiac Life Support.

3. **Provide pharmacologic management to correct dysrhythmias if recommended as the first strategy by ACLS guidelines.**

Management of dysrhythmias is based on providing and/or balancing electrolytes, catecholamines, and other regulators of the cardiac cycle. Provision of antidysrhythmic drugs is done using an antidysrhythmic drug classification system, which has evolved from the original Vaughan Williams classification system. Toxic levels of any antidysrhythmic medication can prompt development of different and sometimes lethal dysrhythmias. All antidysrhythmic agents have the potential for proarrhythmic effects (Box 5-4).

4. **Provide therapy for rapid HRs using current ACLS guidelines to manage ventricular tachycardias (monomorphic and polymorphic), ventricular fibrillation, and supraventricular tachycardias (atrial tachycardia, junctional tachycardia, atrial flutter, or atrial fibrillation).**

Defibrillation and cardioversion: Delivery of electrical shocks to the heart through the chest wall via use of an external defibrillator used to convert symptomatic, rapid atrial, or ventricular rhythms to sinus rhythm. Shocks may be synchronized (cardioversion) with the patient's R waves (QRS complexes) or may be given as random/ unsynchronized (defibrillation) countershocks. The operator must set the desired amount of electricity, apply the defibrillator paddles with conductive gel or hands-free gel patches to the patient's chest, and discharge the device. Defibrillators also provide the ability to provide electrical therapy "hands free." A special cable and multifunction/defibrillator pads are used instead of the conventional paddles.

- The placement of the pads or paddles is critical to deliver the electrical therapy to the heart muscle. The two pads are placed either on the anterior chest with one beneath the right clavicle and one on the left chest near the lower aspect of the heart, or with one pad over the heart anteriorly, and the other on the patient's back over the posterior side of the heart. Pads/paddles should not be placed over the larger bones (sternum and clavicle anteriorly, scapula and spinal column posteriorly), medication patches, or implanted electrical devices, including pacemakers and ICDs. Medication patches should be removed and residual medication wiped off. Defibrillators may use monophasic or biphasic technology. Biphasic defibrillation requires lower energy settings than recommended for monophasic defibrillation. Synchronized cardioversion also requires the additional step of synchronzing the patient's "R" waves with the cardioverter; plus lower energy is required to convert the rhythm to NSR.
- *Defibrillation:* Used for ventricular tachycardias without a pulse and ventricular fibrillation. Patients are in full cardiopulmonary arrest when defibrillation is used. Recommendations change for how electrical therapy should be performed. The energy sequence for biphasic defibrillators is initially 120 to 200 joules (manufacturer guidelines provide recommendations) followed by 2 minutes of CPR, then 300 joules followed by 2 minutes of CPR, then 360 joules (AHA, 2008).

Box 5-4	ANTIDYSRHYTHMIC DRUGS

Class I (sodium channel blockers)

Block the rapid, inward sodium current. Local anesthetics and other drugs that decrease automaticity of ventricular conduction, delay ventricular repolarization, decrease conduction velocity, increase conduction via AV node, and suppress ventricular automaticity. Class IA decreases depolarization moderately and prolongs repolarization. Class IB decreases depolarization and shortens repolarization. Class IC significantly decreases depolarization with minimal effect on repolarization.

Class IA	Class IB	Class IC
Disopyramide (PO)	Lidocaine (IV, IM)	Encainide (PO)
Procainamide (PO, IV, IM)	Mexiletine (PO)	Flecainide (PO)
Quinidine (PO, IV)	Phenytoin (PO)	Propafenone (PO)
	Tocainide (PO)	
	Moricizine (PO)	

Class II (beta adrenergic blockers)

Block stimulation of beta$_1$ and beta$_2$ receptors by catecholamines. Slow sinus node automaticity, slow conduction via AV node, control ventricular response to supraventricular tachycardias, and shorten the action potential of Purkinje fibers.

Acebutolol (PO)	Carvedilol (PO)	Oxyprenolol (PO)*
Atenolol (PO)	Esmolol (IV)	Penbutolol (PO)
Betaxolol (PO)	Labetalol (PO, IV)	Pindolol (PO)
Bisoprolol (PO)	Metoprolol (PO,IV)	Propranolol (PO, IV)
Carteolol (PO)	Nadolol (PO, IV)	Timolol (PO, IV)

Class III (potassium channel/1K1 blockers)

Block the outward current of potassium. Increase the action potential and refractory period of Purkinje fibers, increase ventricular fibrillation threshold, restore injured myocardial cell electrophysiology toward normal, and suppress reentrant dysrhythmias.

Amiodarone (PO, IV)	Bretylium (IV, IM)	Ibutelide (IV)
Azimilide (PO)	Dofetilide (PO)	Sotalol (PO, IV)

Class IV (calcium channel blockers)

Depress automaticity in the SA and AV nodes, block the slow calcium current in the AV junctional tissue, reduce conduction via the AV node, and are useful in treating tachydysrhythmias due to AV junctional reentry.
    Diltiazem (PO, IV)
    Verapamil (PO, IV)

Unclassified

Depress activity of the AV node.
    Adenosine (IV)

AV, atrioventricular; *PO*, by mouth; *IV*, intravenous; *IM*, intramuscular; *SA*, sinoatrial.
*Available in Great Britain.

- *Cardioversion:* Used for all types of tachycardia with a pulse present, when patients have unstable vital signs or a high risk of developing unstable vital signs. Can be scheduled in advance for patients with a high risk of developing unstable vital signs. Short-acting sedation is used prior to discharging the energy, to render the patient unaware of the pain produced by the electrical shock received. The energy sequence may vary slightly for various tachycardias and recommendations change but, in general, it begins with 50 to 100 joules, followed by 200 joules, then 300 joules, then 360 joules. Energy is always increased with subsequent shocks (AHA, 2008).

Defibrillation (Unsynchronized Cardioversion)
Providers must clear the area by shouting "clear" prior to pressing the button to discharge the defibrillator. Ensure no one else is touching patient/bed as shock is delivered to patient. Anyone in contact with the bed is at risk of receiving the electrical shock. All fluids in contact with the patient should be considered electrical conductors. Every attempt must be made to wipe or dry fluids from the area surrounding the patient. It is unsafe to defibrillate or cardiovert a patient who is in a pool of liquid (water, therapeutic fluids, or body fluids) unless the care providers are NOT in contact with the fluids.

Safety Alert

Synchronized Cardioversion
The defibrillator will not discharge the energy until R wave synchronization is achieved, which sometimes takes several seconds. Providers need to exercise extreme caution to remain "clear" and not touch the patient, bed, or anything connected to the patient until the energy is delivered.

- *AED:* Defibrillation technique designed to provide ECG interpretation needed for the device to determine the need for electrical therapy. The device will give a series of voice prompts instructing the operator on how to connect the cable and apply defibrillator pads, assess the patient, and clear the area when the device analyzes the rhythm. When finished analyzing, the device will either automatically discharge if appropriate (fully automatic), or ask the provider to press a button to discharge if appropriate (semiautomatic). When providing basic life support, the sequence of action includes defibrillation as the fourth step, following ensuring a patent airway, providing manual ventilation if breathing is absent, and providing cardiac compressions if the pulse is absent. The operator must be able to assess for pulselessness and apnea, along with applying "hands-free" defibrillator pads in the proper position at the right sternal border and anterior axillary line, fifth intercostal space. If health care providers are using the AED, the anterior-posterior pad position may also be used.

AEDs
Not all AEDs are programmed for current ACLS guidelines. Some still deliver three stacked shocks (per older ACLS guidelines) when it is time to defibrillate, rather than the currently recommended one shock. If a health care provider comes across this type of defibrillator, the provider is generally advised to follow the instructions and not interrupt the cycle. Interruption may cause the device to malfunction, resulting in the patient not receiving any further electrical therapy, or the device ceasing to give associated instructions regarding the proper steps of resuscitation.

- *Life vest "wearable" cardioverter-defibrillator:* The first defibrillator worn outside the body rather than implanted in the chest with continuous cardiac monitoring to detect life-threatening dysrhythmias, including VT and VF. The device uses nonadhesive sensing electrodes. If a life-threatening rhythm is detected, the device alerts the patient prior to delivering the shock, which allows time for a conscious patient to disarm the device prior to the shock. If the patient is conscious, the shock may not be necessary. If the patient is unconscious, the device releases a gel over the therapy electrodes and delivers the shock. The device is designed for home use, rather than as part of hospital management. The device may be used as a "bridge" to ICD implantation while patients are evaluated for appropriateness of the therapy.
- *ICD:* A battery-powered pulse generator (electrical device) implanted into the pectoral area, with a lead system and shocking coil positioned inside the heart and superior vena cava, which can recognize and terminate potentially lethal dysrhythmias. Risks and complications of thoracotomy (T) versus nonthoracotomy (NT) implantation are outlined in Table 5-16. Newer, third-generation devices do not

require thoracotomy for insertion. The devices are smaller and lighter, allowing prepectoral implantation. These devices may also provide antitachycardia pacing (ATP), low-energy cardioversion, high-energy cardioversion, antibradycardia pacing, and high-energy defibrillation along with the ability to score performance data. Algorithms for treatment of recognized dysrhythmias are programmed into the device. Maximal energy output is 30 to 40 joules, which can defibrillate malignant or lethal rhythms such as pulseless ventricular tachycardia and ventricular fibrillation. Magnets may be used for emergency deactivation/activation or suppression of all or part of programmed therapies in newer devices. If the patient has a combination ICD/pacemaker, the magnet will deactive the ICD and will change from demand (discharges electrical impulses or "fires" as needed to maintain the selected HR) pacing to fixed mode (discharges the selected number of impulses per minute, regardless of the patient's underlying heart rhythm). When the device discharges or "fires," the patient's status should be documented in the medical record.

| **Safety Alert** | *Immediate intervention is required for a device that is not delivering appropriate therapy. If the device does not deliver therapy, external cardioversion can be used. A patient with an ICD who has a sustained hemodynamically unstable ventricular rhythm should be treated exactly as one who does not have an ICD. The placement of the external pads should not be over the ICD generator. When inappropriate firing occurs in the absence of a treatable dysrhythmia, there is a high probability that an ICD lead has become dislodged, a connection has become loose, or the device sensitivity setting is too "low," which causes the device to respond "too soon" to certain rhythm changes.* |

- *Catheter ablation:* Prior to ablation, an electrophysiology study (EPS) is done to evaluate the electrical activity of the heart. The "electrical map" guides the placement of the ablation catheters which are placed in the heart during cardiac catheterization. The energy stimulus is then applied to the area in which the dysrhythmia originates or where an accessory pathway (bypasses AV node during conduction) is located. The energy causes controlled, localized necrosis of the area and may be applied via radiofrequency, thermal (heat), or cryo (cold) catheters. Bypass tracts (WPW) that produce AV reciprocating tachycardias and reentrant pathways that produce AV

Table 5-16	**IMPLICATIONS FOR PATIENT CARE AND COSTS: IMPLANTABLE CARDIOVERTER-DEFIBRILLATORS (ICDs)**		
Complication	**Thoracotomy (T)**	**Nonthoracotomy (NT)**	**Patient Care Implications**
Pneumothorax or hemothorax	Higher risk	Lower risk	ICU monitoring required for T. ICU unnecessary for NT. Length of hospital stay decreases with NT.
Pocket hematoma, seroma, wound adhesions	Higher risk	Lower risk	Wound care and home care less complex for NT.
Wound infection	Higher risk	Lower risk	If wound infection, T more likely to require IV antibiotics, which will increase costs and length of hospital stay.
Blood loss/ bleeding	Higher risk	Lower risk	T may need type and screen for blood products. NT does not.
Pneumonia	Higher risk	Lower risk	T may have decreased activity tolerance and requires pulmonary toilet.
Pain	Higher risk	Lower risk	NT requires less analgesia to manage pain.

nodal reentrant tachycardias can be ablated to modify the heart tissue and stop abnormal rapid conduction in these areas, which produces supraventricular tachycardia. Ablation can be done as adjunctive therapy for management of monomorphic VT, following placement of an ICD to enhance rhythm control. Postablation assessment of the patient involves careful monitoring of the cardiac rhythm, vital signs, catherter insertion sites, LOC, and peripheral pulses. Complications include cardiac perforation, cardiac tamponade, coronary artery spasm, cerebral or pulmonary embolus, bleeding, thrombosis, and dysrhythmias including AV blocks.

- *Specific tachycardias:*
  - *Sustained monomorphic VT:* The VT ECG tracing has a regular rhythm, the QRS shape is wide and uniform, and the ventricular rate ranges from 130 to 250 bpm. The impulse is generated either from a single site of increased automaticity on one of the ventricles or is due to reentry. Scarring from prior MI often provides the setup for reentry, as the impulse attempts to travel around the infarcted tissue. Patients may be hemodynamically stable or may be pulseless, so proper assessment is crucial in deciding on therapy. Options for treatment include antidysrhythmic medication (amiodarone 150 mg IV over 10 minutes, repeated once if needed and followed by a continuous IV infusion at 0.5 mg/min; total dose should not exceed 2.2 g in 24 hours). Synchronized cardioversion is used for unstable tachycardia (hypotension or chest discomfort accompanies the rapid HR), and defibrillation if the patient is unconscious, apneic, and pulseless (cardiac arrest), with 120 to 200 joules using a biphasic defibrillator (or 360 joules using a monophasic device), along with CPR and advanced life support measures. See ACLS guidelines for *Tachycardia with Pulses* or *Pulseless Arrest* for specific management algorithms.
  - *Sustained polymorphic VT:* Appears as a series of somewhat irregular, multishaped wide QRS "twisting" around the isoelectric line as seen on the ECG. It is important to try to determine if the patient's QT interval was normal or prolonged just prior to when the tachycardia ensued. If the QT interval was normal before onset of the tachycardia, the rhythm is simply called polymorphic VT. If polymorphic VT is sustained and the patient is symptomatic due to the tachycardia, treat any ischemia, correct electrolyte imbalances, and manage using guidelines for monomorphic VT. If the QT interval was prolonged, the patient has a particular type of polymorphic VT called *torsade de pointes (TdP)*. Abnormal levels of potassium, magnesium, and calcium may contribute. Acquired TdP is usually related to drug toxicity or electrolyte abnormalities, or myocardial ischemia. Many patients with TdP experience cardiac arrest immediately. Regardless, when TdP is sustained and the patient is symptomatic, discontinue any medications (particularly continuous infusions) that may prolong the QT interval; correct electrolyte abnormalities; initially give magnesium sulfate IV if patient is stable; or if the patient is unstable, attempt defibrillation as for VF. These patients may be resistant to defibrillation. If the patient continues to experience TdP, an agent such as isoproterenol may be infused to increase the HR, thereby shortening the QT interval. This may be especially necessary if TdP is caused by medications with a long half-life. Antidysrhythmic drugs including Class 3 amiodarone and sotalol prolong the QT interval and, like Class 1 agents (e.g., quinidine, disopyramide [Norpace]), are proarrhythmic. Initiate a magnesium infusion if not done initially. Other drugs, including certain antibiotics and antihistamines, may promote polymorphic VT, particularly when used in combination. Congenital causes include long-QT syndrome, Brugada syndrome (possibly congenital), and catecholaminergic polymorphic VT.
  - *Atrial fibrillation:* Atrial fibrillation with rapid ventricular response (RVR) may result in progressive ventricular dysfunction and decreased CO. The "quivering" atria are not contracting, so the atrial contribution to ventricular filling is lost. Blood stagnates in the atria, often resulting in clot formation. Platelet activation occurs, making thromboembolic complications possible when the atria once again contract. The goal of therapy is to convert the rhythm to NSR as soon as possible unless the atrial fibrillation is chronic. Those with sustained, new-onset atrial fibrillation who become unstable (signs of decreased CO, CHF, or acute coronary syndrome) or become hemodynamically unstable are generally managed with synchronized cardioversion. Atrial fibrillation may occur post CABG, producing CO compromise and danger of stroke. Rate control to slow the rapid ventricular response can be

achieved by diltiazem (Cardizem). Loading dose is 0.75 mg/kg IV followed by a continous infusion at 5 mg/hr. If atrial fibrillation reoccurs or persists over a 24-hour period, warfarin (Coumadin) anticoagulation for 4 weeks will be needed. For patients with normal QTc interval, immediate chemical conversion might be attained using ibutilide (Corvert) 1 mg diluted in 10 ml IV solution given over 10 minutes, and repeated once if atrial fibrillation has been present for less than 48 hours. Ibutilide is reserved for patients with a normal QTc interval to avoid lethal ventricular dysrhythmias following administration. An alternative is amiodarone (Cordarone) in a loading dose of 150 mg IV over 10 minutes followed by 1 mg/min drip for 6 hours and then 0.5 mg/min drip for 18 hours. For chronic atrial fibrillation patients, conversion to NSR without anticoagulation is not a goal due to the risk of atrial thrombus formation and possible embolization. If synchronized cardioversion is needed during the immediate postoperative period and anticoagulation is not an option, Doppler or transesophageal echocardiography may be used to check for atrial thrombus formation. In addition to cardioversion, other nonpharmaceutical treatments for atrial fibrillation include AV node and focal ablation, surgical correction such as the MAZE procedure, and implanted permanent pacing with atrial fibrillation suppression algorithms.

5. **Provide electrical therapy (cardiac pacing) to support unstable patients with slow HRs, and some rapid HRs if recommended as the most appropriate strategy by current ACLS guidelines**

Management of symptomatic bradycardias includes heart blocks, slow junctional rhythms, and idioventricular rhythms or certain tachycardias (antitachycardia pacing) including atrial flutter, atrial tachycardia, reentrant tachycardias, and WPW. Cardiac pacing can be provided temporarily or permanently.

- *Permanent cardiac pacing:* A battery-powered device is implanted to provide an artificial pacing or electrical pacing stimulus for the heart; used for problems with either automaticity or conduction to either generate an appropriate number of pacing impulses or facilitate conduction of the impulses to all areas of the heart in a coordinated fashion to facilitate increased CO. Most often used for management of symptomatic bradycardias including second- and third-degree heart block, it may be used for patients with ventricular asynchrony (RV and LV contraction is uncoordinated). Specialized devices may also be used to correct rapid atrial and ventricular rhythms via ATP. Third-generation ICDs may also be programmed for cardiac pacing. Pacemakers are named or coded based on the functions they are able to perform (Table 5-17). If CO is disturbed by ventricular asynchrony, biventricular pacing or cardiac resynchronization therapy (CRT) may be used. CRT is recommended for patients with LV ejection fraction less than or equal to 35%, a QRS duration greater than or equal to 0.12 second, and a sinus rhythm. CRT may also have an ICD added for treatment of patients with New York Heart Association functional Class III or ambulatory Class IV HF symptoms.

- *Temporary cardiac pacing:* Temporary pacing can be done using transthoracic, transcutaneous pacing pads applied to the skin on the chest (may be a dual pad used for either pacing or cardioversion [synchronized and unsynchronized]), via transvenous catheter insertion with positioning of leads into the endocardium or via surgically inserting epicardial wires with leads during open heart surgery.

Safety Alert *Patients in the critical care areas often have electrolyte disturbances, receive antidysrhythmic medications, and have acute coronary syndromes, acid-base imbalance, or hypotension/shock states. All of these conditions may alter the ability of the cardiac muscle to repond to a pacing stimulus and loss of capture may occur. Vigilance in watching for proper pacemaker function (pacing, capture, and sensing) is warranted in both temporary or permanent pacing.*

- *Temporary epicardial pacing:* Placement of temporary pacing wires on the epicardial surface of the heart while the chest is open during cardiac surgery so that cardiac pacing can be used in the postoperative period. Usually two atrial and two ventricular wires (pacing and ground wires) are attached to the outside surface of the heart and exit through the skin incision allowing attachment to a temporary pacing generator. The exposed pacing wires may be capped and later connected to a generator if pacing

Table 5-17		NBG PACEMAKER CODES		

The pacemaker code is written in a five-letter format as in the table, using no more letters than necessary. For example, the DDDR pacemaker is a dual-chamber paced, dual-chamber sensed, dual response, rate-modulated device. At least one pacemaker mode, the DVIC mode variation, does not conform to the NBG identification code and may sometimes be written DVI(C).

In the 1970s and 1980s, before the NBG codes came into being, the Inter-Society Commission for Heart Disease (IHCD) established standardized codes for pacemakers. Information on these older pacemaker codes can be found at NASPE.

Chambers Paced (1)	Chambers Sensed (2)	Modes of Response (3)	Programmable Functions (4)	Antitachycardia Functions (5)
V = Ventricle	V = Ventricle	T = Triggered	R = Rate Modulated	O = None
A = Atrium	A = Atrium	I = Inhibited	C = Communicating	P = Paced
D = Dual (A & V)	D = Dual (A & V)	D = Dual Triggered/Inhibited	M = Multiprogrammable	S = Shocks
O = None	O = None	O = None	P = Simple Programmable	D = Dual (P & S)
—	—	—	O = None	—

NASPE, North American Society of Pacing and Electrophysiology; BPEG, British Pacing and Electrophysiology Group, *and generic.* www.MeDiCaLeSe.org/pacemakers.html.

is needed. The end of the leads, connection points and pacing generator terminals should be protected and insulated from electrical micro shock. The temporary pacing wires are removed when no longer needed by slowly and gently pulling them out through the skin. The patient is monitored carefully after the pacing wires are removed for dysrhythmias, cardiac tamponade, hemorrhage, hematoma, and hemodynamic changes. If left in for a prolonged period of time, tissue may adhere to the wires and the provider may elect to cut the external wires at the level of the skin. The skin will then grow over the entry points and heal.

- *Atrial overdrive pacing:* ATP is used to control or terminate supraventricular dysrhythmias including atrial flutter, atrial tachycardia, reentrant tachycardias, and WPW. Atrial flutter and reentrant supraventricular tachycardias often result from electrical pathways or circuits set up around scarred or infarcted tissue. Using atrial pacing wires (transvenous or epicardial) connected to a pulse generator (pacemaker), the atria are rapidly paced by rapid bursts of electrical impulses during a 10- to 30-second period. The pacing rate selected is usually 20% to 30% faster than the rate of the tachydysrhythmia being treated. Successive bursts are performed at gradually increasing rates until termination of the tachycardia is achieved. The short bursts of rapid pacing create refractory cardiac tissue that interrupts the reentry circuit.

Safety Alert *Special care is given to proper connection of the atrial wires and to ensure against microshock. Rapid pacing of the atria can result in VT or VF.*

- *Transcutaneous, transthoracic cardiac pacing:* Cardiac pacing performed with a device that delivers electrical stimulation to the heart via two conductive pads applied to the skin of the chest, positioned either anteriorly or over the anterior and posterior walls of the heart. Certain defibrillators include capability for transcutaneous cardiac pacing. One pad is near the left sternal border and the other is near the left paraspinal line beneath the scapula for anterior-posterior position or in the same areas used for "hands-free" defibrillator pads in the proper position at the right sternal border and anterior axillary line, fifth intercostal space. Resistance of all muscles and bones of the chest wall must be overcome for impulses to reach the heart, requiring a higher milliamphere (mA) to be used. Transcutaneous pacing will cause the muscles of the chest and back to contract, which can be quite uncomfortable for the patient, and sedation may be required.

Safety Alert *The pads cannot both sense and pace; therefore, the device includes an ECG monitor so that efficacy (capture) of pacing can be assessed. Leads should be applied to the chest in addition to the pads to assess capture. Capture should reflect the level electrical stimulation (mA) provided was able to prompt ventricular contraction. The ECG tracing generally becomes larger and wider when capture is achieved. When pacing is effective, the patient's vital signs should improve. If the level of energy needed to achieve capture is uncomfortable, sedation may be necessary for the patient to tolerate transcutaneous cardiac pacing.*

6. **Provide surgical procedures to help control dysrhythmias.**
   - *LV aneurysmectomy and infarctectomy:* Excision of possible focal spots of ventricular dysrhythmias.
   - *Myocardial revascularization:* Performed alone or in conjunction with electrophysiologic mapping, with excision or cryoablation of the dysrhythmia focus. Newer surgical techniques are less invasive than the more standard median sternotomy approach.
   - *Maze procedure:* Surgically placed incisions arranged in a "Maze"-like pattern in the atria to eliminate atrial fibrillation. Some Maze procedure variations use both surgical incisions and ablation of cardiac tissue in the electrophysiology laboratory (convergence procedure).
   - *Stellate ganglionectomy and block:* Alters the electrical stability of the myocardium. Surgical option to treat inherited long-QT interval and predisposition to ventricular dysrhythmias.
7. **Initiate anticoagulation for patients at higher risk for development of blood clots within the heart secondary to dysrhythmias that decrease either atrial or ventricular wall motion.**

Use of warfarin (Coumadin) and/or platelet inhibitors (e.g., ticlodipine, clopidogrel) may be recommended.

8. **Explain the content of dietary guidelines designed to help reduce stimulants normally consumed.**

Patients with recurrent dysrhythmias are usually placed on a diet that restricts or reduces caffeine and sodium and is low in fat and cholesterol (see Tables 5-2, 5-18, and 5-19).

Table 5-18	LOW-CHOLESTEROL DIETARY GUIDELINES
Foods to Avoid	**Foods Allowed**
Egg yolks (no more than 3/wk)	Egg whites; cholesterol-free egg substitutes
Foods made with many egg yolks (e.g., sponge cakes)	Lean, well-trimmed meats; minimize servings of beef, lamb, and pork
Fatty cuts of meat, fat on meats	Fish (except shellfish), chicken, and turkey (without the skim)
Skin on chicken and turkey	Dried peas and beans as meat substitutes
Luncheon meats or cold cuts	Nonfat (skim) or low-fat (2%) milk
Sausage, frankfurters	Low-fat cheese
Shellfish (e.g., lobster, shrimp, crab)	Ice milk, sherbet, low-fat yogurt
Whole milk, cream, whole milk cheese	Monosaturated oils for cooking and food preparation: canola, safflower, olive
Ice cream	Margarines that list one of the above oils as their first ingredients
Commercially prepared foods with hydrogenated shortening, which is saturated fat	Foods prepared "from scratch" with the above suggested oils
Coconut and palm oils and products made with them (e.g., cream substitutes)	Meats (in acceptable quantity) and vegetables prepared by broiling, steaming, or baking (never frying)
Butter, lard, hydrogenated shortening	Spices, herbs, lemon juice, wine, flavored wine vinegars
Meats and vegetables prepared by frying	
Seasonings containing large amounts of sugar and saturated fats	
Sauces and gravies	
Salad dressings containing cream, cheese, or mayonnaise	

Dysrhythmias and Conduction Disturbances

Table 5-19	GUIDELINES FOR A DIET LOW IN SATURATED FAT
Foods to Avoid	**Foods to Choose**
Red meat especially when highly "marbled"; salami, sausages, bacon	Lean cuts of meat, fresh fish, poultry from which skin was removed before cooking; meats that have been grilled
Whole milk, whipping cream	Low-fat or skim milk
Tropical oils (coconut, palm oils; cocoa butter)	Monosaturated cooking oils, such as olive or canola oil
Candy	Fresh fruit, vegetables
Sweet rolls, donuts	Whole grain breads, cereals
Ice cream	Nonfat yogurt, sherbet
Salad dressings	Vinegar, lemon juice
Peanut butter, peanuts, hot dogs, potato chips	Unbuttered popcorn
Butter	Margarine (safflower oil listed as the first ingredient)

CARE PLANS FOR DYSRHYTHMIAS AND CONDUCTION DISTURBANCES

Decreased cardiac output *related to altered rate, rhythm, or conduction or negative inotropic changes secondary to cardiac disease*

GOALS/OUTCOMES Within 15 minutes of development of serious dysrhythmias, patient has adequate CO as evidenced by BP at least 90/60 mm Hg or baseline, HR 60 to 100 bpm, and NSR on ECG. CVP is less than 7 mm Hg, and CO is 4 to 7 L/min.
NOC Circulation Status

Cardiac Care
1. Monitor patient's heart rhythm continuously; note BP and symptoms if dysrhythmias occur or increase in occurrence.
2. If a PA catheter is present, note PAP, PAWP, and RAP; monitor for a reduced CO in response to dysrhythmias.
3. Document dysrhythmias with rhythm strip. Use a 12/15/18-lead ECG as necessary to identify the dysrhythmia.
4. Monitor patient's laboratory data, particularly K^+, Mg^{2+}, glucose, and digoxin levels.
5. Administer antidysrhythmic agents as prescribed; note patient's response to therapy.
6. Provide oxygen as prescribed. Oxygen may be beneficial if dysrhythmias are related to ischemia.
7. Maintain a quiet environment, and administer pain medications promptly. Both stress and pain can increase sympathetic tone and cause dysrhythmias.
8. If life-threatening dysrhythmias occur, initiate immediate unit protocols or standing orders for treatment, as well as CPR and ACLS algorithms as necessary.
9. When dysrhythmias occur, stay with patient; provide support and reassurance while performing assessments and administering treatment.
10. Administer inotropic agents (see Appendix 6) as prescribed to support patient's BP and CO.

NIC Hemodynamic Regulation; Medication Management; Oxygen Therapy; Respiratory Monitoring; Vital Signs Monitoring

Risk for activity intolerance *related to imbalance between oxygen supply and demand secondary to dysrhythmias that reduce cardiac output*

GOALS/OUTCOMES During activity, patient rates exertion less than 3 on a scale of 0 to 10 and exhibits tolerance of the dysrhythmia by an RR less than 20 breaths/min, SBP within 20 mm Hg of baseline, HR within 20 bpm of resting HR, and absence of chest discomfort and/or new dysrhythmias.
NOC Activity Tolerance; Endurance; Energy Conservation

Energy Management
1. Monitor patient's response to activity. Instruct patient to report chest discomfort and SOB. Note new dysrhythmias associated with activity or other stressors.
2. Administer medications as prescribed.
3. Observe and report signs of acute decreased CO, including oliguria, decreasing BP, altered mentation, and dizziness.
4. Monitor BP and other vital signs frequently, and as soon as possible report to the physician changes such as irregular HR, HR greater than 120 bpm, or decreasing BP.
5. Assess integrity of peripheral perfusion by monitoring peripheral pulses, distal extremity skin color, and urinary output. Report changes such as decreased pulse amplitude, pallor or cyanosis, and decreased urine output.

NIC Activity Therapy; Cardiac Care; Surveillance

Deficient knowledge: disease process or other mechanisms by which dysrhythmias occur *related to lifestyle implications*

GOALS/OUTCOMES Within the 24-hour period before discharge from critical care, patient and significant others verbalize knowledge about causes of dysrhythmias and the implications for modification of patient's lifestyle.
NOC Knowledge: Disease Process; Knowledge: Health Promotion; Knowledge: Medication

Teaching: Individual
1. Discuss causal mechanisms for dysrhythmias, including resulting symptoms. Use a heart model or diagrams as necessary.
2. Teach the signs and symptoms of dysrhythmias that necessitate medical attention: unrelieved and prolonged palpitations, chest pain, SOB, rapid pulse (greater than 150 bpm), dizziness, and syncope.
3. Teach patient and significant others how to check pulse rate for 1 full minute.
4. Teach patient and significant others about medications that will be taken after hospital discharge, including drug name, purpose, dosage, schedule, precautions, and potential side effects. Stress that patient will be maintained on long-term antidysrhythmic therapy and that it could be life-threatening to stop or skip these medications without physician approval, because doing so may decrease blood levels required for dysrhythmia suppression.
5. Advise patient and significant others about the availability of support groups and counseling; provide appropriate community referrals. Patients who survive sudden cardiac arrest may experience nightmares or other sleep disturbances at home. Explain that anxiety and fear, along with periodic feelings of denial, depression, anger, and confusion, are normal following this experience.
6. Stress the importance of leading a normal and productive life, even though patient may fear breakthrough of life-threatening dysrhythmias. If patient is going on vacation, advise him or her to take along sufficient medication and to investigate health care facilities in the vacation area.
7. Advise patient and significant others to take CPR classes; provide addresses of community programs.
8. Teach the importance of follow-up care; confirm date and time of next appointment, if known. Explain that outpatient Holter monitoring is performed periodically.
9. Explain that individuals with recurrent dysrhythmias should follow a general low-fat, low-sodium, and low-cholesterol diet (see Tables 5-2, 5-18, and 5-19) and reduce intake of products containing caffeine, including coffee, tea, chocolate, and colas.
10. As indicated, teach patient relaxation techniques or guided imagery, which will reduce stress and enable patient to decrease sympathetic tone (see *Appendix 7*).

NIC Surveillance; Teaching: Prescribed Medication; Vital Signs Monitoring

Ineffective health maintenance *related to ineffective stress management and inability to relax*

GOALS/OUTCOMES Within the 24-hour period after instruction, patient verbalizes and demonstrates the following relaxation technique.
NOC Health Promoting Behavior; Health-Seeking Behavior

Anxiety Reduction

1. Explain that to decrease sympathetic tone, some patients with dysrhythmias may benefit from practicing a relaxation response. Many different techniques can be used, including use of breathing alone or in conjunction with muscle group contraction and relaxation. Other techniques incorporate use of imagery.

2. Teach patient a relaxation technique effective for stress reduction and facilitation of ability to take deep breaths slowly to relax. See Appendix 7 for a sample relaxation technique.

NIC Calming Technique; Meditation; Music Therapy; Simple Guided Imagery; Simple Relaxation Therapy; Teaching: Prescribed Activity/Exercise

For patients with an ICD and/or permanent pacemaker
Deficient knowledge: ICD or pacemaker insertion procedure and follow-up care

GOALS/OUTCOMES Within the 24-hour period before the procedure, patient and significant others describe rationale for the procedure and method of insertion. Within the 24-hour period before discharge from ICU, patient and significant others describe postinsertion care and need for continued physician and nurse follow-up.
NOC Knowledge: Illness Care

Teaching: Procedure/Treatment

1. Assess patient's understanding of his or her medical condition (dysrhythmias) and the amount of detailed information desired.

2. Discuss the following with the patient and significant others:
   - Type of dysrhythmia patient has, using rhythm strip and heart model or drawings/illustrations/ charts to promote understanding.
   - Possible need for temporary transvenous pacemaker insertion before ICD or permanent pacemaker procedure.
   - Use of appropriate anesthesia throughout procedure.
   - Testing of the ability of the device to control lethal dysrhythmias, which will occur in the operating room/ catheterization laboratory after implantation and before the incision is closed.
   - Reassurance that should the mechanism fail to control the dysrhythmia, the device can be adjusted or reprogrammed to do so.
   - Continuous observation of patient in a cardiac care unit for ≈24 hours, with ongoing monitoring of BP, HR, and RR.
   - Importance of deep breathing, coughing (as necessary), and incentive spirometry exercises as appropriate. Explain that patient is at increased risk for respiratory tract and incisional infection if thoracic surgery was done, which tends to cause patient to avoid deep breathing and coughing to guard against pain. Have patient return demonstrations of breathing exercises. Reassure patient that analgesics can be administered before pulmonary toilet exercises, if needed.
   - No lifting of arm above level of shoulder ×4 weeks; may resume showering at 72 hours.
   - *Discharge instructions:* Follow-up visit within 10 to 14 days, need for obtaining an AED/"home defibrillator," and importance of CPR/defibrillator classes for significant others.

3. Describe the procedure should ICD device deliver a "shock." If the patient is aware of the shocks, the physician should be notified as soon as possible that the device is firing. With newer devices, patients may be unaware of shocks but may become symptomatic (e.g., become intolerant of activity, dizzy, have chest discomfort) with prolonged or serious dysrhythmias. Teach patient to record the number of "shocks" experienced.

4. Explain use of the AED/"home defibrillator," which is available commercially from several companies. It is designed to allow the nonmedical person or care providers untrained in dysrhythmia interpretation to effect defibrillation, and its purpose is to convert lethal dysrhythmias should the ICD fail. Provide information on Life Vest (xxx, Zoll).

5. Explain that "shocks" during sinus rhythm may indicate a lead fracture in the ICD system. Usually this is detected while the patient is being monitored (e.g., by ECG in physician's office, by hospital monitor, or by Holter monitor).

NIC Learning Facilitation; Learning Readiness Enhancement; Risk Identification; Teaching: Disease Process; Teaching: Prescribed Medication; Teaching: Psychomotor Skill

Risk for infection *related to invasive procedure into thorax*

GOALS/OUTCOMES Patient is free of infection as evidenced by normothermia, WBC count 11,000/mm^3 or less, negative culture results, and absence of the clinical indicators of infection at the incision site and of the respiratory tract.
NOC Infection Severity

Infection Protection
1. Encourage and assist with deep breathing, coughing (if needed), and incentive spirometry exercises every 2 hours, and encourage early ambulation to the chair. As indicated, assist patient with splinting the incision site with hands or pillow to promote pain control. Administer prescribed analgesics 20 minutes before scheduled breathing exercises. For more information, see this nursing diagnosis in *Acute Pneumonia,* p. 373.
2. Assess incision site every 2 hours for warmth, erythema, swelling, and drainage. The presence of a seroma, which has the same symptoms as incision site infection, is confirmed by decubitus chest radiograph studies or CT.
3. Monitor patient's temperature every 2 to 4 hours, being alert to elevation greater than 38.6°C (101.5°F).
4. Monitor CBC for elevation of WBCs.
5. Consult physician for significant findings.
6. Teach patient and significant others the signs and symptoms of infection, of both the incision site and the respiratory tract: cough, sputum production, fever, dyspnea, chills, headache, myalgia. Explain that the older adult with an infection may be confused and disoriented and may run low-grade fevers even though few other indicators are present.

NIC Infection Control; Cough Enhancement; Exercise Promotion; Surveillance; Medication Prescribing; Home Maintenance Assistance

---

For patients with a pacemaker (temporary or permanent) or patients with third-generation ICDs with cardiac pacing
Decreased cardiac output *related to malfunction of cardiac pacemaker*

GOALS/OUTCOMES Within the 24-hour period preceding hospital discharge or throughout the duration of temporary cardiac pacing, patient has adequate CO as evidenced by SBP at least 90 mm Hg, RR 12 to 20 breaths/min, HR less than 100 bpm, urinary output at least 0.5 ml/kg/hr, warm and dry skin, and ECG indicative of effective capture, sensing, response to sensing, and function of antitachycardia pacing (if operational).
NOC Circulation Status

Cardiac Care: Acute
1. *Recognize and document paced rhythms.* Events to document include the following: (1) recognition of pacing spike preceding P wave and/or QRS complex as appropriate for settings; (2) sensing of patient's inherent pacing; (3) response of pacemaker when triggering and/or inhibiting pacing; (4) response of HR to activity if pacemaker is programmed "rate responsive"; and (5) initiation of antitachycardia pacing or electric shock (with ICD) for dysrhythmias.
2. *Promptly detect problems with pacemaker functions.* Include assessment of potential electromagnetic interference (EMI) (Table 5-20). Ensure that temporary pacemaker battery is still functional or changed as needed, and that cable connectors for temporary pacemakers are appropriately connected to the pulse generator (pacemaker box). For problems with functions of permanent pacemakers and ICDs, the physician should be notified immediately.
3. *Provide electrical safety measures for temporary cardiac pacing* to include proper grounding and protection of exposed catheter tips and/or heart wires. Caregiver must wear rubber/nonconductive gloves when handling pacing lead wires/catheter so that microshocks are avoided. Microshocks can induce lethal dysrhythmias.
4. *Observe for complications of temporary pacing,* which include dysrhythmias, lead displacement or fracture, and lead perforation of the heart that could lead to cardiac tamponade, pericarditis, infection, and bleeding.
5. *Perform threshold checks per hospital policy.*

NIC Dysrhythmia Management; Vital Signs Management; Surveillance; Environmental Management: Safety

Dysrhythmias and Conduction Disturbances

Table 5-20	ELECTROMAGNETIC INTERFERENCE AND THE THIRD-GENERATION ICD AND SOME PROGRAMMABLE PACEMAKERS		
Unsafe Hospital Procedures/Equipment	**Unsafe Home Equipment: Use Caution**	**Safe Home Equipment**
MRI (magnetic resonance imaging)	Large magnets: junkyards, construction sites, other areas that may have large magnets	Microwave ovens
Nerve stimulator	Hand-held wands at airport security	Refrigerator magnets
Electrocautery	Bingo wands	Electric blankets
Diathermy	Certain slot machines	Tanning bed
Lithotripsy	Large stereo speakers (unsafe to carry) Cellular telephones High-tension wires Industrial transformers Robotic jacks Arc welders Power generators in dams Industrial motors Large boat motors	Riding lawnmower Jacuzzi CB radio HAM radio (except for antennas) Table saw Gas welder Electric drill Weed Eater™ Small boat motors

ICD, implantable cardioverter defibrillator.
Magnetic fields are measured in units (Gauss) or 1000th of a gauss, milliGauss (mG). Ten Gauss will affect an ICD or some programmable pacemakers. Common household electrical appliances (interferences) are less than 50 mG. Electrical fields are measured in volts per meter. 750 V is approximately 30 J.

For patients with an ICD
Sexual dysfunction (or risk for same) *related to fear of inducing dysrhythmias during sexual activity*

GOALS/OUTCOMES Within the 24-hour period before discharge from the ICU, patient and significant other verbalize understanding of interventions during and alternatives for sexual intercourse.
NOC Sexual Identity; Role Performance

Sexual Counseling
1. Ask patient to describe any symptoms of dysrhythmias during presurgical sexual experiences.
2. Explain the following interventions or alternatives that can be made if patient continues to experience dysrhythmias during sexual intercourse:
   • Patient may need to take a less active role.
   • Patient may find that taking a prescribed vasodilator before engaging in sexual intercourse will prevent dysrhythmias. Should be advised not to take a vasodilator with NTG.
   • Suggest that during periods when dysrhythmias are a problem, less stressful forms of sexual activity, such as caressing and hugging, are positive alternatives.
3. As appropriate, advise patient that stressful situations, such as extramarital relations or unfamiliar environment/partner, may contribute to symptoms during sexual activity.
4. Explain that the device may "shock" at any time. If the patient's partner is in contact with the patient's body at that time, the shock may be experienced as a tingling sensation by the partner.

NIC Teaching: Sexuality; Anxiety Reduction; Coping Enhancement; Support Group

ADDITIONAL NURSING DIAGNOSES
The patient with ICD is at risk for pneumothorax. As indicated, also see *Pneumothorax*, p. 388, for information related to this disorder. Also see nursing diagnoses and interventions in *Hemodynamic Monitoring* (p. 75) and *Emotional and Spiritual Support of the Patient and Significant Others* (p. 200).

HYPERTENSIVE EMERGENCIES

PATHOPHYSIOLOGY

Hypertension is responsible for more deaths and disease than any other cardiovascular risk factor worldwide. Hypertension causes ventricular remodeling and increases the risk of heart attack, HF, stroke, and kidney failure. The Joint National Committee on Prevention, Detection, Evaluation, and Treatment of High Blood Pressure (JNC-7) defined "hypertension" as a BP of greater than 140/90 mm Hg. At least 73 million adult Americans, nearly 25% of adults in the United States, have hypertension. Prevalence increases with age. Another 25% have "prehypertension," defined as an SBP of 120 to 139 mm Hg or a diastolic BP (DBP) of 80 to 89 mm Hg (Table 5-21).

The guidelines for the treatment of hypertension, the Seventh Report of the JNC-7, were published in 2004. The next report, JNC8, is expected in 2010 and will be available at the National Heart, Lung, and Blood Institute website (www.nhlbi.nih.gov/guidelines/hypertension/index.htm).

JNC-7 recommends that BP is maintained at less than 120/80 mm Hg. The risk of death from ischemic heart disease and stroke increases in tandem with BP. The risk of heart attack or stroke increases several times when hypertension exists with obesity, smoking, high blood cholesterol levels, or diabetes. Patients with comorbidities such as diabetes or chronic kidney disease (CKD) are at higher risk of the cardiovascular complications of hypertension when SBP exceeds 130 mm Hg or DBP exceeds 80 mm Hg.

Elevation of SBP versus DBP is related to age. SBP and DBP rise simultaneously until about 50 years of age, after which SBP continues to increase, while DBP generally decreases. Age also affects the impact of SBP and DBP as risk factors for heart attack and stroke. For persons younger than 50 years, DBP is the main risk factor, while for those older than 60 years, SBP is more important. The mortality rate for both doubles for every 20 mm Hg SBP or 10 mm Hg DBP increase above 115/75 mm Hg. For older adults, controlling SBP and pulse pressure, rather than DBP, is recognized as increasingly important. Pulse pressure is the pressure

Table 5-21	CLASSIFICATION OF BLOOD PRESSURE FOR ADULTS AGE 18 AND OLDER*			
Category	Systolic Pressure (mm Hg)		Diastolic Pressure (mm Hg)	Follow-up
Normal†	<120	and	<80	
Prehypertension‡	130–139	or	80–89	Begin lifestyle modification
Hypertension§				
Stage I	140–159	or	90–99	Begin pharmacologic therapy along with lifestyle change
Stage II	>160	or	>100	Evaluate or refer to source of care within 1 mo

Modified from National Institutes of Health: The Seventh Report of the Joint National Committee on Prevention, Detection, Evaluation, and Treatment of High Blood Pressure (JNCVII), NIH Publication No. 03-5231, May 2003.

*Not taking hypertensive drugs and not actually ill.
†Optimal blood pressure with respect to cardiovascular risk is below 120/80 mm Hg. However, unusually low readings should be evaluated for clinical significance.
‡Begin instructions on lifestyle modification, including:
  Lose weight if overweight.
  Limit alcohol intake <1 oz ethanol/day (24 oz beer, 8 oz wine, or 2 oz whiskey).
  Reduce sodium intake to <100 mmol/day (2.3 g sodium or 6 g sodium chloride).
  Maintain adequate dietary potassium, calcium, and magnesium intake.
  Stop smoking.
  Reduce dietary saturated fat and cholesterol intake for general cardiovascular health.
§Based on the average of two or more readings taken at each of two or more visits.
In the presence of diabetes and chronic kidney disease, treat to a goal at 130/80.

difference (mm Hg) between SBP and DBP values. The pulse pressure represents the force the heart generates during systole/ventricular contraction. There are little data available regarding the effect of antihypertensive drugs on pulse pressure. Several studies indicate increased pulse pressure causes more damage to arteries in hypertensive patients. Elevated pulse pressure also reflects increased stress on the left ventricle during systole.

Hypertensive crisis is seen in about 1% of those with hypertension and is more common among older persons. The JNC-7 guidelines define *hypertensive crisis* as SBP greater than 180 mm Hg or DBP greater than 120 mm Hg. The morbidity and mortality of hypertensive emergencies depend on the extent of end-organ damage when the patient presents and subsequent BP control. Following a crisis, those with BP control and medication compliance have a 10-year survival rate of nearly 70%. A hypertensive crisis is divided into two categories or types: hypertensive urgencies and hypertensive emergencies. The two conditions are differentiated by the presence or absence of end-organ damage (EOD).

Hypertensive urgencies are situations in which there is no evidence of EOD, yet the BP is significantly elevated and must be reduced. Signs and symptoms include severe headache, severe anxiety, and SOB. BP can be reduced within the subsequent 24 to 48 hours following diagnosis. IV treatment of BP is not necessary. Oral treatment is satisfactory.

Hypertensive emergencies are situations in which there is evidence of EOD and the patient requires substantial reduction of BP within 1 hour to avoid the risk of serious complications or death. Hypertensive emergencies encompass a spectrum of clinical presentations where uncontrolled hypertension leads to progressive or impending end-organ dysfunction. The BP should be lowered aggressively over minutes to hours. During a hypertensive emergency, the patient may experience life-threatening signs and symptoms, such as severe pulmonary edema, cerebral edema, ischemia or hemorrhage of the brain, aortic dissection, AMI, and eclampsia (during pregnancy). Immediate vascular necrosis is possible if the diastolic pressure exceeds 120 mm Hg. Necrosis has also manifested with MAPs greater than 150 mm Hg.

Malignant hypertension is BP elevation with encephalopathy or nephropathy with papilledema. Progressive renal failure and permanent blindness can occur if treatment is not provided.

Accelerated hypertension is a recent significant increase in BP from baseline hypertension that is associated with end-organ damage, including optic nerve vascular damage on funduscopic examination. Findings include flame-shaped hemorrhages or soft exudates; both without papilledema.

Hypertensive Emergencies

The pathophysiology of hypertensive emergencies is not well understood. Initially, there is a failure of the normal autoregulation and an abrupt rise in SVR. It is thought that the wall of a stressed vessel causes the release of humoral vasoconstrictors, which increases the SVR. The increased pressure within the vessel then starts a cycle of endothelial damage, local intravascular activation of the clotting cascade, fibrinoid necrosis of small blood vessels, and the release of more vasoconstrictors. The cycle of vascular injury leads to tissue ischemia and autoregulatory dysfunction. Single-organ involvement is found in approximately 83% of patients presenting with hypertensive emergencies. Two-organ involvement is found in 14% of patients, and multiorgan involvement (more than three organ systems) is found in approximately 3% of patients presenting with a hypertensive emergency.

Hypertensive crisis can lead to hypertensive encephalopathy as cerebral blood vessels dilate because of their inability to affect autoregulation. Cerebral autoregulation is the ability of the cerebral vasculature to maintain a constant pressure or CBF. When autoregulation is disrupted, it leads to increased intercranial pressure and cerebral edema. Hallmark signs of hypertensive encephalopathy include cerebral edema and microhemorrhages, altered mental status, and papilledema. Blood flow is increased, and the excessive pressure drives fluid into the perivascular tissue, resulting in cerebral edema. The extreme pressure can cause arteriolar damage, as demonstrated by fibrinoid necrosis of the intima and media of the vessel wall. Although any organ is vulnerable, the eyes and the kidneys are most likely to suffer damage, leading to retinopathy, blindness, and renal failure. Patients with hypertension who are admitted to the ICU may have a rebound elevation of the BP if their usual antihypertensive regimen is interrupted. In addition, a loss of BP control can occur because of the nature of the primary disorder, trauma, or the stress of the ICU.

Patients also have increased cerebrovascular resistance and are more prone to ischemia when the BP decreases. Normotension achieved with BP control measures may result in decreased cerebral blood flow (CBF). Rapid rises in BP can cause hyperperfusion with an increased CBF. The rapidity of the rise in pressure may be more destructive than the level of BP elevation. The 1-year mortality rate is 79% for patients with untreated hypertensive emergencies. The 5-year survival rate among all patients who present with hypertensive crisis is 74%. Progressive stiffness occurs in the arteries, which increases SBP, resulting in a widened pulse pressure, which decreases coronary perfusion pressures, increases myocardial oxygen consumption, and causes the left ventricle to enlarge. The remodeled left ventricle is unable to compensate for an acute rise in SVR, leading to LV failure, pulmonary edema, and myocardial ischemia. Small renal arteries exhibit endothelial dysfunction and impaired vasodilation, which affects renal autoregulation. Once the renal autoregulatory system is disrupted, the intraglomerular pressure varies directly with the systemic arterial pressure. The kidney is no longer protected from fluctuations in perfusion caused by BP changes, resulting in acute renal ischemia during a hypertensive crisis.

ASSESSMENT
Goal of Assessment
The history and physical examination determine the nature, severity, and management of the hypertensive event. Patients should be questioned regarding compliance with antihypertensive drug therapy, intake of over-the-counter (OTC) preparations and sympathomimetic agents, and illicit drug use. Identifying the presence of end-organ dysfunction, particularly renal and cerebrovascular disease, is of paramount importance. Duration and severity of preexisting hypertension and the degree of BP control should be clearly defined by the history.

History and Risk Factors
The most common hypertensive emergency is a rapid unexplained rise in BP in a patient with chronic essential hypertension. Most patients who develop hypertensive emergencies have a history of inadequate hypertensive treatment or an abrupt discontinuation of their medications. Other causes include the following (see also Box 5-5):

- *Coarctation of the aorta*
- *Drugs and drug interactions:* Amphetamines, antidepressants, antihistamines, cocaine, clonidine withdrawal, cyclosporine, diet pills, monoamine oxidase (MAO) inhibitors with tricyclic antidepressants, oral contraceptives, phencyclidine, recreational sympathomimetic drugs, serotonin syndrome, steroid use, tyramine-containing food
- *Endocrine:* Cushing syndrome, pheochromocytoma, primary hyperaldosteronism
- *Hypertension of pregnancy:* Preeclampsia/eclampsia
- *Neurologic disorders:* CNS trauma or spinal cord disorders including Guillain-Barré syndrome

---

Box 5-5   CAUSES OF SECONDARY HYPERTENSION

Renal disease
- Acute glomerulonephritis
- Chronic pyelonephritis
- Hydronephrosis
- Renal tumors
- Renovascular hypertension

Endocrine disorders
- Cushing syndrome
- Pheochromocytoma
- Primary aldosteronism
- Thyroid/parathyroid disease

Congenital disorders
- Adrenal hyperplasia
- Coarctation of the aorta

Pregnancy-induced disorders
- Pregnancy-induced hypertension (PIH)
- Preeclampsia
- Eclampsia

Drug-induced disorders
- Cyclosporine
- Oral contraceptives
- Steroids

Other
- Sleep apnea

- *Postoperative hypertension*
- *Renal parenchymal and renovascular disease:* Chronic pyelonephritis, primary glomerulonephritis, tubulointerstitial nephritis (comprises 80% of all secondary causes); atherosclerosis, fibromuscular dysplasia, polyarteritis nodosa
- *Systemic disorders with renal involvement:* Systemic lupus erythematosus, systemic sclerosis, vasculitis
- *Other factors:* Hypertension is a familial disease; genetic and environmental factors contribute to its etiology. Psychologic stress, a diet high in sodium, and cigarette smoking increase the risk.

Observation

Early indicators: Although most patients are free of symptoms, vague discomfort, fatigue, dizziness, and headache can occur.

Late indicators (nearly always present during a hypertensive crisis): Throbbing suboccipital headache, irritability, confusion, somnolence, stupor, visual loss, focal deficits, and coma. The patient also may have signs of HF, including dyspnea on exertion, orthopnea, and paroxysmal nocturnal dyspnea. If CAD is present, angina may occur as a result of increased myocardial oxygen consumption caused by the high vascular resistance, which is evidenced by high BP. Chest pain may also indicate a dissecting aortic aneurysm. Renal symptoms include hematuria, nocturia, and azotemia. Nausea and vomiting also may occur.

Eye assessment: A funduscopic examination is performed to determine whether hemorrhage, fluffy cotton exudates, or arteriovenous nicking of the vessels has occurred. When these changes occur, visual perception is decreased. Nurses should assess the patient's gross visual acuity by the ability to read and recognize objects and people. Retinal hemorrhages and exudates as well as papilledema may occur.

Neurologic assessment: Assess level of consciousness, visual fields, and focal neurologic signs. May reveal evidence of a residual neurologic deficit from a cerebral infarct or ischemic event, as manifested by a positive Babinski reflex (upgoing toe), hemiparesis, hemiplegia, ataxia, confusion, or cognitive alterations. Assessment should include any onset of headache, nausea, vomiting, lethargy, restlessness, or agitation.

Vital Signs

Blood pressure measurements: An accurate cuff pressure must be obtained after 5 minutes of rest, with two or more measurements taken at least 2 minutes apart. Average these readings unless there is a 5 mm Hg or greater difference. Greater differences warrant additional readings. A well-calibrated manometer with a properly fitting cuff or an automatic BP recorder should be selected for use. The bladder of the cuff must encircle 80% of the arm and cover two-thirds of the length of the upper portion of the arm. BP measurement in both the supine and standing positions (if able) may help in assessment for volume depletion. If a significant difference is noted between the arms, this may be suggestive of an aortic dissection. Note when the patient last smoked or used any nicotine product, how much caffeine was consumed during the previous 4 hours, and whether adrenergic stimulants (e.g., OTC decongestants or bronchodilators) have been used within the past 24 hours, as they elevate BP.

Pheochromocytoma assessment: Paroxysmal elevations of BP associated with palpitations, tachycardia, headache, diaphoresis, pallor, warmth or flushing, tremor, excitation, fright, nervousness, feelings of impending doom, tachypnea, abdominal pain, nausea, and vomiting. Episodes also are associated with hyperglycemia and hypermetabolism. Postural hypotension and paradoxic response to antihypertensive medications may occur.

Palpation

Evaluate for LV hypertrophy: Results from the need of the heart to pump against the high SVR or afterload. A LV heave may be palpated with the palm of the hand at the mitral area (fifth intercostal space [ICS] at the midclavicular line [MCL]). If cardiac failure is present or the left ventricle is enlarged, the apical impulse will be felt nearer to the anterior axillary line (AAL) instead of the MCL.

Peripheral pulses: Pulsus alternans, an alteration in pulse pressure with a regular rhythm, may be palpated at any of the major pulse points. All peripheral pulses should be palpated bilaterally. With coarctation of the aorta, the femoral pulses will be bilaterally weak with a slow upstroke, whereas the radial and brachial pulses will be normal or bounding.

Auscultation

Heart sounds: A fourth heart sound or S_4 gallop may be auscultated in the mitral area with the bell of the stethoscope. In addition, crackles may be auscultated in the presence of cardiac failure along with jugular venous distention and peripheral edema.

DIAGNOSTIC TESTS

The definitive test for hypertension is BP measurement. Once hypertension has been documented, many tests may be performed to determine the amount of end-organ damage or to diagnose the condition responsible for the development of secondary hypertension.

Diagnostic Tests for Hypertensive Urgencies and Emergencies		
Test	Purpose	Abnormal Findings
Noninvasive Cardiology		
Cardiac echocardiography (ECHO)	Assess for mechanical and structural abnormalities related to effective pumping of blood from both sides of the heart.	LVH with or without dilation will be demonstrated on echocardiogram by an increase in the wall thickness with or without increased chamber size; a transesophageal echocardiography may be indicated if aortic dissection is suspected.
Blood and Urine Studies		
Complete blood count	Assesses for anemia	CBC and smear to exclude microangiopathic anemia. The RBC count may fall because of hematuria caused by acute tubular necrosis (ATN).
Electrolytes Potassium (K^+) Magnesium (Mg^{2+}) Calcium (Ca^{2+}) Sodium (Na^+)	Assess for possible causes of dysrhythmias and/or heart failure.	Abnormal levels of K^+, Mg^{2+}, or Ca^{2+} may cause dysrhythmias. Elevation of Na^+ may indicate dehydration (blood is more coagulable); may reveal hyponatremia (dilutional); hypokalemia, which can result from use of diuretics; or hyperkalemia, if glomerular filtration is decreased. Hyperkalemia can also be a side effect of angiotensin-converting enzyme inhibitors (ACEIs) and potassium-sparing diuretics.
Blood urea nitrogen (BUN) and creatinine levels	BUN and serum creatinine levels to evaluate renal impairment	If renal parenchymal disease is present, the patient may have serum creatinine >1.3 mg/dl and BUN >20 mg/dl.
Urinalysis (UA) and urine culture	Detects hematuria or proteinuria; microscopic UA to detect RBCs or RBC casts for renal impairment	Urinalysis results will be normal until hypertension causes renal impairment. Specific gravity may be low (<1.010). Glomerulonephritis is suspected if the urine contains granular or red cell casts or if the patient has hematuria. Pyelonephritis is suspected if there is bacterial growth in the urine.
24-hour urine collection Vanillylmandelic acid (VMA) and urinary catecholamines	Screens for abnormalities of the adrenal glands	Elevations of the 24-hour urine VMA and urinary catecholamines (10–50 times normal) are indicative of pheochromocytoma. The VMA level is elevated only during episodes of hypertension.
Urinary cortisol	Screens for defects in the adrenal cortex	If the patient has Cushing disease, the urine cortisol or adrenocorticotropic hormone (ACTH) level will be elevated.

Hypertensive Emergencies

Continued

Diagnostic Tests for Hypertensive Urgencies and Emergencies—cont'd

Test	Purpose	Abnormal Findings
Radiology		
Chest radiograph (CXR)	Assess size of heart, thoracic cage (for fractures), thoracic aorta (for aneurysm).	Chest radiograph to detect dilation of the left ventricle; if present, the cardiac silhouette will be enlarged. If failure is present, there will be evidence of pulmonary congestion and pleural effusions. Notching of the aorta and a distended aortic root are indicative of coarctation of the aorta. If widening of the mediastinum is seen, a dissection of the aorta is suspected (see Aortic Aneurysm Dissection, p 467). An intravenous pyelogram (IVP) with nephrotomography or CT may identify the adrenal tumor and detect pheochromocytoma. Chest CT scan or aortic angiography is indicated in cases when the patient is being evaluated for aortic dissection.
Brain computed tomography (CT scan) or magnetic resonance imaging (MRI)	Indicated in patients with abnormal neurologic examinations or clinical concern for intracranial bleeding, edema, or infarction	Presence of intracranial bleeding, cerebral edema, or infarction (acute ischemic stroke)
Abdominal aortic angiography or arteriogram	Identifies abnormal vascular anatomy of the aorta and abdominal vessels	Angiography may identify an adrenal medullary tumor.

See diagnostic tests for patients with *Acute Coronary Syndrome* (p. 434), *Aortic Aneurysm/Dissection* (p. 467), *Heart Failure* (p. 421), *Stroke: Acute Ischemic and Hemorrhagic* (p. 674), and *Acute Renal Failure* (p. 584). Additional studies such as a toxicology screen, pregnancy test, and endocrine testing may be necessary.

COLLABORATIVE MANAGEMENT
Care Priorities
In the treatment of hypertensive emergencies complicated by (or precipitated by) CNS injury, IV labetalol or nicardipine may be recommended, since they both are nonsedating and do not cause significant cerebral vasodilation, which can increase intracranial pressure (a potential problem with sodium nitroprusside). In hypertensive emergencies arising from catecholaminergic mechanisms, such as pheochromocytoma or cocaine use, beta-blockers can worsen the hypertension because of unopposed peripheral vasoconstriction; phentolamine may be effective. Labetalol is useful in these patients if the HR must be controlled.

1. **Control the BP within 2 hours during hypertensive crisis:** The initial goal in hypertensive emergencies is to reduce the pressure by no greater than 25% (within minutes to 1 or 2 hours) and achieve a level of 160/100 mm Hg within 2 to 6 hours. Parenteral therapy is indicated in hypertensive emergencies associated with end-organ damage such as encephalopathy or aortic dissection. Constant BP monitoring is necessary. Rapid reductions in pressure may precipitate coronary, cerebral, or renal ischemia. The use of an antihypertensive that is titratable and predictable is preferred.
2. **Manage patients with acute ischemic stroke according to the American Stroke Association (ASA)/AHA guidelines:** With acute ischemic stroke, antihypertensives should only be used if the BP exceeds 220/120 mm Hg, and BP should be reduced cautiously by 10% to 15%. If thrombolytics are to be given, the BP should be maintained at less than 185/110 mm Hg during treatment and for 24 hours following treatment. In hemorrhagic stroke, the aim is to minimize bleeding with a target MAP of less than 130 mm Hg.
3. **Manage patients with acute subarachnoid hemorrhage:** For patients who will not undergo an intervention, the goal is to prevent further bleeding while maintaining cerebral perfusion in the face of cerebral vasospasm.
   - Parenteral antihypertensive therapy:

Nitroprusside: A short-acting, rapid arterial and venous dilator. BP will rise almost immediately if the drip is stopped. The usual initial dose is 0.3–0.5 mcg/kg/minute. AHA guidelines recommend beginning with 0.1 mcg/kg/min and titrate upward every 3 to 5 minutes to desired effect. Usual dose is 3 mcg/kg/min, rarely is greater than 4 mcg/kg/min needed, and maximum dose is 10 mcg/kg/min. Direct arterial pressure monitoring is essential for titration of this drug, with constant vigilance to prevent hypotension. Nitroprusside is metabolized to thiocyanate, a toxin, which can cause fatigue, nausea, tinnitus, blurred vision, and delirium. Serum thiocyanate levels should be drawn after 48 hours of use and regularly thereafter, especially with patients with impaired renal function. Levels of less than 10 mg/dl are considered safe. Concommitant administration of parenteral and oral therapy should be initiated prior to weaning nitroprusside. When oral antihypertensives begin to reduce the BP, weaning is done carefully to prevent hypotensive episodes.

Fenoldopam: A peripherally acting rapid-acting vasodilator and a selective dopamine-1 receptor agonist. Initial dose is 0.1 mcg/kg/min and it can be increased by 0.05 mcg/kg/min; the maximum recommended dose is 1.7 mcg/kg/min with a half-life of 9.8 minutes. The patient must still be kept in the ICU and undergo arterial monitoring with this drug.

Labetalol: A fast-acting alpha/beta-blocking agent, which also can be used to treat the patient in hypertensive crisis. Given slowly by IV push, beginning with a 20- to 80-mg dose, repeated every 10 minutes, or a continuous infusion of 2 to 8 mg/min can be administered. The usual cumulative dose is 50 to 200 mg. Do not exceed a total dose of 300 mg. Keep the patient supine during the injection and until stable. Check BP every 5 minutes and then every 30 minutes. Monitor for bronchospasm, heart block, or orthostatic hypotension.

Esmolol: A short/quick-acting beta-blocker with an onset of action of 1 to 2 minutes and a duration of 10 to 20 minutes. Initial dose is 250 to 500 mcg/kg/min for 1 minute and then 50 to 100 mcg/kg/min for 4 minutes. May repeat the sequence. Observe for hypotension, nausea, vomiting, and, with asthmatics, bronchospasm.

Nicardipine: A potent CCB given at a rate of 5 to 15 mg/hr. When desired BP reduction is achieved, consider reducing to the average maintance dose of 3 mg/hr. When discontinuing, can lose 50% of effect within 30 minutes, but gradually decreased effects persist for up to 50 hours. It may cause tachycardia, headache, and flushing; it has been noted to aggravate angina. Do not exceed 150 ml/hr (15 mg/hr).

Enalaprilat: An ACEI that reduces peripheral arterial resistance. The usual dose is 1.25 to 5 mg by IV bolus, administered over a 5-minute period. Dose may be repeated every 6 hours. Patients on diuretics should receive a lower standard dose. Initial response may take 15 minutes to 1 hour. Peak BP reduction occurs in 1 to 4 hours, and effects last up to 6 hours. Enalaprilat should be used with caution in patients with renal failure or those with bilateral renal artery stenosis (because of high renin states). Avoid in AMI.

Hydralazine: A potent vasodilator administered as a 10 to 20 mg IV bolus or a 10 to 40 mg intramuscular (IM) injection. The onset is 10 to 30 minutes, with a duration of 2 to 6 hours. Adverse effects include tachycardia, headache, vomiting, and aggravation of angina.

Nitroglycerin: A coronary and peripheral vasodilator supplied in a 50 mg vial, which is added to a 250 ml glass bottle of D_5W. The IV infusion may be concentrated to prevent fluid overload if higher doses are needed to control BP. NTG is administered via an infusion pump starting at 5 mcg/min. Onset is rapid, so BP must be monitored closely during titration of the drug. Increase by 5 to 10 mcg every 3 to 5 minutes. Headache is common and controlled with analgesics.

Phentolamine: An alpha adrenergic–blocking agent that reduces afterload and has minimal effect in reducing BP except for secondary hypertension caused by pheochromocytoma. A dose of 5 to 20 mg is administered via IV push. The onset is immediate, and the half-life is approximately 19 minutes. Use with caution in patients with CAD.

- *Oral antihypertensive medications:* Added as soon as the patient responds to oral medications, including captopril, clonidine, and labetalol. These medications are also used for management of hypertensive urgencies.

Safety Alert *Nifedipine is no longer recommended for the management of hypertensive emergencies. Liquid nifedipine had been used for rapid treatment of hypertension by piercing the capsule and squeezing out the contents under the tongue, with the thought that it was rapidly absorbed sublingually. The drug was not absorbed sublingually but rather was swallowed and absorbed in the stomach, producing a quick onset of action. Effects were varying and dangerous. Variations in dosage occurred, since the amount removed from the capsule by squeezing liquid from the small pierced hole was variable, as was the amount actually swallowed, versus that left pooled in the mouth. Serious side effects, including stroke have been reported.*

4. **Facilitate adjustment to a routine antihypertensive regimen:** As the patient is adjusted to a routine antihypertensive regimen, diuretics, ACEIs, CCBs, beta-blockers, alpha blockers, or ARBs may be used in various combinations. For persons with severe hypertension, three to five medications are often needed to achieve normal BP. Resistant hypertension is defined as BP that remains above goal despite the concurrent use of three antihypertensive agents of different classes (Calhoun et al., for AHA, 2008, p. 1403).

5. **Provide patient education regarding lifestyle alterations:** Behavioral changes are the cornerstones of medical treatment for early and established hypertension. Normal body weight should be achieved and maintained. Alcohol consumption should be less than 1 oz ethanol per day. Daily intake of sodium for the average adult should be modified to 2 to 3 g for the person with hypertension. Smoking cessation is imperative (1) to halt the injury to the intima of the coronary and peripheral vessels and (2) to reduce the workload of the heart. A regular aerobic program has been proved beneficial in maintaining better control of BP. This should consist of 30 minutes of exercise three to five times per week at a target HR of 60% to 80% of their anaerobic threshold (determined by an exercise physiologist). Maintenance of adequate potassium, calcium, and magnesium intake is important.

6. **Educate patients regarding ongoing pharmacotherapy:** Maintenance pharmacotherapy for hypertension is now approached by evaluating on an individual basis the best treatment option based on the patient's other disease states or demographic factors. For persons with severe hypertension, three to five medications are often needed to achieve normal BP. Patients must be informed that taking more than one drug is to be expected and not a sign of failure or a worsening of disease. Health care providers must set patient expectations for compliance. This approach has been accepted and promoted by JNC-7 and the AHA. After an adequate trial of the first drug, a second drug from a different category may be tried. (See Figure 5-33 for the algorithm and Table 5-22 for medications, the usual dosage, the schedule, and potential side effects of the antihypertensive agents commonly used.)

7. **Discuss surgical treatment of appropriate conditions that prompt hypertension:** Although there is no surgical intervention for primary hypertension, several forms of secondary hypertension respond well to the surgical correction of the primary problem. A coarctation of the aorta can be repaired by removing the narrowed area of the vessel and inserting a Teflon aortic graft. Renal artery stenosis may be corrected by grafting or by renal artery angioplasty. For patients with pheochromocytoma, surgical removal of the tumor(s) will return the patient to a normotensive state.

CARE PLANS FOR HYPERTENSIVE EMERGENCIES

Ineffective tissue perfusion: cardiopulmonary, cerebral, and renal *related to interruption of arterial flow secondary to vasoconstriction that occurs with interruption of the normal BP control mechanism; interruption of venous flow secondary to vasodilation or tissue edema that occurs with loss of autoregulation*

GOALS/OUTCOMES Tissue perfusion is established within 24 hours as evidenced by systemic arterial BP 110 to 160/70 to 110 mm Hg (or within patient's normal range); MAP 70 to 105 mm Hg; equal and normoreactive pupils; strength and tone of the extremities bilaterally equal and normal for patient; orientation to time, place, and person;

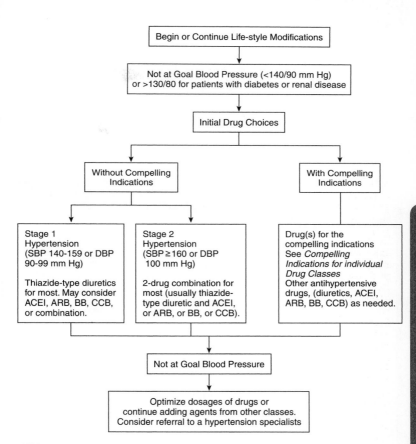

ACE, Angiotensin-converting enzyme; ISA, intrinsic sympathomimetic activity,
* Unless contraindicated.
† Based on randomized controlled trials.

Key: ACEI, angiotensin converting enzyme inhibitor, ALDO ANT, aldosterone antagonist, ARB,
     angiotensin receptor blocker, BB, beta blocker, CCB, calcium channel blocker,
     THIAZ, thiazide diuretics.

Compelling Indications for Individual Drug Classes	Initial Therapy Options
• Heart failure	THIAZ, BB, ACEI, ARB, ALDO ANT
• Post myocardial infarction	BB, ACEI, ALDO ANT
• High CVD risk	THIAZ, BB, ACEI, CCB
• Diabetes	THIAZ, BB, ACEI, ARB, CCB
• Chronic kidney disease	ACEI, ARB
• Recurrent stroke prevention	THIAZ, ACEI

Figure 5-33 Algorithm for the treatment of hypertension. (Modified from the Joint National Committee:
The Seventh Report of the Joint National Committee on Prevention, Detection, Evaluation, and Treatment of
High Blood Pressure [JNC VII], NIH Publication No. 03-5231, May 2003.)

urinary output 0.5 ml/kg/hr or greater; and stable weight. Within 48 hours, SBP is less than 140 mm Hg and diastolic BP is less than 90 mm Hg, with MAP 70 to 105 mm Hg.

NOC Circulation Status

Hemodynamic Regulation

1. Monitor BP and MAP every 1 to 5 minutes during titration of the medications. As patient's condition stabilizes, perform these assessments every 15 minutes to 1 hour. Be alert to sudden drops or elevations in BP. As the oral medications begin to affect BP, gradually wean IV nitroprusside and other potent vasodilators to prevent hypotensive episodes. Continuous monitoring is recommended.
   - Correlate cuff pressure with pressure from arterial cannulation.
   - Determine ideal range for BP control and maximal nitroprusside dose with physician. Usually the following guidelines are used: SBP less than 140 to 160 mm Hg; MAP less than 110 mm Hg; DBP less than 90 mm Hg.
   - If hypotension develops, decrease or stop nitroprusside infusion until the pressure rises.

Table 5-22	MEDICATIONS USED IN THE TREATMENT OF HYPERTENSION		
Drug Type	**Medication**	**Dosage/Schedule**	**Side Effects**
Diuretics			
Thiazides/related compounds	chlorothiazide (Diuril)	12.5–50 mg daily	Hypokalemia and hyperuricemia in thiazides and loop diuretics; hypercholesterolemia, hyperglycemia, increased type 2 diabetes, impotence, indigestion in all categories of diuretics
	chlorthalidone (Hygroton)	12.5–25 mg daily	
	cyclothiazide (Anhydron, Renazide)	1–2 mg daily	
	hydrochlorothiazide (Hydrodiuril)	12.5–50 mg daily	
	hydroflumethiazide (Aldactide)	12.5–50 mg daily	
	indapamide (Lozol)	2.5–5 mg daily	
	methylchlorthiazide (Enduron)	2.5–5 mg daily	
	metolazone (Mykrox) *or*	0.5–1 mg daily	
	metolazone (Zaroxlyn)	2.5–20 mg daily	
	polythiazide (Renese)	2–4 mg daily	
Loop diuretics	bumetanide (Bumex)	0.25–2.5 mg every 12 hr	
	ethacrynic acid (Ethacrynate)	25–200 mg every 12 hr	
	furosemide (Lasix)	20–200 mg every 6–24 hr	
	torsemide (Demadex)	2.5–10 mg every 12–24 hr	
Potassium-sparing agents	amiloride (Midamor)	5–10 mg every 12–24 hr	Hyperkalemia, gynecomastia, menstrual abnormalities
	eplerenone (Inspra)	25–100 mg daily	
	spironalactone (Aldactone)	25–200 mg every 8–24 hr	
	triamterene (Dyrenium)	100–300 mg every12–24 hr	

Table 5-22	MEDICATIONS USED IN THE TREATMENT OF HYPERTENSION—cont'd		
Drug Type	**Medication**	**Dosage/Schedule**	**Side Effects**
Adrenergic-Inhibiting Agents			
β-blockers	atenolol (Tenormin)*	25–100 mg daily	Fatigue, drowsiness, depression, fluid retention, heart failure, impotence, hypoglycemia, flushing, bronchospasm (diminished with cardioselective β_1-blockers)
	betaxolol (Kerlone)*	5–20 mg daily	
	bisoprolol (Zebeta)*	2–20 mg daily	
	metoprolol (Lopressor)*	50–100 mg every 12–24 hr	
	metoprolol extended release (Toprol XL)	50–100 mg daily	
	nadolol (Corgard)	40–120 mg daily	
	nebivolol (Bystolic)	2.5–40 mg daily	
	propranolol (Inderal)	40–160 mg every 12 hr	
	propranolol long–acting (Inderal LA)	60–180 mg daily	
	propranolol long–acting (InnoPran XL)	80–120 mg at bedtime	
	timolol (Blocadren)	20–40 mg every 12 hr	
β-blockers with ISA	acebutolol* (Sectral)	200–800 mg every 12–24 hr	
	carteolol (Cartrol)	2.5–10 mg daily	
	penbutolol (Levatol)	10–40 mg daily	
	pindolol (Visken)	10–40 mg twice daily	
α- and β-blocker	labetalol (Normodyne, Trandate)	200–800 mg twice daily	May cause severe postural hypertension; dose adjustments should be made based on standing BP.
	carvedilol (Coreg)	12.5–50 mg twice daily	
α-receptor blocker	alfuzosin (Uroxatral)	2.5–20 mg twice daily	Hypoglycemia, diarrhea, hypertension, flushing, first-dose syncope, blurred vision
	doxazosin (Cardura)	1–16 mg daily	
	phentolamine (Regitine)	50 mg twice daily	
	prazosin HCl (Minipres)	1–7 mg 3 times daily	
	terazosin (Hytrin)	1–20 mg daily	

Continued

Hypertensive Emergencies

Table 5-22	MEDICATIONS USED IN THE TREATMENT OF HYPERTENSION—cont'd		
Drug Type	**Medication**	**Dosage/Schedule**	**Side Effects**
ACE Inhibitors			
	benazepril (Lotensin)	10–40 mg twice daily	To prevent severe hypotension, reduce dose of diuretic; may cause hyperkalemia in person with renal failure; may cause acute renal failure in bilateral renal artery stenosis; also may cause profound postural hypotension; dose adjustments should be made based on standing BP.
	captopril (Capoten)	25–50 mg twice daily	
	enalapril (Vasotec PO)	2.5–40 mg twice daily	
	enalaprilat (Vasotec IV)	0.625–1.25 mg every 6 hours	
	fosinopril (Monopril)	10–40 mg daily	
	lisinopril (Prinivil, Zestril)	10–40 mg daily	
	moexipril (Univasc)	7.5 mg daily	
	perindopril (Aceon)	4–8 mg twice daily	
	quinapril (Accupril)	10–40 mg daily	
	ramipril (Altace)	25 mg daily	
	trandolapril (Mavik)	1–4 mg daily	
Angiotensin Receptor Blockers (ARBs) (Angiotensin II Antagonists)			
	candesartan (Atacand)	8–32 mg daily	Hepatotoxicity, hyperkalemia, agranulocytosis, leukopenia, neutropenia. Less risk of angioedema and cough than with ACE inhibitors.
	eprosartan (Teveten)	400–800 mg daily; may divide doses	
	irbesartan (Avapro)	150–300 mg daily	
	losartan (Cozaar)	25–100 mg daily; may divide doses	
	olmesartan (Benicar)	20–40 mg daily	
	telmisartan (Micardis)	20–80 mg daily	
	valsartan (Diovan)	80–320 mg daily	
Calcium Channel Blockers (CCBs)			
Nondihydropyridines	diltiazem (Cardizem)	30–90 mg 4 times daily	Constipation, peripheral edema
	verapamil (Calan, Isoptin)	80–120 mg 3 times daily	
Dihydropyridines	amlodipine (Norvasc)	2.5–10 mg daily	Dihydropyridines are more potent peripheral vasodilators and may cause more flushing, peripheral edema, tachycardia, dizziness, and headache.
	felodipine (Plendil)	5–50 mg daily	
	isradipine (DynaCirc)	2.5–10 mg twice daily	
	nicardipine (Cardene)	60–120 mg twice daily	
	nifedipine LA (Procardia XL)	30–60 mg 3 times daily	
	nisoldipine (Sular)	10–40 mg daily	

Table 5-22	**MEDICATIONS USED IN THE TREATMENT OF HYPERTENSION — cont'd**		
Drug Type	**Medication**	**Dosage/Schedule**	**Side Effects**
Direct Renin Inhibitors			
	aliskiren (Tekturna)	Starting dose: 150 mg once daily. May titrate up to 300 mg daily. No dosage adjustment in the elderly. Concomitant use with cyclosporine is not recommended.	Addition of aliskiren to an ACEI (or ARB) and β-blocker had favorable neurohumoral effects in heart failure and appeared to be well tolerated.
Miscellaneous Antihypertensives			
	clonidine (Catapres)	0.2–2.4 mg daily in divided doses	Gradually withdraw over 1 week
	guanabenz (Wytensin)	8–30 mg daily	Orthostatic hypotension, xerostomia
	guanfacine (Tenex)	1–2 mg at bedtime daily	Orthostatic hypotension, xerostomia
	methyldopa (Aldomet)	250–1000 mg daily in 2 divided doses	Peripheral edema; sedation with initial dosing
Combination Type	**Brand Name**	**Fixed-Dose Combinations**	
ACEIs and CCBs	Lotrel	amlodipine/benazepril (2.5/10, 5/10, 5/20, 10/20)	
	Lexxel	enalapril maleate/ felodipine (5/5)	
	Tarka	tradolapril/verapamil (2/180, 1/240, 2/240, 4/240)	
ACEIs and ARBs	Exforge	amlodipine/valsartan (5/160, 10/160, 5/320, and 10/ 320 mg)	
	Exforge HCT	amlodipine/valsartan/ HCTZ (5/160/12.5; 10/160/12.5; 5/160/25; 10/160/25; and 10/320/25)	
	Azor	amlodipine/olmesartan (yellow [5/40 mg, 10/20 mg, 10/40 mg tablets], red [10/20 mg and 10/40 mg], and black [10/20 mg])	

Continued

Hypertensive Emergencies

Table 5-22	MEDICATIONS USED IN THE TREATMENT OF HYPERTENSION—cont'd		
Drug Type	**Medication**	**Dosage/Schedule**	**Side Effects**
ARBs and diuretics	Atacand HCT	candesartan cilexetil/HCTZ (16/12.5, 32/12.5)	
	Teveten/HCT	eprosartan mesylate/HCTZ (600/12.5, 600/25)	
	Avalide	irbesartan/HCTZ (150/12.5, 300/12.5)	
	Hyzaar	losartan potassium/HCTZ (50/125, 100/25)	
	Micardis/HCT	telmisartan/HCTZ (40/12.5, 80/12.5)	
	Diovan/HCT	telmisartan/HCTZ (40/12.5, 80/12.5)	
β-blockers and diuretics	Tenorectic	atenolol/chlorthalidone (50/25, 100/25)	
	Ziac	bisoprolol fumarate/HCTZ (2.5/6.25, 5/6.25, 10/6.25)	
	Inderide	propranolol LA/HCTZ (40/25, 80/25)	
	Lopressor HCT	metoprolol tartrate/HCTZ (50/25, 100/25)	
	Corzide	nadolol/bandrofluthlazide (40/5, 80/5)	
	Timolide	timolol maleate/HCTZ (10/25)	
Centrally acting drug and diuretic	Aldoril	methyldopa/HCTZ (250/15, 250/25, 500/30, 500/50)	
	Diupres	reserpine/chlorothiazide (0.125/250, 0.25/500)	
	Hydropres	reserpine/HCTZ (0.125/25, 0.125/50)	
Diuretic and diuretic	Moduretic	amiloride HCl/HCTZ (5/50)	
	Aldactone	spironolactone/hydro-chlorothiazide (25/25, 50/50)	
	Dyazide, Maxzide	triamterene/HCTZ (37.5/25, 50/25, 75/50)	

Table 5-22	MEDICATIONS USED IN THE TREATMENT OF HYPERTENSION—cont'd		
Drug Type	**Medication**	**Dosage/Schedule**	**Side Effects**
Direct renin inhibitor and diuretic	Tekturna HCT	aliskiren/HCTZ (150/12.5 mg, 150/25 mg or 300/12.5 mg, and 300/25 mg)	
	Valturna	aliskiren/valsartan (150/160 mg or 300/320 mg)	

ACE, angiotensin-converting enzyme; *ACEI*, angiotensin-converting enzyme inhibitor; *ARB*, angiotensin receptor blocker; *BP*, blood pressure; *CCB*, calcium channel blocker; *HCT/HCTZ*, hydrochlorothiazide; *ISA*, intrinsic sympathomimetic activity; *IV*, intravenous; *PO*, by mouth.
Some drug combinations available in multiple fixed doses. Each drug dose is reported in milligrams.
*Cardioselective.

2. Assess patient for neurologic deficit by performing hourly neurostatus checks. Be alert to sensorimotor deficit if MAP is greater than 140 mm Hg. As patient's condition stabilizes and BP becomes controlled, perform neurostatus checks at least every 4 hours.
3. Monitor patient for changes in fundoscopic examination. Consult physician if hemorrhages or fluffy cotton exudates are present.
4. Assess patient for evidence of decreasing renal perfusion by monitoring I&O and weighing patient daily. Consult physician if urinary output is less than 0.5 ml/kg/hr for two consecutive hours or if weight gain is at least 1 kg (2.2 lb). Be alert to azotemia (increasing BUN), decreasing creatinine clearance, and increasing serum creatinine. Optimal laboratory values are BUN 20 mg/dl or less, creatinine clearance 9.5 ml/min or higher, and serum creatinine 1.5 mg/dl or less.

NIC Medication Administration; Cardiac Care; Circulatory Care

Acute pain *related to headache secondary to cerebral edema occurring with high perfusion pressures*

GOALS/OUTCOMES Patient's subjective evaluation of pain improves within 12 to 24 hours, as documented by a pain scale. Nonverbal indicators, such as grimacing, are absent or diminished.
NOC Pain Control

Pain Management
1. Monitor patient for headache pain at frequent intervals. Devise a pain scale with patient, rating discomfort from 0 (no pain) to 10 (severe pain).
3. Provide pain medications as prescribed. A variety of analgesics may be used, ranging from acetaminophen with codeine to morphine, depending on the severity of the symptoms. Assess effectiveness of the pain medication, using the pain scale to determine degree of relief obtained.
3. Use of meperidine should be avoided.

Safety Alert *Concurrent use of meperidine and MAOI may result in hypertensive crisis, hyperpyrexia, cardiovascular collapse, and death.*

4. Teach patient relaxation techniques to use in conjunction with the medications. Guided imagery, meditation, progressive muscle relaxation, and music therapy often are effective. Maintain a quiet, low-lit environment that is free of extensive distraction and stimulation. Limit visitations as indicated.

NIC Analgesic Administration; Environmental Management: Comfort; Progressive Muscle Relaxation

◆◆Disturbed sensory perception *related to decreased visual acuity secondary to retinal damage occurring with high perfusion pressures; pain secondary to cerebral edema*

GOALS/OUTCOMES Within 24 to 48 hours of this diagnosis, patient reads print, recognizes objects or people, and demonstrates coordination of movement.
NOC Vision Compensation Behavior

Environmental Management: Safety
1. Assess patient for signs of decreased visual acuity by monitoring patient's ability to read and recognize objects or people. Evaluate patient's coordination of movement to determine depth perception. Perform a fundoscopic examination per institutional guidelines, if appropriate and allowable.
2. If patient has decreased visual acuity, assist with feeding and other ADLs and keep patient's personal effects within his or her visual field.
3. Reassure patient and significant others that visual problems usually resolve when the BP is lowered sufficiently.

NIC Surveillance: Safety

ADDITIONAL NURSING DIAGNOSES
For other nursing diagnoses and interventions, see the following as appropriate: *Hemodynamic Monitoring* (p. 75) and *Emotional and Spiritual Support of the Patient and Significant Others* (p. 200).

PERIPHERAL VASCULAR DISEASE

PATHOPHYSIOLOGY
Peripheral vascular disease (PVD) includes all vascular disorders of the blood vessel system outside of the heart. Both chronic disease states and acute disorders are included. This chapter discusses care of chronic diseases of the carotid arteries and lower extremity peripheral artery disease (PAD) and the acute development of critical limb ischemia.

Chronic, and many acute, vascular diseases develop from progressive atherosclerotic plaque formation in arterial walls throughout the body. The presence of PAD may indicate presence of cardiovascular disease. *Atherosclerosis*, as defined by the World Health Organization, is a combination of changes in the intimal and medial layers of the vessel wall in which lipids, hemorrhage, fibrous tissue, and calcium deposits occur. The intima is the innermost layer composed of endothelial cells within a matrix of collagen and elastin fibers. The media is the thick middle layer of the vessel composed of varying amounts of smooth muscle, collagen, and elastic fibers. The adventitia is the outermost layer composed of collagen and elastin that make it a key element in providing the strength of the arterial wall.

Atherosclerotic plaque formation occurs in three stages. The early stage is development of fatty streaks during childhood or young adult life. The fatty streaks are formed from lipid-laden macrophages called "foam cells." Low-density lipoprotein cholesterol is the main lipid component of the fatty streaks. The second stage is the appearance of fibrous plaque later in life from progression of the fatty streaks from foam cells to a more permanent fibrous plaque. These plaques are most often found at areas of bifurcation of the arterial vessels. The last stage occurs as the fibrous plaque develops into a complicated lesion with necrosis and ulceration of the plaque surface with exposure leading to thrombogenesis through platelet aggregation and thrombus formation. Elasticity of the arterial wall is lost and there is progressive narrowing of the vessel lumen. The vessel wall may also degenerate and dilate, leading to aneurysmal development.

The primary risk factors known to accelerate this process are smoking, hypertension, hyperlipidemia, and diabetes mellitus. The presence of coronary artery disease and renal artery stenosis has been correlated with carotid artery disease of 50% stenosis or greater. Exercise and modification of risk factors can slow the progression and even promote regression of the fatty streaks.

Symptoms of atherosclerosis emerge over time with the progressive narrowing and occlusion of the arterial bed until the vessel that provides the main perfusion of a limb or tissue is critically narrowed to 50% or more of lumen diameter (noted as a hemodynamically significant stenosis). Symptoms of chronic progressive atherosclerosis include subtle changes in skin appearance, color, and temperature. Other factors, such as length of stenosis, blood viscosity, peripheral resistance, and acute versus chronic development, affect blood flow and tissue perfusion. As plaque progresses along the arterial walls in an uneven pattern, the laminar flow of blood becomes turbulent and can be heard with a stethoscope as a "bruit." Generally, the progressive and chronic development of disease allows for the development of collateral blood flow and perfusion to be maintained at a minimal level for the person at rest without symptoms present at this time. Pain occurs when the tissue needs more oxygen, such as with walking or other exercises.

Autonomic neuropathy, which occurs when blood is shunted away from peripheral cutaneous capillary beds, may occur with PAD alone, or in conjunction with diabetes or other comorbidities. Motor neuropathy causes changes in gait and pressure distribution, which may lead to ulceration. Skin is less elastic with diminished capillary perfusion and reparative mechanisms. Loss of protective sensation and proprioception resulting in increased force with each step can lead to callus formation at pressure areas, which decreases elasticity and increases skin ischemia. Bone and joint changes occurring with comorbidities, such as diabetes, can add additional abnormal weight-bearing mechanisms to the feet, leading to callus and ulcer formation. This can become critical in the presence of PAD and diminished perfusion.

Sudden blockage of an artery presents with an acute onset of symptoms that are more pronounced. An acute blockage of a lower extremity artery (acute limb ischemia [ALI]) may present with pain, pallor, and neurosensory impairment in the lower limb, while an acute occlusion of a cerebrovascular artery may present as a stroke.

Carotid Arterial Occlusive Disease

Fifty percent of TIAs and strokes are caused by significant carotid artery stenosis or ulcerative plaque. In the remaining 50% of cases, the source of stroke may be a thromboembolic source (Box 5-6). The internal carotid artery bifurcates at the common carotid, providing perfusion to the intercerebral circulation (the circle of Willis) and is a common area of plaque formation. Significant stenosis or occlusion of this artery may present with classic symptoms consisting of

---

Box 5-6	**CAUSES OF ACUTE ARTERIAL OCCLUSION**

General pathologic processes
Arterial versus atheroembolization
Thrombosis of a diseased artery (acute-on-chronic disease)
Acute occlusion of a vascular bypass graft
Arterial traumas

Specific sources or processes

Cardiac Causes	**Noncardiac Causes**
Atherosclerotic heart disease (most common cardiac source)	Aneurysms (most common noncardiac source)
Arrhythmias—Atrial fibrillation	• Abdominal aortic aneurysms • Peripheral aneurysms (such as femoral or popliteal)
Myocardial infarction (left ventricular mural thrombus formation) (2nd most common source)	Atherosclerotic plaque ulcers (in aorta or common iliac artery; also source of stroke in carotid artery disease)
Cardiomyopathy	Prosthetic grafts
Left ventricular aneurysms	Iatrogenic sources or arterial trauma (such as catheter-induced thrombus formation)
Endocarditis (valvular vegetation)	Paradoxical sources (secondary to an intracardiac defect and a patent foramen ovale)
Prosthetic cardiac valves	
Rheumatic heart disease	

transient monocular blindness (amaurosis fugax) on the side of the lesion, unilateral neuro-sensory deficits (hemiparesis or hemiparesthesias), or difficulties with speech. The objective of treating significant carotid stenosis is to prevent the disease from progressing from a TIA to a stroke.

Lower Extremity Peripheral Arterial Occlusive Disease: Acute

Acute occlusion of a lower extremity artery may occur from chronic PAD with development of an acute thrombosis, referred to as "acute-on-chronic" disease. When the chronic develop-ment of peripheral arterial occlusive disease in the lower extremity becomes severe, it is re-ferred to as "critical limb ischemia" (CLI) and usually is manifested by rest pain and/or isch-emic ulcers of the foot. Acute thrombosis of sites of stenosis in which the blood flow impairment was hemodynamically significant can occur and present with acute symptoms. However, most often acute limb ischemia (ALI) is due to an embolic source. Cardiac disease is one of the most common embolic sources, with atrial fibrillation being one of the most fre-quent cardiac sources. Aneurysmal disease is another common embolic source. See Box 5-6 for a listing of embolic sources. Diagnostic workup will include looking for a source of emboli, especially ruling out a cardiac or aneurysmal source.

The acute occlusion of a limb presents with a sudden onset of symptoms that are charac-teristic and essential in determining the diagnosis of ALI. These prominent symptoms are re-ferred to as the "6 P's" and include pain, pallor, paresthesias, paralysis, pulselessness, and poikilothermia. The severity of the symptoms depends on a number of factors, such as the acuteness of development of the vessel occlusion, presence of chronic disease with collateral circulation, and duration of the ischemic event. Symptoms of paresthesias and paralysis indi-cate advanced ischemia that is affecting nerve pathways of the extremity. Additionally, the presentation may include decreased sensation along the dorsum of the foot and loss of great toe or ankle dorsiflexion. With acute disease, critical ischemia develops within hours and is associated with irreversible anoxic injury to skeletal muscle or peripheral nerves within 4 to 6 hours. Skin and subcutaneous tissue remain viable for longer periods because of increased tolerance to ischemia. In less than 8 hours' duration of acute ischemia, the limb may appear pale, waxy white with a cadaveric appearance. At 8 to 12 hours, areas of local stasis develop with bluish skin mottling followed by blebs, superficial skin necrosis, and dry gangrene mum-mification of toes.

Evaluation and diagnosis of the cause of ALI are crucial to prevent tissue injury and necro-sis. In general, an onset of symptoms indicative of ALI presenting within the past 14 days is considered acute. Early diagnosis would include duplex ultrasound or vascular noninvasive Doppler studies, angiography, echocardiogram, and possible magnetic resonance angiography (MRA) or computer tomography angiography (CTA). Treatment will include a number of options including anticoagulation, thrombolytic therapy, surgical thromboembolectomy; en-dovascular procedures of stent, angioplasty, or atherectomy, and surgical bypass or amputation of the limb. Complications include those secondary to the treatment, as well as complications related to the acute ischemic event and reperfusion injury. These include catheter-induced vessel injury, bleeding, reocclusion, compartment syndrome, and reperfusion injury.

Compartment syndrome and reperfusion injury occur when ischemia to a limb is absent for an extended period of time. *Compartment syndrome* is defined by the swelling of tissues within closed fascial compartments leading to increased pressure, compression, and further necrosis and nerve injury. In anticipation of this, a fasciotomy of the involved limb may be performed at the time of surgical thromboembolectomy or at a later time. Reperfusion injury also involves the development of severe acidosis, hyperkalemia, renal failure secondary to myoglobinuria, and pulmonary insufficiency (see *Compartment Syndrome Ischemic myositis*, p. 301).

PERIPHERAL VASCULAR ASSESSMENT: ARTERIAL OCCLUSIVE DISEASE
Goal of System Assessment
- Evaluate for decreased blood flow and tissue perfusion so as to evaluate for focal dimin-ished perfusion of the cerebrovascular or lower extremity peripheral arterial systems.

History and Risk Factors
- Family or personal history of tobacco abuse, hyperlipidemia, hypertension, diabetes, obesity, hypertriglyceridemia, stress, sedentary living, cardiovascular disease, renal insuf-ficiency, clotting disorders, foot ulcers, or noncompliance with medical management

(daily aspirin and/or clopidogrel or other platelet inhibitors; other medications to control above risk factors)
- Age less than 50 years, with diabetes and one other atherosclerosis risk factor (smoking, dyslipidemia, hypertension, or hyperhomocysteinemia)
- Age 50 to 69 years and history of smoking or diabetes
- Age 70 years and older
- Leg symptoms with exertion (suggestive of claudication) or ischemic rest pain
- Abnormal lower extremity pulse examination
- Known atherosclerotic coronary, carotid, or renal artery disease

Carotid Arterial Occlusive Disease
- Coronary artery disease and renal artery stenosis greater than 60% are associated with increased risk for carotid disease.
- Retinal ischemic events, especially in the absence of migraine or cardiac embolic events, warrant evaluation for carotid artery disease.
- Significant stenosis may be present without symptoms.
- Symptomatic carotid stenosis or occlusion may present with TIA symptoms.
    - TIA symptoms last less than 24 hours.
    - RIND (reversible ischemic neurologic deficit) symptoms last longer than 24 hours but rapidly resolve completely.
- TIA symptoms indicative of stenosis or occlusion of the internal carotid artery include ipsilateral temporary monocular blindness or amaurosis fugax (usually described as a shade coming down over the eye), contralateral motor and sensory deficits (unilateral hemiparesis or hemiparesthesias), or difficulties with speech (aphasia).
- Atypical symptoms of dizziness, vertigo, syncope, unsteady gate, bilateral paresthesias/paresis may be attributed to other causes, such as cardiac disease, hypovolemia, medication side effects, vertebrobasilar insufficiency, and others.

Peripheral Arterial Occlusive Disease With or Without Distal Limb Involvement, Chronic
- Associated with the presence of CAD
- May be chronic or acute-on-chronic disease
- Intermittent claudication is the most common manifestation of PAD.
    - The calf, thigh, hip, or buttock develops tightening or cramping pain with exertion, such as walking a predictable distance, and is relieved with rest.
    - The site of claudication is indication of the location of occlusion, which will be above the presentation of pain.
- Symptoms may also be described as "fatigue" or "numbness" of the extremity that occurs with walking.
- Nocturnal rest pain indicates a worsening of the disease. It occurs at night and is usually relieved by sitting, standing, or dangling the affected limb to use gravity to increase perfusion.
- Rest pain indicates a critically ischemic limb and is generally present in the distal foot, forefoot, and toes.
- Most common symptoms of rest pain: a burning sensation across the dorsum of the foot
- Chronic symptoms may be masked by the presence of other diseases limiting the ability to walk, such as cardiac or respiratory disease causing fatigue or dyspnea before lower extremity symptoms are present.

Peripheral Arterial Occlusive Disease With or Without Distal Limb Involvement, Acute
- Acute occlusions are commonly associated with a thromboembolic source, which needs to be identified.
- Hallmark signs: The "6 P's" (pain, pallor, pulselessness, paresthesia [numbness], poikilothermia [coldness], and paralysis).
    - Paralysis is a late and grave sign; the limb already has necrotic muscle and will not likely regain function and may require amputation.
- Presence of "blue toe syndrome" is indicated by bluish, mottled spots scattered over the toes.
- Outcome depends on duration of tissue ischemia, site of obstruction, extent of thrombus propagation, adequacy of collateral circulation, and hemodynamic state of the patient.

Observation

Symptoms of PAD may vary depending on the vessels involved and may include intermittent claudication if it involves the limbs or TIAs if it involves the carotid arteries, which provide perfusion to the brain. Most patients with intermittent claudication require no intervention; approximately 20% require surgical reconstruction, and approximately 5% to 10% progress to require an amputation. The presence of pain at rest or a nonhealing necrotic ulcer defines CLI and indicates disease in greater than one artery and impending loss of the limb without treatment. Evaluate blood flow quality and tissue perfusion of cerebrovascular and peripheral vascular vessels:

- Cerebrovascular perfusion
  - Level of consciousness, alertness, speech, responsiveness
  - Neurologic assessment of cranial nerve function
  - Extremity strength, movement
- Lower extremity perfusion
  - Look for decreased hair growth, shiny skin, nail changes, distal joint abnormalities, or skin ulcers.
  - Evaluate for change in skin color in a neutral and dependent position (pallor versus rubor).
  - Neurosensory function of peripheral nerves: sensation, strength

Carotid Artery Occlusive Disease

- Presence of unilateral paralysis, facial features, gait ataxia
- Evaluate for cranial nerve (CN) damage status post carotid procedure.
  - CN IX—taste to posterior third of tongue, gag reflex; injury may cause mild dysphagia or loss of taste.
  - CN VII—facial movement, symmetry of face (as in drooping at the corner of the mouth), unable to smile symmetrically.
  - CN X—palatal, pharyngeal, and laryngeal, gag movement; injury may affect tongue movement, dysphagia, or dystonia.
  - CN XI—sternocleidomastoid, trapezius muscle movement; injury may cause an inability to shrug shoulders or move head side to side against resistance.
  - CN XII—tongue movement; injury may cause an inability to move the tongue from side to side or dysarthria.

Peripheral Artery Occlusive Disease

- Presence of pallor in the foot when the extremity is elevated 30 to 45 degrees for several seconds to a minute
- Presence of dependent rubor (intense red color) in the foot when it is dependent for several minutes
- Presence of bluish, mottled discolorations of the foot or toes
- Ulceration, fissures, or gangrene lesions present at the digits, interdigits, or heel
- Presence of extremity pallor, paralysis, or gait ataxia

Vital Signs

Check temperature, HR, BP, and peripheral pulses to evaluate blood flow quality and tissue perfusion.

- Unequal BP in arms can indicate carotid or subclavian artery disease.
- Obtain an ankle-brachial index (ABI). Decreased ABI can indicate presence of PAD.
- Possible fever if cellulitis or infected wounds are present
- Symptomatic bradycardia may develop post carotid procedure caused by vagal stimulation.
- BP may increase or decrease with stimulation of baroreceptors in the carotid bulb.
- Severe hypertension or hypotension is worrisome for impending stroke or MI and will need immediate attention.
- Monitor for changes in BP, HR, and RR post carotid procedure to assess for increased intracranial pressure secondary to hemorrhage, edema, or ischemia.
  - May also represent reperfusion injury following carotid procedures; hemorrhage or headache may occur with increased blood flow, usually after repair of a high-grade stenosis.
- Unequal arm pressures may be present, indicating a possible subclavian stenosis present on the side with the lower pressure. The higher of the arm pressures should be considered the accurate pressure.
- ABI assesses perfusion in the lower extremities and checks for graft patency.

Palpation

Pulse assessment to evaluate for decreased tissue perfusion.
- Pulse quality and regularity bilaterally (scale of 0 to 4+; 0 = absent pulse to 4+ = bounding pulse)
- Capillary refill
- Increased warmth or coolness of extremity
- Extremity edema (scale 0 to 4+): generally not present unless complication of secondary disease (i.e., skin infection, cardiac failure, liver failure, venous insufficiency)

Pulses and Circulation

- Pulse amplitude may be increased or decreased depending on disease process. Change in pulse is palpable below the level of disease.
- Decrease in pulse quality or absent pulse may indicate occluded or stenotic arteries.
- Bounding pulses may be indicative of aneurysmal development of the artery.
  - Palpate the femoral and popliteal arteries for presence of an aneurysm affecting distal circulation.
  - Aneurysmal arteries have an increased diameter and may have an easily palpable or bounding pulse.
  - Pseudoaneurysm can occur due to injury of artery such as the catheter insertion point for thrombolysis.
- Presence of edema (scale 0 to 4+) of extremities is indicative of other secondary problems (such as HF, liver disease, venous insufficiency, or thrombosis)
  - Edema with erythema may be indicative of infection.
  - Lymphedema may be present post bypass procedure due to disruption of the lymph system when making incision or creating vein graft (not caused by arterial disease).
- Slow capillary refill (greater than 2 seconds) is indicative of sluggish circulation and arterial occlusions.
- Temperature changes with coolness distal to the site of occlusion.
- After repair of an acutely ischemic limb, palpate affected limb for compartment syndrome. Most common site is the anterior compartment of the lower leg. Presents with tightness of the skin and muscle pain to a higher degree than expected.

Auscultation

Listen for presence of bruits, which indicate disturbances in flow (plaque formation).
- Bilateral carotid arteries
- Abdominal aortic and bilateral femoral
- Peripheral pulses with Doppler for quality of pulse signal

Bruits and Doppler Ultrasound

- Bruits in the carotid arteries, the aorta, or the renal arteries may be indicative of stenosis or dilation of arteries.
  - Bruits are high-pitched pulsations (similar to a murmur) best heard with the bell of the stethoscope and correlate with the presence of turbulent flow.
  - Carotid bruits are assessed by auscultating the carotid artery from the base of the neck to the angle of the jaw; they are usually loudest in the upper third of the neck in the area of the carotid bifurcation.
  - Renal and aortic bruits are assessed in the mid-abdominal or epigastric area of the abdomen.
- Doppler auscultation of the peripheral pulses
  - A healthy artery has three phases (sounds) heard when using a Doppler for assessment of pulses. A repaired artery may have one or two phases.
  - A change in the Doppler signal from three (triphasic) or two phases (biphasic) to only one (monophasic) may be indicative of complications.

Screening Labwork

Blood studies can help to determine risk of vascular disease or its complications.
- Chemistries: checking for blood glucose and renal function (↑ creatinine, BUN, potassium)
- CBC: anemia, ↑ or ↓ platelet level evaluating for increased clotting/bleeding propensity

Peripheral Vascular Disease

- Coagulation studies: PT/INR or PTT evaluating for increased clotting/bleeding propensity
- Hgb A1c: evaluating risk factor control (presence of, or uncontrolled diabetes)
- Lipid profile: evaluating for control of risk factor (presence of, or uncontrolled hyperlipidemia)

Postprocedural Screening Labwork

Blood studies can reveal postprocedural or surgical complications such as bleeding, fluid overload, early infection, renal insufficiency, or muscle damage associated with reperfusion injury.

- Complete blood counts: possible anemia related to surgical blood loss or postoperative bleeding; increased WBCs indicating possible infection
- Electrolytes: fluid shift or volume changes with increased use of IV fluids; glucose indicates diabetic control
- Creatinine, BUN: possible changes in perfusion of the kidneys
- Liver enzymes, CPK: possible muscle injury related to reperfusion or compartment syndromes
- Coagulation panel: protime, INR, partial thromboplastin time to evaluate anticoagulation management

Diagnostic Tests for Arterial Stenosis

Test	Purpose	Abnormal Findings
Noninvasive Vascular Studies		
Ultrasound carotid duplex	Assess for presence of, and degree of carotid stenosis, location of bifurcation, and stenotic disease. May be screening or diagnostic.	Symptomatic stenosis of >70% shows a clear benefit for repair. Symptomatic stenosis of >50%–69% shows a marginal benefit of repair with success of results greater for males. Asymptomatic stenosis >60% shows significantly less benefit of repair compared to symptomatic stenosis >70%. In general, symptomatic stenosis >50% and asymptomatic stenosis >60% should be considered for repair based on patient's health status and comorbidities.
Lower extremity (LE) Continuous-wave Doppler ultrasound or duplex ultrasound	Assess PAD anatomy, severity, and progression of disease. Provide quantitative data after a successful LE revascularization; provide graft surveillance.	Stenosis of artery or bypass graft causing symptoms to appear or reappear or a decrease in healing noted
Ankle-brachial index (ABI)	Quick, cost-effective method to establish or refute presence of LE PAD. Surveillance of disease progression before and after intervention.	Normal 1.0–0.95 Mild disease 0.94–0.80 Moderate disease 0.75–0.40 Severe disease <0.40 (<0.40 is indicative of ischemic limb or threatened limb loss.)
Doppler waveforms	Assess for LE stenosis, useful in conjunction with ABIs, especially those >1.0 indicating arterial calcification or noncompressible vessels such as a prosthetic graft.	Normal arteries have a sharp systolic component and one or more diastolic components. As the vessel becomes narrowed, the diastolic components are absent and the systolic component widens. An abnormal waveform indicates disease proximal to the site the signal was obtained.

Diagnostic Tests for Arterial Stenosis—cont'd

Test	Purpose	Abnormal Findings
Measurement of compartment pressures	Assess for swelling within the osteofascial compartments of the legs, which causes increased intracompartmental pressure and results in decreased arterial perfusion.	When the pressure of the compartment exceeds capillary perfusion pressure, blood flow to tissues is compromised. This usually occurs with intracompartmental pressures $>30–40$ mm Hg but may be lower in the presence of hypotension.

Blood Studies

Test	Purpose	Abnormal Findings
Complete blood count (CBC) Hemoglobin (Hgb) Hematocrit (Hct) RBC count (RBCs) WBC count (WBCs) Platelets	Assess for anemia, clotting, or bleeding propensity; presence of infection.	Decreased RBCs, Hgb, or Hct reflects anemia, which affects tissue perfusion; $\downarrow$ or $\uparrow$ platelets reflects risk of clotting or bleeding, which may result in interventional complications. Infected tissue from critical limb ischemia or postoperative wound may increase WBCs.
Chemistries Potassium (K^+) Glucose Creatinine (Cr) Blood urea nitrogen (BUN) Glycosylated hemoglobin (A1c)	Assess for presence of, or control of diabetes; assess renal function.	Increase in glucose may indicate diabetes. Increase of Hgb A1c >6.5 indicates diabetes; >7.0 indicates uncontrolled diabetes. Diabetes increases the risk of PAD and affects healing. Increased K^+, Cr, BUN may reflect renal disease; may also restrict use of iodine-based dyes used for diagnostics.
Liver Enzymes Aspartate aminotransferase (AST) Creatine phosphokinase (CPK) Lactate dehydrogenase (LDH)	Assess for presence of rhabdomyolysis associated with compartment syndrome or reperfusion injuries.	Increased levels may indicate damage to skeletal muscles.
Coagulation profile Prothrombin time (PT) with international normalized ratio (INR) Partial thromboplastin time (PTT)	Assess for causes of bleeding, clotting, and disseminated intravascular coagulation (DIC) indicative of abnormal clotting present in shock or ensuing shock.	Decreased PT with low INR promotes clotting; elevation promotes bleeding.
Lipid profile and lipoprotein-cholesterol fractionation Total cholesterol High-density lipoprotein (HDL) cholesterol Low-density lipoprotein (LDL) cholesterol Very low-density lipoprotein (VLDL) cholesterol Triglycerides	Assess for causes of arterial plaque formation contributing to PAD or carotid stenosis. *Total cholesterol:* Measures circulating levels of free cholesterol and cholesterol esters *Triglycerides:* Assesses storage form of lipids	Elevation of total cholesterol, LDL, VLDL, and triglycerides indicates a greater potential for developing arterial stenosis. Elevated HDL lowers probability of arterial stenosis. Concentrations vary with age. *Total cholesterol:* Many physicians prefer patients to have a total cholesterol level of <200 mg/dl, but if fractionation is used, other risk factors are considered prior to recommending patients lower their cholesterol level if >200 mg/dl.

Continued

Diagnostic Tests for Arterial Stenosis — cont'd

Test	Purpose	Abnormal Findings
Radiology		
Magnetic resonance imaging (MRI) Cerebral MRI	Assesses for presence of old or new signs of stoke	Any signs of intracranial lesions indicating old or new infarcts
Computed tomography (CT) Cerebral CT scan	Assesses for presence of old or new signs of stroke	Any signs of intracranial lesions indicating old or new infarcts
Magnetic resonance angiography (MRA)	Assess vascular anatomy, presence and degree of stenosis or vessel occlusions with reconstruction images of vascular anatomy. Similar to MRI with vascular imaging obtained with gadolinium injected for contrast.	Arterial stenosis or occlusions; may suggest presence of aneurysms (will need to corroborate with CT scan)
CT angiography (CTA)	Assess vascular anatomy, presence and degree of stenosis or vessel occlusions with reconstruction images of vascular anatomy. Provides associated soft tissue diagnostic information, acute emboli or aneurysms. Radiopaque contrast media peripherally injected for vascular imaging.	Arterial stenosis or occlusions; presence of aneurysms; presence of acute emboli
Invasive Vascular Studies		
Contrast angiography with digital subtraction	Assesses for presence and extent of arterial stenosis or occlusions using a radiopaque catheter inserted through a peripheral vessel advanced into the carotid, aortic, or distal arteries; allows direct injection of thrombolytic drugs. Identifies presence of distal vessels necessary for outflow during surgical revascularization.	Arterial stenosis; presence of intracranial, aortic, iliac, femoral, or popliteal aneurysms; presence of arteriovenous malformations or fistulas. Test is used to prescribe the most appropriate treatment: endovascular (including thrombolytic) or surgical.

Carotid Duplex and Arteriogram

Carotid duplex ultrasound (DUS) is used to detect the presence of carotid artery stenosis. At centers where the DUS has been internally validated in comparison with angiography and this level of performance has been documented, surgeons may choose to proceed with surgery based on the DUS without the extra risks of a carotid angiogram. At centers where the DUS results are less reliable, this is used as a screening tool with stenosis greater than 50% indicating the need for an angiogram.

Ankle-Brachial Index

BPs are taken in both arms, with the highest pressure used for calculating indices (unequal arm pressures may indicate the presence of carotid or subclavian artery disease). Segmental pressures are also taken with a thigh cuff placed above the knee for a low thigh pressure and above the ankle to obtain ankle pressures of the dorsalis pedis and posterior tibial artery. A handheld Doppler is used to acquire the dorsalis pedis and posterior tibial pulses. Normally, the pressure in the leg is equal to or slightly higher than brachial pressure. A difference of greater than 30 mm Hg between segments indicates disease of the artery proximal to where the pressure was taken. The ankle pressure is divided by the brachial pressure to obtain the ABI. Calcification of the arterial wall provides a falsely high measurement preventing compression of the vessel to obtain the pressure; this is referred to as a "noncompressible" vessel. A prosthetic graft that is tunneled through soft tissue will also be incompressible. In these patients, diagnosis must be based on waveform analysis.

COLLABORATIVE MANAGEMENT
Care Priorities: Peripheral Arterial Occlusive Disease

Priorities for the care of a patient with chronic peripheral arterial occlusive disease should focus on early identification of disease, prevention of disease progression, disability associated with the disease secondary to ischemic injury, and prevention of thrombotic ischemic events. Prevention of progression of the disease would include the control of risk factors, prevention of thrombus formation (i.e., antiplatelet therapy or other anticoagulants), and management of medications to control risk factors.

To assist and guide the identification and management of patients with PAD, many national organizations have collaborated to produce evidence-based guidelines. Selective recommendations from the guidelines that are related to acute care settings are outlined in the tables below.

GUIDELINES FOR THE MANAGEMENT OF PATIENTS WITH PERIPHERAL ARTERIAL DISEASE (PAD)

In October 2005, the American College of Cardiology (ACC) Foundation Board of Trustees and the American Heart Association (AHA) Science Advisory and Coordinating Committee approved the work of a collaborative effort of multiple vascular-associated organizations in the evaluation of multiple evidence-based studies and trials and development of nationally recognized evidence-based guidelines for the management of patients with PAD. This effort was also endorsed by many additional organizations not able to participate in the development activities.

Lower Extremity (LE) Arterial Occlusive Disease With or Without Symptoms

Intervention	Rationale
Assess for risk and presence of PAD.	History evaluation to include questions regarding presence of risk factors, walking impairment, claudication, ischemic rest pain, and/or nonhealing wounds. Patients with LE PAD have an increased risk for stroke or cardiovascular ischemic events due to coronary artery disease and cerebrovascular disease and are more frequent than ischemic limb events.
Identify *asymptomatic* persons with LE PAD by examination and/or measurement of the ankle-brachial index (ABI), toe-brachial index (TBI), or pulse volume recording (PVR) measurement.	Exercise ABI measurement can be useful to diagnose LE PAD in individuals at risk who have a normal ABI (0.91–1.30) without classic claudication symptoms and no other clinical evidence of atherosclerosis. TBI or PVR measurement can be useful to diagnose LE PAD in individuals at risk with an ABI >1.30 and no other clinical evidence of atherosclerosis.
Evaluate for evidence of other disorders that may cause significant functional impairment (e.g., angina, heart failure, chronic respiratory disease, or orthopedic limitations) before revascularization surgery or endovascular procedures.	Patients with symptoms of intermittent claudication should have significant functional impairment with a reasonable likelihood of symptomatic improvement and absence of other disease that would comparably limit exercise before undergoing revascularization.

Critical Limb Ischemia (CLI) and Acute Limb Ischemia (ALI)

Recommendation	Supporting Data
In patients with CLI, initiate an expedited evaluation and treatment of factors known to increase the risk of amputation: vascular history, ASHD risk factor assessment evaluation for arterial disease in other areas, and specific precipitating factors, trauma, or infection.	The natural history of untreated, severe PAD would lead to major limb amputation within 6 months. Determine the time and course of development of the ischemia. If history and examination suggest rapid progression, early revascularization may be required to prevent further deterioration and irreversible tissue loss. Revascularization of an ischemic extremity may be complicated by reperfusion injury to the damaged tissues and precipitate systemic responses, including cardiac, renal, and pulmonary dysfunction.

Continued

GUIDELINES FOR THE MANAGEMENT OF PATIENTS WITH PERIPHERAL ARTERIAL DISEASE (PAD)—cont'd

Immediately assess patients at risk for CLI who develop acute limb symptoms. Ensure emergent assessment and treatment by a specialist competent in treating vascular disease.	Patients at risk for CLI (patients with diabetes, neuropathy, chronic renal failure, or infection) are at risk to develop vascular emergencies.
Ensure that patients with CLI in whom open surgical repair is anticipated undergo assessment of cardiovascular risk.	Patients with LE PAD and CLI have an increased risk for stroke or cardiovascular ischemic events due to coronary artery disease and cerebrovascular disease. A detailed coronary assessment may be performed in selected patients in whom coronary ischemic symptoms would merit such an assessment if CLI were not present; such assessments should not impede care.
Evaluate all patients with CLI or ALI for aneurysmal disease of proximal arteries.	Patients with CLI or ALI who present with clinical features to suggest atheroembolization should be evaluated for more proximal aneurysmal disease (e.g., abdominal aortic, popliteal, or femoral aneurysms). Atheroembolism is suggested by the onset of signs and symptoms of CLI after recent endovascular catheter manipulation.
Establish regular intervals of direct examination of the feet after successful treatment of CLI or ALI.	Patients at risk of CLI (ABI less than 0.4 in a nondiabetic individual, or any diabetic individual with known LE PAD) should undergo regular inspection of the feet to detect objective signs of recurrent or new CLI.
Promptly initiate systemic antibiotics in patients with CLI, skin ulcerations, and evidence of limb infection.	Patients with CLI, skin ulcerations, and infections are at risk for potential development of vascular emergencies.
In CLI and ALI, perform emergent arterial Doppler/ABI studies and imaging studies, such as angiography, CTA, or MRA with gadolinium enhancement. Document evidence of previous history of contrast reaction or renal insufficiency (elevated serum creatinine above normal) prior to imaging studies and postangiography.	Patients with ALI should undergo an emergent evaluation that defines the anatomic level of occlusion and lead to prompt endovascular or surgical revascularization. If baseline renal insufficiency is present, hydration before undergoing contrast angiography is recommended. Follow-up evaluation postangiography is recommended to evaluate renal function after contrast used.
If not contraindicated, initiate catheter-based thrombolysis in patients with ALI of <14 days duration. Mechanical thrombectomy can be used as an adjunctive therapy for acute peripheral arterial occlusion. Above therapies may be considered in patients with ALI of >14 days' duration.	Analysis of control trials indicate that catheter-based, intra-arterial thrombolytic therapy is effective and beneficial in ALI of <14 days' duration; is comparable to surgery (embolectomy) as a low-risk alternative to open surgery in complex patients with severe comorbidities; and may enhance long-term patency relative to the clearing of intra-arterial thrombus from the distal runoff vessels.
In patients with combined inflow and outflow disease with CLI, inflow lesions should be addressed first with endovascular or surgical approach.	Patients with profound limb ischemia may not tolerate the time required to perform thrombolysis. In infrainguinal or distal arterial occlusions, thrombolysis have worse outcomes than more proximal or iliofemoral occlusions. Mechanical thrombectomy may avert the need for thrombolysis or allow the use of lower doses of thrombolytic drugs. A significant improvement in inflow may diminish the symptoms of rest pain; however, pulsatile flow to the foot may be needed for ischemic ulcers or ischemic gangrene.

GUIDELINES FOR THE MANAGEMENT OF PATIENTS WITH PERIPHERAL ARTERIAL DISEASE (PAD) — cont'd

Surgical revascularization, consisting of bypass with vein or prosthetic conduit, may be considered in patients with CLI and both inflow and outflow blockage to the LE.	Comparative studies of vein to prosthetic conduit (graft) for LE arterial reconstruction demonstrate vein to be superior in patency. Prosthetic conduit (PTFE or Dacron) may be used with acceptable patency rate for above-the-knee bypasses; however, patency is significantly lower when used for below-the-knee reconstruction.
Primary limb amputation may be considered in patients with an unsalvageable limb.	Unsalvageable limb may be considered in a limb with significant necrosis of weight-bearing areas of the foot, uncorrectable flexion contracture, refractory ischemic rest pain, sepsis or presence of significantly limited life expectancy due to comorbid conditions.
Initiate ongoing graft or stent patency surveillance in all patients treated for CLI or ALI.	Long-term patency of bypass grafts and endovascular treatments should be evaluated via a surveillance program at regular intervals (e.g., interval vascular history, resting ABIs, physical examination, and a duplex ultrasound).
Unless contraindicated, initiate a statin medication to lower low-density lipoprotein (LDL) cholesterol. Fibric acid derivative may be used in patients with LE PAD and normal LDL cholesterol but with low high-density lipoprotein (HDL) and elevated triglycerides.	Patients with PAD and LDL cholesterol of ≥100 mg are at greater risk of nonfatal myocardial infarction (MI) or cardiovascular death. An LDL target of 70 mg/dl is suggested for those with very high risk factors (e.g., evidence of PAD, multiple major risk factors including diabetes, severe and poorly controlled risk factors including smoking, metabolic syndrome especially with high triglycerides ≥200 mg/dl, non-HDL cholesterol ≥130 mg/dl and low HDL ≤40 mg/dl, and acute coronary syndromes).
Control hypertension with the following goals: *In nondiabetic*— SBP BP ≤140 mm Hg/DBP ≤90 mm Hg *In diabetic and chronic renal disease*— SBP ≤130 mm Hg/DBP ≤80 mm Hg	Uncontrolled hypertension increases the risk of cardiovascular events (MI, stroke, congestive heart failure). Beta-blockers and/or angiotensin-converting enzyme inhibitors (ACEIs) are acceptable in patients with LE PAD.
Unless contraindicated, initiate antiplatelet therapy in all patients undergoing treatment for CLI or ALI with aspirin 75–325 mg or clopidogrel 75 mg daily.	In patients with LE PAD, antiplatelet therapy is indicated to reduce the risk of MI, stroke, or vascular death.

ABI, ankle-brachial index; *ALI*, acute limb ischemia; *CLI*, critical limb ischemia; *DBP*, diastolic blood pressure; *HDL*, high-density lipoprotein; *LDL*, low-density lipoprotein; *LE*, lower extremity; *PAD*, peripheral arterial disease; *PTFE*, polytetrafluoroethylene; *PVR*, pulse volume recording; *SBP*, systolic blood pressure; *TBI*, toe-brachial index;

Lower Extremity Peripheral Arterial Occlusive Disease: Critical Limb Ischemia

In CLI, rest pain and/or ischemic ulcers are present. For a patient with ischemic ulcers, specific care priorities would include wound care, preventing or treating infection, and protection of the limb to prevent further tissue damage. Additional measures would include:

1. **Relief of ischemic pain:** In general, relieving ischemic pain requires improving perfusion to the limb. However, depending on the length of ischemic time and amount of ischemic nerve injury, administration of a narcotic analgesic is usually required.
2. **Prevention of injury to the ischemic limb:** Pressure to an already ischemic limb diminishes perfusion even further, leading to tissue breakdown. Maintain the heel or other pressure points of the extremity free from sustained pressure.

   In the surgical or endovascular management, care priorities would focus on promoting perfusion to the extremity, prevention of infection, and promoting wound healing. Promotion of perfusion in an extremity includes the prevention of limb edema that could impair graft perfusion and wound healing, maintaining perfusion of the stent or graft, and preventing thrombus or occlusion of the stent or graft. For more information and description of endovascular techniques and instruments, such as intra-arterial stent placement, balloon angioplasty, or atherectomy, see *Acute Coronary Syndromes*, p. 434.

3. **Promoting perfusion of the extremity:** Activities include keeping the extremity warm to prevent vasoconstriction, maintaining hydration, preventing hypotension, and preventing edema to the limb. If a surgical incision has been made to the limb, the limb will have a propensity for edema to develop which not only promotes graft compression, but impairs wound healing. Elevation of the extremity will help prevent or diminish edema.

Safety Alert   *Maintaining hydration and preventing hypotension in a patient who has undergone lower extremity bypass or stent placement are important in the prevention of graft occlusion. Hypotension decreases perfusion to the graft and dehydration increases blood viscosity, leading to thrombosis and graft or stent occlusion.*

---

4. **Prevention of peripheral arterial clot formation:** Antiplatelet therapy is the predominant medication used to prevent thrombus formation. However, unfractionated or low-molecular-weight heparin may be required in those persons with a history of a hypercoagulable state. Antiplatelet therapy includes the use of the following:
   - Aspirin: Low doses of 81 to 325 mg orally are given on a daily basis.
   - *Clopidogrel:* The standard dose is 75 mg daily. If a stent has been placed, clopidogrel is recommended. For patients who have not been on a regimen of daily clopidogrel and are about to undergo a carotid stent, and possibly prior to some peripheral stent placements, a loading dose of 300 mg of clopidogrel prior to stent placement is required.
   5. Provide ticlopidine for patients who are sensitive to other medications:
In patients who are unable to take aspirin or clopidogrel, other antiplatelet drugs will be considered, such as ticlopidine. Ticlopidine is not used as a first-line drug due to the adverse effects of life-threatening neutropenia, agranulocytosis, or thrombotic thrombocytopenia purpura.
6. **Prevent contrast-induced nephropathy secondary to contrast during angiography for endovascular intervention:**
Hydration is paramount and is accomplished with IV fluids. In addition to IV hydration, administration of the following medication is generally used:
   - *Acetylcysteine (Mucomyst):* This medication, generally used in respiratory disease, has proved to be effective in patients with evidence of renal insufficiency and serum creatinine levels greater than 1.4 mg/dl. Acetylcysteine is given at 600 mg as an oral solution or compounded tablet twice daily for four doses. The patient is instructed to start the day prior to the procedure, take the morning of the procedure, and take the last or fourth dose in the evening after the procedure.
   - *Fenaldopam:* Has been used in the past and is administered IV; however, it is no longer considered to be as effective as acetylcysteine.
   7. Provide surgical treatment of CLI using thromboendarterectomy and/or a bypass of the significant arterial stenosis or occlusion by use of a vein or synthetic graft material as a conduit.
   - Thromboendarterectomy or endarterectomy: This procedure is similar to that described above with a carotid endarterectomy (CEA). An incision is made along the length of the artery where the stenosis is located. The plaque is removed and the artery is sewn closed. A vein patch may be placed in the vessel during closure to provide an adequate size for blood flow. This is generally performed on the proximal vessels of the distal aorta, iliac or femoral arteries. A shunt, as may be used in the CEA to ensure cerebral perfusion, is not required in the distal limbs.
   - Surgical placement of a bypass graft or reconstruction: Through surgical incisions, a conduit is surgically attached forming an anastomosis that is end-to-end or end-to side to the artery above the site of an occlusion or hemodynamically significant lesion to provide "inflow" of blood to the extremity. The distal graft is surgically attached below the occlusions to provide "outflow" of blood to the extremity. Synthetic material, such as Dacron or polytetrafluoroethylene (PTFE), is often used as a conduit for bypasses above the knee, since the patency rate is equal to vein. This preserves the vein for future

need. A vein, usually the greater saphenous vein (GSV), is the conduit of choice for a bypass extending below the knee. The patient's vein may be harvested by excising the GSV and placing it in a reversed position to allow blood flow to pass valves. The GSV may also be used in situ, without completely excising, after a valvultome is used to destroy the one-way flow of the valve leaflets.The bypass is referred to by its anatomical placement. For example, an aortobifemoral bypass indicates that the proximal graft is attached at the aorta and bifurcated grafts are inserted bilaterally into each femoral artery. A femoropopliteal bypass indicates that the proximal graft is sewn to the femoral artery and the distal end of the graft is attached at the popliteal artery.

Lower Extremity Peripheral Arterial Occlusive Disease: Acute Limb Ischemia

In ALI resulting from acute arterial occlusion, the care priorities are similar to those of CLI, which would include early identification of an acutely ischemic limb and early intervention to diminish ischemic time and restore blood flow to the ischemic limb. In the limb with an acute arterial occlusion, thrombolysis is the recommended emergent procedure used to dissolve the arterial clot and restore limb perfusion. Time is of great concern in an acute arterial occlusion. Anticoagulation may be initiated with a heparin bolus and continuous infusion. If the patient is unable to undergo thrombolytic therapy, a thromboembolectomy may be performed to treat an acute arterial occlusion to quickly restore perfusion of the limb.

1. **Thrombolysis:** See *Acute Coronary Syndromes*, p 434, for a complete discussion of this procedure and care priorities related to its use. Care priorities for a patient undergoing thrombolysis for an acute peripheral arterial occlusion are essentially the same as in the patient with an acute coronary thrombus.
2. **Thromboembolectomy:** A surgical arteriotomy is performed and an embolectomy balloon catheter is passed past the thrombus, the balloon is inflated, and the clot is extracted. Neighboring arteries are checked for clot. Distal embolization is of great concern with this procedure due to the manipulation of the catheter around the thrombus.

Care priorities for ALI also include monitoring and early recognition of compartment syndrome, thromboembolic injury, and neuromuscular injury. For a full discussion and care priorities of compartment syndrome, see *Compartment Syndrome/Ischemic myositis*, p. 301.

In ALI, care priorities would also include facilitating the identification of the source of emboli. Given that the heart is a common source, an echocardiogram will be performed as soon as perfusion to the limb has been restored. Additional studies that would be considered include an abdominal/pelvic CTA scan or angiogram to look for any aneurysmal source. A lower extremity ultrasound may be performed looking for peripheral aneurysms of the femoral or popliteal arteries.

Safety Alert   *High potential for distal emboli to the foot, referred to as "trashed foot" or "blue toe syndrome." The risk for distal embolism from dislodgment of thrombus or thrombotic plaque is significant in any procedure in which catheters are manipulated around or through the clot causing clot fragmentation, such as with thrombolysis, thromboendarterectomy, angioplasty, or stenting. Incorporate monitoring for distal emboli into care priorities.*

Care Priorities: Carotid Arterial Occlusive Disease

The focus of care is similar to PAD but includes the early recognition and intervention of carotid artery stenosis to reduce progression of disease and to prevent stroke. Patients with a history of ischemic heart disease admitted to critical care are at high risk for carotid artery disease and stroke. The treatment of carotid disease includes medical management and possibly a surgical approach of carotid endarterectomy (CEA) or endovascular placement of a stent. In the general population, 2% to 18% of patients can have carotid artery stenosis yet be completely asymptomatic.

Peripheral Vascular Disease

COLLABORATIVE MANAGEMENT
Care Priorities: Carotid Artery Disease

CLINICAL PRACTICE GUIDELINES FOR THE MANAGEMENT OF ATHEROSCLEROTIC CAROTID ARTERY DISEASE

The Society for Vascular Surgery appointed a committee of experts to formulate evidence-based clinical guidelines for the management of carotid stenosis and published these results in 2008. The committee used systematic reviews to summarize the best available evidence and a grading scheme to grade the quality of evidence. Below are the recommendations from this collaborative committee.

Intervention	Supporting Research
Optimize medical management in patients with asymptomatic carotid stenosis < 60% or symptomatic stenosis < 50%. These include: • Control hypertension—ACEI or ARB are first-line medication in diabetics. • Control glucose—target Hb Alc ≤7% • Hyperlipidemia—target LDL <100 mg/dl in patients with coronary heart disease; <70 mg/dl in patients with multiple risk factors • Increase physical activity • Smoking cessation • Antiplatelet therapy with low-dose aspirin, extended release dipyridamole, or clopidogrel daily	In patients with low-grade carotid stenosis, the risk of disabling stroke or death was increased by 20% in the North American Symptomatic Carotid Endarterectomy Trial (NASCET) and European Carotid Surgery Trial (ECST). The Asymptomatic Carotid Atherosclerosis Study (ACAS) demonstrated that treatment of asymptomatic patients with ≥60% stenosis was of benefit. Asymptomatic patients with <60% stenosis are monitored with a carotid duplex every 3–6 months, and antiplatelet therapy is recommended.
Consider carotid endarterectomy (CEA) and optimal medical therapy in patients with • Symptomatic carotid stenosis ≥50% • Asymptomatic patients with ≥60% stenosis and low perioperative risk • Symptomatic patients with high-grade carotid stenosis of ≥70% • Asymptomatic patients with severe carotid stenosis ≥ 60% and low surgical risk	NASCET patients with 70%– 99% stenosis treated surgically had a cumulative risk of 9% ipsilateral stroke at 2 years compared to 26% of those treated medically. Meta-analysis of randomized trials of 5223 patients with asymptomatic moderate to severe carotid stenosis demonstrated a nonsignificant 30-day perioperative stroke or death rate of 2.8% in the surgical group compared to medical management. The three trials included the Veteran Affairs Cooperative Study (VACS), Asymptomatic Carotid Atherosclerosis Study (ACAS), and Asymptomatic Carotid Surgery Trial (ACST).
Consider carotid artery stenting (CAS) in symptomatic patients with carotid stenosis ≥ 50% and high perioperative risk. High risk includes patients with previous stenosis, prior ipsilateral neck radiation or ablative neck surgery, common carotid artery stenosis below the clavicle, contralateral vocal cord paralysis, and presence of tracheostomy stoma.	Meta-analysis of 10 randomized trials of 3182 patients with >50% stenosis comparing carotid angioplasty and CEA concluded a "nonsignificant" risk reduction of stroke with CAS. Additional high-risk factors may include patients with renal failure on dialysis, extremely low left ventricular ejection fraction, oxygen- or corticosteroid-dependent chronic lung disease, etc. The SAPPHIRE (Stenting and Angioplasty with Protection in Patients at High Risk for Endarterectomy) trial demonstrated that an endovascular approach may be considered in patients at high risk for a surgical approach.
CAS is inappropriate in asymptomatic patients with carotid artery stenosis.	Exceptions include patients with acceptable medical risk and severe carotid artery stenosis of ≥80% and high anatomic risk for CEA and compelling anatomy for CAS.

ACEI, angiotensin-converting enzyme inhibitor; *ARB,* angiotensin receptor blocker; *CAS,* carotid artery stent; *CEA,* carotid endarterectomy; *HDL,* high-density lipoproteins; *LDL,* low-density lipoproteins.

Provide management of patients to help prevent stroke and to manage patients following preventive procedures.

1. **Facilitate recovery from CEA.**
   - Prevent impaired cerebrovascular perfusion secondary to hypotension or hypertension or bradycardia.
   - Prevent respiratory impairment secondary to bleeding or hematoma formation at the incision leading to tracheal deviation and respiratory distress.
2. **Facilitate recovery from an endovascular stenting.**
   - Monitor for potential embolic TIA or stroke, as is done with the surgical approach.
   - Observe for and prevent limb ischemia related to the access site for the endovascular procedure.
   - For patients with a carotid stent: Continue antiplatelet therapy (generally with clopidogrel) to prevent stent occlusion.
3. **Initiate medical management, including antiplatelet medications, for patients with a 100% carotid occlusion of one side.** Postoperative complications of a CEA related to the surgical approach include neurologic deficits, hypertension, bradycardia, neck hematoma with potential for airway obstruction, and local nerve injuries of the laryngeal or hypoglossal nerves that require prompt treatment.

Safety Alert *There is a relationship between the presence of cerebrovascular disease and CAD. The most common cause of mortality following carotid endarterectomy is MI. There is also a relationship between PAD and CAD. The prognosis of patients with lower extremity PAD is characterized by an increased risk for cardiovascular ischemic events due to concomitant CAD and cerebrovascular disease. Cardiovascular ischemic events are more frequent than ischemic limb events in any patient with lower extremity PAD, whether they are asymptomatic, have atypical leg pain, classic claudication, or critical limb ischemia.*

CARE PLANS FOR GENERALIZED PERIPHERAL VASCULAR DISEASE

 Activity intolerance *related to compromised tissue perfusion and pain*

GOALS/OUTCOMES Within the 12- to 24-hour period before discharge from the ICU, the patient exhibits tolerance to increasing levels of activity as evidenced by RR less than 24 breaths/min, NSR on ECG, BP within 20 mm Hg of patient's normal range, HR less than 120 bpm (or within 20 bpm of resting HR for patients on beta-blocker therapy), and generalized pain less than 4 on a 1 to 10 scale.

NOC Endurance; Energy Conservation; Activity Tolerance

Energy Management
1. Determine patient's physical limitations.
2. Determine causes of fatigue and perceived causes of fatigue.
3. Monitor for muscle pain during activity.
4. Reduce all causes of discomfort, including those induced by the patient's environment, such as uncomfortable room temperature or position, thirst/dry mouth, and wrinkled or damp bedding.
5. Provide alternating periods of rest and activity.
6. Assist patient in prioritizing activities to accommodate energy levels.

Self-Care Assistance: Instrumental Activities of Daily Living (IADLs)
1. Determine need for assistance with IADLs including walking, bathing, dressing, cooking, shopping, housekeeping, transportation, and money management.
2. Provide for methods of contacting support of assistance people (such as home health nursing, lifeline services, emergency response services, including readily accessible telephone numbers if patient's area is not within 911 access).
3. Determine financial resources and personal preferences for modifying the patient's home to accommodate any disabilities or assisting with medication costs or other home health care costs.

Deficient fluid volume *related to procedure-related blood loss or inadequate hydration*

GOALS/OUTCOMES Within the 12-hour period before discharge from the ICU, patient exhibits a normal fluid balance as evidenced by normal laboratory results of Hgb, Hct, potassium, sodium, creatinine, BUN; good skin turgor; warm, pink skin; normal level of consciousness (or maintenance of preprocedure level of consciousness if baseline is impaired); normal vital signs and weight.
NOC Fluid Balance

Fluid/Electrolyte Management
1. Maintain adequate fluid volume.
2. Assess urine output, condition of skin, wound drainage, and I&O.
3. Monitor potassium, sodium, creatinine, and BUN; notify physician if abnormal.
4. Monitor vital signs, weight, restlessness, skin temperature, and decreased LOC.

Hemorrhage Control
1. Monitor vital signs, Hgb, and Hct; notify physician if abnormal.
2. Assess for excess drainage from dressing or drains (if present).
3. Assess for restlessness, pallor, skin temperature, decreased capillary refill, or decreased tissue perfusion.
4. Check operative site for bruising or excessive swelling.

Ineffective tissue perfusion: peripheral *related to reduced circulation resulting from vascular disease*

GOALS/OUTCOMES Within 12 to 24 hours of treatment, patient has adequate tissue perfusion as evidenced by warm, dry skin; brisk capillary refill; normal color, temperature, and sensory and motor function; RR less than 24 breaths/min; NSR on ECG; BP within 20 mm Hg of patient's normal range; HR less than 120 bpm (or within 20 bpm of resting HR for patients on beta-blocker therapy).
NOC Circulation Status; Tissue Perfusion: Peripheral

Circulatory Care: Arterial Insufficiency
1. Monitor vital signs.
2. Assess skin color, temperature; peripheral pulses as appropriate.
3. Provide warmth; avoid prolonged exposure to cold temperatures.
4. Promote smoking cessation and decreased caffeine intake.
5. Encourage activity as tolerated; passive and active ROM exercises if confined to bed.

Peripheral Sensation Management
1. Assess neurologic functions; decreased sensations.
2. Avoid constrictive clothing around operative site.
3. Minimize external pressure points.

Deficient knowledge: peripheral vascular disease process *related to lifestyle implications*

GOALS/OUTCOMES Within the 24-hour period before discharge from the hospital, patient verbalizes understanding of his or her disease, as well as the necessary lifestyle changes that may modify risk factors.
NOC Knowledge: Diabetes Management; Knowledge: Diet; Knowledge: Disease Process; Knowledge: Energy Conservation; Knowledge: Health Behaviors; Knowledge: Medication

Teaching: Peripheral Vascular Disease Process
1. Teach patient about arterial stenosis or occlusion and its resultant symptoms such as TIAs, claudication, or rest pain.
2. Discuss the pathophysiologic process underlying the patient's arterial stenosis or occlusion, using drawings as indicated.
3. Assist patient in identifying his or her own risk factors (e.g., cigarette smoking, high-fat diet, hyperglycemia, high-stress lifestyle).
4. Teach patient about risk factor modification:
   - *Smoking cessation:* Teach patient that smoking causes arteries to constrict and increases platelet viscosity, thus decreasing blood flow to the brain, muscles, and tissues.
   - *Hyperglycemia control:* Discuss how high blood sugar levels accelerate the course of atherosclerosis; cause structural changes in the collagen of skin, joint capsules, and tendons leading to limitations of flexion and extension that result in increased foot pressures and risk of ulcerations; are associated with developing neuropathy; and accelerate wound sepsis.

Teaching: Diet and Prescribed Medications

1. *Diet low in cholesterol and saturated fat:* Provide sample diet plan for meals that are low in cholesterol and saturated fat. Teach patient about foods that are high in cholesterol and low in cholesterol and saturated fat. Stress the importance of reading food labels. (See Tables 5-18 and Table 5-19 for more information.)
2. *Blood pressure control:* If patient was found to have hypertension, he or she should be taught the importance of taking appropriate medications to control BP and to follow recommended dietary guidelines to minimize sodium intake. (See Table 5-2 for more information.) Sodium promotes water retention, which can increase BP. High BP may accelerate the process of atherosclerosis.
   - Teach patient about the prescribed medications, including name, purpose, dosage, action, schedule, precautions, and potential side effects.

Teaching: Activity/Exercise

Discharge Instruction:

1. Increase activity slowly; do not push, pull, or lift anything over 10 lb for 2 to 6 weeks. Do not drive until you talk with your practitioner.
2. Try to develop a regular exercise and/or walking program. Start off slowly and build up.
3. Plan for regular rest periods; let your body guide you in decreasing or increasing activities.
4. Inform your practitioner of any changes in activity tolerance, such as the development of new symptoms with the same activity.

NIC Teaching: Disease Process; Teaching: Prescribed Diet and Medications; Teaching: Prescribed Activity/Exercise; Risk Identification

---

CARE PLANS FOR CAROTID ARTERIAL OCCLUSIVE DISEASE

Ineffective tissue perfusion: cerebral *related to cerebral vascular disease*

GOALS/OUTCOMES Within 12 to 24 hours of treatment, patient has adequate cerebral perfusion as evidenced by RR less than 24 breaths/min, NSR on ECG, BP within 20 mm Hg of patient's normal range, HR less than 120 bpm (or within 20 bpm of resting HR for patients on beta-blocker therapy), and cranial nerves II to XII intact or equal to baseline.
NOC Circulation Status; Neurological Status; Tissue Perfusion: Cerebral

Cerebral Perfusion Promotion

1. Monitor vital signs per unit standards.
2. Assess for increased BP, decreased HR, and Cheyne-Stokes respiration (may indicate increased intracranial pressure secondary to hemorrhage).
3. Assess for decreased BP, increased HR, and increased respirations (may indicate cerebral ischemia).
4. Monitor for symptomatic bradycardia caused by vagal nerve stimulation.

Neurologic Monitoring

1. Monitor neurologic checks per unit standards.
2. Assess for presence of a gag reflex, difficulty swallowing, tongue deviation to one side, or biting of tongue when eating.
3. Assess for symmetry of lip movements by having the patient smile or show teeth.
4. Assess speech for hoarseness, assess uvula for symmetry.
5. Assess shoulder alignment, strength of sternocleidomastoid muscle by having the patient shrug his or her shoulders and rotate his or her head to one side then the other while you provide resistance to the head and shoulder movements.

Deficient fluid volume *related to surgical blood loss*

GOALS/OUTCOMES Within 12 to 24 hours of treatment, patient has adequate fluid volume with no signs of hematoma or hemorrhage; normal Hgb and Hct.
NOC Fluid Balance; Electrolyte and Acid-Base Balance

Hemorrhage Control

1. Monitor vital signs, Hgb, and Hct.
2. Monitor dressing and drain (if present) for excessive drainage/output.

3. Assess operative site for bruising or excessive swelling.
4. Monitor airway for any respiratory compromise or tracheal deviation related to cervical hematoma.

CARE PLANS FOR PERIPHERAL ARTERIAL OCCLUSIVE DISEASE

Ineffective tissue perfusion: peripheral *related to decreased circulation resulting from atherosclerotic lower limb vascular disease*

- -

GOALS/OUTCOMES Within 12 to 24 hours of treatment, patient has adequate peripheral perfusion as evidenced by warm, dry skin; normal or improved pedal pulses; normal color and temperature of skin; normal or improved sensory and motor function; and brisk capillary refill.

NOC Sensory Function: Cutaneous; Tissue Integrity: Skin and Mucous Membranes; Tissue Perfusion: Peripheral

Circulatory Care: Arterial Insufficiency
1. Palpate and/or auscultate per Doppler peripheral pulses distal to treatment site (also pulses distal to catheter insertion site for endovascular procedures). Report any decrease in pulse quality or strength immediately.
2. Monitor capillary refill and temperature and color of skin.
3. Position extremity to optimize circulation.
4. Encourage passive and active ROM exercises.
5. Provide warmth and avoid prolonged exposure to the cold.
6. Instruct patient to avoid crossing legs.

Neurologic Monitoring
1. Assess for decreased sensation of extremities and skin (skin immediately surrounding incisions may be numb if a skin nerve is cut during the incision).
2. Ask the patient to wiggle his or her toes and flex and extend foot and knee to assess motor function.

Skin Surveillance
1. Assess skin integrity of both extremities and pressure points, minimize external pressure points.
2. Change patient's position as appropriate.
3. Promote proper foot care for operative leg and opposite foot as opposite foot will be bearing more weight during the convalescence period.
4. Provide pressure-relieving mattress as appropriate.

Impaired skin integrity *related to inadequate perfusion to maintain tissue integrity*

- -

GOALS/OUTCOMES Within 12 to 24 hours of treatment, patient will maintain intact skin surfaces with healing wounds as evidenced by normal skin temperature, color, and sensation (or baseline); if open wound, minimal drainage present without odor; if open wound, granulation tissue will be present; normal vital signs and white blood count.

NOC Tissue Integrity: Skin and Mucous Membranes; Wound Healing: Primary Intention; Wound Healing: Secondary Intention

Pressure Management
1. Assess skin integrity of both extremities and pressure points; minimize external pressure points.
2. Change patient's position as appropriate.
3. Provide pressure-relieving mattress as appropriate.

Wound Care
1. Assess for decreased perfusion of the wound by assessing pain, swelling, erythema, and drainage.
2. Avoid further skin injury by not using tape directly on the skin.
3. Monitor for wound infection by assessing patient's temperature, WBC count, and exposure of bypass graft (if present).
4. Use aseptic technique for all dressing changes and incisional care.
5. Monitor incisions for drainage, erythema, tenderness, or separation of suture/staple sites.
6. Monitor nutritional status: assess weight, albumin, and prealbumin.

CARE PLANS FOR PATIENTS UNDERGOING ENDOVASCULAR REPAIR OF STENOSIS OR OCCLUSION

🔻**Ineffective tissue perfusion: peripheral** *related to presence of a device within the vessel*

GOALS/OUTCOMES See Goals/Outcomes and plan under *Care Plans for Peripheral Vascular Disease*, (p. 561).

Deficient knowledge *related to endovascular procedure and postprocedure care*

GOALS/OUTCOMES Within the 24-hour period before the procedure, patient describes the rationale for the procedure, how it is performed, and postprocedure care. Patient relates discharge instructions within the 24-hour period before discharge from the ICU.

NOC Knowledge: Treatment Procedures; Knowledge: Disease Process; Knowledge: Medication; Knowledge: Prescribed Activity

Teaching: Carotid/Peripheral Arterial Disease Process
1. Discuss location of the patient's disease using drawings as possible.
2. Assess patient's understanding of carotid/PAD and the purpose of the endovascular procedure. Evaluate patient's style of coping and degree of information desired.

Teaching: Procedure/Treatment
As appropriate for coping style, discuss the following with patient and significant others:
1. Use of local anesthesia and sedation during procedure
2. Insertion site of catheter: groin or arm
3. Sensations that may occur: mild pressure; a feeling of heat as the dye is injected
4. Use of fluoroscopy during procedure. Determine patient's history of sensitivity to contrast material, use of medications that may cause complications such as metformin.
5. Ongoing observations made by nurse after procedure: BP, HR, leg or arm pulses, blood tests, observation of insertion site, neuro checks as indicated, ABIs as indicated
6. Importance of lying flat in bed for 6 to 12 hours after procedure unless a vascular closure device is used. Patients are able to get out of bed sooner when a closure device is used.
7. Necessity for nursing assistance with eating, drinking, and toileting needs after procedure while lying flat
8. Need for increased fluid intake after procedure to flush dye from system
9. If patient and significant others express or exhibit evidence of anxiety regarding the procedure, try to arrange for them to meet with another patient who has had a successful angioplasty.

Teaching: Prescribed Medications/Activity
Discharge Instructions:
1. Importance of taking antiplatelet medications to prevent restenosis
2. Avoidance of strenuous activity during the first few weeks at home
3. Follow-up visit with vascular surgeon/internist 1 week after hospital discharge
4. Signs and symptoms to report to physician
   - Any pain or bruising at catheter insertion site
   - Fever or drainage from insertion site
   - Muscular pain or coolness in the extremity used for the catheter insertion, not experienced prior to procedure
   - Any return of symptoms present before procedure

NIC Teaching: Disease Process; Teaching: Prescribed Activity/Exercise; Anxiety Reduction; Infection Protection; Decision-Making Support

ADDITIONAL NURSING DIAGNOSES

Also see nursing diagnoses and interventions as appropriate in *Nutritional Support* (p. 117), *Hemodynamic Monitoring* (p. 75), *Wound and Skin Care* (p. 167), *Pain* (p. 135), *Prolonged Immobility* (p. 149), *Emotional and Spiritual Support of the Patient and Significant Others* (p. 200), *Compartment Syndrome/Ischemic myositis*, (p. 301), *Stroke: Acute Ischemic and Hemorrhagic* (p. 674), and *Bleeding and Thrombotic Disorders* (p. 837).

VALVULAR HEART DISEASE

PATHOPHYSIOLOGY

The four heart valves help to promote "forward flow" of blood through the heart by providing the "gateway" or "doorway" into the next chamber, which opens and then closes after the chamber fills, preventing backflow of blood. Opening and closing of heart valves result from pressure changes within the four cardiac chambers. The two AV valves separate the atria and ventricles, while the two semilunar valves separate the ventricles from the great vessels.

Atrioventricular Valves

AV valves are connected by chordae tendinae to papillary muscles, enabling the valve cusp to point in the direction of blood flow. Papillary muscle contraction holds the AV valves in place, preventing them from being forced into the atria by the increased ventricular pressure during contraction.

- *Mitral:* Has two leaflets/cusps and is located between the left atrium and the left ventricle
- *Tricuspid:* Has three leaflets/cusps and is located between the right atrium and right ventricle

Semilunar Valves

Semilunar describes the half-moon shape of the valves. A stenotic aortic or pulmonic valve results in increased intramyocardial wall tension. The persistent increase in wall tension leads to ventricular hypertrophy as more muscle is needed for the increased work, resulting in ventricular remodeling. The heart remodels to compensate for the work of pumping blood through the highly resistant valve opening.

- *Pulmonic:* The pulmonic valve has three leaflets/cusps and is located between the right ventricle and the pulmonary artery.
- *Aortic:* The aortic valve has three leaflets/cusps and is located between the left ventricle and the aorta.

  Valvular heart disease manifests as either stenosis (difficult to open, resulting in a narrowed diameter for the time the valve is open) or incompetency/insufficiency (failure to close entirely, resulting in some blood flowing backward during systole), which includes prolapse. A heart murmur is most often the initial indication of valve disease. Stenosis is caused by sclerosing, thickening, and calcification of the valve leaflets.

  A stenotic valve obstructs blood flow from the affected atrium or ventricle, which leads to hypertrophy of the chamber. Increased muscle mass is required to pump blood through the narrowed valve. The heart muscle increases in size, leaving less filling space for the blood, which results in insufficient CO. All the blood is ejected during systole, but the amount is often insufficient to meet the body's demand for oxygen and nutrients.

  An incompetent or regurgitant valve may be caused by rheumatic heart disease, dilation of the valve ring, or damage to the nearby valve structures. Regurgitation results in increased volume into the chamber preceding the valve, because during systole, all blood fails to move forward because the "back door" to the chamber remains slightly open. Mitral and tricuspid regurgitation can occur with the remodeling and enlargement of the ventricles.

  Depending on the location of the dysfunctional valve(s), blood "backs up" into the atrium, leading to either pulmonary congestion from LV failure or peripheral edema from RV failure. Ventricular hypertrophy and high intramyocardial wall tension diminish blood flow to the endocardium.

Mitral Valve Disease

- *Mitral stenosis (MS):* Rheumatic heart disease is the most common etiology. The restrictive opening of the mitral valve leaflets is caused by diastolic doming of the anterior leaflet (hockey-stick) deformity and an immobile posterior leaflet giving the valve a fish-mouth appearance. Stenosis occurs many years after acute rheumatic carditis, which leads to the development of many inflammatory foci (Aschoff bodies, perivascular mononuclear infiltrate) in the endocardium and myocardium. Small vegetations on the valve border may be present. Over time, the valve becomes thickened and calcified, commissural adhesions form, and the valve stenoses.
- *Mitral insufficiency/regurgitation (MR):* Can be caused by injury or disruption to any part of the valve including the mitral annulus, the leaflets (a large anterior [aortic] leaflet and

a small posterior [mural] leaflet), the chordae tendinae, and the papillary muscles. The most common etiologies of MR include mitral valve (MVP), rheumatic heart disease, infective endocarditis, annular calcification, cardiomyopathy, and ischemic heart disease. Pure MR is most commonly caused (71%) by a myxomatous (floppy, prolapse) process. Rheumatic heart disease (postinflammatory disease) accounts for 9% of cases. Heart failure may occur acutely following rupture of an infarcted papillary muscle or chronically from papillary muscle fibrosis, hypertrophy, or LV dilatation.

Tricuspid Valve Disease

- *Tricuspid stenosis (TS):* Usually associated with mitral stenosis resulting from rheumatic heart disease. In the absence of mitral stenosis, the possibility of right atrial myxoma (tumor) should be eliminated.
- *Tricuspid regurgitation (TR)/insufficiency (TI):* Two types of patients are noted: those with normal leaflets and those with abnormal leaflets. Functional TR results from annular dilatation secondary to pulmonary hypertension associated with other valvular disorders. Acquired TR is less common, originating from an abnormality of the leaflets due to a variety of disease processes. Medications used to treat migraine (e.g., methysergide), Parkinson disease (e.g., pergolide), and obesity (e.g., fenfluramine) have been associated with TR.

Aortic Valve Disease

- *Aortic stenosis (AS):* A bicuspid (versus tricuspid) aortic valve is congenital, predominantly in males, occurring in 1% to 2% of the population. Most develop stenosis. Acquired nonrheumatic AS results from calcification of the aortic valve and is associated with aging. The increase in LV afterload, progressive LV hypertrophy, and a decrease in systemic and coronary flow as consequences of valve obstruction result in the symptoms including angina, syncope, and congestive HF in patients with aortic stenosis.
- *Aortic insufficiency (AI)/regurgitation (AR):* Acute AR results from a rapid increase in end-diastolic volume caused by regurgitant blood flow from endocarditis or aortic dissection. The left ventricle fills from both the left atrium and retrograde flow from the aorta through the leaky aortic valve. In acute AR, the left ventricle does not have time to dilate in response to the volume load, resulting in chest pain and acute respiratory distress secondary to pulmonary edema. In severe cases, HF may develop and potentially deteriorate to cardiogenic shock. Early surgical intervention should be considered, especially if AR resulted from aortic dissection, wherein surgery should be done immediately. Chronic AI occurs related to gradual dilatation of the left ventricle, with compensatory mechanisms which mask the symptoms.

Pulmonic Valve Disease

- *Pulmonic stenosis (PS):* Obstruction of the RV outflow tract may be acquired or congenital. The diseased valve is most often functionally benign but more susceptible to infective endocarditis.
- *Pulmonic insufficiency (PI)/regurgitation (PR):* Usually associated with pulmonary hypertension. In the absence of pulmonary hypertension, low-pressure PR is congenital. Rarely, the valve is damaged by a pulmonary artery catheter.

ASSESSMENT: VALVULAR HEART DISEASE
Goal of System Assessment

Evaluate for LV and RV failure, decreased CO, and decreased tissue perfusion. Many persons with longstanding valvular disease leading to atrial enlargement develop atrial fibrillation and should be monitored for both the dysrhythmia and HF. Cardiac cachexia may be seen in persons with longstanding valvular dysfunction.

History and Risk Factors

- Rheumatic heart disease (postinflammatory), a congenital disorder, connective tissue disease including Marfan syndrome and systemic lupus erythematosus, rheumatoid arthritis, chronic inflammatory disease (including ankylosing spondylitis and giant cell arteritis), AMI leading to rupture of the papillary muscle, IV drug use, advanced age, mitral valve prolapse (MVP), infective endocarditis, annular calcification, cancer, syphilis, pulmonary hypertension, cardiomyopathy, and ischemic heart disease cause valvular disease. Atrial fibrillation may result from left atrial enlargement, prompting an increased risk for systemic thromboembolism. Use of the diet drug combinations of fenfluramine, dexfenfluramine, and phentermine can cause severe valvular disease.

Mitral Valve Disease

Assessment Findings	Mitral Stenosis	Mitral Insufficiency
Observation	Dyspnea, pulmonary congestion, edema, hemoptysis, slight cyanosis	Dyspnea, pulmonary congestion, edema, symptoms related to left-sided heart failure
Auscultation	Increased amplitude of the first heart sound; opening snap and mid-diastolic murmur at the mitral area	Holosystolic murmur loudest in the mitral area and transmitted to the axilla or left sternal edge
Chest radiograph	Atrial enlargement	Left and right ventricular enlargement
12-Lead ECG	Left atrial abnormality; P "mitral"; right ventricular hypertrophy; S in leads 1 and V_5, R in V_1	Left ventricular hypertrophy; large S in V_1, large R in V_4, and minor atrial abnormality; atrial and ventricular arrhythmias
Hemodynamics	Elevated pulmonary artery occlusive pressure (PAOP), elevated pulmonary artery pressure (PAP), elevated venous pressure, decreased cardiac output (CO), elevated left atrial pressure (LAP). Patients will not experience valve-related symptoms until the valve area is <2–2.5 cm^2, when moderate exercise may cause exertional dyspnea. Severe mitral stenosis (valve area <1 cm^2) results in an increased resting diastolic mitral valve gradient, and increased LAP. Pulmonary hypertension may develop. As PAP increases, the right ventricle (RV) dilates and tricuspid regurgitation may develop, resulting in increased jugular venous pressure, liver congestion, ascites, and pedal edema. LV end-diastolic pressure (LVEDP) and CO are often normal when only the mitral valve is stenosed. With progressive stenosis, the CO becomes subnormal at rest and fails to increase during exercise.	V waves in the pulmonary artery, increased systolic PAP, decreased cardiac output. Acute mitral regurgitation (MR) causes increased preload and decreased afterload with an increase in end-diastolic volume (EDV) and decrease in end-systolic volume (ESV). The total stroke volume (TSV) is markedly increased, but forward stroke volume (FSV) is decreased because much of the TSV regurgitates, resulting in increased LAP. In chronic compensated MR, the left atrium and ventricle dilate to accommodate the regurgitant volume, so LAP may be normal or minimally elevated. In the chronic decompensated phase, muscle dysfunction decreases both TSV and FSV, but EF may be normal. ESV and EDV increase, then LAP and LVEDP increase, pulmonary edema may occur, and if unmanaged, cardiogenic shock ensues.

Pulmonic Valve Disease

Assessment Findings	Pulmonic Stenosis	Pulmonic Insufficiency
Observation	Abnormal venous pulsations and elevated jugular pressure; hepatic tenderness and enlargement from venous congestion due to right ventricular (RV) failure. Very uncommon as acquired heart disease in adults; generally a congenital anomaly.	
Auscultation	Systolic blowing murmur at the second intercostal space, left sternal border which radiates to the neck.	Diastolic murmur at the second intercostal space at left sternal border, which starts later at lower pitch than aortic murmur. The Graham Steell murmur of pulmonary hypertension is a high-pitched, early diastolic decrescendo murmur heard over the left upper-to-left midsternal area.

Assessment Findings	Pulmonic Stenosis	Pulmonic Insufficiency
Chest radiograph	Atrial enlargement	Left and right ventricular enlargement
12-lead ECG	R voltage increased in V_1; or increased S voltage in V_2	
Hemodynamics	Increased RV systolic pressure, mean RAP, PAWP, and mean PAP	Increased RV systolic pressure with wide pulse pressure; LVEDP and CO often normal but may decrease if severe

Tricuspid Valve Disease

Assessment Findings	Tricuspid Stenosis	Tricuspid Insufficiency
Observation	Abnormal venous pulsations and elevated jugular pressure; hepatic tenderness and enlargement from venous congestion due to right heart failure	
Auscultation	Diastolic murmur at the 4th intercostal space, increases with inspiration	Pansystolic murmur at the 4th intercostal space; S_3 gallop is present.
Chest radiograph	Right atrial enlargement	
12-lead ECG	R voltage increased in V_1 or V_2; S voltage increased in V_5 or V_6; sum of R in V_1 or V_2 and S in V_5 or V_6 will be greater than 35 mm.	
Hemodynamics	Increased CVP, accentuated A wave on the right atrial waveform	Increased CVP and prominent V wave on the right atrial waveform

Aortic Valve Disease

Assessment Findings	Aortic Stenosis	Aortic Insufficiency
Observation	Faint slow radial pulse, low blood pressure and pulse pressure, dizziness, fainting, syncope, pallor, chest pain due to coronary insufficiency, irregularly irregular heart sounds, and left heart failure	Dyspnea, pulmonary congestion, edema, symptoms related to left-sided heart failure. Aortic regurgitation is indicated by three findings: *Corrigan's pulse* is a palpated pulse with rapid and forceful distention of the artery followed by quick collapse. *DeMusset's sign* is forward and backward bobbing of the head. *Quincke's sign* is visible pulsation seen with slight compression of nailbeds. *Hill sign* is popliteal cuff systolic blood pressure 40 mm Hg higher than brachial cuff systolic blood pressure.
Auscultation	Increased amplitude of the first heart sound; opening snap and mid-diastolic murmur at the mitral area	Diastolic blowing murmur heard loudest at the second right intercostal space beginning with S_2. *Duroziez sign* is a systolic murmur over the femoral artery with proximal compression of the artery, and a diastolic murmur with distal compression of the artery.
Chest radiograph	Left ventricular enlargement and dilation of the ascending aorta	Left ventricular enlargement
12-lead ECG	Left ventricular hypertrophy; large S in V_2, large R in V_5; strain results in inverted T and depressed ST segments in 1 and 2 and V_4, V_5, and V_6.	Left ventricular hypertrophy; large S in V_2, large R in V_5; strain results in inverted T and depressed ST segments in 1 and 2 and V_4, V_5, and V_6.

Valvular Heart Disease

Continued

Assessment Findings	Aortic Stenosis	Aortic Insufficiency
Hemodynamics	Increased left ventricular pressure, increased pulmonary artery end diastolic pressure and wedge pressure; increased gradient across the aortic valve on pullback from left ventricular end diastolic pressure to aortic pressure; narrow pulse pressure, decreased cardiac output. LV systolic function is preserved and cardiac output is maintained for many years despite an elevated LV systolic pressure. Despite the cardiac output at rest being normal, it fails to increase appropriately during exercise, causing exercise-induced syncope or near syncope. With severe aortic stenosis, atrial contraction is vital to diastolic filling of the LV so atrial fibrillation can be catastrophic to maintaining stroke volume.	Increased left ventricular pressure, increased PAD and PAOP, decreased cardiac output; increased systolic BP and widened pulse pressure. Peripheral pulses are prominent or bounding. Symptoms may result from the elevated stroke volume during systole and the incompetent aortic valve allowing significantly decreased aortic diastolic pressure (often <60 mm Hg), with pulse pressures often >100 mm Hg. During early chronic AR, the LV ejection fraction (EF) is normal or increased. As AR progresses, LV enlargement exceeds preload reserve and the EF decreases to normal and then subnormal levels. The LV end-systolic volume increases and reflects progressive myocardial dysfunction. The LV gradually transforms from an elliptical to a spherical configuration.

Diagnostic Tests for Evaluation of Valvular Disease

Diagnostic testing for the patient with a heart murmur varies considerably depending on when the murmur occurs in the cardiac cycle, the location and possible radiation, and response to selected physiologic maneuvers used during evaluation. The presence/absence of cardiac and noncardiac symptoms, along with other findings on physical examination, will help determine if the murmur is clinically significant. Treatment is based on echocardiographic measurements of left ventricular (LV) size and systolic function. When determining recommendations, the accuracy and reproducibility of results are critical. Surgical recommendations for asymptomatic patients with mitral regurgitation (MR) or aortic regurgitation (AR) are often dependent on the reliability and validity of the measurements.

Test	Purpose	Abnormal Findings
• *Echocardiography* Doppler flow studies • Color flow mapping • Transesophageal echocardiography (TEE) • Dobutamine stress echocardiography	Recommended for evaluation of all patients found with cardiac murmurs. Provides information on valve morphology and function, chamber size, wall thickness, ventricular function, and pulmonary and hepatic vein flow, and estimates of pulmonary artery pressures can be readily assessed.	Abnormal blood flow patterns, resulting in reduced forward flow of blood. *Stenosis*: Blood flow is somewhat occluded. *Incompetency*: Blood flows backward through the valve into the heart chamber preceding the valve. Echocardiography may not be necessary for the evaluation of asymptomatic younger patients with lower grade murmurs. Minimal or physiologic mitral, tricuspid, or pulmonic valve regurgitations may be detected by color flow imaging in many patients who have no heart murmur. Sensitive Doppler ultrasound devices may find trace or mild regurgitation through structurally normal tricuspid and pulmonic valves, as well as through normal left-sided heart valves (especially mitral) in young, healthy patients.
• Doppler flow studies	Continuous-wave or pulsed-wave frequencies used to determine blood flow	
• Color flow mapping studies	Uses colors (red and blue) to enhance the image of blood flowing through the heart	
• Transesophageal echocardiography (TEE)	Uses an endoscope to produce an image unimpeded by the chest wall. The esophagus is close to the heart, so images are clearer or less distorted.	

Diagnostic Tests for Evaluation of Valvular Disease — cont'd

Dobutamine stress echocardiography	Uses a dobutamine infusion to increase heart rate and force of contraction during an echocardiogram to assess for changes in blood flow under more stressful conditions	Flow gradients across disease valves may deteriorate under more stressful conditions. Assists in determining whether valve stenosis is moderate or severe in patients with aortic stenosis.
Chest radiograph	To evaluate the size of the heart to assist with assessment of degree of ventricular remodeling, indicative of possible heart failure	Cardiac enlargement, reflective of ventricular remodeling
Cardiac catheterization	Unnecessary in most patients with cardiac murmurs with normal or diagnostic echocardiograms. Provides information for patients with a discrepancy between the echocardiographic and clinical findings. Gradients across valves can indicate severity of stenosis. Ventriculogram may assist in visualization of blood flow.	Describes presence and severity of valvular obstruction or regurgitation, and intracardiac shunting. Abnormal or giant V wave on the pulmonary artery occlusive pressure (PAOP) waveform (right-sided heart catheterization) is seen with mitral regurgitation. Visualizing the coronary arteries also provides information about concomitant CAD, which may require revascularization at the time of surgical valve repair or replacement.
Cardiac magnetic resonance imaging (MRI)	Used to provide an enhanced evaluation of patients for whom transthoracic Doppler flow studies are inadequate to describe valvular lesions	Abnormal blood flow patterns, valvular stenosis or incompetency
Exercise testing	Provides information for patients whose symptoms are difficult to assess	Ischemic ECG changes associated with exercise
B-type natriuretic peptide (BNP)	Helps to diagnose if valvular disease has reduced cardiac output resulting in heart failure	Elevation may be an early marker of heart failure resulting from the valvular stenosis or regurgitation.

COLLABORATIVE MANAGEMENT
Care Priorities
1. **Consider antibiotic prophylaxis for infective endocarditis and rheumatic fever.** Prophylaxis, which was once mandatory for all patients, is now controversial. Providing prophylactic antibiotics has not been shown to prevent the development of endocarditis valve disease in all patient populations. Varying levels of evidence support the following recommendations from the ACC and AHA:
   - Infective endocarditis prophylaxis for dental procedures is recommended only for patients with heart disease at the highest risk of adverse outcomes from infective endocarditis.
   - Antibiotic prophylaxis should be provided for patients with aortic and mitral stenosis and for those with rheumatic aortic and mitral stenosis for prevention of recurrent rheumatic fever.
   - High-risk patients should receive prophylaxis for dental procedures involving manipulation of the gums or perforation of oral mucosa.
   - Prophylaxis should not be provided solely based on an increased lifetime risk of infective endocarditis. Symptom evaluation is part of the decision to use prophylaxis.
   - Antibiotics are not recommended to prevent endocarditis in patients undergoing GU or GI tract procedures. (See Acute Infective Endocarditis, p. 453.)
2. **Manage aortic stenosis.**
   - *Monitoring:* Frequently for progression of the disease, including asymptomatic patients; stenosis requires initial and serial visits for grading severity and evaluation of symptom.
   - *Hypertension:* Use of antihypertensive agents is done cautiously.
   - *Decision about surgery:* Need is based largely on the patient's symptoms, rather than exclusively on the transvalvular pressure gradient. Angina, syncope, and HF can

develop suddenly, sometimes following a lengthy asymptomatic period. Following onset of symptoms, survival averages 2 to 3 years.

- *Aortic valve replacement (AVR):* Recommended for all symptomatic patients with severe aortic stenosis, and should be considered for patients undergoing myocardial revascularization, surgery on the aorta or other heart valves, and those with an ejection fraction of less than 50% (impending HF).
- *Aortic balloon valvotomy:* May be used as an alternative to valve replacement for patients too unstable to tolerate AVR.

3. **Manage aortic insufficiency/regurgitation.**
- *Crisis:* Can occur acutely resulting in pulmonary edema and/or cardiogenic shock. Death from cardiogenic shock, ventricular dysrhythmias, and PEA is common with acute, severe AR.
- *Urgent surgery:* Inodilators such as milrinone and inamrinone are used to help increase CO. Dopamine and dobutamine may be used to increase contractility and, along with vasodilators such as nitroprusside, reduce LV afterload for preoperative stabilization. Immediate surgery is recommended for symptomatic patients with acute AR resulting from infective endocarditis.
- *Balloon counterpulsation:* NOT recommended for acute AR; may be harmful.
- *Compensatory tachycardia:* Vital for survival in acute AR; beta-blockers must be used with caution; especially when treating aortic dissection.
- *Medications:* Vasodilators are used for those with chronic severe AR who are not surgical candidates. Diuretics, nitrates, and digoxin are sometimes used to help control symptoms, but there are insufficient data to justify recommending or discouraging these therapies.
- *Chronic AR:* Management is based on LV systolic function. If LV systolic dysfunction occurs (a reduced ejection fraction at rest) and cannot be controlled with antihypertensive therapy, patients may require AVR. Initially, the process of ventricular remodeling is reversible with management of afterload (BP/SVR) using vasodilators.

4. **Manage mitral stenosis.**
- *Monitoring:* A progressive, lifelong disease generally resulting from rheumatic fever, often initially stable for years, followed by rapid development of HF later in life. Once symptoms begin, symptoms are often insignificant for up to 10 years. When severe pulmonary hypertension develops, average survival is 3 years.
- *Atrial fibrillation:* Up to 40% of patients develop atrial fibrillation, which should be managed with anticoagulation initially with heparin (bridged to Coumadin) to avoid intramyocardial clot formation with subsequent embolization and rate control for tachycardia using digoxin, calcium channel–blocking agents or beta adrenergic–blocking agents, or amiodarone. Cardioversion may be used to manage atrial fibrillation according to ACLS guidelines.
- *Percutaneous balloon mitral valvotomy (PBMV):* Recommended for symptomatic patients without severe pulmonary hypertension. Moderate to severely symptomatic patients with PA systolic pressure of greater than 60 mm Hg may require a mitral commissurotomy or mitral valve replacement (MVR).

5. **Manage mitral regurgitation.**
- *Crisis:* May occur acutely resulting in severe symptoms. Medical therapy is useful only to stabilize acute MR patients in preparation for surgery. Vasodilators (e.g., nitroprusside) should be used in combination with inotropic agents (e.g., dobutamine or dopamine) to avoid severe hypotension.
- *Balloon counterpulsation therapy:* Provides stabilization by helping to increase forward blood flow, resulting in increased MAP and reducing the volume of regurgitation and LV preload (LV end-diastolic pressure).
- *MVR:* May be necessary for stabilization of severely symptomatic patients.
- *Mitral valve repair:* Recommended for patients with a lesser degree of LV dysfunction.
- *Chronic MR:* Patients may remain in a stable, compensated state for many years. Incidence of sudden death in asymptomatic patients varies widely among documented studies. There is no universally recommended medical therapy.
- *LV systolic dysfunction:* Patients may benefit from ACEIs or beta adrenergic–blocking agents (e.g., carvedilol) and biventricular cardiac pacing to reduce regurgitant volume.

- *Acute atrial fibrillation (AF):* Managed with calcium channel blockers, beta-blockers, digoxin, and sometimes amiodarone to promote control of tachycardia.
- *Chronic AF:* May require a Maze procedure; may be added to mitral valve repair to help prevent stroke. All patients with chronic AF require long-term anticoagulation with warfarin (Coumadin).

6. **Manage tricuspid valve disease.**
   - *Surgery:* Tricuspid valve repair, valve replacement, or annuloplasty for TR often occurs during mitral valve surgery.
   - *Severe TR:* Patients have poor long-term outcomes due to RV dysfunction with or without systemic venous congestion.

7. **Manage pulmonic valve disease.**
   - *Pulmonic valve stenosis:* Pulmonic stenosis is likely congenital and not likely due to acquired heart disease and is managed with percutaneous balloon valvotomy. Most patients undergoing valvotomy for stenosis also have MR.
   - *Pulmonic regurgitation:* Generally not seen unless other valve disease is present and is also likely to be a congenital defect, and is likely to be managed with pulmonic valve replacement if HF is present.

8. **Provide lifelong anticoagulation for patients with prosthetic heart valves.**
   - *Warfarin:* Maintain the international normalized ratio (INR) as follows:
     - *Aortic valve:* INR 2.0 to 3.0 unless at higher risk for thromboembolism, wherein 2.5 to 3.5 may be more appropriate.
     - *Mitral valve:* INR 2.5 to 3.5
   - *Low-dose aspirin:* 80 to 160 mg may be added to warfarin therapy for those at higher risk for thromboembolization.

9. **Provide short-term anticoagulation for patients with biological heart valves.**
   - May require anticoagulation using warfarin for the first 3 months following surgery, unless at higher risk of thromboembolism (e.g., atrial fibrillation, previous thromboembolism, or a hypercoagulable state), wherein anticoagulation may be continued on a lifelong basis.
   - At least two-thirds of patients do not require lifelong anticoagulation.

10. **Reverse excessive anticoagulation.**
    - *INR greater than 5:* Increases the possibility of bleeding and/or hemorrhage
    - *Prosthetic heart valve:* If the patient with an INR 5 to 10 is not bleeding, withholding warfarin and giving vitamin K (phytonadione) 1 to 2.5 mg orally is appropriate. In an emergency, fresh-frozen plasma is recommended over higher-dose parenteral (IV) vitamin K_1, which often results in a hypercoagulable state. Low-dose IV vitamin K (1 mg) has been found to be safer, if needed. Aspirin should also be discontinued.

11. **Manage thrombosis of prosthetic valves.**
    - *Emergency surgery:* May be necessary for patients with left-sided heart valves with NYHA Class III to IV HF and a large clot burden.
    - *Fibrinolytic therapy:* May be appropriate for patients with right-sided valves with Class II to IV HF and large clot burden, or those with left-sided valves with NYHA Class I to II HF and smaller clot burden.

Surgical Interventions

- **Valve replacement:** Procedure with a mortality rate of about 6%, performed in patients with moderate to severe calcification, stenosis with insufficiency, and pure insufficiency. Three types of replacement valves are available: homografts and heterografts, which are tissue grafts, and artificial valves. Homografts are specially treated human cadaver valves. They are seldom used because of a lack of availability. A heterograft is a specially prepared valve from an animal, usually a pig or a cow. These commonly used valves are readily available.

  Artificial or mechanical valves are made from stainless steel, carbon, plastic, and other durable materials. Natural tissue grafts are advantageous because there is less of a tendency for clots to form and adhere to them. Patients do not require anticoagulant therapy, but these valves function for only 5 to 8 years. Clots tend to form on artificial valves, so these patients receive lifelong anticoagulant therapy for valves that function for 10 to 15 years. Postoperative care of the patient who has had valve surgery is similar to that of the patient who has undergone myocardial revascularization for CAD (see *Acute Coronary Syndromes*, p. 434). Patients undergoing valve surgery are at increased risk for thrombosis and embolism (particularly with mechanical mitral valves and in patients with atrial fibrillation) and for valvular endocarditis.

- **Commissurotomy:** A procedure in which the stenotic valve is opened by a dilating instrument. When performed early in the course of the disease, chances of success are good, although the procedure may result in valve regurgitation and recurrent stenosis.
- **Reshaping:** A portion of the diseased valve is removed and the valve is sewn back together to promote more effective closure.
- **Decalcification:** Calcium deposits are removed to allow the smooth surface of the valve to close more effectively.
- **Patching:** Covering damaged portions or "holes" in valves with tissue to promote more effective closure.
- **Surgical valvuloplasty:** Valvular repair may be possible in select patients. In addition, insertion of a valvular ring can improve native valve function.
- **Percutaneous balloon valvuloplasty:** For dilation of stenotic heart valves. Candidates for this procedure may (1) be at high risk for surgery, (2) refuse surgery, (3) be older adults (often greater than 80 years), or (4) be informed of treatment choices and choose this procedure over others. The procedure parallels the technique for percutaneous coronary intervention (see *Acute Coronary Syndromes*, p. 434). The femoral artery and vein are cannulated, and the patient receives anticoagulation therapy. For aortic valve dilation, a catheter is passed into the femoral artery to measure supravalvular and LV pressures before valvuloplasty. A balloon valvuloplasty catheter is then passed over a guidewire into the left ventricle. It is inflated three times for 12 to 30 seconds at a pressure of 12 atm. Additional anticoagulant is administered, and the valve gradient is remeasured. To reach the mitral valve, the balloon valvuloplasty catheter is passed via the femoral vein through the atrial septum to the mitral valve opening. The inflation procedure is the same.

With both aortic and mitral dilation, initial clinical improvement has been demonstrated in the valve gradient and in blood flow across the valve. However, benefits may not be long lasting. Complications include thromboembolization to the brain, disruption of the valve ring, acute valve regurgitation, valvular restenosis, hemorrhage at the catheter insertion site, guidewire perforation of the left ventricle, and dysrhythmias.

CARE PLANS FOR VALVULAR HEART DISEASE
For patients undergoing valve replacement:
Ineffective protection *related to risk of bleeding/hemorrhage secondary to anticoagulation*

Safety Alert *Patients undergoing aortic valve replacement are at a higher risk for postoperative hemorrhage than are those undergoing CABG.*

GOALS/OUTCOMES Throughout hospitalization, patient is free of symptoms of bleeding or hemorrhage as evidenced by RAP 4–6 mm Hg, PAWP 6–12 mm Hg, BP within patient's normal range, CO 4–7 L/min, CI 2.5–4 L/min/m², urine output 0.5 ml/kg/hr or greater, urine specific gravity 1.010 to 1.030, and chest tube drainage 100 ml/hr or less.
NOC Circulation Status

Circulatory Precautions
1. Measure chest tube drainage hourly. Report chest tube drainage greater than 100 ml/hr. Maintain patency of chest tubes at all times.
2. Monitor clotting studies. Be alert to and report prolonged PT, PTT, and ACT and decreased platelet count. Optimal values are as follows: PT 11 to 15 seconds, PTT 30 to 40 seconds (activated), and ACT 120 seconds or less. For patient with prolonged PT, PTT, or ACT, administer IV protamine sulfate as prescribed if heparin was the anticoagulant used. After discharge from the hospital, the INR should be maintained at 2.5.
3. Assess vital signs hourly, and monitor patient for physical indicators of hemorrhage or hypovolemia: RAP less than 4 mm Hg, PAWP less than 6 mm Hg, decreased BP, decreased measured CO/CI, urine output less than 0.5 ml/kg/hr, increased urine specific gravity, and excessive chest tube drainage (more than 100 ml/hr). Be alert to a decreased Hct. Optimal values are Hct greater than 37% (female) and greater than 40% (male).

4. Assess postoperative chest radiograph for a widened mediastinum, which may indicate hemorrhage and possible cardiac tamponade.
5. As prescribed, administer platelets, fresh-frozen plasma, or cryoprecipitate to replace clotting factors and blood volume.
6. Administer packed RBCs as prescribed to replace blood volume, or use chest tube drainage for autotransfusion.
7. To correct hyperfibrinolytic state (increased fibrin degradation products), aminocaproic acid is sometimes given slowly per IV bolus as prescribed (Box 5-7).

NIC Bleeding Reduction; Autotransfusion; Hemorrhage Control

 Decreased cardiac output (or risk for same) *related to negative inotropic changes secondary to intraoperative subendocardial ischemia and administration of myocardial depressant drugs*

Safety Alert *After cardiac surgery, some myocardial depression is always present, usually lasting 48 to 72 hours. Patients with longstanding aortic stenosis or ventricular failure caused by mitral valve disease are at an even greater risk for postoperative low CO.*

GOALS/OUTCOMES Within 48 to 72 hours, patient has adequate CO as evidenced by NSR on ECG; measured CO of 4 to 7 L/min, CI greater than 2.5 L/min/m^2, BP within patient's normal range, PAP 20 to 30/8 to 15 mm Hg, PAWP 6 to 12 mm Hg (or range specified by physician), Svo$_2$ 60% to 80%, SVR 900 to 1200 dynes/sec/cm^{-5}, peripheral pulses greater than 2+ on a 0 to 4+ scale, warm and dry skin, and hourly urine output greater than 0.5 ml/kg/hr. Patient is awake, alert, and oriented.
NOC Cardiac Pump Effectiveness

Shock Prevention
1. Monitor BP, PAP, RAP, Svo$_2$, HR, and heart rhythm continuously. Monitor PAWP, SVR, and CO hourly. Be alert to and report the following: elevated PAWP, decreased CO, decreased Svo$_2$, or elevated SVR.
2. Monitor urinary output, noting output that is less than 0.5 ml/kg/hr for 2 consecutive hours.
3. Monitor peripheral pulses and color and temperature of extremities every 2 hours.
4. Provide oxygen therapy as prescribed.
5. Maintain an adequate preload (i.e., PAWP greater than 10 mm Hg, RAP 10 mm Hg) via administration of IV fluids.

Safety Alert *With aortic stenosis and severe LV hypertrophy, a high filling pressure (i.e., PAWP greater than 18 mm Hg) may be necessary to ensure an adequate CO.*

Box 5-7	**NURSING IMPLICATIONS FOR ADMINISTRATION OF EPSILON-AMINOCAPROIC ACID (EACA)**

- Be aware that rapid administration may induce hypotension, bradycardia, or cardiac dysrhythmias.
- Monitor for and report the following side effects: nausea, cramps, diarrhea, dizziness, tinnitus, headache, skin rash, malaise, nasal stuffiness, postural hypotension.
- Be alert to clotting or thrombosis, which can be precipitated by this medication. Assess for indicators of thrombophlebitis: calf erythema, warmth, tenderness, or increase in size or positive reaction for Homan sign. Provide pneumatic compression stockings as prescribed.
- Assess for indicators of pulmonary emboli: chest pain, dyspnea, fever, tachycardia, cyanosis, falling BP, restlessness, agitation.
- Monitor and report blood levels of EACA via use of chromatography, which is available in some institutions.
- Consult physician promptly for significant findings.

6. Maintain a normal or reduced afterload (SVR less than 1200 dynes/sec/cm^{-5}) by administering prescribed IV vasodilating drugs such as nitroprusside and NTG.
7. Maintain NSR by administering antidysrhythmic agents as prescribed. Atrial fibrillation is common in aortic and mitral valve disease and may result in a 20% to 50% decrease in CO. If a junctional rhythm or bradycardia occurs, a pacemaker may be necessary.
8. Administer inotropic agents as prescribed to maintain CI greater than 2.5 L/min/m^2 and SBP greater than 90 mm Hg. Commonly used agents include dobutamine, dopamine, milrinone, and amrinone. Monitor for side effects, including tachydysrhythmias, ventricular ectopy, headache, and angina.

 Cardiac Care; Hemodynamic Regulation

Ineffective tissue perfusion (or risk for same): cerebral *related to impaired blood flow to the brain secondary to embolization resulting from cardiac surgery*

| **Safety Alert** | *An air embolus, particulate emboli from calcified valves, and thrombotic emboli from prosthetic valves may lodge in the brain, leading to varying degrees of stroke.* |

GOALS/OUTCOMES Throughout hospitalization, patient has adequate or baseline brain perfusion as evidenced by orientation to time, place, and person; equal and normoreactive pupils; and ability to move all extremities, communicate, and respond to requests (or comparable to patient's preoperative baseline).
NOC Neurological Status

Neurologic Monitoring
1. Monitor patient immediately after surgery and hourly for signs of neurologic impairment: diminished LOC, pupillary response, ability to move all extremities, and response to verbal stimuli.
2. Assess patient's orientation and ability to communicate, answer yes-no questions, point to objects, write responses and requests, identify family members, and state his or her location. Inform other health care personnel about patient's LOC and communication deficits.
3. Assess patient's PT, PTT, and INR as heparin is tapered off and coumadin therapy is instituted. Heparin and coumadin may be initiated simultaneously to reduce the time needed to stabilize the lab values.
4. If CNS impairment is noted, report findings to the physician and administer medications for brain resuscitation as prescribed.
5. In the presence of CNS impairment, implement the following measures:
   - Assist patient with turning and moving as needed. Teach patient to use unaffected extremities to assist with moving.
   - Perform ROM to all extremities four times daily. Have patient assist as much as possible.
   - Progress patient's activity level, as tolerated, with the assistance of a physical therapist.
6. Assess patient's ability to swallow food and fluids. If patient's voice is hoarse or patient coughs when swallowing, consult physician. Patient may require nothing-by-mouth (NPO) status and an enteric tube until the swallowing reflex has improved.

NIC Surveillance; Cerebral Perfusion Promotion

Deficient knowledge: Risk of infective endocarditis after valve surgery and preventive strategies

| **Safety Alert** | *All patients with valve surgery are at risk for infective endocarditis (IE) as a result of bacteria entering the bloodstream and traveling to the heart, leading to destruction of a new tissue valve or obstruction of a new artificial valve.* |

GOALS/OUTCOMES Within the 24-hour period before discharge from the CCU, patient verbalizes knowledge about the risk of IE after valve surgery and the precautions that must be taken to prevent it.
NOC Knowledge: Disease Process

Teaching: Disease Process
1. Teach patient about IE (see *Acute Infective Endocarditis*, p. 453), describing what it is, how it develops, and how it may affect the repaired valve.
2. Teach patient to caution dentists and other health care providers so antibiotics can be prescribed to prevent development of endocarditis after valve surgery. Antibiotics must be taken before any dental work or examination by instrument, including teeth cleaning, fillings, extractions, cystoscopy, endoscopy, or sigmoidoscopy.
3. Instruct patient to cleanse all wounds and apply antibiotic ointments to help prevent infection.

NIC Teaching: Prescribed Medication; Surveillance

Deficient knowledge *related to risk of bleeding or clotting caused by excessive or insufficient anticoagulation therapy*

| **Safety Alert** | *Finding and maintaining the dose of warfarin (coumadin) to maintain target INR are difficult. Foods, medications, vitamins, and food supplements can enhance or inhibit the efficacy.* |

GOALS/OUTCOMES Within the 24-hour period before discharge from the hospital, patient or significant others verbalize knowledge about the risk of coumadin therapy after valve surgery and the precautions that must be taken to prevent embolism or hemorrhage.
NOC Knowledge: Treatment Regimen

Teaching: Prescribed Medication
1. Teach patient how to institute bleeding precautions after discharge. Shave with an electric razor. Take care when handling sharp objects. Prevent injury through an annual safety home check. Use soft-bristle toothbrush.
2. Teach patient to call physician if bleeding or bruising is noted.
3. Teach patient and significant others to report all changes in medication to health care provider who is managing coumadin or other anticoagulant therapy.
4. Teach patient and significant others to avoid altering the intake of foods that may be high in vitamin K. Excessive intake of vitamin K can block coumadin and lower the INR.

NIC Teaching: Prescribed Diet; Surveillance

For patients undergoing percutaneous balloon valvuloplasty:
Deficient knowledge *related to procedure for percutaneous balloon valvuloplasty (PBV) and postprocedural assessment*

GOALS/OUTCOMES Within the 24-hour period before PBV, patient verbalizes rationale for the procedure, the technique, and postprocedural care.
NOC Knowledge: Treatment Regimen

Teaching: Preoperative
1. Assess patient's understanding of aortic stenosis and the purpose of valvuloplasty. Evaluate patient's style of coping and the degree of information desired.
2. As appropriate for patient's coping style, discuss with patient and significant others the valvuloplasty procedure, including the following:
   - Location of diseased valve, using heart drawing
   - Use of local anesthesia and sedation during procedure
   - Insertion site of catheter: femoral artery and vein
   - Use of fluoroscopy during procedure. Evaluate patient for a history of sensitivity to contrast material.
   - Postprocedural observations made by nurse: BP, HR, ECG, pulses, and catheter insertion site
   - Importance of lying flat for 6 to 12 hours after the procedure to minimize the risk of bleeding

NIC Teaching: Procedure/Treatment

Valvular Heart Disease

Decreased cardiac output (or risk for same) *related to altered preload and negative inotropic changes associated with valve regurgitation or hemorrhage secondary to PBV; altered rate, rhythm, or conduction associated with dysrhythmias secondary to PBV.*

GOALS/OUTCOMES Throughout the postoperative course, patient has adequate CO as evidenced by NSR, CO 4 to 7 L/min, CI greater than 2.5 L/min/m^2, HR 60 to 100 bpm, RAP 4 to 6 mm Hg, PAWP 6 to 12 mm Hg, PAP 20 to 30/8 to 15 mm Hg, BP within patient's normal range, urinary output greater than 0.5 ml/kg/hr, peripheral pulses greater than 2+ on a 0 to 4+ scale, orientation to time, place, and person; and absence of new murmurs, pulsus paradoxus, or jugular vein distention.

NOC Cardiac Pump Effectiveness

Shock Prevention
1. Monitor ECG continuously after procedure. Document any changes. Consult physician for dysrhythmias, and treat according to hospital protocol.
2. Monitor CO/CI, HR, RAP, PAWP, and PAP hourly or as prescribed. Report a fall in CO/CI, a change in HR, and an increase or decrease in RAP, PAWP, or PAP.
3. Monitor Hct and electrolyte values. Observe for a decrease in Hct or any change in electrolyte levels (particularly potassium) that could precipitate dysrhythmias. Optimal values are Hct greater than 37% (female) or greater than 40% (male) and serum potassium 3.5 to 5 mEq/L.
4. Assess heart sounds immediately after procedure and every 4 hours. Report the development of a new murmur.
5. Monitor patient for evidence of cardiac tamponade: hypotension, tachycardia, pulsus paradoxus, jugular vein distention, elevation and plateau pressuring of PAWP and RAP, and possibly an enlarged heart silhouette on chest radiograph study. For more information, see *Acute Cardiac Tamponade*, p. 257.

NIC Cardiac Care; Hemodynamic Regulation

Ineffective protection *related to risk of hemorrhage or hematoma formation secondary to heparinization with PBV*

GOALS/OUTCOMES Throughout the postoperative course, patient has minimal or absent bleeding or hematoma formation at the catheter insertion site. PTT is within therapeutic anticoagulation range (as prescribed or according to institutional procedure).

NOC Circulation Status

Bleeding Precautions
1. Monitor catheter insertion site for evidence of bleeding. Report hematoma formation, and outline the bleeding on the dressing for subsequent comparison.
2. Keep patient's catheterized leg straight for the prescribed amount of time.
3. Monitor heparin drip as prescribed. Usually heparin drip is maintained until 1 to 2 hours before the sheaths are removed.
4. Monitor PTT for therapeutic range, which is usually 1½ times that of normal.
5. When IV or invasive lines (arterial or venous sheaths) are removed, apply firm pressure either manually or with a mechanical clamp for 30 minutes.

NIC Surveillance; Bleeding Reduction: Wound

ADDITIONAL NURSING DIAGNOSES
Also see *Deficient Knowledge* in *Pulmonary Embolus* (p. 414). Also see *Altered Tissue Perfusion* in *Acute Coronary Syndromes* (p. 434). See all nursing diagnoses in the discussion of *Coronary Artery Bypass Graft* in *Acute Coronary Syndromes* (p. 434). Also see nursing diagnoses and interventions in *Hemodynamic Monitoring* (p. 75), *Prolonged Immobility* (p. 149), and *Emotional and Spiritual Support of the Patient and Significant Others* (p. 200).

SELECTED BIBLIOGRAPHY

Abbott WM, Brewster DC, Cambria RP, et al: Carotid endarterectomy at the millennium: what interventional therapy must match. *Ann Surg* 240(3):535–546, 2004.

Aehlert B: *ACLS study guide*, ed 3. St Louis, MO, 2007, Mosby.

Aehlert B: *ECGs made easy: pocket reference*, ed 2. St Louis, MO, 2002, Mosby.

Alberts MJ, Latchaw RE, Selman WR, et al: Recommendations for comprehensive stroke centers: a consensus statement from the Brain Attack Coalition. *Stroke* 36(7):1597–1616, 2005.

American College of Cardiology; American Heart Association Task Force on Practice Guidelines; American College of Chest Physicians; International Society for Heart and Lung Transplantation; Heart Rhythm Society: ACC/AHA 2005 Guideline Update for the Diagnosis and Management of Chronic Heart Failure in the Adult: A report of the American College of Cardiology/American Heart Association Task Force on Practice Guidelines (Writing Committee to Update the 2001 Guidelines for the Evaluation and Management of Heart Failure): Developed in collaboration with the American College of Chest Physicians and the International Society for Heart and Lung Transplantation: Endorsed by the Heart Rhythm Society. *Circulation* 112:e154–e235, 2005.

American Heart Association: *Heart disease and stroke statistics–2008 update*. Dallas, 2008, American Heart Association.

American Heart Association: Pericardium and pericarditis. Retrieved May 15, 2009, from http://www.americanheart.org/presenter.jhtml?identifier=4683.

Anderson JL, Adams CD, Antman EM: Management of patients with unstable angina/non-ST elevation myocardial infarction. *Circulation* 116:803–877, 2007.

Angeja BG, Grossman W: Clinician update: evaluation and management of diastolic heart failure. *Circulation* 107:659, 2003.

Antman EM, Hand M, et al: 2007 focused update of the ACC/AHA 2004 guideline for the management of patients with ST segment elevation myocardial infarction. *Circulation* 117:296–329, 2008.

Antman EM, et al: ACC/AHA guidelines for the management of patients with ST-elevation myocardial infarction. *Circulation* 110(9):e82, 2004.

Asymptomatic Carotid Atherosclerosis Study (ACAS) Investigators: Clinical advisory: carotid endarterectomy for patients with asymptomatic internal carotid artery stenosis. *Stroke* 25:2523–2525, 1994.

Balady GJ, Williams MA, Ades PA, et al: AHA/AACVPR Scientific Statement: core components of cardiac rehabilitation/secondary prevention programs. *Circulation* 116:2675–2682, 2007.

Bonham PA, Flemister BG: *Guideline for management of wounds in patients with lower-extremity arterial disease*. Mount Laurel, NJ, 2008, Wound, Ostomy and Continence Nurses Society (WOCN), p 63 (WOCN clinical practice guideline series No. 1).

Bonow RO, Chatterjee K, Faxon DP, et al: ACC/AHA 2006 guidelines for the management of patients with valvular heart disease: executive summary. *Circulation* 114: 450–527, 2006.

Bonow R, et al: ACC/AHA clinical performance measures for adults with chronic heart failure. *Circulation* 112:1853–1887, 2005.

Calhoun DA, Jones D, Textor S, Goff DC, et al: Resistant hypertension: diagnosis, management and treatment: a scientific statement from the American Heart Association Professional Education Committee of the Council for High Blood Pressure Research. *Hypertension* 51:1403–1419, 2008.

Chaturvedi S, Madhavan R, Santhakumar S, et al: Higher risk factor burden and worse outcomes in urban carotid endarterectomy patients. *Stroke* 39:2966, 2008.

Cheng MJ, Den Uil CA, Hoeks ES, et al: Percutaneous left ventricular assist devices vs. intra-aortic balloon pump counterpulsation for treatment of cardiogenic shock: a meta-analysis of controlled trials. *Eur Heart J* July, 2009.

Cheung AT, Hobson RE: Hypertension in vascular surgery: aortic dissection and carotid revascularization. *Ann Emerg Med* 51(3):S28–S33, 2008.

Chobanian AV, Bakris GL, Black HR, Cushman WC, Green LA, Izzo JL Jr, et al; the National High Blood Pressure Education Program Coordinating Committee: Seventh report of the Joint National Committee on Prevention, Detection, Evaluation, and Treatment of High Blood Pressure. *Hypertension* 42:1206, 2003.

Cina CS, Clase CM, Radan A: Asymptomatic carotid bruit. In *ACS surgery: principles and practice*, 2004. http://www.webmd.com/heart-disease/carotid-artery-disease-causes-symptoms-tests-and-treatment

Colucci WS: Clinical manifestations and evaluation of the patient with suspected heart failure. www.uptodate.com.

Colucci WS: *Atlas of heart failure cardiac function and dysfunction*, ed 5. New York, 2009, Springer Publishing.

Cooper BE: Review and update on inotropes and vasopressors. *AACN Adv Crit Care* 19(1):5–15, 2008.

Daughenbaugh LA: Cardiomyopathy: an overview. *J Nurse Practitioners* April 2007:248–258.

Den Uil AC, Lagrand KW, Valk SDA, et al: Management of cardiogenic shock: focus on tissue perfusion. *Curr Probl Cardiol* 34:330–349, 2009.

Di Nisto M, Middeldorp S, Buller H: Direct thrombin inhibitors. *N Engl J Med* 353:1028–1040, 2005.

Erbel R, et al: Diagnosis and management of aortic dissection: recommendations of the task force on aortic dissection, European Society of Cardiology. *Eur Heart J* 22:1642–1681, 2001.

Fahey VA, editor: *Vascular nursing*, ed 3. Philadelphia, 2003, WB Saunders.

Fann JI, Ingels NB, Miller DC: Pathophysiology of mitral valve disease. In *Cardiac surgery in the adult*, ed 3. New York, 2008, McGraw-Hill, Chapter 41.

Fattori R, et al: Complicated acute type B dissection: is surgery still the best option? A report from the International Registry of Acute Aortic Dissection. *Cardiovasc Interv* 1(4):395–402, 2008.

Fiore MC, Jaén CR, et al: Clinical practice guideline. Treating tobacco use and dependence: 2008 Update. U.S. Department of Health and Human Services, May 2008. Retrieved January 4, 2009, from http://www.surgeongeneral.gov/tobacco/treating_tobacco_use.pdf

Fraker TD, Fihn SD: 2007 Focused Update of the ACC/AHA 2002 guidelines for the management of patients with chronic stable angina. *Circulation* 116:2762–2772, 2007.

Garcia-Gonzalez MJ, Dominguez-Rodriguez A, Ferrier-Hita JJ, et al: Cardiogenic shock after primary percutaneous coronary intervention: effects of levosimendan compared with dobutamine on hemodynamics. *Eur J Heart Fail* 8:723–728, 2006.

Gerber MA, Baltimore RS, Eaton CB, Gewitz M, Rowley AH, Shulman ST, et al: Prevention of rheumatic fever and diagnosis and treatment of acute streptococcal pharyngitis: a scientific statement from the American Heart Association Rheumatic Fever, Endocarditis, and Kawasaki Disease Committee of the Council on Cardiovascular Disease in the Young, the Interdisciplinary Council on Functional Genomics and Translational Biology, and the Interdisciplinary Council on Quality of Care and Outcomes Research: endorsed by the American Academy of Pediatrics. *Circulation* 119(11):1541–1551, 2009.

Gibler WB, et al: Practical implementation of the guidelines for unstable angina/non–ST-segment elevation myocardial infarction in the emergency department. *Circulation* 111:2699–2710, 2005.

Golomb BA, Dang TT, Criqui MH: Peripheral arterial disease, morbidity and mortality implications. *Circulation* 114:688–699, 2006.

Habib G, Thuny F, Avierinos JF: Prosthetic valve endocarditis: current approach and therapeutic options. *Prog Cardiovasc Dis* 50(4):274–281, 2008.

Hagan PG, et al: International Registry of Acute Aortic Dissection (IRAD): new insights into an old disease. *JAMA* 283:897–903, 2000.

Hazinski MF, et al: 2005 American Heart Association guidelines for cardiopulmonary resuscitation and emergency cardiovascular care. *Circulation* 112(suppl 1):IV-1–IV-203, 2005.

Hazinski MF, Gilmore D: *American Heart Association handbook of emergency cardiovascular care for healthcare providers*. Dallas, 2008, American Heart Association.

Hazinski MF, Nadkarni VM, Hickey RW, O'Connor R, Becker LW, Zaritsy A: The major changes in the 2005 AHA guidelines for cardiopulmonary resuscitation and emergency cardiovascular care. *Circulation* 112:IV-206–IV-211, 2005.

Hershberger R, Lindenfeld J, Mestroni L, Seidman C, Taylor N, Towbin J: Genetic evaluation of cardiomyopathy—a Heart Failure Society of America practice guideline. *J Card Fail* 15(2):83–97, 2009.

Hirsch A, Haskal ZJ, Hertzer NR, et al: ACC/AHA 2005 practice guidelines for the management of patients with peripheral arterial disease (lower extremity, renal, mesenteric, and abdominal aortic): executive summary. *Circulation* 113:e463–e465, 2006. http://circ.ahajournals.org/cgi/reprint/113/11e463

Hobson RW 2nd, Mackey WC, et al: Management of atherosclerotic carotid artery disease: clinical practice guidelines of the Society for Vascular Surgery. *J Vasc Surg* 48(2):480–486, 2008.

Horstkotte D, Follath F, Gutschik E, Lengyel M, Oto A, Pavie A, et al; The Task Force on Infective Endocarditis of the European Society of Cardiology: *Guidelines on prevention, diagnosis and treatment of infective endocarditis*. France, 2004, European Society of Cardiology.

http://circ.ahajournals.org Downloaded on September 11, 2009.

http://circ.ahajournals.org/cgi/content/full/118/8/887 Downloaded on July 17, 2009.

Hunt S, et al: ACC/AHA 2005 Guideline update for the diagnosis and management of chronic heart failure in the adult—summary article. *Circulation* 112:1825–1852, 2005.

Imazio M: Evaluation and management of acute pericarditis. Retrieved June 12, 2009, from http://www.uptodate.com/home/index.html

Imazio M, Negro A, Belli R, et al: Frequency and prognostic significance of pericarditis following acute myocardial infarction treated by primary percutaneous coronary intervention. *Am J Cardiol* 103(11):1525-1529, 2009.

International Liaison Committee on Resuscitation: 2005 International consensus on cardiopulmonary resuscitation and emergency cardiovascular care science with treatment recommendations. *Circulation* 112:III-1-III-136, 2005.

Isselbacher EM: Thoracic and abdominal aortic aneurysms. *Circulation* 111:816-828, 2005.

Jacobs AK, Antman EM, Fason DP, et al: Development of systems of care for ST elevation myocardial infarction patients (executive summary). *Circulation* 116:8 217-230, 2007.

Jaski BE, Romeo A, Ortiz B, Hoagland PM, Stone M, Glaser D, et al: Outcomes of volume-overloaded cardiovascular patients treated with ultrafiltration. *J Card Fail* 14(6):515-520, 2008.

Joint National Committee: The seventh report of the Joint National Committee on Prevention, Detection, Evaluation, and Treatment of High Blood Pressure (JNC-7), NIH Publication No. 03-5231, May 2003. www.nhlbi.nih.gov/guidelines/hypertension/index.htm

Kamalakannan D, Rosman HS, Eagle KA: Acute aortic dissection. *Crit Care Clin* 23:779-800, 2007.

King S, Aversano TA, Ballard WL, et al: ACCF/AHA/SCAI 2007 clinical competence statement on cardiac interventional procedures. *Circulation* 116:98-124, 2007.

King S, Smith SC, Hirshfeld JW, et al: 2007 focused update of the ACC/AHA/SCA 2005 guideline update for percutaneous coronary intervention. *Circulation* 117:261-295, 2008.

Klein DG: Thoracic aortic aneurysms. *J Cardiovasc Nurs* 20(4):245-250, 2005.

Klocke FJ, et al: ACC/AHA guidelines for the clinical use of cardiac radionuclide imaging. *Circulation* 108:1404, 2003.

Krumholz HM, et al: ACC/AHA 2008 performance measures for adults with ST-elevation and non St-Elevation myocardial infarction. *Circulation* 118(24):2596, 2008.

Lange RA, Hillis LD: Clinical practice. Acute pericarditis. *N Engl J Med* 351(21):2195-2202, 2004.

Lewis PA, Aquila A, Walsh ME, editors: *Core curriculum for vascular nursing.* Beverly, MA, 2007, Society for Vascular Nursing.

Libby P, Bonow RO, Mann DL, et al: *Braunwald's heart disease: a textbook of cardiovascular medicine,* ed 8. Philadelphia, 2008, Saunders Elsevier.

Libby P, Bonow RO, Zipes DP, Mann DL: Valvular heart disease. In *Braunwald's heart disease,* ed 8. Philadelphia, 2008, Saunders Elsevier, Chapter 62.

Long JW, Foury AG, Slaughter MS, et al: Long-term destination therapy with the HeartMate XVE left ventricular assist device: improved outcomes since the REMATCH study. *Congest Heart Fail* 11(3):133-138, 2005.

Maisch B, Seferovic PM, Ristic AD, Erbel R, Rienmüller R, Adler Y, et al. Guidelines on the diagnosis and management of pericardial diseases executive summary; the Task Force on the Diagnosis and Management of Pericardial Diseases of the European Society of Cardiology. *Eur Heart J* 25(7):587-610, 2004.

Mancia G, De Backer G, Dominiczak A, Cifkova R, Fagard R, Germano G, et al; The Task Force for the Management of Arterial Hypertension of the European Society of Hypertension (ESH) and of the European Society of Cardiology (ESC). 2007 guidelines for the management of arterial hypertension. *J Hypertens* 25:1105-1187, 2007.

Mariell J, et al: Focused update: ACCF/AHA guidelines for the diagnosis and management of heart failure in adults. *Circulation* 119:1977-2016, 2009.

Maron BJ, Towbin JA, Thiene G, Antzelevitch C, Corrado D, Arnett D, et al: Contemporary definitions and classification of the cardiomyopathies. An American Heart Association Scientific Statement from the Council on Clinical Cardiology, Heart Failure and Transplantation Committee; Quality of Care and Outcomes Research and Functional Genomics and Translational Biology Interdisciplinary Working Groups; and Council on Epidemiology and Prevention. *Circulation* 113:1807-1816, 2006.

Masoudi FA, et al: ACC/AHA statement on performance measurement and reperfusion therapy. *Circulation* 118(24):2649, 2008.

McNamara RL, et al: Management of atrial fibrillation: review of the evidence for the role of pharmacologic therapy, electrical cardioversion and echocardiography. *Ann Intern Medicine* 139 (12): 1018-1033, 2003.

Morton PG, Fontaine DK: *Critical care nursing: a holistic approach,* ed 9. Philadelphia, 2009, Lippincott, Williams and Wilkins.

Mosca L, Banka CL, Benjamin EJ, et al: AHA guideline: evidence-based guideline for prevention of cardiovascular disease in women: 2007 update. *Circulation* 115:1481-1501, 2007.

Moser D, Riegel B: *Cardiac nursing, a companion to Braunwald's heart disease.* St Louis, MO, 2008, Saunders Elsevier.

National Heart Foundation of Australia (National Blood Pressure and Vascular Disease Advisory Committee): Guide to management of hypertension 2008. Quick reference guide for health professionals. http://www.heartfoundation.org.au/Professional_Information/Clinical_Practice/Hypertension/Pages/default.aspx

Nishimura RA, Faxon DP, Lytle BA, et al: ACC/AHA 2008 guideline update on valvular heart disease: focused update on infective endocarditis. *Circulation* 118:887–896, 2008.

North American Symptomatic Carotid Endarterectomy Trial (NASCET) Collaborators: Beneficial effect of carotid endarterectomy in symptomatic patients with high-grade carotid stenosis. *N Engl J Med* 325:445–453, 1991.

Peberdy MA, Ornato JP: Progress in resuscitation: an evolution, not a revolution. *JAMA* 299(10):1188–1190, 2008.

Ristow B, Ali S, Ren X, Whooley MA, Schiller NB: Elevated pulmonary artery pressure by Doppler echocardiography predicts hospitalization for heart failure and mortality in ambulatory stable coronary artery disease: the Heart and Soul Study. *J Am Coll Cardiol* 49(1):43–49, 2007.

Rosamond W, Flegal K, Furie K, et al: Heart disease and stroke statistics: 2008 update. *Circulation* 117:e1–e121, 2008.

Rothwell PM, Gutnikov SA, Warlow CP, et al: Reanalysis of the final results of the European Carotid Surgery Trial. *Stroke* 34:514–523, 2003.

Runge MS, Ohman ME: *Netter's cardiology*, ed 1. Philadelphia, 2004, Elsevier.

Schocken D, et al: Prevention of heart failure. *Circulation* 119:e391–e479, 2009.

Shah PM, Raney AA: Tricuspid valve disease. *Curr Probl Cardiol* 33(2):47–84, 2008.

Singh M, White J, Hasdai D, et al: Long-term outcome and its predictors among patients with ST-segment elevation myocardial infarction complicated by shock: insights from the GUSTO-I trial. *J Am Coll Cardiol* 50:1752–1758, 2007.

Singh N: Atherosclerotic disease of the carotid artery. Retrieved January 4, 2009, from http://www.emedicine.com/med/topic2964.htm#Multimedia#1

Sobieszczyk P, Beckman J: Carotid artery disease. *Circulation* 114:e244–e247, 2006. http://circ.ahajournals.org/cgi/content/full/114/7/e244

Stenting and Angioplasty with Protection in Patients at High Risk for Endarterectomy (SAPPHIRE) Investigators: Protected carotid-artery stenting versus endarterectomy in high-risk patients. *N Engl J Med* 351(15):1493–1501, 2004.

Suzuki D, et al: Diagnosis of acute aortic dissection by D-dimer: The International Registry of Aortic Dissection substudy on biomarkers (IRADBio) experience. *Circulation* 119:2702–2707, 2009.

Swee W, Dake MD: Endovascular management of thoracic dissections. *Circulation* 117:1460–1473, 2008.

The Merck Manuals: Pericarditis. *The Merck Manual for Healthcare Professionals.* Retrieved May 12, 2009, from http://www.merck.com/mmpe/sec07/ch078/ch078a.html

Thomas RJ, King M, Lui K, et al: AACVPR/ACC/AHA 2007 performance measures on cardiac rehabilitation for referral to and delivery of cardiac rehabilitation/secondary prevention services. *Circulation* 116:1611–1642, 2007.

Thygesen K, Alpert JS, White HD: Universal definition of myocardial infarction. *Circulation* 116:2634–2653, 2007.

Topalian S, Ginsberg F, Parrillo JE: Cardiogenic shock. *Crit Care Med* 36:S66–S74, 2008.

Veterans Affairs Symptomatic Carotid Endarterectomy Trial. *N Engl J Med* 328(4):276–279, 1993.

Webb JG, Lowe AM, Sanborn TA, et al: PCI for cardiogenic shock in the SHOCK TRIAL. *J Am Coll Cardiol* 42:1380–1386, 2003.

Wertman BM, Gura V, Schwarz ER: Ultrafiltration for the management of acute decompensated heart failure. *J Card Fail* 14(9):754–759, 2008.

Wilson W, Taubert KA, Gewitz M, et al: Prevention of infective endocarditis: guidelines from the American Heart Association: a guideline from the American Heart Association Rheumatic Fever, Endocarditis, and Kawasaki Disease Committee, Council on Cardiovascular Disease in the Young, and the Council on Clinical Cardiology, Council on Cardiovascular Surgery and Anesthesia, and the Quality of Care and Outcomes Research Interdisciplinary Working Group. *Circulation* 116(15):1736–1754, 2007.

Yadav JS, Wholey MH, Kuntz RE, et al: Protected carotid artery stenting versus endarterectomy in high-risk patients. *N Engl J Med* 351(15):1493–1501, 2004.

GENITOURINARY ASSESSMENT: GENERAL

Goal of System Assessment
Evaluate for decreased renal function and assess the severity of renal dysfunction.

Detailed Health History
- Chronic symptoms of fatigue, weight loss, anorexia, nocturia, and pruritus
- Renal-related symptoms including dysuria, edema, frequency, hematuria, flank pain, pyuria, frothy urine, bloody urine, and renal colic
- Presence of comorbidities: hypertension, congestive heart failure, diabetes, multiple myeloma, chronic infection, and myeloproliferative disorder
- Current medications including over-the-counter medications
- Exposure to chemicals
- Recent trauma or unaccustomed exertion
- Recent diagnostic studies requiring dye administration

Observation
Evidence of chronic versus acute process
- *Skin:* petechiae, purpura, ecchymosis, livedo reticularis, dryness, pallor, yellowness, decreased turgor
- *Eyes:* uveitis, ocular palsy, findings suggestive of hypertension, atheroembolic disease
- Inspection of the *flank area* in a standing and supine position for raised masses or unusual pulsations

Vital Sign Assessment
Evaluate for changes indicative of fluid volume excess or depletion and infection.
- Blood pressure (BP) and pulse both lying and standing
- Respiratory rate (RR)
- Height and weight
- Temperature

Palpation
Abdominal assessment to identify renal pathology
- Costovertebral angle (CVA) tenderness, which may occur with pyelonephritis
- Enlarged liver, which may occur with congestive heart failure
- Kidneys are difficult to palpate because of location. If they are enlarged and palpable, this could represent polycystic kidney disease or hydronephrosis.
- Ascites may occur with liver failure or acute renal failure.
- Lower extremity or sacral edema
- Bladder tenderness and distension

Auscultation
- Cardiac auscultation for the presence of murmurs, pericardial friction rub, S_3, S_4 significant in uremia, and congestive heart failure (CHF)
- Lung auscultation for the presence of pleural rub, rales, decreased breath sounds significant in uremia, and volume excess states

Labwork
Renal dysfunction causes marked changes in fluid and electrolyte balance, acid-base balance, and red cell production, and increased concentrations of blood urea nitrogen and creatinine.
- Complete blood count (CBC) to evaluate anemia
- Electrolytes including calcium, phosphorus, and magnesium
- Blood urea nitrogen (BUN), creatinine
- Estimated glomerular filtration rate (eGFR) to evaluate clearance
- 24-hour urine collection for creatinine clearance, protein, and metanephrines
- Urinalysis
- Urine electrolytes

ACUTE RENAL FAILURE/ACUTE KIDNEY INJURY

PATHOPHYSIOLOGY
Acute renal failure (ARF) is a syndrome traditionally characterized by an abrupt deterioration of renal function, resulting in the accumulation of metabolic wastes, fluids, and electrolytes, and usually accompanied by a marked decline in urinary output. ARF is one of few types of total organ failure that may be reversible with proper treatment. However, the lack of consensus on the quantitative definition of ARF has hindered comparisons between studies in an effort to improve outcomes. In 2004, the Acute Dialysis Quality Initiative (ADQI) was formed by a group of intensivists and nephrologists to develop consensus on the definition of ARF and propose evidence-based guidelines for the treatment and prevention of ARF.

The product of ADQI was a graded definition of ARF designated as the *RIFLE criteria*. This led to the development of the Acute Kidney Injury network. The workings of these groups resulted in the adoption of the term *acute kidney injury* (AKI), which represents the entire spectrum of ARF. The RIFLE criteria are based on three graded levels of injury which reflect serum creatinine or urine output and two outcome measures (Table 6-1). Formation of urine is a three-step process consisting of (1) ultrafiltration of delivered blood by the glomeruli (renal cortex), (2) internal processing of the ultrafiltrate via tubular secretion and reabsorption (renal parenchyma), and (3) excretion of waste products from the kidneys through the ureters, bladder, and urethra. Corresponding to those steps, ARF/AKI is categorized as prerenal, intrarenal, and postrenal (Table 6-2).

Prerenal failure, or azotemia, is the result of decreased blood flow to the kidneys. The events leading to prerenal insults cause decreased renal vascular perfusion and may be associated

Table 6-1	RIFLE CLASSIFICATION FOR ACUTE RENAL FAILURE (ARF)/ ACUTE KIDNEY INJURY (AKI)	
Classification	**GFR Criteria**	**Urine Output Criteria**
Risk	Serum creatinine increased 1.5 times	Less than 0.5 ml/kg/hr for 6 hours
Injury	Serum creatinine increased 2 times	Less than 0.5 ml/kg/hr for 12 hours
Failure	Serum creatinine increased 3 times or greater than 355 μmol/L or mg/dl when there was an acute rise of greater than 44 μmol/L or mg/dl	Less than 0.3 ml/kg/hr for 24 hours or anuria for 12 hours
Loss	Persistent acute renal failure: complete loss of kidney function for longer than 4 weeks	
End-stage renal disease	End-stage renal disease for longer than 3 months	

Table 6-2	CAUSES OF ACUTE RENAL FAILURE		
Prerenal (Decreased Renal Perfusion)	**Intrarenal (Parenchymal Damage; Acute Tubular Necrosis)**		**Postrenal (Obstruction)**
Hypovolemia • GI losses • Hemorrhage • Third-space (interstitial) losses (burns, peritonitis) • Dehydration from diuretic use ***Hepatorenal syndrome*** ***Edema-forming conditions*** • Right ventricular failure • Cirrhosis • Nephrotic syndrome ***Renal vascular disorders*** • Renal artery stenosis • Renal artery thrombosis • Renal vein thrombosis	***Nephrotoxic Agents*** • Antibiotics (aminoglycosides, sulfonamides, methicillin) • Diuretics (e.g., furosemide) • Nonsteroidal anti-inflammatory drugs (e.g., ibuprofen) • Contrast media • Heavy metals (e.g., lead, gold, mercury) ***Organic solvents (e.g., carbon tetrachloride, ethylene glycol)*** ***Infection (gram-negative sepsis), pancreatitis, peritonitis*** ***transfusion reaction (hemolysis)*** • Rhabdomyolysis with myoglobinuria (severe muscle injury) • Trauma • Exertion • Seizures • Drug-related: heroin, barbiturates, IV amphetamines, succinylcholine ***Glomerular diseases*** • Poststreptococcal glomerulonephritis • IgA nephropathy (e.g., Berger disease) • Lupus glomerulonephritis • Serum sickness • Ischemic injury		***Calculi*** ***Tumor*** ***Benign prostatic hypertrophy*** ***Necrotizing papillitis*** ***Urethral strictures*** ***Blood clots*** ***Retroperitoneal fibrosis***

GI, gastrointestinal; IgA, immunoglobulin A; IV, intravenous.

with systemic hypoperfusion. If treated promptly, this form of ARF/AKI is readily reversible. Chronic heart failure, drugs such as nonsteroidal anti-inflammatory drugs (NSAIDs) and angiotensin-converting enzyme (ACE) inhibitors, volume loss, or sequestration and shock states (especially septic shock) all may lead to reduced renal perfusion. If not managed aggressively, parenchymal (intrarenal) involvement, or *acute tubular necrosis (ATN)*, can result. Intrarenal damage may result from a mean arterial pressure less than75 mm Hg. Autoregulation fails; the sympathetic response increases and, with the action of the renin-angiotensin system, results in severe constriction of the afferent arteriole. Glomerular blood flow and hydrostatic pressure are reduced, and the GFR decreases. The amount of cellular damage depends on the duration of ischemia: mild damage (less than 25 minutes), moderate/severe damage (40 to 60 minutes), and irreversible damage (may occur within 60 to 90 minutes).

The most common cause of ARF/AKI is ATN. ATN may be the result of nephrotoxic injury, a prolonged reduction in renal perfusion (ischemic injury), or pigmenturia (myoglobinuria and hemoglobinuria). Prolonged renal hypoperfusion due to shock, particularly septic shock, is a common cause of ATN. Renal ischemia may potentiate the injury produced by nephrotoxins. Toxic ATN, caused by nephrotoxic agents (aminoglycoside antibiotics, radiographic contrast agents), is an insult or injury to the tubular cell. Thrombotic occlusion, malignant hypertension, emboli, thrombotic thrombocytopenic purpura (TTP), hemolytic-uremic syndrome (HUS), and vasculitis can all result in ATN.

RESEARCH BRIEF 6-1

Conclusion: *N*-acetylcysteine (e.g., Mucomyst) is more renoprotective than hydration alone for management of contrast-induced nephropathy. Theophylline may also reduce risk for contrast-induced nephropathy, although the detected association was not significant. The data support the administration of *N*-acetylcysteine prophylaxis, particularly in high-risk patients, given its low cost, availability, and few side effects. Not all agents analyzed had beneficial effects—fenoldopam, furosemide, mannitol, and the combination of furosemide, dopamine, and mannitol had odds ratios greater than 1.

From Kelly AM. Meta-analysis: effectiveness of drugs for preventing contrast-induced nephropathy. *Ann Intern Med* 148:284-294, 2008.

ATN is characterized by tubular cell necrosis, cast formation, and tubular obstruction caused by casts and cellular debris. Therapy is focused on maintenance of renal perfusion pressure, administering renal vasodilators to restore blood flow, and promoting diuresis to "wash out" the intratubular debris. Sometimes ATN is nonoliguric. Oliguria may occur with both toxic ATN and ischemic ATN. Common nephrotoxic agents are found in Table 6-3.

Postrenal failure is the least common cause of ARF/AKI and may be either intrarenal (within the kidney) or extrarenal (outside the kidney in another area of the elimination tract) obstruction. Intrarenal obstruction is often due to crystal deposition caused by medications (e.g., acyclovir, indinavir, sulfonamides, methotrexate) or endogenous substances (oxalate, uric acid). Extrarenal obstruction may be related to bladder outlet problems (prostate and urethral obstruction) or stones, clots, pus, tumor, fibrosis, or ligation of or papilla within the ureters.

Fluid, electrolyte, and acid-base disorders that occur with ARF include hypervolemia, hyperkalemia, hyperphosphatemia, hypocalcemia, hypermagnesemia, and metabolic acidosis (Table 6-4). Phosphate levels rise because of impaired excretion of phosphorus by the renal tubules with continued gastrointestinal (GI) absorption. Hypocalcemia results from the lack of active vitamin D, which is activated by the kidney, which would otherwise stimulate absorption of calcium from the GI tract, or high phosphate levels, which inhibit absorption of calcium. Hypocalcemia triggers the parathyroid glands to secrete parathyroid hormone (PTH), which mobilizes calcium from the bone into the blood. Hypermagnesemia is generally moderate (2 to 4 mg/dl) and is rarely symptomatic unless the patient receives magnesium-containing antacids (e.g., Maalox, Milk of Magnesia).

Table 6-3	COMMON NEPHROTOXIC AGENTS
Drugs	**X-ray Contrast Media**
Antineoplastics Methotrexate Cisplatin *Antibiotics* Cephalosporins Aminoglycosides Tetracycline *Nonsteroidal anti-inflammatory drugs* Ibuprofen Ketorolac	*Biologic substances* Myoglobin Tumor products *Chemicals* Ethylene glycol Pesticides Organic solvents *Heavy metals* Lead Mercury Gold

There are three identifiable stages/phases of ARF:

1. *Oliguric phase*: A drop in the 24-hour urinary output to less than 400 ml lasting approximately 7 to 14 days. About 30% of patients have nonoliguric renal failure.
2. *Diuretic phase*: A doubling of the urinary output from the previous 24-hour total. During this phase the patient may produce as much as 3 to 5 L of urine in 24 hours.
3. *Recovery phase*: A return to a normal 24-hour volume (1500 to 1800 ml). Usually, renal function continues to improve and may take 6 months to 1 year from the initial insult to return to baseline functional status.

Table 6-4	ALTERED ELECTROLYTE BALANCE IN ACUTE RENAL FAILURE (ARF)
Condition/Cause	**Nursing Implications**
Hyperkalemia	

Decreased ability to excrete K^+; K^+ release with catabolism	• Monitor ECG for tall and peaked T waves, loss of P waves, prolonged PR interval, widened QRS when K^+ is greater than 6.5 mEq/L. Cardiac arrest is more likely seen with K^+ greater than 7.5 mEq/L.
	• Monitor serum K^+ levels for values greater than 5 mEq/L.
	• Monitor patient for such indicators as paresthesias, muscle weakness or flaccidity, and HR less than 60 beats/min.
	• Teach patient and significant others the indicators of hyperkalemia and the importance of notifying nurse promptly if they occur.
	• Provide a list of foods high in potassium (see Box 1-5), and stress the importance of avoiding these foods.
	• Implement the following to help minimize the cellular release of potassium:
	  • Ensure that patient consumes only the amount of protein prescribed by physician; enforce sound infection control techniques to minimize risk of infection; and treat fevers promptly. Catabolism of protein, which occurs in these situations, causes potassium to be released from the tissues.
	  • Ensure that patient consumes the allotted amounts of carbohydrates, and limit strenuous patient activity as prescribed, both of which will spare protein.
	• Be aware that hyperkalemia can be a fatal complication, especially during the oliguric phase of ARF, because of its adverse effect on cardiac status. Keep emergency supplies (i.e., manual resuscitator, crash cart, emergency drug tray) readily available.
	• For more information, see *Fluid and Electrolyte Imbalances: Hyperkalemia*, p. 37.

Continued

Table 6-4	ALTERED ELECTROLYTE BALANCE IN ACUTE RENAL FAILURE (ARF)—cont'd
Condition/Cause	**Nursing Implications**
Hypokalemia	
Prolonged, inadequate oral intake; use of potassium-losing diuretics without proper replacement; excessive loss from vomiting, diarrhea, or gastric or intestinal suctioning	• Monitor ECG for prolonged PR interval, flattened or inverted. • T wave, depressed ST segment, presence of U wave, and ventricular dysrhythmias; ECG changes are more likely to occur at serum K^+ levels less than 3 mEq/L. • Be alert to serum K^+ less than 3.5 mEq/L. • Monitor patient for muscle weakness, soft and flabby muscles, paresthesias, decreased bowel sounds, ileus, weak and irregular pulse, and distant heart sounds. • Neuromuscular symptoms are seen at serum levels of approximately 2.5 mEq/L. • Teach patient and significant others the indicators of hypokalemia and the importance of notifying nurse promptly if they occur. • Provide a list of foods high in potassium (see Box 1-5), and assist with planning menus that incorporate them. • Administer potassium-sparing diuretics (e.g., spironolactone, triamterene) as prescribed. • Administer oral or IV potassium supplements as prescribed; for oral route, administer with at least 4 oz water or juice to minimize gastric irritation. • For more information, see *Fluid and Electrolyte Imbalance: Hypokalemia*, p. 37.
Hypernatremia	
Kidneys' inability to excrete excess sodium; decreased water intake; increased water losses via osmotic diuresis; excessive parenteral administration of sodium-containing solutions (e.g., sodium bicarbonate, 3% sodium chloride)	• Monitor serum sodium levels for serum Na^+ greater than 147 mEq/L. • Monitor VS and I&O hourly; weigh patient daily. • Be alert to dry mucous membranes, flushed skin, firm and rubbery tissue turgor, hyperthermia, oliguria, or anuria. • Assess sensorium for restlessness and agitation; institute seizure precautions as indicated. • Administer prescribed IV replacement fluids. • Administer diuretics as prescribed. • For more information, see *Fluid and Electrolyte Imbalance: Hypernatremia*, p. 37.
Hyponatremia	
Loss through vomiting, diarrhea, profuse diaphoresis; use of potent diuretics; salt-losing nephropathies; administration of large amount of sodium-free IV fluids (may be associated with fluid volume excess or postobstructive diuresis)	• Monitor for serum Na^+ less than 137 mEq/L. • Monitor I&O hourly; record weight daily for trend. • Assess patient for abdominal cramps, diarrhea, nausea, dizziness when changing position, postural hypotension, cold and clammy skin, and apprehension. • Provide parenteral replacement therapy as prescribed. • Institute a safe environment for individuals with altered LOC. • For more information, see *Fluid and Electrolyte Imbalance: Hyponatremia*, p. 46.

Table 6-4	ALTERED ELECTROLYTE BALANCE IN ACUTE RENAL FAILURE (ARF)—cont'd
Condition/Cause	**Nursing Implications**
Hypocalcemia	
Poor absorption of dietary calcium; precipitation of calcium out of the tissues in the presence of elevated phosphorus level; inadequate absorption and utilization of calcium occurring with lack of conversion of vitamin D to its usable form	• Monitor for serum Ca^{2+} less than 8.5 mg/dl. • Monitor for numbness and tingling around the mouth, muscle twitching, facial twitching, and tonic muscle spasms. • Assess for Trousseau sign (carpopedal spasm) and Chvostek sign (spasm of lip and cheek). • Administer calcium and vitamin D supplements as prescribed. • Reinforce the necessity of taking these medications as prescribed. • Teach patient and significant others the indicators of hypocalcemia. • Teach the importance of continued medical follow-up to check serum Ca^{2+} levels. • For more information, see *Fluid and Electrolyte Imbalance: Hypocalcemia,* p. 57.
Hyperphosphatemia	
Abnormal retention of phosphates caused by the kidneys' inability to excrete excess phosphorus	• Monitor for serum phosphate greater than 4.5 g/dl. • Although most foods contain generous amounts of phosphate, those especially high in phosphate include beef, pork, dried beans, dried mature peas, and dairy products (see Box 1-6). Monitor patient's diet accordingly. • Administer phosphate binders as prescribed. Assess for constipation, which may result from use of phosphate binders. • Teach patient and significant others the relationship between calcium and phosphate levels in the body. • Emphasize that maintaining good phosphate control and calcium balance may help control itching and prevent future problems with bone disease. • Reinforce the need for follow-up visits to check serum phosphate levels. • For more information, see *Fluid and Electrolyte Imbalance: Hyperphosphatemia,* p. 67.
Hypermagnesemia	
Administration of magnesium-containing medications to patients with impaired renal function	• Monitor serum Mg^{2+} levels greater than 2.5 mEq/L. • Assess for diaphoresis, flushing, hypotension, drowsiness, weak-to-absent DTRs, bradycardia, lethargy, and respiratory impairment. • Teach the above indicators to patient and significant others. • Avoid giving medications that contain magnesium (see Box 1-7). Emphasize to patient that such medications should not be taken without physician's approval. • For more information, see *Fluid and Electrolyte Imbalance: Hypermagnesemia,* p. 73.

Continued

Table 6-4	ALTERED ELECTROLYTE BALANCE IN ACUTE RENAL FAILURE (ARF)—cont'd
Condition/Cause	**Nursing Implications**

Metabolic Acidosis

Kidneys' inability to excrete excess acid produced by normal metabolic processes; marked tissue trauma, infection, and diarrhea may contribute to a more rapid development of acidosis (often associated with K^+ greater than 5 mEq/L)	• Monitor for HCO_3^- less than 22 mEq/L and pH less than 7.35. • Monitor I&O, LOC, and VS. • Be alert to Kussmaul respirations, SOB, anorexia, headache, nausea, vomiting, weakness, apathy, fatigue, and coma. • Institute seizure precautions in the presence of altered LOC. • Administer IV fluids and bicarbonate as prescribed. • Teach patient the importance of dietary restrictions, particularly of protein, and of maintaining adequate carbohydrate intake to prevent worsening acidosis. • Stress that patient should report to physician increased temperature and other signs of infection. • Teach patient the importance of taking sodium bicarbonate as prescribed and of maintaining dialysis schedule (both hemodialysis and peritoneal dialysis help correct acidosis). • For more information, see *Acid-Base Imbalances, Chronic Metabolic Acidosis, p. 20.*

Uremia

Failure of the kidneys to excrete urea, creatinine, uric acid, and other metabolic waste products	• Monitor patient for chronic fatigue, insomnia, anorexia, vomiting, metallic taste in the mouth, pruritus, increased bleeding tendency, muscular twitching, involuntary leg movements, decreasing attention span, anemia, muscle wasting, and weakness. • Teach patient and significant others that the indicators of uremia develop gradually and are very subtle. Explain the importance of notifying nurse of sudden worsening of the symptoms that may be present. • Monitor and record dietary intake of protein, potassium, and sodium. • Use lotions and oils to lubricate patient's skin and relieve drying and cracking. • Provide oral hygiene at frequent intervals, using a soft-bristle toothbrush and mouthwash, to help combat patient's thirst and the metallic taste caused by uremia. Chewing gum and hard candy also may help alleviate thirst and the unpleasant taste. • Encourage isometric exercises and short walks, if patient is able, to help maintain patient's muscle strength and tone, especially in the legs. • Teach significant others that because of patient's decreasing concentration level, they should communicate with patient by using simple and direct statements. • Teach patient to maintain good nutrition by ingesting the allotted amounts of carbohydrates and high-biologic value protein to support cell rebuilding and decrease waste products from protein breakdown. • Explain that profuse bleeding can occur with uremia and that knives, scissors, and other sharp instruments should be used with caution. • Stress that OTC medications such as aspirin and ibuprofen may enhance bleeding tendency. • Emphasize the importance of follow-up visits to evaluate the progression of uremia. • Stress the dialysis schedule should be maintained to decrease the symptoms of uremia and correct many of the metabolic abnormalities that occur.

ARF, acute renal failure; Ca^{2+}, calcium; *DTR*, deep tendon reflex; *ECG*, electrocardiogram; HCO_3^-, bicarbonate; *HR*, heart rate; *I&O*, intake and output; *IV*, intravenous; K^+, potassium; *LOC*, level of consciousness; Mg^{2+}, magnesium; Na^+, sodium; *OTC*, over-the-counter; *SOB*, shortness of breath; *VS*, vital signs.

ASSESSMENT

Goal of Assessment

Evaluate fluid, electrolyte, and acid-base balances to prevent the development of metabolic encephalopathy (see *Genitourinary Assessment: General*, p. 583).

History and Risk Factors

Chronic illness (e.g., hypertension, diabetes, cardiomyopathy, peripheral vascular disease), recent infections or sepsis (e.g., streptococcal), recent episodes of hypotension (e.g., major bleeding, septic shock, major surgery), exposure to nephrotoxins (e.g., carbon tetrachloride, diuretics, aminoglycoside antibiotics, contrast media), recent blood transfusion, urinary tract disorders, toxemia of pregnancy or abortion, recent severe muscle damage (e.g., rhabdomyolysis with myoglobinuria), crush injury, and burn trauma

Prerenal Presentation

- Oliguric or nonoliguric
- Urinary sodium (Na^+) less than 20 mEq/L
- Elevated specific gravity
- Increased urine osmolality
- Normal or mildly abnormal sediment with the presence of hyaline and granular casts
- Elevated plasma BUN/creatinine ratio (greater than 20:1)

Intrarenal Presentation

- Oliguric or nonoliguric
- Urinary Na^+ greater than 20 mEq/L
- Low specific gravity
- Decreased urinary osmolality
- Markedly abnormal sediment with red blood cell (RBC) casts and cellular debris in the urine
- Decreased plasma BUN/creatinine ratio (10:1)
- Most common cause of ARF/AKI

Postrenal Presentation

- Urinary chemical indices are ineffective in determining postrenal failure
- Likely oliguric but may be nonoliguric
- Normal or mildly abnormal sediment (hematuria, pyuria, and crystals)
  - Often associated with urinary tract or pelvic cancer
  - Often associated with renal/ureteral calculi

Vital Signs

- BP may be elevated in states of fluid volume excess or decreased in states of fluid volume deficit.
- Heart rate (HR) may be increased or decreased with abnormal rhythms based on fluid and electrolyte abnormalities.
- Weight may be increased or decreased based on fluid volume status.
- Temperature: May be hyperthermic or hypothermic if patient is septic

Observation

- Peripheral edema and periorbital edema
- Jugular venous distention
- Shortness of breath
- Kussmaul respirations
- Poor skin turgor, flushed skin, and dry mucous membranes
- Pallor
- Purpura
- Weakness
- Altered mental status and disorientation
- Signs of central nervous system depression
- Neuromuscular dysfunction
- Asterixis

Palpation
- Edema (scale 0 to 4+): extremities and sacrum
- Muscle tenderness
- Suprapubic tenderness or distention
- Flank tenderness

Auscultation
- S_3 and S_4 gallops indicative of heart failure
- Pericardial friction rub
- Tachycardia or dysrhythmias
- Pulsus paradoxus in the presence of fluid volume excess
- Crackles
- Bruits over the renal arteries indicative of renovascular disease

Uremic Manifestations
- Accumulation of urea, creatinine, and uric acid
- Anemia and bleeding tendencies
- Fatigue and pallor
- Increased BP
- CHF
- Pericarditis with tamponade
- Pulmonary edema
- Anorexia, nausea, vomiting and diarrhea
- Behavioral changes
- Decreased wound-healing ability
- Increased susceptibility to infection

Screening Labwork
Blood and urine studies will determine the level of renal dysfunction and can provide clues to the cause of ARF/AKI.
- *BUN and creatinine:* Elevations indicative of renal impairment
- *GFR:* Most reliable estimation of renal function using 24-hour creatinine clearance or laboratory estimation, which is part of renal panel in most laboratories
- *Electrolyte levels:* Elevated or decreased potassium, phosphorus, magnesium, sodium
- *Urinalysis:* Presence of sediment including tubular epithelial cells, debris, casts, protein, RBC casts, or myoglobin
- *Urinary sodium:* Prerenal disease results in urinary sodium levels less than 10 mEq/L
- *CBC and coagulation studies (PT, PTT):* Evaluate for hematologic complications.
- *Arterial blood gas (ABG) values:* Evaluate for metabolic acidosis associated with ARF/AKI.

Diagnostic Tests For Acute Renal Failure (ARF)/Acute Kidney Injury (AKI)		
Test	**Purpose**	**Abnormal Findings**
Ultrasonography	Provides general appearance, size and scarring	Small scarred kidneys Renal mass Kidney stones Hydronephrosis
Radionuclide renal scan	Evaluate renal perfusion	Renal thromboemboli Tumors or cysts Asymmetry of blood flow
Magnetic resonance imaging	More specific in detecting renal masses and vessel malformations	Tumors or cysts Vessel malformation

Diagnostic Tests for Acute Renal Failure (ARF)/Acute Kidney Injury (AKI)—cont'd

Test	Purpose	Abnormal Findings
Retrograde or antegrade pyelography	Diagnose partial or complete obstruction	Ureteric or ureteral stenosis or obstruction
Renal angiography	Evaluate renal vessels	Thrombotic, stenotic lesions in the main renal vessels
Renal biopsy	Determine intrarenal pathology	Acute glomerulonephritis, vasculitis, or interstitial nephritis
Blood Studies		
Complete blood count (CBC) Hemoglobin (Hgb) Hematocrit (Hct) RBC count (RBCs) WBC count (WBCs)	Assess for anemia, inflammation, and infection; assists with differential diagnosis of septic cause of ARF/AKI	Decreased RBCs, Hgb, or Hct reflects anemia or recent blood loss.
Coagulation profile Prothrombin time (PT) with international normalized ratio (INR) Partial thromboplastin time (PTT)	Assess for the presence of bleeding or clotting and disseminated intravascular coagulation (DIC)	Decreased PT with low INR promotes clotting; elevation promotes bleeding.
Blood urea nitrogen (BUN) Creatinine Estimated glomerular filtration rate (eGFR)	Assess for the severity of renal dysfunction	Elevation indicates renal dysfunction. Creatinine may be markedly elevated in the presence of massive skeletal muscle injury (e.g., multiple trauma, crush injuries). BUN is influenced by hydration, catabolism, GI bleeding, infection fever, and corticosteroid therapy. The eGFR in ARF/AKI is usually less than 50 ml/min.
Electrolytes Potassium (K^+) Sodium (Na^+) Calcium (Ca^{2+}) Magnesium (Mg^{2+})	Assess for abnormalities associated with ARF/AKI	Increase or decrease in K^+ may cause arrhythmias. Elevated Na^+ may indicate dehydration. Decreased Na^+ may indicate fluid retention. Low Mg^{2+} or Ca^{2+} may cause dysrhythmias.
Arterial blood gases (ABGs)	Assess for the presence of metabolic acidosis	Low $Paco_2$ and plasma pH values reflect metabolic acidosis.
Urinalysis	Assess for the presence of sediment	Presence of sediment containing tubular epithelial cells, cellular debris, and tubular casts supports diagnosis of ARF/AKI. Increased protein and many RBC casts are common in intrarenal disease. Sediment is normal in prerenal causes. Large amounts of myoglobin may be present in severe skeletal muscle injury or rhabdomyolysis
Urinary sodium	Differentiate prerenal from intrarenal cause	Urinary Na^+ is less than 20 mEq/L in prerenal causes. Urinary Na^+ is more than 20 mEq/L in intrarenal causes.

COLLABORATIVE MANAGEMENT
Care Priorities for All ARF/AKI Pathologies

The major priorities for all patients with ARF/AKI regardless of etiology are the assessment of the contributing causes of the initial injury, identification of the clinical course with an emphasis on comorbidities, assessment of volume status, and prevention of further deterioration in renal function (Table 6-5).

1. **Maintain hydration:**
   a. Use of pulmonary artery catheters to measure filling pressures, cardiac output, and systemic vascular resistance to determine volume status
   b. In preoperative patients, to prevent kidney hypoperfusion and ischemia
   c. Adjust dose of nephrotoxic agents based on patient's GFR and serum levels.
   d. Hydration prior to radiographic studies and the use of acetylcysteine (Mucomyst) before and after the administration of contrast. Acetylcysteine is an antioxidant with vasodilatory properties and may minimize vasoconstriction and oxygen free radical generation from radiocontrast materials.
   e. Normal saline administration in patient with rhabdomyolysis to maintain urine output of 200 to 300 ml/hr

Table 6-5	MANAGEMENT CONSIDERATIONS: ACUTE RENAL FAILURE (ARF)/ACUTE KIDNEY INJURY (AKI)
Treatment	**Rationale**
Volume replacement for dehydration	Replacement solutions include free water plus electrolytes lost through urine, wounds, drainage tubes, diarrhea, and vomiting. Usually losses are replaced on a volume-for-volume basis. Maintenance fluid approximately 1500 ml/24 hr. With moderate fluid deficit (5% weight loss), at least 2400 ml/24 hr. Severe deficit (more than 5% weight loss) requires replacement of at least 3000 ml/24 hr.
Forced alkaline diuresis	Use of mannitol or sodium bicarbonate solution to manage pigmenturia (myoglobinuria, hemoglobinuria) due to rhabdomyolysis or severe crush or skeletal muscle injury. In addition, aggressive volume replacement to maintain renal perfusion pressure and reduce cast formation leading to renal tubular obstruction.
Diuretics (furosemide, bumetanide, torsemide, ethacrynic acid)	Decrease filtrate reabsorption and enhance water excretion. Use only after adequate hydration to increase urine output or in an attempt to prevent onset of oliguria. If volume overload is present, they are used to prevent pulmonary edema. Osmotic diuretics such as mannitol may be used to increase intravascular volume, promote renal blood flow, increase glomerular filtration rate, and stimulate urinary output. See Table 6-7.
Dopamine	Controversial treatment: Low doses usually less than 2 mcg/kg/min used to stimulate dopaminergic receptors, encourage renal vasodilatation, and promote renal blood flow. Studies have shown that this approach is ineffective if the patient remains oliguric. Doses of 3-10 mcg/kg/min are used to stimulate beta$_1$ receptors resulting in improved BP, cardiac output, and urine output. Doses greater than 10 mcg/kg/min may cause damaging renal vasoconstriction. May increase urine output in critically ill patients, but it neither prevents nor improves ARF. Increased diuresis may actually increase the risk of ARF in normovolemic and hypovolemic patients. Potentially detrimental effect of dopamine on splanchnic oxygen uptake Decreased GI motility Diminished respiratory drive
Nesiritide	Synthetic BNP (brain natruretic peptide), which results in vasodilatation, natriuresis, diuresis, and decreased renin-angiotensin activity, resulting in lower pulmonary artery occlusive pressure, decreased systemic vascular resistance, and increased cardiac output and cardiac index. Used to manage heart failure associated with prerenal azotemia. Increased cardiac output augments renal perfusion. Meta-analyses have revealed there is increased mortality and increased renal dysfunction with use of nesiritide compared to other medications.

Table 6-5	MANAGEMENT CONSIDERATIONS: ACUTE RENAL FAILURE (ARF)/ACUTE KIDNEY INJURY (AKI)—cont'd
Treatment	**Rationale**
Management of hyperkalemia	Intravenous calcium gluconate 10% or calcium chloride 10% (1 g of calcium chloride does not provide an equivalent dose to 1 g gluconate) (immediate onset) infusion of glucose, insulin, bicarbonate (20- to 60-minute onset) Inhaled albuterol (30- to 60-minute onset), sodium polystyrene sulfonate (Kayexalate) with sorbitol enema (1- to 4-hour onset). Hemodialysis (1- to 3-hour onset) may be used for control of elevated potassium.
Removal or discontinuation of toxin	Agents such as aminoglycoside antibiotics or angiotensin-converting enzyme (ACE) inhibitors used for blood pressure control and heart failure prevention; and nonsteroidal anti-inflammatory drugs (NSAIDs) used for pain management, must be discontinued or removed.
Prevention of contrast-induced nephropathy	Hydration, oral or IV Mucomyst (N-acetylcysteine) may be used before sending borderline or patients with renal insufficiency for radiologic procedures requiring contrast media. Aggressive hydration and possible IV mannitol after the procedure may also assist in clearing contrast from the patient. Intravenous fenoldopam (e.g., Corlopam) is no longer recommended in this setting.
Renal replacement therapy	Maintain homeostasis (see *Continuous Renal Replacement Therapies*, p. 603).
Nutrition therapy	Diet high in carbohydrates and with catabolic patients, essential and nonessential amino acids to prevent endogenous protein catabolism and muscle breakdown; low in sodium for individuals who retain sodium and water, high in sodium for those who have lost large volumes of sodium and water as a result of diuresis or other body drainage; low in potassium if the patient is retaining potassium; and if not catabolic, low in protein to maintain daily requirements while minimizing increases in azotemia. Nutrition is delivered via oral, enteral, or total parenteral nutrition (TPN). (See Box 1-4 for a list of foods high in sodium and Box 1-5 for a list of foods high in potassiums.)
Hematologic problems	Packed RBCs are given to maintain Hct. Anemia caused by decreased erythropoietin, low-grade GI bleeding from mucosal ulceration, blood drawing, and shortened life of the RBCs. Erythropoietin is used for primary prevention and treatment of anemia. Prolonged bleeding time is caused by decreased platelet adhesiveness.
Pharmacotherapy	Antihypertensives (see Table 5-22): phosphate binders (calcium carbonate antacids, calcium acetate) to bind phosphorus and control hyperphosphatemia and hypermagnesemia are given with meals. Sodium bicarbonate is given to control metabolic acidosis and promote the shift of potassium back into the cells. Water-soluble vitamin supplements are given to patients on dialytic therapy.
Relief of obstruction	Achieved via catheterization with indwelling urinary catheter or nephrostomy tube, or ureteral stent to relieve obstruction prior to surgical intervention or lithotripsy to disintegrate stones.

2. **Maintain kidney perfusion:**
   a. Vasoactive agents such as low-dose dopamine are no longer shown to improve kidney function; consider nesiritide (synthetic BNP) infusion.
   b. Debate continues on the effectiveness of crystalloids versus colloids.
   c. *Correction of fluid and electrolyte and acid-base balance (judiciously monitor for hyperkalemia and hyperphosphatemia)*
   d. Consider forced alkaline diuresis for patients with crush injuries or rhabdomyolysis.
3. **Minimize exposure to nephrotoxic agents:**
   a. Antibiotics
   b. Radiocontrast material
   c. NSAIDs

4. **Nutritional support:** Maintain nutrients essential for cellular reproduction and mitigate the response to insult and effects of acute illness.
5. **Continued assessment and monitoring of kidney function and modification of interventions as appropriate decrease the potential for infections:** skin, respiratory, and indwelling line and catheter care.
6. **Initiation of renal replacement therapy:** Renal replacement therapies include hemodialysis and continuous renal replacement therapies.
   a. Refractory fluid overload
   b. Hyperkalemia
   c. Metabolic acidosis
   d. Uncontrolled azotemia
   e. Drug overdose

 Safety Alert *See Table 6-6 for a list of common medications that require dosage modification for patients with ARF/AKI. Drugs that require dosage modification in renal failure are those that are excreted primarily by the kidneys. Dosage must be governed by clinical responses, as well as serum levels, if available. Nephrotoxic drugs should be avoided (Box 6-1). Also avoid drugs that are toxic to other organs if they accumulate—those that aggravate uremic symptoms and those that contribute to metabolic derangements of renal injury. Diuretics must be used judiciously in patients with ARF/AKI. See Table 6-7 for a detailed explanation of the use of diuretics.*

Table 6-6	**DRUGS THAT REQUIRE DOSAGE MODIFICATION IN RENAL FAILURE**			
Antimicrobials	**Cardiovascular Agents**	**Analgesics**	**Sedatives**	**Miscellaneous**
Amikacin	ACE inhibitors	Meperidine	Meprobamate	Cimetidine
Amphotericin B	Digitoxin	Methadone	Phenobarbital	Clofibrate
Chloramphenicol	Digoxin			Glycoprotein IIB, IIIA inhibitors
Ethambutol	Guanethidine			Insulin
Gentamicin	Procainamide			Neostigmine
Kanamycin				NSAIDs
Lincomycin				Platelet inhibitors
Penicillins				Promethazine
Promethazine				
Sulfonamides				
Tobramycin				
Vancomycin				

ACE, angiotensin-converting enzyme; *NSAIDs*, nonsteroidal anti-inflammatory drugs.

Box 6-1	**DRUGS TO AVOID IN RENAL FAILURE**

- Amiloride
- Aspirin
- Cisplatin
- Lithium carbonate
- Magnesium-containing medications (see Table 1-9)
- Nitrofurantoin
- Nonsteroidal anti-inflammatory drugs (e.g., ibuprofen)
- Phenylbutazone
- Spironolactone
- Tetracycline

Table 6-7	DIURETIC USE IN ACUTE RENAL FAILURE	
Types	**Mechanisms of Action**	**Potential Fluid and Electrolyte Abnormalities**
Osmotic Diuretics		
Mannitol Urea	Increase osmotic pressure of the filtrate, which attracts water and electrolytes and prevents their reabsorption	Hyponatremia Hypokalemia Rebound volume expansion
Loop Diuretics		
Furosemide Ethacrynic acid Bumetanide Torsemide	Inhibit reabsorption of Na^+ and Cl^- at the ascending loop of Henle in the medulla; they produce a vasodilatory effect on the renal vasculature	Hypokalemia Hyperuricemia Hypocalcemia Hyperglycemia and impairment of glucose tolerance Dilutional hyponatremia Hypochloremic acidosis
Thiazides		
Bendroflumethiazide Benzthiazide Chlorothiazide sodium Hydrochlorothiazide Hydroflumethiazide Polythiazide Trichlormethiazide	Inhibit Na^+ in the ascending loop of Henle at the beginning of the distal loop	Hypokalemia Dilutional hyponatremia Hypercalcemia Metabolic alkalosis Hypochloremia Hyperuricemia Hyperglycemia and impaired glucose tolerance
Thiazide-like Diuretics		
Chlorthalidone Indapamide Metolazone Quinethazone	Action same as thiazides	Same as thiazides
Potassium-sparing Diuretics*		
Amiloride HCl Spironolactone Triamterene	Inhibit aldosterone effect on the distal tubule, causing Na^+ excretion and K^+ reabsorption	Hyperkalemia Hyponatremia Dehydration Acidosis Transient increase in BUN
Carbonic Anhydrase-inhibitors		
Acetazolamide sodium Dichlorphenamide Methazolamide	Block the action of the enzyme carbonic anhydrase, producing excretion of Na^+, K^+, HCO_3^-, and water	Hyperchloremic acidosis Hypokalemia Hyperuricemia

Note: Loop or osmotic diuretics (or a combination of both) are used in patients with acute renal failure to prevent hypervolemia and to stimulate urinary output.
*Used with caution in patients with oliguria.
BUN, blood urea nitrogen; Cl^-, chloride; HCO_3^-, bicarbonate; K^+, potassium; Na^+, sodium.

CARE PLANS FOR ACUTE RENAL FAILURE/ACUTE KIDNEY INJURY

Excess fluid volume *related to inability of kidney to normally excrete urine*

GOALS/OUTCOMES Within 24 to 48 hours of onset, patient becomes normovolemic as evidenced by balanced intake and output (I&O), urinary output greater than 0.5 ml/kg/hr, body weight within patient's normal range, BP within patient's normal range, central venous pressure (CVP) 2 to 6 mm Hg, HR 60 to 100 beats/min (bpm), and absence of edema, crackles, gallop, and other clinical indicators of fluid overload.

NOC Fluid Overload Severity; Fluid Balance

Safety Alert *Although patient is retaining sodium, his or her serum sodium level may be within normal limits or decreased from baseline because of the dilutional effect of the fluid overload.*

Fluid Management

1. Document I&O hourly. Consult physician or midlevel practitioner if urinary output falls to less than 0.5 ml/kg/hr.
2. Weigh patient daily; consult physician or midlevel practitioner regarding significant weight gain (e.g., 0.5 to 1.5 kg/24 hr.
3. Assess for and document the presence of basilar crackles, jugular vein distention, tachycardia, pericardial friction rub, gallop, increased BP, increased CVP, or shortness of breath (SOB), any of which are indicative of fluid volume overload. Chronic heart failure may require additional support measures to help resolve ARF.
4. Assess for and document the presence of peripheral, sacral, or periorbital edema.
5. Restrict patient's total fluid intake to 1200 to 1500 ml/24 hr or as prescribed. Measure all output accurately, and replace milliliter for milliliter at intervals of 4 to 8 hours or as prescribed.
6. Provide ice chips, chewing gum, or hard candy to help patient quench thirst and moisten mouth.
7. Monitor serum osmolality and serum sodium values. These values may be decreased because of the dilutional effect of fluid overload.
8. Recognize that if it is delivered, total parenteral nutrition (TPN) will provide the largest volume of fluid intake for the patient. If total fluid intake is greater than 2000 ml/day, ultrafiltration (UF) with hemodialysis or continuous renal replacement therapy (CRRT) (continuous venovenous hemofiltration [CVVH], continuous venovenous hemodialysis [CVVHD], continuous venovenous hemodiafiltration [CVVHDF], slow continuous ultrafiltration [SCUF], or continuous arteriovenous hemofiltration [CAVH]) may be necessary to maintain fluid and electrolyte balance (see *Continuous Renal Replacement Therapies*, p. 603).
9. If patient is retaining sodium, restrict sodium-containing foods (see Table 6-8, p. 604) and avoid diluting IV medications with high-sodium diluents. Also avoid sodium-containing medications such as sodium penicillin.

NIC Electrolyte Management: Hypokalemia; Electrolyte Management: Hyponatremia; Fluid/Electrolyte Management; Fluid Management; Fluid Monitoring. Additional, optional interventions include Dysrhythmia Management; Hemodialysis Therapy; Hemodynamic Regulation; Invasive Hemodynamic Monitoring; Medication Management; Positioning; Skin Surveillance; and Weight Management

 Deficient fluid volume *related to overdiuresis and/or dehydration resulting in acute kidney injury*

GOALS/OUTCOMES Within 24 hours of this diagnosis, patient becomes normovolemic as evidenced by balanced I&O, urinary output greater than 0.5 ml/kg/hr, CVP 2 to 6 mm Hg, HR 60 to 100 bpm, BP within patient's normal range, and absence of thirst and other indicators of hypovolemia. Patient's weight stabilizes within 2 to 3 days.

NOC Hydration; Fluid Balance

Hypovolemia Management

1. Weigh patient daily. Consult physician or midlevel practitioner for weight loss of 1 to 1.5 kg/24 hr.
2. Monitor and document I&O hourly. Consult physician if patient's output is less than 0.5 ml/kg/hr. With a deficit, intake should exceed output by 0.5 to 1 L (depending on severity of dehydration).
3. Consult physician or midlevel practitioner for increase in losses from vomiting, diarrhea, or wound drainage or sudden onset of diuresis.

4. Observe for and document indicators of dehydration and hypovolemia (e.g., poor skin turgor, dry and sticky mucous membranes, thirst, hypotension, tachycardia, decreasing CVP, increasing BUN and creatinine).
5. Encourage oral fluids if they are allowed. Ensure that IV fluid rates are maintained as prescribed.
6. Approximately 20% of patients with ARF have GI bleeding. Monitor hemoglobin (Hgb), hematocrit (Hct), and BUN levels. In the presence of bleeding with ARF, Hgb and Hct values will fall steadily, and they will fall rapidly if there is massive bleeding.

 Safety Alert *A patient with ARF may have an Hct in the range of 20% to 30% if prerenal azotemia has occurred over time. Anemia occurs as a result of prolonged renal insufficiency leading to failure. BUN will increase in the presence of GI bleeding without a concomitant rise in serum creatinine level.*

---

7. Test all stools, emesis, and peritoneal dialysate drainage for occult blood. Check urine and dialysate drainage at least every 8 hours.
8. To minimize the risk of bleeding, keep side rails up, minimize invasive procedures, use small-gauge needles for injections, minimize blood drawing, and promote the use of electric razors and soft-bristle toothbrushes. If possible, avoid intramuscular (IM) or subcutaneous injections for 1 hour after hemodialysis. Apply gentle pressure to injection sites for at least 2 to 3 minutes.
9. Inspect gums, mouth, nose, skin, and perianal and vaginal areas every 8 hours for bleeding. Also inspect hemodialysis insertion and/or peritoneal access sites for bleeding every 8 hours. Apply a soft, occlusive, sterile dressing to access sites to protect the skin from irritation and bleeding caused by catheter movement.

Imbalanced nutrition, less than body requirements *related to the adverse effects of acute kidney injury on digestion and absorption of nutrients*

GOALS/OUTCOMES Within 72 hours of this diagnosis, patient has adequate nutritional intake as evidenced by a caloric intake that ranges from 35 to 45 calories (cal)/kg normal body weight, a daily protein intake that consists of 50% to 75% high–biologic value proteins, and a nitrogen intake of 4 to 6 g greater than nitrogen loss (calculated from 24-hour urinary urea excretion and protein intake).
NOC Nutritional Status

Nutrition Therapy
1. Infuse enteral feedings and TPN as prescribed.
2. Assess and document patient's intake of nutrients every shift.
3. Weigh patient daily. Consult physician or midlevel practitioner for significant findings (e.g., loss of greater than 1.5 kg/24 hr).
4. Control nausea and anorexia using small, frequent meals. Present appetizing food in a pleasant atmosphere; eliminate any noxious odors. As indicated, administer medication with prescribed antiemetic 30 minutes before meals.
5. Control catabolism:
   - *Manage fever.* As prescribed, use cooling blanket or antipyretic agents to control fever. Fever increases tissue catabolism, which in turn increases metabolic needs. Critically ill patients are often catabolic and require careful nutritional management, especially when either hemodialysis, peritoneal dialysis, or CRRT is implemented. Supplementation with 10 to 20 g/day essential and nonessential amino acids may be needed. The end products of protein metabolism that accumulate in renal failure are reflected by an increase in BUN level. Ensure intake of protein with high biologic value (e.g., eggs, meat, fowl, milk, fish), which contains essential amino acids necessary for cell building.
   - *Provide adequate calories.* Be sure that caloric intake ranges from 30 to 60 cal/kg normal body weight for a critically ill adult in ARF. The exact amount will vary with age, gender, activity, and the degree of preexisting malnutrition. Foods that may be used to increase caloric intake include fats and concentrated carbohydrates.
6. Manage electrolytes:
   - *Restrict high-potassium foods* such as bananas, citrus fruits, potatoes, fruit juices, nuts, tea, coffee, legumes, and salt substitute. In ARF, the kidneys are unable to excrete potassium effectively.
   - *Assess sodium requirement,* since it will vary greatly. If oliguria is present, sodium intake may be restricted in the diet. If diuresis is present, sodium intake may be increased because of excess sodium loss in the urine. Intervene accordingly.

- *Measure ionized calcium* to avoid inappropriate treatment of malnourished patients whose values may appear falsely low due to serum calcium being bound to albumin, which is decreased in patients with renal failure.
- *Treat hypocalcemia if present early in ARF* as a result of decreased absorption of calcium from the gut and the presence of hyperphosphatemia. Replace calcium orally (e.g., with dairy products, Tums) or intravenously and administer phosphate binders as prescribed.

NIC Nutrition Management; Nutritional Monitoring; Fluid Management; Fluid Monitoring. Additional, optional NIC interventions include: Bowel Management; Energy Management; Enteral Tube Feeding; Exercise Promotion; Gastrointestinal Intubation; Hyperglycemia Management; Hypoglycemia Management; Intravenous Insertion; Intravenous Therapy; Medication Management; Mutual Goal Setting; Phlebotomy: Venous Blood Sample; Positioning; Teaching: Individual; Teaching: Prescribed Diet; Total Parenteral Nutrition Administration; and Venous Access Devices Maintenance.

Risk for infection *related to immunocompromised state associated with renal failure*

GOALS/OUTCOMES At the time of discharge from the intensive care unit (ICU), patient is free of infection as evidenced by normothermia, negative culture results of dialysate and body secretions, and white blood cell (WBC) count less than 11,000/mm³.
NOC Immune Status

Safety Alert *After the initial insult, infection is the primary cause of death in ARF.*

Infection Protection
1. Monitor and record patient's temperature every 8 hours. If it is elevated (i.e., greater than 37°C [98.6°F]), monitor temperature every 4 hours. Because ARF may be accompanied by hypothermia, even a slight rise in temperature of 1° to 2° may be significant especially if on CRRT as it is an extracorporeal therapy.
2. Inspect and record the color, odor, and appearance of all body secretions. Be alert to cloudy or blood-tinged peritoneal dialysate return, cloudy and foul-smelling urine, foul-smelling wound exudate, purulent drainage from any catheter site, foul-smelling and watery stools, foul-smelling vaginal discharge, or purulent sputum.
3. Be aware that uremia retards wound healing; therefore, it is important that all wounds (including scratches resulting from pruritus) be assessed for indicators of infection. Send samples of any suspicious fluid or drainage for culture and sensitivity (C&S) tests as indicated.
4. Monitor WBC count for elevations, and obtain specimens for C&S as prescribed.
5. Use aseptic technique when manipulating central lines, peripheral IV lines, and indwelling catheters. Avoid use of indwelling urinary catheter in patients with oliguria and anuria. The presence of a catheter in these patients further increases the risk of infection.
6. Be aware that catabolism of protein, which occurs with infection, causes potassium to be released from the tissues.
7. Provide oral hygiene every 2 hours to help maintain the integrity of the oral mucous membranes.
8. Reposition patient every 2 to 4 hours to help maintain the barrier of an intact integumentary system. Provide skin care at least every 8 hours.
9. Encourage good pulmonary hygiene by having patient practice deep-breathing exercises (and coughing, if indicated) every 2 to 4 hours.

NIC Infection Control. Additional, optional interventions include Airway Management; Exercise Promotion and Therapy (all listed); Medication Management; Respiratory Monitoring; Teaching: Disease Process; Tube Care: Urinary; and Vital Signs Monitoring.

Deficient knowledge *related to disease process of acute renal failure*

GOALS/OUTCOMES Within 72 hours of admission, patient and significant others verbalize accurate information regarding patient's disease state and the measures that can be taken to prevent its occurrence or minimize its effects.
NOC Knowledge: Disease Process

Teaching: Disease Process

1. Determine patient's and significant others' knowledge about patient's disease process and the biochemical alterations (hyperkalemia, hypokalemia, hypernatremia, hyponatremia, hypocalcemia, hyperphosphatemia, hypermagnesemia, metabolic acidosis, and uremia) that can occur.
2. Teach patient and significant others the signs and symptoms of the biochemical alterations (see Table 6-4 and care plan for *Infection Protection*, p. 600).
3. Provide lists of foods high in potassium (see Box 1-5), sodium (see Box 1-4), phosphorus (see Box 1-6), and magnesium (see Box 1-7), which patient should add or avoid when planning meals. In addition, provide a list of medications that contain magnesium (see Table 1-9), which should not be taken without physician or midlevel practitioner approval.
4. Explain the importance of consuming only the amount of protein prescribed by physician and avoiding exposure to persons with infection or a febrile illness to minimize catabolism of protein, which causes potassium to be released from the tissues. Reinforce that patient should consume the prescribed diet and limit strenuous activity as prescribed, both of which will spare protein and thus minimize potassium release.
5. Teach patient to report to physician or midlevel practitioner an increase in temperature or other signs of infection.
6. Reinforce the importance of taking vitamin D and calcium supplements as prescribed.
7. Teach the relationship between calcium and phosphate levels. Emphasize that maintaining good phosphate control and calcium balance may help control itching and prevent future problems with bone disease.
8. Stress the importance of taking phosphate binders (e.g., Amphojel, Alternagel, PhosLo) as prescribed and to avoid antacids containing magnesium (e.g., Maalox, Milk of Magnesia).
9. Teach patient not to take over-the-counter (OTC) medications without first consulting physician. Aspirin, for example, exacerbates the bleeding tendency caused by uremia.
10. Instruct patient about the importance of maintaining the prescribed dialysis schedule, inasmuch as dialysis will help correct acidosis, uremia, and many of the metabolic abnormalities that occur.
11. Teach patient to use lotions and oils to lubricate skin and relieve drying and cracking.
12. Stress the importance of follow-up monitoring of serum electrolyte levels.

NIC Teaching: Individual; Teaching: Prescribed Medication. Additional, optional interventions include Discharge Planning; Medication Management; and Weight Management.

Acute confusion *related to altered level of consciousness which results from fluid and electrolyte imbalance and/or uremia*

- -

GOALS/OUTCOMES Within 48 to 72 hours of onset, patient verbalizes orientation to time, place, and person and maintains his or her normal mobility.
NOC Neurologic Status

Neurologic Monitoring

1. Monitor patient for the following mentation and motor dysfunctions associated with ARF:
   - *Hyperkalemia* (during oliguric phase): muscle weakness, irritability, paresthesias
   - *Hypokalemia* (during diuretic phase): lethargy; muscle weakness, softness, flabbiness; paresthesias
   - *Hypernatremia:* fatigue, restlessness, agitation
   - *Hyponatremia:* dizziness when changing position, apprehension, personality changes, agitation, confusion
   - *Hypocalcemia:* neuromuscular irritability, tonic muscle spasms, paresthesias
   - *Hyperphosphatemia:* excessive itching, muscle weakness, hyperreflexia
   - *Hypermagnesemia:* drowsiness, lethargy, sensation of heat
   - *Metabolic acidosis:* confusion, weakness
   - *Uremia:* confusion, lethargy, itching, metallic taste, muscle twitching
2. Explain to significant others that patient's decreasing attention level necessitates simple and direct communication efforts.
3. To alleviate unpleasant metallic taste caused by uremia, provide frequent oral hygiene. Because patient with uremia is at increased risk for bleeding, ensure use of soft-bristle brushes.
4. If appropriate, provide chewing gum or hard candy, which may help alleviate the unpleasant metallic taste.
5. Encourage isometric exercises and short walks, if patient is able, to help maintain muscle strength and tone, especially in the legs.
6. Decrease environmental stimuli, and use a calm, reassuring manner in caring for patient.
7. Encourage establishment of sleep/rest patterns by scheduling daytime activities appropriately and promoting relaxation method (see *Appendix 7*).

8. Assess for decreased tactile sensations in the feet and legs, which may occur with peripheral neuropathy. Be alert to the potential for pressure sores and friction burns, which may occur with peripheral neuropathy.
9. Use splints and braces to aid in mobility for patients with severe neuropathic effects.

NIC Additional, optional interventions include Nutrition Management; Nutrition Therapy; Nutritional Counseling; Pressure Management; Pressure Ulcer Prevention; and Teaching: Individual.

Constipation *related to fluid and electrolyte imbalance and reduced activity level*

GOALS/OUTCOMES Within 48 hours of onset, patient has bowel movements of soft consistency.
NOC Bowel Elimination

Constipation/Impaction Management
1. Monitor and record the number and quality of patient's bowel movements.
2. Administer prescribed stool softeners and bulking agents, such as psyllium husks.
3. If these measures fail, administer oil retention or tap water enemas as prescribed. Because excess fluid can be absorbed from the gut, avoid using large-volume water enemas.
4. Encourage moderate exercise on a routine basis.
5. Establish a regular schedule for fluid intake within patient's prescribed limits.
6. Administer metoclopramide as prescribed to increase motility in the presence of autonomic neuropathy.

NIC Additional optional interventions include Exercise Promotion; Medication Administration: Oral; Medication Management; Pain Management; and Skin Surveillance.

Impaired skin integrity *related to uremia*

GOALS/OUTCOMES Patient's skin remains intact.
NOC Tissue Integrity: Skin and Mucous Membranes

Pruritus Management
1. Monitor patient for presence of pruritus with resulting frequent and intense scratching. Pruritus decreases with reduced BUN level and control of hyperphosphatemia. Monitor laboratory values of BUN and phosphorus, and report levels outside the optimal range (BUN greater than 20 mg/dl and phosphorus greater than 4.5 mg/dl or less than 2.6 mEq/L). Pruritus increases in the presence of secondary hyperparathyroidism. Monitor serum calcium and PTH levels, and report elevations (Ca^{2+} greater than 10.5 mg/dL and PTH greater than 30% above the upper limit of the test used).
2. Administer phosphate binders (e.g., Alternagel) as prescribed, and, if possible, reduce patient's dietary intake of phosphorus (see Box 1-6).
3. Ensure that patient's fingernails are cut short and that the nail tips are smooth.
4. Because uremia retards wound healing, monitor scratches for indicators of infection.
5. Because of reduced oil gland activity associated with uremia, the patient's skin may be quite dry. Use skin emollients liberally, and avoid harsh soaps and excessive bathing.
6. Advise patient of the potential for bruising because of clotting abnormality and capillary fragility.
7. Administer oral antihistamine, such as diphenhydramine, to relieve itching as prescribed.

NIC Skin Surveillance; Pressure Ulcer Prevention. Additional, optional interventions include Bathing; Bleeding Reduction; Cutaneous Stimulation; Exercise Promotion and Therapy (all listed); Electrolyte Monitoring; Exercise Promotion: Stretching; Fluid/Electrolyte Management; Infection Control; Infection Protection; Medication Management; Nail Care; Nutrition Management; Perineal Care; Surveillance; and Vital Signs Monitoring.

ADDITIONAL NURSING DIAGNOSES

For patients undergoing dialytic therapy (conventional hemodialysis), see nursing diagnoses and interventions in *Continuous Renal Replacement Therapy*. Also see the following as appropriate: *Nutritional Support* (p. 117), *Prolonged Immobility* (p. 149), and *Emotional and Spiritual Support of the Patient and Significant Others* (p. 200).

CONTINUOUS RENAL REPLACEMENT THERAPIES

The patient with acute kidney injury may progress to a physiologic disequilibrium requiring renal support with a renal replacement therapy to prevent metabolic complications. CRRT has gained acceptance throughout Europe and the United States for the treatment of hemodynamically unstable patients who have not responded to conservative management and pharmacologic interventions. The initiation of this therapy is variable throughout institutions and physician practice. Patient characteristics that are considered include age, severity of illness, and existing comorbidities.

The goals of CRRT include:
1. Prevention of uremic complications
2. Acid-base balance
3. Electrolyte and volume homeostasis
4. Maintenance of cardiopulmonary function and hemodynamics
5. Maintenance of adequate nutritional support

The most common indications for CRRT include:
1. Hyperkalemia and other electrolyte disturbances refractory to medical management
2. Metabolic acidosis unresponsive to medical therapy
3. Intravascular volume excess refractory to diuretics
4. Uremic intoxication
   - Neurologic (encephalopathy)
   - Hematologic (bleeding caused by platelet dysfunction)
   - Gastrointestinal (anorexia, nausea, vomiting)
   - Cardiovascular (pericarditis)
5. Need for removal of dialyzable substances (metabolites, drugs, toxins)

Other indications for CRRT include:
1. Massive fluid overload: CHF, overaggressive fluid resuscitation in multiple trauma
2. Fluid overload in the presence of hemodynamic instability
3. Cardiogenic shock with pulmonary edema
4. Oliguric patient unresponsive to diuretics
5. Patient with anuria who requires large volumes of parenteral fluid: acts as a supplement to hemodialysis to maintain fluid balance

Indications for early initiation of CRRT include:
1. Possible impending electrolyte or acid-base disturbances
2. Presence of oliguria and the need for infusion of large volumes of fluid for medications or nutrition
3. Presence of AKI with a poor prognosis for immediate recovery
4. AKI in the presence of sepsis or systemic inflammatory response syndrome (SIRS)

PATHOPHYSIOLOGY

Historically, CRRT has evolved from an arteriovenous to a venovenous extracorporeal process to achieve solute and fluid removal in the critically ill patient. CRRT has been traditionally limited to the ICU setting based on the requirement for close hourly monitoring and fluid adjustments. The multiple acronyms and description of therapies are available in Table 6-8.

The principles of solute and water removal during CRRT are similar to other methods of renal replacement therapy (e.g., hemodialysis) and include diffusion, ultrafiltration, and convection. These therapies provide solute clearance and fluid removal slowly and continuously. Conventional hemodialysis is more aggressive and may not be tolerated in unstable patients.

Diffusion: Movement of solutes, including high concentrations of waste products and excess electrolytes, from an area of greater concentration to an area of lesser concentration. Diffusion requires a concentration gradient. During CRRT, high concentrations of these excess particles diffuse into the dialysate/effluent, which contains much lower concentrations of these solutes.

Ultrafiltration: Removal of water from the blood compartment of the hemofilter by generating a lower pressure in the effluent compartment. In hemodialysis, lower or negative pressure in the dialysate facilitates the rapid removal of excess water from the blood compartment in which positive or higher pressure exists.

Convection: Removal of a substance with fluid across a semipermeable membrane over time. This occurs in response to the pressure gradient across the membrane. Small molecules

Table 6-8	COMPARISON OF CONTINUOUS RENAL REPLACEMENT THERAPIES			
CAVH	**CAVHD**	**CVVH**	**CVVHD**	**SLEDD**
Access Route				
Arterial and venous catheters. Patient's mean arterial pressure drives flow rate.	Same as CAVH	Double-lumen venous catheter	Pump used to achieve adequate flow rate Pump used to achieve flow rate	Double-lumen venous catheter Same as CVVHD
Semipermeable Membrane				
High-efficiency, high-flux material (polysulfone, polyamide, and polyacrylonitrile)	Same as CAVH	Same as CAVH	Same as CAVH	Same as CAVH
Molecular Movement				
Convection	Convection and diffusion	Convection	Convection and diffusion	Convection and diffusion
Water Removal				
Ultrafiltration-hydrostatic pressure	Same as CAVH	Same as CAVH	Same as CAVH	Same as CAVH
Duration				
Continuous	Continuous	Continuous	Continuous	6 to 12 hours a day, 5 days a week
Efficiency				
High for fluid removal, moderate solute removal	High for fluid and solute removal	Same as CAVH	High for fluid and solute removal	High for fluid and solute removal
Risk of Infection				
High for access infection	Same as CAVH	High for access infection	Same as CAVH	Same as CAVH
Major Problem				
Dehydration and hypotension	Dehydration, hypotension, and electrolyte imbalance	Dehydration and hypotension	Dehydration, hypotension, and electrolyte imbalance	Dehydration, hypotension, and electrolyte imbalance

CAVH, continuous arteriovenous hemofiltration; *CVVH*, continuous venovenous hemofiltration; *CAVHD*, continuous arteriovenous hemodialysis; *CVVHD*, continuous venovenous hemodialysis; *SLEDD*, slow extended daily dialysis.

freely pass into the ultrafiltrate. Large molecule removal is dependent on the pore size of the membrane. However, larger molecules tend to move across these membranes better by convection than diffusion. Some elements in plasma water (e.g., urea) are conveyed across the membrane as a result of the differences in hydrostatic pressure. The removal of large amounts of plasma water results in the removal of large amounts of filterable solutes.

The availability of a wide variety of CRRT therapies, however, has not led to standards for initiation of therapy, dosage, choice of modality, or the intensity and duration of therapy. The use of a highly permeable membrane, the infusion of various types of replacement solution, and the continuous nature of each of the techniques make them highly effective and versatile in managing control of fluids. CRRT techniques can serve as a regulatory system for fluids without compromising metabolic balance. More recent literature suggests use of daily hemodialysis may provide equally effective therapy in AKI patients or for those with more complex disease processes who are unable to receive consistent therapy due to machine problems, including clotting of the hemofilter. Multiple interruptions in therapy can undermine the efficacy of CRRT, as the patient does not receive continuous therapy if the system is frequently alarming, which interrupts diffusion, ultrafiltration, and convection.

ASSESSMENT: PRE-CRRT
Goal of Assessment
Evaluate fluid, electrolyte, and acid-base balances to prevent the development of metabolic complications due to AKI.

History and Risk Factors
Chronic illness (e.g., hypertension, diabetes, cardiomyopathy, peripheral vascular disease), recent infections or sepsis (e.g., streptococcal), recent episodes of hypotension (e.g., major bleeding, septic shock, major surgery), exposure to nephrotoxins (e.g., carbon tetrachloride, diuretics, aminoglycoside antibiotics, contrast media), recent blood transfusion, urinary tract disorders, toxemia of pregnancy or abortion, recent severe muscle damage (e.g., rhabdomyolysis with myoglobinuria), crush injury, and burn trauma

Vital Signs
- BP may be elevated in states of fluid volume excess or decreased in states of fluid volume deficit.
- HR rate may be increased or decreased with abnormal rhythms based on fluid and electrolyte abnormalities.
- Baseline electrocardiogram (ECG) and rhythm
- Hemodynamic parameters of cardiac output (CO), cardiac index (CI), ejection fraction, CVP, and pulmonary artery wedge pressure (PAWP)
- Weight may be increased or decreased based on fluid volume status.
- Temperature: may be hyperthermic or hypothermic if patient is septic
- Pulse oximetry

Observation
- Peripheral edema and periorbital edema
- Jugular venous distention
- SOB
- Kussmaul respirations
- Poor skin turgor, flushed skin, and dry mucous membranes
- Pallor
- Purpura
- Weakness
- Altered mental status and disorientation
- Signs of central nervous system depression
- Neuromuscular dysfunction
- Asterixis
- Mechanical ventilation parameters
- Presence of any assist devices such as extracorporeal membrane oxygenator (ECMO)

Palpation
- Edema (scale 0 to 4+): extremities and sacrum
- Muscle tenderness
- Suprapubic tenderness or distention
- Flank tenderness

Auscultation
- S_3 and S_4 gallops indicative of heart failure
- Pericardial friction rub
- Tachycardia or dysrhythmias

- Pulsus paradoxus in the presence of fluid volume excess
- Crackles
- Bruits over the renal arteries indicative of renovascular disease

Uremic Manifestations
- Accumulation of urea, creatinine, and uric acid
- Anemia and bleeding tendencies
- Fatigue and pallor
- Increased BP
- CHF
- Pericarditis with tamponade
- Pulmonary edema
- Anorexia, nausea, vomiting, and diarrhea
- Behavioral changes
- Decreased wound-healing ability
- Increased susceptibility to infection

Screening Labwork
Blood and urine studies will determine the level of renal dysfunction and can provide clues to the cause of ARF/AKI.
- BUN, creatinine: elevations indicative of renal impairment
- GFR: most reliable estimation of renal function using 24-hour creatinine clearance or laboratory estimation, which is part of renal panel in most laboratories
- Electrolyte levels: elevated or decreased potassium, phosphorus, magnesium, sodium
- Urinalysis: presence of sediment including tubular epithelial cells, debris, casts, protein, RBC casts, or myoglobin
- Urinary sodium: prerenal disease results in urinary sodium less than 10 mEq/L
- CBC and coagulation studies (PT, PTT): evaluate for hematologic complications
- ABG values: evaluate for metabolic acidosis associated with ARF/AKI

Diagnostic Tests Used in Association with Continuous Renal Replacement Therapy
Blood Studies

Test	Purpose	Abnormal Findings
Complete blood count (CBC) Hemoglobin (Hgb) Hematocrit (Hct) RBC count (RBCs) WBC count (WBCs)	Assess for anemia, inflammation, and infection. Assists with differential diagnosis of septic cause of acute renal failure (ARF)/acute kidney injury (AKI).	Decreased RBCs, Hgb, or Hct reflects anemia or recent blood loss.
Coagulation profile Prothrombin time (PT) with international normalized ratio (INR) Partial thromboplastin time (PTT)	Assess for the presence of bleeding or clotting and disseminated intravascular coagulation (DIC).	Decreased PT with low INR promotes clotting. Elevation promotes bleeding.
Blood urea nitrogen (BUN) Creatinine Estimated glomerular filtration rate (eGFR)	Assess for the severity of renal dysfunction.	Elevation indicates renal dysfunction. Creatinine may be markedly elevated in the presence of massive skeletal muscle injury (e.g., multiple trauma, crush injuries). BUN is influenced by hydration, catabolism, GI bleeding, infection fever, and corticosteroid therapy. The eGFR in ARF/AKI is usually <50 ml/min.

Diagnostic Tests Used in Association with Continuous Renal Replacement Therapy Blood Studies—cont'd

Test	Purpose	Abnormal Findings
Electrolytes Potassium (K^+) Sodium (Na^+) Calcium (Ca^{2+}) Magnesium (Mg^{2+})	Assess for abnormalities associated with ARF/AKI.	Increase or decrease in K^+ may cause arrhythmias. Elevated Na^+ may indicate dehydration. Decreased Na^+ may indicate fluid retention. Low Mg^{2+} or Ca^{2+} may cause arrhythmias.
Arterial blood gases (ABGs)	Assess for the presence of metabolic acidosis.	Low $Paco_2$ and plasma pH values reflect metabolic acidosis.
Urinalysis	Assess for the presence of sediment.	Presence of sediment containing tubular epithelial cells, cellular debris, and tubular casts supports diagnosis of ARF/AKI. Increased protein and many RBC casts are common in intrarenal disease. Sediment is normal in prerenal causes. Large amounts of myoglobin may be present in severe skeletal muscle injury or rhabdomyolysis.
Urinary sodium	Differentiate prerenal from intrarenal cause.	Urinary Na^+ <20 mEq/L in prerenal causes. Urinary Na^+ >20 mEq/L in intrarenal causes.

DETERMINING TYPE AND MODALITY OF CRRT USED

The availability in the institution of CRRT and type and brand of equipment are part of the considerations that help determine the modality of CRRT used. Water, solutes, or water and solutes are able to be removed. All modalities use a highly permeable, hollow-fiber filter. Solutes removed are generally unbound substances, including urea, calcium, sodium, potassium, chloride, and vitamins, and unbound drugs with a molecular weight between 500 and 10,000 daltons. Types/modalities of CRRT include (see earlier):

- CVVH
- CVVHD
- CVVHDF
- SCUF
- CAVH
- SLEDD

Advantages and disadvantages of CRRT methods are found in Table 6-9. Complications of CRRT are found in Table 6-10.

CVVH, CVVHD, CVVHDF, SCUF, SLEDD, and CAVH are types of renal replacement therapy performed to manage fluid and solute overload in critically ill patients. Their advantage over conventional dialytic therapies is that ultrafiltration occurs more gradually, thus avoiding drastic volume changes and rapid fluid shifts. Treatment duration may be 6 to 24 hours or several days, depending on the total amount of fluid to be removed. The type best suited for each situation is chosen based on clinical status, including the ability to safely anticoagulate the patient and what type of vascular access is available. Catabolism, for example, causes rapid rises in BUN, creatinine, and potassium values. The patient needs rapid removal of metabolic wastes. These patients may require hemodialysis with supplemental CRRT (see Table 6-8). The use of CAVH requires that the patient have an average mean arterial blood pressure (MAP) of 70 mm Hg. Hypotensive patients will not benefit from CAVH but can benefit from CVVH (or any other venovenous therapy).

Table 6-9	ADVANTAGES AND DISADVANTAGES OF METHODS OF RENAL REPLACEMENT THERAPY	
Advantages		**Disadvantages**
SLEDD		
Very efficient; Modification of intermittent hemodialysis therapy by extending the time and slowing the rate of solute and fluid removal.		Special equipment and trained staff required Heparinization usually required Possible difficulty in maintaining vascular access Risk of blood loss necessitating transfusion
Continuous Arteriovenous Therapies		
Physiologic process Ideal for hemodynamically unstable patient Allows for administration of large volumes of fluid (e.g., TPN) MAP must be greater than 60 mm Hg		Must maintain MAP for effective process Must maintain an arterial and venous access, which becomes a problem in a restless patient Risk of blood loss if arterial line displaced Increased responsibilities for the ICU nurses
Continuous Venovenous Therapies		
Physiologic process ideal for the patient who is hemodynamically unstable Allows administration of large volumes (e.g., TPN) CVVH effective in patients with MAP less than 70 mm Hg		Low-efficiency solute removal unless CVVHD or CVVHDF Large-volume fluid replacement Potential for electrolyte imbalance Increased responsibilities for ICU nurses

Table 6-10	COMPLICATIONS OF RENAL REPLACEMENT THERAPIES
SLEDD	**Hemofiltration**
Hypotension	Bleeding
Air embolus	Infection
Angina and dysrhythmias	Volume depletion
Blood loss (dialyzer rupture)	Blood leakage
Infection	Decreased ultrafiltration
Hemolysis	Filter clotting
Hemorrhage	Electrolyte disturbances
Septicemia	Air embolus with CVVH
Clotting	Poor functioning vascular access
High-output heart failure	Hypothermia

CVVH, continuous venovenous hemofiltration.

Principles Applied to Specific Therapies

Ultrafiltration: For ultrafiltration to occur, there must be a pressure gradient across the membrane that favors filtration. The pressure in the blood compartment must exceed the pressure in the filtrate compartment of the hollow filter. In CAVH or CVVH/other venovenous hemofiltration therapies, this is called *transmembrane pressure (TMP)*. Its major determinants are hydrostatic pressure and oncotic pressure. The higher pressure in the blood compartment is a function of the individual's blood pressure when using CAVH. Pressure in the blood compartment is adequate when the MAP is 50 to 70 mm Hg. Higher pressures enhance ultrafiltration.

Venovenous therapies do not rely on the patient's blood pressure for ultrafiltration. Negative pressure for ultrafiltration can be achieved by lowering the collection container 20 to 40 cm below the hemofilter. The differences in hydrostatic pressure also cause the crossing of some elements, such as glucose and some vitamins. The longer it takes for blood to clear the filter, the more likely it is that intermediate molecules (vitamins, glucose) will be filtered out of the patient's system. Opposing the hydrostatic pressure is oncotic pressure, which is maintained by plasma proteins that do not pass through the membrane. When hydrostatic pressure exceeds oncotic pressure, filtration of water and solutes occurs.

Sieving coefficient (SC): Clearance of medication during CRRT is impacted by the SC of the drug as it passes through the membrane. The SC is equal to the ultrafiltrate concentration of the drug divided by the plasma concentration. Drugs that are more protein-bound have a lower clearance during CRRT. However, due to the long duration of CRRT, more of these drugs may be removed.

The amount of drug removed in milligrams is equal to:

$$\text{Ultrafiltrate concentration (mg/L)} \times \text{Ultrafiltration rate (L/min)} \times \text{Time of procedure (min)}$$

Procedure

The hemofilter and lines are primed with normal saline before the treatment is initiated. CAVH, CAVHD, and CAVHDF require cannulation of both an artery and a vein for blood flow. The femoral artery and vein are commonly used, but the subclavian vein can also be used for venous limb access. For the venovenous therapies (CVVH, CVVHD, CVVHDF, and SLEDD), a large double-lumen catheter is placed in the internal jugular, subclavian, or femoral vein. The catheters must have radiographic confirmation of placement prior to beginning therapy. Blood flows from the "arterial" or proximal limb of the vascular access through the filter and returns through the "venous" or distal limb of the access.

A continuous method of anticoagulation is necessary to prevent clotting in the lines and filter. Blood is driven through the system by the patient's blood pressure with CAVH, so no pump is used. With CVVH/other venovenous therapies, a pump is used to drive the blood flow. As the blood flows through the filter, water, electrolytes, and most drugs not bound to plasma protein diffuse across the membrane and thus become part of the filtrate.

If the objective is the removal of large amounts of fluid and solute (i.e., urea, potassium, creatinine), it is necessary to infuse large volumes of filtration replacement fluid (FRF) or replacement fluid to maintain electrolyte balance. Nursing responsibilities include initiating treatment, monitoring the patient and the system, and discontinuing treatment. Tables 6-9 and 6-10 discuss the advantages, disadvantages, and complications of CRRTs. Table 6-11 discusses troubleshooting major problems with CRRT.

Table 6-11	TROUBLESHOOTING MAJOR PROBLEMS IN CONTINUOUS RENAL REPLACEMENT THERAPY	
Problem	**Cause**	**Intervention**
Hypotension	Cardiac dysfunction Excessive intravascular volume removal	Cardiotonic and pressor support Fluid replacement Recalculate UF rate
Poor ultrafiltration	High Hct Decreased MAP Clotted filter	Predilution fluid replacement Pressor support to increase MAP Flush filter; replace if necessary
Clotted hemofilter	Inadequate anticoagulation Poor blood flow rates Kinks in blood tubing	Check ACT or aPTT hourly, and adjust heparin infusion Pressors or fluid replacement to increase MAP Check tubing hourly to guard against kinks Change filter and restart therapy

ACT, activated clotting time; *aPTT,* activated partial thromboplastin time; *Hct,* hematocrit; *MAP,* mean arterial pressure; *UF,* ultrafiltration.

The current preference of most practitioners is pump-assisted CRRT. The advancements in technology have provided several alternatives for automated devices that monitor system pressures, ultrafiltration rates, dialysate solution rates, and various alarm systems. The systems in use in 2010 include:

1. The Fresenius 2008K with a CRRT option can be used for intermittent hemodialysis, SLEDD, or CRRT (Fresenius Medical Care, Bad Homburg, Germany).
2. The Prisma, and Prismaflex, are automated integrated systems for CRRT and continuous fluid management (Gambro, Stockholm, Sweden).
3. Other integrated systems available in the United States are:
   a. Accura (Baxter Healthcare, Deerfield, IL)
   b. Diapact (B. Braun, Bethlehem, PA)
   c. System One (NxStage Medical, Lawrence, MA)

ANTICOAGULATION

Critically ill patients may have an increased tendency to either coagulation or bleeding. All of the variations of CRRT require that the patient's blood is in contact with artificial tubing and membrane, which stimulates the coagulation cascade. The complement cascade may also be stimulated if a biocompatible membrane is not used. Therefore, the goal of anticoagulation is to prevent clotting in the CRRT circuit, preserve the filter performance, and optimize survival of the circuit. There must be a balance between preventing blood loss in the circuit due to clotting and preventing excessive anticoagulation leading to bleeding. The critically ill patient is at increased risk of bleeding due to coagulopathy and endothelial disruption. ARF may be associated with a procoagulant state because of downregulation of natural anticoagulants and inhibition of fibrinolysis.

Factors that May Contribute to Coagulation

Patient Factors
- Decrease in natural anticoagulants
- Platelet count and function
- Transfusions
- Fibrinolysis inhibition

Vascular Access Factors
- Catheter characteristic (i.e., diameter and length)
- Kinking or malposition
- Patient position change

Treatment Variations
- Intermittent blood flow reductions
- Predilution or postdilution fluid replacement
- Reaction time to alarms
- Blood–air contact in the system

The choice of anticoagulation may depend on the physician preference, patient condition, and the nursing staff comfort with specific regimens. The three factors to maintain a clot-free system include the type of therapy used, the anticoagulant used, and the blood flow rate.

Heparin

Heparin is the most common and least expensive of the choices. It can be administered either systemically or regionally.

Systemic heparinization: Heparin can be infused in a separate IV line for systemic heparinization or into the arterial line of the CRRT device. In addition to the complication of bleeding, heparin-induced thrombocytopenia can occur. This complication has limited the use of heparin in recent years.

Regional heparinization: A relatively uncommon procedure that produces anticoagulation in the circuit but not systemically to the patient. There is little research available on regional heparinization. When done, it requires two infusion devices: one to infuse heparin pre filter (before the hollow fiber filter) and another for protamine, a heparin antagonist that is run post filter into the return line to neutralize the heparin. This process requires determining the aPTT systemically from the patient and post-filter preprotamine infusion. The goal is to heparinize the circuit without systemically heparinizing the patient. This process is labor intensive and requires meticulous monitoring and frequent dose adjustment of both the heparin and protamine. Use of protamine in this fashion is quite uncommon, so few centers engage in this method of anticoagulation.

Direct Thrombin Inhibitors
These agents are used for anticoagulation in patients with heparin-induced thrombocytopenia. The most common agents are Argatroban, bivalirudin (e.g., Angiomax) and lepirudin (e.g., Refludan). Argatroban is eliminated by the liver and is more suitable for most patients on CRRT. Lepirudin is excreted renally and therefore not the choice for patients with AKI. Bivalirudin is not indicated for use in this setting. All of these agents are considerably more expensive than heparin.

Citrate
The other alternative to heparin for regional anticoagulation is citrate. Citrate is infused into the arterial limb of the circuit pre filter, chelates calcium, and prevents clotting. Citrate regional anticoagulation puts patients at risk for severe hypocalcemia. When citrate is used, it is important to infuse calcium systemically post filter, to maintain normal levels of ionized calcium. If dialysate and predilution fluids (FRF or replacement fluid) are used, they should be calcium free to prevent reversal of the citrate effect in the circuit. During citrate anticoagulation, the body metabolizes the citrate into bicarbonate in the liver. Therefore, alkalosis is a potential complication of citrate anticoagulation. Citrate anticoagulation is contraindicated in patients with hepatic failure or lactic acidosis because the liver cannot metabolize the citrate. Treatment of alkalosis includes IV administration of sodium chloride or hydrochloric acid or reduction in the rate of citrate infusion. Monitoring of all laboratory values, including ionized calcium, sodium, and acid-base balance, is essential.

Isotonic Sodium Chloride Solution
If the patient's condition prohibits anticoagulation, this presents a challenge in maintaining circuit patency. The system may need to be flushed with small boluses of isotonic sodium chloride to reduce stagnation of blood in the system. Specific unit protocol may require flushing with 50 to 100 ml every hour to maintain patency and decrease the potential for clotting.

The use of predilution fluid replacement (FRF or replacement fluid) hemodilutes the blood, which decreases the chance for clotting. Predilution also helps separate all solute particles, making it easier for solutes to pass into the filter. The fluid provides continuous flushing of the system. Use of sodium chloride must be done judiciously, with monitoring of acid-base balance and electrolytes. If large amounts of sodium chloride solution are infused, patients can develop hyperchloremic acidosis.

FILTRATION REPLACEMENT FLUID (REPLACEMENT FLUID)
Electrolyte imbalances that may occur with CRRT include hypokalemia, hypocalcemia, hypophosphatemia, and hypoglycemia. Other abnormalities include acid-base imbalance and depletion of free water. The replacement fluid may be infused pre filter or post filter and is tailored to the specific needs of individual patients. Three types of solutions are available: citrate-based, lactate-based, and bicarbonate-based. Citrate and lactate solutions are not used in patients with liver abnormalities or in patients with lactic acidosis.

Approaches to filtration fluid replacement and calculation of FRF rate can be found in Table 6-12 and Box 6-2.

ASSESSMENT: DURING CONTINUOUS RENAL REPLACEMENT THERAPY
Goals of System Assessment
Evaluate hemodynamic stability and maintain homeostasis.

History and Risk Factors

- Events leading to the development of AKI
- Underlying chronic kidney disease
- Presence of cardiovascular disease
- Presence of pulmonary compromise
- Nutritional state
- Neurologic status

Table 6-12	APPROACHES TO CONTINUOUS RENAL REPLACEMENT THERAPY FILTRATION FLUID REPLACEMENT
Predilution: Replacement Fluid Infused Proximal to the Filter	**Postdilution: Replacement Fluid Infused Distal to the Filter**
Patient population: Those with poor blood flow and elevated BUN and Hct levels	*Patient population:* All types
Replacement fluid infused into arterial line	Replacement fluid infused into venous line
Used to enhance urea clearance to ≥18%; decreases oncotic pressure, increasing net TMP; moves urea from erythrocytes into plasma	Used to maintain fluid and electrolyte balance
Increases net fluid removal	Less replacement fluid required
Potentially increases filter life	Simplified clearance determination
*Urea clearance 12.5 ml/min	Urea clearance 10.6 ml/min

BUN, blood urea nitrogen; *Hct*, hematocrit; *TMP*, transmembrane pressure.
*If increased urea clearance is desired, predilution mode of fluid replacement is used.

BOX 6-2	CALCULATION OF FILTRATION REPLACEMENT FLUID (FRF) RATE

Infusion rate
Equals ultrafiltrate plus other losses per hour minus all fluid infused minus net removal rate

Example
Ultrafiltrate = 600 ml/hr + Losses (urine, GI) = 100 ml/hr − TPN (total parenteral nutrition) 100 ml/hr
Vasopressors 50 ml/hr − Net fluid removal rate 150 ml/hr

FRF rate
= (600 + 100) − (100 + 50 + 150)
= 700 − 300

FRF rate
= 400 ml/hr

Vital Signs
- BP may increase or decrease based on fluid volume status
- HR may increase or decrease in response to fluid and electrolyte changes
- Hyperthermia or hypothermia in the presence of sepsis
- Hypothermia is a common complication of CRRT
- Cardiac arrhythmias may occur with hypothermia
- Cold patients are prone to use more energy and increase CO
- PAWP and CVP will change with volume status
- Oxygen saturation to assess respiratory status
- Body weight to assess fluid balance
- Urine output and other fluid losses (blood loss drainage fluid)

Observation
Hourly Monitoring of the CRRT Circuit
- Blood flow rate
- Venous pressure
- Arterial pressure
- Filter pressures (if applicable)

- Balance pressures
- Effluent pressures
- Color of the blood in the circuit
- Presence of air in the system
- Dialysate flow rate (if applicable)
- Transmembrane pressure
- Ultrafiltration rate
- Calculate fluid balance
- Filter patency
- Anticoagulation

Hourly Monitoring of the Vascular Access
- Catheter patency
- Access pressures
- Access site for signs of bleeding or infection

Palpation
- Pulse quality and regularity bilaterally (scale 0 to 4+)
- Vascular access site for tenderness or expression of exudate
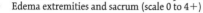• Edema extremities and sacrum (scale 0 to 4+)

Auscultation
- Heart sounds to evaluate for contributors to decreased CO
- Friction rub indicative of pericarditis
• S_3 and S_4 indicative of heart failure
- Pleural rub
- Bowel sounds to evaluate gastric motility

Screening Labwork
- Electrolytes, BUN, and creatinine to determine renal function and effectiveness of CRRT
- CBC to assess for the presence of anemia
- Calcium if using citrate anticoagulation
- Coagulation profile to monitor effects of other anticoagulants

COLLABORATIVE MANAGEMENT
Goal for patients undergoing continuous replacement therapies: venovenous or arteriovenous. The goal is the removal of excess fluid and, with CVVHD/CVVHDF, excess solutes, while maintaining electrolyte balance and adequate fluid intake for homeostasis. In the critically ill adult, catabolic rate is two to three times that of normal.

Key Considerations	Goals
Total parenteral nutrition	Maintain nutritional requirements.
Predilution fluid replacement	Used if increased solute removal is required
Filtration replacement fluid	Used to maintain fluid and electrolyte balance
Anticoagulation	To prevent clotting in the circuit
Vasopressors	Used with CAVH only to maintain arterial pressure
Vascular access	Double-lumen catheter in the subclavian or internal jugular vein for venovenous procedures
	Arterial access needed for CAVH

Care Priorities
Prevention of hemodynamic instability and maintenance of homeostasis are the goals of CRRT. This includes fluid removal and electrolyte replacement. Continuous monitoring and frequent prescription changes based on patient condition and needs are required to meet the goal of therapy. Fluid removal, electrolyte balance, and maintaining nutrition in these critically ill catabolic patients present a major care challenge for the treatment team.

Continuous Renal Replacement Therapies

1. **Maintain hemodynamic stability.** Evaluate the volume status based on weight, PAWP, CO, CVP, and the clinical signs of volume overload. Determine electrolyte balance with particular attention to sodium, potassium, and calcium. Determine the state of catabolism based on the BUN and creatinine levels, along with the presence of metabolic acidosis.

2. **Provide adequate nutrition to promote healing.** Assess the nutritional requirements based on the rate of catabolism, serum albumin, and losses of protein. Most will require enteral feedings or parenteral nutrition to meet nutritional requirements. This is one element that must be accounted for in the calculation of "fluid to be removed" hourly with CRRT, as the volume of all additional intake may need to be removed in the severely fluid-overloaded patient.

3. **Filtration replacement fluids.** Use physiologic solutions (more chemically similar to normal body chemistry) to replace the majority of the filtrate removed hourly, to maintain volume stability and replace electrolyte losses. Use of plain normal saline may not be appropriate for patients with high volume replacement fluid, as electrolyte imbalances or hyperchloremic acidosis may ensue. Determine fluid losses and fluid intake needed hourly to help maintain this stability. Frequent changes in the CRRT prescription (orders) may be necessary based on intake changes. If the patient is receiving citrate-based anticoagulation, replacement fluid must contain calcium to maintain serum calcium levels in the patient. Observe for any signs of hypocalcemia.

4. **Vascular access adequacy.** Maintain adequate flow rates. Assess for alignment and presence of signs of infection. Sterile technique is required when performing access care.

5. **Maintain patency of the CRRT machine circuit.** Monitor coagulation parameters hourly. Check the circuit for any signs of blood stasis in lines or filter. Flush with normal saline for any evidence of clotting. Adjust the rate of the anticoagulant infusion as necessary to maintain regional (circuit) anticoagulation without systemic anticoagulation of the patient.

CARE PLANS FOR CONTINUOUS RENAL REPLACEMENT THERAPY
For patients undergoing continuous renal replacement therapies: venovenous or arteriovenous
Decreased cardiac output *related to fluid overload creating heart failure*

- -

GOALS/OUTCOMES Patient's cardiac output is adequate as evidenced by systolic BP 100 mm Hg or greater (or within patient's normal range), HR 60 to 100 bpm, RR 12 to 20 breaths/min, peripheral pulses >2+ on a 0 to 4+ scale, brisk capillary refill (less than 2 seconds), and normal sinus rhythm on ECG.
NOC Circulation Status

Hemodynamic Regulation
1. Assess and document BP, HR, and RR hourly for the first 4 hours of hemofiltration, and then every 2 hours. Be alert to indicators of fluid volume deficit, manifested by a drop in systolic BP to less than 100 mm Hg, tachycardia, and tachypnea.
2. Assess and document peripheral pulses and color, temperature, and capillary refill in the extremities every 2 hours. Be alert to decreased amplitude of peripheral pulses and to coolness, pallor, and delayed capillary refill in the extremities as indicators of decreased perfusion.
3. Measure and record I&O hourly. Consult physician or midlevel practitioner for a loss of greater than 200 ml/hr over desired loss.
4. Monitor cardiac rhythm continuously; notify physician of decrease in BP greater than 20 mm Hg from baseline, tachycardia, depressed T waves and ST segments, and dysrhythmias, which can occur with hypovolemia, potassium changes, or calcium changes.
5. Ensure prescribed rates of ultrafiltration and replacement fluid infusion (see Box 6-2), and adjust if ultrafiltration rate changes. Use an infusion pump for replacement fluids to ensure precise rate of infusion. Also maintain TPN and IV rates, as well as oral intake, within 50 ml of the values used to calculate the filtration fluid replacement rate. If any parameters change greater than 50 ml, recalculate filtration fluid replacement rate and adjust accordingly.
6. Monitor serum electrolyte values, being alert to changes in potassium, calcium, phosphorus, and bicarbonate. Compare patient's values with the following normal ranges: potassium 3.5 to 5 mEq/L, calcium 8.5 to 10.5 mg/dl, phosphorus 2.5 to 4.5 mg/dl, and bicarbonate 22 to 26 mEq/L (see *Fluid and Electrolyte disturbances*, p. 37, and *Acid-Base Imbalances*, p. 1).

Risk for deficient fluid volume *related to ultrafiltration during CRRT*

GOALS/OUTCOMES Patient is normovolemic as evidenced by gradual weight loss (less than 2.5 kg/day) and urinary output greater than 0.5 ml/kg/hr in nonoliguric patients. Ultrafiltration rate remains within 50 ml of the desired hourly rate.

NOC Fluid Balance

Fluid Monitoring
1. Measure and record I&O every 30 minutes for the first 2 hours and then hourly. Ensure that it is within desired limits.
2. Weigh patient every 8 hours. Be alert to a daily loss of greater than 2.5 kg.
3. Record cumulative ultrafiltrate loss hourly. Measure amount in the ultrafiltrate container. The difference between this value and total hourly intake is the cumulative loss per hour.
4. Check replacement fluid rate hourly to ensure that it is within prescribed limits: usually 25 ml of the calculated rate.
5. Consult physician or midlevel practitioner for unanticipated fluid loss from vomiting, diarrhea, fever, and wound drainage.
6. Consult physician or midlevel practitioner for increased filtration rate, which may occur because of increased BP, or for increased negative pressure, which may be caused by lowering the ultrafiltration collection device.
7. Monitor vital signs hourly; consult physician or midlevel practitioner for increased arterial pressure (greater than 10 mm Hg above baseline), which would increase flow through the hemofilter, thereby increasing the rate of ultrafiltration.
8. Adjust the filtration replacement fluid rate as prescribed when ultrafiltration rate increases.
9. Maintain intake (oral, enteral, IV, TPN) within 25 to 50 ml of the value used to calculate fluid replacement rate. If not possible, fluid replacement rate must be recalculated.

NIC Electrolyte Management: Hyperkalemia; Electrolyte Management: Hypermagnesemia; Electrolyte Management: Hypernatremia; Electrolyte Management: Hyperphosphatemia; Fluid Management; Fluid Monitoring; Hypovolemia Management; Intravenous Therapy. Additional, optional interventions include Dysrhythmia Management; Feeding; Fever Treatment; Gastrointestinal Intubation; Hemodynamic Regulation; Invasive Hemodynamic Monitoring; Medication Management; Nutrition Management; Weight Management; and Phlebotomy: Arterial Blood Sample and Venous Blood Sample.

Excess fluid volume *related to renal insufficiency*

GOALS/OUTCOMES Patient experiences a gradual fluid loss and becomes normovolemic as evidenced by BP remaining at baseline range, system remains patent/no clotting apparent, CVP 4 to 6 mm Hg, HR 60 to 100 bpm, RR 12 to 20 breaths/min, and absence of edema, crackles, and other physical indicators of hypervolemia.

NOC Fluid Overload Severity

Fluid/Electrolyte Management
1. Monitor BP every 30 minutes for the first 2 hours, and then hourly. Consult physician for a 10 mm Hg drop in BP, which would decrease the rate of ultrafiltration significantly.
2. If ultrafiltration rate is decreased to 50% of the baseline, consult physician or midlevel practitioner and decrease FRF rate as prescribed.
3. Check tubes hourly for kinks.
4. Maintain constant heparin infusion per infusion pump to maintain ACT at two to three times that of the baseline value. System must be functional for patient to get the full benefit of CRRT.
5. Monitor clotting time every 2 hours. Use of an ACT device is advisable.
6. Inspect vascular access filter and lines for patency hourly. If clotting or clogging with protein is suspected, flush the system with 50 ml normal saline to check patency.
7. If clots are present, consult physician or midlevel practitioner. As prescribed, change the filter and recheck ACT/PTT to ensure necessary adjustment in heparin infusion rate.
8. On an hourly basis, assess for and document the presence of physical indicators of hypervolemia: CVP greater than 6 mm Hg, BP elevated greater than 20 mm Hg over baseline, tachycardia, jugular venous distention, basilar crackles, increasing edema (peripheral, sacral, periorbital), and tachypnea.

NIC Electrolyte Management: Hypokalemia; Electrolyte Management: Hyponatremia; Fluid/Electrolyte Management; Fluid Management; Fluid Monitoring. Additional, optional interventions include Dysrhythmia Management;

Feeding; Gastrointestinal Intubation; Hemodialysis Therapy; Hemodynamic Regulation; Invasive Hemodynamic Monitoring; Medication Management; Phlebotomy: Arterial and Venous Blood Samples; Positioning; Skin Surveillance; and Weight Management.

Deficient knowledge of CRRT procedure/treatment

GOALS/OUTCOMES Patient or significant other verbalizes accurate information about the CRRT procedure within 24 to 48 hours of the instruction.
NOC Knowledge: Treatment/Procedure

Teaching: Procedure/Treatment
1. Assess patient's knowledge of the procedure, and intervene accordingly.
2. Explain necessity of vascular access and the sensations that can be anticipated during cannula insertion.
3. Explain importance of and rationale for limited movement of the involved extremity after cannula placement.
4. Describe equipment that will be used for the procedure (e.g., CRRT machine, filter, lines, infusion pumps).
5. Explain that vital signs will be assessed and blood tests will be performed at frequent intervals to monitor patient's status during the procedure.
6. Explain to patient that his or her blood will be visible in the filter and lines.
7. Reinforce that a staff member will be close to patient at all times during the procedure and will explain each step as it occurs.
8. Explain that the procedure may require 24 hours or longer to attain fluid balance.
9. Teach patient that the typical access sites are the femoral artery and the femoral vein, or the internal jugular, or the subclavian vein.

NIC Teaching: Disease Process; Teaching: Individual; Teaching: Prescribed Medication. Additional, optional interventions include Discharge Planning; Medication Management; and Weight Management.

Impaired physical mobility *related to weakness ensuing with critical illness*

GOALS/OUTCOMES Patient exhibits ability to move about in bed with assistance without evidence of disruption of hemofiltration equipment. Patient's skin remains intact, and there is no evidence of muscle atrophy or contracture formation caused by imposed immobility.
NOC Mobility

Positioning
1. Secure access catheters with gauze wraps (elastic wrap may compress access site and cause clotting) and tape to ensure safe movement of the involved limb without disruption of access cannula.
2. Explain to patient the need for care and assistance when moving the involved limb.
3. Use soft restraints if movement must be restrained markedly.
4. Turn and reposition patient at least every 2 hours, maintaining good body alignment.
5. Massage bony prominences during every position change to promote comfort and circulation.
6. Support involved extremities with pillows.
7. Teach patient-assisted range-of-motion (ROM) exercises on uninvolved extremities. Encourage isometric, isotonic, and quadriceps-setting exercises on uninvolved extremities, especially for patients whose CAVH or CVVH lasts longer than 24 hours.

NIC Exercise Therapy: Ambulation; Exercise Therapy: Joint Mobility. Additional, optional interventions include Activity Therapy; Body Mechanics Promotion; Circulatory Care; Circulatory Precautions; Fall Prevention; Pain Management; Progressive Muscle Relaxation; Skin Surveillance; and Weight Management.

Risk for injury *related to CRRT equipment*

GOALS/OUTCOMES Patient's CRRT filter and line connections remain intact, and ultrafiltrate test results are negative for blood.
NOC Fluid Balance

Fluid Monitoring
1. Tape and secure all connections within the system.
2. Check connections hourly to ensure that they are secure.
3. Avoid concealing lines, filter, or connections with linen.
4. Position filter and lines close to the access extremity; secure them with gauze wraps and tape to prevent traction on the connections.
5. Inspect ultrafiltrate hourly for any signs of blood. If unsure whether ultrafiltrate contains blood, check the solution for occult blood.
6. If the test is positive for blood, clamp the ultrafiltrate port and consult physician or midlevel practitioner for further interventions.

NIC Electrolyte Management: Hyperkalemia; Electrolyte Management: Hypermagnesemia; Electrolyte Management: Hypernatremia; Electrolyte Management: Hyperphosphatemia; Fluid Management; Fluid Monitoring; Hypovolemia Management; Intravenous Therapy. Additional, optional interventions include Dysrhythmia Management; Feeding; Fever Treatment; Gastrointestinal Intubation; Hemodynamic Regulation; Invasive Hemodynamic Monitoring; Medication Management; Nutrition Management; Weight Management; and Phlebotomy: Arterial Blood Sample and Venous Blood Sample.

ADDITIONAL NURSING DIAGNOSES

For more information about fluid and electrolytes, see *Fluid and Electrolyte Disturbances*, p. 37. Also see *Prolonged Immobility*, p. 149.

SELECTED REFERENCES

American Nephrology Nurses Association: *Core curriculum for nephrology nursing*. Pitman, NJ, 2008, Anthony J. Janetti.

American Nephrology Nurses Association: *Nephrology nursing standards of practice and guidelines for care*. Pitman, NJ, 2005, Anthony J. Janetti.

Bagshaw SM, Berthiaume LR, et al: Continuous versus intermittent renal replacement therapy for acute kidney injury: a meta-analysis. *Crit Care Med* 35(2):610-617, 2008.

Barrett BJ, Pharfrey PS: Preventing nephropathy induced by contrast medium. *N Engl J Med* 354:379-386, 2006.

Bouchard J, Mehta RL: Acid-base disturbances in the intensive care unit: current issues and the use of renal replacement therapy as a customized treatment tool. *Int J Artif Organs* 31(1):6-14, 2008.

Cerda J, Lameire N, Eggers P, et al: Epidemiology of acute kidney injury. *Clin J Am Soc Nephrol* 3:881-886, 2008.

Chrysochoou G, Marcus RJ, et al: Renal replacement therapy in the critical care unit. *Crit Care Nurse Q* 31(4):282-290, 2008.

Molzhan AE, Butera E: *Contemporary nephrology nursing: principles and practice*, ed 2. Pitman, NJ, 2006, Anthony J. Janetti.

Davenport A, Bouman C, et al: Delivery of renal replacement therapy in acute kidney injury: what are the key issues? *Clin J Am Soc Nephrol* 3:869-875, 2008.

Dirkes S, Hodge K: Continuous renal replacement therapy in the adult intensive care unit. History and current trends. *Crit Care Nurse* 27(2):61-80, 2007.

Eknoyan G: Emergence of the concept of acute kidney injury. *Adv Chronic Kidney Dis* 15(3):308-313, 2008.

Ghossein C, Grouper S, Soong W: Renal replacement therapy in the intensive care unit. *Int Anesthesiol Clin* 47(1):15-34, 2009.

Gibney N, Hoste E, et al: Timing of initiation and discontinuation of renal replacement therapy in AKI: unanswered key questions. *Clin J Am Soc Nephrol* 3:876-880, 2008.

Himmelfarb J: Continuous renal replacement therapy in the treatment of acute renal failure: critical assessment is required. *Clin J Am Soc Nephrol* 2:385-389, 2007.

Himmelfarb J, Joannidis M, Molitoris B, et al: Evaluation and initial management of acute kidney injury. *Clin J Am Soc Nephrol* 3:962-967, 2008.

Hoste E, Schurgers M: Epidemiology of acute kidney injury: how big is the problem? *Crit Care Med* 36(4, Suppl):S146-S151, 2008.

Kellum J: Acute kidney injury. *Crit Care Med* 36(4, Suppl):S141-S145, 2008.

Kielstein J, Kretschmer U, et al: Efficacy and cardiovascular tolerability of extended dialysis in critically ill patients: a randomized controlled study. *Am J Kidney Dis* 43(2):342-349, 2004.

Continuous Renal Replacement Therapies

Kyung S, Rosner M, Okusa M: Pharmacologic treatment of acute kidney injury: why drugs haven't worked and what is on the horizon. *Clin J Am Soc Nephrol* 2:356-365, 2007.

Mehta R: Continuous renal replacement therapy in the critically ill patient. *Kidney Int* 67:781-795, 2005.

Mehta R, Kellum J, Shah S, et al: Acute Kidney Injury Network: report of an initiative to improve outcomes in acute kidney injury. *Crit Care* 11:R31, 2007.

Morgera S, Slowirski T, et al: Renal replacement therapy with high-cutoff hemofilters: impact of convection and diffusion on cytokine clearances and protein status. *Am J Kidney Dis* 43(3): 444-453, 2004.

Oudenmans-van Straaten HM, Wester JPJ, et al: Anticoagulation strategies in continuous renal replacement therapy: can the choice be evidence based? *Intens Care Med* 32:188-202, 2006.

Palevsky P: Definition of acute kidney injury (acute renal failure), 2008. www.uptodate.com

Palevsky PM, Baldwin I, et al: Renal replacement therapy and the kidney: minimizing the impact of renal replacement therapy on recovery of acute renal failure. *Curr Opin Crit Care* 11:548-554, 2005.

Palsson R, Laliberte KA, Niles JL: Choice of replacement solution and anticoagulant in continuous venovenous hemofiltration. *Clin Nephrol* 65(1):34-42, 2006.

Pannu N, Klarenbach S, et al: Renal replacement therapy in patients with acute renal failure. A systematic review. *JAMA* 299(7):793-805, 2008.

Price Rabetoy C: Acute renal failure. In Molzahn A, editor: *Contemporary nephrology nursing: principles and practice,* ed 2. Pitman, NJ, 2006, Anthony J. Janetti.

Schrier RW, Wang W: Acute renal factors and sepsis. *N Engl J Med* 351:159-169, 2004.

The VA/NIH Acute Renal Failure Trial Network: Intensity of renal support in critically ill patients with acute kidney injury. *N Engl J Med* 359(1):7-20, 2008.

Vanbiesen W, Vanholder R, Lameire N: Defining acute renal failure: RIFLE and beyond. *Clin J Am Soc Nephrol* 1:1314-1319, 2006.

Venkataraman R: Can we prevent acute kidney injury? *Crit Care Med* 36(4, Suppl):S166-S171, 2008.

Waikar S, Liu K, Chertow G: Diagnosis, epidemiology and outcomes of acute kidney injury. *Clin J Am Soc Nephrol* 13:844-861, 2008.

Zappitelli M, Parikh C, Akcan-Ariken A, et al: Ascertainment and epidemiology of acute kidney injury varies with definition interpretation. *Clin J Soc Nephrol* 3:948-954, 2008.

GENERAL NEUROLOGIC ASSESSMENT

Level of Consciousness

- Assess for orientation, drowsiness, inappropriate use of words, slurred speech, arousability, confusion, and amnesia.
- Close monitoring of level of consciousness (LOC) is essential to assess for determining deterioration, and even a slight change may indicate emergent intervention is needed.
- For specifics of how to assess using levels of stimulation, refer to Appendix 2, Glasgow Coma Scale (GCS).

Vital Signs

Refer to specific sections for key vital sign changes specific for the type of neurologic disorder.

Key Cranial Nerve Assessment

It is not always necessary to assess all 12 cranial nerves (see Appendix 3). Specific neurologic disorders will address cranial nerve impairments.

- Assess the nerves responsible for vision (optic), pupillary response (oculomotor), and eye movements (oculomotor, trochlear, abducens).
- Assess facial/corneal sensation and chewing (trigeminal) and facial muscle movement and taste (facial).
- All functions are evaluated bilaterally (e.g., both eyes, both sides of face, etc.).
- A full examination includes all 12 nerves.

Assess Motor and Cerebellar Function

Evaluate bilaterally (both sides of body, both arms and legs) for muscle size, strength, tone, and coordination. Note muscle atrophy or hypertrophy.

- If patient can walk, assess gait.
- Ask patient to walk heel to toe to check for balance and coordination.
- Perform Romberg test: Ask patient to close eyes and stand with feet close together while you stand nearby in case patient sways/falls (abnormal response indicative of cerebellar dysfunction).
- Ask patient to squeeze your hands and push feet against your hands, to assess if strength is equal on both sides.
- Note any involuntary movements (tremors, jerking, fasciculations) and general posture.
- Move the patient's joints through passive range-of-motion (ROM) exercises, noting any tenderness of involved muscle groups.
- To further evaluate muscle strength, have patient perform active ROM exercises while you apply resistance against the movements. Use the following rating scale for muscle strength:

MUSCLE STRENGTH RATING	
Score	**Description of Strength**
5/5	Patient moves joint with full ROM against normal resistance and gravity
4/5	Patient moves joint with full ROM against mild resistance and gravity
3/5	Patient moves joint with full ROM against gravity only
2/5	Patient moves joints with full ROM but not against gravity
1/5	Patient's muscle contracts in an attempt to move joint; joint does not move
0/5	Patient does not visibly attempt to move; no muscle contraction; paralysis

ROM, Range of motion.

- Assess for abnormal motor movements unilaterally and bilaterally:
  - Decorticate posturing (abnormal flexion)
  - Decerebrate posturing (abnormal extension)
  - Flaccidity

  Motor deficits (weakness or paralysis) are caused by injury or edema to the primary motor cortex and corticospinal (pyramidal) tracts.
- Perform specific testing for abnormalities as appropriate:
  - *Grasp:* Place two fingers within the patient's palm and ask patient to squeeze your fingers. Ask the patient to let go. *Abnormal grasp:* Patient cannot let go once grasp is in progress. May reflect frontal lobe disease; observed occasionally with occipital lobe disease, Alzheimer disease, or bilateral thalamic disease.
  - *Babinski sign:* Upward or dorsiflexion of the big toe when stroking the outer sole and ball of the foot) can indicate a lesion of the pyramidal tract.
  - *Kernig sign:* Painful resistance to full extension of the leg at the knee when the hip is flexed; used in diagnosis of meningitis due to meningeal irritation
  - *Brudzinski sign:* Flexion of the hip and knee involuntarily with neck flexion and used in diagnosis of meningitis due to meningeal irritation

Sensory Assessment

Sensory deficits occur when the primary sensory cortex, the sensory association areas of the parietal lobe, or the spinothalamic tracts are injured or edematous. Sensory deficits include inability to distinguish objects according to characteristics (e.g., size, shape, weight) and inability to distinguish overall changes in temperature, touch, pressure, and position.

- Assess perception of touch, proprioception, pain, temperature, and vibration (if possible). Ask patient to close eyes while you apply stimuli. The patient should not be given the opportunity to anticipate your moves. Compare the same stimulus on the right side of the body to the identical location on the left side of the body. Note if patient perceives stimuli symmetrically and appropriately (sharp versus dull using a needle versus a cotton swab, or hot versus cold). Compare proximal and distal parts of arms and legs when testing pain and touch.
- Superficial and deep reflexes are tested on symmetrical sides of the body and compared noting the strength of contraction.
- Test vibratory sense (with vibrating tuning fork) distally (on the tip of big toe or finger) and ask when patient feels the vibration stop.
- For position sense, move distal joints about using very light touch and ask about the position the patient perceives of the joint.
- Two-point discrimination can be done using a bent paper clip. Note the smallest distance between the two points at which the patient senses two points are pressing on the skin. Document using a dermatome map.

  Improvement in both motor and sensory perception may be seen as cerebral edema subsides.

Fundoscopic Assessment

Generally done by the physician or midlevel practitioner and may reveal retinal hemorrhage(s) at the side of the optic disc. Hemorrhage is caused by blood from the subarachnoid space (SAS) being forced along the optic nerve sheath under high pressure. The patient may complain of blurred vision or blind spots (scotomata). Terson hemorrhage associated with vitreous and/or subhyaloid hemorrhage has been seen as a subarachnoid complication and its presence has been noted with increased mortality and morbidity rates.

Dysphagic Screening

Should be performed early, particularly when stroke has occurred, to prevent complications of aspiration and to initiate appropriate nutritional therapy. People with neurologic dysfunction are poor judges of their own ability to swallow, so a thorough evaluation and intervention by a speech pathologist may be required, following routine screening procedures recommended by institutional protocol.

Diagnostic Tests for Neurologic Disorders

Test	Purpose	Abnormal Findings
Cerebral angiography	Digital subtraction angiography visualizes blood flow. Involves use of intravascular catheter The gold standard for evaluating cerebral vasculature Invasive procedure with minimal risk used to visualize the cerebral blood vessels	Areas of reduced cerebral blood flow, aneurysms, arteriovenous malformations (AVMs), vascular abnormalities Used with interventional neuroradiologic procedures such as coiling, AVM embolization (gluing) Provides specific information on the cause of stroke by identifying the blood vessel involved
Computed tomography (CT) of brain	Performed emergently, is the gold standard of differentiating ischemic from hemorrhagic stroke; may be done at intervals to monitor progress Assess details of structures of bone, tissue, and fluid-filled space. Detects exudate, abscesses, and intracranial pathology (e.g., tumors, brain injury) Assess for hydrocephalus.	Shift of structures due to enlarged mass, edema, exudate, abscesses, fresh hemorrhage, hematomas, infarction, hydrocephalus Can visualize facial skeleton and soft tissue structures for abnormalities (e.g., tumors, brain injury) Within the first few hours after an acute ischemic stroke, the scan may appear normal. Intracranial hemorrhage is easily diagnosed on CT—blood appears as a bright white signal.
Continuous electrocardiographic (ECG) monitoring	Evaluate cardiovascular status, especially during medication administration.	Phenytoin and other AEDs can cause dysrhythmias and hypotension.
CT angiography	Less invasive than cerebral angiography; involves use of contrast media injection into peripheral vein and use of CT scanner	Visualize intra-arterial clot, small intracranial aneurysm, AVM
CT perfusion or CT-xenon scan (CTP)	Provides information related to cerebral blood flow (CBF) and volume Used to guide clinical decision making regarding the use of thrombolysis or interventional procedures	Compromised blood flow; a limited test; cannot detect infarcted tissue
Electroencephalography (EEG)	Evaluate the brain's electrical activity for ongoing seizures, even if there are no clinical signs of seizures.	Diagnosis of seizures and localization of structural abnormalities Also used as element of criteria for brain death

Continued

Diagnostic Tests for Neurologic Disorders—cont'd

Test	Purpose	Abnormal Findings
Electromyography (EMG) or nerve conduction velocity (NCV)	Assesses nerve conduction velocity deficit as a result of the demyelination of peripheral nerves	EMG and NCV demonstrate profound slowing of motor conduction velocities and conduction blocks several weeks into the illness.
Lumbar puncture (LP) with cerebrospinal fluid (CSF) specimen for analysis	Measures CSF pressures and obtains CSF specimen when infection, such as meningitis or neurosyphilis, is suspected May be performed when SAH is suspected and CT is normal	Elevated protein, low glucose, elevated WBC
Magnetic resonance imaging (MRI) of brain	Minute oscillations of hydrogen atoms in brain create graphic image of bone, fluid, and soft tissue Provides a more detailed image MRI is most useful for ischemic patients in identifying the cause and area involved. Provides detailed information regarding the area of injury or its vascular supply (MRA) Diffusion-weighted imaging (DWI) is a measurement of edema, whereas perfusion weighted imaging (PWI) is a measurement of global CBF.	Infarcts, areas at risk or ischemic areas, vascular defects, stenosis, occlusion
Positron emission tomography (PET) and single-photon emission computed tomography (SPECT)	To evaluate brain metabolism and blood flow using three-dimensional imaging produced using a radioactive tracer	Demonstrates abnormal function of the brain by revealing abnormal structures, metabolism, and perfusion Locates areas of brain causing seizures, head injury, and some disorders (e.g., Alzheimer's)
Radioisotope brain scan	Examine areas of blood flow through concentration of isotope uptake in the brain.	Increased or decreased blood flow intraoperatively or assess for postoperative cerebral infarction Lack of uptake may indicate cerebral brain death.
Transcranial Doppler	Noninvasive and can be done serially at the bedside Evaluates the intracranial vessels and assesses the velocity of blood flow in the anterior and posterior cerebral circulation Also used to evaluate vasospasm, to determine brain death via detection of cerebral circulatory arrest, for intraoperative monitoring, and to locate emboli	Arterial narrowing vasospasm, cerebral circulatory arrest, emboli due to vasospasm Can also be used to confirm absent blood flow in brain death

BRAIN DEATH

PATHOPHYSIOLOGY

Brain death is defined as irreversible loss of function of the brain, including the brainstem and respiratory centers. *Cardiac death* is the cessation of mechanical action/pumping of the heart, resulting in absence of pulse, heart sounds, blood pressure, and respirations. Brain death is most frequently the result of increased intracranial pressure (ICP) caused by severe traumatic head injury or hemorrhagic stroke caused by ruptured cerebral aneurysm with subarachnoid hemorrhage (SAH) or intracranial hemorrhage (ICH). A significant number of patients with acute ischemic strokes (AIS) experience cerebral edema and herniation. Hypoxic-ischemic encephalopathy with massive brain swelling after prolonged cardiopulmonary resuscitation or asphyxia and encephalopathy with cerebral edema resulting from fulminant hepatic failure may also result in increased ICP, herniation, and brain death.

If brain death occurs quickly, cardiac death may occur immediately. If brain death occurs more slowly, with time to initiate mechanical ventilation prior to cardiac death, the heart can continue to beat/pump since the cardiac pacing cells operate independently from brain regulation. Mechanical ventilation provides the oxygen necessary to maintain the pacing cells if the patient is circulating adequate amounts of blood cells carrying oxyhemoglobin, acidosis is controlled, and electrolytes are managed. Over time, without a functional hypothalamus and pituitary gland, patients experience further instability of blood pressure due to loss of regulation of the thyroid and adrenal glands. Massive diuresis is common when the posterior pituitary gland ceases to function. If the patient is an organ donor, the organs must be sustained prior to removal, requiring management of all sequelae of brain death. Guidelines for managing brain dead organ donors have common elements internationally, with most controversy stemming from the need to provide additional hormones to help control endocrine-related crises associated with loss of function of the pituitary and hypothalamus and use of prophylactic antibiotics to prevent infection.

Neurologists or neurosurgeons may diagnose brain death approximately two to three times monthly in large referral centers. Herniation, or displacement of a portion of the brain through openings in the intracranial cavity, results from increased ICP. Herniation occurs when there is difference between the cranial compartment pressures above (supratentorial) and below (infratentorial) the tentorium, the rigid membrane that divides the skull. If additional blood or cerebrospinal fluid (CSF), edematous tissue, or tumor occupies space inside the skull, there is little ability to expand to "make room" for anything not normally present. These "mass lesions" or "space-occupying lesions" cause "crowding" within their cavity, which increases the pressure.

When pressure in one of the two compartments (supratentorial or infratentorial) is markedly elevated, the brain structures and blood vessels within the cavity are compressed, resulting in ischemia, hypoxia, and, if uncontrolled, cerebral anoxia. When blood flow is minimal to absent, the hypoxic/anoxic brain tissues become more edematous. Eventually, no space remains for further expansion. The skull cannot expand and the tentorium expands minimally, so the brain is forced through the available openings. The movement or displacement through an opening causes further compression of blood vessels, with possible laceration and destruction, which leads to necrosis of brain tissues and brain death (see *Traumatic Brain Injury, Neurologic Herniation Syndromes*, p. 333).

NEUROLOGIC ASSESSMENT: BRAIN DEATH
Goal of System Assessment
To validate absence of function of the brain and brainstem. According to the American Academy of Neurology (AAN) guidelines, if coma or unresponsiveness, absence of brainstem reflexes, and apnea are present, the patient is dead. If mechanical ventilation is terminated, natural death results. Severity of brain injury should be determined following two expert clinical assessments and diagnostic testing.

History and Risk Factors
- Severe traumatic head injury (motor vehicle accident, gunshot/other assault, recreational/industrial accidents)
- Ruptured cerebral aneurysm with SAH
- ICH resulting in intracerebral hematoma
- Large AIS resulting in massive cerebral edema and/or brain herniation
- Prolonged cardiopulmonary resuscitation
- Asphyxia (asthmatic cardiac arrest, drug overdose, hanging, carbon monoxide poisoning, drowning, meningitis)
- Fulminant hepatic failure

Apnea Test

- Determines absence of respirations when mechanically induced ventilations cease. Must be done carefully to avoid cardiac death during the test. If the patient begins to deteriorate while off the ventilator, the patient should be placed back on the ventilator.

Vital Signs

- *Mild hypothermia*: Core temperature must be greater than 32°C (90°F), but less than 36.5°C (97°F).
- *Hypotension*: With mechanical ventilation in place, blood pressure is greater than 90 mm Hg. Without mechanical ventilation, the heart rate will decrease, resulting in hypotension and eventually asystole.
- *Apnea*: No spontaneous respirations when mechanical ventilation is suspended. A formal apnea test is required to confirm the absence of respirations.

Observation/Inspection/Palpation

- *Coma or unresponsiveness*: Patient does not respond to verbal stimuli, touch, or deep pain induced by pressure exerted on nail beds, the supraorbital area of the skull, or the temporomandibular joint or rubbing the sternum.
- *Brainstem reflexes/cranial nerve function*: Absent
    - *Pupils*: Unresponsive to bright light; size is 4 to 9 mm (dilated) in midposition.
    - *Ocular movement*: No oculocephalic reflex ("doll's eyes" negative). No oculovestibular reflex: no deviation of eyes toward irrigation of ear canal with 50 ml ice cold water within 1 minute following irrigation. Irrigation of each ear canal should be done at least 5 minutes apart (cold caloric test).
    - *Facial sensory and motor responses*: No corneal reflex to touch with a cotton swab, no jaw reflex, no grimacing to deep pain
    - *Pharyngeal and tracheal reflexes*: No coughing or gagging when posterior pharynx is stimulated by a tongue blade; no cough response to bronchial suctioning (See *Appendix 1, Cranial Nerves*.)
- *Apnea*: No spontaneous respirations. Structured testing is required for diagnosis.
- *Euvolemia*: Patient does not exhibit signs of dehydration. If dehydration is present, patient must be hydrated prior to structured apnea testing.

Screening Labwork

- *Toxicology screen*: Evaluates for presence of toxic doses of recreational drugs, medications, or poisons (see *Drug Overdose*, p. 868)
- *Basic metabolic panel/blood chemistry*: Identifies electrolyte imbalance, including hypoglycemia, hyperglycemia, and acidosis (using bicarbonate/CO_2). May also reflect patient's volume status, including dehydration and hypovolemia (see *Fluid and Electrolyte Disturbances*, in p. 37).
- *Arterial blood gas (ABG) analysis*: Evaluates for hypoxia, acidosis, and hypercapnia (see *Acid-Base Balance*, p. 1).

Making the Diagnosis of Brain Death

The three cardinal signs/symptoms in brain deat h are coma, absent brainstem reflexes, and apnea according to the AAN guidelines. Patients must have all three findings to be considered dead (brain dead patients are dead). There should be at least two separate clinical examinations, preferably by a neurologist, with at least 2 hours between examinations. If clinical uncertainty is present, two different physicians, preferably neurologists, should examine the patient following completion of appropriate diagnostic testing to ensure patient has not overdosed on a drug; has ingested a poison; has undiagnosed endocrine system dysfunction, electrolyte imbalance, or dehydration; and is free of untreated significant hypoxia, hypercapnia, or acidosis. Adherence to the AAN guidelines varies among the large medical centers in the United States. Diabetes insipidus, myxedema coma, and adrenal crisis may result from loss of the hypothalamic/pituitary regulatory axis as part of brain death. Large amounts of dextrose-containing IV fluids and insulin resistance may prompt hyperglycemia.

RESEARCH BRIEF 7-1

Guidelines for brain death determination are developed at an institutional level, according to the Uniform Determination of Death Act, which may lead to variability of practice. The authors evaluated the differences in brain death guidelines in major U.S. hospitals with strong neurology and neurosurgery services to determine variation from the guidelines of the American Academy of Neurology (AAN). Results revealed major discrepancies were present among institutions in the guidelines' requirements for performance of the evaluation, prerequisites before testing, techniques used for the brainstem examination and apnea testing, and ancillary tests performed. Major differences exist in brain death guidelines used among the leading neurologic hospitals in the United States. Adherence to the AAN guidelines is variable. There may be substantial differences in practice, which might have consequences for the determination of death and initiation of transplant procedures.

From Greer DM, Varelas PN, Hague S, Wijdicks, EFM: Variability of brain death determination guidelines in leading US neurologic institutions. *Neurology* 70(4):284–289, 2008.

DIAGNOSTIC TESTS FOR BRAIN DEATH

Test	Purpose	Abnormal Findings
Arterial blood gas (ABG) analysis	Assesses for acidosis resulting from abnormal gas exchange or compensation for metabolic derangements	*Low pH*: Acidosis may reflect respiratory failure or metabolic crisis. *Carbon dioxide*: Elevated CO_2 or hypercapnia reflects respiratory failure; decreased CO_2 may reflect compensation for metabolic acidosis. *Hypoxemia*: Pao_2 less than 80 mm Hg *Oxygen saturation*: Sao_2 less than 92% *Bicarbonate*: HCO_3- less than 22 mEq/L *Base deficit*: less than -2
Apnea test • The ventilator is disconnected, the patient placed on 100% oxygen via T-tube and observed for apnea. Vital signs must be stable (mild hypothermia, normotensive BP, euvolemia, with normal Pao_2 and Pco_2) to begin the test. Pao_2, Pco_2, and pH are measured after approximately 8 minutes; the ventilator is reconnected after the ABG sample is drawn.	Validates absence of spontaneous respirations while ventilator is disconnected; test is designed to be completed safely, to avoid inducing cardiopulmonary instability during the procedure: • O_2 saturation is monitored continuously by pulse oximetry. • Ventilator is reconnected if patient becomes unstable (hypoxia, hypotension, or lethal dysrhythmias occur).	**Confirmatory findings** *The apnea test is positive if:* • No spontaneous chest or abdominal excursions that produce reasonably normal, effective tidal volumes occur. • The arterial Pco_2 is either more than 60 mm Hg or increased 20 mm Hg from the baseline Pco_2. • The ventilator must be reconnected before 8 minutes due to instability/intolerance of test. *The apnea test is negative if:* • Effective respiratory movements are observed. • Pco_2 does not increase by 20 mm Hg above baseline or is not more than 60 mm Hg.

Continued

DIAGNOSTIC TESTS FOR BRAIN DEATH—cont'd

Test	Purpose	Abnormal Findings
Note: If the patient has severe facial trauma, preexisting abnormal pupils, sleep apnea, severe lung disease resulting in chronic hypercapnia (CO_2 retention), or toxic levels of any sedative drugs, aminoglycosides, tricyclic antidepressants, anticholinergics, antiepileptic drugs, chemotherapeutic agents, or neuromuscular blocking agents, additional testing may be required to confirm brain death. Additional confirmatory tests are not mandatory if the clinical diagnosis is positive (patient is unresponsive/in a coma, brainstem reflexes are absent, apnea test is positive).		
Cerebral angiography	Assesses if cerebral perfusion is present	*Absent perfusion:* No intracerebral blood filling is present at the level of the carotid bifurcation or circle of Willis.
Electroencephalography (EEG)	Assesses level of electrical activity of the brain (brain wave analysis)	*No signs of viability:* No electrical activity during at least 30 minutes of recording, which meets the minimal technical criteria of EEG recording for brain viability; test adheres to American Electroencephalographic Society criteria for those with suspected brain death.
Transcranial Doppler ultrasonography	Assesses for presence of cerebral perfusion and degree of vascular resistance using Doppler signals Positive findings indicate very high vascular resistance resulting from markedly increased ICP.	*No functional blood flow:* Small systolic peaks corresponding with early systole without diastolic flow or reverberating flow. *Note:* 10% of patients do not have temporal windows appropriate for transmitting ultrasound signals. Initial absence of Doppler signal does not confirm brain death.
Cerebral perfusion scan using technetium-99m hexamethapropyleniamineoxime	Assesses for cerebral circulation and brain cell viability using uptake of isotope as the criteria	*No circulation/no uptake:* No uptake of isotope by brain cells ("hollow skull phenomenon")
Somatosensory evoked potentials	Assesses for normal brain responses to electrical stimulation	*No response:* Bilateral absence of N20-P22 response with median nerve stimulation

COLLABORATIVE MANAGEMENT

ORGAN DONOR MANAGEMENT FOLLOWING BRAIN DEATH

Once brain death has been diagnosed, the organ removal team may begin preparations for organ removal within 5 minutes under ideal conditions. If the death was unanticipated, or organ donation was not discussed or controversial, additional time is needed for approaching the donor's family/significant other(s) regarding donation. The parameters below must be managed in order to provide the best opportunity to recover viable organs from the donor.

From the Australasian Transplant Coordinators Association Inc: *National guidelines for organ and tissue donation*, ed 3. 2006. http://www.atca.org.au/files/ATCAguidelinesonlineoct06.pdf

Physiologic Parameter	Intervention
Maintain blood pressure.	MAP 60 to 70 mm Hg: maintain euvolemia; administer vasopressor agents (e.g., norepinephrine) if needed.
Monitor organ perfusion.	Monitor urine output and lactate level; consider hemodynamic monitoring with a pulmonary artery catheter.
Balance electrolytes.	Monitor electrolytes (Na^+, K^+) every 2 to 4 hours; correct to normal range.

ORGAN DONOR MANAGEMENT FOLLOWING BRAIN DEATH—cont'd

Control diabetes insipidus.	Suspected diabetes insipidus (urine output more than 200 ml/hr, rising serum sodium): administer DDAVP (e.g., 2 to 4 mcg IV in adults) and replace volume loss with 5% dextrose.
Manage hyperglycemia.	Treat hyperglycemia: keep blood glucose 100 to 180 mg/dl.
Control hypothermia.	Keep temp greater than 35°C. Early use of warming blankets to prevent declining temperature is helpful; hypothermia is difficult to reverse once developed.
Ventilate and oxygenate.	Provide ongoing respiratory care: frequent suctioning, positioning/turning, PEEP, alveolar recruitment strategies.
Manage anemia.	Maintain hemoglobin at greater than 8 g/dl.
Control hormonal imbalances causing hemodynamic instability.	Consider hormonal replacement therapy if volume resuscitation and low-dose inotropes are ineffective for maintaining BP and/or if cardiac ejection fraction is less than 45%. Typical regimens include: Triiodothyronine (T$_3$): 4 mcg IV bolus, then 4 mcg/hr by IV infusion Arginine vasopressin (AVP): 0.5 to 2.4 units/hr to maintain MAP 60 to 70 mm Hg Methylprednisolone: 15 mg/kg IV single bolus

Care Priorities

1. **Confirm a clinical diagnosis of brain death:** Unresponsiveness or coma, absence of brainstem reflexes and apnea. Complete additional diagnostics as needed.
2. **Allay doubts about the diagnosis:** When patient manifests the three cardinal findings of brain death recognized by the AAN, the health care team should educate the patient's family members about signs and symptoms that may be present. The following findings commonly cause doubt about the diagnosis of brain death in both care providers and the patient's family:
   - Spontaneous movement of limbs: spinal reflex movements may occur.
   - Respiratory-like movements of the chest and abdomen: shoulder elevation and adduction, back arching, intercostal expansion, which do not produce effective tidal volume
   - Sweating, blushing, and tachycardia: residual autonomic responses
   - Normal blood pressure without vasopressors or sudden increases in blood pressure: residual autonomic responses
   - Absence of diabetes insipidus: does not occur in some patients
   - Reflexes are present: deep tendon, superficial abdominal, triple flexion, Babinski
3. **Discuss organ donation ONLY AFTER the clinical diagnosis of brain death has been made and the family understands the patient is dead.** Contact with the organ procurement organization should be done in a timely manner when death is imminent. Collaborate with the organ procurement organization to enhance the experience of the donation process. Do not broach the subject of donation or hint about donation prior to the time the patient has been pronounced dead, unless the patient had resolved the issue of organ donation with the family prior to death. The subject of organ donation is generally better discussed after the patient has been pronounced dead and the family understands that despite the patient having a beating heart, without mechanical ventilation, cardiac death will ensue. Choose a quiet, private, comfortable place to discuss organ donation, ideally leaving the lead role to a professional from the organ procurement agency. The family requires privacy, so they can express their grief regarding the death and can be left alone to discuss donation, if needed. Ensure all members of the team participating in the discussion are introduced to family members. All family members/significant others should be introduced to the team by name, and their role in the family/life of the deceased should be explained. Only those whom the next of kin requests to be present should participate in the discussion. Adequate time should be given asking/answering questions. The words used during the discussion are very important:
   - *Words to avoid:* harvest, cadaver, remains, breathing, respirator, corpse, or any complex medical terminology
   - *Phrases to avoid:* artificial life support, will live on in others, deeply comatose

- *Words to include*: the deceased patient's name, ventilator, procurement, retrieval, donation, dead
- *Phrases to include*: time of death, wishes regarding organ donation, reasons for declining the opportunity, religious beliefs on organ donation

4. **Maintain organs for donation if the family/significant others agree.** If the family agrees to donation, the next of kin/others chosen by next of kin are interviewed by the organ procurement team regarding the patient's medical and social history. Reassure the family that the patient's body will be handled with utmost care/respect to maintain dignity and will not be visibly disfigured. Offer the opportunity to view the patient's body following donation. Major immediate threats to organ donation are development of pulmonary edema, hypotension, polyuria leading to dehydration from diabetes insipidus, and infection. Initiate measures discussed in the table on p. 626.

5. **Discontinue life support after the family has had time to visit the patient, if the family declines the opportunity to donate the patient's organs.** Weaning of mechanical ventilation and vasoactive drugs is unnecessary because the patient is dead. Reasons for declining donation generally relate to the wishes of the patient, religious convictions, fear of disfigurement/mutilation of the patient's body, and mistrust of the motives or anger with the procurement team members. Mistrust and anger often ensue if the family is improperly approached regarding organ donation. Involving the experienced health care professionals from the organ procurement team has been shown to yield a higher success rate with donation.

CARE PLANS FOR BRAIN DEATH

Decreased intracranial adaptive capacity *related to increased intracranial pressure resulting from imminent brain death. When brain death is imminent, mechanisms that normally compensate for increases in intracranial pressure are failing. When failed, brain herniation occurs.*

GOALS/OUTCOMES Patient is maximally supported for reduction of ICP until efforts are proved futile, when brain herniation ensues, resulting in brain death. Following brain death, hemodynamic status is supported until decisions are made regarding organ donation and/or discontinuation of life support.
NOC Tissue Perfusion: Cerebral; Neurological Status: Consciousness.

Cerebral Perfusion Promotion
1. Consult with physician or midlevel practitioner to determine hemodynamic parameters.
2. Maintain hemodynamics within set parameters.
3. Administer osmotic diuretics/rheologic agents (e.g., mannitol, dextran) as ordered.
4. Administer vasopressin as ordered if diabetes insipidus ensues.
5. Keep blood glucose level within ordered range, avoiding hyperglycemia unless using medications which induce osmotic diuresis.
6. Avoid neck flexion or extreme hip/knee flexion.
7. Consult with physician regarding optimal elevation of the head of bed.

Cerebral Edema Management
1. Monitor neurologic status closely and compare with baseline.
2. Monitor respiratory status: rate, rhythm, depth of respirations, PaO_2, PcO_2, pH, and bicarbonate.
3. Monitor ICP and cerebral perfusion pressure (CPP) at rest and in response to patient care activities. Minimize activities that result in further increases in ICP.

Neurologic Monitoring
1. Monitor pupillary size, shape, symmetry, and reactivity.
2. Assess LOC, orientation, and trend of Glasgow Coma Scale score.
3. Monitor vital signs: temperature, blood pressure (BP), pulse, and respirations (RR).
4. Monitor for corneal reflex, cough and gag reflexes.
5. Monitor EOMs and gaze characteristics.
6. Monitor Babinski response.
7. Monitor for Cushing response; a late indicator of increased ICP.

Decisional conflict *related to the uncertainty regarding the proper course of action related to the discontinuation of life support and possible organ donation following brain death*

GOALS/OUTCOMES Family/support system is maximally supported in making judgments, and choosing between immediate discontinuation of life support, organ donation, or possibly continuing life support until information about brain death can be processed and accepted.

NOC Decision Making; Information Processing; Dignified Life Closure; Acceptance: Health Status

Dying Care
1. If cerebral perfusion promotion measures fail and brain death ensues, provide care appropriate for the dying.
2. Encourage family to share feelings about death.
3. Monitor deterioration of patient's physical (and mental) capabilities.
4. Facilitate obtaining spiritual support for the family/significant others.
5. Facilitate discussion of funeral arrangements.

Coping Enhancement
1. Assess the impact of the patient's life situation on roles and relationships within family/support system.
2. Use a calm, reassuring approach.
3. Provide factual information concerning diagnosis, treatment, and prognosis.
4. Seek to understand the family's perception of the stressful situation.
5. Acknowledge the patient and significant others' religious, spiritual, and cultural beliefs surround death, dying, and organ donation.
6. Encourage gradual mastery of the situation if resistance or denial is impacting the family's ability to accept the diagnosis of brain death.
7. Ensure the family understands brain dead patients are dead. Patients are no longer able to breathe without mechanical ventilation, will experience cardiac death when removed from mechanical ventilation, will never regain consciousness, will never interact with others, and have no ability to experience joy related to human life.
8. Explain the difference between brain death, persistent vegetative state, and cardiac death. The family and significant others may have difficulty understanding why brain dead patients are different than those in coma who can recover from their insult/injury and those in a vegetative state who can recover brainstem function to begin breathing spontaneously. Families may not be able to comprehend why when the brain is dead, the heart still functions unless mechanical ventilation is removed. Guilt may be associated with removal of mechanical ventilation since the patient appears "alive" with mechanical ventilation in place.

NIC Emotional Support; Environmental Management; Fluid/Electrolyte Management; Fluid Monitoring; Hypovolemia Management; Infection Control; Intravenous Therapy; Mechanical Ventilation; Positioning; Surveillance; Respiratory Monitoring; Spiritual Support; Vital Signs Monitoring

ADDITIONAL NURSING DIAGNOSES

As appropriate, see nursing diagnoses and interventions in *Nutritional Support* (p. 117), *Acute Respiratory Failure* (p. 383), *Mechanical Ventilation* (p. 99), *Prolonged Immobility* (p. 149), and *Emotional and Spiritual Support of the Patient and Significant Others* (p. 200).

CEREBRAL ANEURYSM AND SUBARACHNOID HEMORRHAGE

PATHOPHYSIOLOGY

An *aneurysm* is a localized dilation of an arterial lumen caused by weakness in the vessel wall—90% of cerebral aneurysms are berry or saccular, while the other 10% are fusiform, traumatic, septic, dissecting, and Charcot-Bouchard aneurysms. Recent research suggests that cerebral aneurysms result from degenerative vascular diseases complicated by hypertension and atherosclerosis. Aneurysms most often occur at the bifurcation of the blood vessels of the circle of Willis, with 85% in anterior cerebral circulation and 15% in posterior cerebral circulation. Approximately 25% of patients have multiple aneurysms.

The critical care nurse may care for a patient with an unruptured aneurysm or a patient who is post rupture and has a diagnosis of subarachnoid hemorrhage (SAH). Unruptured aneurysms may be asymptomatic, but nearly half of the affected population experiences some warning sign or symptom prior to rupture as a result of expansion of the lesion and compression of cerebral tissue. When rupture occurs, an SAH into the subarachnoid space (SAS) and basal cisterns results. If the patient survives the initial compromise of cerebral circulation from the force of hemorrhaging arterial blood, with sharply increased ICP, the next challenge is the possibility of rebleeding and cerebral arterial vasospasm. The greatest incidence of rebleeding is between 3 and 11 days after SAH, with the peak at day 7. Mortality is about 70% overall from aneurysmal SAH. Theories regarding the cause(s) of rebleeding involve the normal process of clot dissolution coupled with fluctuations in arterial pressure.

The major complication for which the critical care nurse monitors post rupture is the occurrence of delayed cerebral ischemia from cerebral arterial vasospasm, in which the constriction of the arterial smooth muscle layer of the major cerebral arteries causes a dramatic decrease in cerebral blood flow and leads to cerebral ischemia and progressive neurologic deficit. Vasospasm occurs in as many as 60% of patients 4 to 14 days following SAH, with incidence peaking between 7 and 10 days. The pathogenesis of cerebral vasospasm is poorly understood, but ongoing research indicates it may be directly related to the amount of blood in the SAS and basal cisterns. The greater the volume of blood, the more pronounced is the risk of vasospasm. As clots in the basal cisterns begin to hemolyze, substances may be released that precipitate vasospasms. Current treatments include careful fluid balance, "triple H" (hypervolemia-hemodilution-hypertension) therapy, calcium antagonists, balloon or chemical angioplasty, and possibly cisternal fibrinolytic drugs. The patient with a ruptured cerebral aneurysm and SAH is also at risk for communicating or obstructive hydrocephalus, hypothalamic dysfunction, and hyponatremia.

Some patients present with an obstructive hydrocephalus from intraventricular blood, but communicating hydrocephalus develops in approximately 20% of patients with SAH as a result of the presence of blood in the SAS and ventricular system. The hydrocephalus may be acute (occurs within less than 24 hours), subacute (occurs within less than 4 hours to 1 week), or delayed (beginning 10 or more days after SAH). Blood in the SAS and ventricles obstructs the flow of CSF, interferes with circulation and resorption of CSF, and causes increased ICP, with concomitant worsening of neurologic status. In some patients, the hydrocephalus produces minimal symptoms and resolves without medical intervention, while others may require temporary or permanent diversion of CSF circulation to achieve symptom relief.

Hypothalamic dysfunction, seen in approximately one-third of patients with hydrocephalus after SAH, may result from mechanical pressure on the hypothalamus from a dilated third ventricle. The increased pressure causes an increase in the releasing hormones from the hypothalamus, which activates the hypothalamic-pituitary axis of the anterior pituitary as well as stimulating the production of antidiuretic hormone (ADH) by the posterior pituitary gland. The response to the increased adrenocorticotropic hormone (ACTH) from the anterior pituitary gland mimics an exaggerated stress response, which includes a marked increase in serum catecholamines leading to overstimulation of the sympathetic nervous system. The vasoconstrictive response is severe enough in a subset of patients to cause "stunned myocardium," similar to what is seen with an acute myocardial infarction.

The surge of ADH from the posterior pituitary results in SIADH, which may include hyponatremia caused by cerebral salt-wasting syndrome, or a combination of factors influencing sodium and water metabolism (Table 7-1). Fluid management strategies in this patient population may be difficult (see *Syndrome of Inappropriate Antidiuretic Hormone*, p. 734). Hyponatremia may occur in 10% to 50% of patients with SAH. Untreated hyponatremia may lead to intracranial hypertension, cerebral ischemia, seizures, coma, and death.

Note: Both hypothalamic dysfunction and hyponatremia are seen more frequently in patients with extensive SAH and are positively correlated with the subsequent development of cerebral vasospasm.

NEUROLOGIC ASSESSMENT: CEREBRAL ANEURYSM(S) AND SUBARACHNOID HEMORRHAGE
Goal of System Assessment
Evaluate for key nursing diagnoses requiring emergent intervention: alteration in cerebral tissue perfusion due to vasospasm of cerebral vessels and increased ICP due to decreased intracranial adaptive capacity, risk for seizure activity with potential impairment of cerebral tissue perfusion, impaired gas exchange or ineffective airway clearance due to altered level of

Table 7-1	CLINICAL PRESENTATION WITH CEREBRAL SALT-WASTING SYNDROME VS SYNDROME OF INAPPROPRIATE ANTIDIURETIC HORMONE (SIADH)
Cerebral Salt-Wasting Syndrome	**SIADH**
Hypotension	Normotension
Postural hypotension	Normotension
Tachycardia	Normal pulse rate or bradycardia
Elevated hematocrit	Normal or low hematocrit
Decreased glomerular filtration rate	Increased glomerular filtration rate
Normal or elevated BUN and creatinine	Normal or decreased BUN and creatinine
Normal or low urine output	Normal or low urine output
Hypovolemia	Normovolemia or hypervolemia
Dehydration	Normal hydration
True hyponatremia	Dilutional hyponatremia
Hypo-osmolality	Hypo-osmolality
Decreased body weight	Increased body weight

BUN, Blood urea nitrogen.

consciousness, potential need for management of hyperglycemia, and fluid volume imbalance and potential for aspiration.

History and Risk Factors

Research has shown that outcomes for patients with ruptured aneurysms and SAH have predictor indicators such as patient's age, worst clinical grade on the Fisher Scale, the World Federation of Neurosurgeons Scale (WFNS), the Claassen Scale, the Ogilvy and Carter Scale, or the commonly used Hunt and Hess scale (see later). The *Fisher Scale* is predictive of the possibility of vasospasm, which is indicative of the amount of blood in the SAS. *The Claassen grading system* quantifies the risk of delayed cerebral ischemia from vasospasm associated with SAH. Unlike the Fisher scale, the Claassen scale considers the additional risk of SAH and intraventricular hemorrhage (IVH). The Claassen scale has not yet been prospectively validated. The *WFNS grading system* is widely used and includes objective terminology to determine grades. Similar to the Hunt and Hess scale, the data predictive power of the WFNS grades are inconsistent. The *Ogilvy and Carter scale* includes several features that may affect the outcome, including age, Hunt and Hess grade (clinical condition), Fisher grade (SAH volume and vasospasm risk), and aneurysm size, but it is more complicated to administer than Hunt and Hess and has been tested only on patients who have undergone aneurysm surgery. Patient outcomes are also related to aneurysm size, fever post SAH, and hyperglycemia on admission as a new finding affecting outcome. A noncontrast CT scan confirms the diagnosis of SAH by establishing the presence, amount, and location of blood in the SAS, the presence and degree of hydrocephalus, and the presence or absence of IVH or intraparenchymal hemorrhage.

Hunt and Hess classification system: Permits objective evaluation of progression of the patient's initial symptoms. Used to predict clinical outcomes and for choosing treatments. Critical care nurses can benefit from using this grading system. Grading is performed according to symptom presentation and LOC.

Grade I: Asymptomatic, alert, and oriented

Grade II: Alert, oriented, headache, and stiff neck

Grade III: Lethargic or confused; minor focal deficit such as hemiparesis

Grade IV: Stuporous, moderate to severe focal deficits, hemiplegia, possible early decerebrate rigidity, and vegetative disturbances

Grade V: Deep coma, decerebrate rigidity, moribund appearance

The critical care nurse must carefully review the patient's history and diagnostic findings to understand the potential risk for complications. Patients with unruptured aneurysms are at risk for rupture, but this depends on the location and size of the aneurysm. Unruptured aneurysms are usually found during a workup for headaches or other neurologic symptoms but may still produce symptoms of cerebral ischemia. A person with new onset of oculomotor nerve palsy, visual field loss, or lower cranial nerve deficits should be worked up for a potential aneurysm. Patients with unruptured aneurysms are typically encountered in the critical care setting after elective securing of the aneurysm. Additionally, some patients admitted for management of a ruptured cerebral aneurysm have additional unruptured aneurysms, which will be secured at a later date.

The typical distinguishing characteristic of a ruptured aneurysm is a patient who complains of the "worst headache of my life." This is usually accompanied by severe nausea and vomiting, nuchal rigidity, visual disturbances, and photophobia. These patients are at high risk for rebleed within 24 hours. "Sentinel" or warning headaches are associated with an aneurysm that begins leaking days to weeks before rupturing. Very few patients manifest a sentinel headache prior to aneurysm rupture.

Rupture results in hemorrhage producing seizures, neurologic deficits, changes in LOC, and a high rate of mortality.

Vital Signs

BP, heart rate (HR), and RR/pattern may change secondary to altered cerebral tissue perfusion. BP control is essential to prevent rebleeding of an aneurysm and should be monitored intra-arterially. Many patients are hypertensive following the hemorrhage and BP and headache may fluctuate together. Because treatment involving volume expansion intravenously can affect BP, it is not generally instituted until after the aneurysm has been surgically clipped or treated endovascularly. Conversely, hypotension can affect cerebral blood flow and perfusion, so great care should be taken to avoid overaggressive management of hypertension. Temperature should be monitored closely because fever increases cerebral metabolic rate, which can worsen cerebral ischemia if not properly managed and may worsen outcomes post SAH.

Intracranial Pressure

Blood in the SAS can produce acute, subacute, or chronic hydrocephalus by blocking pathways for the resorption of CSF and leading to ventricular enlargement and nonfocal neurologic deterioration. Intraventricular extension at the time of aneurysm rupture can result in symptoms of acute hydrocephalus and will require temporary external ventricular drainage for management. Nuchal rigidity may be present even in the absence of hydrocephalus. Indicators of increased ICP are listed in Box 7-1.

Indicators of Hydrocephalus

- *Acute:* Persistent or sudden onset of coma with loss of pupillary reflexes within 24 hours of SAH
- *Subacute:* Gradual onset of confusion, drowsiness, lethargy, or stupor within 1 to 7 days of SAH
- *Delayed:* Gradual onset of confusion, incontinence, or impaired balance, mobility, and gait; intellectual impairment (slowness, mutism); lack of affect; and presence of the grasp and sucking frontal lobe reflexes (abnormal in adults), at about 10 days following SAH

Observation and Functional Assessment

Diminished level of consciousness: Acute deterioration in a patient's neurologic function may signal re-rupture in a patient with a ruptured but unsecured aneurysm or herald the onset of vasospasm. At the onset of significant hemorrhage, unconsciousness may occur with only reflexive or pathologic motor responses seen. Morbidity and mortality are high in those with massive hemorrhage.

Pupillary changes: Depending on location of the aneurysm, visual changes may vary; assess for visual field loss, oculomotor palsy, diplopia, immobile eye, retro-orbital pain, or hemianopsias.

Motor/sensory assessment: Fluctuating hemiparesis or aphasia with increasing confusion can be clinical symptoms of vasospasm. Hydrocephalus is generally not associated with

Box 7-1	INDICATORS OF INCREASED INTRACRANIAL PRESSURE

- Alterations in consciousness: increasing restlessness, confusion, irritability, disorientation, increasing drowsiness, and lethargy
- Bradycardia
- Increasing systolic blood pressure with a widening pulse pressure
- Irregular respiratory patterns (e.g., Cheyne-Stokes, ataxic, apneustic, central neurogenic, hyperventilation)
- Hemisensory changes and hemiparesis or hemiplegia: caused by involvement of hemispheric sensory and motor pathways
- Worsening headache
- Papillary changes
- Dysconjugate gaze and inability to move one eye beyond midposition: caused by involvement of cranial nerves III, IV, and VI
- Seizures
- Involvement of other cranial nerves: depends on the severity of neurologic insult

Note: If these indicators of increased ICP are left untreated, the patient will undergo irreversible brain damage or death. If these indicators occur suddenly, there will be displacement of brain substance (herniation), which will progress rapidly to permanent brain damage or death. For additional information about herniation syndromes, see *Traumatic Brain Injury* (p. 331). *BP,* Blood pressure.

focal neurologic deficits. Anxiety, confusion, agitation, disorientation, lethargy, stupor, and coma may indicate hydrocephalus, vasospasm, or early hyponatremia. Anorexia, nausea, vomiting, abdominal pain, cold and clammy skin, generalized weakness, and lower extremity muscle cramps are late signs of untreated hyponatremia. Flushing, diaphoresis, pupillary dilation, decreased gastric motility, increased serum glucose, fever, hypertension, tachycardia, cardiac dysrhythmias, ischemia, and infarction can be due to increased circulating catecholamines.

Fundoscopic assessment: See p. 621 under "General Neurologic Assessment."

Screening Labwork

- CSF analysis may be performed to confirm the presence of blood in the CSF in patients with symptoms suggestive of SAH but with no clear abnormalities detected on the CT scan. CSF pressure, normally 0 to 15 mm Hg (75 to 180 mm H_2O), may be elevated. The pressure is proportionate to the amount of bleeding. Protein may increase to 80 to 130 mg/dl (normal is 15 to 50 mg/dl). Note: Performance of lumbar puncture in the patient with SAH and increased ICP carries substantial risk of herniation and rebleeding; thus, it is not a routine study in this patient population. In patients with SAH and an external ventricular drain for the management of hydrocephalus, CSF may be sampled as part of a workup of infectious causes of sustained fever.
- Electrolytes and glucose levels should be monitored at least daily to detect hyponatremia and hyperglycemia. Fluid management in SAH after an aneurysm is secured can be associated with hypokalemia, hypomagnesemia, and hypophosphatemia so these electrolytes should be also monitored on at least a daily basis.
- *ABG analysis:* To detect hypoxemia and hypercapnia and to determine appropriate respiratory therapy.

DIAGNOSTIC TESTING
Refer to *Neurologic Diagnostic Testing,* p. 621.

COLLABORATIVE MANAGEMENT
Care Priorities
1. Pharmacotherapy
   - *Calcium channel blocker:* Nimodipine (Nimotop) inhibits calcium influx across the cell membrane of vascular smooth muscles. The resulting decrease in peripheral vascular resistance and vasodilation is believed to increase perfusion in cerebral vessels. While nimodipine does not prevent vasospasm, its use has been shown to be associated with

improved long-term outcomes in patients who experience vasospasm. Nimodipine is given as 60 mg enterally every 4 hours for 21 days (the recommended course of therapy). Some patients experience significant decreases in BP with nimodipine and may require a dosing schedule of 30 mg every 2 hours. Intravenous (IV) administration of calcium antagonists is not supported in evidence at this time.

- *Antihypertensives:* Antihypertensive therapy is used cautiously in this patient population because allowing hypertension is a significant element of standard therapeutic management in aneurysmal SAH. Hydralazine hydrochloride (Apresoline), labetalol (Normodyne), or nicardipine may be administered to control BP both prior to definitive securing of the ruptured aneurysm and after clipping or coiling to maintain BP in desired parameters.
- *Osmotic diuretics:* Mannitol (Osmitrol), urea (Ureaphil), and glycerin (Glycerol) may be used to reduce ICP and treat cerebral edema via diuresis to remove fluid from the brain. Patients should be monitored for electrolyte imbalances, other systemic side effects, and adverse reactions related to fluid shifting.

HIGH ALERT! With the rapid movement of extracellular fluid from brain tissue to plasma with associated decrease in brain volume, potential for rebleeding may be increased after giving mannitol. Mannitol may cause a rebound increase in ICP 8 to 12 hours after administration, as fluid shifts from cells into the vascular compartment. Furosemide (Lasix) is often used to decrease the rebound effect of mannitol.

- *Loop diuretics:* Furosemide (Lasix) is often used as a sole agent to decrease cerebral edema without causing the rise in intracranial blood volume that occurs with mannitol.
- *Corticosteroids:* Dexamethasone (Decadron) is a controversial medication used to relieve cerebral edema and decrease ICP. Use of dexamethasone is most likely to be seen in the immediate postoperative management of the patient who has undergone surgical intervention to secure the aneurysm. The patient should be monitored carefully for side effects, including GI tract irritation. Medications such as H2-blockers or proton pump inhibitors may be used to reduce the risk of gastritis and ulceration.
- *Antipyretics:* Acetaminophen is used to control fever, which increases cerebral metabolism. Usually aspirin is avoided, because its platelet action impairs clotting and promotes bleeding. In patients requiring multiple interventions to manage increased ICP, sustained fever can compromise outcome and aggressive measures may be required to control the fever. Clinical trials have been conducted to evaluate conventional treatment (use of acetaminophen and cooling blankets) compared to addition of an intravascular catheter–based heat exchange system for patients with temperatures higher than 38°C and have shown the effect to decrease fever.
- *Anticonvulsants:* Patients with aneurysmal SAH are at high risk for seizures so antiepileptic drugs such as phenytoin (Dilantin) or levetiracetam (Keppra) may be used to control or prevent seizures. If phenytoin is used, monitoring of drug levels is required to ensure optimal dosing and avoid toxicity.
- *Analgesics:* Blood in the SAS is very irritating and the headache associated with SAH can be difficult to control. Acetaminophen is commonly used along with a combination of IV and oral narcotic analgesics as necessary. Pain medications should not routinely be withheld solely out of concern for the ability to detect future neurologic deficits. Pain should always be treated. Stress management techniques can be helpful adjuvant therapy. Photophobia may persist for several days after SAH and contribute to patient discomfort. Maintaining a low light environment even after the aneurysm is secured can be helpful with this issue.
- *Stool softeners:* Restrictions in activity related to hospitalization and narcotic analgesic use can predispose the patient to constipation. Docusate sodium (Colace) is the drug of choice for preventing straining, which can increase ICP.
- *Insulin:* Glucose control particularly intraoperatively. More research is needed to determine specific critical timing of stricter glucose controls for patients with aneurysmal SAH.

- *Statins*: The use of statins is a newer therapy supported by meta-analysis, which has indicated that the initiation of statins after SAH reduces the incidence of vasospasm, delays ischemic deficits, and affects mortality. Liver function tests and creatine kinase should be assessed prior to initiation of statin therapy and then monitored on a weekly basis during acute management of aneurysmal SAH. Patients who do not otherwise require statin therapy will require it only during hospitalization.
- *Triple H therapy*: Each of the following therapies may be used singly or in combination.

Safety Alert *Although hypervolemic-hypertensive therapy with hemodilution (triple H therapy) represents standard management in SAH for vasospasm, it carries great risks. The patient's cardiovascular status requires close monitoring, as patients with existing cardiovascular disease may be unable to tolerate the hypervolemia. Additionally, the patient should be very closely monitored to establish whether their neurologic function varies with changes in BP or fluid status. If used before the aneurysm is secured, this modality may precipitate ICP with rerupture of and rebleeding from the aneurysm. When used after definitive intervention, the patient may experience cerebral edema with cerebral ischemia and subsequent neurologic deficit.*

- *Hypervolemia* (saline, whole blood, packed cells, plasma protein fraction, albumin, or hetastarch): increases circulating volume to prevent ischemia caused by vasospasm. The patient's neurologic status is often used to gauge the effectiveness of hypervolemic therapy. If concern exists about the patient's ability to tolerate hypervolemia, noninvasive methods of monitoring cardiac output and index can be employed. Use of central venous catheters and CVP monitoring is restricted to patients with clinical symptoms of vasospasm. Very rarely, invasive hemodynamic monitoring with a pulmonary artery catheter may be required.
- *Hemodilution* (albumin and crystalloid fluids): decreases blood viscosity. CVP greater than 8 mm Hg is usually sufficient to maintain hypervolemia and dilute the hematocrit to less than 35%.
- *Hypertension*: By increasing BP, CPP increases and may help prevent ischemia and infarction. Once the ruptured aneurysm is definitively secured, hypertension is allowed up to systolic BPs (SBPs) of 200 to 220 mm Hg. If a patient develops clinical symptoms of vasospasm, continuous IV vasopressors such as phenylephrine or norepinephrine may be used to assess for clinical improvement with elevation of BP to a maximum systolic pressure of 240 mm Hg. Ideally, BP is maintained 60 mm Hg above baseline.

2. **Surgical/endovascular intervention:** Initial management involves stabilizing the patient and minimizing the risk of re-rupture of the aneurysm. The National Institute of Neurological Disorders and Stroke (NINDS), a division of the National Institutes of Health (NIH), is recognized as the leader in research on the brain and nervous system in the United States. The NINDS sponsored the International Study of Unruptured Intracranial Aneurysms, including greater than 4,000 patients at 61 sites in the United States, Canada, and Europe. Results revealed the risk of rupture for aneurysms less than 7 mm in size is low. The findings provide a comprehensive evaluation of these vascular defects, offering guidance to both patients and health care professionals facing the difficult decision about the best treatment for a cerebral aneurysm.

Advances in imaging, use of microscopes intraoperatively, dedicated neurologic intensive care units, endovascular treatment methods, and aggressive cerebral vasospasm prevention and management have reduced morbidity and mortality. Treatment options depend on assessment of preoperative risk factors, predictive indicators, and location and size of the aneurysm. Successful treatments include endovascular embolization ("gluing"), surgical clipping, and endovascular detachable coiling.

Recent studies confirm improved patient outcomes when the ruptured aneurysm is secured within the first 24 to 72 hours for patients with grade I or II symptoms (Hunt and Hess Scale). Early intervention may prevent rebleeding, an often fatal complication, and allows for the management of vasospasm without risk of rebleeding. Securing of the aneurysm during the time period associated with the highest risk of development of cerebral arterial vasospasm has been shown to be associated with increased morbidity and mortality, so if the aneurysm is not secured within 24 to 72 hours of rupture, repair should be delayed until the peak time for vasospasm (7 to 10 days after SAH) has passed. Patients with grades III to V symptoms are generally considered poor interventional risks, especially in the period immediately after SAH. If these patients are clinically unstable, they may be treated medically until they improve or stabilize enough for endovascular or surgical intervention. Surgery is considered for a patient with a large intracranial clot causing life-threatening, intracranial brain shifting. Intervention is delayed for a patient with cerebral vasospasm until the vasospasm subsides.

While surgical clipping of aneurysms had previously been the only method of intervention available, neurovascular interventionalists can now use an alternative to surgery using Guglielmi Detachable Coils (GDC coils). The overall size and location of the aneurysm and the aneurysmal neck size are evaluated to decide if this option is feasible. GDC coils are microcoils composed of a soft platinum alloy that are placed with use of a microcatheter through the femoral artery. The catheter is advanced into the cerebral circulation using radiographic imaging. Low-voltage current is applied to the guidewire to detach the coil(s) placed into the sac of the aneurysm. Placement of one or more coils fills the sac, reduces the pressure inside, and isolates the aneurysm from normal circulation. When this is performed for the management of unruptured aneurysm, the patient's hospital stay is very brief (24 to 48 hours) unless the aneurysm ruptures or another complication of angiography occurs.. Endovascular treatment complications differ from those associated with surgical clipping and can include arterial dissection, arterial perforation, distal embolization, and groin hematomas. Aneurysmal recurrence has been seen in a small number of cases. However, endovascular methods have become an acceptable alternative to microsurgical clipping in appropriate cases.

Neurovascular interventionalists can also perform cerebral angioplasty for arterial vasospasm to decrease vascular narrowing and reverse ischemia in patients with new-onset vasospasm within 6 to 12 hours of onset. Patient selection for this is limited to those whose vasospasm involves accessible major cerebral vessels; distal cerebral arterial vasospasm is not amenable to angioplasty.

3. **Management of hydrocephalus:**
- *External ventricular drainage (EVD):* Hydrocephalus develops in 20% to 25% of patients with SAH from a ruptured cerebral aneurysm. Patients with symptomatic hydrocephalus generally require placement of an external ventricular drainage system for management of their hydrocephalus. For those with massive hydrocephalus, coma and Hunt-Hess classification of III or IV, placement of an external ventriculostomy drain can decompress the ventricles enough to produce significant improvements in the patient's neurologic function and make the patient a candidate for intervention to secure the ruptured aneurysm.
- *Ventricular shunt:* Most patients do not develop chronic hydrocephalus following SAH. For those who do develop a chronic problem, the percentage of those who initially require extraventricular drainage who progress to needing a shunt is not clearly reflected in the literature. When a shunt is necessary, one end of a small catheter is positioned into a ventricle, with the other end draining into a body cavity or space (e.g., SAS, cistern, peritoneum, vena cava, pleura). Major complications include infection and malfunction. If the shunt has a valve for the purpose of controlling drainage or preventing reflux of CSF, the surgeon may request that the valve be pumped periodically to ensure proper functioning. For nursing interventions after shunt placement, see Box 7-2.

CARE PLANS FOR CEREBRAL ANEURYSM AND SUBARACHNOID HEMORRHAGE

Risk for ineffective cerebral tissue perfusion *related to vasospasm of cerebral vessels and/or decreased intracranial adaptive capacity related to increased intracranial pressure*

- -

GOALS/OUTCOMES Maintain normal ICP and/or minimize clinical effects on cerebral adaptability through preventive measures, aggressive volume management, regulation of cerebral blood flow, and close hemodynamic monitoring.
NOC Circulation Status

Box 7-2   NURSING INTERVENTIONS AFTER SHUNT PLACEMENT

- After the shunting, assess patient for indicators of increased ICP (see Box 7-1) caused by either the disease itself or shunt malfunction.
- Position patient on side opposite the insertion site, either flat or with head elevated slightly (as prescribed) to prevent pressure on shunt mechanism.
- Assess vital signs; LOC (orientation to time, place, and person); papillary light reflex; and motor function.
- Monitor I&O, and limit fluids as prescribed.
- Avoid severe head and neck rotation, flexion, or hyperextension to prevent kinking, compression, or twisting of the shunt catheter, which would impede CSF flow.
- If the shunt has a valve for controlling drainage or preventing reflux of CSF, pump the valve to ensure proper functioning, according to surgeon's directive. Usually the valve is located behind or above the ear and is the approximate diameter of a fingertip. Pumping involves gentle, serial compressions of the tissue over the shunt. If the valve is working properly, the emptying and refilling of the valve will be felt with palpation.
- Assess for indicators of meningitis including peritonitis and sepsis, caused by presence of shunt mechanism. (See *Peritonitis*, p. 805, and *SIRS, Sepsis, and MODS*, p. 924.)

CSF, Cerebrospinal fluid; *ICP,* intracranial pressure; *I&O,* intake and output; *LOC,* level of consciousness.

Cerebral Perfusion Promotion
1. Bed rest, with aneurysm precautions and prevention of ICP
2. Subarachnoid precautions are instituted while the patient is awaiting definitive management of a ruptured cerebral aneurysm. Try to keep patient quiet and calm in a soothing environment, with lowered lights and noise level.
3. Active ROM and isometric exercises are restricted during acute and preoperative stages to prevent ICP.
4. Passive ROM is prescribed to prevent formation of thrombi, with subsequent pulmonary emboli.
5. Bowel management program is essential to prevent straining at stool. Instruct patient to avoid activities using isometric muscle contractions (e.g., pulling or pushing side rails, pushing against the foot board), which raise SBP, with resultant increased ICP.

Instruct patient to avoid coughing because increased intrathoracic pressure increases ICP.

Intracranial Pressure Monitoring
1. Increased ICP is common after SAH, but its manifestations range from minimal (e.g., persistent headache or drowsiness) to severe (e.g., coma or death). Elevated ICP that does not respond to treatment has been associated with poor patient outcomes.
2. In patients who require invasive devices to manage their ICP, the critical care nurse strives to maintain normal ICP (0 to 10 mm Hg with an upper limit of 15 mm Hg) and CPP 60 to 80 mm Hg. Calculate CPP by means of the formula: CPP = MAP (mean arterial BP) − ICP. CPP less than 30 mm Hg causes cerebral anoxia.
3. HOB elevation: A 30- to 45-degree angle facilitates venous outflow from the intracranial cavity and lowers ICP. Head should be kept in straight alignment to prevent increased ICP secondary to obstruction of jugular venous outflow. Values of 180 to 220 mm Hg as prescribed end points.

Impaired gas exchange or ineffective airway clearance due to altered level of consciousness

GOALS/OUTCOMES Effective airway clearance and gas exchange and maintain appropriate $Paco_2$ level, which can affect ICP.

NOC Respiratory Status: Gas Exchange

Ventilation Assistance
1. Supplemental oxygen, maintenance of patent airway, possible intubation and ventilation if needed. Serial ABG tests are performed to identify hypoxemia (Pao_2 less than 80 mm Hg) and hypercapnia ($Paco_2$ greater than 45 mm Hg). Hypercapnia is a potent cerebral vasodilator that can increase ICP in patients who are already at risk.

Oxygen Therapy
2. Avoid vigorous, prolonged suctioning, which precipitates hypoxemia and hypercapnia. Preoxygenation with slight hyperventilation using 100% oxygen helps prevent cerebral vasodilation associated with hypercapnia.

Risk for injury *related to the potential impact of hyperglycemia*

GOALS/OUTCOMES Glucose levels are controlled within normalized parameters throughout all phases of treatment.
NOC Risk Control

Risk Identification
1. Studies have shown that admission hyperglycemia or perioperative hyperglycemia is associated with poor outcome after aneurysmal SAH. Daily glucose monitoring is encouraged. More frequent monitoring and intervention are required in patients with persistent hyperglycemia.
2. Further research is underway to determine the critical timing for strict glucose control, effect on neurological outcome, and how serum glucose levels impact brain glucose concentrations.

Risk for imbalanced fluid volume *related to initiation of measures to maintain hypervolemia*

GOALS/OUTCOMES Adequately managed intake and output with control of fluid volumes affecting systemic and cerebral blood flow and electrolyte levels
NOC Fluid Balance

Fluid/Electrolyte Management
1. Fluid balance is maintained based on CVP, weight, and monitoring of intake/output (I&O) balance.
2. Electrolytes should be replaced on the basis of the patient's laboratory values.
3. *Hyponatremia* is often seen in this patient population. Standard fluid management can make it difficult to determine whether the underlying cause is cerebral salt wasting or SIADH. Regardless of the underlying cause, hyponatremia is treated with salt repletion since the fluid restriction commonly used in other patient populations to manage SIADH is contraindicated in SAH patients who are still at high risk for vasospasm and cerebral ischemia. In mild hyponatremia, initial repletion is oral (e.g., salt tablets with meals). If hyponatremia does not respond to oral replacement, IV use of hypertonic saline (1.8% or 3%) is initiated. Hyponatremia requires frequent monitoring of laboratory values to assess effectiveness of therapy. Once the patient's sodium normalizes, therapy is slowly tapered to assess the patient's ability to maintain a normal serum sodium level.
4. Triple H therapy may lead to fluid volume overload and must be closely monitored. Multiple electrolyte abnormalities are often seen with triple H therapy, and serum magnesium and phosphorus levels should be monitored regularly along with standard blood chemistries.
5. Maintain adequate nutritional intake using enteral feedings, oral intake, parenteral nutrition, or lipid emulsions as indicated by patient's neurologic status. Initially patients may present with severe nausea and vomiting following aneurysmal rupture, but this generally resolves in first 24 hours.

ADDITIONAL NURSING DIAGNOSES

As appropriate, see nursing diagnoses and interventions in *Nutritional Support* (p. 117), *Mechanical Ventilation* (p. 99), *Alterations in Consciousness* (p. 24), *Prolonged Immobility* (p. 119), *Emotional and Spiritual Support of the Patient and Significant Others* (p. 200), *Diabetes Insipidus* (p. 703), and *Syndrome of Inappropriate Antidiuretic Hormone* (p. 734).

CARE OF THE PATIENT AFTER INTRACRANIAL SURGERY

Cranial surgery can be performed to remove a space-occupying lesion such as a tumor, evacuate a hematoma or abscess, or remove a foreign object. A patient may have a surgical repair of a vascular abnormality, such as an aneurysm or arteriovenous malformation (AVM) or to correct skull fractures. Neurosurgeon may elect to perform a procedure as a treatment modality, such as to drain CSF from the ventricular system or to divert CSF to promote dural repair, control seizures or tremors, and reduce pain. Minimally invasive intracranial procedures using stereotactic techniques are used for some biopsies and for implantation of deep brain stimulators for control of essential tremors. Endoscopic and stereotactic aspiration is being performed for noncomatose basal ganglia hemorrhages. The type of surgical approach the neurosurgeon takes depends primarily on the location of the pathologic condition. The *supratentorial* approach is used to remove or correct problems in the frontal, temporal, or occipital lobes, as well as in the diencephalic area (i.e., pituitary, hypothalamus). Lesions of the cerebellum and brainstem usually require an *infratentorial* (i.e., suboccipital) approach. The *transsphenoidal* approach gains access to the pituitary gland to remove a tumor, control bone pain associated with metastatic cancer, or attempt to arrest the progression of diabetic retinopathy in a patient with diabetes mellitus.

NEUROLOGIC ASSESSMENT: POSTOPERATIVE CARE
Goal of System Assessment
Evaluate for several key nursing diagnoses requiring emergent intervention:
- Alteration in cerebral tissue perfusion due to increased ICP or cerebral vasospasm
- Impaired gas exchange and/or ineffective airway clearance due to altered level of consciousness
- Risk of infection at site or due to cerebral spinal fluid leak
- Fluid volume deficit or excess impaired mobility
- Altered sensory perception involving trunk, extremities, or cranial nerves
- Alteration in cardiac output from dysrhythmias
- Adequate control of pain

History and Risk Factors
The critical care nurse caring for a postoperative neurosurgical patient needs to have a thorough understanding of the patient's preoperative history and condition requiring surgical intervention and, most important, knowledge of the patient's baseline or immediate preoperative neurologic assessment findings. It is essential to note any changes in assessment to evaluate for new postoperative neurologic changes due to the surgical intervention. Neurologic assessment data must be closely monitored for new focal changes, noting a trend in assessment data and correlated to the pathophysiologic process to identify appropriate nursing interventions. Three key causes of acute deterioration in a patient's neurologic status in the immediate postoperative period are cerebral edema, hemorrhage into or around surgical site, and seizures.

Vital Signs
- *BP, HR, and RR changes*: May further alter cerebral tissue perfusion. Uncontrolled high BP can lead to ICH; therefore, close monitoring is important to keep the SBP less than 160 mm Hg to prevent bleeding. Hypotension reduces cerebral perfusion and can cause cerebral infarcts. Monitor rate, rhythm, and depth of respirations for changes or abnormal breathing patterns.
- *Hyperthermia*: May be associated with injury or irritation of the hypothalamic temperature-regulating centers, presence of blood in the CSF, or infection. Elevated temperature increases the metabolic needs of the brain, potentially leading to increased blood flow to the area, with concomitant cerebral hyperemia.
- *Intracranial pressure*: If ICP monitoring is utilized, the critical care nurse needs to understand the dynamics of CPP. A postoperative increase in either the volume of brain tissue (e.g., edema), cerebral spinal fluid, or blood or the addition of a hematoma can cause intracranial hypertension. The normal ICP is generally 0–10 mm Hg (up to 15 mm Hg). CPP is inversely related to ICP and in pressures less than 50 mm Hg can lead to cerebral ischemia or infarction: CPP = MAP – ICP.

Observation
- *LOC*: The improvement in the degree of LOC depends on preoperative damage to cerebral tissue. LOC often improves as anesthesia wears off, or as cerebral edema subsides, and then the ICP approaches normal.
- *Pupillary changes*: Pupillary abnormalities can indicate unilateral or bilateral brain dysfunction, interruption of sympathetic or parasympathetic pathways, damage in the brainstem, cranial nerve damage, and herniation.
- *Communicative and cognitive deficits*: The ability to communicate and understand spoken or written words after surgery depends on the level of preoperative dysfunction, the site of the lesion, extent of the procedure, and the degree of postoperative cerebral edema.
  - *Broca* (expressive, motor, nonfluent) aphasia: Inability to communicate verbally or in writing. Can understand situations, follow commands.
  - *Wernicke* (receptive, sensory, fluent) aphasia: Individual does not understand the situation and cannot follow commands appropriately.
- *CSF leakage:* Assess for CSF leakage from the ear (otorrhea), from the nose (rhinorrhea) which is seen particularly with transphenoidal surgery, and also from the surgical site. The leakage of CSF indicates an open pathway to the SAS, which carries a serious risk of infection. Causes specific to craniotomy include the use of an external ventricular

drainage device (which is being used as a treatment modality) and can be a source of entrance of organisms, or remote site infection, and any repeat operation. CSF leak treatment depends upon severity, site, and weighing the risk for infection and may include the use of external CSF drainage (e.g., lumbar subarachnoid drain) to divert CSF flow and thus reduce pressure, keeping patient flat (if not contraindicated), and allowing time for the dural tear to heal. Surgical intervention may be done to seal the dural leak at the origin site.

Observation and Functional Assessment

1. **Assess motor function and sensory responses:**
   - *Motor*: Motor deficits (weakness or paralysis) are caused by injury or edema to the primary motor cortex and corticospinal (pyramidal) tracts.
   - *Sensory*: Sensory deficits occur when the primary sensory cortex, the sensory association areas of the parietal lobe, or the spinothalamic tracts are injured or edematous. Sensory deficits include inability to distinguish objects according to characteristics (e.g., size, shape, weight) and inability to distinguish overall changes in temperature, touch, pressure, and position.

   Improvement in both motor and sensory perception may be seen as cerebral edema subsides.

2. **Assess for cranial nerve impairment:** The degree of cranial nerve deficit(s) depends on site of the lesion, preoperative deficit, degree of postoperative cerebral edema, and surgical approach. Infratentorial surgery for lesions in the posterior fossa (brainstem and cerebellum) involves significant cranial nerve manipulation with high risk of injury to cranial nerves IX, X, and XII, which innervate the pharynx and tongue. Risk of airway obstruction is high. Removal of tumors (i.e., acoustic neuromas) may injure the facial nerve and result in facial paralysis and loss of corneal reflex. The loss of corneal reflex may be caused by surgical trauma to frontal lobe motor pathways or brainstem cranial nerve nuclei. Corneal abrasion, ulceration, and blindness may occur if not recognized and treated promptly. Always prevent corneal abrasion and irritation. Keep cornea moist with prescribed ophthalmic solution and use an eye shield if indicated.

   Cranial nerve deficit(s) may improve as cerebral edema resolves or may be permanent. Nursing assessment of cranial nerve dysfunction is important. For more information about the function of all the cranial nerves, see Appendix 3.

Screening Labwork

- *Sodium levels and osmolality*: Important for management of SIADH and diabetes insipidus. Close monitoring during hyperosmolar therapy is important. Hyponatremia can indicate dehydration and if not managed can produce brain swelling.
- *CSF analysis*: Evaluates the color, white blood cell (WBC) count, differential, glucose content, and protein level, which are important whenever CSF leak develops
- *Complete blood count (CBC), electrolytes, and coagulation studies*: Evaluates for anemia, hypo- or hyperglycemia; potential for hemorrhage or infection
- *Anticonvulsant medication levels*: If patient is receiving anticonvulsant therapy, monitor for subtherapeutic and supratherapeutic levels.

DIAGNOSTIC TESTING

Refer to *Neurologic Diagnostic Testing*, p. 621.

COLLABORATIVE MANAGEMENT AFTER INTRACRANIAL SURGERY
Care Priorities

1. **Respiratory support:** Supplemental oxygen, intubation, and mechanical ventilation as needed. In patients requiring mechanical ventilation who have potential or actual increased ICP, use of hyperventilation needs careful monitoring to avoid cerebral vasoconstriction. The Brain Tumor Foundation standard emphasizes that in absence of increased ICP, chronic hyperventilation ($Paco_2$ less than 25 mm Hg) should not be done the first 24 hours after traumatic brain injury. Use of prophylactic hyperventilation ($Paco_2$ less than 35 mm Hg) should be avoided during the first 24 hours or used only if increased ICP does not respond to other measures such as CSF drainage, sedation, or use of neuromuscular blocking agents.

2. **Positioning:** Head of the bed (HOB) is most often elevated 30 degrees to promote venous drainage, which reduces ICP. Head should be kept in straight alignment with trunk to prevent increased ICP.
   - *In posterior fossa surgery (infratentorial approach),* the supporting muscles of the neck are altered. Patients should be turned with the neck in alignment with the head, with the head, neck, and shoulders supported.
   - *After hemicraniectomy,* to avoid injury, the patient should not be turned to the side from which hemicraniectomy has been removed. Label head dressing, chart, and bed with location of missing bone. A head protective device such as a specially sized helmet should be worn.
   - *After procedures in which a large intracranial space is left after extensive surgery,* to avoid a sudden shift in intracranial contents, with subsequent hemorrhage or herniation, the patient should not be positioned on operative side immediately after surgery.
3. **Manage pain:**
   - *Analgesics:* Clinical trials have shown that the addition of tramadol or nalbuphine to acetaminophen controls pain more adequately in patients who have undergone craniotomy.
   Note: The effect of morphine and tramadol patient-controlled analgesia (PCA) on arterial carbon dioxide tension is still unknown for craniotomy patients.
4. **Reduce cerebral edema:**
   - *Corticosteroids* (e.g., dexamethasone): To decrease cerebral edema
   Note: Research is ongoing to determine whether steroids are effective in the treatment of cerebral edema. They are prescribed for the treatment of vasogenic cerebral edema and edema caused by cerebral tumor.

> **Safety Alert**   *Steroids can cause a hyperosmolar state and dehydration. Monitor serum osmolality and electrolytes and assess fluid status before and after administration.*

   - *Osmotic diuretics* (e.g., mannitol): To control cerebral edema causing increased ICP. Dose is usually 0.25 to 1 g/kg of 20% solution administered over 20 to 30 minutes, and ICP levels should be measured before, during, and after administration of mannitol. When the ICP reaches a desired fixed reduced level (usually within 15 minutes), the dosage of mannitol needs to be gradually reduced.
   - *Fluid and electrolyte management:* To prevent or treat increasing cerebral edema
5. **Perioperative and postoperative deep venous thrombosis (DVT) prevention**

> **Safety Alert**   *A systematic review of literature done for the Agency for Healthcare Research and Quality (AHRQ) showed the risk of neurosurgical patients for deep venous thrombosis (DVT) is 28%. The 5 Million Lives Campaign, National Hospital Quality Measure of The Joint Commission, National Hospital Quality Measure by the CMS, and the National Quality Forum all endorse aspects of DVT prophylaxis. Craniotomy patients without contraindications for anticoagulation should receive DVT prophylaxis using either a low-molecular-weight heparin or low-dose unfractionated heparin (LDUH) given as an alternative. Pharmacologic agents can be used as an adjunct to mechanical prophylaxis using intermittent pneumatic compression, elastic stockings, or both. Venous imaging techniques such as ultrasonography can be used before discharge to detect thrombosis.*

6. **Control seizures:**
   - *Anticonvulsants:* Phenytoin should be considered for prophylaxis of provoked or early seizures occurring within 7 days of surgery. Use of other agents such as carbamazepine, phenobarbital, and valproate remains controversial and in some studies has not shown to reduce postoperative seizures.
7. **Prevent infection:**
   - *Antibiotics:* Prevent postoperative surgical site infection or respiratory or urinary tract infection. Randomized controlled trials have shown that in patients undergoing craniotomy, the use of prophylactic antibiotics reduces the frequency of postoperative meningitis.

Safety Alert *The American Society of Health System Pharmacists and the Centers for Disease Control and Prevention (CDC) have recommended that administration be via the IV route at induction of anesthesia and/or that the bactericidal concentration of the drug be established in the tissues and serum when the incision is made.*

8. **Nutritional support:** The method and type of nutritional support are determined by the patient's condition and may include any of the following: oral feedings, enteral feedings, supplements, or parenteral nutrition (i.e., total parenteral nutrition [TPN], fat emulsion therapy). See *Nutritional Support* (p. 117).

9. **Reduce fever:**
   - *Antipyretics*: Treat elevated temperature, which can increase use of oxygen and glucose supplies.

10. **Prevent gastric ulcers:**
    - *Histamine H2-receptor antagonists/ proton pump inhibitors*: To inhibit gastric secretions and thus prevent or facilitate healing of gastric ulcers and prevent bleeding

11. **Facilitate mobility and return of functions needed for activities of daily living:**
    - *Physical medicine consultation:* To evaluate patient and plan for rehabilitation: physical and occupational therapies for planning return of function

    Speech therapy may be important for dysphagic screening, monitoring for meeting communication needs.

12. **Implement therapeutic hypothermia:** Not routine therapy but can be used. Is generally used according to a research protocol. The effects of cooling of the injured brain continues to be studied to evaluate the effects of mild to moderate hypothermia on protection against ischemic and nonischemic brain hypoxia, traumatic brain injury, and anoxic injury with cardiac arrest. Prophylactically induced hypothermia has yet to be shown as having beneficial effects on outcomes of traumatic brain injury.

CARE PLANS: COMPLICATIONS AFTER INTRACRANIAL SURGERY

Decreased intracranial adaptive capacity *related to possible changes in intracranial fluid or brain tissue volume following surgery*

GOALS/OUTCOMES Maintain normal ICP (0 to 10 mm Hg with upper limit of 15 mm Hg) through regulation of cerebral flow and cerebral spinal circulation.

NOC Neurological status: consciousness

Cerebral Perfusion Promotion

1. *Monitor for increased ICP with potential for herniation:* Cerebral edema, hemorrhage, infection, and surgical trauma can all lead to increased ICP with herniation (see Box 7-1). Some cerebral edema is expected after intracranial surgery, and usually peaks about 72 hours after surgery (see *Traumatic Brain Injury*, p. 331). Postoperative uncontrolled nausea and vomiting can cause high intra-abdominal and also increased intrathoracic pressure (e.g., high PEEP ventilator settings) leading to high ICP.

2. *Monitor for intracranial bleeding:* Postoperative bleeding can be related to the surgical site and may be intracerebral, intracerebellar, subarachnoid, subdural, epidural, or intraventricular. Coagulation profiles and platelet counts should be monitored closely. Bleeding may be caused by the lengthy and extensive surgical procedure, high BP, prolonged anesthesia, preexisting medical problems, or medications. Contusions can develop after evacuation of epidural or subdural hematomas and may create a mass effect.

3. *Control seizures:* Generalized or partial seizures can occur as a result of surgical trauma, irritation of cerebral tissue by the presence of blood, cerebral edema, cerebral hypoxia, hypoglycemia, preexisting seizure disorder, or inadequate anticonvulsant levels. The use of anticonvulsants prophylactically remains controversial.

4. *Monitor for hydrocephalus:* May appear before surgery or occur after surgery as an acute or chronic complication. Usually it is caused by a slowing or complete stoppage of the flow of CSF through the ventricular system secondary to edema, bleeding, scarring, or obstruction. For further discussion, see *Cerebral Aneurysm and Subarachnoid Hemorrhage* (p. 629).

5. *Assess for tension pneumocephalus:* Uncommon but can occur as a result of air entering the subdural, extradural, subarachnoid, intracerebral, or intraventricular spaces and is an emergent situation May be a complication of

infratentorial/posterior fossa craniotomy, burr holes for removal of chronic subdural hematoma, and transsphenoidal hypophysectomy. Rapid decompression is usually required.

Ineffective breathing pattern *related to altered level of consciousness and inability to maintain adequate airway and respiratory rate*

GOALS/OUTCOMES Maintain adequate airway, provide supplemental oxygenation, ventilate patient as necessary to maintain $PaCO_2$ to 35 mm Hg. Increase in $PaCO_2$, hypercapnia, can lead to cerebral vasodilation with a subsequent increase in intracranial volume, and thus increased ICP. A severe drop in $PaCO_2$ can lead to cerebral vasoconstriction and cerebral ischemia.
NOC Respiratory Status: Gas Exchange

Ventilation Assistance
1. Monitor for partial or complete airway obstruction caused by accumulation of secretions, improper positioning, or change in level of consciousness.
2. Assess for increased crackles caused by neurogenic pulmonary edema resulting from a sudden increase in ICP.
3. Assess for changes in level of consciousness caused by cerebral edema that causes compression of brainstem respiratory centers.
4. Discourage vigorous coughing, as it increases ICP.
5. Encourage deep breathing to help prevent atelectasis and pneumonia.
6. Following institutional protocol for venous thromboembolism (VTE)/DVT prophylaxis to help prevent pulmonary embolism.

Risk for infection

GOALS/OUTCOMES Prevent infection at site or secondary infections such as meningitis, encephalitis, or ventriculitis or due to invasive procedures.
NOC Risk Control

Infection Control
1. Monitor for a central nervous system (CNS) infection: can be caused by a preoperative event such as organisms introduced at the time of injury (e.g., gunshot wound) or a break in sterile technique or due to nature of the surgical procedure involving opening of the dura. (See *Meningitis*, p. 644.)
2. Monitor for a ventriculostomy-related infection (VRI): A ventriculostomy may be performed with introduction of an intraventricular catheter to monitor and manage postoperative ICP or to provide external ventricular drainage for CSF diversion secondary to dural leaks. Extended duration of catheterization has been correlated with increasing risk of CSF infections.

Deficient fluid volume or excess fluid volume *related to hormonal or electrolyte imbalances*

GOALS/OUTCOMES Adequately managed I&O, control of fluid imbalances resulting from hormonal or electrolyte disturbances, and prevention of fluid loss.
NOC Fluid Balance

Fluid Management
1. Monitor for sodium imbalance secondary to diabetes insipidus and SIADH: results from disturbance of the hypothalamus or posterior lobe of the pituitary gland. ADH is produced in the hypothalamus and stored in the posterior pituitary.
   - *Diabetes insipidus* (DI) results from decreased ADH production, which leads to excessive urinary output, with potentially serious fluid and electrolyte problems (see *Diabetes Insipidus,* p. 703). DI may result from edema, manipulation, or partial or total removal of the gland.
   - *SIADH*, a less common problem, results from an increase in the release of ADH, which leads to resorption of large amounts of water via the renal tubules with concurrent loss of large amounts of sodium. Like DI, SIADH can cause serious fluid and electrolyte problems (see *Syndrome of Inappropriate Antidiuretic Hormone,* p. 734).
2. Assess for hypovolemic shock: may occur as a result of general fluid loss associated with treatment using osmotic diuretics; therefore, close monitoring is essential. Critical care nurses need to be observing patients for development of DI postoperatively, because severe dehydration and hypovolemic shock can occur if fluid balance is not restored.

3. Monitor for gastrointestinal (GI) bleeding: GI bleeding associated with cerebral trauma and the postoperative period after neurosurgery can cause fluid volume deficit. Although the cause is unclear, stress from the trauma or the surgery can produce continuous vagal stimulation leading to a hyperacidic state resulting in gastric erosion, ulceration, and ultimately hemorrhage. These conditions also result from medications, especially cortico-steroids (see *Acute Gastrointestinal Bleeding*, p. 751). Other GI conditions may occur, such as constipation, after neurologic surgery. Decreased or absent peristalsis results from prolonged anesthesia, immobility, trauma, elec-trolyte deficiencies, and mechanical obstruction (e.g., obstipation).

Impaired physical mobility *related to prolonged bed rest or motor dysfunction*

GOALS/OUTCOMES Prevent vascular complications through appropriate pharmacotherapy and mechanical prophylaxis, and prevent atrophy and/or joint contractures through passive exercises, early mobilization, and activity progression.
NOC Mobility

Exercise Promotion
1. *Thrombophlebitis, DVT, and pulmonary embolism:* May result from prolonged bed rest and immobility after intra-cranial surgery. Other factors such as a prolonged surgical procedure, preexisting hypercoagulable states, and other blood dyscrasias may influence the postoperative complications. VTE is the most frequent complication following craniotomy for removal of brain tumors. Prophylactic management standards have been developed for the prevention of DVT.

Decreased cardiac output *related to unstable blood pressure or cardiac dysrhythmias*

GOALS/OUTCOMES Stabilize BP and HR within normal limits to maintain adequate cardiac output, thereby promoting appropriate cerebral blood flow.
NOC Circulation Status

Cardiac Precautions
1. *Monitor for cardiac dysrhythmias:* May occur as a result of cerebral hypoxia or ischemia, manipulation of the brainstem, or the irritating effects of blood in the CSF (see *Dysrhythmias and Conduction Disturbances*, p. 492).

Pain *related to headache or discomfort secondary to surgical intervention*

GOALS/OUTCOMES Pain and discomfort are controlled as evidenced by patient's self-report response, stable vital signs, and lack of skeletal muscle tension and behavioral signs. Pain and autonomic system stimulation and physical agitation can increase ICP, produce sleep deprivation, and mask neurologic changes and thereby lead to further complications.
NOC Pain Control

Pain Management
1. *Medicate and intervene appropriately to keep patient's pain controlled and maintain comfort level.* Use of an evidence-based pain scale measurement such as a numerical rating scale (1 to 10) or a behavioral pain scale may be appropriate for patients with impaired communication ability.
2. *Assess level of sedation appropriately.* Overmedication with analgesics or sedatives in postoperative patients with altered level of consciousness can produce impaired gas exchange and compromised airway.

ADDITIONAL NURSING DIAGNOSES
See also nursing diagnoses and interventions in *Traumatic Brain Injury* (p. 331), *Cerebral Aneurysm and Subarachnoid Hemorrhage* (p. 629) *Status Epilepticus, Meningitis* (p. 644), *Diabetes Insipidus* (p. 703), *Syndrome of Inappropriate Antidiuretic Hormone* (p. 734), *Nutritional Support* (p. 117), *Prolonged Immobility* (p. 149), and *Emotional and Spiritual Support of the Patient and Sig-nificant Others* (p. 200).

MENINGITIS
■

PATHOPHYSIOLOGY
Meningitis is an inflammation of the brain and spinal cord (CNS) affecting the meninges (i.e., dura, arachnoid, pia), brain surface, and cranial nerves. There are several types of meningitis, broadly classified as bacterial (pyogenic), viral, aseptic, tuberculous, fungal, and parasitic. Menin-gitis is most commonly community acquired or the result of direct contamination. Unfortunately,

the incidence of nosocomial meningitis is on the rise. The causative agent usually travels in the bloodstream from various sources before entering the CSF. The CSF is deficient in mounting any antibacterial response as it lacks immunoglobulins and complement. Therefore, when contamination of the CSF occurs, phygocytosis and opsonization of the bacteria do not occur. Bacterial meningitis, a consequence of bacterial invasion, progresses through four interconnected phases: (1) invasion of host leading to CNS infection, (2) inflammation of the subarachnoid and ventricular space as bacteria multiply, (3) pathophysiologic changes consistent with progression of inflammation, and (4) neuronal damage.

Bacterial Meningitis

The most common form, can be community acquired or associated with prior infection. Other causes include injury (e.g., open/penetrating wounds), facial or basilar skull fractures, shunt occlusion/malfunction, craniotomy, otitis media, sinusitis, or bacteremia (e.g., endocarditis, pneumonia).

Streptococcus pneumoniae, a gram-positive cocci, has been the leading cause of adult meningitis in the United States. Pneumococcal meningitis occurs in crowded conditions and is spread seasonally (fall and winter). This organism is not as prevalent as a cause of meningitis since the development of Pneumovax and Prevnar vaccines. Pneumococcal meningitis may occur following an upper respiratory tract infection (URI) or nasopharyngeal colonization with a pneumococcal strain, is a complication of conditions associated with CSF leaks, is associated with asplenia, and is more prevalent in immunocompromised persons and in older adults.

Neisseria meningitidis, a gram-negative cocci, is the second leading cause of meningitis in adults. Infection is more likely to occur in patients with complement component deficiencies (e.g., congenital or associated with nephrotic syndrome, hepatic failure, systemic lupus erythematosus, multiple myeloma).

Haemophilus influenzae, a gram-negative bacilli, is the most common cause in children; however, it may affect adults. Predisposing factors include URIs, hypogammaglobulinemia, diabetes mellitus, alcoholism, and head trauma. Since 1990, the *H. influenzae* vaccine type B (Hib vaccine) has reduced the incidence of bacterial meningitis substantially in infants and children, making it a disease predominantly of adults. Prior to 1990, *H. influenzae* type b was the leading cause of bacterial meningitis.

Listeria monocytogenes, gram-positive bacilli, is being seen more frequently as a cause of meningitis, especially in immunocompromised patients and those of extreme ages (very young and very old). Outbreaks have been linked to consumption of contaminated dairy products, undercooked chicken, fish, and meats.

Gram-negative species (*Escherichia coli, Klebsiella, Proteus,* and *Pseudomonas*) are increasing in prevalence as a nosocomial cause secondary to trauma or neurosurgical procedures. Spontaneous gram-negative meningitis is found in older adults, the immunocompromised, or persons with underlying conditions such as cirrhosis, diabetes, malignancy, or splenectomy. The urinary tract is the usual portal of entry of bacteria.

Other microbes: *Mycobacterium pneumoniae, B. burgdorferi,* and *Treponema pallidum* are also associated with meningitis.

Other surgical procedures complicated by gram-negative infections are ventriculoperitoneal shunts, craniofacial repair, ventriculostomy, hypophysectomy, reservoir insertion, and myelography.

Tuberculous Meningitis

Mycobacterium tuberculosis is a meningeal infection more common in human immunodeficiency virus (HIV)-infected patients, along with older adults and children living among people with tuberculosis.

Fungal Meningitis

Cryptococcus neoformans, an opportunistic organism seen with acquired immune deficiency syndrome (AIDS), is the leading cause of CNS fungal infection. Other fungi are associated less often.

Viral Meningitis

Enteroviruses are the most common cause of viral meningitis in the spring and fall seasons. The condition generally lasts 7 to 10 days and, although serious, is rarely fatal in people with normal immune systems. Herpesviruses, including herpes simplex viruses (the cause of chickenpox, Epstein-Barr virus, and shingles), measles, and influenza may lead to viral meningitis. Mosquitoes and other insects spread arboviruses, which cause infections that precede viral meningitis.

Aseptic Meningitis Syndrome
In aseptic meningitis, the clinical and laboratory evaluations provide evidence for inflammation, but bacterial cultures are negative. It may be drug induced, related to infection, or unrelated to infection. Aseptic meningitis has been linked to adverse drug reactions with nonsteroidal anti-inflammatory drugs (NSAIDs) and antimicrobials such as trimethoprim-sulfamethoxazole (TMP-SMX).

Noninfectious Causes
Sarcoidosis, leptomeningeal carcinomatosis, systemic lupus erythematosus, Wegener granulomatosis, and Bechet disease

Safety Alert *Acute meningitis may manifest as a community-acquired illness with a negative Gram stain. The pathogen causing the disease may never be determined. Syphilis, bacteremia, and Borrelia burgdorferi (Lyme disease) have been identified in some cases. Variables affecting diagnosis of meningitis include presentation in winter months, age older than 60 years, and comorbid disease, especially immunodeficiency.*

NEUROLOGIC ASSESSMENT: MENINGITIS
Goal of System Assessment
A complete neurologic examination should be performed to establish the patient's baseline neurologic function. One or more tests for meningitis usually are positive (see Table 7-2). Examination of associated systems (head, eye, ear, nose, and throat [HEENT] and pulmonary) provides additional data.

Bacterial meningitis presents with classic symptoms of fever, altered mental status, headache, and nuchal rigidity. Immediate diagnosis and isolation of the organisms are paramount in this life-threatening disease. Delay in obtaining the necessary information needed to diagnosis and treat the underlying organism will increase morbidity and mortality.

History and Risk Factors
- History of present illness
  - Time course for symptom development
  - Recent infection (respiratory/ear)
  - Recent trauma to the head
  - Exposure to meningitis
  - Use of antibiotics
  - Petechial or ecchymotic rash
  - Ear or nose drainage
- Medical /social history
  - Drug allergies
  - Past medical history

Table 7-2	POSITIVE MENINGEAL SIGNS
Test/Description	**Positive Findings**
Stiff neck sign (nuchal rigidity): Raise patient's head by flexing the neck and attempting to make the patient's chin touch the sternum.	Pain and resistance to neck motion
Brudzinski sign: Assess for nuchal rigidity.	Flexion of the hips and knees when the examiner flexes the patient's neck
Kernig sign: Flex the patient's leg at the knee and hip when the patient is supine, and then attempt to straighten the leg.	Pain in the lower back and resistance to straightening the leg

- Recent surgical procedure
- Immunocompromising condition
- IV drug use
- HIV status or risk behavior
- Travel to endemic meningococcal area

Vital Signs

- *BP, HR, and RR changes*: May further alter cerebral tissue perfusion. Monitor rate, rhythm, and depth of respirations for changes or abnormal breathing patterns.
- *Hyperthermia*: May be associated with injury or irritation of the hypothalamic temperature-regulating centers, presence of blood in the CSF, or infection. Elevated temperature increases the metabolic needs of the brain, potentially leading to increased blood flow to the area, with concomitant cerebral hyperemia.

Observation

Meningeal signs (see Table 7-2):

Level of Consciousness (LOC): When assessing LOC it is important to not use subjective terms such as "stupor or lethargy" but rather to assess and communicate clearly the description of the patient's spontaneous activity response, response to verbal stimuli and reaction to painful stimuli, and how this differs from previous assessment. Assess for an acute change in mental status or fluctuation in mental status; various scales can be used that include LOC and other key indicators. Examples are the Richmond Agitation and Sedation Score (RASS) and GCS.

Pupillary changes: Examine pupils for size (in mm), shape, symmetry, reactivity to light, constriction, consensual response, and accommodation. Pupillary abnormalities can indicate unilateral or bilateral brain dysfunction, interruption of sympathetic or parasympathetic pathways, damage in the brainstem, cranial nerve damage, and herniation.

Clinical Presentation

- *S. pneumoniae*: The classic presentation of pneumococcal meningitis is fever, headache, meningismus, and altered mental status that progresses quickly to coma. Nuchal rigidity and Kernig or Brudzinski sign are present. Nausea, vomiting, profuse sweats, weakness, myalgia, seizures, and cranial nerve palsies also may be present.
- *N. meningitidis*: Patients may quickly deteriorate, beginning with fever and early macular erythematous rash that progresses rapidly to petechial and purpuric states, conjunctival petechiae, and aggressive behavior. Dysfunctions of cranial nerves VI, VII, and VIII (see Appendix 4) and aphasia, ventriculitis, subdural empyema, cerebral venous thrombosis, and disseminated intravascular coagulation (DIC) may occur.
- *H. influenzae*: The most distinguishing sign is early development of deafness, which can occur within 24 to 36 hours after onset. A morbilliform or petechial rash may be present.
- *L. monocytogenes*: Seizures and focal deficits such as ataxia, cranial nerve palsies, and nystagmus are seen early in the course of infection. Conclusive diagnosis may require serology testing.
- *Gram-negative species*: In older adults, fever may be absent or low grade and headache may not be reported. Meningeal signs may be subtle, but confusion, severe mental status changes, and pneumonia are commonly reported. Nuchal rigidity in older adults must be differentiated from degenerative changes of the cervical spine.
- *B. burgdorferi*: The symptoms of meningitis may be preceded by symptoms of Lyme disease, which occur in three stages. The first stage is a "bull's eye" rash within a few days of the tick bite followed by headache, stiff neck, lethargy, irritability, and changes in mental status, especially memory loss. Stage two, weeks to months after the tick bite, causes persistent headache, nausea, vomiting, malaise, irritability, cranial nerve deficits, mental status changes, peripheral neuropathies, and myalgias. In the last or third stage, arthritic types of symptoms and brain parenchymal changes are apparent.
- *Acute meningitis with negative Gram stain*: Fever and neck stiffness are the most frequent findings. The Gram stain for bacteria is negative, but CSF WBC count is elevated. Symptoms are similar to those for other types of meningitis.
- *M. tuberculosis*: A slow-onset process that causes neurologic damage before treatment is sought. Symptoms include headache, lethargy, confusion, nuchal rigidity, cranial nerve abnormalities, SIADH, weight loss, and night sweats. Kernig and Brudzinski

signs are present. The chest radiographic results may be clear, and purified protein derivative (PPD) may be nonreactive.

- *Cryptococcus neoformans:* Because the infection is subacute, fever and headache may have a subtle pattern lasting for weeks while other symptoms of meningitis occur, including positive meningeal signs (Table 7-2), alterations in mental status (e.g., hyperactivity, bizarre behavior, emotional lability, poor judgment), photophobia, focal cranial nerve deficits, nausea, vomiting, and (rarely) seizures.
- *Aseptic meningitis syndrome:* Fever, headache, stiff neck, fatigue, anorexia, and altered LOC are seen several hours after ingestion of causative drug. Severity varies with amount of drug taken and previous exposures. CSF glucose may be slightly elevated.

Functional Assessment

1. **Assess motor function and sensory responses.**
   - *Motor:* Assess motor movement in extremities related to strength, symmetry of movement, and coordination. Assess for abnormal motor movements unilaterally and bilaterally, such as decorticate posturing (abnormal flexion), decerebrate posturing (abnormal extension), or flaccidity. Motor deficits (weakness or paralysis) are caused by injury or edema to the primary motor cortex and corticospinal (pyramidal) tracts.
     - *Babinski sign, Kernig sign, & Brudzinski sign:* See page 620 under *General Neurologic Assessment.*
   - *Sensory:* Assess perception of touch, proprioception, pain, temperature, and vibration (if possible). Superficial and deep reflexes are tested on symmetrical sides of the body and compared noting the strength of contraction. Sensory deficits occur when the primary sensory cortex, the sensory association areas of the parietal lobe, or the spinothalamic tracts are injured or edematous. Sensory deficits include inability to distinguish objects according to characteristics (e.g., size, shape, weight) and inability to distinguish overall changes in temperature, touch, pressure, and position. Improvement in both motor and sensory perception may be seen as cerebral edema subsides.
2. **Assess for cranial nerve impairment:** Cranial nerve deficit(s) may improve as cerebral edema resolves or may be permanent. Nursing assessment of cranial nerve dysfunction is important. For more information about the function of all the cranial nerves, see Appendix 3.

Screening Labwork

- *CSF analysis:* Evaluates the color, WBC count, differential, glucose content, and protein level
- *Complete blood count, electrolytes, and coagulation studies:* Evaluate for anemia, hypo or hyperglycemia; potential for hemorrhage or infection.

DIAGNOSTIC TESTS

Bacterial meningitis presents with classic symptoms of fever, altered mental status, headache, and nuchal rigidity. Immediate diagnosis and isolation of the organisms are paramount in this life-threatening disease. Delay in obtaining the necessary information needed to diagnosis and treat the underlying organism will increase morbidity and mortality.

Diagnostic Tests for Meningitis

Test	Purpose	Abnormal Findings
Imaging		
Computed tomography (CT) of brain Do not delay lumbar puncture or administration of antibiotics for the CT scan, especially if the history does not support traumatic injury or an expanding intracranial lesion.	Assess details of structures of bone, tissue, and fluid-filled spaces. Detects exudate, abscesses, and intracranial pathology (e.g., tumors, brain injury). Assess for hydrocephalus.	Shift of structures due to enlarged mass, edema, exudate, abscesses, fresh hemorrhage, hematomas, infarction, hydrocephalus. Can visualize facial skeleton and soft tissue structures for abnormalities (e.g., tumors, brain injury).

Diagnostic Tests for Meningitis—cont'd

Test	Purpose	Abnormal Findings
Magnetic resonance imaging (MRI) of brain	Minute oscillations of hydrogen atoms in brain create graphic image of bone, fluid, and soft tissue. Provide a more detailed image.	Masses Detects exudate, abscesses, and intracranial pathology (e.g., tumors, brain injury).
Laboratory Testing		
Serum CBC with WBC count and differential	Assesses for presence of infection	Elevated WBCs
CSF analysis An LP should not be done following head injury, if focal neurologic deficits or papilledema are present, since these signs indicate increased ICP (see Box 7-1). Antibiotic therapy should not be delayed if CSF samples cannot be obtained. **_Polymerase chain reaction (PCR) assays antibody titers_** A DNA-based CSF test to check for the presence of certain causes of meningitis includes HSV1, HSV2, VZV, HIV, Epstein-Barr virus (EBV), West Nile virus, cytomegalovirus (CMV), HHV-6. **_Other CSF studies_** Venereal Disease Research Laboratories (VDRL) Fluorescent Treponemal Antibody-Absorption (FTA-ABS) (evaluates for syphilis)	The most important laboratory test for diagnosing meningitis. CSF may be obtained through an intraventricular catheter, ventriculostomy and reservoir via cervical approach, or lumbar puncture (LP). Note: Clinical signs of improve-ment rather than repeat CSF analysis is a better indicator of treatment response. However, repeat LP if: 1) there is no clinical improvement within 24–72 hrs after treatment is initiated; 2) it is performed 2-3 days after initiation of treatment if microorganisms are resistant to standard therapy; and 3) fever persists for greater than 8 days.	The CSF is analyzed for cell count with white cell differential, glucose, protein, Gram's stain, acid-fast stain, culture, and sensitivity (Table 7-3). CSF studies include the following: • _Cultures:_ Bacterial, viral, fungal, M. tuberculosis cultures with sensi-tivities, and aerobic and anaerobic cultures • _Latex agglutination:_ For bacterial antigens of N. meningitidis, S. pneumoniae, E. coli, influenza type B (Hib), group B strep • _Antigen:_ Cryptococcal and Histo-plasma polysaccharide antigen (bacterial antigen testing rarely useful) • _Antibodies:_ Coccidioides immitis complement fixation antibodies, herpes simplex virus (HSV), and varicella zoster (VZV) antibodies
Blood, urine, and sputum cultures	Help identify the infecting organ-isms and determine if there is a bacteremia, urinary tract infec-tion, or respiratory infection	Presence of infecting organisms in the bloodstream, urinary tract or lungs/upper airways

COLLABORATIVE MANAGEMENT
Care Priorities
1. **Control infection**
   - _Antibiotic therapy_: There are two major caveats to treating bacterial meningitis. First, the bactericidal agent must be effective against the organism and second, the agent must achieve a bacteriocidal effect within the CSF. Only IV antibiotics should be used, except for rifampin which is useful as a synergistic agent.
   - _Rapid sterilization of the CSF via appropriate pharmacologic therapy_ (Table 7-4): Prophylaxis, using appropriate antimicrobials for people exposed to N. meningitidis (rifampin or spiramycin) or H. influenzae meningitis, is recommended.
2. **Reduce inflammation with adjunctive pharmacologic therapies:** Dexamethasone may decrease inflammation by reducing cytokines produced by bacterial products. In recent study results, improvement in outcome, decrease in neurologic sequelae, and reduction in mortality with the use of dexamethasone have been reported. Recommended dosing is 0.15 mg/kg every 6 hours for 4 days. Start dose with or just prior to first antibiotic dose.

Table 7-3	MENINGITIS: TYPICAL CEREBROSPINAL FLUID FINDINGS		
Findings	**White Cell Count**	**Glucose**	**Protein**
Normal	0 to 5/mm^3 lymphocytes	40 to 80 mg/dl	15 to 50 mg/dl
Bacterial	Predominantly polycytes: 1,000 to 10,000	<40 mg/dl	100 to 500 mg/dl
Viral	Predominantly lymphocytes (may see polycytes initially)	Normal	Slightly elevated
Tuberculous	Elevated lymphocytes: 100 to 400; lymphocyte elevation minimal or absent in immunocompromised patients	<40 mg/dl or 50% of blood sugar drawn simultaneously	100 to 500 mg/dl; may increase gradually with progression of disease
Fungal	Predominantly elevated lymphocytes	Slightly decreased	Elevated
Lyme disease	Mildly elevated lymphocytes	Normal	Mildly elevated
Aseptic (nonbacterial)	Elevated lymphocytes	Normal	50 to 100 mg/dl

Table 7-4	COMMON DRUG THERAPY FOR THE MANAGEMENT OF MENINGITIS	
Causative Agent	**Characteristic**	**Therapy**
Bacterial Meningitis		
S. pneumoniae	Gram-positive cocci	Penicillin (PCN), ceftriaxone, cefotaxime, vancomycin with ceftriaxone if beta-lactam resistance; chloramphenicol for PCN allergies
H. influenzae	Gram-negative bacilli	Cefotaxime or ceftriaxone, add rifampin if pharyngeal colonization
N. meningitides	Gram-negative cocci	Penicillin G, add rifampin, fluoroquinolones, or cephalosporin if pharyngeal colonization; alternative is third-generation cephalosporin (cefotaxime)
L. monocytogenes	Gram-positive bacilli	Penicillin G or ampicillin with gentamycin for synergy; if allergy to PCN, then trimethoprim-sulfamethoxazole
M. tuberculosis	Acid-fast bacteria	Isoniazid, rifampin, ethambutol, pyrazinamide
B. burgdorferi	Spirochete	Ceftriaxone or penicillin G
Fungal		
C. neoformans	Fungus	Amphotericin B + flucytosine, fluconazole, or itraconazole
Cocci		
	Gram-positive	Vancomycin + penicillin G + aminoglycosides
	Gram-negative	Penicillin G
Bacilli		
	Gram-positive	Ampicillin, penicillin + aminoglycosides
P. aeruginosa, Klebsiella, E. coli, Citrobacter, Acinetobacter, Enterobacter, Serratia marcescens	Gram-negative	High doses of third-generation cephalosporins + aminoglycosides

Data from Fekete T, Quagliarello V: Treatment and prevention of bacterial meningitis in adults. *http:www. uptodate.com* ; Friedman N, Sexton D: Epidemiological and clinical features of Gram-negative bacillary meningitis. *http:www.uptodate.com*; and Frankel and Hartman (2004)

3. **Maintain fluid and electrolyte balance:** Overhydration and underhydration can lead to adverse effects. Research supports the use of IV maintenance fluids over fluid restriction during the first 48 hours of treatment of bacterial meningitis. Electrolyte imbalances should be corrected.

4. **Provide adequate nutrition:** Oral feeding should be encouraged when possible. Enteral or parenteral feeding may be initiated. Parenteral nutrition is used if enteral feeding is not tolerated. Hydration should be maintained.

5. **Control seizures with anticonvulsant therapy:** Used prophylactically or if seizures occur. Seizures increase metabolic rate and cerebral blood flow, which may cause deterioration in patients with cerebral edema and intracranial hypertension.

6. **Maintain normothermia/control fever:** Helps prevent intracranial hypertension associated with increased metabolic rate. Fever should be controlled by antipyretics such as acetaminophen or use of other cooling measures such as tepid baths.

7. **Prevent infection:** Vaccines are currently available for meningitis prophylaxis, including the following: (1) influenza type B (Hib), given as a childhood immunization; (2) bacillus Calmette-Guérin (BCG), used for tuberculosis, also prevents tuberculosis meningitis; (3) pneumococcal vaccine recommended for those who are chronically ill and adults over 65 years of age, and (4) *N. meningitides* vaccines for specific or combined prophylaxis for five investigational subgroups. The CDC guidelines recommend Transmission-Based Precautions be implemented until effectiveness of antimicrobial treatment is established.

8. **Facilitate mobility:** Physical therapy (PT), occupational therapy (OT), and speech therapy should be initiated as soon as patient is stable, to minimize physical and cognitive complications.

9. **Evaluate the need for support services:** Evaluate the need for home health care, support groups, and social services.

CARE PLANS: MENINGITIS

Decreased intracranial adaptive capacity *related to altered fluid dynamics secondary to brain and spinal cord inflammation*

GOALS/OUTCOMES Within 72 hours of initiation of antimicrobial therapy, patient's ICP returns to normal range as evidenced by orientation to time, place, and person; bilaterally equal and normoreactive pupils; bilaterally equal strength and tone of extremities; absence of cranial nerve palsies; RR 12 to 20 breaths/min with normal depth and pattern; HR 60 to 100 beats/min (bpm); BP within patient's normal range; and absence of headache, vomiting, papilledema, and other clinical indicators of increased ICP. After instruction, patient verbalizes knowledge of the importance of avoiding Valsalva-like activities.

NOC Neurological Status

Neurologic Monitoring

1. Assess neurologic status at least hourly. Monitor pupils, LOC, and motor activity; perform cranial nerve assessments (see Appendix 3). Early indicators of increased ICP and possible herniation include decreased LOC, changes in pupillary size and reaction, a decreased motor function (weakness, posturing), and cranial nerve palsies.

2. Monitor patient and report physical indicators of increased ICP (see Box 7-2) to the physician.

3. Monitor vital signs at least every 15 minutes if patient has signs of increased ICP. Be alert to changes in respiratory pattern, fluctuations in BP and pulse, widening pulse pressure, and slow HR.

4. Optimize cerebral oxygenation: Keep patient's head in neutral alignment, maintain a patent airway, and provide supplemental oxygen as prescribed. Ensure that patient's neck is not constricted by tracheostomy ties and oxygen tubing.

5. Avoid overhydration, which increases cerebral edema. Ensure precise delivery of IV fluids and timely delivery of medications prescribed for the prevention of sudden increases or decreases in ICP, BP, HR, or RR.

6. Teach patient to avoid activities that increase ICP: coughing, straining, and bending over.

7. If patient shows evidence of increased ICP, implement measures to decrease ICP.

NIC Cerebral Edema Management; Cerebral Perfusion Promotion; Intracranial Pressure (ICP) Monitoring: Neurologic Monitoring

Acute pain *related to headache, photophobia, and fever secondary to meningeal irritation*

GOALS/OUTCOMES Within 2 hours of initiating interventions to relieve pain, patient reports pain relief, as documented by a pain scale.
NOC Comfort Level

Pain Management
1. Monitor patient for pain and discomfort. Devise a pain rating scale with patient. Administer analgesics as prescribed. (See *Pain*, p 135.)
2. Monitor temperature every 2 hours and as needed. Administer tepid baths or cooling blanket and prescribed antipyretics/antibiotics to keep temperature within prescribed limits.
3. Maintain an environment of comfort for each individual patient.
4. Provide care and visiting hours to allow for uninterrupted periods (at least 90 minutes) of rest. If ICP is elevated, clustering care is contraindicated.
5. Darken patient's room or provide blindfold to minimize the discomfort of photophobia.

Risk for infection *related to possible cross-contamination secondary to communicable bacterial and aseptic meningitis*

GOALS/OUTCOMES Other patients, staff members, and patient's significant others do not exhibit evidence of having acquired meningitis: diminished LOC, confusion, fever, headache, nuchal rigidity, and other signs (see previous sections for Meningitis on *Neurologic Assessment,* p. 623, and *Diagnostic Tests,* p. 649).
NOC Infection Severity
For patients with bacterial meningitis:

Infection Control
1. Some forms of bacterial meningitis are transmitted via droplet contact. Provide patient with a private room.
2. Initiate Transmission-Based Precautions: Droplet, on admission, and maintain them for at least 24 hours after start of antimicrobial therapy.
   • Standard Precautions should be instituted to provide safety and protection regardless if infection is bacterial, fungal, or viral. Be alert for airborne pathogens and those in stool or oral secretions.

ADDITIONAL NURSING DIAGNOSES

See *Risk for Trauma (Oral and Musculoskeletal)* in *Status Epilepticus* (p. 672). Because these patients are at risk for SIADH, see *Syndrome of Inappropriate Antidiuretic Hormone,* p. 734. See *SIRS, Sepsis, and MODS,* p. 924, since these patients are at risk for septic shock; *Nutritional Support,* p. 117, *Prolonged Immobility,* p. 149, and *Emotional and Spiritual Support of the Patient and Significant Others* (p. 200).

NEURODEGENERATIVE AND NEUROMUSCULAR DISORDERS

◼ PATHOPHYSIOLOGY

Neurodegenerative diseases are conditions wherein the neurons, or the myelin sheath of the neurons of the brain and spinal cord, are destroyed. Cells of the brain and spinal cord do not effectively regenerate in large numbers, so profound destruction is sometimes devastating. Over time, the progressive destruction leads to dysfunction and disabilities. The disorders are divided into two groups; conditions affecting movements (e.g., ataxia) and conditions affecting memory (e.g., dementia), which are not mutually exclusive. Alzheimer, Pick, Parkinson, Huntington, and Lou Gehrig (amytrophic lateral sclerosis [ALS]) diseases, prion diseases (Cruetzfeldt-Jakob [CJD]), and multiple sclerosis are a few of the more commonly recognized conditions. Some of the diseases are genetic, while alcoholism, cancer, and vascular disease are associated with other conditions. Environmental toxins, chemicals, or viruses may cause other disorders. Neurodegeneration often begins long before the patient manifests symptoms. Treatments vary with each disorder.

Neuromuscular disorders include the neurodegenerative diseases, which affect voluntary movements. Communication between the nervous system and muscles is not possible when nerves are destroyed. Muscles weaken and atrophy due to disuse. Weakness may also be associated with muscle twitching, cramps, and pain, along with joint and movement deficits. These disorders may affect the heart and respiratory muscles. Many neuromuscular disorders are genetic, while others are immune mediated, associated with an immunologic disorder. *Myasthenia gravis* (MG) Guillain-Barré Syndrome (GBS) and *muscular dystrophy* are several of the more commonly recognized conditions. Most of the diseases are incurable. The goal of treatment is to improve symptoms, increase mobility, and lengthen life. Patients with MG may experience difficulties with medication management resulting in a crisis, which is rather easily corrected with the proper medication adjustment. Patients with other neuromuscular disorders may require more elaborate treatments including high-dose corticosteroids, plasmapheresis, and more prolonged hospitalization.

Diagnosis of neuromuscular diseases depends on identification of a specific defect of neuromuscular function. The functional defect can sometimes be inferred by a physical examination done by a physician or midlevel practitioner coupled with laboratory testing of blood and possibly CSF. A more extensive diagnostic process evaluates the function of nerves, muscles, and the connections between them by using two complementary techniques—nerve conduction velocity testing (NCVs) and electromyography (EMGs).

Care of critically ill patients may involve managing patients with respiratory failure and cardiovascular instability related to exacerbations of neuromuscular disorders. Patients at this stage of instability may be terminally ill. Patients with either MG or GBS (GBS) may be treated and fully recovered. The chapter will focus on MG and GBS; however, the nursing diagnoses, interventions, and outcomes are common to most neurodegenerative and neuromuscular disorders.

MYASTHENIA GRAVIS

PATHOPHYSIOLOGY

MG is a chronic, progressive autoimmune disorder causing weakness and abnormal fatigability of the voluntary striated skeletal muscles. MG usually affects women between 20 and 40 years of age and men after age 40; the peak incidence for women is during the second and third decades and for men during the sixth decade. The overall ratio of affected women to men is 3:2. Of patients with MG, 85% to 90% have an anti–acetylcholine receptor (AChR) antibody (immunoglobulin). MG is associated with other autoimmune disorders. The thymus gland undergoes pathologic changes in 80% of MG patients and may produce anti-AChR antibodies when exposed to inflammation. The course of the disease depends on the muscle groups involved and the degree of their involvement.

MG causes changes in the structural integrity of the postsynaptic membrane at the neuromuscular junction by markedly reducing the number of AChRs. Acetylcholine (ACh), a neurotransmitter, is synthesized and stored in the terminal expansion of motor nerve axons. ACh is released into the synaptic cleft. The attachment of ACh to AChR on the postsynaptic membrane activates muscle action potential, resulting in muscle contraction. Contraction terminates when ACh is deactivated by acetylcholinesterase in the neuromuscular junction.

Patients may experience remissions and exacerbations. Many medications can increase the weakness associated with MG, including several commonly administered antibiotics (erythromycin, aminoglycosides, and azithromycin) and cardiac medications such as magnesium or antidysrhythmic agents including procainamide, beta adrenergic–blocking agents, and quinidine. Paradoxical weakness may occur when a patient receives an excessive dose of anticholinesterase medications (cholinesterase inhibitors such as physostigmine or neostigmine), which are used to treat MG. Distinguishing worsening MG from side effects from prescribed medication effects can be difficult. Exacerbations can be profound, and thus are called crises.

A *myasthenic* or *cholinergic crisis* may occur rapidly or incipiently. *Myasthenic crisis* can occur as part of the natural course of myasthenia gravis or may result from other factors, including infection, tapering of immunosuppressive medications, administration of various other medications, pregnancy, childbirth, or following a surgical procedure, ultimately resulting in respiratory failure from weakness of the respiratory muscles. Severe weakness of the oropharyngeal muscles (bulbar signs) is often associated with respiratory muscle weakness, resulting in dysphagia and aspiration. Endotracheal (ET) intubation with mechanical ventilation may be needed. A *cholinergic crisis* results from excessive dosing of anticholinesterase medications and rarely occurs if the dose of medications remains within the normally prescribed range. The patient is acutely aware of all sensations. Crisis is dramatic and frightening.

ASSESSMENT
Goal of Assessment
To differentiate between acute and chronic neurologic assessment findings. Signs of myasthenic and cholinergic crises may be subtle. Increasing anxiety, apprehension, or insomnia may indicate the onset of crisis.

History and Risk Factors
History of rheumatoid arthritis, systemic lupus erythematosus, thyrotoxicosis, Sjögren syndrome, polymyositis, ulcerative colitis, Hashimoto thyroiditis, and pernicious anemia. Recent infection, trauma, surgery, temperature extremes, stress, endocrine imbalance, or intake of medications with neuromuscular-blocking properties, such as sedatives, tranquilizers, opiates, or antibiotics (e.g., neomycin, kanamycin, gentamicin, streptomycin, tetracycline), may prompt crisis.

Vital Signs
- Findings vary significantly, depending on whether patient is experiencing a crisis.
- RR may be normal or slightly tachypneic.
- Tachycardia may be present with impending respiratory failure.

Observation
- Patients may be asymptomatic or have mild symptoms if crisis develops slowly.
- Weakness and abnormal fatigability of skeletal muscles, which worsens with sustained efforts.

Symptom Progression
Ocular muscle group: First muscle group to be affected in 65% of patients. During course of disease, 90% will have ocular involvement. Eye signs include ptosis (drooping of one or both eyelids), diplopia (double vision), and inability to maintain upward gaze.
Muscles of face, neck, and oropharynx with bulbar signs: Second area of involvement. Bulbar signs are present, with increased risk of aspiration due to difficulty chewing, dysphagia, dysarthria, inability to close mouth, nasal regurgitation of fluids, mushy and nasal tone to voice, neck-muscle weakness with head bob, inability to raise chin off chest, and loss of facial expression.
Muscles of limbs and trunk: Weakness is greater in proximal muscles than distal. Strength is decreased in all extremities, with inability to maintain position without support. Diaphragmatic and intercostal weakness, dyspnea, ineffective cough, and accumulation of secretions are present, which increases the risk for respiratory arrest.
Myasthenic and cholinergic crises: Increasing anxiety, apprehension, or insomnia may indicate the onset. ABG values may be normal. Note subtle decreases in chest expansion and air movement and increased dysphagia, dysarthria, and dysphonia. Accumulation of oropharyngeal secretions increases the risk of aspiration.
- *Myasthenic crisis*: Occurs when the patient needs increased medication as a result of drug tolerance or an exacerbation of the disease. Signs and symptoms: Increasing muscle weakness despite normal or increased drug dosage, increasing anxiety and apprehension, severe ocular and bulbar weakness, with rapid onset of respiratory muscle weakness, which can lead to respiratory arrest.
- *Cholinergic crisis*: Results from an overdose of anticholinesterase medication, causing a depolarizing neuromuscular blockade. Signs and symptoms: Increasing muscle weakness, increasing anxiety and apprehension, fasciculations (twitching) around the eyes and mouth, diarrhea and cramping, sweating, pupillary constriction, sialorrhea (excessive salivation), and difficulty breathing and swallowing.

Auscultation
- Breath sounds may reflect reduced movement of air or shallow breaths.

Diagnosis of Myasthenic or Cholinergic Crisis

Test	Purpose	Abnormal Findings
Tensilon (edrophonium) test With MG, weakness and muscle fatigue will improve within 30 to 60 seconds of receiving IV Tensilon injection (2 to 10 mg), and improvement will last up to 5 minutes.	Identifies the type of crisis. Tensilon is a short-acting anticholinesterase agent that delays hydrolysis of acetylcholine, permitting the acetylcholine released by the nerve to act repeatedly over a longer period.	*Myasthenic crisis:* Weakness improves with edrophonium chloride (Tensilon) versus *Cholinergic crisis:* Symptoms worsen with Tensilon. Test is done by a neurologist who assesses the patient's immediate response.
Caution: Have atropine sulfate at the bedside during Tensilon test to reverse the effects of Tensilon if the patient is in cholinergic crisis.		
Serum antibody titer Correlation between titer and disease severity and course has not been proved.	Assesses for presence of serum antibodies against acetylcholine receptors	Elevated serum antibodies against are present in 80% to 90% of cases of generalized MG.
Electromyography (EMG) Muscle action potentials are recorded from selected skeletal muscles.	Tests muscle action potentials, reflective of ability to contract	The amplitude of the evoked muscle action potentials falls rapidly in persons with MG.
Mediastinal magnetic resonance imaging (MRI) of the thymus gland or mediastinoscopy	To evaluate for thymic abnormalities, present in 80% of patients with MG	65% to 90% have thymic hyperplasia, whereas 10% to 15% have gross or microscopic thymomas.
Thyroid studies Thyroid abnormalities are often present in young women.	Evaluate for hyperthyroidism.	MG is associated with Hashimoto thyroiditis, an autoimmune thyroid disorder.
Other laboratory studies: Creatine phosphokinase (CPK), erythrocyte sedimentation rate (ESR), and antinuclear antibody levels: There is a frequent concurrence of other immunologic disorders with MG.		

COLLABORATIVE MANAGEMENT
Care Priorities for Patients with Myasthenia Gravis

1. **Manage respiratory failure:** ET intubation with mechanical ventilation may be necessary, depending on the degree of involvement of the respiratory muscles. (See *Mechanical Ventilation,* p. 99.) Bilevel positive pressure ventilation (BiPAP) may also be used effectively in a subset of patients, if able to breathe somewhat effectively.
2. **Provide emergency interventions for myasthenic or cholinergic crisis:** Once the patient is stabilized in the intensive care unit (ICU), the type of crisis is identified, and specific treatment is begun. Anticholinesterase medications may be withheld or reduced temporarily. A "drug holiday" will improve subsequent patient responsiveness to medication. With the resumption of anticholinesterase medications, dosage, timing, and combinations of medications will need readjustment. In severe MG, plasmapheresis (see later) may hasten improvement of signs and symptoms.
3. **Initiate nutritional support:** If patient has dysphagia, enteral or parenteral feedings may be needed. (See *Nutritional Support,* p. 117.)
4. **Manage pharmacotherapy during noncrisis periods:** Medications must be given on time to maintain therapeutic effects. Drug combinations are patient-specific.
   - *Cholinesterase inhibitors:* Pyridostigmine bromide (Mestinon), neostigmine bromide (Prostigmin), and ambenonium chloride (Mytelase) are used to inhibit the hydrolysis of ACh by acetylcholinesterase at the neuromuscular junction. Pyridostigmine is often used, since it has fewer side effects and is longer acting. The patient is given a dose every 3 hrs during the day, and the dose is adjusted based on effects. Sustained-release preparations usually are given at bedtime to maintain the patient's strength throughout the night and early morning hours.

- *Immunosuppression*: Glucocorticosteroids (e.g., ACTH and prednisone) and other immunosuppressive agents: Glucocorticosteroids are used alone or in conjunction with anticholinesterase drugs. They provide clinical improvement for 70% to 100% of patients with MG who refuse thymectomy and have weakness uncontrolled by anticholinesterase drugs. Although the mechanism of action of steroids is uncertain, studies indicate they directly influence neuromuscular transmission, suppress the action of the immune system by decreasing the size of the thymus gland and lymphatic tissue, decrease circulating lymphocytes, and decrease antireceptor reactivity of peripheral lymphocytes. Treatment is continued indefinitely. Glucocorticosteroids produce favorable results in all patients with muscle involvement, from ocular to severe respiratory impairment. Azathioprine (Imuran) may be used alone or in combination with other therapies in situations in which response to steroids is poor. Side effects of azathioprine include toxic hepatitis, thrombocytopenia, leukopenia, leukemia, lymphoma, infections, vomiting, and teratogenic effects.
- *Immune globulin*: Routine use of human immune globulin (IG) is not recommended, but administration of IV immunoglobulin (IVIg) may be considered in patients with severe MG for whom other treatments have been unsuccessful or are contraindicated.

5. **Consider plasmapheresis:** A complete exchange of plasma with removal of abnormal circulating antibodies that interfere with acetylcholine receptors. Box 7-3 describes potential complications, nursing assessments and interventions. (For additional information, see *Fluid and Electrolyte Disturbances*, p. 37.)
6. **Carefully consider thymectomy:** Removal of the thymus gland may prompt clinical improvement in 70% of patients, particularly newly diagnosed females with hyperplasia of thymic tissue. A suprasternal approach, a transsternal approach with sternal splitting, or the minimally invasive technique called video-assisted thoracic surgery (VATS) may be used. Plasmapheresis sometimes is used before surgery to increase strength and allow for a decrease in medication dosage.

Box 7-3	NURSING INTERVENTIONS FOR COMPLICATIONS OF PLASMAPHERESIS

Hypovolemia

Can result from rapid removal of up to 3 L of body fluid during plasmapheresis with volume replacement that is too slow during the procedure

- Perform a baseline assessment of patient's weight, skin turgor, and VS before the procedure is begun. During plasmapheresis, monitor patient for thirst, poor skin turgor, dizziness, confusion, nausea, and flattened neck veins. Assess VS continuously for evidence of hypovolemia, including decreased BP and increased HR. Monitor Hct for elevation, which occurs with hypovolemia. Weigh patient after procedure. Remember that L of fluid equals 1 kg; thus hypovolemia can be reflected readily in weight changes.
- Provide fluids during plasmapheresis as prescribed, via oral, enteral, or IV access.
- Monitor and record I&O throughout the procedure. Be alert to oliguria (urinary output less than 30 ml/hr for 2 consecutive hours).
- Protect patients who are dizzy or confused by keeping side rails up and the bed in its lowest position.

Clotting Abnormalities

Can result from removal of clotting factors during plasmapheresis

- Assess PT, PTT, and platelet count before and after procedure. Be alert to PT and PTT greater than those of control values and to increased platelet count. Normal ranges are as follows: PT 11 to 15 seconds, PTT 30 to 40 seconds, and platelet count 150,000 to 400,000/mm^3.
- Be alert to signs of impaired clotting, such as oozing from arterial puncture, venous access, or IV sites. Monitor patient for epistaxis or other signs of hemorrhage, such as elevated pulse rate, decreased BP, or changes in patient's mental status.

Box 7-3	NURSING INTERVENTIONS FOR COMPLICATIONS OF PLASMAPHERESIS—cont'd

- Apply firm, continuous (e.g., for 10 minutes) pressure to the arterial puncture site once the catheter or needle is removed. A pressure dressing is recommended.
- Check gastric aspirate and stools for occult blood.
- Instruct patient to alert staff to the presence of bleeding from puncture and other sites.

Hypokalemia
Can result from removal of potassium during the plasma exchange
- Assess serum potassium before, during, and after plasma exchange. Be alert to decreasing levels (less than 3.5 mEq/L).
- Monitor for physical signs of hypokalemia, including bradycardia, fatigue, leg cramps, nausea, and paresthesias.
- Observe cardiac monitor for signs of cardiac dysrhythmias: ST-segment depression, flattened T wave, presence of U wave, and ventricular dysrhythmias. Report abnormal cardiac rhythms to physician.
- During reinfusion of blood, administer potassium as prescribed to prevent hypokalemia and dangerous dysrhythmias. If prescribed, administer antidysrhythmic agents.

Hypocalcemia
Can result from binding of calcium to ACD, the anticoagulants used during plasmapheresis
- Assess serum calcium levels before, during, and after plasmapheresis. Be alert to decreasing levels (less than 8.5 mg/dl).
- Monitor patient for signs of hypocalcemia, such as numbness with tingling of fingers and circumoral area, hyperactive reflexes, muscle cramps, tetany, paresthesia, Chvostek sign, diffuse irritability, emotional instability, impaired memory, and confusion.
- Observe cardiac monitor for evidence of hypocalcemia: prolonged QT interval caused by elongation of ST segment.
- Encourage patient to drink milk before and during the plasma exchange.
- As prescribed, administer calcium gluconate during plasmapheresis if indicators of hypocalcemia occur.

Myasthenic Crisis
Can result from removal of circulating anticholinesterase drugs during plasmapheresis

Cholinergic Crisis
Can result from removal of antibodies and decreased need for anticholinesterase drugs after plasmapheresis
- In the event of either crisis, have the following available: IV infusion apparatus, medications (edrophonium chloride [Tensilon], neostigmine bromide, atropine, and pralidoxime chloride [Protopam Chloride]), manual resuscitator, oxygen, suction equipment, and intubation tray if intubation is not already in place.
- Monitor patient for evidence of crisis, such as decreased vital capacity (less than 1 L), inability to swallow, ptosis, diplopia, dysarthria, dysphonia, dyspnea, muscle weakness, and nasal flaring. Stay with patient if these signs appear, and notify physician promptly.

Caution: Patients on prednisone or digitalis therapy are at increased risk for hypokalemia and should be monitored closely for its occurrence.
ACD, Acid-citrate-dextrose; *PT,* prothrombin time; *PTT,* partial thromboplastin time; *VS,* vital signs.

CARE PLANS FOR MYASTHENIA GRAVIS

Impaired gas exchange *related to altered oxygen supply associated with decreases in chest expansion and air movement secondary to weakness and abnormal fatigability of pharyngeal, diaphragmatic, intercostal, and accessory muscles of respiration*

GOALS/OUTCOMES Within 12 to 24 hours of initiation of treatment, patient has adequate gas exchange as evidenced by orientation to time, place, and person; RR less than 20 breaths/min with normal depth and pattern (eupnea); Pao_2 greater than 80 mm Hg; $Paco_2$ less than 45 mm Hg; and oxygen saturation greater than 95%.
NOC Respiratory Status: Gas Exchange; Respiratory Status: Ventilation; Mechanical Ventilation Response: Adult

Respiratory Monitoring
1. Assess patient for indicators of impending respiratory failure or hypoxia: diminished or adventitious breath sounds; changes in rate, rhythm, or depth of respirations; pallor; nasal flaring; use of accessory muscles; and restlessness, irritability, confusion, or somnolence.
2. Monitor ventilatory capability via pulmonary function tests. Vital capacity less than 75% of predicted value, tidal volume less than 1000 ml (or patient's normal/baseline volume), and RR greater than 34 breaths/min are signals of need for assisted ventilation.
3. Monitor ABG and pulse oximetry results. Falling Pao_2 (less than 60 mm Hg), rising $Paco_2$ (greater than 50 mm Hg), and falling oxygen saturation, coupled with changes in vital capacity, tidal volume, and increasing RR, indicate the need for additional respiratory support.
4. Provide pulmonary toilet every 2 hours when patient is awake and as needed. In addition, turn patient after each physiotherapy session to facilitate lung expansion, decrease risk of atelectasis, and prevent consolidation of secretions.

> **Safety Alert** *If mechanical ventilation already is in place, ventilator settings will vary, depending on patient's size and ABG results. Check ventilator settings at set intervals. Consult with an intensivist, pulmonologist, associated midlevel practitioner, and/or respiratory therapy staff members regarding setting changes as patient's needs change.*

NIC Airway Management; Coping Enhancement; Acid-Base Monitoring; Oxygen Therapy; Mechanical Ventilation Response: Adult

Ineffective airway clearance *related to ineffective cough; decreased energy; abnormal fatigability of diaphragmatic, intercostal, pharyngeal, and accessory muscles of respiration*

GOALS/OUTCOMES Within 24 to 48 hours of intervention/treatment, patient's airway is clear as evidenced by absence of adventitious breath sounds.
NOC Aspiration Prevention; Respiratory Status: Airway Patency

Airway Management
1. Assess breath sounds, effectiveness of patient's cough, and the quality, amount, and color of sputum. Consult physician or midlevel practitioner for significant findings, including patient's inability to raise secretions; for secretions that are tenacious, thick, or voluminous.
2. Suction secretions as indicated, using hyperoxygenation before and after procedure.

> **Safety Alert** *To prevent aspiration of secretions, always suction the trachea and mouth before deflating endotracheal or tracheostomy cuff. Consider use of ET tube with continuous supraglottic suction, if available. This is especially important because of the increase in saliva.*

3. Place patient in semi-Fowler's to high Fowler's position to facilitate chest excursion and decrease risk of aspiration. Fully elevate HOB during feedings.
4. Assess vital signs for indicators of atelectasis and upper respiratory infection (see *Risk for Infection*, which follows). Report significant findings to physician or midlevel practitioner.

5. Increase activity as tolerated to minimize stasis of secretions and to facilitate lung expansion.
6. Administer or assist with noninvasive BiPAP as needed.
7. Keep a tracheostomy tube and obturator at the bedside in the event of inadvertent extubation.

NIC Artificial Airway Management; Cough Enhancement: Oxygen Therapy; Ventilation Assistance

Risk for infection *related to inadequate primary defenses (stasis of secretions); inadequate secondary defenses (suppressed inflammatory response); invasive procedures (e.g., insertion of ET tube); chronic disease*

GOALS/OUTCOMES Patient is free of infection as evidenced by normothermia; HR 60 to 100 bpm; pulmonary secretions that are clear, thin in consistency, and odorless; and WBC count less than 11,000/mm³.
NOC Immune Status

Health Screening
1. Monitor for temperature greater than 37.7°C (100°F), tachycardia, and diaphoresis.
2. Assess color, consistency, amount, and odor of secretions. Report changes in sputum color to the physician. Obtain sputum specimens for culture as indicated.
3. Monitor CBC results for elevation of WBC count (greater than 11,000/mm³).
4. Administer antibiotics as prescribed.
5. Protect patient from persons with infection, particularly URI.
6. Turn and reposition patient at least every 2 hours to prevent stasis of secretions.

Impaired swallowing *related to decreased or absent gag reflex; decreased strength or excursion of muscles involved in mastication; facial paralysis; mechanical obstruction (tracheostomy tube)*

GOALS/OUTCOMES Before oral foods and fluids are given or reintroduced, patient demonstrates capability for safe and effective swallowing as evidenced by presence of gag reflex and adequate strength and excursion of muscles involved in mastication.
NOC Aspiration Prevention; Swallowing Status

Aspiration Precautions
1. Assess patient for the presence of the gag reflex, ability to swallow, and strength and excursion of muscles involved in mastication. As indicated, consult with a speech therapist to determine patient's ability to swallow.
2. If patient cannot swallow, confer with physician regarding alternate method of nutritional support, such as enteral or parenteral nutrition (see *Nutritional Support,* p. 117).
3. After patient's gag reflex and ability to swallow return, begin oral feedings cautiously.
   - When reinstating oral intake, offer a few ice chips to help stimulate the swallowing reflex, progress to semisolid foods (e.g., textured food, applesauce) and then to solid foods. Confer with speech/swallowing therapist regarding a dysphagia diet and teaching swallowing techniques.
   - Elevate HOB greater than 70 degrees to facilitate gravity flow through the pylorus and to minimize regurgitation and aspiration.
   - Provide small feedings at frequent intervals (e.g., every 4 hours while patient is awake).
   - Avoid cold foods and beverages, which cause bloating and upward pressure on the diaphragm.
   - Keep suction equipment at the bedside; suction excess secretions as necessary after each feeding. Inspect the mouth for residual food after meals. Provide for oral hygiene after every meal.
4. If patient begins oral feedings with a tracheostomy tube in place, elevate HOB greater than 70 degrees. Inflate tracheostomy tube cuff for 30 minutes before and after feeding to prevent aspiration. Progress the diet slowly, as described in the previous intervention.
5. If patient is unable to communicate verbally, be alert to signs of severe aspiration: dyspnea, tachypnea, restlessness, agitation, pallor, and presence of adventitious breath sounds. If these signs occur, discontinue feeding immediately; elevate HOB; and provide oxygen. If a tracheostomy tube is in place, suction to remove food or secretions obstructing the airway.

NIC Swallowing Therapy; Positioning; Nutrition Management

Disturbed sensory perception (visual) *related to altered sensory perception associated with diplopia or ptosis*

GOALS/OUTCOMES Within 48 to 72 hours of this diagnosis, patient relates that vision is adequate to perform activities of daily living (ADLs).
NOC Neurological Status: Cranial/Sensory/Motor Function

Environmental Management: Safety
1. Assess for and document signs of weakness of the ocular muscles (i.e., diplopia, ptosis, incomplete closure of the eye).
2. Provide an eye patch or frosted lens for the patient with diplopia; alternate the patch or lens to the opposite eye every 2 to 3 hours during patient's waking hours.
3. Provide eyelid crutches for the patient with ptosis, or loosely tape eyelids open but only when providing direct care.
4. Administer artificial tears in each eye at least every 4 to 6 hours to lubricate and protect corneal tissue.
5. As indicated, provide assistance with ADLs and ambulation to protect patient from injury.
6. Keep patient's environment consistent to facilitate location of desired objects.

NIC Communication Enhancement: Visual Deficit; Environmental Management; Fall Prevention; Surveillance: Safety

Deficient knowledge *related to thymectomy procedure, including preoperative and postoperative care*

GOALS/OUTCOMES Before surgery, patient verbalizes understanding of the surgical procedure, including preoperative and postoperative care.
NOC Knowledge: Treatment Procedure(s)

Teaching: Procedure/Treatment
1. Explain thymectomy and its relationship to myasthenia gravis.
2. Provide information about preoperative routine. Discuss medications, application of antiembolic hose, the potential for postoperative discomfort, and the availability of analgesic agents. Advise patient that medications may change after surgery, as the patient may improve. With a thoracotomy approach, explain postoperative chest tubes. With a transcervical approach, a wound drainage system (e.g., Hemovac) is used.
3. Teach coughing and deep-breathing techniques used after surgery.
4. Explain that plasmapheresis may be performed preoperatively to improve the patient's clinical state. (See *Deficient Knowledge: Purpose and Procedure for Plasmapheresis,* which follows.)
5. Explain that pulmonary function and ABG studies will be performed preoperatively and postoperatively to assist in determining the patient's respiratory status.
6. Explain the possibility of tracheostomy with assisted ventilation to prevent respiratory problems that can occur from stresses of surgery or myasthenic or cholinergic crisis.
7. Explain that results of a thymectomy vary and may not be apparent for several months to years.

Deficient knowledge *related to purpose and procedure for plasmapheresis*

GOALS/OUTCOMES Before the first plasma exchange, patient verbalizes knowledge of the purpose and procedure for plasmapheresis.
NOC Knowledge: Treatment Procedure(s)

Teaching: Procedure/Treatment
1. Assess patient's previous experience with and knowledge of plasmapheresis.
2. As appropriate, teach patient the following about plasmapheresis: (1) blood is withdrawn via an arterial catheter, anticoagulated, and then passed through a cell separator; (2) the plasma portion of the blood that contains the AChR antibodies is removed; (3) red blood cells (RBCs), WBCs, and platelets are mixed with saline, potassium, and plasma protein fraction and then are returned to the body.
3. Advise patient that plasmapheresis is generally performed to control severe symptoms until other modalities (i.e., medications, thymectomy) take effect, when other treatments have failed, or to increase patient's strength and improve general status before surgery.
4. Explain that the nurse will make assessments before, during, and after plasmapheresis (see Box 7-3).
5. Advise patient that the procedure takes several hours and may be performed daily.
6. Explain that the degree of weakness may increase during and after the procedure because of the removal of plasma-bound medications (corticosteroids, anticholinesterase agents). Reassure patient that he or

she will be monitored closely during the procedure and will receive appropriate medication after plasmapheresis.

Deficient knowledge *related to signs and symptoms of myasthenic and cholinergic crises*

GOALS/OUTCOMES Within 24 hours of stabilization of respiratory status, patient and significant others verbalize the signs and symptoms of impending myasthenic and cholinergic crises.
NOC Knowledge: Disease Process

Teaching: Disease Process
1. Assess patient's/family's knowledge of myasthenic and cholinergic crises.
2. Explain the differences between myasthenic crisis: an exacerbation of the myasthenic symptoms, frequently triggered by an infection; and cholinergic crisis: an episode triggered by toxic levels of anticholinesterase medication. The crisis, regardless of type, may manifest similar symptoms, including abdominal cramping, diarrhea, generalized weakness, increased pulmonary secretions, and impaired respiratory function.
3. Advise patient/family to immediately report signs and symptoms of crisis.
4. Prepare patient for potential discharge when stabilized and consider the use of home health services for follow-up after discharge.
5. Teach patient and significant others how to use emergency respiratory support equipment (resuscitator bag and suction apparatus) and facilitate it being available in the home if patient has a history of crisis events.
6. Advise patient to carry an identification card with diagnosis, medications, medication contraindications, and physician's name and phone number.
7. Provide contact information for Myasthenia Gravis Foundation of America, Inc. 222 South Riverside Plaza, Suite 1540, Chicago, IL 60606; 800-541-5454, 312-258-0522; fax: 312-258-0461; website: www.Myasthenia@myasthenia.org).

ADDITIONAL NURSING DIAGNOSES

See also *Nutritional Support* (p. 117), *Mechanical Ventilation* (p. 99), and *Emotional and Spiritual Support of the Patient and Significant Others* (p. 200).

GUILLAIN-BARRÉ SYNDROME

PATHOPHYSIOLOGY

GBS is a disorder wherein the immune system mistakenly attacks the peripheral nervous system, causing weakness and paresthesias of the lower extremities. Symptoms can intensify and ascend toward the head, resulting in loss of ability to use all muscles. When severe, the patient is totally paralyzed and the disorder is life threatening, with impending respiratory muscle paralysis and cardiovascular instability. GBS is not considered a classic neuromuscular or neurodegenerative disorder, as the onset is sudden, with rapid progression, and once peaked, patients have the potential for a complete recovery.

This disorder is an acute inflammatory, immune-mediated, demyelinating polyneuropathy of the peripheral nervous system, affecting 1.5 to 2 individuals per 100,000 population.

GBS affects mainly the Schwann cell, which synthesizes and maintains the peripheral nerve myelin sheath. Studies suggest that macrophages penetrate the basement membrane and strip apparently normal myelin from intact peripheral nerve axons, causing the characteristic signs and symptoms of GBS. The ventral (motor) root axons of the anterior horn cells, which innervate voluntary skeletal muscles, are primarily involved. Dorsal (sensory) root axons of the posterior horn are not as affected. Recovery of neurologic function depends on proliferation of Schwann cells and remyelination of axons. Recovery can be expected in 80% to 90% of cases, with minor residual deficits in less than half of the patients, and 2% to 5% experiencing recurrence after complete recovery.

ASSESSMENT: GUILLAIN-BARRÉ SYNDROME
Goal of Assessment

Identify the extent of current neurologic deficits, compared to the baseline, and intervene in profound deterioration. There are several clinical variations of signs and symptoms: ascending, descending, the Miller Fisher variant, or pure motor. The disease generally has three phases: (1) acute phase of 1 to 3 weeks after onset of the first symptom; (2) plateau phase beginning with no further clinical deterioration and lasting several days to weeks; and (3) recovery phase, which can last 4 months up to 2 years and correlates with the remyelination and axonal regrowth process.

History and Risk Factors
Respiratory or GI illness 10 to 14 days before onset of the neurologic symptoms, in which (1) a viral agent such as parainfluenza 2 virus, measles, mumps, rubella, varicella, or herpes zoster is present (50% of cases); (2) recent vaccination (15% of cases), such as for influenza; and (3) recent surgical procedure (5% of cases). Miller Fisher syndrome, an acute axonal variant of GBS, has been shown to follow infection with *Campylobacter jejuni*.

Vital Signs
- *Autonomic nervous system involvement (a type of autonomic dysreflexia):* Occurs in most patients with GBS: sinus tachycardia, bradycardia, orthostatic hypotension, hypertension, excessive diaphoresis, bowel and bladder dysfunction, loss of sphincter control, increased pulmonary secretions, SIADH, and cardiac dysrhythmias (a common cause of death)

Observation
- Ascending flaccid motor paralysis is the most common presenting sign and is associated with the early loss of deep tendon reflexes (DTRs).
- Symmetric motor weakness, decreased or absent DTRs, hypotonia or flaccidity of affected muscles, presence of respiratory abnormalities (e.g., nasal flaring, hypoventilation), facial paralysis
- Weakness, usually preceding the paralysis, is symmetrical, begins in distal muscle groups, and ascends to involve more proximal muscles.
- Muscles of respiration (intercostals and diaphragm) are frequently involved. Approximately half of all patients will require mechanical ventilation.
- Complaints of distal paresthesias are common. In more serious or prolonged cases, proprioceptive and vibratory dysfunctions are present. Sensory complaints usually appear first, with muscle weakness developing rapidly over 24 to 72 hours. About 90% of patients reach the peak of dysfunction within 2 weeks.
- Loss of pain and temperature sensations in a glove-and-stocking distribution has been reported.
- *Cranial nerve involvement:* All cranial nerves except I and II may be involved. See Appendix 3.

Diagnosis of Guillain-barré Syndrome

The diagnosis for Guillain-Barré Syndrome (GBS) is based on clinical presentation, history of antecedent illness, and cerebrospinal fluid (CSF) findings. A detailed neurological examination must be done as a baseline to assess for any changes as the disease progresses.

Test	Purpose	Abnormal Findings
Lumbar puncture (LP) and CSF analysis The CSF findings may be due to deposits of immunoglobulins IgG, IgM, and IgA localized to the nerve roots.	Assesses for abnormalities in CSF that distinguish GBS from other neurodegenerative disorders. CSF protein, normally between 15 and 45 mg/dl, may peak 4 to 6 weeks after onset of GBS to levels of several hundred mg/dl.	CSF analysis usually shows albumino-cytologic dissociation: an elevated protein, without increase in WBCs. This dissociation may be noted during the course of GBS and is helpful in differentiating GBS from other central nervous system (CNS) disorders.
Electromyography (EMG) or nerve conduction velocity (NCV)	Assesses nerve conduction velocity deficit as a result of the demyelination of peripheral nerves.	EMG and NCV demonstrate profound slowing of motor conduction velocities and conduction blocks several weeks into the illness.
Pulmonary function studies	Assesses for respiratory insufficiency during initial diagnostic evaluation	Vital capacity (VC) of less than 1 L indicates a possible need for assisted ventilation and should be assessed every 2 to 4 hours during the early acute phase.

Diagnosis of Guillain-barré Syndrome—cont'd		
Arterial blood gas analysis (ABGs)	Assesses for respiratory failure. Performed if VC drops below 1 L or if patient is dyspneic, confused, restless, has nasal flaring, use of accessory muscles of respiration, or is breathless	A decrease in Pao_2 greater than 10 to 15 mm Hg or an increase in $Paco_2$ of 10 to 15 mm Hg over baseline or normal value signals the need for immediate intubation or tracheostomy.

COLLABORATIVE MANAGEMENT
Care Priorities

1. **Provide respiratory support:** ET intubation with assisted mechanical ventilation, as necessary
2. **Perform plasmapheresis:** Involves a complete exchange of plasma with the removal of abnormal circulating antibodies that affect the peripheral nerve myelin sheath. Removal of these autoantibodies may lessen the duration and severity of GBS. For nursing interventions for complications of plasmapheresis, see Box 7-3.
3. **Administer IVIG (IV Immunoglobulin G or IVIgG):** IVIG given at 0.4 mg/kg/body weight/day for 5 days has been recommended as an alternative to plasma exchange in children and adults with GBS.
4. **Support cardiovascular function and carefully monitor for dysrhythmias:** Continuous cardiac monitoring may be initiated to assess for dysrhythmias, which are a common cause of death; arterial pressure monitoring may be used to evaluate hypertension or hypotension; and antihypertensive agents or vasopressors may be administered to maintain BP within normal levels.
5. **Manage bowel and bladder dysfunction:** Some patients may experience a paralytic ileus. Nasogastric suction and parenteral infusion may be started; stool softeners and laxatives may be given for constipation. A urinary catheter may be inserted in patients with urinary retention.
6. **Provide nutritional support:** Parenteral feedings are given until return of peristalsis. Tube feedings or gastrostomy feedings are used for patients with severe dysphagia. With recovery of gag reflex and swallowing ability, the diet will progress to semisolid and solid foods, which are more readily swallowed than are liquids.
7. **Rehabilitation:** Active and passive ROM exercises are performed at frequent intervals during all phases of GBS. Activity must be balanced with caloric intake to prevent muscle wasting. As the patient's condition stabilizes, a physiatrist consultation to plan rehabilitation with physical and occupational therapy should be done while the patient is in critical care. The primary goal is to pace recovery to obtain maximum mobility, promote self-care, and adapt to changes in body image. Rehabilitation does not improve nerve regeneration.

Safety Alert   *ROM is done gently during the acute phase. Overly aggressive exercise may exacerbate weakness and accelerate the demyelinating process.*

CARE PLANS FOR GUILLAIN-BARRÉ SYNDROME

Impaired gas exchange *related to altered oxygen supply associated with decreased lung expansion secondary to weakness or paralysis of intercostal and diaphragmatic muscles*

GOALS/OUTCOMES Within 12 to 24 hours of this diagnosis, patient has adequate gas exchange as evidenced by orientation to time, place, and person; RR 12 to 20 breaths/min with normal pattern and depth; HR less than 100 bpm; BP within patient's normal range; Pao_2 greater than 80 mm Hg; $Paco_2$ less than 45 mm Hg; and oxygen saturation greater than 94%.

NOC Respiratory Status: Gas Exchange; Respiratory Status: Ventilation; Mechanical Ventilation Response: Adult

Respiratory Monitoring

1. Monitor for respiratory distress. Report adventitious breath sounds (crackles, rhonchi); decreased or absent breath sounds; temperature greater than 37.7°C (100°F); increased HR and BP; tidal volume or vital capacity decreased from baseline; decreased PaO_2 or $PaCO_2$ increased by greater than 10 to 15 mm Hg from baseline; abnormal respiratory rate or rhythm; increasing restlessness, anxiety, or confusion.
2. Assess for weakness hourly, or as often as needed. Ascending motor and sensory dysfunctions usually occur rapidly (over 24 to 72 hours) and can lead to respiratory arrest.
3. Prepare to assist with intubation for respiratory failure.
4. Maintain mechanical ventilation as indicated. (See *Mechanical Ventilation,* p. 99).
5. Monitor ABG results and pulse oximetry. Consult physician for continued abnormalities.

NIC Airway Management; Acid-Base Monitoring; Oxygen Therapy; Mechanical Ventilation, Respiratory Status: Ventilation

Ineffective airway clearance *related to ineffective cough; decreased energy; increasing paralysis of respiratory, pharyngeal, and facial muscles; absence of the gag reflex*

GOALS/OUTCOMES Within 12 to 24 hours of this diagnosis, patient's airway is clear as evidenced by absence of adventitious breath sounds; HR 60 to 100 bpm; BP within patient's baseline range; RR 12 to 20 breaths/min with normal depth and pattern; tidal volume within baseline parameters; PaO_2 greater than 80 mm Hg; $PaCO_2$ less than 45 mm Hg.
NOC Aspiration Prevention; Respiratory Status: Airway Patency

Airway Management

1. Monitor for crackles, rhonchi, and decreased or absent breath sounds; increased HR and BP; tidal volume or vital capacity decreased from baseline; abnormal respiratory rate or rhythm; decrease in PaO_2 or increase in $PaCO_2$; and increasing restlessness or anxiety.
2. Suction the airway as need is determined by auscultation findings. As the paresis or paralysis subsides (usually after 2 to 4 weeks), cranial nerve function will begin to return (i.e., gag reflex, swallowing, coughing). Evaluate patient's ability to cough, whether or not he or she has been placed on mechanical ventilation. Assess for the presence of adventitious sounds to determine effectiveness of patient's cough.
3. Deliver oxygen and humidification as prescribed.
4. Maintain mechanical ventilation as prescribed. (See *Mechanical Ventilation,* p. 99.)
5. Maintain adequate hydration to minimize thickening of pulmonary secretions.
6. Turn and reposition patient at least every 2 hours to prevent stasis of secretions.

NIC Positioning; Airway Suctioning; Respiratory Monitoring; Cough Enhancement; Aspiration Precautions: Positioning

Risk for disuse syndrome *related to ascending flaccid paralysis and paresthesias*

GOALS/OUTCOMES Patient maintains baseline/optimal ROM of all joints and baseline muscle size and strength; no evidence of deep vein thrombosis (DVT).
NOC Endurance

Energy Management

1. Assess neurologic function hourly or as often as indicated. Ascending motor and sensory dysfunction usually occurs rapidly (over 24 to 72 hours). When neurologic dysfunction is progressing in GBS crisis, assess motor and sensory deficits by starting with the lower extremities and working upward.
    *   Assess muscle symmetry by using a side-to-side comparison.
    *   Assess for deep vein thrombus. Monitor for Homan sign, fever, and calf tenderness. Apply antiembolic stockings as prescribed to help promote tissue perfusion.
    *   Assess muscle strength: For lower extremities: have patient pull heel of foot toward the buttocks as you provide resistance by holding onto the foot. For upper extremities: have patient extend and flex the wrists and arms against your resistance.
    *   Assess DTRs of the Achilles, patellae, biceps, triceps, and brachioradialis. Normal response is $+2$; report decreased $(+1)$ or absent (0) response.

- Assess for paresthesia, including the location, degree, and whether it is ascending.
- Assess position sense by moving patient's big toe or thumb up and down while patient's eyes are closed. Note vibratory sense by placing a vibrating tuning fork over bony prominences.
- Assess response to light touch or pinprick by starting at the feet and working upward to determine the level of dysfunction. *Note:* Sensory symptoms are usually milder than motor complaints, with vibration and position sensations affected most often. However, about 25% of affected patients will experience pain, requiring analgesia. When light touch, pinprick, and temperature sensations are affected, they most often are found in a glove-and-stocking distribution. Patients frequently experience muscle tenderness and sensitivity to pressure.
- Assess for cranial nerve dysfunction (see Appendix 3).
2. Turn and record and report sensorimotor deficit, including degree of involvement.
3. Reposition patient in correct anatomic alignment every 2 hours or more often if requested by patient. Support patient's position with pillows and other positioning aids.

Activity Therapy
1. To maintain patient's muscle function and prevent contractures, ensure that active or passive ROM exercises are performed every 2 hours during all phases of GBS. Involve significant others in exercises, if appropriate.
2. Obtain a physical therapy referral, and begin rehabilitation planning process during the early stages of the disorder.
3. As indicated, apply splints to hands-arms and feet-legs to help prevent contracture; alternate splints so that they are on for 2 hours and off for 2 hours.
4. Specialty beds may be used to manage the respiratory, integumentary, autonomic, and musculoskeletal problems.

NIC Neurologic Monitoring; Exercise Therapy (all); Exercise Promotion; Positioning

Autonomic dysreflexia (AD) (or risk for same) *related to excessive or inadequate activity of the sympathetic or parasympathetic nervous system*

GOALS/OUTCOMES Patient has no symptoms of AD as evidenced by normal T-wave configuration on ECG, HR 60 to 100 bpm, BP within patient's normal range, cool and dry skin, patient's normal strength, and absence of headache and chest and abdominal tightness.

NOC Neurological Status: Autonomic; Symptom Severity; Vital Signs

Dysreflexia Management
1. Assess for signs of AD: cardiac dysrhythmias; HR less than 60 bpm or greater than 100 bpm; elevated and sustained BP (greater than 250 to 300/150 mm Hg); facial flushing; increased sweating, possibly caused by loss of thermal regulation; extreme generalized warmth; profound weakness; and complaints of severe headache or tightening in the chest and abdomen.
2. Place patient on cardiac monitor as prescribed.

| **Safety Alert** | *Because of the risk of fatal cardiac dysrhythmias in GBS, continuous cardiac monitoring is recommended for the first 10 to 14 days of hospitalization.* |

3. Monitor patient carefully during activities that are known to precipitate AD: position changes, vigorous coughing, and suctioning. Patient should be taught to avoid straining with bowel movements.
4. Be aware of and implement measures to prevent and intervene immediately to remove causes that may precipitate AD such as the following:
   - *Bladder stimuli:* urinary tract infection, cystoscopy, urinary catheter insertion, clogged urinary catheter, urinary calculi
   - *Bowel stimuli:* fecal impaction, rectal examination, enemas, suppositories. Ensure patient is well hydrated and has stool softeners and laxatives prescribed to reduce the chance of constipation.
   - *Sensory stimuli:* pressure caused by tight clothing, dressings, bed covers, thigh straps on urinary drainage bags; prolonged pressure on skin surface or over bony prominences; temperature changes, such as exposure to a cool breeze or draft

5. If indicators of AD are present, implement the following:
   a. Elevate HOB or place patient in a sitting position to promote decrease in BP.
   b. Monitor BP and HR every 3 to 5 minutes until patient's condition stabilizes.
   c. Determine and remove offending stimulus:
      - For example, if patient's bladder is distended, catheterize cautiously, using sufficient lubricant.
      - If patient has an indwelling urinary catheter, check for obstruction such as granulation in catheter or kinking of tubing. As indicated, irrigate catheter, using no greater than 30 ml normal saline. If infection is suspected, obtain a urine specimen for culture and sensitivity testing once crisis stage has passed.
      - Carefully check for fecal impaction. Perform the rectal examination gently, using an ointment that contains a local anesthetic (e.g., Nupercainal).
      - Check for sensory stimuli, loosen clothing, bed covers, or other constricting fabric as indicated.
6. Consult a physician or midlevel practitioner if symptoms do not abate within 15 to 30 minutes, especially elevated BP. This may lead to seizures, subarachnoid or intracerebral hemorrhage, or other stroke.
7. As prescribed, administer antihypertensive agents and monitor effectiveness.

NIC Neurologic Monitoring; Vital Signs Monitoring; Urinary Elimination Management

Decreased cardiac output (or risk for same) *related to decreased afterload secondary to reduced peripheral vascular tone. Normovolemic patients may have a decreased cardiac output as a result of vasodilation. This is similar to the vascular response seen in distributive (e.g., anaphylactic, septic) shock.*

GOALS/OUTCOMES Patient has adequate cardiac output as evidenced by BP within patient's normal range; HR 60 to 100 bpm; urinary output greater than 0.5 ml/kg/hr; peripheral pulses greater than 2+ on a 0 to 4+ scale; orientation to time, place, and person; central venous pressure (CVP) 4 to 6 mm Hg, pulmonary artery wedge pressure (PAWP) 6 to 12 mm Hg; systemic vascular resistance (SVR) 900 to 1200 dynes/sec/cm^{-5}; cardiac output (CO) 4 to 7 L/min; and normal sinus rhythm.
NOC Tissue Perfusion: Peripheral; Tissue Perfusion: Cerebral

Hemodynamic Regulation
1. Monitor patient for indicators of decreased cardiac output: drop in SBP greater than 20 mm Hg from baseline, SBP less than 80 mm Hg, or a continuing drop in SBP of 5 to 10 mm Hg with every assessment; HR greater than 100 bpm; irregular HR; restlessness, confusion, and dizziness; warm and flushed skin; edema; and decreased urinary output less than 0.5 ml/kg/hr for 2 consecutive hours. Monitor hemodynamic pressures, particularly PAWP, CO, and SVR.
2. Assess and report changes in cardiac rate and rhythm.
3. Implement measures to prevent decreased cardiac output caused by orthostatic hypotension:
   - Change patient's position slowly.
   - Perform ROM exercises every 2 hours to prevent venous pooling.
   - Apply elastic antiembolic hose as prescribed to promote venous return.
   - Keep patient's legs straight. Do not use pillows or "gatch" the knees on the bed.
   - Collaborate with physical therapist to use a tilt table to help stand the patient.
4. As prescribed, administer fluids to treat the hypotension.
5. Administer a vasopressor (e.g., norepinephrine) to counteract peripheral vasodilation.

NIC Cardiac Care: Acute; Circulatory Precautions; Resuscitation; Shock Prevention

Sensory/perceptual alterations (or risk for same) *related to altered sensory transmission secondary to cranial nerve involvement with GBS*

GOALS/OUTCOMES Patient reports normal vision and exhibits normal pupillary and gag reflexes, intact corneas, ability to masticate, and full ROM of head and shoulders.
NOC Neurological Status: Cranial/Sensory/Motor Function

Environmental Management: Safety
1. Assess cranial nerve function (see Appendix 3).
   - If patient experiences a deficit, place objects where patient can see them and assist with ADLs.

- Cover one eye with a patch or frosted lens if patient has diplopia; alternate patch or lens every 2 to 3 hours during patient's waking hours.
- Use eyelid crutches for patients with ptosis.
- Assess patient for corneal irritation or abrasion. Apply artificial tear drops or ointments as prescribed. Secure the eyelid in a closed position if corneal reflex is diminished or absent.
- Suction during oral hygiene. Do not feed patient an oral diet until the gag reflex returns.
- Position patient's head in a position of comfort and proper anatomic alignment.

NIC Neurological Monitoring; Peripheral Sensation Management; Surveillance: Safety

---

Constipation *related to hypoperistalsis or paralytic ileus associated with neuromuscular impairment*

GOALS/OUTCOMES Within 3 to 5 days of this diagnosis, patient has a bowel movement.
NOC Bowel Elimination; Hydration

Bowel Management

1. Assess patient's GI status: bowel sounds, abdominal distention, nausea, vomiting, and abdominal discomfort. In the presence of hypoperistalsis or paralytic ileus, patient will exhibit (1) high-pitched, tinkling sounds that will be heard early in obstruction or ileus or (2) a decrease or absence of sounds occurring with complete obstruction or paralytic ileus.
2. If patient is having bowel movements, determine the amount, consistency, and frequency. Question patient about his or her usual pattern of bowel elimination.
3. Provide 2 to 3 L/day of fluid to prevent dehydration and constipation. This may be contraindicated for patient with impaired renal or cardiac status.
4. Begin bowel training program based on patient's needs and status of dietary intake:
   - Provide a high-fiber diet if patient is able to chew and swallow without difficulty.
   - If patient is bed bound, bulk-forming laxatives should be avoided.
   - Give patient prune juice every evening.
   - Establish a regular time for elimination and have a bed pan readily available.
   - Facilitate patient's normal bowel habits; ensure privacy.
   - Administer stool softeners (e.g., docusate sodium).
   - Carefully administer prescribed medicated suppositories.

 Safety Alert *Care must be taken to avoid stimulation of autonomic dysreflexia by using generous amounts of anesthetic ointment and ensuring gentle insertion when giving suppository or enema.*

---

5. See *Risk for Disuse Syndrome* (p. 664), for neuroassessment parameters. Also see Box 7-3 for the following complications: hypovolemia, clotting abnormalities, hypokalemia, and hypocalcemia.

NIC Constipation/Impaction Management; Fluid Monitoring; Nutrition Management

---

Resources for Education

GBS/CIDP Foundation International
Address: The Holly Building 104 1/2 Forrest Ave, Narberth, PA 19072
info@gbs-cidp.com
http://www.gbs-cidp.org
Tel: 610-667-0131; 866-224-3301
Fax: 610-667-7036
For more information on neurological disorders or research programs funded by the National Institute of Neurological Disorders and Stroke, contact the Institute's Brain Resources and Information Network (BRAIN) at:
BRAIN
P.O. Box 580
Bethesda, MD 20824
(800) 352-9424
http://www.ninds.nih.gov

ADDITIONAL NURSING DIAGNOSES

See also *Urinary Retention* in *Acute Spinal Cord Injury* (p. 276). See *Deficient Knowledge: Related to Post-Organ Transplant Care* (p. 923). For other nursing diagnoses and interventions, see the following as appropriate: *Nutritional Support* (p. 117), *Mechanical Ventilation* (p. 99), *Prolonged Immobility* (p. 149), and *Emotional and Spiritual Support of the Patient and Significant Others* (p. 200).

STATUS EPILEPTICUS

PATHOPHYSIOLOGY

Status epilepticus (SE) is a state of recurring or continuous seizures of at least 30 minutes' duration, in which the patient does not return to full consciousness from the postictal state before another seizure occurs. If possible, treatment should be initiated immediately to prevent neuronal injury, which may begin within 20 to 30 minutes of the onset of SE. The mortality rate for SE is estimated to be from 12% to 25%.

A practical definition of SE may be revised to include seizures of only 5 to 10 minutes' duration, because of a high likelihood that they will continue. There are two major types of SE: convulsive and nonconvulsive. Another classification is based on Gastaut and used by Engel in which *generalized SE* includes convulsive SE (generalized tonic-clonic seizures) and partial SE. Convulsive SE is more common and is considered a life-threatening medical emergency, because the hypoxia and metabolic exhaustion of neuronal tissue may cause neuronal death. *Partial SE* includes simple partial SE (focal motor or epilepsia partialis continua) and complex partial SE (temporal or nontemporal seizures). The term "nonconvulsive status" may also be used to describe absence, complex partial SE, and simple partial SE. It is hard to determine the type of nonconvulsive seizure activity clinically.

SE in persons with epilepsy is often due to noncompliance with medications or a drop in anticonvulsant serum levels caused by alcohol abuse or infection. Other causes for individuals with and without preexisting epilepsy include acute metabolic disturbances (e.g., hypoglycemia, hyponatremia, hypocalcemia), stroke, CNS infection (e.g., meningitis, encephalitis), CNS trauma or tumors, hypoxia, and alcohol or drug abuse. Prompt treatment may prevent complications including cardiac dysrhythmias, hyperthermia, aspiration, hypertension or hypotension, anoxia, hyperglycemia or hypoglycemia, dehydration, rhabdomyolysis, myoglobinuria, and oral and/or musculoskeletal injuries. The prognosis of SE is thought to be related to the etiology.

ASSESSMENT

Goal of System Assessment

Evaluate for cessation of seizures, return to baseline neurologic function, and to determine cause of seizures.

History and Risk Factors

Epilepsy, drug or alcohol abuse, recent head injury, infection, headaches. If the patient is taking anticonvulsant medications, note the following: drug name, dosage, time last taken, length of time drug has been taken, and any recent medication changes. Determine if patient is taking any other medications, including name, dose, and time last taken. Some medications may lower the seizure threshold.

Vital Signs

Changes resulting from the massive sympathetic nervous system response to continuous, generalized seizures include hypertension, tachycardia, dysrhythmias, tachypnea, and hyperthermia.

Observation and Seizure Assessment

Evaluate for ongoing seizures.

- Changes in mental status such as confusion, dreamy state, stupor
- Automatisms
- Lipsmacking, chewing, swallowing
- Speech difficulty
- Twitching of the face, hand, arm, leg (focal motor seizures)

- Mild clonic movements (e.g., fluttering of the eyelids)
- Tonic-clonic activity of all extremities

Screening Labwork:
Blood studies can reveal causes of seizures.
- *Blood chemistries*: Electrolyte imbalance or metabolic disturbance
- *CBC*: Elevated WBCs may indicate infection as cause.
- *Anticonvulsant blood levels*: Decreased or low levels may be cause of return of seizures.
- *Serum drug screen*: Rule out drug or alcohol intoxication.
- *ABGs*: Obtain baseline levels and state of oxygenation.

Electroencephalography
Continuous electroencephalographic (EEG) monitoring is used to determine whether the patient is still in SE even though there are no clinical signs or very subtle clinical signs and for those patients who are placed in medication-induced coma for refractory SE.

Diagnostic Tests for Status Epilepticus		
Test	**Purpose**	**Abnormal Findings**
Electrolytes Sodium Calcium Magnesium Glucose	Assess for possible causes of status epilepticus (SE)	Hyponatremia, hypocalcemia, hypoglycemia
CBC	Assess for infection	Infection may be a precipitant for SE
Serum drug screen	Assess for drug and/or alcohol intoxication	May be a precipitant for SE
Antiepilepsy drug (AED) levels	Determine amount of drugs in the system	Low levels may be cause of SE
Arterial blood gases (ABGs)	Obtain baseline levels and determine oxygen saturation	Decreased oxygen saturation due to convulsive SE and medication administration
Continuous ECG monitoring	Evaluate cardiovascular status, especially during medication administration	Phenytoin and other AEDs can cause dysrhythmias and hypotension
EEG	Evaluate the brain's electrical activity for ongoing seizures even if there are no clinical signs of seizures	Epileptiform discharges and seizure activity
CT brain scan	Evaluate for any brain abnormalities responsible for the SE	Space-occupying lesions

COLLABORATIVE MANAGEMENT
Care Priorities
1. **Support of ventilation and perfusion:** Cardiopulmonary function and vital signs are closely monitored. Measures should be initiated to maintain a patent airway, including intubation, as well as ventilatory and cardiovascular support. The increased metabolic rate and oxygen demands are high during constant seizures, which prompts tachycardia to try to meet the demand. The patient may need support to try to augment the cardiac output if the response is insufficient to meet the demand. Cardiac dysrhythmias, hypertension or hypotension, and dehydration are common complications of SE. More

extensive evaluation for muscle damage should be done if lengthy tonic-clonic seizures continue or occur frequently. Patients can develop rhabdomyolysis, which may lead to acute renal failure if not appropriately managed.

2. **Establish IV access:** For medication administration, fluid resuscitation, and to draw blood for needed labwork

3. **Pharmacotherapy**

Prevention of Wernicke-Korsakoff syndrome: 100 mg IV thiamine and 50 ml of 50% glucose are administered if chronic alcohol ingestion or hypoglycemia is suspected.

Administration of fast-acting anticonvulsant: Given to quickly achieve high serum and brain concentrations. Not used as long-acting anticonvulsant. First-line agents are the benzodiazepines. Treatment is most effective when started promptly. *Midazolam (Versed)* has recently been used more commonly in children.

- Lorazepam (Ativan)
  - Preferred by most epileptologists
  - 0.1 mg/kg, up to 8 mg, given IV. Do not infuse faster than 2 mg/min.
  - Monitor respiratory and cardiovascular status continuously.
  OR
- Diazepam (Valium)
  - 0.2 mg/kg, up to 20 mg, given IV.
  - Do not infuse faster than 5 mg/min to avoid respiratory depression, which may occur with faster infusion rate.

Administration of long-acting anticonvulsant

- Fosphenytoin (Cerebyx)
  - Usual IV loading dose is 20 mg/kg PE (phenytoin equivalents). Infusion rate is 100 to 150 PE/min. Most IV solutions are compatible with fosphenytoin, including dextrose solutions. Phlebitis and soft tissue damage at IV site are not seen as frequently with fosphenytoin.
  - Monitor vital signs closely. Hypotension and cardiac dysrhythmias may develop.
  - If status persists after 20 mg/kg, an additional 5 to 10 mg/kg may be given, up to a maximal total dose of 30 mg/kg.
  OR (if fosphenytoin is not used)
- Phenytoin (Dilantin)
  - Usual loading dose is 18 to 20 mg/kg given IV. Do not infuse faster than 50 mg/min to avoid serious dysrhythmias, including asystole.
  - Phlebitis and soft tissue damage at IV site may occur.
  - Flush line with normal saline only. Microcrystallization, which occurs when phenytoin is used with dextrose, may also occur when it is used in saline as a continuous drip.
  - Monitor closely for hypotension and dysrhythmias.

 Safety Alert *High doses of phenytoin can cause seizure activity; therefore greater than 30 mg/kg is not recommended.*

- If seizures persist after 20 mg/kg dose, an additional 5 to 10 mg/kg may be given, up to a maximal total dose of 30 mg/kg.

Administration of IV phenobarbital: Used if patient is allergic to phenytoin

- Usual dosage is 20 mg/kg. Do not infuse faster than 50 to 75 mg/min.

Safety Alert *If given simultaneously with or after lorazepam or diazepam, respiratory depression and hypotension can occur, possibly necessitating ventilatory support.*

- Aggressive treatment is required for refractory SE that continues despite administration of benzodiazepines, phenytoin or fosphenytoin, and phenobarbital. Consider deep sedation/general anesthesia using propofol, midazolam, or pentobarbital.

Continuous EEG monitoring is required for patients in refractory SE to determine effectiveness of treatment. There are no current studies comparing these agents to help determine which is the most effective in the treatment of refractory SE.

Administration of Levetiracetam (Keppra)

- Not the drug of choice for patients actively seizing, but an appropriate choice for long-term management of epilepsy. Usual initial dose is 500 mg orally every 12 hours. Drug can be increased by 100 mg/day every 2 weeks up to a maximum of 300 mg/day.

4. **General anesthesia, neuromuscular blockade and/or heavy sedation**

Pentobarbital coma

- Given only if administration of fast-acting anticonvulsant, long-acting anticonvulsant, or IV phenobarbital is ineffective in stopping the seizure activity.
- Loading dose is 5 mg/kg. Maintenance dose is 0.5 to 3 mg/kg/hr to stop seizures.
- Monitor respiratory and cardiovascular activity continuously.
- Mechanical ventilation and vasopressors are usually required.
- Periodic tapering of pentobarbital is done to see if seizures have remitted.
- Patient may be in a coma for days to weeks.

- *Propofol*
  - Given for refractory SE
  - Loading dose is 1 to 2 mg/kg given IV. Initial maintenance dose of 2 to 10 mg/kg/hr to stop seizure activity. Adjust dose according to EEG findings.
  - Monitor respiratory and cardiovascular activity continuously.
  - Mechanical ventilation and vasopressors are required.
  - Periodic tapering of propofol is done to see if seizures have remitted.

- *Midazolam*
  - Given for refractory SE
  - Loading dose is 0.2 mg/kg given by IV. Maintenance of 0.75 to 1 mcg/kg/min to stop seizure activity. Maintenance dose is adjusted according to EEG findings.
  - Monitor respiratory and cardiovascular activity continuously.
  - Mechanical ventilation and vasopressors are usually required.
  - Periodic tapering of midazolam is done to see if seizures have remitted.

Safety Alert   *Intravenous valproic acid (Depacon) and levetiracetam (Keppra) are being used more frequently in the treatment of status, and studies are being done to evaluate their effectiveness in status. Other agents that can be used in refractory status are paraldehyde, lidocaine, or neuromuscular blockade. Neuromuscular blockade stops only movements (not brain electrical activity) and should be administered only when continuous EEG monitoring is available.*

---

5. **Nutritional support:** Enteral or parenteral nutrition may be necessary, depending on the duration of the status epilepticus and patient's underlying nutritional state.

CARE PLANS FOR STATUS EPILEPTICUS

Impaired gas exchange *related to altered oxygen supply associated with hypoventilation and bradypnea secondary to depressant effect of seizures and medications on respiratory center*

GOALS/OUTCOMES Within 1 hour of treatment/intervention, patient has adequate gas exchange as evidenced by Pao$_2$ greater than 80 mm Hg, Paco$_2$ 35 to 45 mm Hg, pH 7.35 to 7.45, and RR 12 to 20 breaths/min with normal depth and pattern.

NOC Respiratory Status: Ventilation

Respiratory Monitoring

1. Monitor for respiratory distress. Note RR, depth, and rhythm and skin color. Report use of accessory muscles, rapid or labored respirations, and cyanosis.
2. Monitor ABG values to assess oxygenation. Be alert to hypoxemia (Pao$_2$ less than 80 mm Hg) and respiratory acidosis (Paco$_2$ greater than 45 mm Hg; pH less than 7.35).
3. Keep intubation equipment ready for airway and ventilation assistance.

4. Position an oral airway to help maintain open airway. Suction as necessary.
5. Keep patient turned to the side to allow secretions to drain.
6. Administer oxygen as prescribed.
7. Administer antiepilepsy medications within prescribed criteria to avoid further depression of respiratory center.

NIC Airway Management; Oxygen Therapy; Aspiration Precautions

Altered tissue perfusion: cerebral and cardiopulmonary *related to altered blood flow during continuous seizure activity or vasodilatory effects of specific antiepilepsy medications. Note: Metabolic demands of the brain and heart are increased greatly during seizure activity; adequate cerebral perfusion is essential to maintain brain function.*

GOALS/OUTCOMES Within 1 hour of treatment/intervention, patient has adequate cerebral and cardiopulmonary perfusion as evidenced by orientation to time, place, and person; normal sinus rhythm on ECG; BP within patient's normal range; RR 12 to 20 breaths/min with normal depth and pattern (eupnea); and absence of headache, papilledema, and other clinical indicators of increased ICP.
NOC Tissue Perfusion: Cerebral; Tissue Perfusion: Cardiac

Cerebral Perfusion Promotion
1. Support ventilation and perfusion for maximal delivery of oxygen to the brain. Monitor vital signs every 2 to 4 minutes. Respiratory depression, decreased BP, and dysrhythmias can occur with rapid infusion of diazepam and phenytoin. BP must be maintained within normal limits for optimal brain perfusion.
2. Monitor for dysrhythmias, especially during medication administration.
3. Ensure safe administration of antiepileptic drugs: diazepam at 5 mg/min; lorazepam at 2 mg/min; phenobarbital at 50 to 100 mg/min; or phenytoin at 50 mg/min.
4. Perform baseline and serial neurologic assessments to determine the presence of focal findings that suggest an expanding lesion.

NIC Cerebral Perfusion Promotion; Neurologic Monitoring; Seizure Management; Cardiac Care: Acute

Risk for trauma (oral and musculoskeletal) *related to seizure activity*

GOALS/OUTCOMES Patient's mouth and extremities are not injured during the seizure.
NIC Tissue Integrity: Skin and Mucous Membranes

Environmental Management: Safety
1. Keep side rails padded and up at all times, with bed in the lowest position.
2. Perform protective measures during the seizures:
   - Put a soft object such as a flat pillow under patient's head.
   - Move sharp or potentially dangerous objects away from patient.
   - Loosen any tight clothing.
   - Avoid restraining patient. The force of tonic-clonic movements may cause strains and fractures of extremities if thrashing occurs with restraints in place.
   - Avoid forcing airway into patient's mouth when jaws are clenched. Force could break teeth, and patient could swallow or aspirate them.
   - Avoid use of tongue blade, which could splinter and cut the mouth.
   - Stay with patient; assess and record seizure type and duration. Record any automatic behavior (e.g., lip smacking, chewing movements), motor activity, incontinence, tongue biting, and postictal state.
3. After seizure, reorient and reassure patient.

NIC Environmental Management: Safety; Positioning; Seizure Precautions; Seizure Management

Noncompliance with prescribed medication regimen *related to misunderstanding health care recommendations, not understanding importance of following medication schedule, running out of medication, stopping medication intentionally*

GOALS/OUTCOMES Within the 24-hour period before discharge from the critical care unit, patient verbalizes understanding of the rationale and importance of taking the medication as prescribed, as well as the consequence of noncompliance.

NOC Compliance Behavior

Mutual Goal Setting
1. Once a diagnosis of noncompliance with the medication regimen has been established, determine patient's reason for noncompliance.
2. Assess patient's understanding of epilepsy and its treatment.
3. Ensure that patient is aware that stopping the antiepilepsy medication can result in serious problems, including SE. If patient plans to stop the medication for any reason, he or she should consult with the physician.
4. Evaluate the effect epilepsy has on patient's lifestyle.
5. Once the cause of noncompliance is identified, work to find a solution. If the patient has side effects from the medication, such as gastric upset, suggest that patient try taking the medication after meals. If the gastric upset is a result of increasing the medication, advise patient to increase the dose more slowly.
6. Refer patient to regional epilepsy support groups and the Epilepsy Foundation of America (EFA), including regional affiliate and national headquarters.
7. As appropriate, refer patient to nurse specialist or social worker at regional center for individual counseling.

NIC Teaching: Prescribed Medication; Decision-Making Support; Coping Enhancement; Values Clarification

Deficient knowledge *related to disease process, treatment, and lifestyle changes that epilepsy necessitates*

GOALS/OUTCOMES Within the 24-hour period before discharge from the critical care unit, patient verbalizes understanding of epilepsy, including its etiology and pathophysiology and seizure classification, as well as its treatment and the lifestyle changes it necessitates.

NOC Knowledge: Disease Process

Teaching: Disease Process
1. Assess knowledge level and provide necessary information about epilepsy.
2. Ask patient to describe seizure(s) in detail, including warning signals (aura) at the beginning of seizures. Explain that the aura or warning signals onset of seizures and that patient should lie down or get into a safe position to prevent injury.
3. Assess patient's knowledge of antiepilepsy medications, including name(s), purpose, schedule, dosage, precautions, and side effects. Reinforce importance of maintaining a constant blood level of medication by taking it as prescribed. Explain if the medication is missed or taken erratically, he or she cannot attain the blood level needed to prevent seizure breakthrough. If a dose of medication is missed, instruct patient to notify his or her physician.
4. Emphasize to the patient that a normal life is possible.
5. Insure patient knows sleep deprivation can precipitate SE. Every patient must know his or her own limits. Having epilepsy does not mean it is necessary to get more sleep than do persons who do not have epilepsy.
6. Teach patient/significant others the importance of safety measures used during a seizure. Emphasize how to ease patient to the floor and turn him or her to a side-lying position.
7. Inform patient of your local driving regulations/laws for persons with epilepsy.
8. Teach patient the importance of avoiding dangerous machinery and heights if his or her seizures are not being controlled adequately by medications.

NIC Teaching: Individual; Support Group

Ineffective coping *related to frustration secondary to unpredictable nature of the disease*

GOALS/OUTCOMES Within 24 to 48 hours of this diagnosis, patient verbalizes feelings, identifies strengths and ineffective coping behaviors, and understands responsibility for self-care.

NOC Coping

Coping Enhancement
1. Assess patient's knowledge of the disease and its treatment. See preceding diagnosis, *Deficient Knowledge.*
2. Encourage patient to express feelings so areas of major concern are known.
3. Involve patient in decisions regarding care so he or she has more sense of control over life (e.g., encourage patient to participate in the decision for scheduling the medications). Problem solve for major concerns.
4. Help patient set realistic goals for employment and living arrangements. Refer patient to regional or local EFA as appropriate.
5. Encourage patient to educate others in what to do should a seizure occur.
6. Encourage involvement in support groups; coping strategies can be learned from other persons with seizures.

NIC Coping Enhancement; Crisis Intervention; Emotional Support; Support System Enhancement

ADDITIONAL NURSING DIAGNOSES

For other nursing diagnoses and interventions, see the following as appropriate: *Mechanical Ventilation* (p. 99) and *Emotional and Spiritual Support of the Patient and Significant Others* (p. 200).

STROKE: ACUTE ISCHEMIC AND HEMORRHAGIC

PATHOPHYSIOLOGY

The term *stroke* refers to an acute brain injury which results from interruption in blood flow; also referred to as a "brain attack." Stroke was termed a cerebrovascular accident (CVA) in the past. Stroke is the third-leading cause of death in the United States. The AHA estimates approximately 600,000 new and 180,000 recurrent strokes occur annually. Fourteen percent of patients with new stroke will have a recurrent stroke within the first year. The overall mortality rate was 273,000 in 2007. Eighty-seven percent are ischemic strokes, 10% are intracranial hemorrhages (ICH), and the remaining 3% are subarachnoid hemorrhages (SAH). Women experience 60,000 more strokes each year than do men. Subcategories are shown in Figure 7-1. Each stroke type is defined by the pathophysiologic event. *Acute ischemic stroke (AIS)* and *intracranial hemorrhage (ICH)* are discussed here. Subarachnoid hemorrhage (SAH) from cerebral aneurysmal rupture was discussed in an earlier section of this chapter (see *Cerebral Aneurysm and Subarachnoid Hemorrhage*, p 629). A *transient ischemic attack (TIA)* is a loss of localized cerebral perfusion lasting less than 24 hours. Although not considered a stroke, a TIA may precede an AIS by hours to years. A TIA generally lasts 5 to 10 minutes and is most often caused by a cerebral thrombus. A *reversible ischemic neurological deficit (RIND)* is a term which has been used for a type of TIA that lasts longer than 24 hours.

Prior to the introduction of thrombolytic therapy, a stroke was not always viewed as a medical emergency, as there was little to offer patients to stop the process. As therapies evolved, an acute ischemic stroke became an emergency since treatment with thrombolytics must be provided within the first 4.5 hours to be effective (ideally within the first hour of arrival in a hospital/stroke center), while hemorrhage might be managed using an immediate treatment intervention to reduce ICP, such as inserting a ventriculostomy to drain CSF.

AIS results from atherosclerosis of the blood vessels which perfuse the brain. Approximately 20% of AIS results from extracranial vascular disease of the carotid or vertebrobasilar arteries, while 25% results from diseased penetrating, small intracranial arteries which result in lacunar or subcortical strokes. Another 20% results from low to absent cerebral perfusion caused by cardiogenic emboli, most often resulting from atrial fibrillation. Cardiac disease is the most common cause of cerebral embolism. Cerebral emboli may be formed in the heart and travel to the brain or be formed in the carotid or other cerebral arteries and migrate to occlude a smaller artery in the brain. The remaining 30% are cryptogenic, and include critically ill patients in shock experiencing systemic hypoperfusion. A thrombus is a clot formed in the artery, usually in branches with low flow due to plaque. Thrombotic strokes are usually caused by local atherosclerosis of large vessels (e.g., internal cerebral artery [ICA] or middle cerebral artery [MCA]) related to occlusion of small, perforating vessels. Characteristic deficits are produced, depending on the artery involved (Table 7-5).

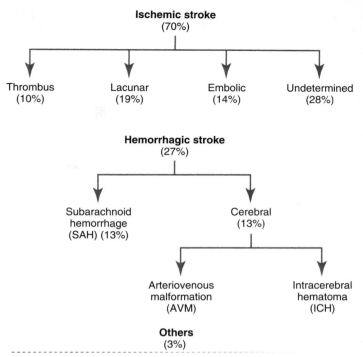

Figure 7-1 Stroke classification.

Table 7-5	CEREBRAL PERFUSION NEUROANATOMY RELATED TO NEUROLOGIC DEFICIT	
Vessel	**Area Supplied**	**Deficit**
Internal carotid artery	Right or left hemisphere	Contralateral motor or sensory deficit, aphasia with dominant hemisphere, neglect with non-dominant hemisphere, contralateral visual field deficit (hemianopia), contralateral eye deviation
Middle cerebral artery	Right or left convex surface of the brain, most of the basal ganglia, internal capsule, putamen, and globus pallidus	Contralateral hemiplegia (arm and face > leg), sensory involvement, aphasia of dominant hemisphere, neglect of nondominant hemisphere (denial of weakness), homonymous hemianopia
Anterior cerebral artery	Right of left frontal lobe, corpus callosum, caudate nucleus, internal capsule	Weakness or sensory loss of contralateral leg and proximal arm; behavior disturbance: abulia, confusion, memory loss, urinary incontinence
Posterior cerebral artery	Midbrain thalamus, choroid plexus, occipital lobe, and medial temporal lobe	Contralateral visual field deficit, color blindness, impaired depth perception, occasional sparing of central vision, memory loss, sensory loss, nystagmus, pupillary abnormalities, ataxia
Vertebral artery	Medulla and/or cerebellum	Face, nose, or eye ipsilateral numbness with contralateral body numbness, facial weakness, vertigo, ataxia, nystagmus, dysphagia, dysarthria
Basilar artery cerebellum	Pons, midbrain, and/or locked-in syndrome (pons)	Quadriplegia or hemiplegia/paresis, dysarthria, dysphagia, ataxia, nystagmus, vertigo, coma

Cerebral ischemia disrupts the sodium/potassium (Na^+/K^+) pump, leading to neuronal depolarization and neurotransmitter release, followed by a massive flux of ions and water resulting in brain cell edema. Extracellular K^+ and intracellular calcium (Ca^{2+}) increase. Brain cells deprived of oxygen begin anaerobic metabolism. The resulting lactic acidosis and high concentration of intracellular Ca^{2+} lead to cellular death.

Lactic acidosis prompts the CNS *ischemic response*: The vasomotor center is stimulated, which causes vasoconstriction with marked elevation in blood pressure. Systolic pressures less than 220 mm Hg and diastolic BPs (DBPs) less than 110 mm Hg are not treated, since this is a natural response to perfuse the ischemic brain. If thrombolytic therapy is to be initiated, the blood pressure is slowly lowered to less than 185/105 mm Hg. The CNS ischemic response is seen during the acute phase of stroke, but is most pronounced during the Cushing response before herniation.

Intracranial hemorrhage (ICH) resulting in hemorrhagic stroke, may occur anywhere in the brain (Table 7-6), resulting in an intracerebral hematoma. Although various pathophysiologic events can result in ICH, the most common cause is hypertension, usually resulting in the rupture of a small penetrating artery in the subcortical region. Other causes include bleeding disorders, abnormal vasculature, alcohol abuse and liver disease. Damage occurs as accumulated blood destroys and displaces the brain tissue. Disrupted tissue and the ruptured vessel reduce normal blood flow to the area that surrounds the already injured brain tissue, resulting in even greater ischemic injury. Intracerebral blood may rupture into the lateral ventricle, creating risk for communicating hydrocephalus. Lobar hemorrhages are less common and in older persons are often caused by cerebral amyloid angiopathy. Other common causes of hemorrhage include vascular anomalies such as arterial venous malformations (AVMs), arterial venous fistulas (AVFs), vasculitis, neoplasms, hematologic disorders, and stimulant abuse (e.g., cocaine, amphetamines).

ASSESSMENT OF STROKE: AIS AND ICH
Goal of System Assessment
During the hyperacute phase, determine stroke type, cause, location, and eligibility for thrombolytic therapy. Thrombolysis must be initiated within 4.5 hours of symptom onset. Then, evaluate for risk factors of stroke extension or secondary neurologic injury.

History and Risk Factors
Evaluation can provide valuable clues that help facilitate the diagnosis of stroke. The CT brain scan, screening for bleeding risk, and initiation of thrombolytic therapy must be done within the first 4.5 hours. ICH may also have improved outcomes with timely management of increased ICP.

- *Risk factors commonly associated with AIS:* Hypertension, smoking, diabetes mellitus, hypercholesterolemia, atrial fibrillation, sick sinus syndrome, hormone replacement therapy, oral contraceptives, dilated cardiomyopathy, ventricular thrombus after acute myocardial infarction (MI), valvular disease, sedentary lifestyle, aging, obesity, previous history of TIA or stroke, ethnicity including Native American, Alaska Native, African American, or Hispanic origins, previous MI, or family history of stroke or TIA. Other risk factors for women:
  - Women with a waist measuring greater than 35 inches between the ages of 45 and 55 are at highest risk of stroke.

Table 7-6	HEMORRHAGIC LOCATIONS AND SYNDROMES
Area	**Syndrome**
Putamen	Contralateral hemiplegia, hemisensory loss, hemianopia, slurred speech
Thalamic	Contralateral hemiplegia; hemisensory loss; small, poorly reactive pupils; decreased level of consciousness
Pontine	Locked-in syndrome (awake, aware, unable to verbally communicate, quadriplegia), coma
Cerebellar	Occipital headache, ataxia, dizziness, headache, nausea, vomiting
Lobar	Mimics cerebral infarct (e.g., contralateral motor and sensory signs)

- Waist size greater than 35 inches increases risk in all age groups of women.
- Pregnancy: primarily during delivery and post partum
- *Risk factors commonly associated with ICH*: Hypertension, smoking, African American ethnicity, aging, excessive alcohol consumption, bleeding disorders, and liver dysfunction, in addition to known underlying vascular anomalies.

Vital Sign Assessment
- Measure BP frequently.
- Document MAP and track trends; titrate medications to maintain parameters.
- Respiratory status: Rate, rhythm quality, and breath sounds; proper positioning and turning to maintain adequate oxygenation
    - Maintain Pao_2 greater than 95% for adequate oxygenation to the brain.
    - Implement continuous cardiac monitoring, observe for dysrhythmias including QT prolongation, ST-segment depression, T-wave inversion, U waves, and ventricular ectopy.
    - Dysrhythmias after stroke may be caused by release of catecholamines, causing hypertension, cardiac irritability, and/or muscle damage. Individuals with new ECG changes have a less favorable prognosis.
    - ECG monitoring for the first 24 to 72 hours is recommended.
    - Monitor for hyperthermia and hypothermia: maintain normal thermal temperature.

Neurological Evaluation: Observation
General Presentation: AIS and ICH   Sudden onset of weakness/numbness of the face/arm and/or leg, one-sided facial droop, blurred or loss of vision in one eye, inability to produce or understand speech, fixed gaze to the right or left side, change in level of consciousness, hemisensory loss on right or left side, neglect or ignoring of one side, paralysis of right or left side, ataxia, possible headache
- Use a recognized Stroke Assessment Scale to identify deficits and the time of onset: Several stroke assessment scales are available, including the FAST (Face, Arm, Speech, Time), the Cincinnati Prehospital Stroke Scale, the Los Angeles Prehospital Stroke Scale, and Melbourne Prehospital Stroke Scale.
- Rate stroke severity: Use the NIH Stroke Scale (NIHSS) or shortened prehospital version (sNIHSS) or the Los Angeles Motor Scale.
- Perform a complete neurologic assessment to establish baseline status (see *Neurological Assessment,* p. 619).
- *Obtain* information regarding baseline neurologic function (e.g., dementia, prior stroke, and neuropathy) and *identify* risk factors associated with stroke.

Clinical Presentation: AIS (Table 7-5)
- Sudden or acute onset of symptoms. Although both thrombotic and embolic strokes can begin abruptly, the former are more likely to evolve over several hours and may fluctuate over several hours or days.
- Those with AIS do not usually experience pain other than a headache, nor do they have altered LOC unless the stroke causes mass effects as a result of swelling or involves the brainstem or thalamic regions bilaterally.
- Women more often report stroke symptoms such as face and limb pain, hiccups, nausea, general weakness, chest pain, palpitations, fainting, SOB, and seizures. Further research is being conducted to better understand the gender differences related to stroke.
- *Embolic stroke*: The deficit caused is usually maximal at onset and often occurs during activity.
- *Ischemic stroke caused by MCA occlusion in the dominant hemisphere*: Patients are usually awake with hemiparesis, aphasia, visual field cut, and sensory loss.
- *Acute hemispheric infarction*: People have elevated arterial BP and often appear drowsy even in the absence of swelling.

Clinical Presentation: ICH (Table 7-6)
- Severe headache, altered LOC, vomiting, very high BP, and increased ICP
- Symptoms of ICH depend on the size and location of the hematoma. A relatively small hemorrhage into the brainstem may produce quadriplegia and coma, whereas a hematoma of similar size in the basal ganglia may produce hemiparesis without altered LOC. A larger hematoma (as measured by CT brain scan) may indicate a poorer prognosis.
- The neurologic deficit may evolve over minutes to a few hours.

Screening Neurologic Imaging

CT brain imaging is diagnostic and guides decision making for treatment.
- Prepare to transfer patient to radiology for immediate acute imaging of the brain.
- Continue aggressive monitoring of vital signs and neurologic status while maintaining safety of patient during transport.

Screening Labwork

- Biochemical profile: Evaluates for abnormal glucose and electrolyte imbalances
- Coagulation profile to determine risk for bleeding and/or clotting
- CBC with differential: Evaluates for abnormal platelets, sepsis, and anemia
- Creatine phosphokinase–myocardial band (CK-MB) isoenzymes
- Drug screen may be used to determine if drugs may be related to neurological changes.

Diagnosis of Acute Ischemic Stroke vs Hemorrhagic Stroke

Test	Purpose	Abnormal Findings
Imaging		
Computed tomography (CT) brain scan	Performed emergently, is the golden standard of differentiating ischemic from hemorrhagic stroke; may be done at intervals to monitor progress	Within the first few hours after AIS, the scan may appear normal. ICH is easily diagnosed on CT— blood appears as a bright white signal.
CT angiogram (CTA)	To visualize the vascular system of the brain	Vascular anomalies, narrowing, or occlusion
CT perfusion or CT-xenon scan (CTP)	Provides information related to cerebral blood flow and volume; used to guide clinical decision making regarding the use of thrombolysis or interventional procedures	Compromised blood flow; a limited test; cannot detect infarcted tissue
Magnetic resonance imaging (MRI) and magnetic resonance arteriogram (MRA)	MRI is most useful for ischemic patients in identifying the cause and area involved. Provides detailed information regarding the area of injury or its vascular supply (MRA).	Infarcts, areas at risk or ischemic areas, vascular defects, stenosis, occlusion *Diffusion weighted imaging (DWI)* is a measurement of edema, while *Perfusion weighted imaging (PWI)* is a measurement of global CBF.
Positron emission tomography (PET) and single-photon emission computed tomography (SPECT)	To evaluate brain metabolism and blood flow using 3D imaging produced using a radioactive tracer	Demonstrates abnormal function of the brain by revealing abnormal structures, metabolism, and perfusion
Cerebral angiography	The golden standard for evaluating cerebral vasculature; invasive procedure with minimal risk used to visualize the cerebral blood vessels	Provides specific information on the cause of stroke by identifying the blood vessel involved

Diagnosis of Acute Ischemic Stroke vs Hemorrhagic Stroke—cont'd

Test	Purpose	Abnormal Findings
Doppler Studies		
Transthoracic echocardiogram (TTE) or transesophageal echocardiogram (TEE)	Evaluates heart structure and function	Extremely useful in detecting blood clots, masses, and tumors that are located inside the heart; determines severity of certain valve problems and helps detect infection of heart valves, atrial septal defect (ASD), or patent foramen ovale (PFO). All can lead to clot formation and emboli causing thromboembolic stroke.
Carotid Doppler or duplex	Evaluates blood flow and presence or degree of stenosis in the extracranial carotid arteries	Carotid stenosis or clot formation in the carotid artery
Transcranial Doppler	Evaluates the intracranial vessels and assesses the velocity of blood flow in the anterior and posterior cerebral circulation; also used to evaluate vasospasm, to determine brain death via detection of cerebral circulatory arrest, for intraoperative monitoring, and to locate emboli	Vasospasm, cerebral circulatory arrest, emboli
Laboratory Studies		
Hematology profile or complete blood count (CBC) with differential	Screens for anemia (may alter CBF), determines status of platelets. 2010 ICH guidelines recommend replacement of platelets as soon as possible in those with thrombocytopenia	If the number of platelets is too low, excessive bleeding can occur. If the number of platelets is too high, blood clots can form. Anemia decreases oxygens-carrying capacity and increases cerebral velocities.
Biochemical profile	Helps determine fluid and electrolyte balance	Hyponatremia, hyperosmolality, elevated or hypoglycemia
Coagulation profile	Detects hypercoagulable or hypocoagulable blood. May include levels of homocysteine, proteins C and S. Warfarin may prolong INR.	Anticoagulation proteins may be deficient in the young (<45 years) stroke patient. Deficient coagulation factors may prompt ICH.
Less Commonly Done Tests		
Lupus anticoagulant, Anticardiolipin antibody, and Hemoglobin electrophoresis	Screens for possible causes of stroke and to assess presence of sickle cell disease (Hgb electrophoresis)	Outside normal range indicating possible risk factor or cause
Syphilis (e.g., Venereal Disease Research Laboratory [VDRL], rapid plasma reagin [RPR], fluorescent treponemal antibody [FTA]); sedimentation rate	To assess for infection or vasculitis	Positive results
Drug screen (e.g., cocaine, amphetamine)	Assesses for presence of drugs which may alter level of consciousness	Positive results, indicating the patient has the drugs in the bloodstream and/or urine

Continued

Diagnosis of Acute Ischemic Stroke vs Hemorrhagic Stroke—cont'd

Test	Purpose	Abnormal Findings
Lumbar Puncture (LP)	Measures CSF pressures and obtains CSF specimen when infection, such as meningitis or neurosyphilis is suspected; may be performed when SAH is suspected and CT is normal	Elevated protein, low glucose, elevated WBC
Electroencephalogram (EEG)	Although rarely done, brain activity or seizure activity	Possible slowing or low voltage over the infarct, except in lacunar infarcts, where results are usually normal

COLLABORATIVE MANAGEMENT

AHA/ASA GUIDELINES FOR ACUTE ISCHEMIC STROKE AND HEMORRHAGIC STROKE MANAGEMENT ARE THE MOST REFERENCED PUBLICATIONS FOR SETTING THE STANDARDS OF PRACTICE

The Joint Commission (TJC) developed its program on the basis of these guidelines. Effective January 1, 2008, all organizations seeking Joint Commission Disease-Specific Care (DSC) certification for stroke must use a set of 10 standardized performance measures to meet the performance measurement requirements for certification. Detailed information on TJC's DSC stroke measure set is available in the Disease-Specific Care Certification Program stroke performance measurement implementation guide, ed 2, version 2.a., updated October 2008.

Website: http://www.jointcommission.org/CertificationPrograms/PrimaryStrokeCenters/stroke_pm_edition_2_ver_2a.htm

The TJC quality indicators for AIS are:

1. *Deep Vein Thrombosis (DVT) Prophylaxis
2. Discharged on Antithrombotics
3. Patients with Atrial Fibrillation Receive Anticoagulation Therapy
4. Thrombolytic Therapy Administered (in eligible patients)
5. Antithrombotic Therapy by End of Hospital Day Two
6. Discharged on Statin Medication
7. *Dysphagia Screening
8. *Stroke Education
9. *Smoking Cessation/Advice Counseling
10. *Assessed for Rehabilitation

The TJC quality indicators for ICH are:

1. Deep Vein Thrombosis (DVT) Prophylaxis
2. Dysphagia Screening
3. Stroke Education
4. Smoking Cessation/Advice Counseling
5. Assessed for Rehabilitation

*Indicators for both AIS and ICH.

Care Priorities

Goals of management are to prevent secondary neurologic damage and secondary complications and to promote optimal functional outcome. Early detection via accurate neurologic examination and immediate medical or surgical intervention help prevent stroke extension, increased brain edema, and hydrocephalus. Medical and nursing interventions are guided by the findings derived from the physical examination. The Joint Commission requires the following list of interventions for certified stroke centers: initiation of DVT prophylaxis, discharge on antithrombotic medications, patients with atrial fibrillation receive anticoagulation therapy, thrombolytic therapy is administered, antithrombotic therapy is begun by the end of the second hospital day, dysphagia screening is completed, stroke education is provided, smoking cessation counseling is initiated, and assessment for rehabilitation is done.

1. **Rapidly evaluate patients for type of stroke and minimize brain damage:**
Medical Therapies
- *Oxygen therapy:* Maintain oxygen saturation of at least 92% using 2 to 3 L nasal cannula oxygen. Maximizing oxygenation is of paramount importance for all stroke patients.
- *Hydration:* IV fluids (initially without dextrose), infusing at 75 mL/hour help to maintain adequate circulating blood volume.
- *For intracranial hemorrhage:* Replace platelets or coagulation factor if needed. If INR is elevated, hold warfarin and treat with vitamin K.

Acute Ischemic Stroke (AIS)
- *Thrombolysis:* Clots are "dissolved" using IV recombinant tissue plasminogen activator (rtPA). The window of treatment for *ischemic stroke* has been extended from 3 hours to 4.5 hours after onset of symptoms. Stroke centers strive to provide rtPA within one hour of arrival. Vital signs and neurologic assessments should be performed every 15 minutes during rtPA infusion. Following infusion, BP should be monitored every 30 minutes for 6 hours and then every hour for 16 hours to complete the initial 24-hour period following the stroke. Heparin, aspirin, clopidogrel, dipyridamole, or warfarin should *NOT* be given for 24 hours, after which these antithrombotic agents should be started as prescribed. Imaging with CT brain scan or MRI should be done immediately following rtPA infusion. Monitor for major and minor bleeding complications during and following the infusion. Continuous cardiac monitoring should remain in place for at least 72 hours.

HIGH ALERT! If the patient experiences profound deterioration in status during rtPA infusion, a hemorrhagic transformation may have ensued, wherein rtPA causes an ICH. *If suspected, the rtPA infusion should be discontinued immediately.* Subsequent measures include vital signs and neurological assessments every 15 minutes, and consideration of hyperventilation, mannitol infusion, administration of blood products (cryoprecipitate, FFP, platelets, factor VIIa, and PRBCs), possible initiation of hemodynamic monitoring, and further neurodiagnostic testing and laboratory studies to evaluate the potential for further bleeding.

Antithrombotic Therapy: Antithrombotics should be ordered within the first 24 hours of admission for those who are ineligible for thrombolysis. Continuous cardiac monitoring should be provided for up to 48 hours for patients ineligible for thrombolysis.
- *Anticoagulation:* IV heparin may be indicated for patients with progressing stroke or unstable signs and symptoms of stroke such as TIAs and for cardioembolic stroke. If long-term anticoagulation is planned, the patient is converted to oral warfarin (Coumadin) therapy. Newer anticoagulants, including direct thrombin inhibitors, may be used.
- *Antiplatelet therapy:* Used to reduce risk of stroke and decrease frequency of TIAs. Aspirin (30 to 1300 mg/day dosage range) is the most common agent, usually given 75 to 325 mg four times daily. *Aspirin/ extended-release dipyridamole 25/200 mg* (Aggrenox) is given twice daily and has the best stroke risk reduction, but 40% of patients who take it have headaches. However, the dose may be titrated to reduce this side effect. *Ticlopidine* (Ticlid) reduces the overall risk for fatal and nonfatal strokes by nearly 25% when compared with aspirin but is now rarely used due to the side effects. *Clopidogrel* (Plavix) is the most common drug used for patients at risk for ischemic events (myocardial, cerebrovascular, peripheral vascular). Plavix 75 mg four times daily to total 300 mg may be given as a loading dose followed by 75 mg daily for first-line therapy with or without aspirin or as a second-line therapy when aspirin has failed.

Interventional approaches for AIS
- *Intra-arterial (IA) thrombolysis using rtPA* has a 6-hour window in which to implement the therapy directly into the cerebral vasculature. This approach is much more successful with large-vessel strokes than with small-vessel strokes.
- *Mechanical disruption* of the clot is faster with intra-arterial rtPA. Two devices currently being used are the Merci catheter (8-hour window to implement) and the penumbra system. The Merci is a "corkscrew" catheter that is embedded in the clot; then the catheter is pulled back to remove the clot. The penumbra is a suction device that breaks down and sucks the

clot back through the catheter. Both have a good result of establishing TIMI flow in the cerebral vessel. There are no comparison studies to indicate which interventional approach is superior. Both devices may dislodge and migrate distally.

- *Carotid stenting:* Stents may be used for carotid stenosis, and this is currently done in the United States under a registry protocol. Patients who meet criteria include those who are not surgical candidates and are symptomatic from their carotid stenosis.

Endovascular Surgery: **Interventional approaches for ICH** (see July 22, 2010 AHA/ASA Spontonecus ICH guidelines)

- Patients may have an AVM or AVF as an underlying cause for hemorrhage. These lesions are embolized as a single therapy or as adjunctive therapy prior to surgical removal of the vascular anomaly or use of radiosurgery. Embolization may be achieved using either a polymer or "glue," or Guglielmi Detachable Coils (GDC coils) are placed to occlude the malformation (see *Cerebral Aneurysm and Subarachnoid Hemorrhage*, p. 629).

2. **Manage hypertension and stabilize vital signs:** Antihypertensives are frequently used in the stroke population to control hypertension. BP should be controlled prior to initiating a reperfusion strategy. Frequency of BP measurements should be increased to at least every 15 minutes if SBP remains greater than 180 mm Hg or DBP is greater than 105 mm Hg during and following the therapy. For long-term management, antihypertensive agents are selected based on the individual's medical history. Those belonging to ethnic groups with higher risk of stroke may receive more aggressive therapy. Long-term therapy may be prescribed based on the National Heart, Lung, and Blood Institute (NHLBI) algorithm (Table 7-7). Systolic BP is often elevated in the acute phase and requires vasoactive IV medications such as sodium nitroprusside (Nipride) or labetalol (Normodyne). Nicardipine (Cardene IV) is the NINDS recommendation for managing hypertension in AIS. Hypotension is a concern, especially in the patient with ICP, because MAP is decreased. If MAP is decreased in the presence of a normal or elevated ICP, a decrease in CPP results, further compromising neurologic status. Vasopressors and/or inotropes may be titrated to keep MAP high enough to maintain CPP greater than 60 mm Hg.

Intracranial Hemorrhage (ICH): The American Heart Association and American Stroke Association (AHA/ASA) recommend the following for management of BP in patients with ICH/acute cerebral hemorrhage:

- If the SBP is greater than 200 mm Hg or MAP is greater than 150 mm Hg, aggressive BP reduction should be considered.
- If SBP is greater than 180 mm Hg or MAP is greater than 130 mm Hg with possibly elevated ICP, reduction of BP with concurrent ICP monitoring should be considered to assist in keeping CPP at 60 to 80 mm Hg.
- If SBP is greater than 180 mm Hg or MAP is greater than 130 mm Hg and there is no suspicion of increased ICP, reduction of MAP to 110 mm Hg or 160/90 (a moderate reduction) should be considered.

Acute Ischemic Stroke (AIS)

- *Patients eligible for a reperfusion strategy* (including tPA) with SBP of greater than 185 mm Hg or DBP greater than 110 mm Hg should have the blood pressure reduced to less than 185 mm Hg and DBP to less than 110 mm Hg prior to beginning the reperfusion strategy. TPA is contraindicated if the BP cannot be reduced to these parameters. For at least 24 hours after reperfusion, SBP for those who were initially hypertensive should be maintained at less than 180 mm Hg with DBP less than 105mm Hg. The physician or midlevel practitioner should be notified of an SBP greater than 185 mm Hg or less than 110 mm Hg, DBP greater than 105 mm Hg or less than 60 mm Hg, HR less than 50 bpm or greater than 110 bpm, RR greater than 24 breaths/min, temperature greater than 99.6°F, or a deterioration in neurologic status.
- *Patients who have concomitant medical problems that require management of hypertension* should be provided with aggressive BP reduction.
- *Patients who are not eligible for thrombolytic therapy* should have BP reduced by 15% within the first 24 hours following the stroke, or SBP reduced to less than 220 mm Hg, with DBP reduced to less than 120 mm Hg. The physician or midlevel practitioner should be called if the SBP is greater than 220 mm Hg or less than 110 mm Hg, the DBP is greater than 120 mm Hg or less than 60 mm Hg, HR is less than 50 bpm or greater than 110 bpm, RR is greater than 24 breaths/min, temperature is greater than 99.6°F, or if there is a deterioration in neurologic status.

Table 7-7   CLASSIFICATION AND MANAGEMENT OF BLOOD PRESSURE FOR ADULTS*

BP Classification	SBP,* mm hg	DBP,* mm hg	Lifestyle Modification	Initial Drug Therapy	
				Without Compelling Indication	With Compelling Indications
Normal	<120	and <80	Encourage	No antihypertensive drug indicated	Drug(s) for compelling indication‡
Prehypertension	120 to 139	or 80 to 89	Yes	Thiazide-type diuretics for most; May consider ACEI, ARB, BB, CCB, or combination	Drug(s) for the compelling indications‡; Other antihypertensive drugs (diuretics, ACEI, ARB, BB, CCB) as needed
Stage 1 hypertension	140 to 159	or 90 to 99	Yes		
Stage 2 hypertension	≥160	or ≥100	Yes	Two-drug combination for most† (usually thiazide-type diuretic and ACEI, ARB, BB, or CCB)	

Seventh Report of the Joint National Committee on Prevention, Detection, Evaluation, and Treatment of High Blood Pressure (JNC 7). Bethesda, MD, 2003. National High Blood Pressure Education Program; National Heart, Lung, and Blood Institute; U.S. Department of Health and Human Services, National Institutes of Health. NIH Publication No 03-5231.

*Treatment determined by highest BP category.

†Initial combined therapy should be used cautiously in those at risk for orthostatic hypotension.

‡Treat patients with chronic kidney disease or diabetes to BP goal of 130/80 mm Hg.

ACEI, angiotensin-converting enzyme inhibitor; ARB, angiotensin receptor blocker; BB, beta-blocker; BP, blood pressure; CCB, calcium channel blocker; DBP, diastolic blood pressure; SBP, systolic blood pressure.

- Hypotensive patients should be evaluated and treated for the cause of low BP, including hypovolemia and dysrhythmias. Vasopressors may be used if absolutely necessary to raise BP to improve cerebral blood flow.

3. **Monitor ICP and manage CPP:** CPP = MAP − ICP (keep CPP greater than 60 mm Hg). Invasive monitoring may be necessary for patients with increased infarct size, increased edema, and hydrocephalus. Patients with increased ICP may receive mannitol, which lowers ICP by reducing water within brain cells. Careful monitoring of ICP for rebound effect is necessary after mannitol infusion. Patients should remain on bedrest until stabilized. Serum osmolality should be assessed to prevent excessive dehydration. Patients with hydrocephalus often require a ventriculostomy. For more information about ICP monitoring and CPP management, see *Traumatic Brain Injury*, p. 331.
   - *Invasive monitoring:* Assessment and maintenance of neurologic monitors is an essential part of the neurologic assessment.
   - *ICP monitoring:* Ensure an adequate wave form, zero balance equipment, and patency of tubing (if applicable), and maintain sterility of system. Increased ICP is due to extension of the infarct or hematoma and its associated edema. May cause midline shift and herniation; increased ICP is associated with hydrocephalus after ICH; seizures generally occur within the first 24 hours but may present at any time
   - *Extraventricular drainage (EVD):* Maintain sterility of system and proper positioning for drainage. Maintain patency. Observe/document color consistency and amount of CSF.

4. **Prevent stroke extension:** The opportunity to prevent further stroke depends on adequate perfusion of the penumbra, which is the ischemic brain tissue surrounding the initial infarct that is at immediate risk of infarction. Perfusing the penumbra decreases the potential infarct size and optimizes patient outcome. Controlling arterial BP is essential in limiting the infarct size. Close monitoring and use of potent vasoactive medications achieve BP control. A "normal" BP may be too low, causing further ischemia and infarct by decreasing cerebral perfusion. Arterial BP should not be lowered abruptly in patients with AIS. At times, maintenance of a somewhat elevated BP may be warranted, depending on the underlying vascular and brain pathology. In contrast, with ICH many practitioners believe that an elevated BP should be reduced aggressively. The best approach is unclear, and therefore the treatment of increased BP in ICH requires individual consideration (Table 7-7).

   Choose evidence-based tools for monitoring neurologic changes:
   - *NIH Stroke Scale (NIHSS)* (Table 7-8): Provides a better measurement of deficits and is easy to use. It also guides the examiner in evaluating cognitive, language, and motor deficits that are unique to stroke. A comprehensive neurologic assessment assists the critical care nurse in detecting changes in neurologic status and the response to interventions.
   - *Glasgow Coma Scale (GCS)* (see Appendix 2): Used to measure changes in level of consciousness in those who cannot participate in NIHSS.

Table 7-8	**NATIONAL INSTITUTES OF HEALTH STROKE SCALE (NIHSS)**

Patient Identification __ __.__ __ __.__ __ __
Pt. Date of Birth __ __/__ __/__ __
Hospital _____ (__ __.__ __)
Date of Exam __ __/__ __/__ __

Interval: [ ] Baseline   [ ] 2 hours post treatment [ ] 24 hours post onset of symptoms ±20 minutes
[ ] 7–10 days [ ] 3 months [ ] Other _____(____ ____)
Time: ____ ____:____ ____ [ ] am [ ] pm
Person Administering Scale _____

Administer stroke scale items in the order listed. Record performance in each category after each subscale exam. Do not go back and change scores. Follow directions provided for each exam technique. Scores should reflect what the patient does, not what the clinician thinks the patient can do. The clinician should record answers while administering the exam and work quickly. Except where indicated, the patient should not be coached (i.e., repeated requests to patient to make a special effort).

Table 7-8	NATIONAL INSTITUTES OF HEALTH STROKE SCALE (NIHSS)—cont'd	
Instructions	**Scale Definition**	**Score**
1a. Level of Consciousness: The investigator must choose a response if a full evaluation is prevented by such obstacles as an endotracheal tube, language barrier, orotracheal trauma/bandages. A 3 is scored only if the patient makes no movement (other than reflexive posturing) in response to noxious stimulation.	0 = **Alert**; keenly responsive. 1 = **Not alert**; but arousable by minor stimulation to obey, answer, or respond. 2 = **Not alert**; requires repeated stimulation to attend, or is obtunded and requires strong or painful stimulation to make movements (not stereotyped). 3 = **Responds** only with reflex motor or autonomic effects or totally unresponsive, flaccid, and flexic.	_____
1b. LOC Questions: The patient is asked the month and his/her age. The answer must be correct—there is no partial credit for being close. Aphasic and stuporous patients who do not comprehend the questions will score 2. Patients unable to speak because of endotracheal intubation, orotracheal trauma, severe dysarthria from any cause, language barrier, or any other problem not secondary to aphasia are given a 1. It is important that only the initial answer be graded and that the examiner not "help" the patient with verbal or non-verbal cues.	0 = **Answers** both questions correctly. 1 = **Answers** one question correctly. 2 = **Answers** neither question correctly.	_____
1c. LOC Commands: The patient is asked to open and close the eyes and then to grip and release the non-paretic hand. Substitute another one-step command if the hands cannot be used. Credit is given if an unequivocal attempt is made but not completed due to weakness. If the patient does not respond to command, the task should be demonstrated to him or her (pantomime), and the result scored (i.e., follows none, one or two commands). Patients with trauma, amputation, or other physical impediments should be given suitable one-step commands. Only the first attempt is scored.	0 = **Performs** both tasks correctly. 1 = **Performs** one task correctly. 2 = **Performs** neither task correctly.	_____
2. Best Gaze: Only horizontal eye movements will be tested. Voluntary or reflexive (oculocephalic) eye movements will be scored, but caloric testing is not done. If the patient has a conjugate deviation of the eyes that can be overcome by voluntary or reflexive activity, the score will be 1. If a patient has an isolated peripheral nerve paresis (CN III, IV, or VI), score a 1. Gaze is testable in all aphasic patients. Patients with ocular trauma, bandages, pre-existing blindness, or other disorder of visual acuity or fields should be tested with reflexive movements, and a choice made by the investigator. Establishing eye contact and then moving about the patient from side to side will occasionally clarify the presence of a partial gaze palsy.	0 = **Normal.** 1 = **Partial gaze palsy;** gaze is abnormal in one or both eyes, but forced deviation or total gaze paresis is not present. 2 = **Forced deviation,** or total gaze paresis not overcome by the oculocephalic maneuver.	_____

Continued

Table 7-8   NATIONAL INSTITUTES OF HEALTH STROKE SCALE (NIHSS)—cont'd

3. **Visual:** Visual fields (upper and lower quadrants) are tested by confrontation, using finger counting or visual threat, as appropriate. Patients may be encouraged, but if they look at the side of the moving fingers appropriately, this can be scored as normal. If there is unilateral blindness or enucleation, visual fields in the remaining eye are scored. Score 1 only if a clear-cut asymmetry, including quadrantanopia, is found. If patient is blind from any cause, score 3. Double simultaneous stimulation is performed at this point. If there is extinction, patient receives a 1, and the results are used to respond to item 11.	0 = **No visual loss.** 1 = **Partial hemianopia.** 2 = **Complete hemianopia.** 3 = **Bilateral hemianopia** (blind including cortical blindness).
4. **Facial Palsy:** Ask or use pantomime to encourage the patient to show teeth or raise eyebrows and close eyes. Score symmetry of grimace in response to noxious stimuli in the poorly responsive or noncomprehending patient. If facial trauma/bandages, orotracheal tube, tape, or other physical barriers obscure the face, these should be removed to the extent possible.	0 = **Normal** symmetrical movements. 1 = **Minor paralysis** (flattened nasolabial fold, asymmetry on smiling). 2 = **Partial paralysis** (total or near-total paralysis of lower face). 3 = **Complete paralysis** of one or both sides (absence of facial movement in the upper and lower face).
5. **Motor Arm:** The limb is placed in the appropriate position: extend the arms (palms down) 90 degrees (if sitting) or 45 degrees (if supine). Drift is scored if the arm falls before 10 seconds. The aphasic patient is encouraged using urgency in the voice and pantomime, but not noxious stimulation. Each limb is tested in turn, beginning with the non-paretic arm. Only in the case of amputation or joint fusion at the shoulder, the examiner should record the score as untestable (UN), and clearly write the explanation for this choice.	0 = **No drift;** limb holds 90 (or 45) degrees for full 10 seconds. 1 = **Drift;** limb holds 90 (or 45) degrees, but drifts down before full 10 seconds; does not hit bed or other support. 2 = **Some effort against gravity;** limb cannot get to or maintain (if cued) 90 (or 45) degrees, drifts down to bed, but has some effort against gravity. 3 = **No effort against gravity;** limb falls. 4 = **No movement.** UN = **Amputation** or joint fusion, explain: _____ **5a. Left Arm** **5b. Right Arm**
6. **Motor Leg:** The limb is placed in the appropriate position: hold the leg at 30 degrees (always tested supine). Drift is scored if the leg falls before 5 seconds. The aphasic patient is encouraged using urgency in the voice and pantomime, but not noxious stimulation. Each limb is tested in turn, beginning with the non-paretic leg. Only in the case of amputation or joint fusion at the hip, the examiner should record the score as untestable (UN), and clearly write the explanation for this choice.	0 = **No drift;** leg holds 30-degree position for full 5 seconds. 1 = **Drift;** leg falls by the end of the 5-second period but does not hit bed. 2 = **Some effort against gravity;** leg falls to bed by 5 seconds, but has some effort against gravity. 3 = **No effort against gravity;** leg falls to bed immediately. 4 = **No movement.** UN = **Amputation** or joint fusion, explain: _____ **6a. Left Leg** **6b. Right Leg**

Table 7-8	NATIONAL INSTITUTES OF HEALTH STROKE SCALE (NIHSS) — cont'd

7. Limb Ataxia: This item is aimed at finding evidence of a unilateral cerebellar lesion. Test with eyes open. In case of visual defect, ensure testing is done in intact visual field. The finger-nose-finger and heel-shin tests are performed on both sides, and ataxia is scored only if present out of proportion to weakness. Ataxia is absent in the patient who cannot understand or is paralyzed. Only in the case of amputation or joint fusion, the examiner should record the score as untestable (UN), and clearly write the explanation for this choice. In case of blindness, test by having the patient touch nose from extended arm position.	0 = **Absent.** 1 = **Present in one limb.** 2 = **Present in two limbs.** UN = **Amputation** or joint fusion, explain: _____
8. Sensory: Sensation or grimace to pinprick when tested, or withdrawal from noxious stimulus in the obtunded or aphasic patient. Only sensory loss attributed to stroke is scored as abnormal, and the examiner should test as many body areas (arms [not hands], legs, trunk, face) as needed to accurately check for hemisensory loss. A score of 2, "severe or total sensory loss," should only be given when a severe or total loss of sensation can be clearly demonstrated. Stuporous and aphasic patients will, therefore, probably score 1 or 0. The patient with brainstem stroke who has bilateral loss of sensation is scored 2. If the patient does not respond and is quadriplegic, score 2. Patients in a coma (item 1a = 3) are automatically given a 2 on this item.	0 = **Normal;** no sensory loss. 1 = **Mild-to-moderate sensory loss;** patient feels pinprick is less sharp or is dull on the affected side; or there is a loss of superficial pain with pinprick, but patient is aware of being touched. 2 = **Severe-to-total sensory loss;** patient is not aware of being touched in the face, arm, and leg.
9. Best Language: A great deal of information about comprehension will be obtained during the preceding sections of the examination. For this scale item, the patient is asked to describe what is happening in the attached picture, to name the items on the attached naming sheet, and to read from the attached list of sentences. Comprehension is judged from responses here, as well as to all of the commands in the preceding general neurological exam. If visual loss interferes with the tests, ask the patient to identify objects placed in the hand, repeat, and produce speech. The intubated patient should be asked to write. The patient in a coma (item 1a=3) will automatically score 3 on this item. The examiner must choose a score for the patient with stupor or limited cooperation, but a score of 3 should be used only if the patient is mute and follows no one-step commands.	0 = **No aphasia;** normal. 1 = **Mild-to-moderate aphasia;** some obvious loss of fluency or facility of comprehension, without significant limitation on ideas expressed or form of expression. Reduction of speech and/or comprehension, however, makes conversation about provided materials difficult or impossible. For example, in conversation about provided materials, examiner can identify picture or naming card content from patient's response. 2 = **Severe aphasia;** all communication is through fragmentary expression; great need for inference, questioning, and guessing by the listener. Range of information that can be exchanged is limited; listener carries burden of communication. Examiner cannot identify materials provided from patient response. 3 = **Mute, global aphasia;** no usable speech or auditory comprehension.

Continued

Table 7-8	NATIONAL INSTITUTES OF HEALTH STROKE SCALE (NIHSS) — cont'd	
10. **Dysarthria:** If patient is thought to be normal, an adequate sample of speech must be obtained by asking patient to read or repeat words from the attached list. If the patient has severe aphasia, the clarity of articulation of spontaneous speech can be rated. Only if the patient is intubated or has other physical barriers to producing speech, the examiner should record the score as untestable (UN), and clearly write an explanation for this choice. Do not tell the patient why he or she is being tested.	0 = **Normal.** 1 = **Mild-to-moderate dysarthria;** patient slurs at least some words and, at worst, can be understood with some difficulty. 2 = **Severe dysarthria;** patient's speech is so slurred as to be unintelligible in the absence of or out of proportion to any dysphasia, or is mute/anarthric. UN = **Intubated** or other physical barrier, explain:	
11. **Extinction and Inattention (formerly Neglect):** Sufficient information to identify neglect may be obtained during the prior testing. If the patient has a severe visual loss preventing visual double simultaneous stimulation, and the cutaneous stimuli are normal, the score is normal. If the patient has aphasia but does appear to attend to both sides, the score is normal. The presence of visual spatial neglect or anosagnosia may also be taken as evidence of abnormality. Since the abnormality is scored only if present, the item is never untestable.	0 = **No abnormality.** 1 = **Visual, tactile, auditory, spatial, or personal inattention** or extinction to bilateral simultaneous stimulation in one of the sensory modalities. 2 = **Profound hemi-inattention or extinction to more than one modality;** does not recognize own hand or orients to only one side of space.	_____

5. **Prevention of recurrent stroke:**
   - Reduction of BP using antihypertensive medications is recommended for prevention of stroke and other vascular problems. BP should be monitored every 15 minutes initially, then every 30 minutes for 6 hours, and then every hour for 16 hours to complete the initial 24-hour period following the stroke. For those with AIS, treatment is begun following the initial or hyperacute stroke period.
   - Target BP should be individualized to each patient. Patients with moderate hypertension may benefit from a drop of 10 mm Hg systolic and 5 mm Hg diastolic.
   - Lifestyle changes should be part of all stroke prevention programs.
   - The JNC-7 (or when available, the JNC-8) report should be used to guide the choice of antihypertensive medications. Ideal choices remain uncertain. A diuretic coupled with an angiotensin-converting enzyme (ACE) inhibitor is acceptable. For some patients, the choice of a specific class of antihypertensive medication is clearer (see Table 7-7).
6. **Manage agitation.**

Safety Alert Use of Sedation
A thorough neurologic evaluation to rule out organic causes of agitation is indicated. Sedation may be used as adjunctive therapy for patients with increased ICP to reduce the risk of extending the stroke, which in the worst case scenario, may result in permanent loss of ability to interact with the environment or death. Benzodiazepines, fentanyl (Sublimaze), or morphine sulfate are effective. Propofol (Diprivan) is a short-acting, IV hypnotic agent that is also cautiously used for sedation. Pentobarbital coma is occasionally used for patients who experience high ICP that does not respond to other forms of therapy. (See Sedation and Neuromuscular Blockade, p. 158.)

7. **Optimize regulatory functions:** To prevent secondary complications, see *Summary* (Table 7-9). In general, patients with stroke need adequate cerebral blood flow and perfusion with adequate glucose and oxygenation. Nursing interventions help facilitate optimal cerebral perfusion.

Table 7-9	**MAINTENANCE OF NORMAL REGULATORY FUNCTIONS IN STROKE**	
Function	**Goal/Rationale**	**Intervention(s)**
Optimal body position	*Facilitate cerebral blood flow:* An ideal position has not been determined. Patient response determines the best position. Arterial perfusion improves with head down, while venous drainage improves with head elevated.	Keep HOB elevated 25–30°. Lower HOB to flat to increase cerebral perfusion. HOB should be elevated to decrease ICP in patients with hemorrhagic strokes. Keep neck neutral; avoid bending at the waist.
Temperature	*Maintain normothermia:* Decreases metabolic demands and ICP	Temperature greater than 99.6°F should be treated with acetaminophen.
Breathing and patent airway	*Maximize oxygenation:* Optimizes O_2 delivery to the brain, prevents atelectasis and pneumonia; Reducing intrathoracic and intra-abdominal pressures helps to prevent increased ICP; Pt may be unable to protect his or her airway, resulting in aspiration of secretions.	Administer O_2, individualize positioning, pulmonary toilet; Suctioning: No longer than 10 seconds in duration; preoxygenate with 100% for full 2 minutes between each attempt; his or her do not provide overly aggressive manual ventilation when suctioning.
Circulation	*Control dysrhythmias and promote electrolyte balance:* Normal sinus rhythm optimizes CO to promote perfusion to the brain; Hemorrhagic strokes are more likely to cause dysrhythmias. *Promote hydration:* Helps maintain normal circulating blood volume	Monitor dysrhythmias for at least 24 hours; Cardiac monitoring should be continued for 72 hours if thrombolytics were used. Manage fluid and electrolyte imbalances. Administer IV fluids at 75ml/hour during the first 1 to 3 days, depending on patient's initial hydration status.
Digestion and bowel elimination	*Prevent aspiration pneumonia:* Swallowing dysfunction may be present. *Reduce incidence of stress ulcers and constipation:* Straining with bowel movements increases ICP.	NPO until ability to swallow has been evaluated within the 24 hours of hospitalization. Bedside swallow may precede modified barium swallow. Initiate H_2 blockers and a bowel program.
Cellular glucose supply	*Maintain a normal blood glucose level:* Optimizes brain cell function by ensuring adequate intracellular supply of glucose	Aggressively manage blood glucose to control hyperglycemia and prevent/treat hypoglycemia; Avoid glucose-containing IV solutions in the Emergency Dept.
Nourishment	*Maintain an anabolic state; prevent catabolism:* Promote optimal healing opportunity and prevent recurrent stroke by controlling CVD/ASHD risk factors.	Initiate nutrition ASAP; enteral feeding, then long-term diet to meet caloric needs; low-Na+, low-fat, weight reduction if needed
Urinary continence	*Prevent urinary tract infection and skin breakdown:* Removal of foley catheter may prompt skin breakdown if patient is incontinent.	Prevent unnecessary use of urinary foley catheter; remove within 48 hours if possible; bladder training ASAP
Mobility and endurance	*Promote proper body alignment and muscle strengthening:* Prevents contractures, DVT, and complications of immobility	Perform ROM exercises, regular repositioning; Increase activity as tolerated; Use mobility beds if needed. Initiate DVT prophylaxis.
Skin integrity	*Prevent skin breakdown and dependent edema*	Keep skin clean and dry; Use pressure relief surfaces.

Continued

Table 7-9	MAINTENANCE OF NORMAL REGULATORY FUNCTIONS IN STROKE—cont'd	
Function	Goal/Rationale	Intervention(s)
Communication	Develop appropriate communication techniques; Promotes sense of well-being and facilitates more timely response to patient needs when requests are understood	Provide pictorial board so patient can point at needs, ask yes and no questions which do not require long answers, provide pencil and paper for those who can write; Ensure glasses and hearing aides are in place for those who use them.

CO, cardiac output; *GI*, gastrointestinal; *GU*, genitourinary; *ICP*, intracranial pressure; Na^+, sodium; *NPO*, nothing by mouth; O_2, oxygen; *ROM*, range of motion; *UTI*, urinary tract infection; *DVT*, deep vein thrombosis.

8. **Provide rehabilitation:** Should begin immediately once stabilized. Consults to physiatrist, physical therapist, occupational therapist, and speech therapist should be made within the first 24 hours. Death within the first month after stroke is commonly caused by myocardial infarction (MI), pneumonia, and sepsis, which can result from inactivity. Pulmonary embolism, deep vein thrombosis, skin breakdown, and depression are also common.

9. **Manage seizures:** Anticonvulsant therapy is used for seizures in the acute phase. Generally the patient is given a loading dose of phenytoin (Dilantin) or fosphenytoin (Cerebyx), followed by a maintenance dose. Benzodiazepines (e.g., Ativan) may be used initially. Phenobarbital may be used if the patient is in SE. Temperature greater than 99.6°F should be treated with acetaminophen.

10. **Surgical management:**
    - *Carotid endarterectomy:* Carotid endarterectomies, surgical removal of plaque in the obstructed carotid artery to promote blood supply to the brain, may be performed immediately following stroke. Considered treatment of choice for patients with greater than 70% carotid stenosis.
    - *Craniotomy:* Often young patients with AIS need to be watched carefully for signs of increased ICP and pending herniation due to the lack of space in the cranium. A craniotomy with a dural incision or temporal lobectomy may be considered as a preventative measure. Hematoma evacuation may be performed by aspiration through a burr hole or clot evacuation by craniotomy for patients who have expanding clot or uncontrolled ICP, edema, or mass effect.

NURSING CARE PLANS: AIS AND ICH

Decreased intracranial adaptive capacity *related to interrupted blood flow secondary to thrombus or embolus*

GOALS/OUTCOMES Within 72 hours of diagnosis, patient has adequate cerebral tissue perfusion, as evidenced by no decrease in LOC; no deterioration in motor function on affected side; and no new or further deterioration of language, cognition, or visual field per NIHSS (see Table 7-8).
NOC Neurological Status

Neurologic Monitoring
1. Assess for neurologic changes hourly in the acute phase. Use NIHSS to record and monitor neurologic changes after stroke.
2. Maintain ICP less than 15 mm Hg and CPP greater than 60 mm Hg: CPP = MAP − ICP.
3. Position patient to maintain adequate cerebral perfusion. Keep HOB at 25–30° or less as tolerated for patients with ischemic stroke. Keep HOB raised at 30 degrees as tolerated for patients with hemorrhagic stroke. Avoid extreme hip flexion. When positioning, monitor tolerance to position change.
4. Maintain Spo₂ of at least 92%. Consider ICP effects of respiratory care. Suction only if needed. Assess breath sounds frequently. Avoid activities that can increase ICP (e.g., excessive coughing). Avoid hypercapnia and hypoxia.

5. Maintain adequate SBP. Higher pressures (140 to 180 mm Hg) may be necessary to perfuse an area of brain at risk of infarction if ischemia is present. For patients with hemorrhagic stroke, maintain adequate BP. Use vasodilators or vasopressors as necessary to optimize BP and maintain CPP at greater than 60 mm Hg for all stroke patients. For AIS patients, lower HOB to flat to promote cerebral perfusion.
6. Notify the physician or midlevel practitioner of deterioration in neurological status or the vital sign changes as described in *Collaborative Management*.
7. Use sedation as prescribed and monitor response: effects of sedation and changes in ICP.

NIC Cerebral Perfusion Promotion; Positioning: Neurologic; Neurologic Monitoring

---

Impaired physical mobility *related to decreased motor function of upper and/or lower extremities and trunk after stroke*

GOALS/OUTCOMES At time of discharge from ICU, patient has no complications of immobility such as skin breakdown, contracture formation, pneumonia, or constipation.
NOC Mobility Level

Exercise Promotion: Strength Training
1. Turn and position frequently as tolerated. Transfer toward unaffected side.
2. Teach methods for turning and moving using stronger extremity to move weaker extremity.
3. Position weaker extremities to avoid contracture formation, frozen shoulder, or foot drop.
4. Begin passive ROM within 24 hours of admission. Modify exercises if BP or ICP increases.
5. Obtain PT and OT referrals as soon as possible to establish appropriate therapy.
6. Have patient cough and breathe deeply as tolerated at scheduled intervals.

NIC Positioning; Exercise Therapy: Joint Mobility; Self-Care Assistance

---

Impaired verbal communication *related to aphasia secondary to cerebrovascular insult*

GOALS/OUTCOMES At a minimum of 24 hours before discharge from ICU, patient demonstrates improved self-expression and relates decrease in frustration with communication.
NOC Communication Ability

Communication Enhancement: Speech Deficit
1. Evaluate for aphasia: partial or complete inability to use or comprehend language and symbols. Assess nature and severity of aphasia: ability to point to and name specific objects, follow simple directions, understand "yes/no" and complex questions, repeat simple and complex words and sentences, relate purpose or action of the objects, fulfill written request, write request, and read. May occur with dominant (left) hemisphere damage.
   - *Receptive aphasia* (e.g., Wernicke, sensory): inability to comprehend spoken words. Patient may respond to nonverbal cues.
   - *Expressive aphasia* (e.g., Broca, motor): difficulty expressing words or naming objects. Gesture, groans, swearing, or nonsense words may be helpful. Use of a picture or word board may be helpful.
2. Assess for dysarthria, which signals risk for aspiration resulting from ineffective swallowing and gag reflexes. Consult with speech therapist to assess ways to promote independence and facilitate swallowing.
3. Decrease environmental distractions, such as television or others' conversations. Fatigue affects ability to communicate; plan adequate sleep/rest.
4. Communicate frequently as follows: face patient, establish eye contact, speak slowly and clearly, give patient time to process information and give answer, keep messages short and simple, stay with one clearly defined subject, avoid questions with multiple choices, and instead phrase questions that can be answered "yes" or "no," and use the same words each time when repeating a statement or question. If patient does not understand after repetition, try different words. Use gesture, facial expressions, and pantomime to supplement and reinforce message.
5. Help patients regain use of symbolic language: start with nouns and progress to more complex statements. Keep a record at the bedside of words to be used (e.g., "pill" rather than "medication"). Treat patient as an adult. Do not speak louder unless patient is hard of hearing. Be respectful.
6. Facilitate verbal expression and naming objects: encourage patient to repeat words after you say them to practice verbal expression. Expect labile emotions, because patients are frustrated and emotional about impaired

speech. Patients who cannot monitor their speech may not speak sensible language but may think they are making sense.

7. Avoid labeling patient "belligerent" or "confused" when the problem is aphasia and frustration. Patients with nondominant (right) hemisphere damage may speak well, but may give overly detailed information, or get off on tangents. Redirect by saying, "Let's go back to what we were talking about."

8. Ensure that call light is available and patient knows how to use it. If patient is unable to use call light, check frequently and anticipate needs to ensure safety and trust.

NIC Communication Enhancement: Speech, Visual, Hearing Deficits; Active Listening: Anxiety Reduction; Touch

ADDITIONAL NURSING DIAGNOSES

See care of the patient after *Intracranial Surgery* (p. 638), *Cerebral Aneurysm and Subarachnoid Hemorrhage* (p. 629), *Risk for Trauma (Oral and Musculoskeletal)* in *Status Epilepticus* (p. 672), *Traumatic Brain Injury* (p. 331), *Prolonged Immobility* (p. 149).

SELECTED REFERENCES

Adams HP Jr, del Zoppo G, Alberts MJ, et al: Guidelines for the early management of adults with ischemic stroke: a guideline from the American Heart Association/American Stroke Association Stroke Council, Clinical Cardiology Council, Cardiovascular Radiology and Intervention Council, and the Atherosclerotic Peripheral Vascular Disease and Quality of Care Outcomes in Research Interdisciplinary Working Groups: the American Academy of Neurology affirms the value of this guideline as an educational tool for neurologists [published corrections appear in *Stroke* 38:e38, 2007, and 38:e96, 2007]. *Stroke* 38:1655–1711, 2007.

Albers GW, Amarenco P, Easton JD, et al: Antithrombotic and thrombolytic therapy for ischemic stroke: American College of Chest Physicians Evidence Based Guidelines (8th ed). *Chest* 133(6) suppl: 630S-669S, June 2008.

Alshekhlee A, Miles JD, Katirji B, et al: Incidence and mortality rates of myasthenia gravis and myasthenic crisis in US hospitals. *Neurology* 72:1548, 2009.

American Academy of Neurology: Practice parameters: determining brain death in adults (Summary Statement). Report of the Quality Standards Subcommittee of the American Academy of Neurology. *Neurology* 45:1012–1014, 1995. http://www.aan.com/professionals/practice/guidelines/pda/Brain_death_adults.pdf

Arif H, Hirsch LJ: Treatment of status epilepticus. *Semin Neurol* 28(3):342–354, 2008.

Australasian Transplant Coordinators Association Inc: *National guidelines for organ and tissue donation*, ed 3. 2006. http://www.atca.org.au/files/ATCAguidelinesonlineoct06.pdf

Barker FG II: Efficacy of prophylactic antibiotics against meningitis after craniotomy: a meta-analysis. *Neurosurgery* 60:887–894, 2007.

Bartholomew LK, Cushman WC, Cutler JA, et al: Getting clinical trial results into practice: design, implementation, and process evaluation of the ALLHAT Dissemination Project. *Clin Trials* 6(4):329–343, 2009.

Beckham JD, Tyler KL: Initial management of acute bacterial meningitis in adults: summary of ISDA guidelines. *Rev Neurol Dis* 3(2): 57–60, 2006 Spring.

Bederson JB, Connolly ES Jr, Batjer HH, et al: Guidelines for the management of aneurysmal subarachnoid hemorrhage: a statement for healthcare professionals from a special writing group of the Stroke Council, American Heart Association. *Stroke* 40: 994–1025, 2009.

Bleck TP: Intensive care unit management of patients with status epilepticus. *Epilepsia* 48(suppl 8): 59–60, 2007.

Carter BL, Rogers M, Daly J, et al: The potency of team-based care interventions for hypertension: a meta-analysis. *Arch Intern Med* 169(19):1748–1755, 2009.

Chaudhuri A, Martinez-Martin P, Kennedy PG, et al; EFNS Task Force: EFNS guideline on the management of community-acquired bacterial meningitis: report of an EFNS Task Force on acute bacterial meningitis in older children and adults. *Eur J Neurol* 15(7):649–659, 2008.

Chobanian V: Impact of nonadherence to antihypertensive therapy. *Circulation* 120(16):1558–1560, 2009.

Choi EK, Fredl and V, Zachodni C, et al: Brain death revisited: the case for a national standard. *J Law Med Ethics* 36(4):824–836, 2008.

Claassen J, Hirsch LJ, Emerson RG, et al: Treatment of refractory status epilepticus with pentobarbital, propofol, or midazolam: a systematic review. *Epilepsia* 43(2):146–153, 2002.

Claassen J, Lokin JK, Fitzsimmons BF, et al: Predictors of functional disability and mortality after status epilepticus. *Neurology* 58:139–142, 2002.

Cummings B, Noviski N, Moreland MP, et al: Circulatory arrest in a brain-dead organ donor: is the use of cardiac compression permissible? *J Intens Care Med* 24(6):389–392, 2009.

De Marco M, de Simone G, Roman MJ, et al: Cardiovascular and metabolic predictors of progression of prehypertension into hypertension: the Strong Heart Study. *Hypertension* 54(5):974–980, 2009.

Deghmane AE, Alonso JM, Taha MK: Emerging drugs for acute bacterial meningitis. *Exp Opin Emerg Drugs* 14(3):381–393, 2009.

Dorhout Mees SM, Luitse MJ, van den Bergh WM, et al: Fever after aneurismal subarachnoid hemorrhage: relation with extent of hydrocephalus and amount of extravasated blood. *Stroke* 39(7):2141–2143, 2008.

Engel J Jr: A proposed diagnostic scheme for people with epileptic seizures and with epilepsy: report of the ILAE Task Force on Classification and Terminology. *Epilepsia* 42(6):796–803, 2001.

Fitz Maurice E, Wendell L, Snider R, et al: Effect of statins on intracerebral hemorrhage outcome and reoccurrence. *Stroke* 39(7):2151–2154, 2008.

Fountas KN, Kapsalaki EZ, Lee GP, et al: Terson hemorrhage in patients suffering aneurismal subarachnoid hemorrhage: predisposing factors and prognostic significance. *J Neurosurg* 109(3): 439–444, 2008.

Friedman N, Sexton D: Epidemiological and clinical features of Gram-negative bacillary meningitis. http:www.uptodate.com

Gastaut H: Classification of status epilepticus. *Adv Neurol* 34:15–35, 1983.

Greer DM, Varelas PN, Hague S, et al: Variability of brain death determination guidelines in leading US neurologic institutions. *Neurology* 70(4):284–289, 2008. http://www.ncbi.nlm.nih.gov/pubmed/18077794?dopt=Abstract

Heurer GG, Smith MJ, Elliott JP, et al: Relationship between intracranial pressure and other clinical variables in patients with aneurismal subarachnoid hemorrhage. *J Neurosurg* 101(3):408–416, 2004.

Honda H, Warren DK: Central nervous system infections: meningitis and brain abscesses. *Infect Dis Clin North Am* 23(3):609–623, 2009.

Hsieh ST, Wijdicks EFM: Brain death worldwide: accepted fact but no global consensus in diagnostic criteria. *Neurology* 67(5):919, 2006.

Hughes RA, Wijdicks EF, Barohn R, et al: Practice parameter: immunotherapy for Guillain-Barré syndrome: report of the Quality Standards Subcommittee of the American Academy of Neurology. *Neurology* 61(6):736–740, 2003.

Johnson R: Aseptic meningitis in adults. http:www.upto   date.com

Juel VC: Myasthenia gravis: management of myasthenic crisis and perioperative care. *Semin Neurol* 24:75, 2004.

Knake S, Gruener J, Hattemer K, et al: Intravenous levetiracetam in the treatment of benzodiazepine refractory status epilepticus. *J Neurol Neurosurg Psychiatry* 79:588–589, 2008.

Lozier AP, Sciacca RR, Romagnoli MF, et al: Ventriculostomy-related infections: a critical review of the literature. *Neurosurgery* 51(1):170–181, 2002.

Machado C, Lin KC, Kuo JR, et al: Variability of brain death determination guidelines in leading US neurologic institutions. *Neurology* 71(14):1125–1126, 2008.

McGirt MJ, Woodworth GF, Ali M, et al: Persistent perioperative hyperglycemia as an independent predictor of poor outcome after aneurismal subarachnoid hemorrhage. *J Neurosurg* 107(6): 1080–1085, 2007.

Misra UK, Kalita J, Patel R: Sodium valproate versus phenytoin in status epilepticus: a pilot study. *Neurology* 67:340–342, 2006.

Mocco J, Ransom ER, Komotar RJ, et al: Preoperative prediction of long-term outcome in poor-grade aneurismal subarachnoid hemorrhage. *Neurosurgery* 59(3):529–538, 2006.

Qui W, Zhang Y, Sheng H, et al: Effects of mild hypothermia on patients with severe traumatic brain injury after craniotomy. *J Crit Care* 22(3):229–235, 2007.

Rahman S, Hanna MG: Diagnosis and therapy in neuromuscular disorders: diagnosis and new treatments in mitochondrial diseases. *J Neurol Neurosurg Psychiatry* 80(9):943–953, 2009.

Rhoney D, Peacock WF: Intravenous therapy for hypertensive emergencies, part 1. *Am. J. Health Syst Pharm* 66(15):1343–1352, 2009.

Rinkel GH, Feigin VL, Algra A, et al: Calcium antagonists for aneurismal subarachnoid hemorrhage. *Cochrane Database Syst Rev* (4):CD00027, 2002.

Rosamond W, Flegal K, Furie K, et al: Heart disease and stroke statistics: 2008 update: a report from the American Heart Association Statistics Committee and Stroke Statistics Subcommittee. *Circulation* 117:e25–e146, 2008.

Rosen DS, Macdonald RL: Subarachnoid hemorrhage grading scales: a systematic review. *Neurocrit Care* 2:110, 2005.

Seneviratne J, Mandrekar J, Wijdicks EF, et al: Predictors of extubation failure in myasthenic crisis. *Arch Neurol* 65:929, 2008.

Seventh Report of the Joint National Committee on Prevention, Detection, Evaluation, and Treatment of High Blood Pressure (JNC 7). Bethesda, MD, 2003, National High Blood Pressure Education Program; National Heart, Lung, and Blood Institute; U.S. Department of Health and Human Services, National Institutes of Health. NIH Publication No 03-5231.

Sexton D: Dexamethasone to prevent neurological complications of bacterial meningitis in adults. http:www.uptodate.com.

Sharar E: Current therapeutic options in severe Guillain-Barré syndrome. *Clin Neuropharmacol* 29(1):45–51, 2006.

Smith ML, Grady MS: Neurosurgery. In Brunicardi FC, editor: *Schwartz's principles of surgery*, ed. 8. New York, 2005, McGraw-Hill.

Stecker MM, Kramer TH, Raps EC, et al: Treatment of refractory status epilepticus with propofol: clinical and pharmacokinetic findings. *Epilepsia* 39(1):18–26, 1998.

Summers D, Leonard A, Wentworth D, et al; on behalf of the American Heart Association Council on Cardiovascular Nursing and the Stroke Council: Comprehensive overview of nursing and interdisciplinary care of the acute ischemic stroke patient: a scientific statement from the American Heart Association. *Stroke* 40:2911–2944, 2009.

Swartz MN: Meningitis: bacterial, viral, and other. In Goldman L, Ausiello D, editors: *Cecil Medicine*, ed 23. Philadelphia, PA, 2007, Saunders Elsevier.

Tempkin NR: Antiepileptogenesis and seizure prevention trials with antiepileptic drugs: meta-analysis of controlled trials. *Epilepsia* 42:515–524, 2001.

Treatment of convulsive status epilepticus. Recommendations of the Epilepsy Foundation of America's Working Group on Status Epilepticus. *JAMA* 270:854–859, 1993.

Treiman DM, Meyers PD, Walton NY, et al: A comparison of four treatments for generalized convulsive status epilepticus. Veterans Affairs Status Epilepticus Cooperative Study Group. *N Engl J Med* 339:792–798, 1998.

Verchere E, Grenier G, Mesli A, et al: Postoperative pain management after supratentorial craniotomy. *J Neurosurg Anesthesiol* 14:96–101, 2002.

Walker MC: Status epilepticus on the intensive care unit, *J Neurol* 250:401–406, 2003.

Wijdicks EFM: The diagnosis of brain death. *N Engl J Med* 344(16):1215–1221, 2001.

Wijdicks EFM, Rabinstein AA, Manno EM, et al: Pronouncing brain death: contemporary practice and safety of the apnea test. *Neurology* 71(16):1240–1244, 2008.

Working Group on Status Epilepticus: Treatment of convulsive status epilepticus: recommendations of the Working Group on Status Epilepticus. *JAMA* 270(7):854–859, 1993.

Endocrinologic Disorders

ENDOCRINE ASSESSMENT

Assessment of the endocrine system is complex when assessing the system as a whole because it regulates all body functions in conjunction with the nervous system. Focusing on assessment appropriate to critically ill patients, the following principles should be considered:

1. Critical illness initiates the stress response.
2. The stress response increases the metabolic rate.
3. The hypothalamic-pituitary axis (Figure 8-1) regulates the metabolic rate. The thyroid and adrenal glands are extremely stressed by the stimulus of critical illness to maintain the increased metabolic rate, along with meeting the energy demands at the cellular level. Hypofunction of the thyroid and adrenals requires assessment of not only the primary glands, but also the hypothalamus (produces releasing factors) and anterior pituitary (produces stimulating hormones.) The hypothalamic-pituitary-target organ feedback loop must be fully intact to maintain normal metabolism.
4. The stress response markedly increases endogenous glucocorticoids, which increase blood glucose. The pancreas may not be able to produce sufficient insulin to manage the glucose level, resulting in hyperglycemia. Insulin may be required to manage hyperglycemia until the stress of illness resolves. People with diabetes mellitus are always challenged with hyperglycemia, and with additional illness, can experience the crisis states of diabetic ketoacidosis (DKA) and hyperosmolar hyperglycemic syndrome (HHS).
5. Under prolonged extreme stress, both the adrenal glands and thyroid may be unable to sustain hormone production to support the stress level. Supplemental glucocorticoids (corticosteroids) and thyroid hormones may be needed.
6. The assessment of the critically ill patient should focus on the signs of failure of the endocrine system to support the stress response. Signs of hypofunction are explained the sections on hyperglycemia, adrenal crisis, and myxedema coma. Patients with adequate function of the pancreas, thyroid, and adrenal glands under normal conditions may not be able to maintain balance when exposed to the stress of critical illness. Those with underlying hypofunction are more likely to experience crises.
7. Hyperthermia and cardiac symptoms can make diagnosis of thyroid storm difficult, as the crisis mimics other cardiac crises and infection. Thyroid storm results from underlying Graves' disease/hyperthyroidism; not a complication of critical illness.
8. Assessment of the causes of unusual fluid and electrolyte imbalances should include evaluation of posterior pituitary function, in addition to screening for renal dysfunction. Posterior pituitary dysfunction may result in abnormal levels of antidiuretic hormone (ADH) and may be a complication of critical illness, or result from hypothalamic or pituitary disease. Diabetes insipidus (DI) produces dehydration and Syndrome of Inappropriate ADH (SIADH) produces hyponatremia, which can reach critical states if not properly addressed. Nephrogenic DI results from failure of the kidneys to respond to ADH. The elderly are at higher risk of complications with DI as a result of age-related changes to the thirst mechanism and renal function.

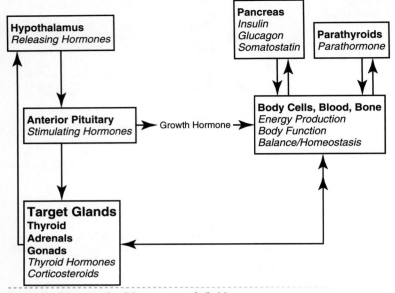

Figure 8-1 Endocrine system: hypothalamic-pituitary axis feedback loop.

9. Medication noncompliance for management of existing endocrine disease must be assessed. People with lower income are at higher risk of crisis due to inability to purchase medications and teenagers may not practice meticulous management; particularly those with diabetes mellitus. Elders may not take medications appropriately due to lack of understanding or mis-dosing due to deteriorating short-term memory.

ACUTE ADRENAL INSUFFICIENCY (ADRENAL CRISIS)

PATHOPHYSIOLOGY

Acute adrenocortical insufficiency, also known as adrenal crisis and Addisonian crisis, is a life-threatening condition that manifests as shock with profound, refractory hypotension. Severe sepsis with pituitary suppression and steroid withdrawal are the most common causes of acute adrenal insufficiency in critically ill patients. Adrenal crisis also results from acute exacerbation of chronic adrenocortical insufficiency in patients who become stressed by sepsis, surgery, adrenal hemorrhage (septicemia-induced Waterhouse-Friderickson syndrome from meningococcemia), and anticoagulation complications. There are approximately 50 total hormones produced by the adrenal glands, with cortisol and aldosterone being by far the most abundant.

The function of the adrenal cortex is dependent on the hypothalamic-pituitary axis. The normal relationship occurs as the hypothalamus secretes releasing factors, which:

1. Stimulate the pituitary to secrete stimulating hormones (adrenocorticotropic hormone [corticotropin] [ACTH]), which in turn
2. Stimulates the adrenal glands to secrete glucocorticoids (cortisol) and mineralocorticoids (aldosterone), which in turn
3. Facilitates cellular functions throughout the body (metabolism), which in turn
4. Creates signals back to the hypothalamus from the cells to increase or decrease releasing hormones (see Figure 8-1).

If *primary adrenal insufficiency* is the cause of the crisis, the adrenal glands are the root cause of the problem. *Addison disease* manifests when the entire adrenal cortex is destroyed, which stops the production of glucocorticoids (cortisol) and mineralocorticoids (aldosterone).

Glucocorticoids are essential hormones produced by the adrenal cortex that help maintain vascular tone and cardiac contractility, facilitate wound healing, and support immunity. Cortisol deficiency intensifies the clinical effects of hypovolemia by promoting a decrease in vascular tone, which is partially related to unopposed endothelial production of nitric oxide, and a decreased vascular response to the catecholamine hormones epinephrine and norepinephrine. Relative hypoglycemia may be present, as the breakdown of stored glycogen is not possible without cortisol. Mineralocorticoid hormones are primary regulators of fluid and electrolyte balance, and when unavailable, patients experience hyponatremia, hypovolemia, hyperkalemia, and metabolic acidosis. Large amounts of sodium and water are excreted in the urine. Severe hypotension, shock, and eventually death may occur without intravenous adrenocortical hormone and fluid replacement. In patients with chronic primary adrenocortical insufficiency or Addison disease, acute crises may be prevented by tripling hormone replacement doses during periods of stress.

Primary adrenal insufficiency is relatively rare, can be acute or chronic, and is most often caused by autoimmmune-mediated, idiopathic atrophy. Other causes include tuberculosis, fungal infection, hemorrhage, congenital adrenal hyperplasia, enzyme inhibitors (e.g., metyrapone), cytotoxic agents (e.g., mitotane), and other diseases infiltrating the adrenal glands.

Secondary adrenal insufficiency is relatively common and caused by a failure of either the pituitary gland or hypothalamic-pituitary axis to provide appropriate signals to the adrenal glands to secrete cortisol. Exogenous glucocorticoids (e.g., hydrocortisone) administered elevate the circulating level and the hypothalamic-pituitary-adrenal axis is no longer functional. The adrenal glands do not receive signals to produce endogenous cortisol because the circulating level remains high while the glucocorticoid therapy continues. When glucocorticoid therapy is abruptly discontinued, the adrenal gland cannot immediately respond and the patient experiences adrenal crisis. Secondary adrenocortical insufficiency also manifests when inflammatory mediators or trauma suppress or damage the hypothalamus or pituitary. Pituitary or other tumors may impair pituitary function or, in rarer cases, produce glucocorticoids, which suppress the hypothalamic-pituitary axis.

In patients with possible pituitary suppression from severe sepsis, glucocorticoid replacement for *relative adrenal insufficiency* remains controversial. Relative adrenal insufficiency is not readily identified by all practitioners. Patients with pituitary dysfunction generally do not require mineralocorticoid replacement because the release of aldosterone is dependent on release of angiotensin II rather than ACTH from the pituitary.

RESEARCH BRIEF 8-1

Sprung and colleagues published a multicenter, double-blind, randomized clinical trial in 2008. Fifty-two ICUs enrolled 500 patients who were older than 18 years with onset of septic shock within the previous 72 hours (SBP less than 90 mm Hg systolic despite fluids or need for vasopressors for *longer than* 1 hour). An ACTH 250 µg Stimulation Test was performed on all patients meeting criteria. Nonresponders were those patients whose serum cortisol level rose less than 9 µg/dl after stimulation. All of these patients then received hydrocortisone dosing or placebo. Hydrocortisone was administered in the following pattern of deceleration:

1. 50 mg IV every 6 hours × 5 days
2. 50 mg IV every 12 hours on days 6 to 8
3. 50 mg IV every 24 hours on days 9 to 11 and then stopped

The results were dismal in terms of mortality reduction because there was little difference from placebo. Of note, however, was that the group receiving hydrocortisone spent less time in shock by the prior mentioned definition.

From Sprung CL, Annane D, Keh D, et al: Hydrocortisone therapy for patients in septic shock. *N Engl J Med* 358(2):111–124, 2008.

ENDOCRINE ASSESSMENT ADRENALS
Goal of System Assessment:
To evaluate for severe hypotension, refractory to volume and vasopressor administration

History and Risk Factors
- Extreme emotional or physiologic stress, which increases the need for adrenocortical "stress" hormones to mediate the stress response
- Patients previously receiving glucocorticoids (steroids) who may be abruptly withdrawn from steroids or are not given sufficient steroids to manage additional stress
- Adrenalectomy, hypophysectomy, sepsis, human immunodeficiency (HIV) disease
- Other medications: beta adrenergic blockers, diuretics, angiotensin-converting enzyme (ACE) inhibitors, angiotensin release blockers (ARBs), nitrates, aspirin, and other platelet inhibitors

Observation and Vital Signs: Primary (First-Degree) and Secondary (Second-Degree) Insufficiency
- Refractory, severe hypotension resulting from vascular collapse
- Acute abdomen assessment findings: abdominal pain, distention
- Tachycardia and tachypnea
- Hyperpyrexia, with temperatures often reaching in excess of 105°F
- Cyanosis, confusion; may be comatose
- Relative hypoglycemia: tremors, diaphoresis, tachycardia, tachypnea

Observation and Vital Signs: Primary (First-Degree) Insufficiency Only
- Prominent nausea and vomiting
- Weakness
- Signs of dehydration: poor skin turgor, sunken, soft eyeballs, weight loss
- Bronze hue to the skin secondary to excess production of ACTH
- Hyperkalemia, which may be associated with metabolic acidosis: peaked T waves, widening QRS complex, prolonged PR interval, flattened-to-absent P wave

Screening Labwork
For Suspected Acute Adrenal Crisis
- *Random plasma cortisol level:* Drawn prior to initiating hydrocortisone replacement but must be interpreted with caution in critically ill patients, because greater than 90% of circulating cortisol is protein bound. When patients are hypoproteinemic, with serum albumin less than 2.5 g/dl, low values may be gleaned from *all* cortisol testing in patients who have normal adrenal function. A random plasma cortisol level of greater than 25 mcg/dl excludes both primary and secondary adrenal insufficiency.
- *Free cortisol level:* Done in the setting of hypoproteinemia to better determine the cortisol level. An abnormal test may require a complete endocrinology assessment when the patient stabilizes.

For Noncritical Adrenocortical Insufficiency
- *Corticotropin (ACTH) stimulation test:* The goal is to differentiate primary from secondary adrenocortical insufficiency or to assess if the adrenal cortex is capable of producing cortisol. Testing of the hypothalamic-pituitary-adrenal axis using this test can differentiate primary from secondary insufficiency. Baseline plasma cortisol level is drawn immediately prior to ACTH administration.
  1. A dose of 250 mcg synthetic ACTH is given IM or IV.
     - *Low-dose protocol:* Doses as low as 1 mcg/kg of ACTH have been used to more closely mimic the amount of normal physiologic ACTH released.
  2. Within 15 to 30 minutes of receiving ACTH, the normal adrenal cortex releases two to five times the baseline or basal plasma cortisol level.
  3. Thirty or 60 minutes following the ACTH injection, another cortisol level is drawn. *If the low-dose protocol was used, only the 30-minute cortisol level is accurate.*
  4. If evaluating for primary adrenal insufficiency, aldosterone levels are drawn with the cortisol levels. *The 30-minute aldosterone level is more accurate than the 60-minute level.*

- Adrenal insufficiency is diagnosed when:
  - *Cortisol level*: Does not increase at least a total of 9 mg/dl at 30 or 60 minutes following ACTH administration. Typically will rise to above 20 to 30 mg/dL.
  - *Aldosterone level (if testing specifically for primary insufficiency)*: An initial value of less than 5 ng/100 ml that fails to double or increase by at least 4 ng/100 ml at 30 minutes following ACTH administration.

Diagnostic Tests for Acute Adrenal Insufficiency

Test	Purpose	Abnormal Findings
Noninvasive		
Chest radiograph	Assess for heart size and presence of opportunistic infections (primary)	The chest radiogram may be normal but often reveals a small heart. Stigmata of earlier infection or current evidence of tuberculosis (TB) or fungal infection may be present when this is the cause of Addison disease.
Computed tomography (CT) scan of abdomen	Assess abdominal organs, size, presence of blood (primary)	Abdominal CT scan may be normal but may show bilateral enlargement of the adrenal glands in patients with Addison disease because of TB, fungal infections, adrenal hemorrhage, or infiltrating diseases involving the adrenal glands. In Addison disease due to TB or histoplasmosis, evidence of calcification involving both adrenal glands may be present. In idiopathic autoimmune Addison disease, the adrenal glands usually are atrophic.
Blood Studies		
Complete blood count (CBC) Hemoglobin (Hgb) Hematocrit (Hct) RBC count (RBCs) WBC count (WBCs)	Assess for anemia, inflammation and infection (primary and secondary)	CBC count may reveal a normocytic normochromic anemia, which, upon initial presentation, may be masked by dehydration and hemoconcentration. Relative lymphocytosis and eosinophilia may be present.
Electrolytes Potassium (K^+) Sodium (Na^+)	Assess for abnormalities of aldosterone (primary)	Elevation in K^+ may cause dysrhythmias; decrease of Na^+ may indicate fluid retention and/or concomitant heart failure.
Serum glucose	Assess for relative hypoglycemia (primary and secondary)	Hypoglycemia may be present in fasted patients, or it may occur spontaneously. It is caused by the increased peripheral utilization of glucose and increased insulin sensitivity. It is more prominent in children and in patients with secondary adrenocortical insufficiency.
Thyroid-stimulating hormone	Assess for thyroid dysfunction (primary and secondary)	Increased thyroid-stimulating hormone, with or without low thyroxine, with or without associated thyroid autoantibodies, and with or without symptoms of hypothyroidism, may occur in patients with Addison disease and in patients with secondary adrenocortical insufficiency due to isolated ACTH deficiency. These findings may be reversible with cortisol replacement.

COLLABORATIVE MANAGEMENT

DIAGNOSIS AND MANAGEMENT OF CORTICOSTEROID INSUFFICIENCY IN CRITICALLY ILL PATIENTS

Recommendations for the diagnosis and management of corticosteroid insufficiency in critically ill adult patients: consensus statements from an international task force by the American College of Critical Care Medicine.

From Marik PE, Pastores SM, Annane D, et al: *Crit Care Med* 36(6):1937–1949, 2008.

In 2008, an interdisciplinary, multispecialty task force of experts in critical care medicine was convened from the membership of the Society of Critical Care Medicine and the European Society of Intensive Care Medicine. In addition, international experts in endocrinology were invited to participate. The goal was to develop a strategic tool for defining and treating critical illness acute adrenal insufficiency.

Treatment	Rationale
Moderate dose of hydrocortisone (200–300 mg/day) for critically ill patients with septic shock.	Six randomized control trials demonstrate significant and greater shock reversal in patients who received hydrocortisone although no difference in mortality.
Moderate dose of hydrocortisone in the management of severe early ARDS (PF ratio <200) instituted before day 14.	Five randomized studies evaluated moderate hydrocortisone administration in ARDS from various origins. Consistent improvement was reported in the PF ratio, inflammatory markers were reduced, and both ventilator days and ICU length of stay were reduced.
In patients with septic shock, intravenous hydrocortisone should be given in a dose of 200 mg/day in four divided doses or as a bolus of 100 mg followed by a continuous infusion at 10 mg/hr (240 mg/day).The optimal initial dosing regimen in patients with early severe ARDS is 1 mg/kg/day methylprednisolone as a continuous infusion.	Multiple clinical trials, both randomized and not, as well as prospective and retrospective of patients in severe sepsis and ARDS.
Glucocorticoid (GC) treatment should be tapered slowly and not stopped abruptly.	Abruptly stopping hydrocortisone will likely result in a rebound of proinflammatory mediators, with recurrence of the features of shock (and tissue injury).
Treatment with dexamethasone has previously been suggested in patients with septic shock until an ACTH stimulation test is performed, this approach can no longer be endorsed	Physiologic and pathologic understanding that dexamethasone leads to immediate and prolonged suppression of ACTH.

Care Priorities

1. **Correct hypovolemia** Initiate replacement of intravascular fluid volume. Rapid volume replacement is essential, using normal saline crystalloid IV solution. Administer 1 L over the first hour, followed by an additional 1 to 2 L over the next 6 to 8 hours. If hypovolemia persists, colloid/volume-expanding IV solutions may be necessary.

2. **Manage hypotension** Use vasopressors if intravascular volume replacement fails to effectively increase BP (see Appendix 6). Response to catecholamine infusions (epinephrine, norepinephrine, dopamine) is reduced in adrenal insufficiency; higher-than-normal doses may be needed to manage refractory hypotension.

3. **Replace cortisol** During stressful situations, the normal adrenal gland output of cortisol is approximately 250 to 300 mg over 24 hours. IV hydrocortisone should be given only to adult septic shock patients after it has been confirmed their BP is poorly responsive to fluid resuscitation and vasopressor therapy.
   - Administer 100 mg of hydrocortisone in 100 ml of normal saline solution by continuous IV infusion at a rate of 12 ml/hr. Infusion may be initiated with 100 mg of hydrocortisone as an IV bolus.
   - A continuous infusion method maintains plasma cortisol levels effectively if the stress level is steady or constant, particularly in patients who rapidly metabolize the drug. Rapid metabolizers have a greater likelihood of having low plasma cortisol levels between IV boluses.

- An alternative method of hydrocortisone administration is 50-75 mg IV every 4-6 hours for 5 days.
- Improvement in BP and other vital signs should be evident within 4 to 6 hours of hydrocortisone infusion. If not, the diagnosis of adrenal insufficiency is questionable.
- After 2 to 3 days, the stress hydrocortisone dose should be reduced to 100 to 150 mg, infused over a 24-hour period regardless of the patient's status. In addition to helping with adrenal recovery, lower doses may help abate gastrointestinal (GI) bleeding.
- As the patient improves and the clinical situation allows, the hydrocortisone infusion can be gradually tapered over the following 4 to 5 days to daily replacement doses of approximately 3 mg/hr (72 to 75 mg over 24 hours) and eventually to daily oral replacement doses when oral intake is possible.
- If the patient receives at least 100 mg of hydrocortisone in 24 hours, no mineralocorticoid replacement is necessary, because the mineralocorticoid activity of hydrocortisone in this dosage is sufficient.
- As the hydrocortisone dose continues to be weaned, mineralocorticoid replacement should begin in doses equivalent to the daily adrenal gland aldosterone output of 0.05 to 0.1 mg daily or every other day.

4. **Maintain normal blood glucose level:** If patient is initially hypoglycemic, 50% dextrose may be needed to correct hypoglycemia. When hydrocortisone or other cortisol replacement is initiated, hyperglycemia may result. An insulin infusion may be needed to control the blood glucose (see *Hyperglycemia, p 711*).

Safety Alert   *The need for aggressive insulin titration is reduced if the patient is managed using a continuous (24-hour) infusion of cortisol replacement rather than bolus doses every 6 hours.*

CARE PLANS FOR ADRENAL INSUFFICIENCY

Deficient fluid volume   *related to failure of regulatory mechanisms secondary to impaired secretion of aldosterone, causing increased sodium excretion with resultant diuresis*

GOALS/OUTCOMES Within 12 hours of initiating treatment, patient is moving toward normovolemia as evidenced by BP approaching normal range; heart rate (HR) 60 to 100 beats/min (bpm); respiratory rate (RR) 12 to 20 breaths/min with normal pattern and depth, or if on the ventilator, weaning from the ventilator; central venous pressure (CVP) 2 to 6 mm Hg; if hemodynamic monitoring is in place, pulmonary artery wedge pressure (PAWP) approaching 6 to 12 mm Hg; normal sinus rhythm on electrocardiogram (ECG); and improvement in level of consciousness (LOC).

NOC Fluid Balance

Fluid and Electrolyte Management
1. Monitor vital signs and hemodynamic measurements every 15 minutes until stabilized for 1 hour. Consult physician or midlevel practitioner promptly for deterioration in vital signs or hemodynamics.
2. Administer IV fluids to replace fluid volume. Initially, rapid fluid replacement is essential.
3. Maintain accurate input and output (I&O) record. Weigh patient daily.
4. Monitor for electrolyte imbalance. Imbalances associated with adrenal insufficiency include the following:
   - *Hyponatremia:* Headache, malaise, muscle weakness, abdominal cramps
   - *Hyperkalemia:* Lethargy, nausea, hyperactive bowel sounds with diarrhea, numbness or tingling in extremities, muscle weakness. Be aware hyperkalemia will worsen in the presence of metabolic acidosis.
5. Monitor ECG continuously; observe for potassium-related changes. Increased ventricular irritability may signal hypokalemia. (See *Fluid and Electrolyte Disturbances, Hypokalemia, p 52.*)
6. Monitor laboratory results. With appropriate treatment, serum sodium levels should rise to normal and serum potassium levels should fall to normal. Prevent rapid correction or overcorrection of hyponatremia. Serum sodium levels should not be allowed to increase greater than 12 mEq/L during the first 24 hours of treatment because of the risk of neurologic damage. (See *Fluid and Electrolyte Disturbances, Hyponatremia, p 46,* or *Syndrome of Inappropriate ADH, p 734.*)
7. Assess mental and respiratory status at frequent intervals. Institute safety measures as indicated. Reorient and reassure patient as needed.

Acute Adrenal Insufficiency (Adrenal Crisis)

8. Encourage oral fluid intake as patient's condition stabilizes. Add sodium-rich foods (see Box 8-1) as tolerated. Begin oral glucocorticoid replacement therapy as prescribed.
9. Consult physician or midlevel practitioner if signs and symptoms of fluid and/or electrolyte imbalance persist or worsen.

NIC Fluid Monitoring; Neurologic Monitoring; Hypovolemia Management; Electrolyte Management: Hyponatremia; Electrolyte Management: Hyperkalemia

Risk for injury *related to potential for acute regulatory dysfunction (cortisol and aldosterone deficiency) secondary to increased psychological, emotional, or physical stressors with increased hormonal demand and inadequate adrenal reserves*

GOALS/OUTCOMES Patient does not manifest symptoms of sepsis; is able to verbalize orientation to time, place, and person, has stable weight, urine output less than 80 to 125 ml/hr, HR 60 to 100 bpm, BP within patient's normal range, and normothermia.

NOC Immune Status; Infection Status; Energy Conservation

Energy Management
1. Monitor and report signs of increasing crisis: urinary output increased from usual amount, changes in LOC, orthostatic hypotension, nausea, vomiting, and tachycardia.
2. Provide a quiet, nonstressful environment. Adjust lighting to meet needs of individual activities, avoiding direct light in the eyes. Control noise when possible. Prevent unnecessary interruptions, and allow for rest periods. Limit the number of visitors and the length of time they spend with patient. Speak softly and reassuringly to patient.
3. Monitor for and manage hyperthermia using tepid baths, antipyretics, and cooling blankets.

Box 8-1	PATIENT AND FAMILY EDUCATION CONCERNING GLUCOCORTICOID AND MINERALOCORTICOID REPLACEMENT

Glucocorticoids (e.g., Cortisone, Acetate, Prednisone)

- Take medication in a diurnal pattern to mimic normal secretion (i.e., two thirds of dose in the morning and one third of dose in the afternoon).
- Take steroids with food to decrease gastric irritation.
- Weigh self regularly, and report to physician gains of greater than 2 lb/wk.
- Avoid exposure to infection, and be alert to indicators of infection (e.g., fever, nausea, diarrhea, malaise).
- Contact physician promptly during periods of physical or emotional stress; dosages will require adjustment at these times.
- Indicators of overreplacement: weight gain (moon face, truncal obesity); edema, thin, fragile skin (striae, easy bruising); slow wound healing; chronic fatigue; emotional lability
- Indicators of underreplacement: weight loss, hyperpigmentation, skin creases, anorexia, nausea, abdominal discomfort, chronic fatigue, depression, irritability

Mineralocorticoids (e.g., Fludrocortisone, Desoxycorticosterone Acetate)

- As prescribed, modify diet with liberal amounts of sodium (see Box 1-4), protein, and carbohydrates.
- Weigh self regularly, and report to physician sudden gains or losses greater than 2 lb/wk.
- Contact physician promptly during periods of physical or emotional stress; dosages will require adjustment at these times.
- Indicators of overreplacement: edema, muscle weakness, hypertension
- Indicators of underreplacement: excessive urination, weight loss, decreased skin turgor

4. Maintain a cool environmental temperature. Maintain strict environmental asepsis, and monitor patient carefully for signs of infection. Avoid exposing patient to staff members or visitors who have colds or infections.

NIC Fluid Monitoring; Environmental Management; Infection Protection

Deficient knowledge: illness care *related to prevention of adrenal crisis in patients with chronic adrenal insufficiency or those undergoing steroid therapy*

GOALS/OUTCOMES Before discharge from the intensive care unit (ICU), patient understands factors that increase the risk of adrenal crisis, how to avoid adrenal crisis, precautions that must be taken, and when to notify physician or midlevel practitioner.

NOC Knowledge: Disease Process; Knowledge: Energy Conservation; Knowledge: Medication

Teaching: Disease Process
1. Teach patient about prescribed medications, including purpose, dosage, route of administration, and potential side effects (Box 8-1). Medication administration should mimic normal diurnal pattern of plasma cortisol levels (e.g., two thirds in the morning and one third in late afternoon).
2. Provide dietary instruction: dietary sodium and potassium may need to be adjusted on the basis of the patient's clinical condition and drug therapy (see discussions of sodium and potassium in *Fluid and Electrolyte Disturbances*, p. 37).
3. Explain the importance of controlling stress, both emotional and physiologic, which increases adrenal demand. Teach patient to seek medical intervention during times of increased stress (e.g., fever, infection), inasmuch as medication dosages may need to be increased.
4. Teach indicators of overreplacement and underreplacement of steroids, which require prompt medical attention (see Box 8-1).
5. Stress the importance of never abruptly discontinuing use of any steroid preparation. Use must be tapered to avoid precipitation of crisis.
6. Remind patient of the importance of continued medical follow-up.
7. Explain the procedure for obtaining a medical-alert bracelet or card.

NIC Teaching: Prescribed Medication; Emotional Support

DIABETES INSIPIDUS

PATHOPHYSIOLOGY

Diabetes insipidus (DI) is a metabolic disorder that affects total body free water regulation, resulting in an abnormally high output of extremely dilute urine, increased fluid intake, and constant thirst. The volume of hypotonic urine excreted is 3-20L/day. Vasopressin (antidiuretic hormone [ADH]) is a key component in the regulation of fluid and electrolyte balance, through direct effects on renal water regulation. Vasopressin is produced in the hypothalamus, is stored in the posterior pituitary gland, and exerts action in the kidneys for water regulation. Three subtypes of receptors respond to the effects of vasopressin (Table 8-1).

Table 8-1	LOCATIONS AND ACTIONS OF VASOPRESSIN RECEPTORS		
	V1a	**V1b**	**V2**
Location	Central nervous system Vascular smooth muscle Liver Platelets	Anterior pituitary gland	Distal nephron
Physiologic effects	Neurotransmitter and autonomic neuroregulation Smooth muscle contraction Stimulation of glycogenolysis Increased platelet adhesion	Increased ACTH release	Increased production and action of aquaporin-2

Diabetes Insipidus

When any aspect of water regulation fails, if free water is lost, the extracellular fluid volume rapidly decreases, causing plasma osmolality and serum sodium to rise. Plasma osmolality is the main determinant of vasopressin secretion from the posterior pituitary. The osmoregulatory systems for thirst and vasopressin secretion, and the actions of ADH on renal water excretion, maintain plasma osmolality between 284 and 295 mOsmol/kg. Thirst and drinking are key processes in the maintenance of fluid and electrolyte balance. Thirst perception and the regulation of water ingestion involve complex neural and neurohormonal pathways. Thirst occurs when plasma osmolality rises above 281 mOsm/kg, similar to the threshold for ADH release. The osmoreceptors regulating thirst are located in the hypothalamus. Situations that alter the balance between plasma osmolality and vasopressin concentration include:

- *Rapid changes of plasma osmolality*: Rapid increases in plasma osmolality result in an abnormal increase in ADH/vasopressin release.
- *Drinking fluids*: Oral fluid consumption rapidly suppresses the release of ADH, through afferent pathways originating in the oropharynx.
- *Pregnancy*: The osmotic threshold for ADH release is lowered in pregnancy.
- *Aging*: Plasma vasopressin concentrations increase with age, together with enhanced ADH responses to osmotic stimulation. Age-related changes in ADH production can result in blunting of the thirst response, decreased fluid intake, impaired ability to excrete a free water load, and reduced ability of the kidneys to concentrate urine. These changes predispose the elderly to both hypernatremia and hyponatremia.

There are *four major subtypes of DI*, based on which mechanism involved with concentrating urine has failed:

- *Central, hypothalamic or pituitary DI (neurogenic DI)* is the most common type and is caused by lack of vasopressin (ADH) production by a diseased or destroyed posterior pituitary gland. Lack of ADH results in massive diuresis, because ADH normally prompts the kidney to concentrate the urine. Approximately 50% of central DI is idiopathic, as diagnostic testing does not reveal a cause. Central DI is usually permanent, but the signs and symptoms (i.e., thirst, drinking fluids, and urination) are controlled by daily use of synthetic vasopressin.
- *Nephrogenic DI (NDI)* is caused by inability of the kidneys to respond to normal amounts of ADH, resulting from a variety of drugs or kidney diseases including genetic predisposition. The collecting tubules have decreased permeability to water caused by decreased response to vasopressin by the nephrons. NDI does not improve with synthetic vasopressin and may not improve when probable causes are managed. Familial NDI requires lifelong management. Treatments partially relieve the signs and symptoms. Medications, including lithium, amphotericin B, and demeclocycline can induce NDI. Hypercalcemia can sometimes prompt NDI.
- *Gestational* or *gestogenic DI* results from a lack of vasopressin that develops during the third trimester of pregnancy if the pregnant woman's thirst center is abnormal, causing a blunted thirst response, and/or the placenta destroys vasopressin too rapidly. The placenta may increase the action of vasopressinase, the enzyme that breaks down vasopressin. The condition is controlled using synthetic vasopressin until the DI resolves. Vasopressin can generally be discontinued 4 to 6 weeks after delivery. Signs and symptoms of DI will recur with subsequent pregnancies.
- *Dipsogenic DI* or *primary polydipsia* results from vasopressin suppression caused by excessive fluid intake. Primary polydipsia is most often caused by an abnormality in the thirst center of the brain. Unquenchable thirst results in water intoxication. Dipsogenic DI is differentiated from central (pituitary) DI using the water deprivation test. There is no cure for dipsogenic DI at present, but symptoms can be safely relieved. *Psychogenic polydipsia* is another subtype due to psychosomatic causes that has no treatment that is recognized as consistently effective.

The most common presentation of DI is following head trauma or intracranial surgery. When a person cannot adequately respond to stimulation of the thirst center by drinking fluids, extracellular and intracellular dehydration may result. Electrolyte imbalance, primarily hypernatremia, may produce neurologic symptoms ranging from confusion, restlessness, and irritability to seizures and coma. DI sometimes occurs in brain-dead organ donors and must be managed to effectively preserve organs.

In normal individuals, a more concentrated circulating volume stimulates ADH release through activation of osmoreceptors that monitor serum osmolality. ADH is also released as part of the renin-angiotensin-aldosterone mechanism as a result of hypotension sensed by the juxtomedullary apparatus located outside the glomerulus of the kidney. A 5% to 10% decrease in arterial BP is necessary to increase circulating vasopressin concentrations. Progressive hypotension in healthy individuals results in an exponential increase in plasma ADH via baroreceptor stimulation, while osmoregulated ADH release in response to dehydration is more linear. If the hypothalamus is damaged, production of ADH may not be possible and both the ability to regulate circulating volume and vascular tone may be affected.

In addition to the pharmacologic use of vasopressin in managing DI, exogenous vasopressin also has a role in responding to changes in cardiovascular status and is used as an alternative to epinephrine in resuscitation following cardiac arrest. Exogenous vasopressin administration is used to manage vasodilated shock because ADH is also a potent vasopressor agent with actions mediated through receptors (V_1R) located in vascular smooth muscle cells. Although systemic effects on arterial BP are only seen at high concentrations, ADH is also important in maintaining BP in mild volume depletion.

RESEARCH BRIEF 8-2

Vasopressin is used an alternative to epinephrine management of cardiovascular collapse during cardiopulmonary resuscitation. The authors randomly assigned adults with an out-of-hospital cardiac arrest to receive two injections of either 40 IU of vasopressin or 1 mg of epinephrine, followed by additional treatment with epinephrine if needed. The primary end point was survival to hospital admission, and the secondary end point was survival to hospital discharge. Among 1186 patients, 589 were assigned to receive vasopressin and 597 to receive epinephrine. The two treatment groups had similar clinical profiles. There were no significant differences in the rates of hospital admission between the vasopressin group and the epinephrine group either among patients with ventricular fibrillation. Among patients with asystole, however, vasopressin use was associated with significantly higher rates of hospital admission. Cerebral performance was similar in the two groups. The effects of vasopressin were similar to those of epinephrine in the management of ventricular fibrillation and pulseless electrical activity, but vasopressin was superior to epinephrine in patients with asystole. Vasopressin followed by epinephrine may be more effective than epinephrine alone in the treatment of refractory cardiac arrest.

From Wenzel V, Krismer AC, Arntz HR, Sitter H, et al: A comparison of vasopressin and epinephrine for out of hospital cardiopulmonary resuscitation. *N Engl J Med* 350(2):105–113, 2004.

Larger pharmacologic doses of vasopressin exert powerful vascular effects in the regulation of regional blood flow. The sensitivity of vascular smooth muscle to the vasoconstrictive effects of ADH varies with each vascular bed and within various parts of each bed. Vasoconstriction of splanchnic, hepatic, and renal vessels occurs at ADH concentrations close to the normal range. Selective actions within the kidney blood vessels lead to redistribution of blood flow from the renal medulla to the cortex. Baroregulated (pressure response) release of vasopressin is a key physiologic mediator in an integrated hemodynamic response to volume depletion.

ENDOCRINE ASSESSMENT: DIABETES INSIPIDUS
Goal of Assessment

The clinical presentation of DI is dependent on the overall health of the patient and the primary cause. Evaluate for degree of dehydration and its effects on overall hemodynamics, heart rate/rhythm, and mental status. Generally, DI is recognized and managed prior to resulting in serious complications. Practitioners working with brain dead organ donors must be particularly alert to the occurrence of DI. Severe, unmanaged or under managed dehydration in cases of DI may cause hemoconcentration, which may predispose the patient to thrombosis. Dehydration and electrolyte imbalance must be prevented or managed immediately to avoid possible organ damage.

History and Risk Factors

Central/Hypothalamic/Pituitary DI: Brain tumors, especially in the hypothalamus or pituitary region; neoplasms such as leukemia or breast cancer; surgery in the area of the pituitary gland; intracranial hemorrhage; brain death; head injury, especially to the base of the brain; meningitis or encephalitis; any disorder that causes increased intracranial pressure (ICP); cerebral hypoxia; and various inheritable defects. Those with genetic defects have the onset in early childhood. Genetic predisposition is revealed by family history.

NDI: From medications (e.g., lithium, demeclocycline, glyburide, phenytoin); insufficient dose prescribed of ADH: ethanol abuse; chronic hypercalcemia; hypokalemia; osmotic diuresis; congenital disorder of defective expression of renal vasopressin V2 receptors; or patients with polycystic kidney disease, pyelonephritis, renal amyloidosis, myeloma, Sjögren syndrome, or sickle cell anemia.

Gestational DI: Seen in patients during the last trimester of pregnancy who have oligohydramnios, preeclampsia, and/or hepatic dysfunction. In addition to the blunted thirst response associated with pregnancy, these patients break down only endogenous vasopressin (ADH) and can be managed with synthetic vasopressin (desmopressin).

Dipsogenic DI: Unquenchable thirst with massive water intake; psychogenic causes may be associated with patients with a history of mental illness. Water intoxication from massive fluid intake presents with headache, loss of appetite, lethargy, and nausea and signs such as an abnormally large decrease in the plasma sodium concentration (hyponatremia).

Vital Signs

- Tachycardia and tachypnea are present with dehydration.
- Diuresis alone may have no effect on vital signs if the patient is able to drink enough fluids.
- Orthostatic hypotension if dehydration is present

Observation

- Polyuria with dilute urine; 3-20 L/day of urine may be excreted, with specific gravity of 1.000 to 1.005.
- History may include nocturia (getting up frequently at night to urinate) and/or enuresis (bed wetting).
- Extreme thirst
- *Dehydration:* Poor skin turgor, dry mucous membranes, sunken eyes, slow capillary refill
  1. *Electrolyte imbalance:* Generalized weakness, possible exhaustion, nausea and vomiting, impaired vision and leg cramps may be present; patients may become unable to get out of bed.
  2. *Urine output:* More than 200 ml/hr for 2 consecutive hours or greater than 500 ml/hr, especially if risk factors are present.
  3. *Hemodynamics:* CVP less than 2 mm Hg; PAWP less than 6 mm Hg. It is not routine practice to use hemodynamic monitoring solely to manage DI, but if DI develops in a critically ill patient, readings typically reflect hypovolemia.
- *Altered mental status:* Serum hyperosmolality and hypernatremia affect consciousness and behavior. Changes may also be related to the underlying disease.
  1. Cranial nerve examination may be abnormal, with nerve palsies present.
  2. Altered level of consciousness (confusion, disorientation, agitation) is more common with older adults; in extreme unmanaged cases, coma and seizures are possible.

Auscultation

- In rare cases, Bowel sounds may be lessened if hypovolemic shock has reduced abdominal vessel perfusion.

Screening Labwork

- Point-of-care (POC) capillary blood glucose to rule out hyperglycemia as the cause for diuresis
- Fluid and electrolyte imbalance screening:
  1. *Electrolyte panel:* To assess for hypernatremia and concentrations of other electrolytes associated with hemoconcentration
  2. *Urinalysis/specific gravity:* Assesses for dilute, poorly concentrated urine
  3. *Urinary and serum osmolality:* Values may become similar. When kidneys properly concentrate urine, urine osmolality is generally 4 times the value of serum osmolality.

Differential Diagnosis of Diabetes Insipidus

Test	Purpose	Abnormal Findings
Urine osmolality	Assesses for decreased concentration or dilute urine	Decreased to <200 mOsm/kg; may be higher if volume depletion is present
Urine specific gravity	Assesses for dilute urine	Specific gravity: <1.005 Normal is 1.010–1.025
Serum osmolality	Assesses for concentrated blood/hemoconcentration	Increased to >290 mOsm/kg
Serum sodium	Monitors for hypernatremia	Increased to >147 mEq/L
Plasma ADH level (vasopressin level)	Assesses if vasopressin is elevated or decreased	*Central DI:* Decreased *Nephrogenic DI:* Normal or increased *Gestational DI:* Decreased *Dipsogenic DI:* Decreased
Water deprivation test (Miller-Moses Test) Dehydration should prompt the kidneys to concentrate urine.	To distinguish between the types of DI. Assesses for changes in weight, serum and urine osmolality, and specific gravity when fluid intake is prohibited.	Differentiates psychogenic polydipsia from DI. Central DI and NDI are unaffected by this test.
ADH (Vasopressin) test ADH administration will correct the problem if ADH was lacking.	Assesses if the kidneys begin to concentrate urine when ADH is administered. Distinguishes NDI from other types of DI.	Corrects central/neurogenic DI, wherein ADH is lacking. NDI is unaffected by ADH administration, since the problem is unrelated to lack of ADH.
Brain or Pituitary magnetic resonance imaging **(MRI)**	MRI scan used to identify pituitary lesions that may have caused the DI.	If the patient has the "bright spot" or hyperintense emission from the posterior pituitary gland, the patient likely has primary polydipsia. If the "bright spot" is small or absent, the patient likely has central DI.

COLLABORATIVE MANAGEMENT
Care Priorities
1. **Rehydrate If Dehydration and/or Hypovolemia are Present**
   - Place at least two large-bore IV lines, or have a central line inserted.
   - Administer hypotonic IV fluids (5% Dextrose solution, 0.45% saline.). Hyperglycemia and volume overload should be avoided.
   - Avoid overly aggressive correction of hypernatremia. Do not decrease sodium level by more than 5mEq/L per hour or 12 mEq/L within 24 hours..
   - Patient may be allowed to drink fluids, with the volume accurately recorded
   - Monitor urine output judiciously. Total water deficit may be estimated by assuming body water composes approximately 60% of total body weight in kg.
   - Monitor continuous ECG for tachycardia and dysrhythmias.
   - Evaluate basic ABCs: airway, breathing, and circulation if the patient becomes hypotensive.
2. **Administer Exogenous ADH (Vasopressin)**
   - Use of desmopressin acetate (DDAVP) is popular because it produces fewer side effects (Table 8-2).
   - Several preparations are available, and dosage is adjusted to patient response to DI management. Vasopressin's potential vasoconstrictive effects occur rarely with appropriate dosing for management of DI. Excessive dosing of ADH may cause hypertension and cardiac symptoms; other side effects include abdominal cramping and increased peristalsis.
3. **Manage Electrolyte Imbalances, Focusing on Hypernatremia**
   - Prior to rehydration, patients are hypernatremic. Hypernatremia should resolve with aggressive hydration.

Table 8-2	VASOPRESSIN PREPARATIONS					
Generic Name	**Trade Name**	**Route**	**Onset**	**Duration**	**Total Daily Dose**	**Comments**
Desmopressin acetate	DDAVP Stimate Minirin	Intranasal	1–2 hr	8–12 hr	10–40 mcg daily	Administered by nasal spray or rhinal tube applicator. Action decreased by nasal congestion/discharge or atrophy of nasal mucosa. Stored in refrigerator. Drug of choice for chronic CDI.
		Subcutaneous	Within 1/2 hr	1.5 – 4 hr	0.1–2 mcg daily in 2 divided doses	Keep refrigerated. More potent than intranasal route.
		Intravenous	Within 1/2 hr	1.5– 4 hr	0.1–2 mcg daily in 2 divided doses	Keep refrigerated. More potent than intranasal route.
		Oral tablets	1–2 hr	8–12 hr	100–1000 mcg daily in 2–3 divided doses	Simple to use. More consistent absorption and few side effects.
Vasopressin	Pitressin	Subcutaneous	1–2 hr	2–8 hr	5–10 units (20 units/ml)	Used primarily to confirm the diagnosis, differentiate between CDI and NDI, and treat acute situations.
		Intramuscular	1–2 hr	2–8 hr	5–60 units daily given in 2–4 divided doses	
Lysine vasopressin	Diapid	Intranasal	Within 1 hr	3–8 hr	7–14 mcg in 4 dose (q6h)	Lower cost than DDAVP for patients with partial CDI who require 1–2 daily doses.

CDI, Central diabetes insipidus; NDI, nephrogenic diabetes insipidus.

4. **Identify and Manage the Precipitating Cause**
   - As dehydration is managed, efforts should be under way to identify the cause of DI, if not initially known, using the water deprivation test and ADH test. Subsequent diagnostics may be needed to identify additional disease processes which may have resulted in DI.

5. **Manage NDI (ADH insensitive) with pharmacotherapy**
   - Thiazide diuretics (e.g., hydrochlorothiazide [HCTZ]) in combination with a low-sodium diet are the major form of therapy for NDI, to reduce the loss of free water in the urine.
   - Chlorpropamide stimulates the release of ADH and facilitates the renal response to ADH.
   - Amiloride hydrochloride (a potassium-sparing diuretic) is the medication of choice for the treatment of lithium-induced NDI.
   - Nonsteroidal anti-inflammatory drugs (NSAIDs) such as indomethacin have been used as adjunctive therapy in NDI.

CARE PLANS FOR DIABETES INSIPIDUS

Deficient fluid volume *related to diuresis secondary to ADH deficiency or altered ADH action*

GOALS/OUTCOMES Within 12 hours of initiating treatment, patient is euvolemic reflected by BP 90/60 mm Hg or greater (or within patient's normal range), mean arterial pressure (MAP) 70 mm Hg or greater, HR 60 to 100 bpm, CVP 2 to 6 mm Hg, urinary output 0.5 to 1.5 ml/kg/hr, intake equal to output plus insensible losses, firm skin turgor, pink and moist mucous membranes, and stable weight. ECG exhibits normal sinus rhythm. Electrolyte values are serum sodium 137 to 147 mEq/L, serum osmolality 275 to 300 mOsm/kg, urine osmolality 300 to 900 mOsm/24 hr, and urine specific gravity 1.010 to 1.030.

NOC Fluid Balance, Electrolyte and Acid-Base Balance, Hydration

Hypovolemia Management
1. Monitor vital signs every 15 minutes until patient is stable for 1 hour. Monitor CVP, MAP, and, if hemodynamic monitoring was in place, pulmonary artery pressure (PAP), and pulmonary capillary wedge pressure (PCWP), if ordered. Consult physician or midlevel practitioner for the following: HR greater than 140 bpm or BP less than 90/60 or decreased 20 mm Hg or greater, or MAP decreased 10 mm Hg or greater from baseline, CVP less than 2 mm Hg, and PAWP less than 6 mm Hg. Manage judiciously in all patients, including brain-dead organ donors.
2. Monitor hydration status: mucous membranes, pulse rate and quality, and BP. Excessive water intake may result in fluid overload, particularly in elders and children.
3. Administer hypotonic solutions (e.g., D_5W, $D_50.25$, or 0.45 NaCl) for intracellular rehydration. Usually, fluids are administered as follows: 1 ml IV fluid for each 1 ml of urine output. In patients with brain injury, moderate diuresis may be permitted to avoid the need for administering osmotic diuretics. Hypernatremia, if present, must be corrected slowly (at a rate no greater than 0.5 mEq/L/hr or 12 mEq/L/day) to prevent cerebral edema, seizures, permanent neurologic damage, or death.
4. Administer vasopressin (DDAVP) as ordered. Observe for and document effects. Also be alert to side effects of therapy: hypertension, cardiac ischemia, and hyponatremia.
5. Weigh patient daily, at the same time and using the same scale and garments to prevent error. Consult physician or midlevel practitioner for weight loss greater than 1 kg/day.
6. Observe for indications of dehydration (e.g., poor skin turgor, delayed capillary refill, weak/thready pulse, dry mucous membranes, hypotension).
7. Monitor for fluid overload, which can occur as a result of rapid infusion of fluid or excessive fluid intake in patients with heart failure: jugular vein distention, dyspnea, crackles (rales), and CVP greater than 12 mm Hg.
8. If urinary catheter has been removed, observe for resolution of nocturia (waking up at night to urinate) and enuresis (bed wetting) as treatment progresses.

Fluid/Electrolyte Management
1. Monitor laboratory studies, observing for an appropriate response to treatment, including a decrease in serum sodium, increase in serum and urine osmolality, and increase in urine specific gravity.
2. Monitor urine specific gravity hourly to evaluate response to therapy. Patients may be allowed to develop hypotonic polyuria between doses of vasopressin to demonstrate persistence of DI when transient DI is suspected.
3. Report lack of improvement or deterioration to the physician or midlevel practitioner. Urine output greater than 200 ml/hr for 2 consecutive hours, or 500 ml/hrs in the presence of risk factors should be reported.

4. Instruct patients with permanent DI to wear a medical-alert bracelet labeled with DI. Immediate family members should be familiar with the patient's current treatment plan in case they are contacted in an emergency.

NIC Fluid Monitoring; Intravenous (IV) Therapy; Invasive Hemodynamic Monitoring; Electrolyte Management: Hypernatremia

Disturbed sensory perception (visual and auditory) *resulting from hyperosmolality, dehydration, or hypernatremia*

GOALS/OUTCOMES Patient verbalizes orientation to time, place, and person; patient is protected from unnecessary complications and bodily injury.
NOC Cognitive Orientation

Surveillance
1. Monitor neurologic status frequently. Notify physician or midlevel practitioner of deterioration.
2. Keep bed in lowest position with side rails raised, if patient is confused.
3. Consider nasogastric tube with suction for comatose or brain-dead organ donor patients to decrease likelihood of aspiration.
4. Elevate head of the bed (HOB) to 30 degrees to minimize the risk of aspiration.

NIC Neurologic Monitoring

Risk for infection *related to inadequate primary defenses secondary to incisional opening into sella turcica for patients who have undergone transphenoidal hypophysectomy*

GOALS/OUTCOMES Patient is free of infection as evidenced by normothermia; verbalization of orientation to time, place, and person; and absence of cerebrospinal fluid (CSF) leakage or nuchal rigidity. HR 100 bpm or less, BP within patient's normal range, white blood cell (WBC) count 11,000/mm^3 or less, and negative culture results.
NOC Infection Severity, Immune Status

Infection Protection
1. *For patients who have undergone transphenoidal hypophysectomy,* inspect nasal packing often for frank bleeding or evidence of CSF leak. If glucose is detected in clear nasal drainage (tested using a glucose reagent stick), CSF is leaking, which indicates a flaw in cranial bone integrity. (See *Care of the Patient After Intracranial Surgery,* p 638.)
2. Elevate the HOB to minimize the chance of bacterial migration into the brain if CSF leak is suspected. Consult physician or midlevel practitioner promptly.
3. Monitor for infection, including elevated temperature, nuchal rigidity, and altered LOC.
4. Monitor for increased WBC count, which initially may reflect dehydration or the stress response.
5. Since patient is at higher risk for bacterial infection, invasive lines should be managed carefully to avoid bloodstream infection (BSI). Central lines should be removed as soon as possible.
6. To prevent injury and contamination of operative site, patients should not brush their teeth until instructed to do so by physician. Provide sponge-tipped applicators for oral hygiene.

NIC Incision Site Care; Infection Protection; Neurologic Monitoring

Deficient knowledge: Illness Care *related to the need to manage transient to permanent DI and possible management of additional hormonal imbalance if anterior pituitary was damaged or removed; care after transphenoidal hypophysectomy*

GOALS/OUTCOMES Before discharge from ICU, patient verbalizes understanding of the basics of DI management and care after transphenoidal hypophysectomy, if appropriate.
NOC Knowledge: Illness Care; Knowledge: Medication; Knowledge: Treatment Regimen

Teaching: Procedure/Treatment
1. Teach patient appropriate administration of exogenous vasopressin and its side effects.
2. Explain exogenous hormone replacement if the anterior pituitary gland was damaged or removed during surgery. If patient is also experiencing anterior pituitary dysfunction (panhypopituitarism), teach the indicators of hormone replacement excess or deficiency.
   - *Adrenal hormone excess:* weight gain, moon face, easy bruising, fatigue, polyuria, polydipsia
   - *Adrenal hormone deficiency:* weight loss, easy fatigability, abdominal pain, excess pigmentation
   - *Thyroid hormone excess:* heat intolerance, irritability, tachycardia, weight loss, diaphoresis
   - *Thyroid hormone deficiency:* bradycardia, cold intolerance, weight gain, slowed mentation
   - *Androgen replacement deficiency:* some degree of sexual dysfunction, ranging from menstrual irregularities to infertility and impotence
3. Demonstrate the method for accurate measurement of urine specific gravity and the importance of keeping accurate records of test results.
4. Teach when to seek medical attention, including signs of dehydration (hypernatremia) and water intoxication (hyponatremia).
5. Explain the importance of obtaining a medical-alert bracelet and identification (ID) card.
6. Stress the importance of continued medical follow-up.
7. For patients with permanent need for hormone replacement, explain the method for obtaining a medical-alert bracelet and ID card outlining diagnosis and appropriate treatment in the event of an emergency.

NIC Teaching: Disease Process; Teaching: Prescribed Medication; Emotional Support

ADDITIONAL NURSING DIAGNOSES
If patient has developed DI following a transphenoidal hypophysectomy, see *Decreased intracranial adaptive capacity, Ineffective breathing pattern, Risk for infection,* and *Pain* in *Care of the Patient After Intracranial Surgery,* p. 638; also see *Hypernatremia* and *Hyponatremia* in *Fluid and Electrolyte Disturbances,* p 37.)

HYPERGLYCEMIA

PATHOPHYSIOLOGY
Management of hyperglycemia (elevated blood glucose level) in hospitalized patients has been a key factor in collaborative care since late in 2001, when a landmark study by Van den Berghe and colleagues resulted in dramatic improvement in outcomes of postoperative cardiovascular surgical intensive care patients when glucose was maintained within normal range (80 to 110 mg/dl) using an IV insulin infusion. The practice of normalizing blood glucose was termed "tight glycemic control." Values in excess of 110 mg/dl were regarded as hyperglycemia after the study, versus the previously accepted value of 126 mg/dl, the threshold fasting blood sugar level associated with a diagnosis of diabetes mellitus. A subset of patients *without* diabetes mellitus are hyperglycemic as a result of an exaggerated stress response. Prior to 2001, most care providers were prompted to manage hyperglycemia solely in patients with diabetes mellitus.

Patients in the Van den Berghe study who received tight glycemic control for new-onset hyperglycemia realized a much greater improvement in outcomes than did patients with diabetes mellitus, a particularly difficult concept for the medical community to accept. A subset of those with "new-onset" hyperglycemia were found to be undiagnosed diabetics, which prompted a recommendation that all patients undergo glycohemoglobin screening (hemoglobin A1c) performed on hospital admission. Assessment of glycemic control prior to hospitalization helps care providers anticipate whether patients will need insulin following hospitalization. Those with diabetes mellitus may be discharged on oral hypoglycemic agents or insulin. "Stress responders" without diabetes generally do not require insulin following hospitalization, because the stress of their illness or procedure resolves.

Hyperglycemia

RESEARCH BRIEF 8-3

This prospective, randomized, controlled study involved 1548 adults admitted to a surgical intensive care unit receiving mechanical ventilation. On admission, patients were randomly assigned to receive intensive insulin therapy (blood glucose level maintained at 80 to 110 mg/dl) or conventional treatment of blood glucose levels greater than 215 mg/dl lowered to target 180 to 200 mg/dl. After 12 months of study, intensive insulin therapy reduced ICU mortality to 4.6% from 8.0% with conventional therapy ($p < 0.04$ with adjustment for sequential analyses). For patients who remained in the unit longer than 5 days, mortality using intensive insulin therapy was reduced to 10.6% from 20.2% using conventional therapy. Total in-hospital mortality of the study population was reduced by 34%, bloodstream infections by 46%, acute renal failure requiring dialysis or hemofiltration by 41%, the median number of red blood cell transfusions by 50%, and critical illness polyneuropathy by 44%. The greatest reduction in mortality involved deaths due to multiple organ failure with a proven sepsis focus.

From Van den Berghe G, et al: Intensive insulin therapy in critically ill patients. *N Engl J Med* 345(19):1359-1367, 2001.

Care providers aware of the evolving research began practicing tight glycemic control. Organizations not traditionally focused on blood glucose control, including the Society of Critical Care Medicine, the American Association of Critical Care Nurses, and corresponding international societies, were challenged by the problem of hyperglycemia. Normalization of blood glucose was considered "best practice." Numerous studies ensued to discern how glucose control was suddenly thrust into the forefront of management of hospitalized patients. Despite recommendations by numerous professional societies, to date, less than 10% of hospitals have implemented glycemic control programs for all patients.

Ongoing studies have yielded variable findings using tight glycemic control. Favorable results include a reduction in morbidity and mortality, decreased incidence of sepsis and wound infections, decreased need for blood transfusions, and lower incidence of acute renal failure requiring hemodialysis. Tight glycemic control has been shown in selected studies to reduce morbidity associated with stroke, acute coronary syndromes, vascular disease, community-acquired pneumonia, and other medical-surgical diagnoses. Without glucose control, many patients studied had longer length of hospital stay and increased morbidity and mortality compared with those with tight glycemic control.

There is no question that controlling glucose in hospitalized patients improves outcomes, but defining a safe target range has been challenging. The range of control has undergone rigorous debate, and has become the focal point of studies, without regard to the different IV insulin dosing regimens used for each study. Rather than focusing on how insulin should be dosed for differing patient populations, an ongoing debate ensued regarding whether 80 to 110 mg/dl was a safe goal for all critically ill patients, because along with positive results, many studies resulted in increased incidence of hypoglycemia. Exploring the efficacy of various insulin dosing regimens in controlling hyperglycemia while avoiding life-threatening hypoglycemia (less than 40 mg/dl) has not been a priority. Researchers have sought a universally accepted, safe range of blood glucose control that can be attained using all dosage protocols in all patient populations without adverse effects. To compound the difficulty of this monumental task, the definition of hypoglycemia has been inconsistent.

Physicians create insulin titration regimens, because no one method of insulin dosing has been universally accepted. Unlike the frequent titration of medications used to manage hypotension or hypertension, most dosage adjustments of IV insulin infusions are done hourly, because a continuous reading of glucose level is not possible. Dose responses are more difficult to assess. Few protocols individualize dosing based on insulin sensitivity or resistance. Individualization increases the complexity of care if nurses must perform mathematical calculations to make dosing adjustments.

Technology has evolved in response to research supporting tight glycemic control. Several computerized IV insulin dosing systems are available to lessen the burden of mathematical calculations being done by nurses. With the raging debate regarding safety of tight glycemic control in all patient populations, less than 5% of hospitals in the United States have been comfortable investing in the equipment.

In early 2009, the NICE SUGAR trial highlighted that the incidence of hypoglycemia was unacceptably high when tight control was used in many studies. The American Diabetes Association (ADA) and American Association of Clinical Endocrinologists (AACE) moved away from recommending tight glycemic control for hospitalized patients and created a less stringent guideline recommending that critically ill patients be controlled to blood glucose values of 140 to 180 mg/dl. For more stable hospitalized patients who are eating meals, the recommendation became for premeal blood glucose values to be less than 140 mg/dl. The change prompted confusion and controversy within hospitals with a low incidence of hypoglycemia using tight glycemic control. Centers that realized improved outcomes using tight control may not embrace the new guidelines, while others may compromise, using a target range such as 90 to 140 mg/dl.

Krinsley's research revealed that extreme variations in glucose are associated with poorer outcomes. Insulin dosing regimens with little ability to be individualized have caused severe drops in glucose, prompting administration of 50% dextrose solution to recover patients. Patients with hyperglycemia due to an exaggerated stress response often respond to insulin differently than do patients with diabetes mellitus already receiving either insulin or oral hypoglycemic agents. Many insulin dosing protocols failed to consider patient condition and other care environment variables, and thus were more likely to result in hypoglycemia. A myriad of factors impact glucose control.

Varying methods are used by care providers who may lack the knowledge of how to appropriately monitor blood glucose when insulin is given. Some centers rely on laboratory glucose readings instead of POC testing. POC testing can be done more frequently, with timelier availability of results, affording a better opportunity for insulin dosage adjustments. Several studies have cast doubt on the accuracy of POC testing systems, because hemoglobin level has been shown to affect results. Those with higher hematocrit readings may have lower glucose readings.

Hospitals also struggle with the logistics involved with safe blood glucose control. Staffing, skill level, movement of patients around the hospital for procedures, adjustments in diet, delivery of meal trays, medication delivery systems, ability to perform POC glucose testing, and other factors impact the ability to control hyperglycemia. Hyperglycemic and hypoglycemic emergencies result.

Although both quality organizations and insurers acknowledge the challenges of glycemic control, as of October 2009, the occurrences of hypoglycemia, diabetic ketoacidosis (DKA), and hyperglycemic hyperosmolar syndrome (HHS) have been considered "never events" for hospitalized patients. Hospital-acquired conditions that are considered preventable are termed "never events" for hospitalized patients. If patients are admitted with the conditions present, the hospital is paid if they recur, but if the same conditions occur in patients without a history, the events are considered preventable. Careful admission screening of all patients related to past experience with both hyperglycemia and hypoglycemia is of paramount importance to realize payment for treatment of the patients. Despite the difficulties, hospitals must prevent both hyperglycemic and hypoglycemic crises or risk not being paid for care associated with managing the crises and sequelae.

DIABETIC KETOACIDOSIS

PATHOPHYSIOLOGY

DKA is a life-threatening complication of diabetes mellitus characterized by hyperglycemic crisis, ketosis, acidosis, hypovolemic shock due to dehydration, and electrolyte imbalance involving potassium. Progressive hyperglycemia occurs due to inadequate circulating insulin, preventing cellular uptake of glucose and resulting in a state of starvation at the cellular level. Starvation prompts glucagon secretion from the pancreas and release of other stress hormones including catecholamines, cortisol, and growth hormone (GH), which facilitate glycogenolysis and gluconeogenesis, further raising plasma glucose. Proteolysis and lipolysis ensue, forming free fatty acids, which are converted to ketoacids (acetoacetate, beta-hydroxybutyrate, and acetone), due to lack of intracellular glucose required for normal metabolic conversion of the acids.

Accumulation of ketones creates a metabolic acidosis. The excessive glucose and ketones in the blood cause severe osmotic diuresis as intracellular fluids move into the vascular compartment to dilute the blood; however, the excess fluid is eliminated by the kidneys, which also lose the ability to effectively eliminate excess glucose. A vicious cycle of progressive metabolic disruption begins and will continue until hydration, insulin, and additional management of acidosis/fluid and electrolyte imbalance are provided. Osmotic diuresis causes loss of sodium, potassium, phosphorus, magnesium, and body water, which leads to dehydration and, possibly, hypovolemic shock. Increased blood viscosity and platelet aggregation can result in thromboembolism.

Despite significant loss of potassium in the urine, the patient may initially manifest normal or elevated plasma potassium because of the dramatic shift of potassium out of the cells secondary to insulin deficiency, acidosis, and tissue catabolism. Dehydration lowers BP and decreases tissue perfusion, and cells begin anaerobic metabolism. The resulting lactic acid waste products worsen acidosis. Low pH stimulates the respiratory center, producing deep, rapid, *Kussmaul* respirations. Abundant plasma ketones cause fruity or acetone breath. If not managed, elevated serum osmolality, acidosis, and dehydration depress consciousness to a coma state. Death can result.

The cause of death in patients with DKA and the other hyperglycemic emergency, HHS, rarely results from the metabolic complications of hyperglycemia or metabolic acidosis. Death is related to the underlying medical illness that caused the metabolic decompensation. Successful treatment depends on a prompt and careful evaluation for the precipitating cause(s). The clinical symptoms of DKA generally appear within 24 hours of failure to manage hyperglycemia.

HYPERGLYCEMIC HYPEROSMOLAR SYNDROME

PATHOPHYSIOLOGY

HHS is a life-threatening emergency created by a relative insulin deficiency and significant insulin resistance, resulting in severe hyperglycemia, with profound osmotic diuresis leading to life-threatening dehydration and hyperosmolality. HHS is also known as hyperosmolar hyperglycemic state, hyperosmolar nonketotic syndrome (HONK), hyperosmolar nonketotic state (HNS), hyperglycemia hyperosmolar nonketotic syndrome (HHNS) and, traditionally, hyperosmolar hyperglycemic nonketotic coma (HHNK). HHNK, HHNS, HNS, and HONK are somewhat incorrect titles for the syndrome, as recent evidence reveals a mild degree of ketosis is often present with HHS, and true coma is uncommon. The mortality rate of HHS ranges from 10% to 50%, higher than that for DKA (1.2% to 9%). Mortality data are difficult to interpret because of the high incidence of coexisting diseases or comorbidities.

Historically, HHS and DKA were described as distinct syndromes, but one third of patients exhibit findings of both conditions. HHS and DKA may be at opposite ends of a range of decompensated diabetes, differing in time of onset, degree of dehydration, and severity of ketosis. HHS occurs most commonly in older people with type 2 diabetes, but with the recent obesity epidemic, occasionally obese children and teenagers with both diagnosed and undiagnosed type 2 diabetes manifest HHS. The cascade of events in HHS begins with osmotic diuresis. Glycosuria impairs the ability of the kidney to concentrate urine, which exacerbates the water loss. Normally, the kidneys eliminate glucose above a certain threshold and prevent a subsequent rise in blood glucose level. In HHS, the decreased intravascular volume or possible underlying renal disease decreases the glomerular filtration rate (GFR), causing the glucose level to increase. More water is lost than sodium, resulting in hyperosmolarity. Insulin is present, but not in adequate amounts to decrease blood glucose levels, and with type 2 diabetes, significant insulin resistance is present. DKA and HHS are compared in Table 8-3.

Primary causes of HHS include infections, noncompliance with a diabetes management regimen, undiagnosed diabetes, medications, substance abuse, and coexisting diseases. Infections are the leading cause (57% of patients); pneumonia (often gram negative) is the most common, followed by UTI and sepsis. Lack of compliance with diabetic medications or other aspects of diabetes management may be a frequent cause (21%). Undiagnosed diabetes prompts a failure to recognize early symptoms of the complications of unmanaged hyperglycemia. Acute coronary syndrome (MI), stroke, pulmonary embolus, and mesenteric thrombosis have caused HHS. In urban populations, at least one study revealed the three leading causes to be lack of

Table 8-3	COMPARISON OF DIABETIC KETOACIDOSIS (DKA) AND HYPERGLYCEMIC HYPEROSMOLAR SYNDROME (HHS)	
Criterion	**DKA**	**HHS**
Diabetes type	Type 1	Type 2; rarely, Type 1
Typical age group	More common in young children and adolescents than adults	57-69 yrs, with average age 60 yrs
Signs and symptoms	Polyuria, polydipsia, polyphagia, weakness, orthostatic hypotension, lethargy, changes in LOC, fatigue, nausea, vomiting, abdominal pain	Same as DKA, but slower onset Also, very commonly, neurologic symptoms predominate
Physical assessment	Dry and flushed skin, poor skin turgor, dry mucous membranes, decreased BP, tachycardia, altered LOC (irritability, lethargy, coma), Kussmaul respirations, fruity odor to the breath	Same as DKA, but no Kussmaul respirations or fruity odor to the breath; instead, occurrence of tachypnea with shallow respirations
History and risk factors	Recent stressors such as surgery, trauma, infection, MI; insufficient exogenous insulin; undiagnosed type 1 diabetes mellitus	Undiagnosed type 2 diabetes mellitus; recent stressors such as surgery, trauma, pancreatitis, MI, infection; high-calorie enteral or parenteral feedings in a compromised patient; use of diabetogenic drugs (e.g., phenytoin, thiazide diuretics, thyroid preparations, mannitol, corticosteroids, sympathomimetics)
Monitoring parameters	*ECG:* Dysrhythmias associated with hyperkalemia: peaked T waves, widened QRS complex, prolonged PR interval, flattened or absent P wave. Hypokalemia (K^+ <3 mEq/L), which may produce depressed ST segments, flat or inverted T waves, or increased ventricular dysrhythmias	ECG evidence of hypokalemia as listed with DKA *Hemodynamic measurements:* CVP >3 mm Hg below patient's baseline; PADP and PAWP >4 mm Hg below patient's baseline
Diagnostic tests	*Serum glucose:* Greater than 250 mg/dl	Greater than 600 mg/dl
	Serum ketones: Large presence	Usually absent to mild presence due to dehydration
	Urine glucose: Positive	Positive
	Urine acetone: "Large"	Usually Negative
	Serum osmolality: Greater than 290 mOsm/L	Greater than 320 mOsm/L
	Bicarbonate: Less than 15 mEq/L	Greater than 15 mEq/L
	Serum pH: <7.2	Normal or mildly acidotic (pH < 7.4)
	Anion Gap: Elevated greater than 13	Normal
	Serum potassium: normal or elevated >5.0 mEq/L initially and then decreased	Normal or <3.5 mEq/L
	Serum sodium: elevated, normal, or low	Elevated, normal, or low
	Serum Hct: elevated because of osmotic diuresis with hemoconcentration	Elevated because of hemoconcentration
	BUN: elevated >20 mg/dl	Elevated
	Serum creatinine: >1.5 mg/dl	Elevated

Hyperglycemia

Continued

Table 8-3	COMPARISON OF DIABETIC KETOACIDOSIS (DKA) AND HYPERGLYCEMIC HYPEROSMOLAR SYNDROME (HHS)—cont'd	
Criterion	**DKA**	**HHS**
	Serum phosphorus, magnesium, *chloride:* decreased	Elevated
	WBC: elevated, even in the absence of infection	Normal unless infection present
Onset	A few days	Days to weeks
Mortality	1-10%	14%–58% because of age group and complications such as stroke, thrombosis, renal failure

BP, Blood pressure; *BUN,* blood urea nitrogen; *CVP,* central venous pressure; *DKA,* diabetic ketoacidosis; *ECG,* electrocardiogram; *Hct,* hematocrit; *HHS,* hyperglycemic hyperosmolar syndrome; *LOC,* level of consciousness; *MI,* myocardial infarction; *PADP,* pulmonary artery diastolic pressure; *PAWP,* pulmonary artery wedge pressure; *WBC,* white blood cell count.

compliance with medications, drinking alcohol, and use of cocaine. Chronic use of steroids and gastroenteritis are commonly associated with HHS in children.

The blood glucose level is higher with HHS than with DKA. A global electrolyte loss is present. Sodium and potassium levels vary at diagnosis, but deficiencies of both are present. Magnesium, calcium, phosphate, and chloride deficiencies evolve. Patients may lose from 15% to 25% of total body water or approximately 100 to 200 ml/kg. Fluids are drawn from cells to dilute the concentrated bloodstream. Significant intracellular dehydration results. Neurologic deficits occur in response to severe dehydration and hyperosmolality. The blood is highly viscous, and flow slows, increasing risk for the formation of thromboemboli. Increased cardiac workload and decreased renal and cerebral blood flow may result in MI, renal failure, and stroke.

Unlike DKA, wherein acidosis produces severe symptoms, HHS develops slowly, and frequently symptoms are nonspecific. Polyuria and polydipsia occur but may be ignored. Neurologic deficits may be mistaken for senility. Similarity of symptoms to other disease processes in older adults may delay diagnosis and treatment, allowing the process to progress.

METABOLIC ASSESSMENT: HYPERGLYCEMIA
Goal of Metabolic Assessment
Evaluate for degree of hyperglycemia and its effects on overall hemodynamics, respiratory rate/pattern, and mental status. Hyperglycemia may be asymptomatic or, with DKA, result in hypotension causing decreased perfusion, increased work of breathing with Kussmaul respirations, ineffective breathing patterns, abdominal pain, and neurologic deficits including coma and/or strokelike symptoms. HHS findings are similar but are more likely to result in neurologic changes, cause abdominal pain less often, and almost never cause compensatory Kussmaul respirations, because acidosis is mild, if present at all. Dehydration, hyperglycemia, and acidosis must be managed immediately. Associated electrolyte imbalances may be managed as the patient's glucose level normalizes and hydration is provided.

History and Risk Factors
Hyperglycemia manifests more commonly in hospitalized patients with diabetes mellitus or impaired glucose tolerance than in normal patients with an exaggerated response to stress. Obese patients are more likely to have insulin resistance associated with metabolic syndrome, impaired tolerance for glucose, or undiagnosed type 2 diabetes mellitus. Type 2 diabetic patients generally manifest HHS when hyperglycemia is ineffectively managed. Rarely, a type 2 patient will manifest DKA. The majority of patients with DKA have type 1 diabetes mellitus. The type 1 patient will die without adequate insulin administration.

Recent stressors that prompt DKA in patients with diabetes mellitus include:

- *Infection (20% to 55%):* May be overestimated because DKA may prompt leukocytosis and vasodilation, which mimic sepsis.
- *Inadequate insulin/noncompliance (15% to 40%):* Teenagers may be at higher risk for noncompliance; all illnesses increase stress, which increases the need for insulin. Type 1 patients are totally reliant on administration of exogenous insulin to control hyperglycemia, because without functional beta islet cells in the pancreas, they have no ability to produce insulin.
- *Undiagnosed diabetes (10% to 25%):* Onset of type 1 diabetes is generally preceded by a significant illness—often a viral infection or childhood disease.
- *Other medical illness (10% to 15%):* Pneumonia, urinary tract infection, ischemic bowel, pregnancy, hypothyroidism, pancreatitis, pulmonary embolism, surgery, and new medications (notably corticosteroids, sympathomimetics, alpha and beta blockers, fluoroquinolone antibiotics [Levaquin], and diuretics)
- *Cardiovascular disease (3% to 10%):* Significant cardiovascular disease may be the result of diabetes mellitus, and subsequently, unstable patients may experience variable stress levels making control of hyperglycemia difficult. Vascular events such as MI, cerebrovascular accident (CVA), or ischemic bowel may precipitate or worsen DKA.
- *Cause unknown (5% to 35%):* Any physiologically stressing illness or event has the potential to cause the condition. Certain women are more likely to go into DKA at the time of menstruation. Severe emotional stress is associated with onset of DKA.

Recent stressors that prompt HHS in patients with diabetes mellitus:

- *Diabetes:* First symptomatic presentation of undiagnosed hyperglycemia; poor control of hyperglycemia (noncompliance, inadequate resources, abuse or neglect of patient by caregivers or self-inflicted, accidental omission of medication, or ingestion of excessive carbohydrates)
- *Associated medical conditions*
  1. Infection: urinary tract, pneumonia, cellulitis, sepsis, dental infection/abscess
  2. MI or other acute coronary syndromes
  3. Stroke or intracranial hemorrhage
  4. Temperature alteration: hyperthermia or hypothermia
  5. Mesenteric ischemia: intestinal/bowel ischemia or bowel infarction
  6. Pancreatitis
  7. Pulmonary embolism
  8. Acute abdomen
  9. Acute renal failure or decompensated chronic renal failure ("acute on chronic")
  10. Burns
  11. Hyperthyroidism
  12. GI bleeding
  13. Cushing syndrome or other ACTH-secreting tumor
- *Medication related*
  14. Beta blockers (metoprolol, atenolol, inderal)
  15. Carbonic anhydrase inhibitors (diazoxide)
  16. Calcium channel blockers (diltiazem, verapamil)
  17. Chlorpromazine or other antipsychotics (olanzepine)
  18. Diuretics (*loop:* furosemide, bumetanide; *thiazide:* HCTZ)
  19. Glucose-containing fluids (total parenteral nutrition, tube feedings, dialysis solutions)
  20. Glucocorticoid/steroids (cortisone, hydrocortisone, prednisone)
  21. H_2-receptor antagonists (ranitidine, cimetidine)
  22. Phenytoin or other anticonvulsants
  23. Substance abuse: alcohol, amphetamines, cocaine, MDMA ("ecstasy")

Vital Signs

- Findings vary significantly, depending on patient's situation.
- Hyperglycemia alone may have no effect on vital signs.
- Tachycardia and tachypnea are present if a hyperglycemic crisis (DKA, HHS) is present.
- Hypotension is present with DKA and HHS.
- Hypovolemia alone may prompt tachycardia.

Observation

- Hyperglycemia alone may not cause overt physical assessment changes.
- Skin should be examined for lesions, rashes, cellulitis, and other signs of possible infection.
- If patient presents to the emergency department, observe for signs of recent alcohol consumption.
- *With DKA:* Kussmaul respirations (rapid, deep) are present to exhale CO_2 as a compensatory response to relieve metabolic acidosis; may appear fatigued, with or without diaphoresis from Kussmaul breathing
- *With DKA and HHS:*
  1. Significant abdominal pain is present in at least 40% of patients; paralytic ileus or gastroparesis may be present, but will resolve when hyperglycemia and dehydration are managed.
  2. Ashen, pale or gray/blue facial color, lip color, or nail beds from severe hypotension and hypoperfusion due to dehydration
  3. Signs of dehydration: poor skin turgor, dry mouth/lips, sunken eyes, slow capillary refill
  4. Generalized weakness, possible exhaustion, nausea and vomiting, impaired vision and leg cramps may be present; patients may become unable to get out of bed.
  5. Cranial nerve examination may be abnormal, with nerve palsies present.
  6. Altered LOC (confusion, disorientation, agitation) is more common with older adults; strokelike symptoms may be present; coma is present in about 10% of patients presenting with HHS; seizures are present in 25% of HHS patients.
  7. If severe shock has ensued, agitation is more commonly associated with hypoxemia, while somnolence is associated with hypercarbia (elevated carbon dioxide level) and acidosis.
  8. Associated findings: patient may manifest symptoms of heart failure, pneumonia, and other risk factors if hyperglycemic crisis is present.

Auscultation

- Hyperglycemia does not change baseline physical assessment unless it has progressed to crisis level (DKA, HHS).
- Clear breath sounds with DKA and HHS because dehydration is present.
- Bowel sounds may be absent if paralytic ileus and gastroparesis are present with DKA and HHS.
- Heart sounds may reflect heart failure with DKA and HHS.

Palpation

- *For DKA:* Abdomen may be palpated if abdominal pain is present.

Percussion

- *For DKA and HHS:* Lung percussion may reveal presence of consolidation or fluid (dullness) indicative of a pulmonary infection.

Screening Labwork

- POC capillary blood glucose (bedside glucose monitoring)
- If POC glucose is elevated, a plasma glucose sample should be drawn.
- In addition, if DKA or HHS is suspected:
  1. *ABG analysis:* Done promptly to evaluate for acidosis, hypoxemia, and hypercapnia
  2. *CBC:* Evaluates for elevated WBCs indicative of infection
  3. *Sputum and urine culture and sensitivity:* Identifies infecting organism
  4. *Blood culture and sensitivity:* If positive, indicates organism has migrated into the bloodstream to cause a systemic infection

Diagnostic Tests for Hyperglycemia and Hyperglycemic Emergencies

Test	Purpose	Abnormal Findings
Hemoglobin A1c (HbA1c) or glycosylated hemoglobin Performing this test more frequently than every 6–8 weeks does not yield useful information about blood glucose control	Assesses for control of blood glucose for the 6 to 8 weeks preceding the test. Recommended screening for all hospitalized patients so poorly controlled blood glucose readings can be addressed immediately to avoid development of DKA (diabetic ketoacidosis) or HHS (hyperglycemia hyperosmolar syndrome)	HbA1c >7 reflects poor control. AACE and ADA guidelines have varied; stricter guidelines recommend patients with HbA1c >6 have inadequate control. If a patient with diabetes mellitus who has been managing at home presents with an elevated value, home management and medications should be adjusted. If a patient without diabetes has an elevated value, the patient should undergo a full evaluation for presence of undiagnosed diabetes.
Fasting blood glucose (FBG) Test is performed in the morning after fasting all night and prior to consuming breakfast	Evaluates the effectiveness of basal insulin dosage by assessing for presence of hyperglycemia or hypoglycemia; used for daily screening of blood glucose control during hospitalization	<40 mg/dl: Severe hypoglycemia 41–69 mg/dl: Hypoglycemia 70–110mg/dl: Normoglycemia 111–125mg/dl: Borderline hyperglycemia 126–180mg/dl: Hyperglycemia 181–220mg/dl: Significant hyperglycemia >220 mg/dl: Possible impending DKA or HHNS if glucose is not managed
Mealtime blood glucose Generally, a point-of-care (POC) reading is done either 15 to 30 minutes prior to a meal, or as the meal begins.	Assesses blood glucose control with existing hyperglycemia management program	If reading is <140 mg/dl (2009 AACE and ADA recommendation), no mealtime, short acting, subcutaneous insulin is needed. The recommendations have not been universally accepted. Thresholds for supplemental insulin vary with each hospital and sometimes, each physician.
Postprandial blood glucose May be done 1 or 2 hours following meals using serum glucose or point of care capillary glucose readings	Evaluates ability of glucose to normalize following a meal. Readings may be done 1 or 2 hours following the meal.	>180 mg/dl: If glucose is >180 at 1 hour following a meal, the patient is unable to produce enough insulin, or has not received enough mealtime insulin, or may be insulin resistant, or may require initiation of mealtime insulin. >140 mg/dl: If glucose is >140 at 2 hours following a meal, the patient is unable to produce enough insulin or may be insulin resistant.
Oral glucose tolerance test (OGTT) Following at least 8 hours of fasting, oral glucose is consumed by the patient to determine how quickly it is cleared from the blood.	Used to test for diabetes, insulin resistance, and reactive hypoglycemia. Fasting blood glucose (FBG) is used at the beginning of the test. Additional readings are done 2 hours later. Fasting readings are compared to 2 hours post glucose ingestion to determine extent of glucose intolerance.	FBG >126 mg/dl with 2-hour reading >200 mg/dl: Confirms diagnosis of diabetes mellitus (DM) FBG 111–125 mg/dl with 2-hour reading >140 mg/dl: Patient has impaired glucose tolerance (IGT) FBG 111–125mg/dl with 2-hour reading <140 mg/dl: Patient has impaired fasting glucose (IFT)

Continued

Hyperglycemia

Diagnostic Tests for Hyperglycemia and Hyperglycemic Emergencies — cont'd

Test	Purpose	Abnormal Findings
Arterial blood gas analysis (ABG) Done promptly, following confirmation of hyperglycemia to assess for DKA and HHS.	Assess for abnormal gas exchange or compensation for metabolic derangements in patients in hyperglycemic crisis; profound acidosis can indicate DKA is present, since HHS typically presents with minimal to mild acidosis unless prolonged, severe hypovolemic shock is present.	pH changes: With DKA, may be 6.8–7.2; acidosis results from ketosis or lactic acidosis Carbon dioxide: With DKA, decreased CO_2 reflects tachypnea and Kussmaul respirations Hypoxemia: With DKA or HHS, PaO_2 <80 mm Hg may indicate pneumonia precipitated the crisis Oxygen saturation: If pneumonia or heart failure is present, SaO_2 may be <92% Bicarbonate: HHS: HCO_3^- 15-22 mEq/L; DKA: HCO_3^- may be <15 mEq/L Base deficit: HHS <−2; with DKA, <−10
Complete blood count (CBC)	Evaluates for presence of infection	Increased WBC count: >11,000/mm³ is seen with bacterial pneumonias, urinary tract infections and other infections.
Sputum Gram stain, culture and sensitivity	Screens for pneumonia, a common underlying cause of hyperglycemic crisis; identifies infecting organism	Gram stain positive: Indicates organism is present; Culture: Identifies organism Sensitivity: Reflects effectiveness of drugs on identified organism.
Blood culture and sensitivity	Screens for sepsis, a common underlying cause of hyperglycemic crisis Identifies whether an organism has become systemic	Secondary bacteremia: a frequent finding; patients with bacteremia are at higher risk for developing respiratory failure.
Blood chemistry	Screens for electrolyte imbalances; potassium imbalances may create potentially dangerous dysrhythmias	DKA and HHS: Hypernatremia is present: BUN, creatinine, and K^+ may be elevated, normal, or low. Anion gap DKA: >13 Anion gap HHS: 10–12
Plasma osmolality	Screens for elevated osmolality associated with severe hyperglycemia	Osmolality is increased more with HHS than with DKA. DKA: 290–320 mmol/L HHS: >320 mmol/L
Urine ketones	Screens for the presence of ketones to confirm diagnosis of DKA; HHS does not cause ketonuria.	DKA: Ketones strongly positive HHS: Ketones negative, or mildly positive
12-Lead ECG	Used to rule out myocardial infarction as the cause of HHS or DKA	Tall, peaked T waves if ↑K^+ is present prior to management of hyperglycemia, hypovolemia and acidosis; VPCs/ventricular irritability is seen with ↓K^+ seen as insulin normalizes glucose.
Chest radiograph	Screens for pneumonia and acute respiratory distress syndrome, which may prompt DKA and HHS	"Fluffy whiteness" may not initially be present due to dehydration, but may appear as patient is rehydrated revealing pneumonia or ARDS
Computed tomography (CT) brain scan	Screens for ischemic and hemorrhagic stroke, which may prompt DKA and HHS	Generally not done until patient has had at least 1 hour of rehydration and insulin therapy to see if symptoms resolve spontaneously.

COLLABORATIVE MANAGEMENT

When approaching how to manage hyperglycemia in hospitalized patients, the following key elements should be considered when evaluating current management blood glucose control strategies:

1. Oral hypoglycemic agents are not recommended for use in acutely ill or unstable hospitalized patients because the response to therapy is unpredictable. If further glucose control is needed, the use of insulin superimposed on oral hypoglycemic agents may prompt episodes of hypoglycemia.
2. Guidelines should be evidence based and parallel the recommendations of the recognized expert organizations (ADA and AACE).
3. Protocols/order sets must be "user-friendly" and clearly written with minimal abbreviations and strive to keep mathematical calculations to a minimum.
4. A system should be in place to identify patients who need insulin or adjustment in an existing insulin regimen.
5. Variations in nutritional requirements/nutritional support should be identified, recognized, and included in the planning of any insulin dosing regimen for patients with varying levels of stability as they move through the hospital.
6. Requirements for safe insulin administration, including availability of point of care testing, IV pumps that can deliver volumes less than 1 ml accurately, and staffing with competent nurses must be considered prior to implementation of a glycemic control program.
7. Expert nurse consultants and/or certified diabetes educators who can provide diabetes patient education should be available to both patients and staff nurses.
8. An interdisciplinary team should be formed to address the following questions about the hospital's hyperglycemia management practices:
   A. Does the current insulin dosing regimen:
      1) Assume all patients can be placed into one of a few subgroups for dosage adjustment?
      2) Take into consideration the patient's insulin sensitivity and/or insulin resistance when titrating toward the target level?
      3) Provide small, incremental dosage changes to keep the patient safely within the target range without causing extreme fluctuations in glucose (hypoglycemia, when treated, resulting in hyperglycemia)?
      4) Have equipment/infusion reconstitution available for insulin dosage adjustments of 0.1 unit/hr, which several best practice dosing regimens require?
   B. Has the total hyperglycemia management approach been proved to be effective and safe and meet current evidence-based guidelines? Has data been gathered on the patients to measure both glucose control and incidence of hypoglycemia?
   C. Can nurses throughout the hospital safely implement the insulin dosing regimen? During IV insulin infusions and when patients are transitioned from IV to subcutaneous insulin, nurses must be appropriately educated and have sufficient staffing to safely manage the patients.

Care Priorities

1. **Resuscitate patients with severe dehydration in hypovolemic shock:**
   - Evaluate basic ABCs: airway, breathing, and circulation.
   - Intubate and ventilate patients with hypoxemia/decreasing oxygen saturation.
   - Place at least two large-bore IV lines, or have a central line inserted.
   - Monitor continuous ECG, pulse oximetry, and frequent, if not constant, BP.
   - Apply oxygen, or set oxygen appropriately if mechanical ventilation is used.
   - Insert a urinary catheter and monitor urine output judiciously.
   - Consider inserting a nasogastric tube if high risk for aspiration.
2. **Provide aggressive rehydration to replace fluid loss from polyuria:**
   - *HHS:* Large amounts of isotonic IV fluids (normal saline, sometimes greater than 9 L) may be required to rehydrate the patient. Half normal saline is sometimes used. Fluids should not include dextrose. Osmotic diuresis causes a 100 to 200 ml/kg fluid loss. At least 1 L of saline should be administered during the first hour of therapy. Hemodynamic or CVP monitoring may be needed to provide aggressive rehydration, as large amounts of fluids may not be well tolerated in older adults. The remaining 8 L should

ideally be infused within the next 24 hours. Highly viscous blood is prone to thrombosis. Patients are at risk of developing thrombotic complications before, during, and after a severe hyperglycemic crisis.

- *DKA*: Large amounts of nondextrose, isotonic IV fluids are needed. Half normal saline is sometimes used. From 1 to 2 L may be needed over the first 60 to 90 minutes. Approximately 4 L should be infused over the first 5 hours, and then the patient should be reevaluated for need for further hydration. Older patients or those with comorbidities that complicate therapy may require hemodynamic or CVP monitoring to guide fluid replacement. Rehydration improves perfusion, which improves oxygen delivery and thus helps to reestablish aerobic metabolism. As cellular metabolism normalizes, lactic and ketotic acidosis resolve.

3. **Support hemodynamics/perfusion:** Hemodynamic monitoring may be useful in guiding fluid replacement tolerance and efficacy and may help recognize the patient's response to the effects of other comorbidities. Although hypovolemic shock is the primary problem associated with hyperglycemia, cardiogenic shock may ensue if the patient has had an MI, or septic shock is possible if severe infection is present. Use of catecholamine infusions and steroids should be avoided, if possible, until hyperglycemia is resolved.

4. **Control hyperglycemia:** IV insulin infusion may be the most efficacious insulin delivery system to manage hyperglycemia. Insulin dosing should be done taking into consideration the patient's insulin sensitivity or degree of insulin resistance. Type 2 diabetes is associated with significant insulin resistance, while type 1 patients are less likely to be insulin resistant. Insulin-resistant patients will require more insulin than normal patients to resolve hyperglycemia. Highly insulin-sensitive patients may require less. Insulin dosing should strive to reduce the blood glucose at least 15% hourly until the blood glucose approaches 250 mg/dl, when the insulin dosage should be reevaluated. Glucose-containing solutions (5% dextrose), with 20 mEq of added potassium should be initiated to help avoid hypoglycemia and hypokalemia. High doses of insulin facilitate the transport of both glucose and potassium across the cell membrane into the cells from the bloodstream. The probability of both hypoglycemia and hypokalemia is increased as glucose normalizes. The 2009 AACE/ADA recommended glucose target range for critically ill patients is 140 to 180 mg/dl. Once the target range is attained, small incremental doses of insulin should be provided to sustain the patient within the target range. Blood glucose is generally measured hourly as long as aggressive insulin therapy is in progress. Once hyperglycemia is controlled, a recalculated dose of basal (long acting) and mealtime (bolus) subcutaneous insulin should be initiated. Blood glucose levels should be maintained at less than 140 mg/dl prior to meals. If blood glucose levels exceed 140 mg/dl prior to meals, supplemental short-acting insulin is given in addition to mealtime insulin.

5. **Manage electrolyte imbalances, focusing on potassium imbalances:** Prior to rehydration, patients are hypernatremic and may be hyperkalemic. Those with DKA are more likely to be hyperkalemic due to the presence of metabolic acidosis, during which hydrogen ions force K^+ (potassium ions) out of the cells into the bloodstream. As hydration progresses, perfusion improves, acidosis resolves, and potassium moves back into the cells, with a high probability of creating hypokalemia. Potassium replacement should begin, as mentioned in the previous section, when glucose reaches 250 mg/dl, wherein 20 mEq K^+ is added to IV solutions. Replacement of calcium, magnesium, and phosphates may be done as needed. Chlorides are replaced by the normal saline IV solutions. Use of bicarbonate for management of acidosis is not recommended unless the acidosis does not respond to hydration and insulin or when essential medications needed for support of hemodynamics fail to work in the acidotic environment (e.g., if catecholamines are needed to support BP).

6. **Identify and manage the precipitating cause:** As hyperglycemia is managed, further efforts should be under way to identify the cause of the hyperglycemic crisis. A robust listing of risk factors and probable causes was included earlier, with infections and cardiac and vascular occlusive events as the most likely precipitating events for the hyperglycemic crisis. If the pH and anion gap fail to improve with hydration and insulin, other causes of shock and acidosis should be evaluated and managed accordingly.

CARE PLANS FOR HYPERGLYCEMIA

Glucose, risk for unstable blood *related to hyperglycemia resulting from the stress response associated with critical illness, and in those who have or may be at risk for diabetes mellitus*

GOALS/OUTCOMES Patient is free of hyperglycemia reflected by normoglycemia and normovolemia; pH and serum osmolality are within normal limits.

NOC Blood Glucose Level, Hydration

Hyperglycemia Management

- Monitor blood glucose levels as ordered or according to protocol.
- Facilitate patient having HbA1c measured to assess for glycemic control prior to hospitalization. If patient has been transfused, HbA1c is no longer a reliable measure of blood glucose control, as patient is circulating blood that includes another person's glycohemoglobin.
- Assess for signs and symptoms of hyperglycemia including polyuria, polyphagia, blurred vision, headache, change in LOC, weakness, and lethargy.
- Monitor for urine ketones if patient has type 1 diabetes, is a ketosis-prone type 2 diabetic, or manifests severe hyperglycemia.
- Monitor ABGs in severely hyperglycemic patients to assess if acidosis is present.
- Identify possible causes of hyperglycemia and work with physicians to construct an individualized management plan.
- Evaluate hydration status if patient has been hyperglycemic with polyuria due to osmotic diuresis.
- Encourage oral noncaloric fluid/water intake.
- Monitor for potassium imbalance, with awareness that hyperglycemic patients can experience wide variation in potassium when IV insulin therapy is used to control hyperglycemia. As glucose normalizes, hypokalemia may be present and should be managed with careful potassium replacement.
- Instruct patient and significant others on how to prevent, recognize, and manage hyperglycemia.
- Encourage patient to participate in POC testing to assist in refining testing techniques if needed.
- Discuss the need to count and control ingested carbohydrates to provide the best opportunity for glycemic control. Explain the difference in simple (bad) and complex (good) carbohydrates and how they are metabolized.
- Ensure patient understands the need for adherence to the prescribed diet and exercise regimen.
- Assess whether patient has the financial means to procure the proper food and medications to control hyperglycemia following discharge from the hospital.

Hypoglycemia Management

1. Identify patients at increased risk for hypoglycemia.
2. Monitor blood glucose levels carefully as ordered, especially if insulin is used to manage hyperglycemia.
3. Assess for signs and symptoms of hypoglycemia, including changes in personality, irritability, shakiness or tremors, sweating, nervousness, palpitations, tachycardia, nausea, headache, dizziness, weakness, faintness, blurred vision, difficulty concentrating, confusion, coma, or seizures.
4. Maintain IV access for more precise management of hypoglycemia using IV 50% dextrose, rather than glucagon for instances of severe hypoglycemia that render patient unable to take glucose tablets, juice, or milk.
5. Ensure patient is given IV fluids containing 5% dextrose when glucose approaches 250 mg/dl if receiving an IV insulin infusion for management of severe hyperglycemia.
6. Keep patient NPO or on a no-calorie liquid diet while receiving an insulin infusion. If patients receive meals while insulin is infusing, additional mealtime subcutaneous insulin should be given, rather than adjusting IV insulin to cover glucose increases resulting from meals. If the IV insulin infusion is titrated upward throughout the day for meals, when the patient stops eating meals at night, the probability of hypoglycemia is high.
7. Instruct patient and significant others regarding the signs, symptoms, and management of hypoglycemia.
8. Collaborate with patient and care team members to make changes in insulin regimen if hypoglycemic episodes occur more than occasionally.

Fluid volume, deficient *related to hyperglycemia-induced dehydration and osmotic diuresis*

GOALS/OUTCOMES Within 12 hours of initiating treatment, patient is euvolemic as evidenced by BP 90/60 mm Hg or greater (or within patient's normal range), MAP 70 mm Hg or greater, HR 60 to 100 bpm, CVP 8 to 12 mm Hg, balanced I&O, urinary output 0.5 ml/kg/hr or greater, firm skin turgor, and pink and moist mucous membranes. ECG exhibits normal sinus rhythm.

NOC Fluid Balance, Electrolyte and Acid-Base Balance, Hydration

Hypovolemia Management

1. Monitor vital signs every 15 minutes until patient is stable for 1 hour. Monitor CVP, MAP, and possibly PAP and PCWP, if ordered. Consult physician or midlevel practitioner for the following: HR greater than 140 bpm or BP less than 90/60 or decreased 20 mm Hg or greater, or MAP decreased 10 mm Hg or greater from baseline, CVP less than 4 mm Hg, and PAWP less than 6 mm Hg.
2. Monitor hydration status: mucous membranes, pulse rate and quality, and BP.
3. Monitor I&O. Decreased urine output may indicate inadequate fluid volume or impending renal failure. Consult physician for urine output less than 0.5 ml/kg/hr for 2 consecutive hours.
4. Replace volume with IV fluids. Monitor for fluid overload, which can occur as a result of rapid infusion of fluids: jugular vein distention, dyspnea, crackles (rales), and CVP greater than 6 mm Hg.

Fluid/Electrolyte Management

1. Monitor for abnormal electrolyte levels as ordered.
2. Note an increase in anion gap (greater than 14 mEq/L), signaling increased production or decreased excretion of acids. Anion gap should decrease steadily with successful treatment of DKA.
3. Monitor for symptomatic cardiac dysrhythmias. (See *Fluid and Electrolyte Disturbances*, p. 37.)
4. Observe for clinical signs of electrolyte imbalance associated with DKA and its treatment:
   - *Hypokalemia:* Ventricular dysrhythmias, muscle weakness, anorexia, and hypoactive bowel sounds
   - *Hypophosphatemia:* Muscle weakness, malaise, confusion, respiratory failure, decreased oxygen delivery, and decreased cardiac function
   - *Hypomagnesemia:* Anorexia, nausea, vomiting, lethargy, weakness, personality changes, tetany, tremor or muscle fasciculations, seizures, confusion, and difficulty managing hypokalemia
5. Weigh patient daily, and monitor trends.

NIC Fluid Monitoring; Invasive Hemodynamic Monitoring; Acid-Base Management: Metabolic Acidosis; Electrolyte Management: Hypokalemia

---

Risk for infection *related to inadequate secondary defenses (suppressed inflammatory response) due to protein depletion and hyperglycemia*

GOALS/OUTCOMES Patient is free of infection as evidenced by normothermia; HR 100 bpm or less, BP within patient's normal range, WBC count 11,000/mm³ or less, and negative culture results.
NOC Infection Severity, Immune Status

Infection Protection

1. Monitor for signs of infection. Fever may be suppressed secondary to acidosis. Monitor for increased WBC count, which initially may reflect dehydration or the stress response.
2. Since patient is at higher risk for bacterial infection, invasive lines should be managed carefully to avoid bloodstream infection (BSI). Central lines should be removed as soon as possible.
3. Manage urinary catheters meticulously to prevent UTI.
4. Maintain skin integrity. Assess for areas of decreased sensation.

NIC Skin Surveillance

Confusion, Acute *related to hyperosmolality, dehydration, or hypoglycemia*

GOALS/OUTCOMES Patient verbalizes orientation to time, place, and person; patient is protected from unnecessary complications and bodily injury.
NOC Cognitive orientation

Neurologic Monitoring

1. Monitor neurologic status frequently. Notify physician or midlevel practitioner of deterioration.
2. Keep bed in lowest position with side rails raised, if patient is confused.
3. Consider nasogastric tube with suction for comatose patients to decrease likelihood of aspiration.
4. Elevate HOB to 30 degrees to minimize the risk of aspiration.
5. Monitor blood glucose hourly while on insulin infusion. Consult physician or midlevel practitioner if blood glucose drops faster than 100 mg/dl/hr or if it drops to less than 250 mg/dl. Obtain prescription for

glucose-containing IV solution to prevent hypoglycemia and allow the continued administration of insulin necessary to correct acidosis.

NIC Hyperglycemia Management; Hypoglycemia Management

🔻Deficient knowledge *related to new-onset diabetes or misunderstanding of the causes and prevention of DKA or HHS*

GOALS/OUTCOMES By discharge from the ICU, patient can explain causes, symptoms, and prevention of hyperglycemic crises.
NOC Knowledge: Illness Care; Knowledge: Medications; Health-seeking behavior

Teaching: Disease process
1. Consider referral to diabetes educator for new-onset diabetes or if patient has not managed condition well in the past. Provide instructions simply, incorporating patient teaching into patient care routines.
2. Explain the relationship of DKA or HHS to illness and stress. Emphasize importance of adhering to the diabetes regimen, including meal planning, medication, exercise, and monitoring.
3. Review illness guidelines for individuals with diabetes (i.e., need for increased fluid and insulin with illness) with patient and significant others.
4. Provide hospital and community resources for diabetes education and support.
5. Provide address and websites for the American Diabetes Association (ADA): American Diabetes Association, Inc., 18 East 48th Street, New York, NY 10017; www.ada.org and www.diabetes.org

NIC Teaching: Disease Process; Teaching: Prescribed Diet; Teaching: Prescribed Medication; Teaching: Prescribed Activity/Exercise; Emotional Support

ADDITIONAL NURSING DIAGNOSES
See also nursing diagnoses and interventions in *Hyperkalemia, Hypokalemia,* and *Hypovolemia* in *Fluid and Electrolyte Disturbances, p 37; Alterations in Consciousness, p 24; Prolonged Immobility* (p. 149); and *Emotional and Spiritual Support of the Patient and Significant Others* (p. 200).

MYXEDEMA COMA

PATHOPHYSIOLOGY
Myxedema coma is a life-threatening condition that occurs when hypothyroidism is untreated or when a stressor such as infection affects an individual with known/unknown hypothyroidism. The clinical picture of myxedema coma includes exaggerated hypothyroidism, with decreased mental status or coma, hypoventilation, hypothermia, hypotension, seizures, and shock. Myxedema coma usually develops slowly, has a greater than 50% mortality rate, and requires prompt, aggressive treatment. Even with early diagnosis and treatment, mortality is nearly 45%.

Hypothyroidism is a common endocrine disorder reflecting inadequacy of production or uptake of the thyroid hormone. Localized disease of the thyroid gland that results in decreased thyroid hormone production is the most common cause of hypothyroidism. Normally, the thyroid gland releases 100 to 125 nmol of thyroxine (T_4) daily and only small amounts of triiodothyronine (T_3). T_4 is a prohormone functioning as a reservoir for the more metabolically active form of the thyroid hormone, T_3. Primary conversion occurs in the peripheral tissues via 5′-deiodination. Decreased production of T_4 and failure of deiodinization to T_3 causes an increase in the secretion of thyroid-stimulating hormone (TSH) by the functional pituitary gland. TSH stimulates hypertrophy and hyperplasia of the thyroid gland and an increase in thyroid T_4-5′-deiodinase activity. Early in the disease process, compensatory mechanisms maintain T_3 levels; however, this compensatory mechanism may be short lived.

Individuals who are acutely or critically ill may have an extreme disruption of the normal hypothalamic–anterior pituitary–thyroid axis, particularly related to the nocturnal surge that is normally seen with thyrotropin. These patients will have a low T_3 level even after the TSH is restored to normal and are commonly referred to as presenting with low T_3 syndrome. Patients with poor heart function or more intense inflammatory reaction show more pronounced downregulation of the thyroid system. During sepsis, the pituitary gland is activated via blood-borne proinflammatory cytokines and through a complex interaction between the autonomic nervous system and the immune cells. Sepsis elicits a pattern of pituitary hormone dysfunction which may cause a significant decrease in the secretion of TSH.

Hypothyroidism results in inadequate amount of circulating thyroid hormone, causing a decrease in metabolic rate that affects all body systems.

Primary hypothyroidism, the most common presenting form of thyroidal disorders, is caused by thyroid suppression for any direct reason (i.e., cancer, radiation, autoimmune dysfunction).

1. *Autoimmune:* The most frequent cause of acquired hypothyroidism is autoimmune thyroiditis (Hashimoto thyroiditis). The body recognizes the thyroid antigens as foreign, and a chronic immune reaction ensues, resulting in lymphocytic infiltration of the gland and progressive destruction of functional thyroid tissue. Most affected individuals have circulating antibodies to thyroid tissue.

2. *Postpartum thyroiditis:* 10% of postpartum women develop lymphocytic thyroiditis 2 to 10 months after delivery. The frequency may be 5% in women with type 1 diabetes mellitus. The condition may only last 2 to 4 months but usually requires treatment with levothyroxine; however, postpartum patients with lymphocytic thyroiditis are at increased risk of permanent hypothyroidism. The hypothyroid state may be preceded by a short thyrotoxic state.

3. *Subacute granulomatous thyroiditis:* Inflammatory conditions or viral syndromes may be associated with transient hyperthyroidism followed by transient hypothyroidism. This presentation is linked to fever, malaise, and a painful and tender gland.

Secondary hypothyroidism results from inadequate secretion of TSH from the anterior pituitary gland. The cause of the deficiency is not always clear but is often associated with surgery, trauma, or radiation therapy. If TSH level is inadequate, the thyroid lacks the proper stimulus to produce T_4.

Tertiary hypothyroidism is related to hypothalamic dysfunction and is diagnosed by the release of thyrotropin-releasing hormone (TRH). Other causes are listed in Box 8-2.

Because all metabolically active cells require thyroid hormone, the effects of hormone deficiency vary. Systemic effects are due to either derangements in metabolic processes or direct effects by myxedematous infiltration in the tissues. The patient's presentation may vary from asymptomatic to, rarely, coma with multisystem organ failure (myxedema coma). *Hypothyroidism is eight times more likely to occur in women than in men, and it frequently presents in the later years of life; older women are the most likely candidates to present with myxedema.*

Box 8-2	COMMON CAUSES OF ACUTE HYPOTHYROIDISM

Primary hypothyroidism
- Hashimoto thyroiditis (autoimmune)
- Surgical removal of thyroid gland
- Ablation with radioactive iodine
- External irradiation
- Defective iodine organification
- Thyroid tumor
- Drug related
    - Lithium
    - Interferon
    - Amiodarone

Secondary hypothyroidism
- Pituitary or hypothalamic disease

Safety Alert *Euthyroid sick syndrome (ESS) may manifest as a low T_3, low T_4, low TSH, or all three. ESS results from inactivation of 5'-deiodinase, resulting in conversion of FT_4 to rT_3 (a reverse form of T_3 that is not metabolically active). ESS may occur in critically ill patients without any known cause but may also present in patients who have diabetes mellitus, malnutrition, or iodine loads or as the result of medications (amiodarone, PTU, glucocorticoids).*

ESS should be considered when TSH and/or T_4 are normal, T_3 is low, and the patient presents with symptoms that suggest hypothyroidism.

ENDOCRINE ASSESSMENT: MYXEDEMA COMA
Goal of System Assessment
Evaluate for end-organ effects of hypothyroidism, including altered mental status, hypothermia, hypoglycemia, hypotension, bradycardia, and hypoventilation. Not all patients have noticeable myxedema (polysaccharide accumulation).

History and Risk Factors
Signs and symptoms may be life-threatening in a patient with history of hypothyroidism who has experienced a recent stressful event. Undiagnosed patients may report early fatigue, weight gain, anorexia, lethargy, cold intolerance, menstrual irregularities, constipation, depression, and muscle cramps. Family may report depression, psychosis, cognitive dysfunction, or poor memory.

 Safety Alert *A change in mental status may be the most compelling sign to assist in making the diagnosis.*

Vital Signs
Cardinal signs and symptoms of myxedema coma include hypothermia (may be less than 80°F), hypoventilation, hypotension, and bradycardia, as well as hyponatremia and hypoglycemia. The presentation of any three of these signs and symptoms together should be considered in differential diagnosis as signs of acute hypothyroidism until proven otherwise.

Safety Alert *The presence of a normal temperature in a patient who appears to present with acute hypothyroid dysfunction is abnormal and should be considered an indicator of infection.*

Observation
Cardiac: Nonspecific ECG changes, prolonged conduction times, prolonged QT syndrome. Cardiac enlargement, possible effusion. If hypotensive, may be refractory to volume and vasopressors until thyroid hormone given.

Respiratory: Respiratory depression from reduced hypoxic drive and decreased ventilatory response and increasing CO_2. The increase in CO_2 is a major factor in the induction of coma. May also have edema of the conducting airways.

Gastrointestinal: Anorexia, nausea, abdominal pain, and constipation. Quiet abdomen, ileus, and megacolon not uncommon.

Hypothyroidism
- Possible presence of obesity and/or weight gain from fluid retention
- The skin may be dry, cool, and coarse, and the hair may be thin, coarse, and brittle. The tongue may be enlarged (macroglossia), and the reflexes may be slowed. Periorbital edema may be noted.
- There may be a surgical scar or a goiter when evaluating the neck. Nodules may be palpated.

- The patient may have muscle weakness, memory and mental impairment, and constipation.
- Polysaccharide substances may be deposited beneath the skin (myxedema), which may prompt hypovolemia.

 Safety Alert *A change in mental status may be the most important sign. It is commonly noted first to be lethargy, then stupor, and ultimately coma.*

Screening Labwork
Blood studies may reveal the presence of thyroid dysfunction. Expected abnormalities include (see also Figure 8-2):
- TSH increased or normal (chronic thyroiditis)
- T_4 decreased
- Hypercholesterolemia

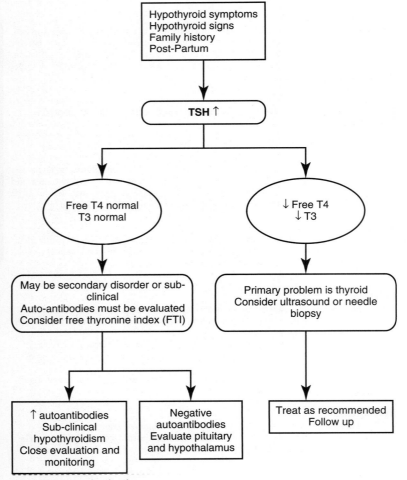

Figure 8-2 Diagnosing hypothyroidism.

- Elevated serum lactate
- Hypoglycemia
- Hyponatremia
- Hypoxemia
- Hypercapnia

Common Diagnostic Tests for Hypothyroid Crisis: Myxedema Coma

Test	Purpose	Abnormal Findings
Blood Studies		
Thyroid-stimulating hormone (TSH) Standard normal: 0.4–4.5 mIU/L Revised normal: 0.4–2.5 mIU/L TSH >2.5 mIU/L from the NAHAMES III study indicated hypothyroidism.	Measures TSH output from the anterior pituitary. Completes a negative feedback loop with the thyroid. When thyroid hormone level decreases, TSH level should increase.	Elevated unless hypothyroidism is longstanding or severe. When TSH is higher than 2.5 mIU/L in the presence of clinical symptoms, the diagnosis of hypothyroidism will be considered positive until proved otherwise. Always beneficial to also evaluate T_4 at the same time. If TSH is higher than 4.5, the diagnosis of hypothyroidism is considered positive.
Thyroperoxidase antibodies	Assesses for thyroid antibodies	Positive test signals chronic autoimmune thyroiditis.
Free T_4 or free thyroxine index (FTI) Normal: 60–170 nmol/L	Measures the level of primary thyroid hormone May be unreliable in the face of critical illness	Decreased. When levels are below normal, diagnosis of hypothyroidism is made. If the TSH is high, diagnosis would be a primary hypothyroidism, If TSH is normal or low and T_4 is low, the problem is in the hypothalamic-pituitary response to elevated circulating thyroid levels (secondary hypothyroidism). However if the T_3 is also low, this may signify euthyroid sick syndrome.
T_3 (triiodothyronine) Normal: 0.8–2.7 nmol/L	Measures the more metabolically active form of the thyroid hormone.	Controversial regarding value of treatment of low levels, since it has a higher frequency of adverse cardiac events and is generally reserved for patients who are not improving clinically on LT_4.
Thyroid-binding globulin (TBG)	To measure the level of the protein that binds with circulating thyroid hormones. Abnormal T_4 or T_3 measurements are often due to binding protein abnormalities rather than abnormal thyroid function.	Total T_4 or T_3 must be evaluated with a measure of thyroid hormone binding such as T_3 resin uptake or assay of thyroid-binding globulin. These methods are known as free T_4 or free T_3 even though they do not measure free hormone directly.
Electrolytes Potassium (K^+) Magnesium (Mg^{2+}) Calcium (Ca^{2+}) Sodium (Na^+)	Assess for possible abnormalities	Frequently, abnormalities of calcium are related to parathyroid disorders exist concurrently with thyroid dysfunction.
Radiology/Imaging		
Thyroid scan with radioactive iodine uptake[123]I or ^{99m}Tc pertechnetate	To identify thyroid nodules	Not beneficial in hypothyroidism as uptake of radioactive iodine may not occur

Myxedema Coma

Continued

Common Diagnostic Tests for Hypothyroid Crisis: Myxedema Coma—cont'd		
Test	**Purpose**	**Abnormal Findings**
Thyroid scan ^{131}I and radioactive iodine uptake	To identify thyroid nodules	In primary hypothyroidism, will be less than 10% in a 24-hour period. In secondary hypothyroidism, uptake increases with administration of exogenous TSH.
Chest radiograph	Assess size of heart, and presence of pericardial or pleural effusion	Cardiac enlargement or fluid around the heart is common with myxedema
Ultrasound	Assess size and presence of nodules and goiter	Abnormal thyroid is unusual in Hashimoto disease.
Fine needle biopsy	Evaluate suspicious nodes	Cancerous cells indicate thyroid cancer

COLLABORATIVE MANAGEMENT
Care Priorities
1. Stabilize the patient:
   - *Perform emergent endotracheal intubation and provide mechanical ventilation support:* Required to relieve or prevent profound hypoxemia and CO_2 narcosis detected by SpO_2 and $ETCO_2$ monitoring. Monitoring of arterial blood gas is done periodically to validate SpO_2, $ETCO_2$ and to monitor pH.
   - *Treat hypothermia:* Although the hypothermia will be addressed ultimately by the institution of thyroid hormone, it may take several days. Extreme caution must be taken when re-warming (only passive techniques should be used) in order to avoid uncompensated vasodilation and profound hypotension.

   - *Treat hypotension:* Prior to institution of even passive re-warming, careful volume resuscitation should occur. Administer of IV isotonic fluids (normal saline and lactated Ringer's solution). Hypotonic solutions, such as 5% dextrose in water (D_5W), are contraindicated because they decrease serum Na^+ levels further. These patients respond poorly to vasopressors because of alteration in sympathetic response. Consider IV vasopressin or IV corticosteroids.
2. **Administer IV thyroid hormone as soon as possible:** **Patients may die without prompt treatment.** The best dose or approach to rapidly returning the circulating and active hormones to normal is uncertain, and therefore recommendations tend to be empiric at best. Practitioners often initially administer T_4 (levothyronine [LT_4]). An effective approach is to use intravenous LT_4 at a dose of 4 mcg/kg of lean body weight, or approximately 200 to 250 mcg as a bolus in a single or divided dose, depending on the patient's risk of cardiac disease (if at risk, give ½ the dose) followed by 100 mcg 24 hours later for stabilization; then 50 mcg IV or PO daily, given with IV or PO glucocorticoids.

RESEARCH BRIEF 8-4

A recent meta-analysis of randomized controlled trials of thyroxine-triiodothyronine combination therapy ($T_4 + T_3$) versus thyroxine monotherapy (T_4) for treatment of clinical hypothyroidism found no difference in the effectiveness of the combination versus monotherapy in bodily pain, depression, fatigue, body weight, anxiety, quality of life, total cholesterol, LDL-C, HDL-C, and triglyceride levels. T_4 monotherapy was recommended as the treatment of choice for hypothyroidism.

From Grozinsky-Glasberg S: Thyroxine-triiodothyronine combination therapy versus thyroxine monotherapy for clinical hypothyroidism: meta-analysis of randomized controlled trials. *J Clin Endocrinol Metab* 91(7):2592-2599, 2006.

Thyroid Hormone Supplementation

Use of IV triiodothyronine (LT$_3$): Controversial therapy, because it has a higher frequency of adverse cardiac events and is generally reserved for patients who are not improving clinically on LT$_4$. LT$_3$ can be given initially as a 10 mcg IV bolus and repeated every 8 to 12 hours until the patient can take maintenance oral doses of T$_4$.

Oral thyroid hormone (i.e., levothyroxine): This is not the avenue of choice in myxedema coma. It is given early in treatment for primary hypothyroidism. To prevent hyperthyroidism caused by too much exogenous hormone, patients are started on low doses that are increased gradually, based on serial laboratory tests (TSH and T$_4$) and adjusted until the TSH is in a normal range. This therapy is continued for the patient's lifetime. For patients with secondary hypothyroidism, thyroid supplements can promote acute symptoms and therefore are contraindicated.

Safety Alert *Rapid IV administration of thyroid hormone should be done with careful monitoring, as this may cause hyperadrenalism. Concomitant administration of IV hydrocortisone helps prevent adrenal problems but may cause hypoadrenalism if not carefully monitored.*

3. **Manage hyponatremia:** If serum Na$^+$ is greater than 120 mEq/L, fluids are restricted. If serum Na$^+$ is less than 120 mEq/L, consider administration hypertonic (3%) saline followed by water diuresis.
4. **Manage hypoglycemia:** IV solutions containing glucose or 50% dextrose (D$_{50}$)
5. **Manage Associated Illnesses Such as Infections**
6. **Administer stool softeners:** To minimize constipation owing to decreased gastric secretions and peristalsis
7. **Avoid barbiturates:** Because of alterations in metabolism, patients with hypothyroidism do not tolerate barbiturates and sedatives, and therefore CNS depressants are contraindicated.

CARE PLANS FOR MYXEDEMA COMA

Ineffective protection (myxedema coma) *related to inadequate response to treatment of hypothyroidism or stressors such as infection*

GOALS/OUTCOMES Patient is free of symptoms of myxedema coma as evidenced by HR greater than 60 bpm, BP greater than 90/60 mm Hg (or within patient's normal range), RR greater than 12 breaths/min with normal depth and pattern, and orientation to person, place, and time.
NOC Risk Control

Risk Identification
1. Monitor vital signs frequently and note bradycardia, hypotension, or decrease in RR. Report systolic BP greater than 90 mm Hg, HR less than 60 bpm, or RR less than 12 breaths/min.
2. Monitor patient for hypoxia. Report significant findings to physician.
3. Monitor serum electrolytes and glucose levels. Note decreasing Na$^+$ (less than 137 mEq/L) and glucose (less than 60 mg/dl).
   - Restrict fluids or administer hypertonic saline as prescribed to correct hyponatremia. Do not correct too rapidly, to avoid central pontine myelinolysis.
   - In chronic, severe symptomatic hyponatremia, the rate of correction should not exceed 0.5 to 1 mEq/L/hr, with a total increase not to exceed 12 mEq/L/day. It is necessary to correct the hyponatremia to a safe range (usually to no greater than 120 mEq/L) rather than to a normal value.
4. Administer IV thyroid replacement hormones with IV hydrocortisone and IV glucose to treat hypoglycemia.
5. Monitor for heart failure: jugular vein distention, crackles (rales), shortness of breath (SOB), peripheral edema, weakening peripheral pulses, and hypotension. Notify physician of any significant findings.
6. Keep an oral airway and manual resuscitator at the bedside in the event of seizure, coma, or the need for ventilatory assistance.

NIC Vital Signs Monitoring; Respiratory Monitoring; Shock Prevention; Cardiac Care: Acute

Ineffective breathing pattern *related to enlarged thyroid gland and/or decreased ventilatory drive caused by greatly decreased metabolism*

GOALS/OUTCOMES Patient maintains effective breathing pattern as evidenced by RR 12 to 20 breaths/min with normal depth and pattern, normal skin color, oxygen saturation greater than 95%, and absence of adventitious breath sounds. If ineffective breathing pattern occurs, it is reported and treated promptly.
NOC Respiratory Status: Ventilation; Vital Signs

Respiratory Monitoring
1. Assess rate, depth, and quality of breath sounds. Monitor for inadequate ventilation: changes in respiratory rate or pattern, falling SpO_2, pallor, or cyanosis. Report findings to physician or midlevel practitioner promptly, including presence of adventitious sounds (e.g., from developing pleural effusion) or decreasing or crowing sounds (e.g., from swollen tongue or glottis).
2. Measure SpO_2 intermittently or continuously in patients with decreased ventilatory drive.
3. Teach patient coughing, deep breathing, and use of incentive spirometer. For respiratory distress, assist physician with intubation or tracheostomy and maintenance of mechanical ventilatory assistance. Suction upper airway as needed.

NIC Airway Management

Excess fluid volume *related to compromised regulatory mechanisms occurring with associated adrenal insufficiency*

GOALS/OUTCOMES By a minimum of 24 hours before hospital discharge, patient is normovolemic as evidenced by urinary output greater than 0.5 ml/kg/hr, stable weight, nondistended jugular veins, presence of eupnea, and peripheral pulse amplitude 2+ or greater on a 0 to 4+ scale.
NOC Fluid Balance

Hypervolemia Management
1. Monitor I&O hourly for evidence of decreasing output.
2. Weigh patient at the same time every day, using the same scale. Monitor for the following indicators of heart failure: jugular vein distention, crackles (rales), SOB, dependent edema of extremities, and decreased pulse amplitude. Report significant findings to physician.
3. Restrict fluid and Na^+ intake as prescribed.

NIC Fluid Management; Electrolyte Monitoring

Activity intolerance *related to weakness and fatigue secondary to slowed metabolism and decreased cardiac output caused by pericardial effusions, atherosclerosis, and decreased adrenergic stimulation*

GOALS/OUTCOMES During activity patient rates perceived exertion at 3 or less on a 0 to 10 scale and exhibits cardiac tolerance to activity as evidenced by HR 20 bpm or less over resting HR, systolic BP 20 mm Hg or less over or under resting systolic BP, warm and dry skin, and absence of crackles (rales), murmurs, chest pain, and new dysrhythmias.
NOC Activity Tolerance; Endurance; Energy Conservation

Energy Management
1. Monitor vital signs frequently for hypotension, slow pulse, dysrhythmias, complaints of chest pain or discomfort, decreasing urine output, and changes in mentation. Promptly report significant changes to physician.
2. Balance activity with adequate rest to decrease workload of the heart.
3. Administer IV isotonic solutions such as normal saline to help prevent hypotension.

NIC Activity Therapy; Exercise Promotion: Strength Training

Risk for infection *related to compromised immunologic status secondary to alterations in adrenal function*

GOALS/OUTCOMES Patient is free of infection as evidenced by normothermia, absence of adventitious breath sounds, normal urinary pattern and characteristics, and well-healing wounds.
NOC Status; Infection Severity

Infection Protection
1. *Monitor for infection:* fever, erythema, swelling, or discharge from wounds or IV sites; urinary frequency, urgency, or dysuria; cloudy or malodorous urine; presence of adventitious sounds on auscultation of lung fields; and changes in color, consistency, and amount of sputum. Minimize risk of UTI by providing care of catheters.
2. Provide care to maintain skin integrity and prevent pressure ulcers.
3. Advise visitors who have contracted or been exposed to a communicable disease not to enter patient's room without appropriate infection control precautions.

NIC Identification; Infection Protection

Risk for imbalanced nutrition: more than body requirements *related to slowed metabolism*

GOALS/OUTCOMES Patient does not gain weight. Within the 24-hour period before hospital discharge, patient verbalizes understanding of the rationale and measures for the dietary regimen.
NOC Status: Food and Fluid Intake; Weight Control

Nutritional Management
1. Provide a diet that is high in protein and low in calories and sodium.
2. Encourage foods that are high in fiber content (e.g., fruits with skins, vegetables, whole grain breads and cereals, nuts) to improve gastric motility and elimination.
3. Administer vitamin supplements as prescribed.

NIC Counseling; Weight Management

Constipation *related to inadequate dietary intake of roughage and fluids, bed rest, and/or decreased peristalsis secondary to slowed metabolism*

GOALS/OUTCOMES Within 48 to 72 hours of admission, patient resumes normal pattern of bowel elimination.
NOC Elimination

Bowel Management
1. Monitor bowel function; report problems to the physician. Note decreasing bowel sounds, distention, and increased abdominal girth (may indicate ileus or an obstruction).
2. Encourage patient to maintain a diet with adequate roughage and fluids. Ensure that fluid intake in persons without underlying cardiac or renal disease is at least 2 to 3 L/day.
3. Administer stool softeners and laxatives as prescribed.

> **Safety Alert** *Suppositories may be contraindicated because of the risk of stimulating the vagus nerve (decreases HR and BP).*

NIC Constipation/Impaction Management; Fluid Management

Deficient knowledge: Illness Care *related to management of hypothyroidism*

GOALS/OUTCOMES Within the 24-hour period before hospital discharge, patient verbalizes knowledge of potential side effects of prescribed medications, dietary guidelines, signs and symptoms that require medical attention, and importance of following the prescribed medical regimen.
NOC Knowledge: Disease Process

Myxedema Coma

Teaching: Disease Process
1. Provide teaching about medications including drug name, purpose, dosage, schedule, precautions, drug-drug and food-drug interactions, and potential side effects. Remind patient that thioamides, iodides, and lithium are contraindicated because they decrease thyroid activity. Be sure patient is aware that thyroid replacement medications are to be taken for life.
2. Review dietary requirements and restrictions, which may change as hormone replacement therapy takes effect.
3. Explain expected changes with hormone replacement therapy: increased energy level, weight loss, and decreased peripheral edema. Neuromuscular problems should improve.
4. Stress the importance of continued, frequent medical follow-up.
5. Discuss importance of avoiding physical and emotional stress, and ways for patient to maximize coping mechanisms for dealing with stress.
6. Review signs and symptoms that require medical attention: fever or other symptoms of upper respiratory, urinary, or oral infections and signs and symptoms of hyperthyroidism, which may result from excessive hormone replacement.

NIC Management; Exercise Promotion; Teaching: Prescribed Diet; Teaching: Disease Process; Anxiety Reduction

SYNDROME OF INAPPROPRIATE ANTIDIURETIC HORMONE
PATHOPHYSIOLOGY
Syndrome of inappropriate antidiuretic hormone (SIADH) or syndrome of inappropriate antidiuresis (SIAD) is a condition of abnormal release of antidiuretic hormone (ADH, vasopressin) in response to changes in plasma osmolality that results in hyponatremia. Hyponatremia is defined as an excess of water in relation to the amount of sodium in the extracellular fluid. SIADH is the most frequent cause of hyponatremia, the most common electrolyte imbalance in hospitalized patients. Mild hyponatremia (serum sodium, less than 135 mEq/L) occurs in 15% to 22% of hospitalized patients and 7% of ambulatory patients, while moderate hyponatremia (serum sodium, less than 130 mEq/L) occurs in 1% to 7% of hospitalized patients. Hyponatremia is often caused by extracellular fluid volume depletion associated with many diuretics, which cause a significant loss of sodium along with water. Hyponatremia is important to manage because of potential morbidity and should be recognized as an indicator of underlying disease.

ADH (vasopressin) is produced in the hypothalamus and stored in the posterior pituitary and regulates free water volume in the kidney. Hyponatremia resulting from chronic SIADH is not always caused by reduced water excretion or volume overload. Plasma ADH level may not be high and measurement is often not helpful in establishing the diagnosis. Findings may reflect dilute (hypo-osmolar) plasma and hyponatremia with a normal circulating blood volume. Morbidity and mortality of hyponatremia associated with SIAD stem from cerebral edema and abnormal nerve function. Values of serum sodium 100 mEq/L or less are life-threatening. Four patterns of abnormal vasopressin secretion have been identified in Table 8-4. The disorders and medications associated with SIAD are listed in Table 8-5.

Table 8-4	SYNDROME OF INAPPROPRIATE ANTIDIURESIS (SIAD): FOUR TYPES	
	Characteristics	**Prevalence**
Type A	Large fluctuations in plasma ADH concentration independent of osmolality	35%
Type B	Subnormal osmotic threshold for ADH release Osmoregulation is set around a subnormal threshold	30%
Type C	ADH is not suppressed when plasma osmolality is low Normal response to osmotic changes	~25%
Type D	Normal osmoregulated ADH release Unable to excrete excess body water.	<10%

Table 8-5	MEDICATIONS AND DISEASES ASSOCIATED WITH SIADH AND HYPONATREMIA	
Cancer Related		**Pulmonary Disorders**
Carcinoma (bronchus, duodenum, pancreas, bladder, ureter, prostate) Carcinoid bronchial adenoma Ewing sarcoma Lymphoma, leukemia Mesothelioma Thymoma		Aspergillosis Cystic fibrosis Empyema Pneumothorax Pneumonia Tuberculosis
Brain/Nervous System		**Medications and Recreational Drugs**
Alcohol withdrawal syndrome Brain abscess or tumor Cavernous sinus thrombosis Cerebellar and cerebral atrophy Cerebral hemorrhage/stroke Guillain-Barré syndrome Head injury, neurosurgery Hydrocephalus Meningitis, encephalitis Peripheral neuropathy Shy-Drager syndrome Seizures Subdural hematoma		ACE inhibitors Alkylating agents and Vinca alkaloids Angiotensin II receptor antagonists (ARBs) Anticonvulsants Carbamazepine Carboplatin Chlorpropamide Cisplatin Clofibrate Cyclophosphamide DDAVP Dopamine antagonists Ifosfamide MAO inhibitors MDMA ("ecstasy") NSAIDs Opiates Selective serotonin reuptake inhibitors (SSRIs) Sodium valproate Sulphonylureas Thiazides & Loop diuretics Tricyclic antidepressants Venlafaxine Vinblastine Vincristine
Other		
Abdominal surgery Hyperglycemia Idiopathic Porphyria Psychosis		

ADH is a key component in the regulation of fluid and electrolyte balance, through direct effects on renal water regulation. Water is reabsorbed in the distal nephron, where the kidney both concentrates and dilutes urine in response to the ADH level. Vasopressin (VP) stimulates the nephron to produce aquaporin (AQP), a specific water channel protein, on the surface of the interstitial cells lining the collecting duct. The presence of AQP in the wall of the distal nephron allows resorption of water from the duct lumen according to the osmotic gradient, and excretion of concentrated urine.

Hyponatremia resulting in SIAD is often drug induced, reflecting either direct stimulation of ADH/VP release from the hypothalamus, indirect stimulation of ADH action on the hypothalamus, or abnormal resetting of the hypothalamic osmotic threshold that governs release of ADH. The prevalence of hyponatremia in patients taking high-dose dopamine antagonists is greater than 25% and is associated with more than one class of these drugs. Hyponatremia secondary to antidepressants is common, occurring with most selective serotonin reuptake inhibitors (SSRIs). Patients receiving concurrent diuretic therapy are at high risk, indicating that hypovolemia contributes to the hyponatremia. Loop diuretics promote both sodium and water loss. Anticonvulsants commonly cause hyponatremia, which prompts SIAD. Patients treated with carbamazepine have a 5% to 40% incidence of SIAD.

RESEARCH BRIEF 8-5

Hyponatremia is a predictor of death among patients with chronic heart failure and cirrhosis. At present, therapy for acute and chronic hyponatremia is often ineffective and poorly tolerated. The authors investigated whether tolvaptan, an oral vasopressin V_2-receptor antagonist that promotes aquaresis (excretion of electrolyte-free water), helped in management of hyponatremia. Results revealed serum sodium concentrations increased more in the tolvaptan group than in the placebo group during the first 4 days ($p < 0.001$) and after the full 30 days of therapy ($p < 0.001$). The condition of patients with mild or marked hyponatremia improved ($p < 0.001$ for all comparisons). During the week after discontinuation of tolvaptan on day 30, hyponatremia recurred. Side effects associated with tolvaptan included increased thirst, dry mouth, and increased urination. A planned analysis that combined the two trials showed significant improvement from baseline to day 30 in the tolvaptan group according to scores on the Mental Component of the Medical Outcomes Study 12-item Short-Form General Health Survey.

From ClinicalTrials.gov numbers, NCT00072683 [ClinicalTrials.gov] [SALT-1] and NCT00201994 [ClinicalTrials.gov] [SALT-2].

ENDOCRINE ASSESSMENT: SYNDROME OF INAPPROPRIATE ANTIDIURESIS
Goal of Endocrine Assessment
To differentiate between SIAD and a compensatory response of ADH release in patients with chronic, mild volume depletion/dehydration. Urine osmolality is generally higher than plasma osmolality in both. Plasma vasopressin levels may be normal or elevated in both. Neither finding alone is diagnostic of SIAD. Diagnosis is often made when urine excreted is not maximally diluted when plasma is dilute (i.e., urine concentration greater than 100 mOsm/kg). Urinary sodium excretion should be greater than 20mEq/L to make the diagnosis. If urinary sodium is less than 20 mEq/L, volume depletion is more likely. SIADH is often associated with urine sodium concentrations greater than 60 mEq/L.

History and Risk Factors
See Table 8-5.

Vital Signs
- Findings vary significantly, depending on the degree of hyponatremia and fluid overload.
- Hyponatremia alone may have no affect on vital signs if the patient is able to achieve brain and CNS compensation.
- Tachycardia and tachypnea are present with fluid overload.
- Pulse may be irregular if hypokalemia has caused dysrhythmias.
- Mild elevation in BP is possible.
- Hypotension may be present with heart failure.
- Weight gain; slightly elevated BP
- CVP less than 6 mm Hg in the absence of underlying cardiac or pulmonary disease

Observation
- Patients may be asymptomatic or have mild symptoms if hyponatremia is less severe and develops slowly.
- Lesser symptoms reflect adaptation of the brain and CNS.

- Oliguria with concentrated urine; urine output less than 0.5 ml/kg/hr with specific gravity greater than 1.030 in the presence of adequate fluid intake
- Headache, difficulty concentrating, impaired memory, altered taste sensation
- *Electrolyte imbalance*: Generalized weakness, possible exhaustion, nausea and vomiting, impaired vision, and leg cramps may be present from hyponatremia or hypocalcemia; patients may become unable to get out of bed; dysrhythmias result from hypokalemia.
- *Altered mental status*: Serum hypo-osmolality and hyponatremia affect consciousness and behavior. Changes may also be related the underlying disease.
  1. Cranial nerve examination may be abnormal, with nerve palsies present.
  2. Altered LOC (confusion, disorientation, agitation) is more common with older adults; coma, hallucinations, decerebrate posturing, seizures, and respiratory arrest are possible.

Auscultation

- Heart sounds may reflect heart failure if fluid overload exceeds the ability of the pumping action of the heart. Only a subset of these patients has fluid overload.

Screening Labwork

- *Biochemical panel*: To assess for hyponatremia and altered concentrations of other electrolytes associated with hemodilution. Decreased blood urea nitrogen (BUN) with a urinary sodium level greater than 40 mmol/L in patients with hyponatremia suggests SIADH but is not diagnostic.
- *Plasma and urine osmolality*: Assesses for plasma hypo-osmolality in the presence of urine hyperosmolality
- *Urine sodium level*: Increased
- *Urinalysis/specific gravity*: Assesses for highly concentrated urine

Differential Diagnosis of SIADH

Test	Purpose	Abnormal Findings
Urine osmolality	Assesses for increased concentration of urine	Must exceed 100 mOsm/kg water when the plasma osmolality is low *Normal:* 300–1090 mOsm/kg
Urine specific gravity	Assesses for concentrated urine.	*Specific gravity:* >1.030 *Normal:* 1.010–1.025
Urine sodium	Assesses for excessive loss of sodium in the urine	Increased to >20 mEq/L; increases to >60 mEq/L are common
Serum osmolality	Assesses for dilute blood/hemodilution	Decreased to <275 mOsm/kg *Normal:* 275–300 mOsm/kg
Serum sodium	Monitors for hyponatremia	Decreased to <130 mEq/L *Normal:* 137–147 mEq/L
Serum arginine vasopressin (VP) level (ADH level) See Table 8-4.	Assesses whether vasopressin is elevated or decreased in relation to serum osmolality *VP/ADH level may be done with the water load test to provide specific information about VP secretion in response to the water load.	*Type A:* Wide fluctuations *Type B:* Normal or increased *Type C:* Normal or increased *Type D:* Normal or increased *Not recommended for routine screening; urinary osmolality >100 mOsm per kilogram of water indicates excessive VP.

Continued

Syndrome of Inappropriate Antidiuretic Hormone

Differential Diagnosis of SIADH—cont'd		
Test	**Purpose**	**Abnormal Findings**
Water load test The test is not required for diagnosis; can be useful in the management of chronic or recurrent hyponatremia	Abnormal ADH/VP secretion resulting in hyponatremia is diagnosed by assessing excretion of a standard water load over 4 hours. Urine output, urine and plasma osmolality are measured hourly. Plasma sodium is measured 2 hours following test completion, and the next morning, along with plasma osmolality.	Excretion of water or urine output may be reduced to 30% to 40% of the ingested load in the presence of VP production. Normal urine output is 78% to 82% of the ingested water load during the 4-hour test. In SIADH, low plasma osmolality is present with highly concentrated urine, with decreased plasma sodium indicating abnormal secretion of ADH/VP.
Urinary aquaporin-2 (AQP-2) Test provides limited information; role in diagnosis remains unclear	May be useful in the differentiation of SIADH from other causes of hyponatraemia	There is a positive correlation between plasma VP concentration and urinary excretion of AQP-2, but urinary AQP-2 cannot clearly diagnose hyponatremic states associated with significant VP/ADH production. SIAD and chronic hypovolemia may generate similar plasma VP concentrations and similar urine AQP-2 levels.

COLLABORATIVE MANAGEMENT
Care Priorities

 Safety Alert CNS Demyelination

Rapid correction of sodium level with gradual development of hyponatremia (with brain/CNS adaptation) may lead to significant changes in brain volume as the osmolar gradient across the blood and brain changes. Brain edema is limited by the loss of sodium, which complicates the management of hyponatremia. The blood-brain barrier may be altered, triggering CNS demyelination, a rare complication of hyponatremia. The phenomenon begins within 1 to 4 days of rapid (greater than 12 mEq each day) correction of plasma sodium, regardless of the method of treatment and has also occurred with less aggressive sodium correction. Demyelination of the pons and adjacent brain structures begins with lethargy and changes in affect, following initial improvement of neurologic symptoms with treatment. Difficulty speaking, swallowing, and weakness, may be seen. Comorbidities affecting fluid and electrolyte balance, such as hepatic failure, hypokalemia, and malnutrition, may increase susceptibility.

1. **Correct acute, symptomatic hyponatremia.**
   - *Key considerations*: The patient's symptoms, severity, and duration of hyponatremia. Electrolytes should be measured every 4 hours. The approximate sodium deficit can be estimated using the following formula:

     $$Na^+ \text{ deficit} = (\text{Desired } Na^+ - \text{Measured } Na^+) \times 0.6 \times (\text{Weight in kg})$$

   - *Treatment goal*: Increase serum sodium level by 1 to 2 mEq/L/hr using an IV 3% saline infusion; aim for resolution of major neurologic symptoms (i.e., seizures) and then decrease the correction rate. An increase in serum sodium levels of less than 10 mEq/L reduces the symptoms while preventing complications. The approximate volume of 3% saline needed:

     $$\text{Volume of 3\% saline needed} = Na^+ \text{ Deficit}/513 \text{ mEq Na/L}$$

   - *Rate of sodium correction*: The rate of correction **should not exceed 0.5 mEq/L/hr.** Correction during the first 24 hours of treatment should be an increase of 8 to 12 mEq/L and no greater than 18 to 25 mEq/L during the first 48 hours, regardless of the severity of hyponatremia:

$$\text{Time needed for correction} = (\text{Desired Na} - \text{Measured Na})/(5 \text{ mEq/L/hr})$$

- *Hypertonic (3%) saline infusion*: The best method for calculating the initial infusion rate remains controversial. The rate of infusion may be calculated:

$$(\text{Volume of 3\% saline needed})/(\text{Time needed for correction}).$$

- *If calculations are not used*: 3% saline may be infused at a rate of 1 to 2 ml/kg of body weight/hr. The serum sodium level will increased by 1 to 2 mmol/L/hr. The rate may be doubled (2 to 4 ml/kg/hr) for a short time in patients with coma or seizures; half the rate (0.5 ml/kg/hr) is used if symptoms are mild.
- *Diuretics*: Consider concomitant use of IV furosemide (1 mg/kg); experts disagree on use. Some recommend avoiding or using it exclusively for those with fluid overload/extracellular-fluid volume expansion. Once renal function normalizes, correct K^+ level.

2. **Manage chronic (or uncertain duration) hyponatremia.**
   - *Occurrence out of hospital*: Most patients have chronic hyponatremia with few symptoms. Severe symptoms seen in marathon runners, users of the street drug 3,4-MDMA (ecstasy), and those who drink excessive amounts of water usually indicate acute hyponatremia and require rapid correction.
   - *Symptomatic hyponatremia of unknown duration*: A correction of 8 mEq/L in 24 hours or 18 mEq/L in 48 hours is recommended; Serum sodium levels may be measured every 2 to 3 hours to avoid overcorrection.
   - *Asymptomatic patients with chronic hyponatremia*: Fluid restriction is used to correct the sodium level slowly while avoiding osmotic demyelination. Maximum fluid intake tolerated depends on the oral osmotic load, so adequate intake of protein and salt should be encouraged. Oral intake of urea (30 grams daily) is effective but poorly tolerated.
   - *Demeclocycline*: A dose of 300 to 600 mg twice daily may decrease urinary osmolality while increasing serum sodium levels; effects are variable and treatment may prompt nephrotoxicity.
   - *Lithium*: No longer recommended

3. **Vasopressin-receptor antagonist therapy**
   - *Conivaptan (Vaprisol)*: A vasopressin-receptor antagonist approved by the Food and Drug Administration in 2005 for the treatment of euvolemic hyponatremia and in 2007 for the treatment of hypervolemic hyponatremia. Intravenous conivaptan is used to treat hospitalized patients with symptomatic moderate-to-severe hyponatremia without seizures, delirium, or coma, who are candidates for hypertonic saline.
   - *Tolvaptan*: Oral vasopressin receptor–selective V_2 receptor antagonist used to increase serum sodium in SIAD patients. The appropriate role for vasopressin antagonist therapy continues to be studied and evaluated. These agents cause dry mouth and thirst, which prompts water intake, thus slowing the rise in serum sodium levels. Use of this agent in practice requires close monitoring of serum sodium levels.
   - *Hemodynamic monitoring*: May be useful in guiding fluid management strategies and efficacy and may help recognize the patient's response to the effects of nonselective vasopressin receptor blockade if shock symptoms occur. Distributive shock has not been reported, but is a possibility with use of these agents. Euvolemic patients may be at higher risk of hypotension.

4. **Identify and manage the precipitating cause:** SIADH associated with surgery, trauma, or drugs is usually temporary and self-limiting. If chronic, the focus is to treat the underlying cause.

5. **Differentiate SIAD from Cerebral Salt Wasting:** SIAD is often difficult to distinguish from cerebral salt wasting, a condition associated with patients with disease, an event or trauma of the CNS. Cerebral salt wasting is consistently associated with extracellular fluid volume depletion, but clinical assessment of volume status is difficult. Many physicians use saline infusion rather than fluid restriction for patients who have hyponatremia with subarachnoid hemorrhage, because of the risks associated with volume depletion in these patients. (See *Cerebral Aneurysms and Subarachnoid Hemorrhage, Table 7-1*, p 631.)

6. **Monitor for signs of osmotic demyelination:** Several case reports have revealed this rare event resulting from too rapid correction of hyponatremia may be managed with

IV vasopressin administration, which lowers the sodium level prompting improvement in neurological symptoms.

7. **Manage postoperative hyponatremia:** Patients undergoing a surgical procedure have been found to have an elevated level of vasopressin. Use of normal saline may be advantageous over use of hypotonic IV solutions for perioperative fluid replacement to avoid hyponatremia.

CARE PLANS FOR SYNDROME OF INAPPROPRIATE ANTIDIURESIS
Decreased intracranial adaptive capacity with alteration in neurologic function *related to management of hyponatremia*

- -

GOALS/OUTCOMES Within 72 hours of initiating treatment, patient verbalizes orientation to time, place, and person. CVP and BP are within patient's normal range. Patient remains free of signs of neurologic deficits with normalization of sodium level.

NOC Fluid Balance, Electrolyte and Acid-Base Balance (Serum Sodium)

Electrolyte Management: Hyponatremia
1. Assess LOC, vital signs, hemodynamic measurements, and I&O hourly; weigh patient daily. Monitor for decreased LOC; elevated BP, CVP, and PAWP; urine output less than 0.5 ml/kg/hr; and weight gain.
2. Monitor for changes in neurologic/neuromuscular symptoms of hyponatremia: lethargy, coma, seizures, headache, confusion, and weakness. Sodium levels of less than 120 mEq/L can cause life-threatening symptoms.
3. Obtain laboratory specimens to assess sodium levels (e.g., serum and urine sodium, serum and urine osmolality, urine specific gravity). Monitor for decreased serum sodium and plasma osmolality, urine osmolality that is disproportionately elevated compared to plasma osmolality, and increased urine sodium. Consult physician or designee for significant findings.
4. Administer hypertonic sodium chloride (3% saline infusion) as prescribed. Rate of administration is usually based on serial serum sodium levels. To minimize the risk of too-rapid correction of hyponatremia, ensure that laboratory specimens are drawn on time. *Serum sodium should not be allowed to increase greater than 12 mEq/L in 24 hours* because of the risk of neurologic damage (osmotic demyelination), particularly if the hyponatremia is chronic rather than acute. Monitor for indications of fluid overload (e.g., crackles, elevated CVP or PCWP, edema) as appropriate. Consult physician or designee promptly for significant findings.
5. Institute seizure precautions. These include padded side rails, supplemental oxygen, bite block, and oral airway at the bedside. Side rails should remain up when a staff member is not present.
6. Restrict fluids if ordered. Explain treatment to patient and significant others. Do not keep water or ice chips at the bedside. Give IV solutions with an infusion pump.
7. Elevate HOB no greater than 20 degrees to promote venous return and thus reduce ADH release. Decreased venous return is a stimulus to the release of ADH.
8. Administer demeclocycline, conivaptan, tolvaptan, and furosemide as prescribed; carefully observe and document patient's response.
9. Provide care calmly and gently to minimize discomfort, which increases ADH release.

NIC Fluid/Electrolyte Management; Neurologic Monitoring; Seizure Precautions

---

ADDITIONAL NURSING DIAGNOSES
See also *Hyponatremia* in *Fluid and Electrolyte Imbalances* (p. 46).

THYROTOXICOSIS CRISIS (THYROID STORM)

PATHOPHYSIOLOGY
Thyroid storm is a *medical emergency* caused by uncontrolled hyperthyroidism. Patients occasionally present with cardiovascular collapse and shock. Hyperthyroidism or thyrotoxicosis is a condition of increased circulating thyroid hormone. The crisis results from a surge of thyroid hormones into the bloodstream, which results in profound stimulation of the sympathetic nervous system, with marked increases in body metabolism. The hypothalamus, anterior pituitary, and thyroid normally work together to balance the level of circulating thyroid hormone. Hyperthyroidism may be caused by an increased synthesis and secretion of thyroid

hormones (thyroxine [T_4] and triiodothyronine [T_3]) from the thyroid or from increased secretion of TSH from the anterior pituitary, possibly by an increase in TRH from the hypothalamus or by autonomous thyroid hyperfunction. Symptoms of hyperthyroidism can also result from excessive release of thyroid hormone from the thyroid without increased synthesis. Such release is commonly caused by the destructive changes of various types of thyroiditis. Thyrotoxicosis crisis may also follow subtotal thyroidectomy because of manipulation of the gland during surgery. *Various clinical syndromes also produce hyperthyroidism, but thyroid storm is most often associated with Graves' disease, also known as diffuse toxic goiter.* Causes of acute hyperthyroid states are listed in Box 8-3. Not all conditions listed are associated with thyroid storm.

 Treatment with amiodarone (a common K^+ antagonist used for dysrhythmia management) may cause either hyperthyroidism OR hypothyroidism and must be considered when evaluating either condition.

 Low TSH may also indicate euthyroid sick syndrome (ESS). When serum thyrotropin is decreased or suppressed by severe or critical illness or by medications, particularly high doses of glucocorticoids and dopamine, this abnormality may be the diagnosis.

 Life-threatening illness in patients with preexisting thyroid disorders may be precipitated by extremes of the primary disorder. These conditions present with exaggerated nonspecific signs and symptoms of the underlying thyroid dysfunction.

 Exacerbated hyperthyroidism occurs in 1 in 500 pregnancies and is second in frequency only to diabetes as an endocrine disorder of pregnancy. During pregnancy, thyroid storm is seen most often in patients with undertreated or undiagnosed hyperthyroidism. As many as 20% to 30% of cases may result in maternal and fetal mortality.

Abnormal laboratory analysis of thyroid function provides a relatively definitive diagnosis. Initial serum measurements should include a free T_4 and TSH, but concerns regarding thyroidal dysfunction should be referred to an endocrinology specialist for a more thorough and evaluative diagnostic panel. Calcium regulation may also be affected by thyroid disease if there is a problem with the level of thyrocalcitonin, a third thyroid hormone that is stimulated by increased calcium levels to help lower the calcium level. Recent diagnostic tests have isolated a long-acting thyroid stimulator, suggesting the disease is an autoimmune response. An acute decrease in thyroxine-binding globulin (inactivating or binding thyroid hormone) facilitates high levels of free and metabolically active hormone. The increased circulating levels of active thyroid hormone increase the response of beta adrenergic receptors (sympathetic stimulation increase) and also increase the system responsiveness to catecholamines.

Box 8-3	COMMON CAUSES OF ACUTE HYPERTHYROID STATES

- Graves' disease
- Toxic multinodular goiter
- Solitary hyperfunctioning nodules
- Autoimmune and subacute postpartum thyroiditis
- Thyrotropin-secreting tumors
- Iodine-induced hyperthyroidism
- Excessive pituitary thyroid-stimulating hormone or trophoblastic disease
- Excessive ingestion of thyroid hormone

ENDOCRINE ASSESSMENT: HYPERTHYROIDISM

Goal of System Assessment

Evaluate for end organ effects of hyperthyroidism. Thyroid hormones work with adrenal glucocorticoid hormones to facilitate carbohydrate, fat, and protein metabolism; work with insulin and growth hormone to promote growth; increase HR and the force of contraction; help to regulate respiratory drive; help increase production of red blood cells (RBCs); and increase metabolism.

History and Risk Factors

A patient with a history of hyperthyroidism resulting from Graves' disease, thyroid nodules, or toxic goiter who has undergone a recent stressful experience including severe infection, trauma, major surgery, thromboembolism, DKA, or preeclampsia, pregnancy, labor, and/or delivery. Complaints include night sweats, unexplained weight loss, rapid gastric turnover with increased bowel movements or diarrhea, feelings of impending doom, rapid heart rate, and sleep disturbances. (*See SIRS, Sepsis, and MODS, p. 924, Hyperglycemia, p. 711, High-Risk Obstetrics, p. 882.*)

Vital Signs

- May have hyperpyrexia (fever)
- Acute exacerbation of tachycardia, palpitations, or new-onset atrial fibrillation with chest discomfort in a patient with enlargement of the thyroid gland
- Both hypertension and widened pulse pressure are common.

Observation

- Confused, possibly psychotic, disoriented person with CNS irritability
- Hyperreflexia and fine tremor may be present.
- Coma, heart failure, and generalized muscle weakness may be present.
- Possible recent weight loss
- Patients with Graves' disease (only in this form of thyrotoxicosis) have significant immune system components that may express as soft tissue swelling around the eye orbit, causing the protrusion of the eyes (exopthalmos), stare, and/or lid lag.
- Males often have gynecomastia. Many patients have fine hair and thin skin.
- Dependent lower extremity edema, alteration in appetite, change in vision, and fertility or menstrual dysfunctions are possible.

Palpation

- The thyroid gland in Graves' disease will usually be enlarged, soft, and symmetrical, although occasionally it may be firm and irregular.
- Older patients may not have enlarged thyroid glands, which may lead to dismissal of the diagnosis.
- Palpation is not the definitive method to evaluate thyroid dysfunction.

Screening Labwork

- *TSH level*: Any type or cause of hyperthyroid disease (except when the cause is secondary excessive TSH production) will create a suppression of TSH. The development of TSH sensitive testing has made the diagnosis of thyroid dysfunction much simpler.
- *T4 level*: Unstable patients who have been diagnosed previously and/or are treated for thyroid disorders require a serum thyroxine (T_4), which will be significantly more valuable in diagnosis. See Figure 8-1 for diagnostic principles.

Common Diagnostic Tests for Thyrotoxic Crisis

Blood Studies

Test	Purpose	Abnormal Findings
Thyroid-stimulating hormone (TSH) TSH is produced by the anterior pituitary gland in response to decreased T_4 level. The hypothalamus, anterior pituitary gland and thyroid are connected in an "axis" of function. *Normal/standard*: 0.4 and 4.5 mIU/L	To assess if TSH level is normal. TSH is decreased when T_4 level is increased. If T_4 is constantly increased, the TSH level is suppressed (low or decreased) by the high level of T_4. Normally, TSH release is needed to stimulate the thyroid to produce additional T_4.	When TSH is low in a patient with symptoms of thyroid storm, the diagnosis of hyperthyroidism will be considered positive until proven otherwise. If TSH is not prompting the increase in T_4, the thyroid has started generating T_4 abnormally. It is always beneficial to also evaluate T_4 at the same time. If the TSH is low while the T_4 is high, the patient is diagnosed with *primary hyperthyroidism.*
Free T_4 (thyroxine) *Normal*: 60–170 nmol/L	Measures the primary thyroid hormone	When levels are above normal, diagnosis of hyperthyroidism is made. If TSH and T_4 are both high, the problem is in the hypothalamic-pituitary response to elevated circulating thyroid levels (*secondary hyperthyroidism*).
T_3 (triiodothyronine) Normal: 0.8–2.7 nmol/L	Measures the more metabolically active form of the thyroid hormone.	Controversial
Thyroid-binding globulin (TBG)	To measure the level of the protein that binds with circulating thyroid hormones. Abnormal T_4 or T_3 measurements are often due to binding protein abnormalities rather than abnormal thyroid function.	Total T_4 or T_3 must be evaluated with a measure of thyroid hormone binding such as T_3 resin uptake or assay of thyroid-binding globulin. These methods are known as free T_4 or free T_3 even though they do not measure free hormone directly.
Radioactive iodine uptake	Differentiates the cause of thyroid disorder	May identify "hot" or "cold" nodules
Cholesterol analysis	Routine screening in biochemical profile	Hypercholesterolemia
Glucose	Routine screening in biochemical profile	Hyperglycemia; patients also have an impaired glucose tolerance test.
Electrolytes Potassium (K^+) Magnesium (Mg^{2+}) Calcium (Ca^{2+}) Sodium (Na^+)	Assess for possible abnormalities	Frequently, abnormalities of calcium are related to parathyroid disorders that exist concurrently with thyroid dysfunction.

Radiology

Thyroid scan ^{123}I (preferably) or ^{99m}Tc pertechnetate	Assess size of heart, thoracic cage (for fractures), thoracic aorta (for aneurysm), and lungs (pneumonia, pneumothorax) Assists with differential diagnosis of chest pain	Scan is done to help determine the cause of the hyperthyroidism. The scan may also be useful in assessing the functional status of any palpable thyroid irregularities or nodules associated with a toxic goiter.

Thyrotoxicosis Crisis (Thyroid Storm)

COLLABORATIVE MANAGEMENT
Care Priorities
1. **Stabilize the patient.**
   - *Reduce the stress response with beta adrenergic–blocking agents (e.g., esmolol, metoprolol, propranolol):* Control tachycardia, manage atrial fibrillation if present, anxiety, heat intolerance, and tremor. Does not decrease the metabolic rate and has a mild effect on global oxygen consumption. DO NOT ASSUME improvement in the thyroid disorder itself, only its symptoms. Calcium channel blockers may be used if beta blockers are contraindicated.
   - *Oxygen:* Used per nasal cannula or mask as needed to maintain SpO_2 greater than 90%.
   - *Control fever:* Antipyretic medications (i.e., acetaminophen) or hypothermia blanket is used. Aspirin is contraindicated, as it worsens thyroid crisis.
   - *Rehydrate using intravenous fluids:* Fever and rapid metabolism can lead to dehydration.
   - *Correct electrolyte imbalance:* Various imbalances may occur. Replace electrolytes as appropriate.
   - *Glucocorticoids:* Administered to help inhibit conversion of thyroxine (T_4) to T_3 and prevent adrenal insufficiency.
   - *Minimize anxiety with mild tranquilizers:* Also promote rest.
2. **Treat the thyroid with antithyroid agents (thioamides):** Noninvasive, relatively cost-effective therapy with low risk of permanent hypothyroidism and a low cure rate.
   - *Propylthiouracil (PTU)* has been the first line of treatment and is more effective in thyroid storm than methimazole. Can be used in pregnant patients. If the patient is unable to swallow, the medication is given using a nasogastric tube. Iodides (potassium iodide or Lugol's solution) are given several hours after PTU to avoid a buildup of hormones stored in the thyroid gland.
   - *Methimazole* may also be used. Both thioamides may cause leukopenia, rash, urticaria, fever, arthralgias, and, rarely, agranulocytosis. Methimazole may have a lower rate of these effects. Agranulocytosis (complete lack of granulocytes) causes fever and sore throat. If agranulocytosis is confirmed by complete blood count (CBC), the thioamide should be stopped.
   - *Iodides (SSKI):* Sodium or potassium iodide drops may be given to help inhibit the release of thyroid hormone or to help abate accumulation of hormones stored in the thyroid. May stain the teeth.
3. **Cure the thyroid with radioactive iodine:** It is the most cost-effective and commonly used agent. Use usually results in hypothyroidism, requiring replacement therapy. Cannot be used for the pregnant patient, as the thyroid gland of the fetus may also be destroyed. Usually reserved for the following indications:
   - Failure to respond to antithyroid drugs
   - Relapse after 1 to 2 years of therapy
   - Toxic multinodular goiter
   - Solitary toxic nodules
   - Noncompliant patients
4. **Perform a subtotal thyroidectomy to provide a rapid, effective, curative therapy:** Most invasive and expensive therapy; hypothyroidism is inevitable. Surgical removal of part of the gland often is the best treatment for patients with extremely enlarged glands or multinodular goiter. Surgery is avoided in the pregnant patient due to risk of miscarriage or preterm delivery. The patient is prepared with antithyroid agents until normal thyroid function is achieved (usually 6 to 8 weeks). The most frequent postoperative complication is hemorrhage at the operative site. The following complications are rare but can be extremely serious: hypoparathyroidism, laryngeal nerve injury, and tetany from damage to the parathyroid glands.

CARE PLANS FOR THYROID STORM

Ineffective protection *related to potential for thyrotoxic crisis (thyroid storm) secondary to emotional stress, trauma, infection, pregnancy (especially labor and delivery), or surgical manipulation of the gland*

GOALS/OUTCOMES Patient is free of symptoms of thyroid storm as evidenced by normothermia, BP 90/60 mm Hg or greater (or within patient's baseline range), HR 100 bpm or less, and orientation to person, place, and time. If thyroid storm occurs, it is noted promptly and reported immediately.

NOC Immune Hypersensitivity Response

Risk Identification
1. Measure and report rectal or core temperature greater than 38.3°C (101°F): often the first sign of impending thyroid storm.
2. Monitor vital signs hourly for evidence of hypotension and increasing tachycardia and fever.
3. Monitor patient for signs of congestive heart failure, which occurs as an effect of thyroid storm: jugular vein distention, crackles (rales), decreased amplitude of peripheral pulses, peripheral edema, and hypotension. Immediately report any significant findings to physician, and prepare to transfer patient to ICU if they are noted. Maternal and fetal monitoring is initiated on pregnant patients.
4. Provide a cool, calm, protected environment to minimize emotional stress if possible. Reassure patient, and explain all procedures. Limit the number of visitors.
5. Ensure good hand washing and meticulous aseptic technique for dressing changes and all procedures. Advise visitors who have contracted or been exposed to a communicable disease either not to enter patient's room or to use appropriate infection control precautions.
6. Administer acetaminophen to decrease temperature.

Safety Alert   *Aspirin is contraindicated because it releases thyroxine from protein-binding sites and increases free thyroxine levels.*

---

7. Provide cool sponge baths or apply ice packs to patient's axilla and groin areas to decrease fever. If high temperature continues, obtain a prescription for a hypothermia blanket.
8. Administer PTU as prescribed to prevent further synthesis and release of thyroid hormones.
9. Administer beta blockers as prescribed to block sympathetic nervous system (SNS) effects.
10. Administer IV fluids as prescribed to provide adequate hydration and prevent vascular collapse. Fluid volume deficit may occur because of increased fluid excretion by the kidneys or excessive diaphoresis. Carefully monitor I&O hourly to prevent fluid overload or inadequate fluid replacement. Decreasing output with normal specific gravity may indicate decreased cardiac output, whereas decreasing output with increased specific gravity can signal dehydration.
11. Administer iodides as prescribed, 1 hour after administering PTU.

Safety Alert   *If given before PTU, iodides can exacerbate symptoms in susceptible persons.*

---

12. Administer small doses of insulin as prescribed to control hyperglycemia. Hyperglycemia can occur as an effect of thyroid storm because of the hypermetabolic state.
13. Administer prescribed supplemental oxygen to support increased metabolism.

NIC Cardiac Care: Acute; Surveillance: Late Pregnancy; Fluid/Electrolyte Management; Hyperglycemia Management; Energy Management; Nutritional Monitoring; Vital Signs Monitoring

Impaired swallowing (or risk for same)   *related to edema or laryngeal nerve damage resulting from surgical procedure*

GOALS/OUTCOMES Patient reports swallowing with minimal difficulty, has minimal or absent hoarseness, and is free of symptoms of respiratory dysfunction as evidenced by RR 12 to 20 breaths/min with normal depth and pattern and absence of inspiratory stridor. Laryngeal nerve damage, if it occurs, is detected promptly and reported immediately.
NOC Aspiration Prevention, Swallowing Status

Aspiration Precautions
1. Monitor respiratory status for signs of edema (i.e., dyspnea, choking, inspiratory stridor, inability to swallow). Assess patient's voice. Slight hoarseness is normal after surgery. Persistent hoarseness indicates laryngeal nerve damage. If bilateral nerve damage is present, upper airway obstruction can occur. Report findings to physician promptly.

2. Elevate HOB 30 to 45 degrees to minimize edema and incisional stress. Support patient's head with flat or cervical pillows so that it is in a neutral position.
3. Keep tracheostomy set and oxygen equipment at the bedside at all times. Suction upper airway as needed, using gentle suction to avoid stimulating laryngospasm.
4. To minimize pain and anxiety and enhance patient's ability to swallow, administer analgesics promptly and as prescribed.

NIC Management; Nutrition Therapy; Respiratory Monitoring; Swallowing Therapy

Anxiety *related to SNS stimulation*

GOALS/OUTCOMES Within 24 hours of hospital admission, patient is free of harmful anxiety as evidenced by a HR 100 bpm or less, RR 12 to 20 breaths/min with normal depth and pattern, and absence of or decreases in irritability and restlessness. Patient and significant others verbalize knowledge about the causes of the patient's behavior.
NOC Anxiety Level, Anxiety Self-Control

Anxiety Reduction
1. Assess for anxiety; administer short-acting sedatives (e.g., lorazepam) as prescribed.
2. Provide a quiet, stress-free environment away from loud noises or excessive activity.
3. Limit number of visitors and the amount of time they spend with patient. Advise significant others to avoid discussing stressful topics and to refrain from arguing with the patient.
4. Administer beta blockers as prescribed to reduce anxiety, tachycardia, and heat intolerance.
5. Reassure patient that anxiety is related to the disease and that treatment decreases severity.
6. Inform significant others that the patient's agitated behavior should not be taken personally.

NIC Coping Enhancement; High-Risk Pregnancy Care

Imbalanced nutrition: less than body requirements *related to hypermetabolic state and/or inadequate nutrient absorption*

GOALS/OUTCOMES By a minimum of 24 hours before hospital discharge, patient has adequate nutrition as evidenced by stable weight and a positive nitrogen balance.
NOC Nutritional Status

Nutrition Therapy
1. Provide foods high in calories, protein, carbohydrates, and vitamins.
2. Administer vitamin supplements as prescribed, and explain their importance to patient.
3. Administer prescribed antidiarrheal medications, which increase absorption of nutrients from the GI tract.
4. Weigh patient daily, and report significant losses to physician.

NIC Weight Management; Weight Gain Assistance; Nutritional Counseling

Disturbed sleep pattern *related to accelerated metabolism*

GOALS/OUTCOMES Within 48 hours of hospital admission, patient relates the attainment of sufficient rest and sleep.

Sleep Enhancement
1. Adjust care activities to patient's tolerance.
2. Provide frequent rest periods of at least 90-minute duration. If possible, arrange for patient to have bed rest in a quiet, cool room.
3. Administer short-acting sedatives (e.g., lorazepam) as prescribed to promote rest.

NIC Anxiety Reduction; Meditation Facilitation

Impaired tissue integrity of the cornea *related to dryness that can occur with exophthalmos in persons with Graves disease*

GOALS/OUTCOMES Within 24 hours of admission, patient's corneas are moist and intact.
NOC Tissue Integrity: Skin and Mucous Membranes

Eye Care
1. Teach patient to wear dark glasses to protect the cornea.
2. Administer lubricating eye drops as prescribed to supplement lubrication and decrease SNS stimulation, which can cause lid retraction.
3. If appropriate, apply eye shields or tape the eyes shut at bedtime.
4. Administer thioamides as prescribed to maintain normal metabolic state and halt progression of exophthalmos.

NIC Skin Care: Topical Treatments

Deficient knowledge: Medications *related to the potential for side effects from iodides and thioamides or stopping thioamides abruptly*

GOALS/OUTCOMES Within the 24-hour period before hospital discharge, patient verbalizes knowledge about potential side effects of prescribed medications, signs and symptoms of hypothyroidism and hyperthyroidism, and the importance of following the prescribed medical regimen. Patient understands that he or she must be seen within 4 months for endocrine follow-up.
NOC Knowledge: Medications; Knowledge: Illness Care

Teaching: Individual
1. Explain importance of taking antithyroid medications daily, as prescribed.
2. Teach indicators of hypothyroidism (e.g., early fatigue, weight gain, anorexia, constipation, menstrual irregularities, muscle cramps, lethargy, inability to concentrate, hair loss, cold intolerance, and hoarseness), which may occur from excessive antithyroid medication, and the signs and symptoms that necessitate medical attention, including cold intolerance, fatigue, lethargy, and peripheral or periorbital edema.
3. Teach side effects of thioamides and symptoms that require medical attention: appearance of a rash, fever, or pharyngitis, which can occur in the presence of agranulocytosis and require prompt medical intervention.
4. Discuss signs of worsening hyperthyroidism including high body temperature, palpitations, rapid HR, irritability, anxiety, and feelings of restlessness or panic.
5. Explain importance of continued and frequent medical follow-up.
6. Indicators that require medical attention: fever, rash, or sore throat (side effects of thioamides), and symptoms of hypothyroidism or worsening hyperthyroidism.
7. For patients receiving radioactive iodine, explain the importance of not holding children to the chest for 72 hours following therapy, because children are more susceptible to the effects of radiation. Explain that there is negligible risk for adults.
8. Stress the importance of avoiding physical and emotional stress early in the recuperative stage and maximizing coping mechanisms for dealing with stress.

NIC Learning Facilitation; Health Education; Teaching: Disease Process; Teaching: Prescribed Medication; Teaching: Activity/Exercise

ADDITIONAL NURSING DIAGNOSES

See *Compromised Family Coping,* in *Oncologic Emergencies,* p. 893; *Nutritional Support,* p. 117; *Alterations in Consciousness,* p. 24; *Emotional and Spiritual Support of the Patient and* Significant *Others,* p. 200; *Dysrhythmias and Conduction Disturbances,* p. 492; *Heart Failure,* p. 421.

SELECTED REFERENCES

AACE Thyroid Task Force. American Association of Clinical Endocrinologists: Medical guidelines for clinical practice for the evaluation and treatment of hyperthyroidism and hypothyroidism: (2006 amended version). *Endocr Pract* 8(6):457-469, 2002. http://www.aace.com/pub/pdf/guidelines/hypo_hyper.pdf

Aghar A, Thornton E, et al: Posterior pituitary dysfunction after traumatic brain injury. *J Clin Endocrinol Metab* 89:5987-5992, 2004.

Albright TN, Zimmerman MA, Selzman CH: Vasopressin in the cardiac surgery intensive care unit. *Am J Crit Care* 11:326-330, 2002.

Ball SG, Bayliss PH: Normal and abnormal physiology of the hypothalamus-posterior pituitary (including DI and SIADH). Chapter 2, Endotext.org downloaded June 15, 2009. http://www.endotext.org/neuroendo/neuroendo2/neuroendoframe2.htm

Bornstein SR: Predisposing factors for adrenal insufficiency. *N Engl J Med* 360:2328-2339, 2009.

Cathie K, Levin M, Faust SN: Drug use in acute meningococcal disease. *Educ Pract* 93:151-158, 2009.

Cohen J, Ward G, Prins J, et al: Variability of cortisol assays can confound the diagnosis of adrenal insufficiency in the critically ill population. *Intens Care Med* 32:1901-1905, 2006.

Daley MR, Seam N, Luboshitzky R; the CORTICUS Study Group: Corticosteroids for septic shock. *N Engl J Med* 358:2068-2071, 2008.

Dunser MW, Hasibeder WR: Sympathetic overstimulation during critical illness: adverse effects of adrenergic stress. *J Intens Care Med* 24:293-316, 2009.

Ellison DH, Berl T: The syndrome of inappropriate antidiuresis. N Engl J Med 356:2064-2072, 2007.

Eskes S, Wiersinga WM: Amiodarone and thyroid. *Clin Endocr Metab* 23(6):735-751, 2009.

Grozinsky-Glasberg S, Fraser A, Nahshoni E: Thyroxine-triiodothyronine combination therapy versus thyroxine monotherapy for clinical hypothyroidism: meta-analysis of randomized controlled trials. *J Clin Endocrinol Metab* 91(7):2592-2599, 2006.

Hamrahain AH, Osenis TS, Arafah BM: Measurements of serum free cortisol in critically ill patients. *N Engl J Med* 350:1629, 2004.

Hollowell JG, Staehling NW, Flanders WD, et al: Serum TSH, T(4), and thyroid antibodies in the United States population (1988 to 1994): National Health and Nutrition Examination Survey (NHANES III). *J Clin Endocrinol Metab* 87(2):489-499, 2002. http://www.endotext.org/neuroendo/neuroendo2/neuroendoframe2.htm.

Krinsley JS: Effect of an intensive glucose management protocol on the mortality of critically ill adult patients. *Mayo Clin Proc* 79:992-1000, 2004.

Ladenson P, Kim M: Thyroid. In Goldman L, Ausiello DA, editors: *Cecil Medicine,* ed 23. Philadelphia, Saunders Elsevier: 1698-1712, 2007.

Langouche L, Van den Berghe G: The dynamic neuroendocrine response to critical illness. Endocrinol Metab Clin North Am 35(4):777-791, ix, 2006.

Lazar HL, McDonnell M, Chipkin SR, et al: The Society of Thoracic Surgeons practice guideline series: blood glucose management during adult cardiac surgery. *Ann Thorac Surg* 87(2):663-669, 2009.

LeBeau SO, Mandel SJ: Thyroid disorders during pregnancy. *Endocrinol Metab Clin North Am* 35(1):117-136, vii, 2006.

Lee CR, Watkins M, Patterson JH, et al: Vasopressin: a new target for the treatment of heart failure. *Am Heart J* 146:9-18, 2003.

Marik PE: Critical illness-related corticosteroid insufficiency. *Chest* 135:181-193, 2009.

Marik PE, Pastores SM, Annane D, et al: Recommendations for the diagnosis and management of corticosteroid insufficiency in critically ill adult patients: consensus statements from an international task force by the American College of Critical Care Medicine. *Crit Care Med* 36(6):1937-1949, 2008.

Moghissi ES, Korytkowski MT, Dinardo N, et al: American Association of Clinical Endocrinologists and American Diabetes Association consensus on inpatient diabetes control. *Endocr Pract* 15(4):1-16, 2009.

Moliach ME, : *Anterior Pituitary.* In Goldman L. & Ausiello DA, editors: **Cecil Medicine,** 23rd ed. Philadelphia, PA: Saunders Elsevier: 1674 -1691, 2007.

Moliach ME: *Neuroendocrinology and the neuroendocrine system.* In Goldman L & Ausiello DA, editors: *Cecil Medicine,* ed 23, Philadelphia, PA: Saunders Elsevier: 1664-1674, 2007.

Navak B, Hodak SP: Hyperthyroidism. *Endocrinol Metab Clin N Am* 36(3):617-656, 2007.

O'Connor KJ, Wood KE, Lord K: Intensive management of organ donors to maximize transplantation. *Crit Care Nurse* 26:94-100, 2006.

Osburne RC, Cook CB, Stockton L, et al: Improving hyperglycemia management in the intensive care unit preliminary report of a nurse-driven quality improvement project using a redesigned insulin infusion algorithm. *Diabetes Educator* 32(3):394–403, 2006.

Reid JR, Wheeler SF: Hyperthyroidism: diagnosis and treatment. *Am Fam Phys* 2:623–630, 2005.

Schrier RW, Gross P, Gheorghiade M, et al: Tolvaptan, a selective oral vasopressin V2-receptor antagonist, for hyponatremia. *N Engl J Med* 355:2099–2112, 2006.

Sprung CL, Annane D, Keh D, et al: Hydrocortisone therapy for patients with septic shock. *N Engl J Med* 358:111–124, 2008.

The NICE SUGAR Study Investigators: Intensive vs conventional glucose control in critically ill patients. *N Engl J Med* 360(13):1283–1297, 2009.

Wartofsky L: Myxedema coma. *Endocrinol Metab Clin North Am* 35(4):687–698, vii–viii, 2006.

Wartofsky L, Dickey RA: Controversy in clinical endocrinology: The evidence for a narrower thyrotropin reference range is compelling. *J Clin Endocrinol Metab* 90:5483–5488, 2005.

Wilson M, Weinreb J, Hoo GWS: Intensive insulin therapy in critical care: a review of 12 protocols. *Diab Care* 30(4):1005–1011, 2007.

Gastrointestinal Disorders

GASTROINTESTINAL ASSESSMENT: GENERAL

Goal of System Assessment
Evaluate for dysfunctional ingestion and digestion of food and elimination of waste products.

Vital Sign Assessment
- Heart rate (HR), blood pressure (BP), and peripheral pulses to identify volume status as significant fluid losses can occur with gastrointestinal (GI) bleeding or diarrhea.
- Note temperature, because infections of the GI tract are common.

Observation
Observe the abdomen for distention and skin color changes, which may be signs of other system disorders.
- Cullen sign (bluish umbilicus)—intra-abdominal hemorrhage
- Turner sign (bruising on the flanks)—indicates retroperitoneal hemorrhage
- Visible, torturous, dilated abdominal veins may indicate inferior vena cava obstruction.
- Cutaneous abdominal angiomas may indicate liver disease.

Auscultation
Evaluate bowel sounds in each of the quadrants in a systemic fashion.
- Hyperactive bowel sounds—may indicate diarrhea or early intestinal obstruction
- Hypoactive to absent bowel sounds—may indicate paralytic ileus or peritonitis
- High-pitched rushing sounds—may indicate intestinal obstruction
Evaluate for systolic bruits (humming, swishing, or blowing sounds) over:
- Abdominal aorta—partial arterial obstruction
- Renal artery—renal artery stenosis
- Iliac artery—hepatomegaly

Palpation
The normal abdomen should be soft and nontender to palpation. Palpate for liver enlargement and tenderness. The spleen is not normally palpable. If found palpable, the spleen is enlarged. Further palpation must be discontinued as it may cause splenic rupture.

> **Safety Alert** *If the abdomen is rigid, do not palpate; it is a sign of peritoneal inflammation. Palpation could cause rupture of the inflamed organ.*

Nutritional Assessment
Evaluate for risk factors and indications of malnutrition for which critically ill patients are at risk. Malnutrition may occur due to negative caloric intake with concomitant GI obstruction, malabsorption syndromes, infectious diseases, certain medications, and surgical treatment.

Table 9-1	GENERAL SIGNS OF MALNUTRITION	
Body System	**Signs**	**Deficiency**
Skin, nails	Dry skin Brittle nails; spooned-shaped nails	Vitamin deficiency Iron deficiency
Mouth	Cracks; beefy, red tongue	Vitamin deficiency
Stomach	Decreased gastric acidity Delayed gastric emptying	Protein deficiency
Intestines	Decreased motility and absorption Diarrhea	Protein deficiency Altered normal flora
Liver/biliary	Hepatomegaly Ascites	Decreased absorption of fat-soluble vitamins, Protein deficiency
Cardiovascular	Edema Tachycardia; hypotension	Protein deficiency Fluid volume deficiency
Musculoskeletal	Decreased muscle mass Subcutaneous tissue loss	Protein, carbohydrate, and fat deficiency

Additionally, caloric needs are greatly increased in the critically ill as a result of hypermetabolic states produced by trauma, fever, sepsis, and wound healing.
- Evaluate for general signs of malnutrition (Table 9-1).
- Evaluate weight for increases and decreases.
- Determine elimination patterns: constipation; diarrhea; ↓ urine output.
- Laboratory identification of malnutrition:
  - Serum albumin less than 3 g/dl
  - Serum transferrin less than 200mg/dl
  - Serum prealbumin less than 16.0 mg/dl
  - Total lymphocyte count ↓
  - Triglycerides ↓

Screening Labwork
- Serum electrolytes levels
- Complete blood count (CBC)
- Serum amylase
- Serum lipase
- Liver function tests (LFTs)

ACUTE GASTROINTESTINAL BLEEDING

PATHOPHYSIOLOGY
Bleeding can occur at any point along the alimentary tract; however, an upper GI (UGI) bleed is 5 times more common than a lower one. Together they account for significant morbidity, with a mortality rate of 8% to 10% that has not changed over the past 30 to 40 years. For an acute UGI bleed, mortality can be greater than 40% in patients with liver disease or other serious illness. Severity of blood loss can be as great as 25% of intravascular volume. The following overview presents common GI bleeding sites and occurrences.

Upper Gastrointestinal Bleeding
Esophagus Esophageal varices secondary to alcoholism are the most common cause of massive and persistent esophageal hemorrhage. Esophagitis, esophageal ulcers, and tumors also can cause acute bleeding but occur less frequently. Maneuvers that increase intra-abdominal pressure (e.g., retching, vomiting, straining, coughing) can lead to Mallory-Weiss tear (a laceration at the esophagogastric junction), which can also result in massive bleeding.
Stomach and Duodenum The most common cause of hematemesis and melena is gastroduodenal ulcer disease, accounting for half of massive UGI bleeding (UGIB) disorders. *Peptic ulcers* are chronic, usually solitary, lesions that are most prevalent in the stomach and duodenum.

These lesions breach the protective mucosa of the GI tract extending deep into the submucosa, exposing tissue to gastric acids with eventual autodigestion. Bleeding occurs when the ulcer erodes into a blood vessel. *Helicobacter pylori* (*H. pylori*) is strongly associated with the pathogenesis of peptic ulceration, much more so than gastric hyperacidity. The toxins and enzymes released by the *H. pylori* organism are believed to cause ulceration through proinflammatory processes and by decreasing duodenal mucosal bicarbonate production. Infection with *H. pylori* is present in almost all patients with duodenal ulcers and 70% of patients with gastric ulcers. In contrast, hyperacidity is present in a minority of patients with gastric ulcers and even less in those with duodenal ulcers. Bleeding occurs in 10% to 20% of patients with peptic ulceration, and perforation occurs in about 5%. Another cause of peptic ulceration is *Zöllinger-Ellison Syndrome* (ZES). In ZES, ulcerations occur in the stomach, duodenum, and jejunum due to excess gastrin secretion by a tumor, resulting in hyperacidity with mucosal erosion. *Stress ulceration* is a common and potentially life-threatening phenomenon that occurs in critically ill patients, especially those who are mechanically ventilated. Stress ulcers, also known as erosive gastritis, tend to be multiple lesions, located mainly in the stomach and occasionally in the duodenum, primarily resulting from stress-related hyperacidity and mucosal ischemia. Stress ulcers occurring in the proximal duodenum are called *Curling ulcers*. They are associated with deep mucosal invasion and are seen in patients with major burn injury or major trauma. *Cushing ulcer* is a related condition occurring in patients who have sustained serious head injury, major surgery, or critical central nervous system (CNS) disorder that raises intracranial pressure. *Gastritis*, another common cause of peptic ulceration, usually occurs as slow, diffuse oozing that is difficult to control. *Benign or malignant gastric tumors* may initiate severe bleeding episodes, especially tumors located in the vascular system that supplies the GI tract.

Ulcer bleeding from the UGI tract is usually self-limiting. However, patients with continued or recurrent bleeding are associated with a poorer prognosis.

Lower Gastrointestinal Bleeding

Small Intestine Only structures distal to the ligament of Treitz (a thin muscular band that wraps around the small intestine where the duodenum and jejunum meet) are involved. These areas of the small intestine account for only a small portion of GI bleeding episodes. Diverticular disease, arteriovenous malformation, intussusception of the small bowel, acute superior mesenteric artery occlusion, and Crohn disease are some of the possible causes for bleeding.
Large Intestine A major cause of significant LGI bleeding (LGIB) is colonic diverticula. Arteriovenous malformation of the ascending colon and the cecum is also a usual cause of massive colonic bleeding. Inflammatory bowel diseases such as ulcerative colitis and Crohn disease result in friable intestinal mucosa, which can lead to massive hemorrhage and other serious complications, including bowel obstruction and perforation. In addition, diverticular disease can cause serious, intermittent bleeding episodes. Other causes include benign or malignant neoplasms and congenital malformation such as hemangioma or telangiectasia.
Rectum Hemorrhoids and neoplasms frequently cause LGIB but are usually hemodynamically insignificant.

Neighboring Organs

Pancreas and Vascular Grafts Acute pancreatitis (see p. 762) and pancreatic pseudocyst are disorders associated with hemorrhage. Persons with intra-abdominal vascular grafts are at risk for the development of aortoenteric fistulas with massive GI hemorrhage.
Systemic Organ Diseases Hypoperfusion associated with decreased cardiac output or volume depletion can lead to GI ischemia, resulting in necrosis and hemorrhage. A high incidence of GI bleeding is associated with uremia in renal failure patients because of platelet dysfunction. Collagen diseases can result in thrombosis of small vessels in the small intestine, eventually leading to ulceration. Many blood dyscrasias (e.g., disseminated intravascular coagulopathy [DIC], thrombocytopenia) are associated with hematemesis and melena caused by decreased clotting ability.

Medications

Longstanding use of aspirin, corticosteroids, or anticoagulants is associated with serious GI bleeding. Ethanol may cause or potentiate ulcer bleeding as it induces gastric mucosal injury. Nonsteroidal anti-inflammatory drugs (NSAIDs) cause increased risk of serious GI bleeding, ulceration, and perforation of the stomach and intestines. Traditional NSAIDs are nonselective inhibitors of both cyclooxygenase-1 (COX-1) and cyclooxygenase-2 (COX-2) enzymes.

COX-1 enzymes regulate gastroduodenal mucosal protective mechanisms. COX-2 enzymes are involved in inflammatory and pain responses. The newer COX-2 selective inhibitors were believed to block pain and inflammation while leaving protective mucosal mechanisms intact, thereby significantly lowering the incidence of GI ulceration and bleeding compared with traditional NSAIDs. However, the COX-2 inhibitors were shown to increase the risk of cardiovascular disease, especially in older adults, resulting in the removal of two of three COX-2 agents from the market. Currently, celecoxib is the only COX-2 selective inhibitor available in the United States. This COX-2 inhibitor is still associated with an increased risk for GI bleeding, while to a lesser degree than traditional NSAIDS; additionally, it does not appear to pose any greater risk for cardiovascular disease than traditional NSAIDs.

Other Trauma

In addition to major abdominal trauma (see p. 245), foreign bodies such as razors, screws, or nails, may lacerate gastric or intestinal mucosa, causing bleeding.

GASTROINTESTINAL ASSESSMENT: ACUTE GASTROINTESTINAL BLEEDING
Goal of Assessment

Evaluate patients for severity of active bleeding, shock states, or risk of rebleeding.

History and Risk Factors

History and risk factors include critical illness, especially that caused by major injury, surgery, CNS disorder, or burns; prolonged shock or hypoperfusion; organ failure; esophageal varices, excessive alcohol, NSAIDs, or corticosteroid ingestion; inflammatory bowel disease; foreign body ingestion; hiatal hernia; hepatic, pancreatic, or biliary tract disease; blood dyscrasias; penetrating or blunt trauma; familial cancer; recent abdominal surgery; and the presence of *H. pylori*, found in greater than 90% of patients with duodenal ulcers and 70% of those with gastric ulcers. Identification of those at risk for recurrent bleeding is essential to guide therapy and prevent poor outcomes. Risk factors associated with rebleeding are listed in Box 9-1.

Vital Sign Assessment

- Systolic BP less than 90 to 100 mm Hg with an HR greater than 100 beats/min (bpm) in a previously normotensive individual signals a 20% or greater reduction in blood volume.
- Orthostatic hypotension signs will be positive revealing a decrease in systolic BP greater than 10 mm Hg with an increase in HR of 10 bpm. Orthostatic hypotension is indicative of recent blood loss of at least 1000 ml in the adult.
- Respiratory rate will be mildly elevated as a response to the diminished oxygen-carrying capacity of the blood. If abdominal pain is present, ventilatory excursion may be limited.
- Urine output will be decreased due to volume depletion.

Blood Loss

- The amount of blood lost and rate of bleeding will have varying effects on cardiovascular and other body systems.
- Blood loss of 1000 ml within 15 minutes usually produces tachycardia, hypotension, nausea, weakness, and diaphoresis. Adults can lose up to 500 ml of blood in 15 minutes and remain free of associated symptoms.
- Massive hemorrhage, which is generally defined as loss of greater than 25% of total blood volume or a bleeding episode that requires transfusion of 6 units of blood in a 24-hour period, can occur.

Box 9-1	RISK FACTORS TO PREDICT RECURRENT BLEEDING

- Large-volume blood loss on admission with transfusion of greater than 6 units
- Shock
- Age greater than 60 years
- Hematemesis as the initial sign of hemorrhage
- Stigmata of ulcer bleeding as identified endoscopically
- Bleeding that occurs while hospitalized for another problem

Acute Gastrointestinal Bleeding

- Syncope associated with hypotension also may occur.
- Sequestration of fluid into the peritoneum and interstitium further depletes intravascular volume.
- Severe hypovolemic shock and decreased cardiac output can lead to ischemia of various organs, especially the brain and kidneys.

Abdominal Pain
- Mild to severe epigastric pain is often associated with gastroduodenal ulcerative or erosive disease. The pain is described as dull or gnawing.
- As blood covers and protects the eroded tissue, pain may disappear.
- Blood can irritate the bowels, thereby increasing transit time in the lower GI tract, causing diarrhea.

Observation
- Extremities are cool and diaphoretic.
- Pallor or cyanosis may be present.
- Alterations in LOC with restlessness and confusion.
- Emesis or gastric aspirate contains obvious whole blood or old blood that resembles coffee grounds.
- Hematemesis usually occurs with UGIB from above the ligament of Treitz. Bleeding originating below the level of the duodenum is not usually associated with hematemesis.
- Stool
  - *Melena* (black, tarry, shiny, stools containing blood, with a distinctive fetid odor) is usually present with UGIB. May also be present with bleeding from the small intestine or proximal large intestine.
  - *Hematochezia* (dark-red stool containing fresh blood) is usually present with LGIB.
  - Massive LGIB is associated with dark red "currant jelly" stools or passing fresh blood with clots.
- Jaundice, vascular spiders, ascites, and hepatosplenomegaly suggest liver disease.

Auscultation
- Auscultation of the abdomen may reveal hyperactive bowel sounds caused by mucosal irritation by blood.
- A silent abdomen suggests serious complications such as ileus, perforation, or vascular occlusion.

Palpation
- Palpation may reveal epigastric tenderness, which is expected in peptic ulceration.
- An epigastric mass or enlarged lymph nodes may indicate gastric malignant disease.
- Decreased peripheral pulses, delayed capillary refill (greater than 2 seconds)

Nutritional Assessment
- Evidence of malnutrition will be noted in the presence of chronic liver disease or active, excessive alcohol use.

Screening Labwork
- CBC: decreased hemoglobin (Hgb), decreased hematocrit (Hct)
- Liver function tests (LFTs): may be elevated if advanced liver disease is present
- Serum chemistry: increased blood urea nitrogen (BUN) and creatinine
- Radiologic tests: upper endoscopy, colonoscopy

Hemodynamic Measurements
- Hypovolemic shock usually reveals a decreased central venous pressure (CVP), pulmonary artery pressure (PAP), central venous oxygen saturation (ScVO2) and cardiac output (CO) and an increased stroke volume variation (SVV) and systemic vascular resistance (SVR).
- After major abdominal surgery, a hyperdynamic state may exist similar to that seen in early septic shock, with an increased CO and decreased SVR (see *SIRS, Sepsis and MODS*, p. 924).

Diagnostic Tests for Acute Gastrointestinal Bleeding

Test	Purpose	Abnormal Findings
Blood Studies		
Complete blood count (CBC) with differential Hemoglobin (Hgb) Hematocrit (Hct) RBC count (RBC) WBC count (WBC) Platelet count	Serial Hgb and Hct values monitor the amount of blood lost. Total counts monitor hematologic function, except for platelets, which may be nonfunctional despite normal number present.	Hgb <10 g/dl correlates with increased rebleeding and mortality rates. The first Hct value may be near normal ~45% because the ratio of blood cells to plasma remains unchanged initially. However, the Hct is expected to fall dramatically ~27% as volume is restored and extravascular fluid mobilizes into the vascular space (hemodilution). Hct < 24% generally requires transfusion. Platelet count rises within 1 hour of acute hemorrhage. Leukocytosis occurs frequently following acute hemorrhage.
Serum chemistry BUN Creatinine BUN:creatinine (Cr) ratio Serum chloride Serum potassium Serum glucose Liver function tests (LFTs): Total bilirubin Ammonia	To assess fluid and electrolyte status. LFTs monitor for hepatic involvement.	BUN will be elevated due to dehydration. Creatinine may be mildly elevated due to ↓ GFR secondary to hypovolemia. BUN:Cr ratio will be elevated >33:1 mg/dl in the patient with upper GI bleed. Hypochloremia, hypokalemia and ↑serum bicarbonate will be noted with excessive vomiting or gastric suction. Mild hyperglycemia is the result of the body's compensatory response to a stressful stimulus. Hyperbilirubinemia is caused by the breakdown of reabsorbed RBCs and blood pigments. Ammonia levels are usually elevated in patients with hepatic disease. Plasma protein levels may rise in response to increased hepatic production.
Arterial blood gas (ABG)	Assesses acid-base status. Lactic acid levels may be drawn separately, and may be available on certain ABG analyzers.	If the shock state is severe, lactic acidosis occurs, reflected by low arterial pH and serum bicarbonate levels and the presence of an anion gap. With a low perfusion state, hypoxemia may be present.
Coagulation studies	Assess for preexisting hypocoagulable disease; liver disease; anticoagulant or antiplatelet therapy for cardiac disease. Large blood volume transfusions may lead to the development of coagulopathies.	Elevation of fibrinogen levels, fibrin split products (FSP), PT, PTT, INR may be seen.
12-Lead ECG	Monitor for severe cardiac ischemia findings as a result of hypoperfusion.	Ischemic changes include T-wave depression or inversion.
Radiologic Procedures		
Esophagogastroduodenoscopy (EGD)	To accurately assess the source of upper GI ulcer bleeding. To locate the ulcer, visualize and implement endoscopic therapy, such as sclerosing bleeding vessels.	Endoscopic ulcer findings (endoscopic stigmata) include: Clean ulcer base Adherent clot Visible vessel Active bleeding

Continued

Diagnostic Tests for Acute Gastrointestinal Bleeding — cont'd		
Test	**Purpose**	**Abnormal Findings**
Plain films Abdominal radiograph Chest radiograph	To identify the presence of dilated bowel or free air. A chest x-ray is taken to establish baseline pulmonary status.	Free air seen under the diaphragm, suggests perforation.
Barium studies	Usually are reserved for nonemergent situations to verify the presence of tumors or other large GI lesions.	Not usually used for acute GI bleeding as this procedure does not allow for the provision of endoscopic therapy.
Colonoscopy	Direct visualization of the rectum and sigmoid colon through an endoscope for diagnosis and triage of lower GI bleeding.	Mucosal bleeding, polyps, hemorrhoids, and other lesions may be identified. Biopsy specimen may be obtained. Emergent colonoscopy is difficult due to length of time for adequate bowel preparation.
Angiography	The visualization of active bleeding from an arterial site or from a large vein in the lower GI tract. Bleeding flow rate must be at least 0.5–1.0 ml/min to be visualized by this test.	Clearly identifies bleeding GI arterial systems. Therapeutic arterial embolization or vasopressin infusion may be performed to stop the bleeding during angiography. Complications include dye-induced renal failure, arterial dissection and occlusion, bowel infarction, and MI with vasopressin infusion.
Nuclear medicine Technetium-labeled red blood cell scan	To detect low-flow rate bleeding in the lower GI tract. Usefulness is controversial.	Identifies low-flow bleeding rates of 0.1–0.5 ml/min in the lower GI tract. Accuracy remains questionable.

Blood Urea Nitrogen–to–Creatinine Ratio

Elevated BUN:creatinine ratio (33:1 to 36:1 mg/dl) reflects a disproportionate increase in BUN compared to a mild increase in serum creatinine with UGIB resulting from RBCs that have bled and pooled in the UGI tract being consumed and digested by duodenal/proximal small intestinal bacteria. The resulting urea is absorbed. The BUN increases without a corresponding increase in creatinine. BUN increases are NOT seen with bleeding from the colon or the lower portion of the small intestine. Dehydration contributes to the increased BUN and total protein levels. Mild reduction in glomerular filtration rate (GFR) from volume depletion causes a mild creatinine elevation.

Esophagogastroduodenoscopy

Esophagogastroduodenoscopy (EGD) is the most accurate means of determining the source of UGI ulcer bleeding. Visualization of the esophagus, stomach, and duodenum using a fiberoptic endoscope passed through the mouth is usually performed within the first 12 hours after the patient's admission to identify the exact source of bleeding and characteristics of ulcers, if present. Endoscopic ulcer findings are referred to as *endoscopic stigmata*. Stigmata indicative of bleeding ulcers, bleeding esophageal varices, or ulcers at risk for rebleeding are identified in Box 9-2, *Stigmata of Active or Recent Hemorrhage (SARH)*. SARH findings are helpful in determining the course of direct therapy as well as providing prognostic information. Antacids and sucralfate should be withheld until after the procedure, because they can alter the appearance of lesions. *Gastric biopsy* is usually obtained with endoscopy for *H. pylori* diagnosis as well as to exclude gastric malignancy.

Electrocoagulation, injection therapy (epinephrine), laser, hemoclips, and other therapeutic techniques such as scleral therapy and variceal ligation (banding) may be used during this procedure to stop current bleeding or prevent further bleeding from esophageal varices or ulcers.

| Box 9-2 | STIGMATA OF ACTIVE OR RECENT HEMORRHAGE (SARH) |

Endoscopic ulcer findings from active or recent upper gastrointestinal hemorrhage:
* Active arterial spurting
* Oozing of blood
* Nonbleeding visible vessel or pigmented protuberance (red, blue, or purple elevated mound protruding from the base of the ulcer)
* Adherent or overlying clot without oozing
* Flat, dark slough or spot on the ulcer base

These findings are indicative of high risk for continued bleeding or rebleeding, requiring more aggressive therapy. For patients who do not exhibit these findings, the risk of rebleeding is significantly lower.

Colonoscopy

Colonoscopy is highly diagnostic for patients with LGIB for identification of bleeding stigmata visualized in the colon and the provision of direct therapy including laser therapy, heater probes, electrocoagulation, injection, and argon plasma coagulation. Diagnostic usefulness depends on the ability of the endoscopist.

COLLABORATIVE MANAGEMENT

Acute GI bleeding can occur from various lesions or sites in the GI tract. The amount of blood loss can vary from minor to massive (Table 9-2) depending on the cause, resulting in hypovolemic shock with significant associated mortality. The patients requiring intensive care management are those with moderate to massive bleeding, advanced age and significant comorbidities such as end-stage renal disease (ESRD), hepatic disease, or cardiovascular disease. Therefore, collaborative management focuses on cessation of active bleeding, identification and treatment of the underlying pathophysiology, and the prevention of rebleeding. Some patients develop GI bleeding during hospitalization for another reason as in the case of stress ulceration. Stress ulcer prophylaxis has been included in the management of mechanically ventilated, critically ill patients but is currently controversial.

Care Priorities

An immediate priority in the acute phase of GI bleeding is the assessment of bleeding severity and the restoration of hemodynamic stability. Intensive care unit monitoring is necessary to reduce morbidity and mortality. Once stabilized, care priorities will shift to the identification and management of the bleeding source.

1. **Fluid and electrolyte management:** Volume replacement in acute GI bleeding must be performed as quickly as possible. Large-bore IV lines should be placed and rapid fluid resuscitation initiated. Volume replacement should include a combination of crystalloid and blood products. Unstable patients who show signs of poor tissue perfusion are generally

Table 9-2	SEVERITY OF BLOOD LOSS	
Severity of Bleed	**Percent of Intravascular Blood Loss**	**Blood Pressure (BP) and Heart Rate (HR) Findings**
Massive	20%–25%	Systolic BP < 90 mm Hg HR >100 beats/min
Moderate	10%–20%	Orthostatic hypotension HR >100 beats/min
Minor	<10%	Normal BP HR <100 beats/min

Adapted from Rockey DC: Gastrointestinal bleeding. In Sleisenger MH, Feldman M, Fordtran JS, et al., editors: *Sleisenger & Fordtran's Gastrointestinal and liver disease: pathophysiology, diagnosis, management*, ed 8. Philadelphia, 2006, Saunders.

transfused. Packed cells and fresh-frozen plasma should be balanced to provide for both the replacement of cells and clotting components. Large transfusions will cause Ca^{-+} to bind with the citrate (the preservative in stored blood) and deplete free Ca^{-+} levels. In addition, large-volume blood transfusions can lead to coagulopathy disorders. Vasopressors and inotropic agents should be used *only* if tissue perfusion remains compromised despite adequate intravascular volume replacement. Hemodynamic monitoring is essential for continuous evaluation of the patient's volume status, especially in patients older than 50 years or those with chronic illnesses such as cardiovascular, pulmonary, renal, or hepatic disease. Overaggressive volume resuscitation may result in fluid volume excess with complications of cardiac failure and pulmonary edema. Electrolyte levels should be closely monitored, especially in patients with renal or hepatic disease.

2. **Respiratory support.** Due to the decrease in oxygen-carrying capacity of the RBC with massive blood loss, oxygen therapy by nasal cannula or face mask is initiated. Continuous or frequent pulse oximetry monitoring is recommended in actively bleeding patients to monitor oxygen saturation, but arterial blood gas (ABG) analysis may be needed to check oxygen if the patient is markedly anemic. Saturation alone is adequate to measure stability because the patient has lost oxygen-carrying capacity by loss of hemoglobin, which may not be compensated effectively by an increased oxygen saturation on the hemoglobin remaining. More aggressive ventilatory support may be required for patients with persistent hypoxemia, evidence of early respiratory failure, or impending ARDS, as well as for patients who were overaggressively volume resuscitated.

3. **Nutritional support.** As soon as the patient's hemodynamic status stabilizes, nutritional support must be considered. Total parenteral nutrition (TPN) is used for patients likely to remain NPO for days to weeks. Enteral or oral feedings are started when there is no further evidence of GI hemorrhage and bowel function has returned.

4. **Gastric intubation.** Gastric intubation is often necessary, especially with UGIB. Gastric lavage is performed using room-temperature saline to clear blood and clots from the stomach and to allow for estimation of ongoing blood loss. A lavage free of blood suggests a lower GI source of bleeding. There is no evidence that lavage stops the bleeding. Gastric intubation is avoided if esophageal varices are the suspected bleeding source, unless balloon tube tamponade is attempted to stop variceal bleeding.

5. **Endoscopic therapies.** Endoscopic modalities including laser, heater probe, and injection therapy are generally effective in stopping bleeding for both UGIB and LGIB. Early endoscopy increases diagnostic accuracy, reduces the risk of rebleeding, and decreases the length of hospitalization. Complications include perforation and Mallory-Weiss tears.

6. **Pharmacotherapy.** Pharmacotherapy including vasopressin and nitroglycerin, is only available for the management of UGIB. No pharmacologic therapies for LGIB are currently available. In the upper GI tract, increased gastric acidity is believed to retard blood clotting, while gastric alkalination may facilitate platelet aggregation thus promoting acid-lowering pharmacotherapies. Pharmacologic agents involved in ulcer treatment include antacids, H_2-receptor antagonists, proton-pump inhibitors prostaglandin analogues, somatostatin, and octreotide.

Antacids (aluminum hydroxide, calcium carbonate, citrocarbonate, magaldrate, magnesium hydroxide, simethicone): Oral antacids raise gastric pH levels and decrease the corrosiveness of gastric acid. They may relieve dyspepsia but have no effect on bleeding ulcers.

Histamine H_2-receptor antagonists (e.g., famotidine, ranitidine, cimetidine, nizatidine): Inhibit gastric acid and pepsin secretion are useful in the treatment of ulcerative disease and for stress ulcer prophylaxis. Their use in ulcer bleeding, is unsupported. They provide inferior acid inhibition to proton-pump inhibitors. Cimetidine is avoided in critically ill patients because it inhibits certain liver enzymes, resulting in potential drug interactions.

Proton-pump inhibitors (PPI) (e.g., esomeprazole, lansoprazole, omeprazole, pantoprazole, rabeprazole): Proton-pump inhibitors deactivate the enzyme system that pumps hydrogen ions from parietal cells thereby inhibiting gastric acid secretion. They have become the preferred agent for erosive ulcer disease with bleeding. Their acid-inhibitory effects are significantly stronger than H_2-receptor antagonists. Intravenous (IV) PPIs or high-dose oral PPIs following a bleeding episode are effective in reducing rebleed, the number of transfusions, and the need for further endoscopic therapy.

Prostaglandin analogues (e.g., misoprostol [Cytotec]): Synthetic prostaglandin E_1 enhances the body's normal mucosal protective mechanisms by stimulating mucosal blood flow and bicarbonate secretion, and reducing mucosal cell turnover. They are useful in reducing the incidence of ulcer development in patients taking NSAIDs.

Vasoconstrictors: Vasopressin or Terlipressin help slow variceal bleeding.

Somatostatin and octreotide: These agents have been shown to reduce rebleeding in ulcer patients but with no improvement in mortality.

Sucralfate (Carafate): Oral sucralfate may be prescribed for patients with gastric erosions. The sucralfate combines with gastric acid and forms an adhesive protective coating over damaged mucosa. It has no effect on gastric pH. It frequently causes constipation and should be avoided in patients with chronic renal insufficiency.

Pharmacotherapy for H. pylori: Eradication of *H. pylori* is effective with combination therapies. *"Triple therapy"* includes two antibiotics (clarithromycin and amoxicillin or metronidazole) and a PPI. *"Quadruple therapy"* includes bismuth salicylate, metronidazole, tetracycline, and a PPI or H_2 blocker. There are several triple therapy combination preparations available to allow the patient to receive the combination in one pill.

7. **Gastric pH monitoring:** Performed to assess the pH of gastric contents (intraluminal pH) or of gastric mucosal tissue (intramural pH). The goal of therapy is to maintain gastric pH within a given range, usually 4.0 to 5.0. Intraluminal pH is measured by aspirating gastric secretions and testing the aspirate with a pH indicator paper. An electronic pH meter is attached to the distal end of a gastric tube that permits continuous monitoring of intraluminal pH. Because the gut is especially vulnerable to ischemia associated with hypoperfusion and shock states, the intramural pH may be a valuable predictor of intestinal ischemia, sepsis, and multisystem organ dysfunction. Its usefulness is significantly reduced due to early initiation of stress ulcer prophylaxis, which results in pH elevation; as well as early implementation of enteral feeding.

8. **Surgical management:** Many surgical techniques are used for both acute UGIB and LGIB, depending on the location and severity of the lesion. Esophageal varices are best managed with endoscopic ligation (banding) or sclerotherapy. Ulcerative disease requires surgery if the lesion continues to bleed despite aggressive medical and endoscopic therapy or if complications such as perforation or obstruction develop. Oversewing of the bleeding vessel usually is followed by an acid-reducing procedure such as *antrectomy*, which removes acid-secreting cells, or *vagotomy*, which denervates the acid-producing fundic mucosa. *Pyloroplasty* is performed if there is impairment of gastric emptying. In the patient whose condition is unstable, both vagotomy and pyloroplasty are performed. Antrectomy and vagotomy may be performed in patients whose condition is more stable with anastomosis of the stomach to the duodenum (*Billroth I* procedure). Also common is the *Billroth II* procedure for duodenal ulcers involving antrectomy with gastrojejunostomy. Massive LGIB is difficult to control and may require aggressive surgical procedures such as a colectomy with the creation of a permanent ileostomy or internal ileal pouch.

CARE PLANS FOR ACUTE GASTROINTESTINAL BLEEDING

Deficient fluid volume *related to active loss secondary to hemorrhage from the GI tract*

GOALS/OUTCOMES Within 8 hours of this diagnosis, patient becomes normovolemic as evidenced by mean arterial pressure (MAP) greater than 70 mm Hg, HR 60 to 100 bpm, CVP 2 to 6 mm Hg, PAOP 6 to 12 mm Hg, cardiac index (CI) greater than 2.5 L/min/m², Hgb approximately 10 g/dl or greater, and urinary output greater than 0.5 ml/kg/hr.

NOC Electrolyte and Acid-Base Balance; Fluid Balance

Fluid Management

1. Monitor BP every 15 minutes during episodes of rapid, active blood loss or unstable vital signs. Be alert to MAP decreases of greater than 10 mm Hg from previous reading.

2. Monitor postural vital signs on patient's admission, every 4 to 8 hours, and more frequently if recurrence of active bleeding is suspected: measure BP and HR with patient in a supine position, followed immediately by measurement of BP and HR with patient in a sitting position (as tolerated). A decrease in systolic BP greater

than 10 mm Hg or an increase in HR of 10 bpm with patient in a sitting position suggests a significant intravascular volume deficit, with approximately 15% to 20% loss of volume.

3. Monitor HR, ECG, and cardiovascular status hourly, or more frequently in the presence of active bleeding or unstable vital signs. Be alert to a sudden increase in HR, which suggests hypovolemia.

4. Measure central pressures and thermodilution CO every 1 to 4 hours. Be alert to low or decreasing CVP, PAOP, and CO. Calculate SVR every 2 to 4 hours, or more frequently in patients whose condition is unstable. An elevated HR, decreased PAOP, decreased CO (CI less than 2.5 L/min/m^2), and increased SVR suggest hypovolemia and the need for volume restoration.

5. Measure urinary output hourly. Be alert to output less than 0.5 ml/kg/hr for 2 consecutive hours. Increase fluid intake or consider fluid bolus if decreased output is caused by hypovolemia and hypoperfusion.

Fluid Resuscitation

1. Obtain two large-bore IV lines (16- or 18-gauge) and central venous access.

2. Initiate crystalloid replacement therapy with a combination of normal saline and lactated Ringer. Fluid should be warmed to prevent hypothermia.

3. Administer packed red blood cells (PRBCs) for persistently low Hct (less than 20% to 25%). Anticipate Hct will increase by 3% following 1 unit of PRBCs.

4. Fresh-frozen plasma is required after 10 units of packed RBCs is infused.

5. Monitor prothrombin time (PT) and partial thromboplastin time (PTT); administer fresh-frozen plasma (FFP) to maintain normal levels.

6. Monitor ionized calcium levels closely because of calcium's tendency to bind with citrate. Administer calcium gluconate for ionized calcium levels less than 4.4 mg/dl.

7. Prepare for platelet transfusion if platelets fall below 50,000 or following 10 units of packed RBCs.

Shock Management

1. Initiate fluid replacement (see **Fluid and Electrolyte Disturbances**, p. 37).

2. Collaborate with physician or midlevel practitioner to administer vasoactive medication if shock persists with volume resuscitation.

3. Monitor for cerebral ischemia or indications of insufficient cerebral blood flow.

4. Monitor renal function (BUN and creatinine levels for elevations) as intravascular volume depletion can lead to prerenal azotemia.

5. Monitor tissue oxygenation using ABG, Svo$_2$, central venous oxygen saturation (Scvo$_2$) monitoring if available, and serum lactate measurements.

6. Monitor ECG for ST-segment depression and T-wave inversion, which may be seen as a result of the shock state.

Bleeding Reduction: Gastrointestinal

1. Administer proton-pump inhibitors IV at least 3 days in patients whose endoscopic stigmata suggest a high risk of rebleeding. Vasopressin (Pitressin), or Terlipressin (Glypressin) may help slow variceal bleeding.

2. Measure and record all GI blood losses from hematemesis, hematochezia, and melena.

3. Check all stools and gastric contents for occult blood.

4. Ensure proper function and patency of gastric tubes. Do not occlude the air vent of double-lumen tubes, because this may result in vacuum occlusion. Confirm placement of gastric tube at least every 8 hours, and reposition as necessary. Inflated esophageal balloon tubes used for tamponade of varices must be secured and stable.

5. Initiate nasogastric lavage to clear the stomach of blood. Gastric lavage does not slow or stop bleeding as once thought but is necessary prior to endoscopy for optimal visualization.

6. Teach patient signs and symptoms of actual or impending GI hemorrhage: pain, nausea, vomiting of blood, dark stools, lightheadedness, and passage of frank blood in stools. Reinforce the importance of seeking medical attention promptly if signs of bleeding occur.

7. Teach patient the importance of avoiding medications/agents with the potential for gastric irritation: aspirin, NSAIDs, ethanol.

NIC Blood Products Administration; Hemodynamic Regulation; Gastrointestinal Intubation; Bleeding Precautions; Teaching: Individual; Surgical Preparation

---

Decreased cardiac output *related to decreased preload secondary to acute blood loss*

GOALS/OUTCOMES Within 8 hours of this diagnosis, CO approaches normal limits with adequate tissue perfusion as evidenced by CI greater than 2.5 L/min/m^2, MAP greater than 70 mm Hg, CVP 2 to 6 mm Hg, urinary output greater

than 0.5 ml/kg/hr, normal sinus rhythm on ECG, distal pulses greater than 2+ on a 0 to 4+ scale, and brisk capillary refill (less than 2 seconds).
NOC Blood Loss Severity

Hemodynamic Regulation
1. Administer vasopressors and inotropic agents as prescribed if tissue perfusion remains inadequate following intravascular volume replacement.
2. Monitor ECG for evidence of myocardial ischemia (i.e., T-wave depression, QT prolongation, ventricular dysrhythmias).
3. Monitor for physical indicators of diminished cardiac output, including pallor, cool extremities, capillary refill greater than 2 to 3 seconds, and decreased or absent amplitude of distal pulses.
4. Monitor vital signs and CO, and replace volume as indicated (see *Fluid and Electrolyte Disturbances*, p. 37).
5. Monitor for oliguria hourly; report urine output less than 0.5 ml/kg/hr for 2 consecutive hours.

Respiratory Monitoring
1. Administer oxygen via nasal cannula or facemask to facilitate maximal oxygen delivery.
2. Monitor pulse oximetry and ABG values for hypoxemia. Report arterial Pao_2 less than 80 mm Hg and oxygen saturation below 92%.
3. Prepare for endotracheal intubation and mechanical ventilation if patient is distressed with oxygen saturation *less than* 90% with supplemental oxygen.
4. Monitor for respiratory crackles, which can result from overaggressive fluid resuscitation.

NIC Cardiac Care: Acute; Oxygen Therapy; Invasive Hemodynamic Monitoring; Dysrhythmia Management

---

Acute pain *related to chemical or physical injury of GI mucosal surfaces caused by digestive juices and enzymes or tissue trauma*

GOALS/OUTCOMES Within 2 hours of this diagnosis, patient's subjective evaluation of discomfort improves, as documented by a pain scale. Nonverbal indicators of discomfort, such as grimacing, are absent.
NOC Comfort Level; Pain Control

Pain Management
1. Monitor and document presence of abdominal pain or discomfort. Devise a pain scale with patient. Pain may disappear during a bleeding episode since blood covers and protects eroded tissue.
2. Administer gastric alkalizing agents and sucralfate as prescribed to relieve pain caused by upper GI disorders. Hold these agents prior to endoscopy.
3. Measure gastric pH at least every 4 hours. For gastric aspirate, use a clean syringe and discard the first aspirate to ensure accuracy. Some may use nasogastric (NG) tonometer to measure gastric mucosal pH.
4. Adjust gastric alkalizing therapy to maintain pH of 4.0 to 5.0 or other prescribed range. Avoid excessive alkalization, which is associated with increased risk of nosocomial pneumonia.
5. Administer opiate analgesics with caution to hypovolemic patients to avoid hypotension and respiratory depression.
6. Supplement analgesics with nonpharmacologic maneuvers to aid in pain reduction. Patients who have pain associated with gastric reflux may be more comfortable with the head of the bed (HOB) elevated, if this position does not compromise hemodynamic status. Reflux may prompt variceal bleeding.

NIC Analgesic Administration; Distraction; Environmental Management; Vital Signs Monitoring

---

Diarrhea *related to irritation and increased motility secondary to the presence of blood in the GI tract*

GOALS/OUTCOMES By the time of hospital discharge, patient's stools are normal in consistency and frequency and negative for occult blood.
NOC Fluid Balance; Bowel Elimination; Electrolyte and Acid-Base Balance

Diarrhea Management
1. Monitor and record the amount, frequency, and character of patient's stools.
2. Provide or have bedpan or bedside commode (only for hemodynamically stable patients) readily available. Consider use of a contained stool management device (e.g., Flexiseal.)

3. Minimize embarrassing odor by removing stool promptly and using room deodorizers.
4. Use matter-of-fact approach when assisting patient with frequent bowel elimination. Reassure patient that frequent elimination is a common problem for most patients with GI bleeding.
5. Evaluate bowel sounds every 4 to 8 hours. Anticipate normal to hyperdynamic bowel sounds. Absence of bowel sounds (especially in association with severe pain or abdominal distention) may signal serious complications such as ileus or perforation.
6. Report abnormal serum sodium, potassium, and calcium levels to physician or midlevel practitioner.

NIC Electrolyte Monitoring; Fluid/Electrolyte Management

Imbalanced nutrition: less than body requirements *related to inability to ingest or digest food secondary to vomiting, mucosal ulceration, ileus or active GI bleeding*

GOALS/OUTCOMES Within 7 days of this diagnosis (or by the time of hospital discharge) patient has adequate nutrition as evidenced by stable weight, thyroxine-binding prealbumin 20 to 30 mg/dl, and a state of nitrogen balance on nitrogen studies.
NOC Nutritional Status

Nutrition Management
1. Collaborate with physician, midlevel practitioner, dietitian, and pharmacist to estimate patient's individual metabolic needs on the basis of activity level, underlying disease process, and nutritional status before hospitalization.
2. Provide parenteral nutrition during acute phase of the bleeding, as prescribed.
3. Begin enteral therapy when acute hemorrhagic episode has subsided and bowel function has returned.
4. Monitor thyroxine-binding prealbumin, and report decreasing levels.
5. Weigh patient daily at the same time of day, using the same scale. Weight can be a practical indicator of nutritional status if patient's weight changes are interpreted on the basis of the following factors: fluid shifts (edema, diuresis, third spacing), surgical resection, and weight of dressings and equipment.

NIC Nutritional Monitoring; Total Parenteral Nutrition (TPN) Administration; Enteral Tube Feeding; Aspiration Precautions

- For additional information, see *Nutritional Support*, see p. 117.

ADDITIONAL NURSING DIAGNOSES
See other nursing diagnoses and interventions as appropriate: *Hemodynamic Monitoring* (p. 75), *Prolonged Immobility* (p. 149), and *Emotional and Spiritual Support of the Patient and Significant Others* (p. 200).

ACUTE PANCREATITIS

PATHOPHYSIOLOGY
Acute pancreatitis (AP) is an autodigestive process of the pancreas and surrounding tissue by its own enzymes. AP may be clinically classified as mild or severe. In cases of mild acute pancreatitis, there is local inflammation, minimal interstitial edema, and no infection or organ system failure. Patients usually improve in 48 to 72 hours with supportive care. This form accounts for the majority of cases with mortality being less than 1%. *Severe acute pancreatitis* (SAP) is a life-threatening condition that is accompanied by necrosis and possibly infection, with mortality rates between 20% and 50%. It should be recognized that 1 in 5 patients with AP will develop SAP.

Normally, pancreatic acinar cells produce and secrete proteolytic enzymes in their inactive form. These proenzymes travel through the pancreatic duct safely until reaching the duodenum, where they are converted to active form by other enzymes found in the intestinal brush border. In AP, the proenzyme trypsinogen is prematurely activated to the proteolytic enzyme trypsin within the acinar cells of the pancreas. Once secreted into the pancreatic duct, trypsin converts other proenzymes into active forms, resulting in enzymatic autodigestion of the pancreas. The exact mechanisms by which trypsin becomes prematurely activated remains unanswered. Activated digestive enzymes within the pancreas not only digest pancreatic tissue, leading to inflammation, capillary leakage, and necrosis, but also digest elastin in blood vessel walls, causing vascular injury and hemorrhage. Inflammatory mediators (kinins, complement, coagulation factors) released at the site of tissue and vessel injury cause further edema, inflammation, thrombosis, and hemorrhage.

The most common causes of AP are alcoholism and gallstones (75% of all cases). Alcohol may have a direct toxic effect on the pancreatic acinar cells or may cause inflammation of the sphincter of Oddi, resulting in the retention of enzymes in the pancreatic duct. In patients with gallstones, the hypothesized mechanism is obstruction of the pancreatic duct by gallstones, as the pancreatic duct and the common bile duct share the same outlet into the duodenum. This obstruction causes bile to reflux into the pancreatic duct. Hypercalcemia, hyperlipidemia, hypertriglyceridemia, and hypothermia are all associated with the development of acute pancreatitis. Other causes or associations of AP include endoscopic retrograde cholangiopancreatography (ERCP) procedure, blunt or penetrating trauma, metabolic factors, infectious agents, and certain drugs (Box 9-3). Recently, the Food and Drug Administration (FDA) issued information for health care professionals identifying occurrences of AP in type 2 diabetic patients using the antidiabetic drug exenatide. The FDA is working to include stronger and more prominent warnings on the label. The cause of AP remains unknown in about 15% of all cases even with thorough investigation.

In SAP, significant pancreatic edema leads to rupture of the pancreatic ducts and spillage of pancreatic enzymes into the peripancreatic tissue, resulting in necrosis. The spread of inflammatory mediators to distant sites results in a systemic inflammatory response syndrome (SIRS), shock, and eventual multiple organ dysfunction syndrome (MODS). SAP is an inflammatory process that is nonbacterial or is considered sterile necrosis. Bacterial infection is an added complication found in one third of patients with SAP. Infected pancreatitis should be considered with the worsening of pain, fever, and leukocytosis 1 to 2 weeks after admission. Infection produces abscesses, localized collections of pus, that must be surgically drained and treated with antibiotics. Unfortunately, infective pancreatitis often leads to sepsis as bacteria translocate the poorly functioning gut, carrying a high mortality rate.

It is important to identify those patients at risk for SAP to rapidly implement appropriate recourses. Ranson criteria provide a scale of severity for acute pancreatitis based on age and laboratory studies. Pancreatitis is classified as severe when three or more of Ranson criteria are met during the first 48 hours following presentation (Box 9-4). Mortality is

---

Box 9-3   PRECIPITATING FACTORS FOR ACUTE PANCREATITIS

Mechanical blockage of pancreatic ducts
- Biliary tract disease (e.g., gallstones)
- Structural abnormalities (e.g., pancreas divisum)
- Preceding ERCP

Toxic/metabolic factors
- Alcohol
- Hyperlipidemia
- Hypertriglyceridemia
- Hypercalcemia (e.g., hyperparathyroidism)
- Pregnancy

Infection
- Viral (e.g., mumps, Coxsackie virus B, hepatitis B, HIV, CMV)
- Bacterial (e.g., *Mycoplasma pneumoniae*, *Salmonella typhi*)

Trauma
- External
- Surgical

Ischemia
- Prolonged/severe shock
- Vasculitis

Tumors

Drugs
- NSAIDs
- Estrogens
- Corticosteroids
- Thiazides
- Tetracycline
- Sulfonamides

ERCP, Endoscopic retrograde cholangiopancreatography; *NSAIDs,* nonsteroidal anti-inflammatory drugs.

Acute Pancreatitis

Box 9-4	RANSON CRITERIA FOR CLASSIFYING THE SEVERITY OF PANCREATITIS

At presentation
- Age >55 years
- WBCs >16,000/µl
- Glucose >200 mg/dl
- AST >250 units/L
- LDH >350 units/L

After initial 48 hours
- Base deficit >4 mEq/L
- BUN increased >5 mg/dl

- Fluid sequestration >6 L
- Serum Ca^{2+} >8 mg/dl
- Hematocrit decrease >10%
- Po_2 (from ABG) >60 mm Hg

Ranson's Criteria Scoring Mechanism
Score 0–2—minimal mortality rate
Score 3–5—10% to 20% mortality rate
Score >5—50% mortality rate

ABG, Arterial blood gas; *AST*, aspartate aminotransferase; *BUN*, blood urea nitrogen; *Ca^{2+}*, calcium; *LDH*, lactate dehydrogenase; *Po_2*, partial pressure of oxygen; *WBCs*, white blood cells.

approximately 16% to 20% with 3 or 4 positive criteria, 40% with 5 or 6 positive criteria, and 100% with 7 or 8 criteria. A contrast-enhanced CT scoring system is also available to assist with diagnosis, in which the severity is graded using CT findings. The Acute Physiology and Chronic Health Evaluation (APACHE) II scoring system (Table 9-3) is another tool to determine severity. An APACHE II point score of less than 8 within the first 48 hours coincides with survival. Higher scores during this time interval reflect increased morbidity and mortality rates. These multiple factor scoring systems do carry a false-positive rate and should be used in conjunction with ongoing clinical findings and other laboratory data.

Complications

A major complication of SAP is marked depletion of intravascular plasma volume, the result of fluid sequestration into the interstitium, retroperitoneum and the gut. Massive, life-threatening hemorrhage from rupture of necrotic tissue results in serious blood volume depletion. SIRS ensues, wherein inflammatory mediators trigger vasodilation and increased capillary permeability, which further contributes to severe hypovolemia and hypotension. Hypoalbuminemia is frequently present, which prompts intravascular fluids to move through the permeable capillaries more rapidly since oncotic pressure is reduced. Severe hypotension may persist despite volume repletion. If hypovolemia is not adequately corrected promptly, acute renal failure may develop, as the patient progresses through the stages of systemic inflammatory response syndrome (SIRS) and organs begin failing (see *SIRS, Sepsis and MODS*, p. 924).

Mild-to-severe respiratory failure with hypoxemia is common, as is the case with all patients with SIRS. Respiratory complications are related to right-to-left vascular shunting within the lung and alveolar-capillary leakage caused by the circulating inflammatory mediators resulting in acute respiratory distress syndrome (ARDS) (see *Acute Lung Injury and Acute Respiratory Distress Syndrome*, p. 365). In addition, elevation of the diaphragm, atelectasis, and pleural effusion caused by subdiaphragmatic inflammation of the pancreas and surrounding tissues can compromise ventilation further. Inflammatory mediators and vascular injury can also cause intravascular coagulopathy, resulting in life-threatening complications such as major thrombus formation, disseminated intravascular coagulopathy (DIC), and pulmonary emboli. The circulatory and respiratory failure that ensue are often the cause of death in these patients.

Hypocalcemia is a complication attributed to calcium-binding in areas of fat necrosis within the pancreas and small intestine. Hypocalcemia occurs between the third and tenth days of illness. If there is associated hypomagnesemia, the hypocalcemia may be refractory because normal magnesium levels are needed for parathyroid function. Calcium levels may fall low enough to cause tetany, seizures, coma, and laryngospasm.

The formation of pancreatic pseudocysts (encapsulated fluid collections with high enzyme content) is common in SAP patients monitored by CT scans. Pseudocysts can appear anywhere but are usually found within or adjacent to the pancreas. Pseudocysts frequently become infected requiring drainage or they may become hemorrhagic.

ASSESSMENT
Goal of System Assessment: Acute Pancreatitis
Evaluate for organ and systemic involvement of dysfunctional pancreatic secretions.

History and Risk Factors
- Excessive alcohol ingestion; biliary tract disease; recent ERCP, high cholesterol levels; use of drugs such as steroids, furosemide, thiazides, and NSAIDs; viral infections (HIV); penetrating and blunt injuries to the pancreas; pregnancy; primary hyperparathyroidism; uremia

Vital Sign Assessment
- Tachycardia and decreased BP result from the massive intravascular losses.
- Increased temperature greater than 38.3°C and tachycardia are associated with an inflammatory response.

Abdominal Pain
- Sudden onset of abdominal pain (often after excessive food or alcohol ingestion) lasting 12 to 48 hours, described as mild discomfort to severe distress, and located from the midepigastrium to the right upper quadrant (RUQ). Occasionally pain is reported in the left upper quadrant.
- The pain is typically described as boring and deep.
- The pain may radiate to the back.
- Nausea, vomiting, and restlessness typically accompany the pain; diarrhea, melena, and hematemesis may also be present.

Observation
- Mild-to-moderate ascites is present.
- Dyspnea and cyanosis may be observed if ARDS is present (see *Acute Lung Injury and Acute Respiratory Distress Syndrome*, p. 365).
- Jaundice may be present with biliary tract disease.
- Grey Turner sign (flank discoloration) and Cullen sign (umbilical area discoloration) occur in about 1% of cases and are associated with a poor prognosis.
- With severe hypocalcemia, Chvostek sign (facial twitching after a facial tap) or Trousseau sign (hand spasms when BP cuff inflates) may be elicited. Hypocalcemia causes numbness or tingling in the extremities that progresses to tetany if calcium is severely depleted.

Auscultation
- Diminished or absent bowel sounds reflective of GI dysfunction and paralytic ileus.
- Breath sounds may be decreased or absent, suggesting focal atelectasis or pleural effusion. Effusions are usually left-sided but can be bilateral. Auscultation of crackles reflects hypoventilation caused by pain, early ARDS, or microemboli.

Palpation
- Abdominal tenderness is common.
- Abdominal palpation will reveal localized tenderness in the RUQ or diffuse discomfort over the upper portion of the abdomen without rigidity or rebound.
- An upper abdominal mass may be palpated due to the inflamed pancreas or a pseudocyst.
- In the presence of hemorrhage or severe hypovolemia, hands are cool and sweaty to touch.
- Peripheral pulses will be diminished and capillary refill delayed with hemorrhage or severe hypovolemia.

Nutritional Assessment
- Malnutrition may be present especially if there is a history of alcoholism (see Table 9-1).

Screening Labwork
- Serum electrolytes levels: hypocalcemia, hypokalemia
- CBC: leukocytosis
- Serum amylase ↑↑↑

Table 9-3　THE ACUTE PHYSIOLOGY AND CHRONIC HEALTH EVALUATION (APACHE) II SCORING SYSTEM

Feature	+4	+3	+2	+1	0	+1	+2	+3	+4
Acute Physiology Score (APS)									
Temperature	≥41	39–40.9		38.5–38.9	36–38.4	34–35.9	32–33.9	30–31.9	≤29.9
Mean arterial BP	≥160	130–159	110–129		70–109		50–69		≤49
Heart rate	≥180	140–179	110–139		70–109		55–69	40–54	≤39
Respiratory rate	≥50	35–49		25–34	12–24	10–11	6–9		<5
A–aPO2†	≥500	350–499	200–349		<100				
PO2*					>70	61–70		55–60	<55
Arterial pH	≥7.7	7.6–7.69		7.5–7.59	7.33–7.49		7.25–7.32	7.15–7.24	<7.15
Serum bicarbonate‡	≥52	41–51.9	32–40.9		23–31.9		18–21.9	15–17.9	<15
Serum sodium	≥180	160–179	155–159	150–154	130–149		120–129	111–119	≤110
Serum potassium	≥7	6–6.9		5.5–5.9	3.5–5.4	3–3.4	2.5–2.9		<2.5
Serum creatinine	≥3.5	2–3.4	1.5–1.9		0.6–1.4		<0.6		
Hematocrit	≥60		50–59.9	46–49.9	30–45.9		20–29.9		<20
WBC count	≥40		20–39.9	15–19.9	3–14.9		1–2.9		<1

BP, blood pressure; $A - aPO_2$, alveolar-arterial oxygen pressure; PaO_2, partial pressure of oxygen in arterial blood; WBC, white blood cell.
*Use if percentage of inspired oxygen (FiO_2) >50 percent.
†Use if FiO_2 <50%.
‡Use only if no arterial blood gas measurements are available.

Age Points (AP)		Chronic Health Problems (CHP)	Scoring
Age	Points	For patients with history of severe organ system insufficiency or immunocompromise, assign points as follows:	APS + AP + CHP = total score
≤44	0	Nonoperative or emergency postoperative: 5 points Elective postoperative: 2 points	
45–54	2		
55–64	3		
65–74	5		
≥75	6		

Scores indicating abnormal reading: on admission, >9; after 24 hours, >10; after 48 hours, >9.

From Knaus WA, Draper EA, Wagner DP, Zimmerman JE: APACHE II: a severity of disease classification system. *Crit Care Med.* Oct;13(10):818-29, 1985.

- Serum lipase ↑↑↑
- LFTs: Elevated with alcoholic or biliary involvement.

Hemodynamic Measurements for Complications of SAP
- *Hypovolemic shock:* Decreased CVP and CO from hemorrhage or dehydration
- *SIRS:* CO may be elevated and SVR decreased initially. Urine output decreases as the body attempts to conserve intravascular volume
- *ARDS or pulmonary emboli:* Increase in pulmonary vascular resistance (PVR)

Diagnostic Tests for Acute Pancreatitis (AP)

Test	Purpose	Abnormal Findings
Blood Studies		
Complete blood count (CBC) White blood cell (WBC) count Red blood cell (RBC) count Hemoglobin (Hgb) Hematocrit (Hct) Platelets	Assess for inflammation and infection. Platelets may be consumed if inflammation is severe enough to prompt DIC. Reflective of volume status and oxygen carrying capacity.	Leukocytosis with a WBC count of 11,000–20,000/mm³ is reflective of the acute inflammatory process and not bacterial infection. Bacterial infection may ensue in a small percentage of patients reflecting a WBC count >20,000/mm³. Hct and Hgb levels vary, depending on the presence of hemorrhage (decreased) or dehydration (increased).
Serum amylase Serum lipase	Cardinal finding consistent with AP, although not diagnostic. Amylase rises almost immediately but can return to normal within 48–72 hours. Lipase remains elevated for 14 days and is a more sensitive test than amylase.	Serum elevations in amylase or lipase levels >3 times the upper normal limit, in the absence of renal failure, are most consistent with acute pancreatitis. Serum lipase is more specific for AP and is preferred.
Serum calcium	Assesses for hypocalcemia. Some calcium is protein-bound; serum levels depend on albumin levels. As serum albumin levels decrease with intravascular fluid losses, reductions in serum calcium levels will follow.	Calcium levels may fall to <8 mg/dl predisposing the patient to tetany and other complications of hypocalcemia. In SAP, serum calcium levels may decrease dramatically as calcium binds with free fatty acids released during lipolysis of peripancreatic fat tissue.
Serum glucose	Assesses for hyperglycemia as a determinant of injury to pancreatic islet cells.	Blood glucose values are commonly >200 mg/dl.
Serum triglyceride	Assess for possible cause of AP.	Serum triglyceride levels >1000 mg/dl are found to be a causative factor of AP.
Serum creatinine	Evaluates renal function	Levels >1.5 mg/dl are seen in patients with acute renal failure.
Electrolytes Serum potassium Serum magnesium Serum bicarbonate	Assess levels closely during fluid resuscitation.	Hyperkalemia is present initially due to significant cellular damage releasing large amounts of K⁺ into circulation and increases with acidosis associated with shock. Increased serum bicarbonate and hypokalemia values reflect metabolic alkalosis later, usually the result of fluid therapy, vomiting or gastric suctioning. Hyponatremia and hypomagnesemia will be seen with vomiting and fluid sequestration.

Diagnostic Tests for Acute Pancreatitis (AP) — cont'd

Test	Purpose	Abnormal Findings
Liver function tests (LFTs) Serum bilirubin Alkaline phosphatase (ALP) Aspartate aminotransferase (AST)	Assesses liver involvement and distinguish between alcohol-induced and gallstone induced disease.	Persistent elevation of liver enzymes suggests hepatic inflammation caused by alcohol ingestion or viral hepatitis. Elevated total bilirubin levels and ALP value >150 IU/L are suggestive of biliary disease.
C-reactive protein (CRP)	Assesses for severe inflammation. CRP is a nonspecific acute-phase reactant of inflammation that is suggestive of severe acute pancreatitis	A CRP level >150 mg/L at 48 hours after disease onset is suggestive of pancreatic necrosis.
Coagulation studies	Assesses the extent of coagulopathic involvement as inflammatory mediators trigger the coagulation cascade. In SAP, DIC may develop.	Decreases in platelets and fibrinogen will be present as they are rapidly consumed. Elevations in circulating levels of fibrin are associated with microthrombi in the pancreas and other tissues.
Arterial blood gas (ABG)	Assesses oxygenation status and acid-base balance	Decreased arterial oxygen tension is a common finding and may be present without other symptoms of pulmonary insufficiency. Early hypoxia produces a mild respiratory alkalosis. Arterial oxygen saturation may be diminished.
Nutrition profile Serum albumin Serum transferrin serum Prealbumin Total lymphocyte count (TLC)	Assesses nutritional status to identify preexisting malnutrition and to guide nutrition replacement therapy.	Decreased albumin, transferrin, and TLC are indicative of malnutrition and seen in patients with alcoholic disease. Prealbumin levels will rise with effective therapy.
Noninvasive Cardiology		
ECG	Assess and monitor for cardiac rhythm disturbances.	ST-segment depression and T-wave inversion may be seen as a result of the shock state, the severe pain that causes coronary artery spasm, or the effect of trypsin and bradykinins on the myocardium. Hypocalcemia results in widening of the ST segment.
Radiology		
Radiography Abdominal radiograph Chest radiograph	*Abdominal x-rays* assess for bowel dilation. *Chest x-rays* identify pulmonary involvement.	Abdominal radiograph identifies dilation of the bowel and ileus. Chest radiograph distinguishes effusions from atelectasis and identifies characteristic infiltrates consistent with ARDS.
Computed tomography (CT) scan	Estimates size of the pancreas; identifies fluid collection, cystic lesions, abscesses, and masses; visualizes biliary tract abnormalities; and monitors inflammatory swelling of the pancreas. The CT scan can determine the presence or extent of necrosis, and thus serves as an indicator of disease severity.	Enlarged pancreas, dilation of the common bile duct and evidence of gallstones when present. CT confirms the diagnosis of AP.

Continued

Acute Pancreatitis

Diagnostic Tests for Acute Pancreatitis (AP) — cont'd		
Test	**Purpose**	**Abnormal Findings**
Endoscopic ultrasonography	Used to visualize the opening to the pancreas when a biliary cause of AP is suspected, to observe for swelling, ductal abnormalities, and presence of tumors or stones.	If these conditions are present, ERCP should not be used as it may worsen the condition.
Endoscopic retrograde cholangiopancreatography (ERCP)	Used to relieve obstruction caused by stone impaction	Not indicated for diagnosis of SAP as it may aggravate inflammation

Serum Lipase and Amylase

Serum lipase has become the primary diagnostic marker for AP. Serum amylase is insensitive in cases of delayed clinical presentation; pancreatitis caused by hypertriglyceridemia; and in patients with chronic pancreatitis experiencing an acute attack. Prolonged clamp time with CABG or valve replacement can lead to acute pancreatitis in which only amylase is elevated.

COLLABORATIVE MANAGEMENT

Management includes monitored supportive care, efforts to prevent, limit and treat complications, and recurrences. The American Gastroenterological Association (AGA)'s guidelines "Management of Acute Pancreatitis" frame the care priorities. Because AP is a disease of significant variability, there is a paucity of large randomized controlled trials. The AGA recommendations (Box 9-5) are therefore based on available scientific studies and evidence with expert opinion.

Care Priorities for Severe Acute Pancreatitis

A team approach is necessary to optimize the management of the patient with SAP. Care priorities reflect adequate fluid resuscitation, the correction of electrolyte and metabolic abnormalities, effective pain control, provision of nutrition, and the prevention of complications and recurrences.

1. **Provide vigorous fluid resuscitation.** The inflammatory process results in fluid sequestration and extensive intravascular volume loss into the pancreas and abdomen leading to hypovolemia and hemoconcentration. Vomiting, gastric suctioning, and hemorrhage contribute to the hypovolemic state. The hypovolemia and hemoconcentration lead to shock wherein the capillary beds are poorly perfused. Colloids and crystalloids are administered to replace volume losses and minimize interstitial edema. Crystalloids reduce hemoconcentration and improve perfusion. Albumin may be considered for serum albumin less than 2 g/dl, but the proteins may leak from capillaries and increase interstitial edema. Packed RBCs may be transfused for Hct less than 25%. Fresh-frozen plasma may be needed for evidence of coagulopathy. Peritoneal and interstitial fluid sequestration continues throughout the acute phase. Volume replacement is essential. CVP monitoring may assist fluid management. PAP, MAP and ScVO2 monitoring and pressors may be needed. Fluid overload is a concern, especially in patients with cardiovascular dysfunction and/or ARDS.
2. **Support ventilation and oxygenation.** In SAP-related pulmonary congestion, pleural effusion and atelectasis result in respiratory insufficiency or failure. Abdominal distention and retroperitoneal fluid sequestration cause diaphragmatic elevation and ventilatory restriction. Oxygen administration is initiated if hypoxemia is present. Early respiratory failure is detected by a decrease in Pao_2 with increase in $Paco_2$. If severe pulmonary insufficiency develops, intubation and positive pressure ventilation is required. Mechanical ventilation is frequently necessary for the patient with SAP. ARDS is a complication found in 20% of patients with SAP. IV fluids are given cautiously to prevent fluid overload resulting in cardiopulmonary compromise.
3. **Correct electrolyte and metabolic abnormalities.** *Hypocalcemia* commonly occurs in patients with SAP and is a marker of poor prognosis. Ionized levels should be monitored,

Box 9-5	AMERICAN GASTROENTEROLOGY ASSOCIATION (AGA) RECOMMENDATIONS FOR ACUTE PANCREATITIS (AP)

Diagnosis
- Establish the diagnosis of AP within 48 hours of admission.
- Consider a diagnosis of AP for patients admitted with unexplained MODS or SIRS.
- Confirm the diagnosis of AP with CT scan of the abdomen using IV contrast.

Assessment of Severity
- Severe disease is defined by mortality, the presence of organ failure, and/or local pancreatic complications (pseudocyst, necrosis, abscess).
- Prediction of severe disease is achieved with the combination of clinical assessment, a multiple factor scoring system and imaging studies. The Acute Physiology and Chronic Health Evaluation (APACHE) II System is preferred.
- If severe disease is predicted, a contrast-enhanced CT should be performed at 72 hours to assess the degree of pancreatic necrosis.

Determination of Etiology
- Establish etiology in at least three-fourths of all patients.
- Admission labs should include amylase, lipase, triglycerides, calcium, and liver chemistries. Ultrasonography should be performed for biliary disease.
- For patients with unexplained pancreatitis less than 40 years of age, extensive or invasive testing is not recommended.

Management
- Provide vigorous fluid resuscitation, supplemental oxygen, correction of electrolyte and metabolic abnormalities, pain control, and nutritional support.
- ERCP should be performed early in patients with gallstone pancreatitis with cholangitis. ERCP should only be performed by endoscopists with appropriate training.
- No recommendation for antibiotic prophylaxis can be made for sterile necrosis. If used, antibiotics should be restricted for only patients with pancreatic necrosis of greater than 30% of the gland by CT.
- Fluid collections and pseudocysts require no therapy unless infected.
- Consider surgical therapy and antibiotics for infected necrosis.

Prevent Recurrences by Referring those with Alcoholic Pancreatitis to Counseling and Patients with Gallstone Pancreatitis for Surgical Removal.

Data from the American Gastroenterology Association (AGA) Institute: Medical position statement on acute pancreatitis. *Gastroenterology* 132:2019–2021, 2007.

since with low albumin levels, the amount of measured protein-bound calcium is falsely low. If levels are low or if the patient develops signs of neuromuscular instability, replace with calcium chloride. Because hypercalcemia is a cause of AP, calcium replacement is prescribed cautiously. Ensure magnesium and albumin levels are adequate.

Hyperglycemia is also included as a poor prognostic marker. Hyperglycemia and glycosuria are consequences of glucagon release in the patient with SAP as a response to stress. Hyperglycemia is also related to the decreased release of insulin by impaired pancreatic islet cells. Hyperglycemia can worsen neutrophil function, increasing the risk of secondary pancreatic infection. Insulin should be administered intravenously and titrated to keep glucose less than 180 mg/dl. Meticulous serum glucose control management facilitates control of serum triglycerides.

4. **Provide effective pain control.** Acute abdominal pain is caused by peritoneal irritation from the inflamed pancreas. Opioid analgesics are administered for relief of severe pain. Continuous or intermittent IV therapy is used, depending on the severity of the pain. Patient-controlled analgesia (PCA) is a helpful mode of delivery. Morphine has been implicated in the past as causing spasm of the sphincter of Oddi, thus worsening the pancreatitis. However, no evidence has been found to demonstrate this in humans. Meperidine was the analgesic of choice but has an active neurotoxic metabolite that

accumulates with long-term use, causing agitation, seizures, and muscle fibrosis. Because of these side effects, many hospitals have limited the availability of IV meperidine. Hydromorphone is the preferred alternative, recommended by the AGA.

Safety Alert *While short-term meperidine can be used safely, use of longer than a few days, at doses exceeding 100 mg every 3 hours must be avoided.*

5. **Initiate nutritional support.** Nutritional supplementation should be considered early to promote tissue repair in patients with SAP as they are unable to tolerate eating for several days. Enteral feedings are preferred over TPN today. Enteral nutrition (EN) may be started within the first 48 hours of admission for the patient with or predicted SAP. Pancreatic secretions are not stimulated with the delivery of enteral elemental nutrition into the mid or distal jejunum, so jejunal feedings are possible for patients with SAP. Weighted NG tubes or NJ tubes should be positioned beyond the ligament of Treitz. The ligament of Treitz is a musculofibrous band that extends from the ascending part of the duodenum and jejunum to the right crus of the diaphragm and tissue around the celiac artery. Nasojejunal feedings are tolerated in most patients with meticulous attention to feeding tolerance and consulting with dieticians and nutritional support pharmacists regarding elemental feedings (see *Nutritional Support*, p. 117). Feeding into the stomach should be avoided, as this modality is associated with more pulmonary complications and more complications overall. If enteral feedings are not tolerated despite trying elemental feedings into the jejunum, TPN may be required, necessitating insertion of a central IV catheter. TPN continues to be associated with significant complications from the catheter, ranging from catheter-related sepsis, local abscess, localized hematomas, pneumothorax, venous thrombosis, venous air embolism, and metabolic complications such as hyperglycemia and electrolyte imbalance. Low-fat oral feedings are begun after the initial episode subsides and bowel function returns.

6. **Suppress pancreatic secretions.** Patients should receive nothing by mouth, and there should be no feedings into the stomach and duodenum to rest the pancreas. Mid to distal jejunal feedings do not stimulate pancreatic secretions. NPO status prevents stimulation of pancreatic secretions, which reduces inflammatory processes and allows the pancreas to heal. In the patient with SAP, all oral feedings, including water, are withheld. Aspiration of gastric secretions via NG suction demonstrated no benefit in patients with mild to moderate AP and is therefore not recommended in these cases. NG suction is only useful for cases of SAP with unremitting vomiting, abdominal distention, or pain not relieved by analgesia. Reducing gastric acidity by administering histamine H_2-receptor antagonists or proton-pump inhibitors may help to prevent stress ulceration. Agents that suppress pancreatic secretions such as somatostatin and octreotide have generally produced disappointing results in human studies and are no longer recommended. Peritoneal lavage has been used in the past to remove toxic necrotic compounds present in peritoneal exudates. This procedure has not been shown to reduce mortality or morbidity in patients with SAP and is no longer recommended.

7. **Manage medically vs. surgically.** In general, SAP is managed medically. Surgery is not necessary for patients with sterile necrosis. Surgery is indicated only for infected necrosis, abscesses or pseudocysts. Patients with necrosis and aspirates positive for bacteria on Gram stain or culture should undergo percutaneous drainage of pancreatic fluid, fine needle aspiration, or débridement of infected areas. Multiple percutaneous drains are sometimes required. Surgery within the first 14 days should be avoided as it is associated with increased mortality.

8. **Prevent infection; possibly with prophylactic antibiotics.** *The use of prophylactic antibiotics to prevent the development of infected necrosis is controversial. The AGA cannot recommend for or against its use.* If antibiotics are to be used, they should be restricted to patients with necrosis involving more than 30% of the pancreas evidenced by CT scan and administered for no longer than 14 days. Antibiotic choice must provide adequate penetration of necrotic tissue, such as imipenem-cilastatin, meropenem, or a combination of a quinolone and metronidazole. For infected necrosis, pseudocysts or abscesses, the antibiotic should be tailored to the infecting organism.

9. **Prevent recurrence.** Patients with alcohol-related pancreatitis should be referred to counseling services. Alcohol cessation, though, has an unpredictable effect on further attacks. Patients with gallbladder-related pancreatitis should undergo cholecystectomy and endoscopic sphincterotomy if medically cleared for these procedures. Avoid the use of ERCP as a diagnostic tool to investigate unexplained abdominal pain to reduce the risk of post-ERCP pancreatitis. Pancreatitis is the most common complication of ERCP.

CARE PLANS FOR ACUTE PANCREATITIS

Deficient fluid volume *related to decreased intake, vomiting, nasogastric suction, fluid loss into the pancreas and abdomen or with SAP, massive fluid sequestration within the peritoneum and retroperitoneal space; hemorrhage associated with tissue necrosis; systemic vasodilation and increased capillary permeability from inflammatory mediators*

GOALS/OUTCOMES Within 24 hours of this diagnosis, patient becomes normovolemic as evidenced by MAP greater than 70 mm Hg, HR 60 to 100 bpm, normal sinus rhythm on ECG, CVP 2 to 6 mm Hg, CO greater than 4 to 6 L/min, brisk capillary refill (less than 2 sec), peripheral pulses at least 2+ on a 0 to 4+ scale; urinary output greater than 0.5 ml/kg/hr.

NOC Electrolyte and Acid-Base Balance; Fluid Balance

Fluid Management
1. Administer crystalloids, colloids, or a combination of both as prescribed.
2. Monitor BP every 1 to 4 hours if losses are caused by fluid sequestration, inadequate intake, or slow bleeding. Monitor BP continuously with arterial line, or hourly and increase to every 15 minutes if patient has active blood loss or massive fluid sequestration.
3. Monitor HR and cardiovascular status at least every 2 to 4 hours, and more often with SAP.
4. Measure urinary output hourly. Report output less than 0.5 ml/kg/hr for 2 consecutive hours. Evaluate intravascular volume and cardiovascular function, and increase fluid intake promptly if decreased urinary output is caused by hypovolemia and hypoperfusion.
5. Monitor for indicators of hypovolemia, including cool extremities, delayed capillary refill (more than 2 seconds), and decreased amplitude of or absent distal pulses.
6. Estimate ongoing fluid losses. Measure all drainage from tubes, catheters, and drains. Note the frequency of dressing changes because of saturation with fluid or blood. Compare 24-hour urine output with 24-hour fluid intake, and record the difference.
7. Administer room temperature IV fluids. Aggressive IV hydration with volumes of 250 to 300 ml/hr of crystalloids may be necessary in patients with no cardiac history.
8. Continuously monitor HR and ECG. Be alert to increases in HR, which suggest hypovolemia.
9. Monitor cardiovascular status hourly including CVP.
10. Measure hemodynamic parameters (i.e., CVP, CO) and thermodilution CO every 1-4 hours or continuously using an arterial based system (e.g., Flotrac or PICO). Be alert to low or decreasing CVP, and CO in patients with borderline cardiac function or respiratory function. An elevated HR, decreased CVP, and decreased CO (CI less than 3 L/min/m^2) suggest hypovolemia.
11. Consider fluid bolus for urine output less than 0.5 ml/kg/hr for 2 consecutive hours. If SAP is present, initiate fluid resuscitation and shock management.

Fluid Resuscitation
1. Obtain and maintain large-bore IV and central venous access.
2. Administer IV fluids; crystalloids are preferred (see *Fluid Management*, above).
3. Administer PRBCs for Hct less than 25%. Anticipate an Hct increase of 3% following 1 unit of PRBCs.
4. Consider administering albumin for serum albumin less than 2 g/dl, but observe for worsening of edema if capillary leak is severe.
5. Monitor coagulation studies and CBC.
6. Administer fresh-frozen plasma for coagulopathy and to replace lost circulating proteins.
7. Assess for signs of overaggressive fluid resuscitation (see *Fluid Volume Excess*, p. 776).
8. Weigh patient daily, using the same scales and method. Weight may increase due to significant capillary leak and anasarca with intravascular volume depletion.
9. Evaluate character of all fluids lost. Note color and odor. Be alert to the presence of particulate matter, fibrin, and clots. Test GI aspirate, drainage, and excretions (including stool) for the presence of occult blood.

Shock Management
1. Monitor fluid status (see *Fluid Management, Fluid Resuscitation*, p. 773).
2. Collaborate with physician or midlevel practitioner to administer vasoactive medication if shock persists with volume resuscitation.
3. Monitor for cerebral ischemia or indications of insufficient cerebral blood flow.
4. Monitor renal function (BUN and creatinine levels for elevations) as intravascular volume depletion can lead to prerenal azotemia.
5. Monitor tissue oxygenation using arterial blood gas, Svo_2 or $Scvo_2$ monitoring and serum lactate measurements.
6. Monitor ECG for ST-segment depression and T-wave inversion, which may be seen as a result of the shock state.

Electrolyte Management
1. Monitor for manifestations of electrolyte imbalance. Calcium, sodium, magnesium, and potassium are lost with fluid sequestration and vomiting.
2. Maintain IV solutions containing electrolytes at a constant rate.
3. Continuously monitor ECG for alterations related to electrolyte imbalances.
4. Monitor ionized calcium. Widening of the QT interval suggests severe hypocalcemia. Hypocalcemia may produce numbness or tingling in the extremities that can progress to tetany.
5. Administer calcium gluconate or calcium chloride for low ionized calcium (less than 4.4 mg/dl). Calcium chloride will provide a higher level of calcium replacement given the strength and chemical composition.
6. Monitor T wave as a sign of alterations in serum potassium levels.

NIC Fluid/Electrolyte Management; Fluid Monitoring; Hemodynamic Regulation; Hypovolemia Management; Invasive Hemodynamic Monitoring; Shock Prevention; Bleeding Precautions; Bleeding Reduction; Hypervolemia Management

Decreased cardiac output *related to myocardial depression secondary to circulating vasoactive amines or hypocalcemia with SAP; decreased preload secondary to hypovolemia*

GOALS/OUTCOMES Within 12 hours of this diagnosis, cardiac output becomes adequate as evidenced by CI greater than 2.5 L/min/m², brisk capillary refill (less than 2 seconds), peripheral pulses greater than 2+ on a 0 to 4+ scale, urinary output greater than 0.5 ml/kg/hr, and warm skin.
NOC Circulation Status

Hemodynamic Regulation
1. Restore acceptable preload by correcting hypovolemia (see preceding nursing diagnosis, *Fluid Volume Deficit*).
2. Administer inotropic agents. Consider dobutamine for myocardial contractile support. Monitor hemodynamic parameters carefully to observe for vasodilation if dose of dobutamine is low.
3. Space out procedures and treatments to allow long periods (at least 90 minutes) of uninterrupted rest.
4. Minimize anxiety-producing situations, and assist patient with reducing anxiety.

NIC Care: Acute; Shock Management; Cardiac: Dysrhythmia Management; Anxiety Reduction; Energy Management

Acute pain *related to chemical injury to the pancreas and peripancreatic tissue secondary to release of pancreatic enzymes*

GOALS/OUTCOMES Within 2 to 4 hours of this diagnosis, patient's subjective evaluation of discomfort improves, as documented by a pain scale. Ventilation and hemodynamic status are uncompromised as evidenced by MAP greater than 70 mm Hg, HR 60 to 100 bpm, and respiratory rate (RR) 12 to 20 breaths/min with normal depth and pattern (eupnea).
NOC Pain Control; Pain Level; Comfort Level

Analgesia Administration
1. As prescribed, administer IV opiate analgesic before pain becomes severe.
2. Meperidine may be used initially for up to 3 days, but should not be administered long-term due to metabolite accumulation which can cause neurological adverse effects. Meperidine is avoided in SAP patients, since analgesia is needed for more than 3 days. Hydromorphone may be a better alternative.
3. Monitor HR and BP at least every 4 hours, and at least every 2 hours with SAP patients. Opiates cause vasodilation and can add to the serious hypotension SAP patient with volume depletion. Monitor every

15 minutes if severe pain is uncontrolled. Consult with physician or midlevel practitioner for changes in analgesic medications and dosages.

4. Evaluate effectiveness of medication, and consult physician or midlevel practitioner for dose and drug manipulation.
5. Consider continuous infusion or PCA for more effective pain control.
6. Consider epidural route if IV route is ineffective.
7. If medications are not effective, prepare patient for splanchnic block or other pain-relieving procedure.
8. Assess for anxiety and consider sedatives in conjunction with analgesia.

Safety Alert *Opioid analgesics decrease intestinal motility and delay return to normal bowel function.*

---

9. Monitor respiratory pattern and level of consciousness (LOC) closely because both may be depressed by the large amounts of opiate analgesics usually required to control pain.

Pain Management

1. Pancreatitis can be very painful. Prepare significant others for personality changes and behavioral alterations associated with extreme pain and opiate analgesia. Family members sometimes misinterpret patient's lethargy or unpleasant disposition and may even blame themselves. Reassure them that these are normal responses.
2. Supplement analgesics with nonpharmacologic maneuvers to aid in pain reduction. Modify patient's body position to optimize comfort. Many patients with abdominal pain find a dorsal recumbent or lateral decubitus bent-knee position most comfortable.
3. Consider cultural influences on pain response.
4. Because anxiety reduction contributes to pain relief, ensure consistency and promptness in delivering analgesic.
5. Patients and family members sometimes are distressed at the health team members' inability to relieve pain. Provide continual reassurance that all possible measures are being implemented.

NIC Patient-Controlled Analgesia (PCA) Assistance; Environmental Management: Comfort; Coping Enhancement; Teaching: Prescribed Medication; Simple Guided Imagery; Respiratory Monitoring

Impaired gas exchange *related to atelectasis and ARDS; elevation of the diaphragm and pleural effusion caused by subdiaphragmatic inflammation of the pancreas, and with SAP, alveolar-capillary membrane changes secondary to microatelectasis, inflammatory mediators and pulmonary fluid accumulation*

GOALS/OUTCOMES Within 4 hours of this diagnosis, patient has adequate gas exchange as evidenced by SaO_2 greater than 92%; PaO_2 greater than 80 mm Hg; $PaCO_2$ 35 to 45 mm Hg; RR 12 to 20 breaths/min with normal depth and pattern; orientation to time, place, and person; and clear and audible breath sounds.
NOC Respiratory Status: Gas Exchange; Respiratory Status: Ventilation

Airway Management

1. Administer oxygen via nasal cannula to maintain an oxygen saturation greater than 95%. Check oxygen delivery system at frequent intervals to ensure proper delivery.
2. Monitor and document respiratory rate every 1 to 4 hours as indicated. Note pattern, degree of excursion, and whether patient uses accessory muscles of respiration. Consult physician for significant deviations from baseline.
3. Auscultate both lung fields every 4 to 8 hours. Note presence of abnormal sounds (crackles, rhonchi, wheezes) or diminished sounds.
4. Be alert to early signs of hypoxia, such as restlessness, agitation, and alterations in mentation.
5. Monitor SaO_2 via continuous pulse oximetry or frequent ABG values during the first 48 hours. Many patients with pancreatitis do not have obvious clinical symptoms of respiratory failure, and a decreased arterial oxygen tension may be the first sign of ARDS or failure. Consult physician or midlevel practitioner if PaO_2 is less than 60 to 70 mm Hg or if oxygen saturation falls below 92%.
6. Maintain a body position that optimizes ventilation and oxygenation. Elevate HOB 30 degrees or higher, depending on patient's comfort. If pleural effusion or other defect is present on one side, position patient with the unaffected lung dependent to maximize the ventilation-perfusion relationship.
7. If patient fails to stabilize, prepare for endotracheal intubation and mechanical ventilation.
8. Monitor SaO_2 via continuous pulse oximetry and frequent ABG values during the first 48 hours. Hypoxemia in the absence of preexisting pulmonary disease may be an early sign of ARDS.

9. Pulmonary hypertension is anticipated in patients with ARDS with normal PAOP values.
10. Avoid overaggressive fluid resuscitation (see *Fluid Volume Excess, below*).

NIC Acid-Base Management; Airway Management; Oxygen Therapy; Respiratory Monitoring; Positioning; Fluid Monitoring; Hypervolemia Management
See *Acute Lung injury and Acute Respiratory Distress Syndrome*, p. 365, for additional information.

Excess Fluid volume *related to excessive intake secondary to overaggressive fluid resuscitation*

GOALS/OUTCOMES Within 24 hours of this diagnosis, patient becomes normovolemic as evidenced by MAP greater than 70 mm Hg, HR 60 to 100 bpm, RR 12 to 20 breaths/min with normal pattern and depth, and absence of adventitious breath sounds and S_3 gallop.
NOC Fluid Overload Severity; Fluid Balance; Electrolyte and Acid-Base Balance

Hypervolemia Management
1. Evaluate patient every 1 to 2 hours for clinical indicators of fluid volume excess: dyspnea, orthopnea, increased respiratory rate and effort, S_3 gallop, or crackles. Document and report changes and new findings.
2. Consider administering furosemide (Lasix) or other diuretic as prescribed to promote diuresis, but only after volume status has been carefully evaluated. Patients may be intravascularly hypovolemic despite significant weight gain resulting from third spacing of fluids. Diuresis may not prove to be beneficial. Document response to diuretic therapy by noting onset and amount of diuresis.

NIC Fluid/Electrolyte Management, Fluid Monitoring, Hemodynamic Regulation

Risk for infection *related to tissue destruction, if bacteria is involved tissue necrosis with SAP and multiple invasive procedures*

GOALS/OUTCOMES Patient remains free of infection as evidenced by no abscess formations, core or rectal temperature less than 37.8°C (less than 100°F), negative culture results, HR 60 to 100 bpm, RR 12 to 20 breaths/min, BP within patient's normal range, CO 4 to 6 L/min/m², CVP 2 to 6 mm Hg, and orientation to time, place, and person.
NOC Infection Severity; Immune Status

Infection Protection
1. Check temperature every 4 hours for increases. Be aware that hypothermia may precede hyperthermia in some patients.
2. Temperature may be slightly elevated due to the inflammatory process. If temperature remains elevated for longer than 1 week suspect the patient may have developed bacterial necrosis.
3. If temperature suddenly rises, obtain specimens for culture of blood, sputum, urine, and other sites as prescribed. Monitor culture reports, and report positive findings promptly.
4. Evaluate orientation and LOC every 2 to 4 hours. Report significant deviations from baseline.
5. Monitor BP, HR, RR, CO, and CVP every 1 to 4 hours. An elevated CO and decreased CVP suggest systemic inflammatory response or sepsis. Be alert to increases in HR and RR associated with temperature elevations.
6. Monitor WBC and anticipate a mild leukocytosis of 11,000 to 20,000/mm³ due to the inflammatory response of SAP. If WBC count is greater than 20,000/mm³, suspect infected pancreatitis. If total WBC count is elevated, monitor WBC differential for an elevation of bands (immature neutrophils).
7. Prophylactic antibiotics are NOT recommended for sterile pancreatitis unless the pancreas is greater than 30% necrosed as evidenced by CT scan.
8. If prescribed, administer parenteral antibiotics in a timely fashion. Reschedule antibiotics if a dose is delayed for more than 1 hour. Recognize that failure to administer antibiotics on schedule can result in inadequate blood levels and treatment failure.
9. Do not administer prophylactic antibiotics for SAP for longer than 14 days.
10. Patients with infected pancreatitis evidenced by aspirates positive for bacteria on gram stain or culture require antibiotic therapy and may undergo surgical debridement.

NIC Medication Management; Vital Signs Monitoring; Temperature Regulation; Intravenous (IV) Therapy

Imbalanced nutrition: less than body requirements *related to decreased oral intake secondary to nausea, vomiting, and nothing-by-mouth (NPO) status; increased need secondary to tissue destruction*

GOALS/OUTCOMES Patient maintains baseline body weight and demonstrates a positive nitrogen balance.
NOC Nutritional Status; Nutritional Status: Food and Fluid Intake

Nutritional Management
1. Collaborate with physician, dietitian, and pharmacist to estimate patient's individual metabolic needs, based on activity level, presence of infection or other stressor, and nutritional status before hospitalization. Overuse of calcium supplements can cause AP; this mechanism should be added as noted above. Develop a plan of care accordingly.
2. Determine preexisting malnutrition with a nutritional assessment.
3. If the patient's condition improves after 48 hours of resting the bowel, oral intake of clear liquids can be slowly started. Mild to moderate increases in serum amylase and lipase may be noted. Feedings should continue unless these elevations are threefold above normal range.
4. If the patient's condition does not improve after 48 hours of bowel rest, administer elemental enteral feedings via NJ feeding tube or jejunostomy as prescribed. Pancreatic secretions are not stimulated with the delivery of enteral elemental nutrition into the mid or distal jejunum. Ensure tube placement beyond the ligament of Treitz.
5. Monitor bowel sounds every 4 hours. Document and report deviations from baseline. Withhold jejunal feedings if bowel sounds are absent unless elemental feedings are used.
6. Monitor blood glucose levels every 4 to 8 hours or as prescribed. Treat blood glucose levels greater than 180 mg/dl with insulin therapy.
7. If enteral feedings are not tolerated, begin TPN as prescribed. Monitor closely for evidence of hyperglycemia (e.g., Kussmaul respirations; rapid respirations; fruity, acetone breath odor; flushed, dry skin; deteriorating LOC), which commonly is associated with pancreatitis. Administer insulin as prescribed.
8. Monitor blood glucose levels every 4 to 8 hours or as prescribed. Consult physician or midlevel practitioner for blood levels greater than 180 mg/dl.
9. Begin low-fat oral feedings when acute episode has subsided and bowel function has returned. This may take several weeks in some patients.

NIC Enteral Tube Feeding; Aspiration Precautions; Total Parenteral Nutrition (TPN) Administration; Venous Access Devices (VAD) Maintenance; Hyperglycemia Management; Hypoglycemia Management
For additional detail, see *Nutritional Support*, p. 117.

Deficient knowledge *related to lack of exposure to health care information*

GOALS/OUTCOMES Within the 24-hour period before hospital discharge, patient verbalizes knowledge regarding availability of alcohol rehabilitation programs, prescribed medications, importance of a low-fat diet, indicators of actual or impending GI hemorrhage, indicators of infection, and the importance of seeking medical attention promptly if signs of recurring pancreatitis appear.
NOC Knowledge: Disease Process; Knowledge Treatment: Regimen

Teaching: Disease Process
1. Inform patients whose pancreatitis is caused by excessive alcohol intake about the availability of alcohol rehabilitation programs.
2. Teach patient about prescribed medications including drug name, dosage, purpose, schedule, precautions, and side effects.
3. Advise patient about the importance of adhering to a low-fat diet if prescribed.
4. Instruct patient about the indicators of actual or impending GI hemorrhage: nausea, vomiting blood, dark stools, lightheadedness, passing frank blood in stools.
5. Teach the indicators of infection: fever, unusual drainage from surgical incisions or peritoneal lavage site, warmth or erythema surrounding surgical sites, and abdominal pain. Have patient demonstrate oral temperature-taking technique using the type of thermometer that will be used at home.
6. Stress the importance of seeking medical attention promptly if signs of recurrent pancreatitis (i.e., pain, change in bowel habits, passing blood in the stools, or vomiting blood) or infection (see *Risk for Infection*, p. 776) appear.

NIC Prescribed Activity Exercise, Prescribed Diet, Prescribed Procedure/Treatment, Prescribed Medication; Behavior Modification

Acute Pancreatitis

ADDITIONAL NURSING DIAGNOSES

As appropriate, see nursing diagnoses and interventions in the following: *Acute Respiratory Distress Syndrome* (p. 365), *Acute Renal Failure* (p. 584), and *SIRS, Sepsis and MODS*, p. 924. Also see *Prolonged Immobility* (p. 149) and *Emotional and Spiritual Support of the Patient and Significant Others* (p. 200).

ENTEROCUTANEOUS FISTULA

PATHOPHYSIOLOGY

Enterocutaneous fistulas (ECFs) are formed when trauma, surgery, infection, neoplastic disease, or other pathologic condition results in a gastrointestinal-cutaneous communication. They can be classified as spontaneous (15% to 25%) or postoperative (75 to 85%). Spontaneous fistulas occur in patients with cancer, inflammatory bowel disease (IBD), diverticular disease, appendicitis, perforated bowel disease, or ischemic bowel or those receiving radiation treatment. Postoperative fistulas account for the majority of ECFs and are observed most commonly following procedures for the treatment of malignancy, IBD, emergency surgery with inadequate bowel preparation, trauma surgery with missed injuries, or those requiring damage control operations, where the abdomen is left open due to packing, or where the bowel is so edematous it is unable to be closed, and for reoperative procedures involving extensive lysis of adhesions.

Fistulas can be classified as high output (greater than 500 ml/day), moderate output (200 to 500 ml/day), and low output (less than 200 ml/day). High-output proximal small bowel fistulas are the most difficult to manage. Drainage from proximal fistulas is hypertonic; rich in enzymes, electrolytes, and proteins; thin in consistency and tends to be copious. Losses as high as 2 L/24 hr are not uncommon. Extensive skin and tissue breakdown often occur because of the presence of activated pancreatic enzymes in fistula drainage. Electrolyte and protein loss is great with high-output proximal fistulas. Drainage from distal sites, such as the ileum and colon, is thick and of less volume than is proximal fistula drainage.

Three factors are associated with mortality in patients with ECFs: (1) fluid and electrolyte imbalance, (2) malnutrition, and (3) sepsis. Fluid, potassium, sodium, proteins, and bicarbonate may be lost in great quantities. Replacement by enteral nutrition (EN) or parenteral nutrition (TPN) is complex, and proper balance often is difficult to achieve. Sepsis is frequently associated with bowel fistulization, as either a cause or a result of anastomotic breakdown or as a result of local wound contamination or inadequate drainage. Hypercatabolism and malnutrition are associated with both sepsis and fistulization, creating a great demand for calories and protein. Aggressive nutritional support and meticulous local wound management are critical to patient survival.

GASTROINTESTINAL ASSESSMENT: ENTEROCUTANEOUS FISTULA

Goal of Assessment: Enterocutaneous Fistula

Evaluate the functional integrity of the intestinal tract.

History and Risk Factors

- Direct trauma to the GI system, especially to the bowel
- Infection of surgical wound, drainage tract, or peritoneum
- Prolonged catabolic state in association with bowel injury, GI neoplasm, GI abscess, or severe inflammatory bowel disease
- Complex GI surgical procedures, such as lysis of adhesions for intestinal obstruction or complicated intestinal anastomosis

Vital Sign Assessment

- Increased temperature and tachycardia due to infection or dehydration
- Irregular heart rate if hypokalemia is present
- Decreased urinary output with increased specific gravity due to excessive fluid loss

Abdominal Pain

- Tenderness, erythema, and possibly pain at the incision/fistula site caused by irritation from fistula output or infection
- Muscle weakness from hypokalemia

Abdominal Drainage
- Discharge of obvious bile, enteric contents, or gas through a surgical incision
- Sudden increase in the amount of drainage from a surgical incision or drainage catheter
- A change in the nature of drainage from serous or serosanguineous to yellow, green, brown, or foul-smelling
- A change in pancreatic drainage to milky white suggests a pancreatic fistula.

Observation
- Mental confusion is often present as a result of electrolyte imbalance, dehydration, or early sepsis.
- Sunken eyes, poor skin turgor, and dry oral mucosa, associated with dehydration
- Peripheral edema and muscle wasting related to protein loss
- Erythema, maceration, and edema may be present on the abdomen because of irritating fistula drainage.

Auscultation
- Diminished or absent bowel sounds if peritonitis or ileus is present

Palpation
- Discomfort and guarding on abdominal palpation over an abdominal mass (abscess) or near a drain site or surgical incision

Nutritional Assessment
- Weight loss and loss of muscle mass due to protein losses and hypercatabolism
- Decreased serum albumin and serum transferrin both indicate malnutrition.

Screening Labwork
- Serum electrolytes levels: depleted due to external losses through the fistula
- CBC: Anemia may be present reducing oxygen delivery.

Hemodynamic Measurements
- Decreased BP, PAP, and CO if severe dehydration is present.
- If early sepsis is present, expect elevated CO and decreased SVR.
- Oxygen demand is increased and may exceed supply. Svo_2 will fall without aggressive pulmonary and cardiovascular support.
- The patient will exhibit general hemodynamic instability until fluid balance, inflammation, and infection are controlled.

Diagnostic Tests for Enterocutaneous Fistula		
Test	**Purpose**	**Abnormal Findings**
Blood Studies		
Complete blood count (CBC) White blood cell (WBC) count	Assess for inflammation, infection, and sepsis	Leukocytosis with WBC count >12,000/mm^3. Leukopenia with WBC count <4,000/mm^3. Normal WBC with >10% bands.
Red blood cell (RBC) count Hemoglobin (Hgb) Hematocrit (Hct)	Reflective of volume status and oxygen carrying capacity	Hct and Hgb levels will be elevated due to the presence of significant dehydration. Anemia is present due to the prolonged period of illness.
Electrolytes Serum potassium Serum magnesium Serum calcium Serum bicarbonate	Determine accurate electrolyte levels to dictate appropriate replacement as large quantities may be lost through fistula drainage.	Hypokalemia Hypocalcemia Hypomagnesemia Metabolic acidosis

Continued

Diagnostic Tests for Enterocutaneous Fistula—cont'd

Test	Purpose	Abnormal Findings
Nutrition profile Serum albumin Serum transferrin Serum prealbumin	Evaluate nutritional status and initiate aggressive nutritional support early.	These labs will vary in individual patients. Serum transferrin levels >140 mg/dl have been shown to correlate with the spontaneous closure of enterocutaneous fistulas thereby reducing mortality among these patients. Levels <140 is a poor prognostic finding. Serum albumin 3 g/dl or less at the time of fistula presentation is a poor prognostic indicator. Prealbumin levels will rise with effective nutritional therapy.
Noninvasive Cardiology		
ECG	Assess and monitor for cardiac rhythm disturbances related to hypokalemia, hypocalcemia, and hypomagnesemia	Hypokalemia may result in flattening of the T-wave or U-wave development. Hypocalcemia, hypokalemia and hypomagnesemia can result in widening of the QT interval.
Radiology		
Fistulogram Water-soluble contrast medium injected into the suspected fistula	To identify the anatomy and characteristics of the fistula tract	Radiographs will confirm anatomic site of origin and fistula tract.
Computed tomography (CT) scan	CT may be used to identify abscesses associated with fistulization.	Confirmation of intraperitoneal abscess is made. Percutaneous drainage may be performed.
Upper GI series	An upper GI series may be indicated if the suspected fistula is proximal to the intestines.	Upper GI series may reveal esophageal, gastric, or duodenal fistulas.

Nonradiographic Evaluation

Bedside maneuver: An external fistula can be simply confirmed without radiology by the oral administration of charcoal. The visible presence of dye in the drainage confirms the presence of a fistula.

Biopsy: In patients with neoplastic disease, a biopsy specimen of the fistula tract may be obtained to determine the presence of malignancy within the tract.

Culture: Fistula effluent from the stomach, duodenum, biliary tree, and pancreas may be cultured for evidence of infection. Small and large bowel fistulas are generally not cultured because of the expected presence of bacteria.

COLLABORATIVE MANAGEMENT

Early management of ECF presents a considerable challenge requiring advanced support of a multidisciplinary team in a surgical intensive care unit setting. The patient with ECF is typically malnourished with a recent history of malignancy, inflammatory or infectious disease, postoperative or traumatic bowel injury, dehiscence, or inadvertent enterotomy. Their physiologic and nutritional reserves are significantly compromised. This complex set of circumstances are usually complicated by sepsis and the metabolic and fluid derangements caused by the fistula. Early fistula identification is imperative in order to implement appropriate management strategies. Management strategies include patient stabilization, investigation of the fistula, evaluation of surgical need, and the promotion of healing.

Care Priorities

Once the fistula is diagnosed, immediate management should focus on fluid restoration and the correction of electrolyte abnormalities. The control of sepsis and septic complications, nutritional support, and fistula management are key components to positive outcomes and should be addressed concurrently.

1. **Fluid and Electrolyte Replacement** Crystalloid resuscitation with normal saline IV solutions that contain added potassium are administered to maintain fluid and electrolyte balance. Often, the amount to be delivered is prescribed in direct relation to fistula output, especially when the output is widely variable. Effluent from each fistula is measured separately for accurate estimation of specific electrolyte and fluid losses. In general, fistulas that are more proximal result in greater fluid, electrolyte, and protein losses than those that are distal.

2. **Control of Sepsis** Sepsis is the often seen in the patient with postoperative ECF following a bowel procedure where bowel contents escape into the peritoneum. All team members should participate in the evaluation of a septic foci. Blood, wound, fistula drainage, sputum, and venous catheter tips should be cultured. Empiric antibiotic therapy is indicated with diagnosis of sepsis followed by specific therapy. Intraperitoneal abscesses should be drained cautiously as manipulation of the septic foci may lead to its spread. If no evidence of sepsis is observed, antibiotic therapy should be withheld in the postoperative period. In patients with ECF, indiscriminate antibiotic use will lead to the emergence of highly resistant bacteria.

3. **Nutritional Support** Fistula patients are typically malnourished due to their postoperative NPO status, the hypercatabolism of sepsis, and the protein- and mineral-rich intestinal fluid loss from the fistula. Both TPN and EN can be used to manage patients with ECF based on a thorough nutritional assessment.

   EN is currently advocated over TPN as EN enhances mucosal proliferation, promotes villus growth, improves hepatic protein synthesis, and stimulates the enterocyte, while TPN has been shown to cause intestinal mucosal atrophy. However, TPN remains a valuable therapeutic modality for patients who cannot tolerate EN and in combination with EN for patients who are unable to absorb sufficient calories from enteral feedings alone. Enteral feedings can be initiated by weighted nasoduodenal intestinal feeding tube if there is sufficient ($\approx$4 feet) functioning small bowel length between the ligament of Treitz (a thin muscle that wraps around the small intestine where the duodenum and jejunum meet) and the fistula. Enteral feedings can be optimized in patients with a feeding jejunostomy (that was placed at the time of their surgery) distal to the fistula, as is the case of many postoperative ECFs. In some cases, enteral feedings may be infused into the fistula itself. The volume and concentration of enteral feedings are started low and increased incrementally; supplementation with TPN is necessary to meet caloric and protein requirements during this time. For some patients, TPN supplementation is needed throughout the duration of care. Enteral feedings are slowed or discontinued if fistula output increases after initiation of feedings.

   Patients with proximal small bowel fistulas, prolonged ileus, or extensive intra-abdominal sepsis usually require TPN. Optimizing nutritional status will enhance the immune system, preserve lean cell mass, and promote wound healing. Improved nutritional status correlates with spontaneous fistula closure.

4. **Fistula Management** Ideally, drainage from each fistula is collected separately to assess individual fistula activity and healing. Individualized systems of gravity or gentle suction drainage and barrier skin protection are devised for each patient. Good local management reduces the incidence of wound-related bacteremias and increases the rate of wound healing. Vacuum-assisted closure (VAC) systems may be used for difficult to manage fistula wounds. The system consists of a porous foam pad that connects to subatmospheric suction under an occlusive dressing. VACs divert fistula drainage away from the wound by providing continuous negative pressure suction to the wound surface. VACs protect the skin and reduce patient discomfort from multiple dressing changes as they require changes only once every 2 to 3 days. This system effectively promotes wound healing by increasing the rate of tissue granulation and augmenting wound contracture.
   Somatostatin and Octreotide: Both somatostatin and its analog octreotide inhibit gastric secretions and thus should decrease fistula output. However, neither drug has shown

significant improvement on fistula closure rate or improvement in mortality rates. Additionally, somatostatin is associated with a frequent incidence of hyperglycemia and both drugs are associated with an increased incidence of cholelithiasis. These drugs are therefore not indicated for routine use in patients with ECF. Octreotide alone however, may have limited application in patients with high-output fistulas.

✼ **Surgery:** *Spontaneous fistula closure occurs in about 30% of patients with ECF with adequate nutritional support and successful treatment of sepsis. If spontaneous closure does not occur after 4 weeks of management, surgical resection is considered.* Surgery is indicated in the following instances: (1) to close fistulas that continue to drain significant amounts despite absence of infection and appropriate nutritional support; (2) to explore and drain fistula tracts that could not be identified or drained by less invasive techniques; and (3) if overwhelming sepsis fails to respond to antibiotics and supportive therapy. Persistently draining fistulas are surgically closed with a procedure involving resection with end-to-end anastomosis. Postoperatively, parenteral nutrition and antibiotic coverage are continued. A gastrostomy usually is created to allow for prolonged intestinal decompression and drainage. The patient may remain NPO for 1 to 2 weeks after surgery, depending on the rate of healing and the return of bowel function. An alternate feeding strategy is initiated during this time.

CARE PLANS FOR ENTEROCUTANEOUS FISTULA

Deficient fluid volume *related to the active loss of intestinal fluids rich in electrolytes, minerals, and protein through fistula output*

GOALS/OUTCOMES Within 8 hours of this diagnosis, patient becomes normovolemic as evidenced by balanced daily input and output, urinary output greater than 0.5 ml/kg/hr, moist mucous membranes, good skin turgor, HR less than 100 bpm, CVP 2 to 6 mm Hg, and PAOP 6 to 12 mm Hg.
NOC Fluid Balance

Fluid/Electrolyte Management
✼ 1. Evaluate patient's fluid balance by calculating and comparing daily intake and output. In patients with high-output fistulas, evaluate total intake and output every 8 hours. Record all sources of output, including drainage from each fistula.
2. Administer IV crystalloids to replace fistula output. Generally, fistula output is iso-osmotic with high potassium content. Thus, normal saline with potassium is a common choice.
3. Administer albumin for serum albumin less than 2 g/dl. Albumin will assist in restoring plasma oncotic pressure but should be used with caution as it may accumulate in the pulmonary interstitium if the patient has sepsis-induced increased capillary permeability.
4. Consider administering PRBCs for Hct less than 25% unless patient is asymptomatic. Transfusion should be based on the symptoms of the patient. Transfusion of PRBCs will improve oxygen-carrying capacity. Anticipate an Hct increase of 3% following 1 unit of PRBCs.
5. Measure urine output every 1-2 hours. Consult physician or midlevel practitioner if urine output is less than 0.5 ml/kg/hr or if specific gravity increases and urine volume decreases.
6. Assess and document condition of mucous membranes and skin turgor. Dry membranes and inelastic skin indicate inadequate fluid volume and the need for increase in fluid intake (PO or IV route).
7. Measure and evaluate vital signs, CVP, and PAP (when available) every 1 to 4 hours, depending on hemodynamic stability. Be alert to increasing HR, decreasing CVP, and decreasing PAP, which indicate inadequate intravascular volume. Encourage increased oral intake (if possible), or consult with physician regarding increase in IV fluid intake.
8. Control sources of insensible fluid loss by humidifying oxygen, maintaining comfortable environment, and controlling fever (if present) with antipyretics such as acetaminophen.
9. Monitor for manifestations of electrolyte imbalance, most commonly hypokalemia, hypocalcemia, and hypomagnesemia that are lost through fistula output.
10. Monitor ECG for T-wave flattening or the presence of a U wave, both of which are signs of hypokalemia.
11. Monitor ECG for prolongation of the QT interval, a result of hypokalemia, hypocalcemia, and hypomagnesemia.

NIC Fluid Monitoring; Hemodynamic Regulation; Hypovolemia Management; Invasive Hemodynamic Monitoring; Shock Prevention

Infection, risk for and actual *related to inadequate primary defenses (altered integumentary system, disruption in continuity of GI system), hypercatabolic state, presence of invasive lines, protein loss/malnutrition, and gut contamination of bowel contents*

GOALS/OUTCOMES Patient remains free of infection as evidenced by core or rectal temperature less than 37.8°C (100°F), negative culture results, HR 60 to 100 bpm, RR 12 to 20 breaths/min, BP within patient's normal range, and orientation to time, place, and person.
NOC Wound Healing: Secondary Intention

Infection Control
1. Check rectal or core temperature every 2 hours for increases or decreases.
2. If temperature suddenly rises, assess patient for potential sources, noting presence of purulent secretions; erythema around wound, drain, or fistula site; and pain, tenderness, or masses with abdominal palpation. Consult physician for temperature elevation and assessment findings. Obtain specimens for culture of likely sites for infection as prescribed by physician or unit protocol.
3. Evaluate orientation and LOC every 2 hours. Document and report significant deviations from baseline values.
4. Monitor BP, HR, RR, CO, and SVR every 2 hours. Be alert to increases in HR and RR associated with temperature elevations. As available, monitor Svo_2 continuously or at scheduled intervals. An elevated CO and a decreased SVR suggest early septic shock (see *SIRS, Sepsis and MODS*, p. 924).
5. Administer parenteral antibiotics in a timely fashion. Reschedule antibiotics if a dosage is delayed for greater than 1 hour. Recognize that failure to administer antibiotics on schedule can result in inadequate blood levels and treatment failure.
6. Optimize gravity drainage of fistula by prone or upright positioning as tolerated by patient.
7. Wear gloves when contact with drainage is possible. Prevent transmission of potentially infectious agents by washing hands thoroughly before and after caring for patient and carefully disposing of dressings and drainage.
8. See *SIRS, Sepsis and MODS* care plans, p. 933.

NIC Medication Management; Hemodynamic Regulation; Vital Signs Monitoring; Temperature Regulation; Intravenous (IV) Therapy; Wound Care

Imbalanced nutrition: less than body requirements *related to decreased intake, protein loss via fistula output, disruption of GI tract continuity, and the hypercatabolism of sepsis*

GOALS/OUTCOMES By the time of hospital discharge, patient has adequate nutrition as evidenced by food intake that increases to his or her recommended daily allowance, and body weight that returns to baseline or within 10% of patient's ideal weight.
NOC Nutritional Status: Nutrient Intake

Nutrition Management
1. Collaborate with physician or midlevel practitioner, dietitian, and pharmacist to estimate patient's metabolic needs on the basis of activity level, estimated metabolic rate, and baseline nutritional status.
2. Determine preexisting malnutrition.
3. Monitor nutrition labs. Serum albumin and serum transferrin are good prognostic indicators for mortality, morbidity and spontaneous fistula closure.
4. Monitor for the presence of bowel sounds every 2 hours. If bowel sounds are absent, consider duodenal or jejunal elemental feedings.
5. If fistula output increases in response to enteral feedings, slow the rate of infusion or reduce the strength of the feeding. If the patient tolerates oral feedings but they increase fistula output, increase the frequency of the feedings and decrease the amount consumed at each feeding.
6. Be aware, when the entire intestine is not available for normal absorption, elemental feeding formulas may be more readily absorbed.
7. Prepare patient for parenteral feedings if enteral feedings are inadequate for patient's requirements.
8. Apply nasogastric suction only in the presence of obstruction or prolonged ileus. In their absence, NG drainage shows little benefit. They may inappropriately contribute to complications such as patient discomfort, sinusitis, pulmonary aspiration and gastroesophageal reflux.

NIC Nutritional Monitoring; Fluid/Electrolyte Management; Total Parenteral Nutrition (TPN) Administration; Enteral Tube Feeding

Enterocutaneous Fistula

For additional information, see *Nutritional Support*, p. 117.

Impaired tissue integrity *related to chemical trauma, infection, and malnutrition*

GOALS/OUTCOMES Within 72 hours of this diagnosis, patient's tissue adjacent to the fistula is free of erythema, excoriation, and edema.

NOC Wound Healing: Secondary Intention; Tissue Integrity: Skin and Mucous Membranes

Wound Care
1. Assess the extent of the local problem (Box 9-6). Consult physician for signs of extensive damage to the tissue adjacent to the fistula (i.e., severe local erythema, excoriation, edema, maceration).
2. Establish drainage and collection system for each fistula (Box 9-7). Consult physician regarding use of continuous wound suction device(s).
3. Note character, color, odor, and volume of output from each fistula. Consult physician for significant changes in any of these indicators.
4. If increased fistula output results from oral or enteral feedings, eliminate or modify the feedings as prescribed.
5. Consult ostomy nurse or enterostomal therapist for recommendations in pouching complex or multiple fistulas.
6. Consider wound management with a vacuum-assist closure (VAC) system — currently used to effectively divert intestinal output to its suction device, thereby preventing spillage into tissue adjacent to the fistula.
7. Change VAC dressing every 2 to 3 days as prescribed. With this frequency of dressing change, the surrounding skin is protected and patient discomfort is decreased.

NIC Ostomy Care; Tube Care; Fluid/Electrolyte Management

Box 9-6   NURSING ASSESSMENT OF ENTEROCUTANEOUS FISTULA

- Evaluate size, shape, and location of the fistula. Reposition or lift skin folds as necessary.
- Identify any potential leakage tracks created by skin folds or body hollows.
- Examine the condition of adjacent skin and tissue. Note the presence and spread of both erythema and excoriation, which suggest leakage tracks.
- Note the consistency and character of fistula output.
- Assess each fistula separately.

Document all findings, and compare them with baseline assessment made at the time of initial evaluation.

Box 9-7   RECOMMENDATIONS FOR CONTAINING FISTULA DRAINAGE

- Clean the intact skin surrounding the fistula with a nonirritating antibacterial cleanser.
- Clip body hair (if present) around the fistula.
- Remove pooled drainage from the wound and surrounding area by using sterile absorbent pads or gentle suction. The help of an assistant may be necessary to maintain a dry field during application of the collection device.
- Apply a barrier powder (e.g., karaya or Orahesive) to excoriated skin. A flexible transparent dressing (e.g., Op-Site) can be used to protect intact skin.
- Use a skin paste (e.g., Stomahesive or karaya) to fill in any grooves surrounding recessed fistulas.
- Apply a sized barrier sheet (e.g., Stomahesive, HolliHesive) to the surrounding skin, being careful not to overlap the fistula.
- Attach a collecting bag to the barrier sheet base. For high-output fistulas, a urostomy bag and collecting system may be necessary. Transparent appliances enable observation of drainage. Devices that have a drainage opening permit emptying and measurement of output.

Reposition the patient frequently to optimize gravity of fistula output. For example, it sometimes is necessary to use a rotating bed frame or a bed modified with foam blocks to facilitate prone positioning.

Disturbed body image   *related to biophysical change secondary to presence of external fistula*

GOALS/OUTCOMES By the time of hospital discharge, patient acknowledges body changes as evidenced by viewing fistula and not exhibiting preoccupation with or depersonalization of fistula.
NOC Body Image

Body Image Enhancement
1. Evaluate the patient's reaction to the fistula by observing and noting evidence of body image disturbance.
2. Anticipate feelings of shock and repulsion initially. Be aware that the development of an external fistula usually is an unanticipated complication and patients are not emotionally prepared for the disfigurement.
3. Anticipate and acknowledge normalcy of feelings of rejection, isolation, and uncleanliness (because of odor and possible presence of feces).
4. Offer patient opportunity to view fistula/wound as desired. Use mirrors if necessary.
5. Encourage patient and significant others to verbalize feelings regarding fistula/wound.
6. If possible, offer the patient an opportunity to participate in wound care. Patient may be able to perform simple tasks, such as holding the bag into which you will deposit the soiled dressing or applying the pouch that collects drainage.
7. Convey an accepting attitude toward the patient. Many fistulas that require critical care involve open and infected wounds. If the attending nurse is inexperienced in dressing these complex wounds, another, more experienced nurse should be present during the initial dressing change.
8. Reassure patient that the fistula is not permanent. Acknowledge that a scar will be visible but the fistula will close with appropriate care.

NIC Coping Enhancement; Self-Care Assistance; Support System Enhancement

Impaired oral mucous membrane   *related to prolonged NPO status*

GOALS/OUTCOMES Within 24 hours of this diagnosis, patient's oral mucosa is intact, moist, and free of pain and oral lesions.
NOC Oral Hygiene; Tissue Integrity: Skin and Mucous Membranes

Oral Health Maintenance
1. Inspect the patient's oral cavity, noting the degree of moisture, inflammation, bleeding, or lesions. Consult physician for open lesions and bleeding.
2. Assist patient with brushing teeth with a soft-bristle toothbrush. Irrigate the oral cavity with a solution of 500 ml normal saline and 15 ml sodium bicarbonate. Provide mouth care every 4 hours.
3. For patients with altered LOC, massage gums and teeth with saline-moistened, sponge-tipped applicator and brush teeth gently if there is no evidence of bleeding. Place patient in a side-lying position, and irrigate the mouth with small amounts of a saline and bicarbonate solution (per second entry). Carefully suction the solution from the oral cavity throughout the procedure with a Yankauer tonsil suction device.
4. Keep the lips moist with emollients such as lanolin or Eucerin cream. Take care to apply emollient to external tissue only. Oil-containing emollients are harmful if aspirated or otherwise introduced into the respiratory tract.

NIC Oral Health Promotion

ADDITIONAL NURSING DIAGNOSES
See *Nutritional Support* (p. 117) for additional information about the patient with extra nutritional needs. See *Emotional and Spiritual Support of the Patient and Significant Others* (p. 200) for psychosocial nursing diagnoses and interventions. Also see nursing diagnoses and interventions related to sepsis under *SIRS, Sepsis and MODS*, (p. 924).

HEPATIC FAILURE

PATHOPHYSIOLOGY
There are various manifestations of chronic and acute liver failure (ALF). Fluid retention, edema, and ascites are common to acute and chronic hepatic failure and are attributed to (1) intrahepatic vascular obstruction with transudation of fluid into the peritoneum;

(2) defective albumin synthesis, resulting in decreased colloid osmotic pressure with failure to retain intravascular fluid; and (3) disturbances of various hormones, including renin, aldosterone, and renal prostaglandins, resulting in sodium and water retention. Massive ascites is usually the result of cirrhosis. Regardless of whether it is acute or chronic, hepatic failure affects the physiologic status of virtually every organ system. Failure of other organs can often be linked to liver dysfunction. An interdisciplinary health care team is needed to vigilantly manage these complex patients.

Acute Liver Failure

ALF is defined as a severe, sudden loss of hepatocytes and hepatic function in someone without a prior history of liver disease. There are approximately 2,000 cases per year in the United States. Acetaminophen overdose was the leading etiology (46%) in adults between 1998 and 2007. Outcomes have improved considerably in the last decade, since the diagnosis can be made more quickly. Placing patients in a hepatic intensive care unit of a liver transplant center has helped improve survival. Specialized centers are familiar with appropriate crisis management, including palliative, non–disease specific treatments (i.e., N-acetylcysteine [NAC]). Only 25% of hospitalized patients receive a liver transplant. The outcomes of the Acute Liver Failure study revealed those with slowly evolving etiologies have a poorer prognosis than patients whose ALF developed hyperacutely (within less than 1 week).

Chronic Liver Failure (End-Stage Liver Disease)

Loss of hepatocytes, abnormal microcirculation, and impaired function of 6 months or longer duration are hallmarks of ESLD. Chronic liver disease is associated with widespread tissue necrosis, fibrosis, liver nodule formation, and cirrhosis, ultimately resulting in hepatic failure. The usual causes are long-term alcohol ingestion, chronic viral hepatitis, prolonged cholestasis, and metabolic disorders.

Transfer to an Appropriate Transplant Center

While only 25% of those patients with ALF go on to receive a liver transplant, it is important for patients to be treated at a hospital with a liver transplant program, with specialized intensive care units for those with ESLD. Specialized interdisciplinary collaboration provides rapid evaluation for etiology, severity of liver damage, and listing for and receiving a liver transplant.

Organ Failure Linked to Liver Disease

Hepatorenal syndrome (HRS) is defined by the International Ascites Club as renal impairment or failure that occurs in patients with advanced chronic liver disease, liver failure, and portal hypertension. Patients have marked abnormalities in the arterial circulation and activity of the endogenous vasoactive systems.

Significant renal vasoconstriction results in low glomerular filtration rate (GFR), while arterial vasodilation in the extrarenal circulation results in reduction of systemic vascular resistance and hypotension. Factors that reduce renal perfusion in persons with chronic liver disease are dehydration, lactulose therapy, NSAID use, hemorrhage, and paracentesis.

Heart failure may result from circulatory abnormalities associated with liver disease. Increased nitric oxide activity is present, which causes systemic arterial, venous, and pulmonary vasodilation leading to right-to-left shunting of deoxygenated blood into the arterial circulation. Initially, hyperdynamic systemic circulation, with decreased SVR and increased CO, is present. As the condition progresses, dysrhythmias result from reduced beta adrenergic receptor signal transduction, defective cardiac excitation-contraction coupling, and conduction abnormalities. Right heart failure ensues and causes venous engorgement resulting in hepatic congestion. The decreased forward flow of blood from the failing right to the left heart circulation results in reduced CO. Decreased hepatic blood flow, with congestion of the vena cava from blood "backing up" from the failing right heart, impedes the emptying of the portal vein into the vena cava.

Heart failure progressively damages the hepatocytes due to hypoxia resulting from circulatory impairment. The portal vein supplies up to 83% of the blood flow to the liver, with the hepatic artery supplying up to 34% (varies from person to person by approximately ±17%). In the final stages of ALF, profound peripheral vasodilation results in severe vascular congestion and third spacing of intravascular fluids including ascites, which causes hemodynamic collapse. Hypotension, tachycardia, heart murmur, warm extremities, an exaggerated precordial impulse, palmar erythema, and/or spider angiomas are present. Peritoneovenous shunting (PVS) and transjugular intrahepatic portocaval shunting (TIPS) are useful for treating portal hypertension associated with refractory ascites and esophageal varices in the cirrhotic patient with ESLD. Studies have revealed an increased association of hepatic encephalopathy following TIPS without significant improvement in survival. The hyperdynamic circulatory state worsens for 1 to 3 months after a TIPS procedure, and therefore TIPS is to be used only with caution in carefully selected patients.

Many patients with microvascular (capillary) vasodilation have *hepatopulmonary syndrome (HPS)*, while others have arteriolar vasoconstriction leading to *portopulmonary hypertension (PPH)*. These pulmonary complications are seen in up to 70% of patients with chronic liver disease. Both conditions can make a patient ineligible for a liver transplant. In HPS, spider angioma, platypnea (orthostatic dyspnea), digital clubbing, and cyanosis are common findings. Patients progressively worsen as intrapulmonary vasodilation develops and gas exchange deteriorates. Liver transplantation is the only strategy proven to help HPS in most patients. Although a significant improvement in gas exchange is observed after transplantation, it may take up to 1 year for arterial hypoxemia to normalize.

PPH is defined by the National Institutes of Health Patient Registry for the Characterization of Primary Pulmonary Hypertension as mean PAP greater than 25 mm Hg and a pulmonary capillary wedge pressure (PCWP) lower than 15 mm Hg in the setting of portal hypertension. Symptoms include fatigue, dyspnea, peripheral edema, syncope, chest pain, and a systolic murmur. The ECG in 90% of patients reflects right bundle branch block, right-axis deviation, or a right ventricular hypertrophy. These patients are controversial liver transplant patients because PPH has a 40% postoperative mortality rate and is irreversible with transplantation. Treatment for most PPH patients is palliative. Several different approaches including channel blockers, oral vasodilators, and chronic IV use of epoprostenol and isosorbide mononitrate have prolonged survival up to 5 years.

Spontaneous bacterial peritonitis (SBP) is a spontaneous infection that affects up to a third of patients with ESLD. The most common organism found in the peritoneal fluid of patients with SBP is *Escherichia coli*, believed to be due to translocation of the bacteria from the intestinal lumen. Mortality in patients with cirrhotic ascites has been reduced due to prophylactic therapy using third-generation cephalosporins.

HEPATIC ASSESSMENT
Goal of System Assessment
A thorough physical assessment along with an accurate history should produce a correct liver disease diagnosis in 85% of cases. Evaluate for cause of and subsequent hepatic and multisystem effects of ALF, because severe liver damage has usually occurred by the time the patient presents for care.

History and Risk Factors
Evaluate for family/personal history of liver disease, exposure to toxins, exposure to complementary and alternative medications, street or prescription drug use, acetaminophen use and abuse, alcohol use and abuse, exposure to *Bacillus cereus* toxin (through food ingestion), and *Amanita phalloides* mushroom poisoning.
- Inquire about compliance with taking antibiotics for spontaneous bacterial peritonitis prophylaxis, diuretics, beta-blockers (for control of portal hypertension), lactulose (to keep ammonia level from rising, thereby preventing hepatic encephalopathy), and any nonprescribed or non–physician-recommended over-the-counter medications.
- Inquire about depression, recent travel abroad, and prescription, over-the-counter, and street drug use.

Vital Sign Assessment
- Neurologic assessment, including Glasgow Coma Scale score, an ICP monitor, and an arterial line may be needed for severely ill patients.
- HR (preferably apical), heart rhythm, and BP to evaluate if liver disease is affecting CO and perfusion; risk of hemorrhage is also a complication.
- Normal to bounding pulses, low to normal BP, elevated CO associated with decreased peripheral vascular resistance and expanded total blood volume

- Take BP while patient is lying down, sitting up and standing (if able)—this also helps to observe for platypnea.
- Take temperature; if elevated may be due to an acute bacterial, viral, or fungal process that may be affecting the liver.
- If the temperature is low, hypothermia may herald the onset of hepatic encephalopathy.

Observation
- Evaluate for pallor, jaundice, and scleral icterus and signs of coagulopathies.
- Note spider angioma, skin excoriation, ecchymosis, petechiae, prominent abdominal collateral veins, palmar erythema, gynecomastia, testicular atrophy, jugular vein distention, Dupuytren contracture, needle marks, loss of body hair, loss of muscle mass, peripheral edema, obvious ascites, eye signs mimicking hyperthyroidism, exertional dyspnea, digital clubbing, cyanosis of the nail beds, and umbilical hernias.
- Note muscle weakness and tenderness; a common finding in ESLD from alcohol (EtOH). Measure abdominal girth.
- Note if asterixis (brief periods of "flapping" or irregular flexion of the hands at the wrist) is present.
- Observe for signs of respiratory distress, impaired renal function, and bacterial, viral, and fungal infections.
- Note if questions are answered appropriately and if patient is AAO × 3, disoriented, or confused.
- Fetor hepaticus may be present (pungent breath odor in some cirrhotic patients).
- In the presence of tense ascites (which increases intra-abdominal pressure), impaired right ventricular filling with decreased stroke volume and decreased CO may be evident.
- If patient has had a massive variceal hemorrhage or is in septic shock, pulses will be diminished and BP will be low, reflecting circulatory collapse.

Palpation
Liver palpation can aid in diagnosis of liver disease etiology and confirm cirrhosis.
- Examine abdomen; palpate all nine sections of the abdomen, palpate the liver and spleen, and assess for abdominal masses.
- Palpate liver and other abdominal organs (i.e., spleen). Note liver firmness, size, edges, and possible pain with palpation. Hepatomegaly may be evident. Many times in liver disease, splenomegaly is also appreciated. Gallbladder (if not previously removed) may be palpated (and if palpable and/or painful may be due to stones or infection); also assess for the presence of any abdominal masses.
- Note pulse quality and regularity bilaterally (scale 0 to 4+), as bilateral lower extremity edema is common in ESLD and can obscure pulses.
- Ascites can be diagnosed if not obvious with palpation and observation of an abdominal fluid wave upon palpation.
- Assess for lymphadenopathy.

Auscultation
- Listen to the heart, carotid artery, lungs, and abdomen.
- Listen to abdominal sounds in all nine sections of the abdomen.
- Bruits and/or rubs may be present (liver disease–related abdominal bruits can be caused by hepatocellular carcinoma, portosystemic shunt, hepatic artery aneurysm, or alcoholic hepatitis).
- Abdominal friction rub, although rare, is reflective of peritoneal inflammation and may be diagnostic for infection (liver abscess), infarction of the liver, or tumor (hepatocellular carcinoma/liver metastasis).
- Listen for inspiratory crackles in lungs, particularly at the bases, and end-expiratory wheezing and egophony (if effusions are present).
- Note if second heart sound and right ventricular heave are present together.

Screening Labwork
Bloodwork may differentiate between ALF and chronic liver disease, as well as aid in diagnosing the severity of liver injury and degree of liver function/dysfunction.

- Elevated liver function tests: ALT, AST, GGT, bilirubin, alkaline phosphatase, with decreased albumin to check for hepatocyte injury, or a cholestatic cause for liver disease
- Viral hepatitis studies, drug panel to check for drug-induced liver injury, EtOH level to screen for alcoholic liver disease
- Coagulation studies: elevated INR, PT, and PTT herald a failing liver.
- Alpha-fetoprotein: nonspecific cancer marker to screen for hepatocellular carcinoma (HCC) as a potential cause of liver disease.
- Electrolytes to monitor for hyponatremia, hypokalemia
- Chemistry profile to monitor glucose and renal function tests
- Street and therapeutic drug levels
- Acetaminophen levels

Liver Biopsy
Useful in acute liver disease for diagnosis and valuable in chronic liver disease for staging and grading. Invaluable when used serially (i.e., every 3 to 5 years) in untreated chronic hepatitis to monitor fibrosis progression.

Other Studies
Chest radiography, Doppler echocardiography, and ABGs are useful in the diagnoses of HPS and PPH.

Diagnostic Tests for Acute and Chronic Hepatic Failure

Test	Purpose	Abnormal Findings
Noninvasive Testing		
Electrocardiogram (ECG) 12-Lead ECG: must be obtained upon admission to ICU	To assess for cardiac dysrhythmias related to end-stage liver disease	Hypokalemia, acidosis, or hypoxia may cause cardiac dysrhythmias. Abnormal rate, rhythm may be part of hepatopulmonary syndrome, or portopulmonary hypertension.
Electroencephalogram (EEG)	For the diagnosis and quantification of hepatic encephalopathy	Often abnormal if hepatic encephalopathy present. Some correlation with ammonia levels and stage of encephalopathy has been reported.
Neuropsychological testing	To establish a baseline at admission (if patient is not in a hepatic coma)	A battery of six tests, called psychometric hepatic encephalopathy score (PHES). A normal score is 0.5 ± 1.83. Those scoring beyond -4 are considered abnormal.
Blood Studies		
Liver function tests	Assess for enzyme changes indicative of hepatic damage	Elevated enzymes reflect liver damage.
Alanine aminotransferase (ALT) Aspartate Aminotransferase (AST)	ALT useful in determining whether jaundice is caused by liver disease or has a hemolytic cause.	Values >300 U/L are present with acute liver failure. Found primarily in the liver ALT is the primary marker of hepatic damage AST: present in organs with high metabolic activity. Damage to the hepatocytes will cause a rise in AST 12 hours after injury and levels will remain elevated for 4–6 days. Levels 10–100 times normal are not unusual in liver disease.
Alkaline phosphatase (Alk Phos)		Alk Phos: found in almost all tissue, but most elevations can be localized to the liver or bone. Alk Phos is elevated to varying degrees in various liver diseases.

Continued

Hepatic Failure

Diagnostic Tests for Acute and Chronic Hepatic Failure—cont'd

Test	Purpose	Abnormal Findings
Bilirubin	To assess the ability of the liver to process bilirubin, which helps with differential diagnosis and to predict the prognosis.	Bilirubin: Total bilirubin is a byproduct of hemolysis. Elevations occur with excessive RBC destruction or when the liver is unable to process normal amounts of bilirubin. Elevations commonly occur in viral hepatitis and cirrhosis. Consistently elevated levels are a poor prognostic sign.
Gamma-glutamic trans-peptidase (GGT/GGTP)	To assist with diagnosing liver disease is present	Present in numerous tissues, but highest in liver disorders. This test can be used to confirm that Alk Phos is elevated due to a hepatic-related condition. Usually elevated in cholestatic liver disease, cirrhosis, alcoholic liver disease, and metastasis to the liver.
Albumin	To assess the ability of the liver to synthesize albumin, which helps predict the prognosis.	Synthesized in the liver, maintains blood oncotic pressure and coagulation proteins needed to form a fibrin clot. Low levels are found in altered synthetic liver function. Decreased levels are seen with ascites and severe liver function, and persistently low levels suggest a poor prognosis.
Glucose	To assess possible cause for altered mentation and lethargy	Impaired gluconeogenesis and glycogen depletion in the cirrhotic liver cause hypoglycemia, which is usually present in severe or terminal liver dysfunction, causing altered mentation and/or lethargy.
Blood urea nitrogen (BUN) and serum creatinine (Cr)	To assess kidney function/presence of hepatorenal syndrome	In liver failure, the BUN is decreased. However, if the patient has bleeding or has renal insufficiency (impending or actual hepatorenal syndrome), the BUN:Cr is elevated.
Ammonia	To rule out hepatic encephalopathy, or other causes of altered mentation	Increased due to the failing liver's inability to clear nitrogenous and other waste products. GI bleeding or an increase in intestinal protein from dietary intake can increase ammonia levels.
Electrolytes		
Sodium (Na$^+$)	To differentiate between potential diagnoses	Decrease in sodium seen in patients with cirrhosis, tense ascites, hepatorenal syndrome.
Potassium (K$^+$)		Decreased potassium observed in those with liver disease accompanied by ascites and in those with alcoholic liver disease. In hepatorenal syndrome, hyperkalemia is observed.
Hematologic Tests		
Hemoglobin (Hgb) Hematocrit (Hct)	To assess if anemia is present	GI bleeding may be present with a decreased Hgb/Hct. The anemia seen in hepatic failure is termed macrocytic (due to increase in mean corpuscular volume [MCV]) and normochromic (normal Hgb)
Platelets (Plts)	To evaluate for the possibility of bleeding	Low due to platelet destruction and malfunctioning hepatic synthesis of platelets.

Diagnostic Tests for Acute and Chronic Hepatic Failure—cont'd

Test	Purpose	Abnormal Findings
White blood count (WBC)	To evaluate for possible infection and inflammation	Elevated if sepsis is present
Coagulation Profile		
Prothrombin time (PT) with international normalized ratio (INR) Partial thromboplastin time (PTT)	Useful prognostic indicators in liver disease	A prolonged PT/INR/PTT is an ominous sign in liver failure patients, particularly in acetaminophen overdose, or unknown causes of liver failure (Box 9-8)
Urinalysis (UA)	Monitors for development of hepatorenal syndrome (HRS)	Decreased urine sodium excretion, with normal urinary sediment is a sign of HRS. In the presence of ascites, the 24-hour urine volume will be decreased and the 23-hour sodium value will be reduced sometimes to <5 mEq/day in severe cases.
Radiology		
Chest x-ray (CXR)	Assesses for any pathology in the lungs and chest cavity, confirm diagnosis of portopulmonary hypertension, hepatopulmonary syndrome	Tumors, lymph nodes, atelectasis, cardiomegaly, infiltrates, tortuous cardiac vessels, diaphragm elevation (bilateral or unilateral)
Magnetic resonance imaging (MRI) Hepatic MRI	Assesses liver size, morphology, function, presence of cirrhosis, steatosis, lesions. Used to characterize known lesions and status of hepatic circulation. Can produce a sharp contrast between tissues and water and/or fat. Can image in transverse, longitudinal, coronal, or oblique planes.	Enlarged liver, cirrhosis, tumors, cysts, hemangiomas, steatosis, macronodular lesions, hemochromatosis (if large iron stores are present), sarcoid nodules, biliary cystadenomas, adenomas, focal nodular hyperplastic nodules, cholangiocarcinoma (CCA), abscesses, thromboses, hepatic congestion
Computed tomography (CT) Hepatic CT scan	Assesses liver size, presence of cirrhosis, look for the presence of lesions, to characterize known lesions and status of hepatic circulation Oral or IV contrast can be administered to help distinguish the bowel lumen and blood vessels and tissue, respectively.	Enlarged liver, cirrhosis, tumors, cysts, hemangiomas, steatosis, macronodular lesions, hemochromatosis (if large iron stores are present), sarcoid nodules, biliary cystadenomas, adenomas, focal nodular hyperplastic nodules, CCA, abscesses, thromboses, hepatic congestion
Ultrasound Hepatic ultrasound	Assess for fluid-filled lesions, vascular abnormalities. Also used to "mark the spot" prior to liver biopsy. *Note:* ultrasound is best suited to thinner patients	Main anatomic features of the liver can be identified, as well as cysts, infections, abscesses, steatosis, hemangiomas, malignant neoplasms, adenomas, hyperplastic lesions, lymphomas, increased echogenicity, hydatid cysts, amebiasis, and fungal disease
Cerebral CT (CCT)	Used for diagnosis when a subdural hematoma or doubt about etiology of altered consciousness in the ESLD patient is in question	Cortical and subcortical atrophy, benign, neoplastic and metastatic lesions, hemorrhaging, aneurysms, hematomas
Brain flow studies Technetium scan of brain	To confirm brain death when patient is in a hepatic coma when EEG is not confirmatory	Brain death as evidenced by lack of blood flow into the brain

Hepatic Failure

Continued

Diagnostic Tests for Acute and Chronic Hepatic Failure—cont'd		
Test	**Purpose**	**Abnormal Findings**
Radioisotope liver scan Injection with radioactive compound and scanned with a scintillation camera or radiography	To determine the presence of three-dimensional lesions in the liver	Hepatocellular carcinoma, melanoma, Hodgkin and non-Hodgkin lymphoma
Invasive Testing		
Liver biopsy (can be percutaneous at the bedside, or transvenous in interventional radiology)	Used as a diagnostic and prognostic tool. Can grade and stage liver disease. Can differentiate between various liver diseases. Can be used to follow the progression of liver diseases.	Inflammation, fibrosis, cirrhosis, hepatocellular carcinoma, regenerative changes, apoptosis, necrosis, iron, complex carbohydrates, steatosis, copper, granulomas, hepatitis B surface antigen, Mallory bodies, talc crystals, inflammatory cells, microabscesses, Cowdry type A inclusions, etc.

Liver Function Tests

LFTs are nonspecific for diagnosing any particular liver disease or measuring efficacy of liver function but rather identify hepatocyte damage or biliary abnormalites (e.g., stasis). Once a liver dysfunction diagnosis is established, tests monitor the progression, stabilization, or improvement of liver damage. In treatable liver diseases, such as hepatitis, the tests monitor effectiveness of treatment. Testing is often done serially to increase specificity and sensitivity.

Alanine aminotransferase (ALT) and aspartate aminotransferase (AST): These enzymes are the most frequently measured indicators of liver dysfunction, since values are elevated in all liver disorders. While the enzymes are also present in the brain, kidneys, and skeletal and cardiac muscles, the concentration is highest in the liver. Values elevate most markedly in acute hepatitis and liver injury from exposure to hepatoxins. ALT seems to be the more sensitive enzyme specific to hepatocyte damage.

Serum bilirubin (bili): Bilirubin in the urine is usually diagnostic for biliary liver disease. Up to 80% of bilirubin comes from the breakdown of hemoglobin, while the other 20% comes from prematurely destroyed cells found in bone marrow and from hemoproteins throughout the body. Bilirubin alone is not diagnostic for determining the cause of jaundice

---

Box 9-8	**KING'S COLLEGE HOSPITAL CRITERIA**

ALF from acetaminophen

- pH <7.30 (24 hours after ingestion and after adequate fluid resuscitation)—irrespective of coma grade
- PT* >100 seconds or INR >6.5 with
- Serum creatinine >3.4 mg/dl in grade 3 or 4 encephalopathy

ALF from other causes

- PT >100 seconds (INR >6.5)—regardless of coma grade or any three of the following regardless of encephalopathy grade:
  1. Age <10 years
  2. Age >40 years
  3. Drug toxicity, indeterminate cause of ALF
  4. Duration of jaundice before onset of coma of >7 days
  5. PT >50 seconds (INR ≥ 3.5)
- Serum bilirubin >17.5 mg/dl

*PT is the most sensitive prognostic marker.
INR, International normalized ratio.

in a patient. Usually bilirubin levels are higher in a neoplastic process in the liver, than in other causes of liver disease.

Alkaline phosphatase (Alk Phos):   Like the other "liver function" tests, Alk Phos is found in many parts of the body. The liver and bone appear to be the main sources of this enzyme. Elevation of this enzyme is usually seen in hepatobiliary diseases.

Serum albumin: Albumin levels tend to be normal regardless of the cause of liver disease. Hypoalbuminemia is usually found in patients with ESLD and/or cirrhosis where decreased albumin synthesis, ascites, and severe liver damage are present.

Prothrombin time: The liver synthesizes 11 blood coagulation proteins. While a prolonged prothrombin time is not specific in diagnosing diseases of the liver, it is prognostic in outcomes in acetaminophen overdose and in patients with alcoholic steatonecrosis, fulminant hepatic necrosis, and acute hepatocellular disease.

Liver Biopsy

Liver biopsy is the "gold standard" of testing used to diagnose the type of liver disease, screen for familial disease, monitor and stage the disease, evaluate the degree of hepatocellular injury, evaluate effectiveness of treatment, and confirm rejection episodes in the transplanted liver.

Safety Alert   *Risk of death from a liver biopsy complication is estimated to be 0.0088% to 0.3%. The patient MUST be adequately prepared for the liver biopsy procedure and the aftercare to minimize potential complications and prevent mortality.*

Before Biopsy

- Explain the procedure to patient and significant others. The patient must be able to demonstrate they can exhale and hold their breath during needle insertion.
- Patient should sign informed consent for procedure before sedation is administered.
- Prothrombin time, INR, and platelet count values must be less than 1 month old.
- Ensure patient has not had salicylates (e.g., aspirin or bismuth) or NSAIDs (e.g., ibuprofen, naproxen) for 7 days before the biopsy.
- All anticoagulants must be stopped 72 hours before the biopsy.
- Patient should not have eaten for 4 to 8 hours prior to the procedure.

During Biopsy
- Assist patient with proper positioning and with remaining motionless during procedure.
- Coach the patient to exhale and hold their breath during the procedure (or manually ventilate intubated patient to prevent lung inflation during puncture) to avoid movement of the lung and possible resulting pneumothorax.

After Biopsy
- Apply direct pressure to biopsy site for 15 minutes followed by a pressure dressing.
- Auscultate breath sounds immediately after the procedure and at 1- to 2-hour intervals until patient discharge to detect pneumothorax or hemothorax (unlikely but serious complications). Diminished sounds on the right side and tachypnea suggest one of these conditions.
- Position patient on the right side for a minimum of 2 hours after the biopsy to tamponade the puncture site to minimize the risk of hemorrhage.
- Monitor hemoglobin and hematocrit to screen for intraperitoneal bleeding.
- Assess for signs/symptoms of peritonitis and intraperitoneal bleeding: severe abdominal pain, abdominal distention and rigidity, rebound tenderness, nausea, vomiting, tachycardia, tachypnea, pallor, decreased BP, and rising temperature.
- If bleeding is suspected, contact physician or midlevel practitioner to obtain an abdominal/liver ultrasound study.
- Remind the patient that mild shoulder pain may persist for 24 to 48 hours after the biopsy.

COLLABORATIVE MANAGEMENT

HEPATIC FAILURE MANAGEMENT GUIDELINES

Care of patients with end-stage liver disease (ESLD) with acute (ALF) or chronic liver failure requires a multidisciplinary approach. While every liver transplant center has its own protocols for the care of these complex patients, all closely follow evidence-based guidelines. Acute liver failure is relatively rare, so attaining an appropriate study sample size has been difficult and prolonged. The Acute Liver Failure Study Group started in 1998, coupled with a study and workshop that were both sponsored by the National Institutes of Health, led by Dr. William H. Lee. It has produced the largest body of knowledge regarding ALF and is considered the benchmark of care. American Association for the Study of Liver Diseases (AASLD) practice guidelines and position papers guide the care of pretransplant, ALF, and chronic liver failure patients as well. The guidelines and position papers are prepared by the experts in that particular area of liver disease and its management.

All guidelines and position papers are available on the AASLD website: www.aasld.org

Interventions	Rationale
Head-to-toe assessment, history, transfer to a transplant center, or if at a transplant center, admission to ICU	With a thorough examination, and history, can find cause in 85% of cases. The quicker a diagnosis is made, the sooner treatment can begin.
Laboratory evaluations	Need to be extensive to evaluate etiology and severity of liver disease. Key laboratory tests include: ALT, AST, bilirubin, GGT, Alk Phos, drugs of abuse profile, acetaminophen level, CBC with platelets and differential, comprehensive chemistries to include BUN/creatinine, AFP and CEA-19.
Liver biopsy	Can confirm a diagnosis, rule out a diagnosis, and may assist in deciding whether to list patient for transplant.
Use of endoscopy, banding, beta-blockers for bleeding from esophageal varices	Variceal bleeding in cirrhotic patients has a 30% to 50% mortality rate associated with each bleeding episode. Endoscopy with subsequent banding, or sclerotherapy and use of nonselective beta-blockers can be used to drastically reduce this risk. Beta-blockers should be titrated to decrease resting heart rate by 25% and systolic blood pressure by $\geq$90 mm Hg.
Encephalopathy and cerebral edema	Patients with encephalopathy need to be placed in ICU. ICP monitor may be necessary once patient has grade III encephalopathy (which is marked by incoherent speech, sleeping the majority of the time but arousable to loud vocal stimuli and when awake is confused).
Diagnostic imaging; US, CT scan, MRI, MRA, and ERCP	US, CT scan, and/or MRI to assess for tumors, hepatic obstruction, and to grade/stage a liver disease/pathology MRA to assess hemodynamics, and ERCP to assess biliary status
Nutritional balance	Protein calorie malnutrition is seen in 60% of patients with ESLD. It is a predictor for first bleeding episode from varices, and is seen in patients with refractory ascites. Patients need to eat 6–8 meals per day to improve nitrogen balance and prevent catabolism of muscles. Zinc supplements have been shown to improve encephalopathy.
Controlling ascites	Give prophylactic antibiotics, perform paracentesis with albumin infusion and analyze ascitic fluid, give diuretics, and consider a TIPS placement.
Monitoring for HRS, HPS, PPH — all of which can complicate care, outcomes, and transplant status	Hemodialysis may be required for HRS, as may a liver-kidney vs. a liver transplant; HPS and PPH may keep a patient from receiving a transplant

Care Priorities

Hepatic failure may develop suddenly in a patient with compensated liver disease. Sustained hypoxia or hypotension from any cause can aggravate hepatocellular failure and must be corrected promptly. EtOH, hepatotoxic drugs, and hepatotoxic alternative therapies are eliminated. Sedatives and tranquilizers may contribute to hepatic encephalopathy and should be discontinued.

1. **Manage fluid and electrolyte imbalance:** Free water clearance is affected in ALF, causing hyponatremia despite increased total body sodium. If hyponatremia is profound, sodium-containing fluids are avoided to reduce ascites and peripheral edema and help avoid renal insufficiency. D_5W generally is used for fluid resuscitation to prevent hypernatremia. Mannitol or albumin is given to increase intravascular oncotic pressure and maintain intravascular volume. Potassium is decreased with the use of mannitol. Hypokalemic alkalosis can worsen encephalopathy and precipitate dysrhythmias. Fresh frozen plasma may be used if clotting factors are deficient, but infusions of large amounts can lead to hypernatremia. Packed RBCs are given if there is brisk bleeding or a low Hct. Variceal bleeding is managed endoscopically. CVP or PAP monitoring may be initiated to ensure adequate tissue perfusion without fluid overload. Hyperdynamic circulation is supported by fluid administration and sympathomimetic agents (e.g., dopamine). ICP monitoring may be necessary to monitor for cerebral edema. Bed rest is necessary to reduce metabolic demands placed on the liver during normal daily activity.

Safety Alert *Accurate measurements and careful interpretation of hemodynamic parameters are essential because fluid balance is delicate in critically ill patients with hepatic failure. Hemodynamic measurements can be difficult to interpret because circulation is hyperdynamic. Svo_2 or $ScVO2$ monitoring is helpful in evaluating the adequacy of tissue oxygenation.*

---

2. **Provide nutritional therapy:** The catabolic rate in acute liver failure increases 4 times over normal and is associated with negative nitrogen balance. To ensure tissue repair, a high-calorie, 80- to 100-g protein-containing diet of dairy products and vegetables is indicated for *patients without encephalopathy,* since the liver is capable of significant regeneration under optimal circumstances. Sodium is moderately restricted unless significant ascites and peripheral edema are present, wherein a less than 500-mg sodium diet is prescribed. If GI function is impaired and the patient is unable to tolerate enteral feedings, parenteral nutrition is initiated. Total caloric intake should be 2500 to 3000 per day.

   For the patient *with acute hepatic encephalopathy, protein is eliminated from the diet* until recovery. During recovery, vegetable protein (preferred over animal protein) is gradually reintroduced at 10 to 20 g every 48 to 72 hours and increased to 40 g/day, which prevents tissue catabolism. Some advocate use of enteral or parenteral branched-chain amino acid supplements to correct the amino acid imbalance common among patients with encephalopathy. Potassium loss must be replaced by potassium-rich foods or supplements. Blood sugar levels should be kept above 100 mg/dl and monitored every 2 to 4 hours. Parenteral lipid replacement should be used with caution as fatty liver (steatosis) has been reported to have developed after their use.

3. **Provide pharmacotherapy that will minimize or avoid further liver dysfunction:** Some commonly used drugs are hepatotoxic (Box 9-9). There are numerous medications necessary for the management of liver failure.
   - **Sedatives:** Avoided if possible because they can precipitate or contribute to encephalopathy. If sedative use is necessary, oxazepam (Serax) is acceptable because it is eliminated safely by patients with hepatic disease. Other sedatives may be used cautiously and in reduced dosages.
   - **Histamine H_2-receptor antagonists:** Prophylactic H_2-receptor antagonists are prescribed to block acid secretion and prevent gastric erosions, which are common in patients with chronic or severe hepatic failure. Famotidine, ranitidine hydrochloride, and nizatidine are competitive blockers of histamine, and thereby inhibit all phases of gastric acid secretion.
   - **Sucralfate (Carafate):** Binds to gastric erosions, aiding in healing established ulcers, and coats the gastric/duodenal mucosa, thereby preventing stress ulcers.

| Box 9-9 | DRUGS AND SUBSTANCES WITH HEPATOTOXIC POTENTIAL |

- Acetaminophen
- Allopurinol
- Amiodarone
- Amoxicillin-clavulanate
- Amphetamines
- Ampicillin
- Antidepressants
- Carbamazepine
- Carbenicillin
- Carbon tetrachloride
- Chloramphenicol
- Chlorpromazine
- Clindamycin
- Cocaine
- Dantrolene
- Dapsone
- Diadanosine
- Diclofenac
- Disulfiram
- Efavirenz
- Ethanol
- Etoposide
- 5-Fluorouracil deoxyribonucleoside (FUDR-[intra-arterial])
- Flutamine
- Gemtuzumab
- Halothane
- Hydrochlorothiazide
- Imipramine
- Isoflurane
- Isonazide
- Ketoconazole
- Labetalol
- Lisinopril
- Metformin
- Methotrexate
- Methyldopa
- Monoamine oxidase (MAO) inhibitors
- Nefazodone
- Nicotinic acid
- Nonsteroidal anti-inflammatory drugs (NSAIDs)
- Ofloxacin
- Oral contraceptives
- Penicillin
- Phenytoin
- Propylthiouracil
- Pyrazinamide (PZA)
- Quetiapine
- Rifampin
- Rifampin-isoniazide
- Salicylates
- Statins
- Sulfonamides
- Tetracyclines (especially parenteral)
- Tolcapone
- Trimethoprim-sulfamethoxazole
- Troglitazone
- Valproic acid
- Yellow phosphorus
- Numerous complementary and alternative (CAM) medications

- **Dextrose:** Moderate to severe hypoglycemia can occur because of impaired gluconeogenesis and impaired insulin degradation. Checks of blood sugar levels every 2 to 4 hours are necessary to detect hypoglycemia. In the event of hypoglycemia, a bolus of 50% dextrose or continual infusion of a 10% solution is indicated.
- *N-Acetylcysteine (NAC):* Administering NAC protects the liver against free radical injury and is useful in acetaminophen overdose and carbon tetrachloride or trichloroethylene exposure. NAC helps replace glutathione stores in the liver, protecting hepatocytes. It can be administered orally at 140 mg/kg or parenterally 140 mg/kg in 5% dextrose with subsequent doses at 70 mg/kg. Careful observation is necessary during IV administration, as an anaphylaxis-like reaction has been observed.
- **Penicillin/silibinin:** Used commonly as an antidote in Europe for *Amanita phalloides* poisoning; penicillin 300,000 to 1,000,000 units/kg/day and silibinin 20 to 50 mg/kg/day given intravenously is alleged to be hepatocyte-protective if treatment is started within 24 hours of ingestion. This combination protects as-yet-unaffected hepatocytes, thereby preventing further hepatocyte necrosis.
- **Zinc:** In malnourished individuals, it is useful not only as mineral replacement therapy but also to reduce the chance for, or severity of, encephalopathy as it increases hepatic urea synthesis. In other countries, the use of ornithine-aspartate is advocated to improve hepatic and muscular ammonia elimination.
4. Manage accumulation of ascites: Fluid intake and physical activity are restricted. Dietary restrictions, therapeutic paracentesis, and diuretics are commonly used, while TIPS or PVS are placed for refractory ascites.

- **Sodium:** If ascites causes discomfort or dyspnea, sodium is limited to less than 500 mg/day.
- **Diuretics:** If more conservative measures are ineffective in controlling ascites, spironolactone (Aldactone), an aldosterone antagonist with weak diuretic action and potassium conservation, or amiloride, another potassium-sparing diuretic, may be used. If ineffective, more potent diuretics such as furosemide (Lasix) or thiazides are added with concurrent use of potassium supplement. For severe ascites, mannitol may be added to the regimen.
- **Paracentesis:** Patients with severe ascites are managed with diuretics and large-volume (greater than 5 L) therapeutic paracentesis with or without infusion of albumin or another plasma volume expander. Repeated removal of 4 to 8 L/week of ascitic fluid may be attempted as a temporary measure to relieve refractory ascites. An increase in CO is noted immediately after the procedure. Once discharged from the ICU, if patients cannot make frequent trips to the hospital, TIPS or PVS is indicated unless the Childs score is 12 or greater, in which case PVS is a better option.
- **Transjugular Intrahepatic Portosystemic Shunt (TIPS):** A non-surgical, invasive radiology procedure done using a stent to create a new circulatory pathway for blood to flow around the liver back to the heart to help relieve portal hypertension.
- **Peritoneovenous Shunt (PVS):** First introduced in 1974, PVS (e.g., LeVeen or Denver shunt) is placed surgically for refractory or life-threatening ascites. PVS helps expand circulating volume, improve response to diuretics, improve circulation, and prevent HRS. A long, perforated catheter connected to a pressure-sensitive valve drains into the superior vena cava. Fluid can flow in only one direction, from the peritoneum into the bloodstream. A common complication is frequent obstruction, which requires reoperation. Fluid overload, infection, DIC, and peritonitis are possible. A rapid increase in intravascular volume has caused variceal hemorrhage. Patients awaiting liver transplantation should not undergo this procedure. See Box 9-10 and *Fluid Volume Excess*, p. 799, for nursing implications.

5. **Eliminate or correct the precipitating factors of encephalopathy:** Up to 80% of patients with cirrhosis and liver failure have cerebral dysfunction or encephalopathy. The causes and precipitating factors include changes in the permeability of the blood-brain barrier, an increase in endogenous benzodiazepines, impairment of neuronal membrane sodium-potassium adenosine triphosphatase (ATPase), abnormal neurotransmitter balance, GI bleed, increased dietary protein, and electrolyte disturbance.
   - **Restrict physical activity:** Permits less stress on all the organs of the body. Less activity reduces the number of metabolites that must be processed by the liver.
   - **Restrict or eliminate dietary protein:** Can be reintroduced if symptoms improve preferably dairy and vegetable proteins.
   - *Manage bleeding complications:* Fresh-frozen plasma and platelets are given to correct abnormal clotting factors and thrombocytopenia. Vitamin K helps correct bleeding tendencies. Serious coagulopathies require specialized component therapy (see *Bleeding and Thrombotic Disorders: Disseminated Intravascular Coagulation*, p. 837).
   - **Clear the bowel:** *Early and thorough catharsis by magnesium citrate or tap water enema helps* eliminate blood from any GI bleeding and eliminates protein lingering in the bowel from ileus, constipation, or other causes.
   - **Administer antibiotics:** Bacterial translocation is problematic in the chronic hepatic failure patient as a result of preexisting cirrhosis. Patients who develop infections have a higher mortality rate. A 5- to 7-day course of prophylactic, broad-spectrum antibiotics (i.e., from the fluoroquinolone class) is recommended.
   - **Administer lactulose:** A synthetic disaccharide that contains both galactose and lactose decreases the pH of the colon by its conversion into lactic, acetic, and formic acids. The unmetabolized lactulose left in the colon causes osmotic diarrhea and migration of ammonia from the blood to the colon. The dose is adjusted to produce two to three semiformed stools/day.

Safety Alert *Lactulose may worsen hypernatremia and promote cerebral edema and should be used with extreme caution.*

Box 9-10	NURSING CARE AFTER PERITONEAL VENOUS SHUNT (PVS) SURGERY

Measure urinary output hourly and CVP or PAP every 1 to 2 hours.
- Anticipate rapid fluid mobilization, as evidenced by increased CVP and increased urinary output.
- Notify physician of abnormal CVP or PAP or lack of diuresis. Failure to mobilize ascitic fluid may signal shunt occlusion or failure.
- Report lessening of urinary output, since renal function may diminish after this procedure.

Administer IV diuretics as prescribed; monitor K^+ levels; and administer K^+ supplements as prescribed.
- Anticipate prescribed K^+ supplements during the first 24 hours after surgery.
- Be aware that furosemide (Lasix), which is frequently prescribed, may cause K^+ depletion. Likewise, the anticipated diuresis depletes K^+.

Instruct and coach patient in the use of the incentive spirometer or similar hyperinflation device.
- Devices that create inspiratory resistance and encourage deep inspiration promote negative inspiratory pressure and facilitate flow of ascitic fluid.
- Encourage patient to cough hourly.

Apply elastic abdominal binder.
- This intervention facilitates the flow of ascitic fluid by increasing the pressure gradient externally.

Monitor for evidence of variceal bleeding; report evidence of bleeding to physician.
- Expanded blood volume may increase variceal pressure, resulting in bleeding. Bleeding is evidenced by a sudden decrease in hematocrit (a mild dilutional decrease is anticipated in the immediate postoperative period), unexplained nausea, lightheadedness, dark stools, or hematemesis.

Monitor for evidence of peritonitis, endocarditis, or other infection.
- Infection occurs frequently. Anticipate antibiotic coverage during the immediate postsurgical period. Assess abdominal incision for leakage of peritoneal fluid, which commonly occurs. Change the dressing immediately if leakage is detected.

Monitor for evidence of postshunt coagulopathy.
- See *Ineffective Protection Care Plan in Hepatic Failure*, p. 803, for details.
- Monitor for other postshunt complications.

Assess for lower extremity edema. After some shunting procedures, none of the venous blood passes through the liver and protein end products are not completely detoxified. These patients are usually placed on a low-protein diet.

CVP, Central venous pressure; *Hct*, hematocrit; *IV*, intravenous; *K+*, potassium; *PAP*, pulmonary artery pressure.

- **ICP monitoring:** Brain damage may occur quickly and without obvious symptoms when ICP exceeds 20 mm Hg. ICP monitoring may be needed for the most critically ill patients awaiting orthotopic liver transplant to detect cerebral edema and guide pharmacologic management (e.g., mannitol, furosemide) and other therapeutic measures. See discussion in *Traumatic Brain Injury*, p. 331.
- **Manage respiratory failure:** Intubation or mechanical ventilation may be indicated when gag reflex is impaired by advanced encephalopathy, if gastric contents are aspirated, or ventilation is impaired by ascites. Frequent assessments and continuous pulse oximetry are used to monitor those at high risk for respiratory failure. Adequate tissue oxygenation is crucial since hepatic hypoxia significantly contributes to hepatic failure.
6. **Hepatic transplantation:** The orthotopic liver transplant survival rate is greater than 90% for the first year after transplant. In cases of chronic progressive or acute hepatocyte damage, it is the only treatment available. Because organs are in such limited supply, adult living donor liver transplantation is being used in those recipients whose diagnosis

necessitates a liver, but whose model for end-stage liver disease (MELD) scores are not high enough to place them at the top of the list. New methods are being sought to extend the life of the native liver until a donor liver becomes available. Auxiliary liver transplantation allows the native liver to remain in the recipient, which will allow it to regenerate. This procedure is only used in potentially reversible conditions. Hepatocyte transplantation, bioartificial liver support, extracorporeal whole-organ perfusion, and other methods such as stem cell transplantation and xenotransplantation are being explored as tools to bridge and increase waiting time to transplantation.

CARE PLANS FOR HEPATIC FAILURE

Deficient fluid volume *related to intravascular volume depletion resulting from third-spaced fluids*

GOALS/OUTCOMES Within 24 hours of this diagnosis, patient becomes normovolemic as evidenced by MAP greater than 70 mm Hg, HR 60 to 100 bpm, brisk capillary refill, distal pulses greater than $2+$ on a 0 to $4+$ scale, CVP 2 to 6 mm Hg, PAP 20 to 30/8 to 15 mm Hg, PAWP 6 to 12 mm Hg, CI greater than $3L/min/m^2$, SVR 900 to 1200 dynes/sec/cm^{-5}, urinary output greater than 0.5 ml/kg/hr, and orientation to person, place, and time.
NOC Risk Control: Fluid Volume Deficit, Fluid Balance, Fluid Status, Electrolyte and Acid-Base Balance

Fluid Management
1. Monitor and record vital signs and central pressures from hemodynamic monitoring at least hourly.
2. Be alert to increases in HR suggestive of hypovolemia or circulatory decompensation. HR increases may also be caused by fever related to infection or cerebral edema.
3. Monitor for dysrhythmias from electrolyte imbalances secondary to diarrhea, gastric suctioning, or diuretic therapy.
4. Be alert to low or decreasing CVP, PAWP, and CO. Calculate SVR at least every 8 hours. An elevated HR, decreased PAWP, CO less than baseline, or CI less than 3, along with decreased urinary output, suggest hypovolemia. Because of altered vascular responsiveness, the SVR may not be increased in patients with hypovolemic hepatic failure. Be aware that a "normal" CO value may actually be too low for these patients. A hyperdynamic circulatory state should be supported. Monitor Svo_2 as possible to evaluate the adequacy of tissue oxygenation.
5. Measure and record urinary output hourly. Be alert to output less than 0.5 ml/kg/hr for 2 consecutive hours. Consider cautious increases in fluid intake (e.g., 50 to 100 ml/hr), and then reevaluate volume status as already described. Use extreme caution in administering potent diuretics, as they may precipitate encephalopathy or renal disease from rapid diuresis and electrolyte changes.
6. Estimate ongoing fluid losses. Weigh patient daily. Measure all drainage from peritoneal or other catheters every 2 to 4 hours. Weight loss should not exceed 0.5 kg/day because more rapid diuresis can lead to intravascular volume depletion and impair renal function.
7. Consult physician or midlevel practitioner if serum albumin and total protein are reduced.

NIC Cerebral Edema Management; Electrolyte Management; Fluid Management; Electrolyte Management: Hypokalemia; Electrolyte Management: Hyponatremia

Excess Fluid volume *related to significant third spaced fluids resulting in total body weight gain*

GOALS/OUTCOMES Within 48 hours of this diagnosis, patient becomes normovolemic as evidenced by CVP 2 to 6 mm Hg, PAWP 6 to 12 mm Hg, HR 60 to 100 bpm, RR 12 to 20 breaths/min with normal depth and pattern, decreasing or stable abdominal girth, and absence of crackles, edema, uncomfortable ascites, and other clinical indicators of fluid volume excess.
NOC Risk Control: Fluid Volume Deficit, Fluid Balance, Fluid Status, Electrolyte and Acid-Base Balance

Hemodynamic Regulation
1. Monitor and record vital signs and central pressures from hemodynamic monitoring at least hourly. Measure more frequently if patient is undergoing ultrafiltration or other continuous renal replacement therapy and immediately after VPS surgery. Consult physician or midlevel practitioner for CVP greater than 8 mm Hg or PAWP greater than 12 mm Hg.
2. Monitor for peripheral edema. Note severity and location. Jugular vein distention at a 45-degree HOB elevation may indicate fluid overload or decreased cardiac output.

Fluid Management
1. Consult physician or midlevel practitioner for fluid overload: presence of dyspnea, tachypnea, rhonchi, orthopnea, basilar crackles that do not clear with coughing, labored and/or shallow breathing, elevated BP, or S_3 heart sound.
2. Use minimal amounts of fluids necessary to administer IV medications and maintain IV catheter patency.
3. If fluids are restricted, offer mouth care and/or ice chips (included as part of oral fluid measurement).
4. Measure and record abdominal girth daily. Be aware that abdominal girth measurements are subject to error and great care is necessary to ensure accuracy. Measure at the widest point, and mark this level for subsequent measurements with a permanent marker. Measure in the supine position if tolerated. If not tolerated, measure patient in the same position each time. Weigh daily at the same time, in the same clothing, using the same scale and method.

Electrolyte Management: Hypernatremia
1. Consult physician or midlevel practitioner for significantly abnormal serum electrolyte levels, especially sodium and potassium.
2. Ensure proper functioning of peritoneal-venous shunt and TIPS in patients after surgery (see Box 9-10).

Imbalanced nutrition: Less than body requirements *related to inability to digest food secondary to anorexia, nausea, and medically prescribed dietary restriction; decreased absorption of nutrients secondary to decreased intestinal motility, altered portal blood flow, decreased intestinal absorption of vitamins and minerals, altered protein metabolism; and the diseased liver's inability to utilize nutrients*

GOALS/OUTCOMES Patient has adequate nutrition as evidenced by a state of nitrogen balance as shown by daily fecal excretion of 2 to 3 g of nitrogen and 13 to 20 g of urinary nitrogen, thyroxine-binding prealbumin 200 to 300 mcg/ml, and retinol-binding protein 40 to 50 mcg/ml. Blood glucose levels remain within an acceptable range of 100 to 160 mg/dl.
NOC Nutritional Status; Biochemical Measures

Nutritional Monitoring
1. Confer with physician, dietitian, and pharmacist (if parenteral feedings are necessary) to estimate patient's current nutritional and metabolic needs, based on anthropometric data, creatinine excretion, albumin, and transferrin, as well as presence of encephalopathy, chronic hepatic disease, infection, and nutritional status before hospitalization. For general information, see *Nutritional Support*, p. 117.
2. Consult physician or midlevel practitioner regarding administration of parenteral or enteral nutrients. If insertion of a feeding tube becomes necessary, use caution to minimize the risk of rupturing gastroesophageal varices. If parenteral feedings are being administered, monitor IV site for infection and other complications.
3. Note, monitor, and record food/fluid ingested and daily caloric intake.
4. Administer prescribed vitamin supplements, particularly those fat-soluble.
5. Encourage food to be brought from home if desired by patient, and ensure it meets prescribed dietary restrictions.

Energy Management
1. Encourage bed rest to reduce metabolic demands on the liver and to promote hepatic regeneration. Increase patient's activity levels gradually as condition improves.

Hypoglycemia Management
1. Monitor blood glucose levels every 4 to 8 hours or as prescribed. Monitor patient for clinical indicators of hypoglycemia: altered mentation, irritability, diaphoresis, anxiety, weakness, and tachycardia. Clinical signs of hypoglycemia can be confused with hepatic encephalopathy. Validate clinical signs with blood glucose levels. Administer D_{10} or D_{50} as prescribed for hypoglycemia. Mild elevations in blood sugar are anticipated in some patients with chronic liver disease. Administer hypoglycemic agents as prescribed for blood glucose levels greater than 180 mg/dl.

Impaired gas exchange *related to altered oxygen supply secondary to arteriovenous shunting, ventilation-perfusion mismatch, and diaphragmatic limitation associated with ascites, hydrothorax, or central respiratory depression occurring with encephalopathy*

GOALS/OUTCOMES Within 4 hours of this diagnosis, patient has adequate gas exchange as evidenced by Pao_2 greater than 80 mm Hg, $Paco_2$ less than 45 mm Hg, RR 12 to 20 breaths/min with normal depth and pattern, oxygen saturation greater than 95% with or without oxygen supplementation or mechanical ventilation, and orientation to person, place, and time.

NOC Respiratory Status: Gas Exchange; Respiratory Status: Ventilation

---

| **Safety Alert** | *Level of consciousness is difficult to evaluate in the presence of moderate to severe hepatic encephalopathy, and obtaining a baseline level of consciousness is imperative.* |

Oxygen Therapy
1. Monitor and document respiratory rate every 1 to 4 hours. Note pattern, excursion, depth, and effort.
2. Administer supplemental oxygen as prescribed to enhance cerebral and hepatic oxygenation. Continuous pulse oximetry should be in use.
3. Maintain body positions that optimize ventilation. Elevate HOB 30 degrees or higher, depending on patient comfort and hemodynamic status.
4. Monitor ABGs and electrolytes as available.
5. Consult physician or midlevel practitioner for abnormal PaO_2, $PaCO_2$, and oxygen saturation.

Aspiration Precautions
1. Assess patient every 4 to 8 hours for atelectasis, hydrothorax (e.g., diminished breath sounds, dullness to percussion), and pulmonary infection. Consult physician or midlevel practitioner if physical assessment findings suggest respiratory complications.
2. Evaluate obtunded patient for presence of gag reflex. Consult speech pathologist for swallowing evaluation. Keep NPO with HOB elevated until patient's risk for aspiration is fully evaluated. If severe, consult physician or midlevel practitioner regarding need for ET intubation. Suction mouth frequently; offer/assist with frequent mouth care.

Disturbed sensory perception *related to endogenous chemical alteration (accumulation of ammonia or other central nervous system [CNS] toxins occurring with hepatic dysfunction), therapeutically restricted environment, sleep deprivation, hypoxia, sensory overload (noise, personnel) in ICU, and medication (side effects, toxic levels from liver's inability to detoxify appropriately)*

GOALS/OUTCOMES By the time of hospital discharge, patient exhibits stable personality pattern, age-appropriate behavior, intact intellect appropriate for level of education, distinct speech, and coordinated gross and fine motor movements. Handwriting is legible, and psychometric test scores are improved from baseline range.

NOC Distorted Thought Self-Control, Information Processing, Neurological Status: Consciousness

Fluid and Electrolyte Management
1. Avoid or minimize precipitating factors for hepatic encephalopathy (Box 9-11).
    a. Help patient keep circadian rhythms in sync (e.g., keep lighting in room appropriate for the time of day, correlate activities of daily living [ADLs] to the correct time of day).
    b. Check gastric secretions, vomitus, and stools for occult blood. Evaluate Hct and Hgb for evidence of bleeding. Consult physician or midlevel practitioner for low values that deviate from baseline. Anticipate mild-to-moderate anemia.
    c. Evaluate serum ammonia levels (normal levels are 40 to 110 mg/dl). Report significant elevations from baseline. Ammonia values and their measurement vary greatly and do not always correlate directly with encephalopathy.
    d. Be alert to potential sources of electrolyte imbalance (e.g., diarrhea, vomiting, occult bleeding).
        1) If patient is pulling out tubes, apply mitts rather than restraints.
        2) Avoid use of conventional and alternative drugs that are hepatotoxic (see Box 9-9).
        3) Correct hypoxemia; administer supplemental oxygen as necessary (see *Impaired Gas Exchange*, p. 800).
2. Evaluate patient for CNS effects such as personality changes, childish behavior, intellectual impairment, slurred speech, ataxia, and asterixis.
3. Administer daily handwriting or psychometric tests (if appropriate for patient's level of consciousness) to evaluate mild or subclinical encephalopathy. Report significant deterioration in handwriting or in test scores.
4. Consult physician or midlevel practitioner for abnormal EEG reports.
5. Administer neomycin as prescribed to reduce intestinal bacteria, which contribute to the production of cerebral intoxicants. Monitor patient for evidence of ototoxic effects (i.e., decreased hearing) and nephrotoxic effects (e.g., urinary output less than 0.5 ml/kg/hr, increased creatinine levels) of neomycin use. Avoid neomycin administration for patients with renal insufficiency.

| **Box 9-11** | **FACTORS THAT CONTRIBUTE TO HEPATIC ENCEPHALOPATHY** |

Chronic factors
- Portal-systemic shunting (entry of portal blood into systemic veins without being metabolized by the liver): may occur via damaged liver, collateral vessels, or surgically created portacaval anastomosis
- Dietary protein intake
- Intestinal bacteria
- Acid-base imbalance
- Progressive hepatic insufficiency

Precipitating factors
- Dehydration/electrolyte imbalance: may occur with overdiuresis, diarrhea, vomiting, or other factors
- Excessive paracentesis
- Surgery in a cirrhotic patient
- Excessive alcohol ingestion
- Sedatives/hypnotics
- Infection
- Constipation
- Extrahepatic bile duct obstruction
- Acute hepatocellular damage
- Viral hepatitis
- Alcoholic hepatitis
- Drug/chemical reactions (see Box 9-9)
- Drug overdose

6. Protect the confused or unconscious patient from injury.
   a. Enlist the aid of family or friends to watch patient during confused or restless periods.
   b. Have call light within patient's reach at all times.
   c. Tape all catheters and tubes securely to prevent dislodgment.
7. Consider possibility of seizures in the patient with severe encephalopathy; have airway management equipment readily available.
8. Minimize unnecessary noise, lights, and other environmental stimuli.
9. Monitor ICP and cerebral perfusion pressure (CPP). For patients with increased intracranial pressure (IICP), position carefully (HOB less than 20 degrees) and avoid fluid overload, hypercarbia, and hypoxemia. Administer mannitol and furosemide (Lasix) as prescribed. Sedation or coma induction may be indicated if cerebral edema does not respond to the measures just mentioned.

NIC Environmental Management; Delirium Management; Intracranial Pressure Monitoring

Risk for infection *related to inadequate secondary defenses (impaired reticuloendothelial system phagocytic activity and portal-systemic shunting); multiple invasive procedures; chronic malnutrition in the individual with cirrhosis*

GOALS/OUTCOMES Patient is free of infection as evidenced by normothermia, HR less than 100 bpm, RR less than 20 breaths/min, negative culture results, WBC count less than 11,000/mm^3, clear urine, and clear, thin sputum.
NOC Immune Status

Infection Protection
1. Monitor vital signs for evidence of infection (e.g., increases in temperature, heart and respiratory rates). Avoid measuring temperatures rectally in the patient with rectal varices.
2. If temperature or WBC elevation is sudden, obtain specimens for blood, sputum, and urine cultures or from other sites as prescribed. Consult physician or midlevel practitioner for positive culture results.
3. Be aware that a normal or mildly elevated leukocyte count may signify infection in patients with hepatic failure since patients with chronic liver disease often have leukopenia (WBC counts less than 3000/mm^3).

4. Evaluate secretions and drainage for evidence of infection (e.g., sputum changes, cloudy urine).
5. Evaluate IV, central line, and paracentesis site(s) for evidence of infection (erythema, warmth, unusual drainage). It is normal for a paracentesis puncture site to have a small amount of drainage immediately after the procedure. Prolonged or foul-smelling drainage can signal infection.
6. Teach significant others and visitors proper hand-washing technique. Restrict visitors with evidence of communicable disease.

Ineffective protection *related to clotting anomaly; thrombocytopenia; itching; disorientation*

GOALS/OUTCOMES Patient's bleeding, if it occurs, is not prolonged. Patient's skin is not damaged from scratching. Patient's confusion (if present) and level of consciousness will not lead to injury (see *Alterations in Consciousness*, p. 24).
NOC Blood Coagulation

Bleeding Precautions
1. Avoid giving intramuscular (IM) injections. If they are necessary, use small-gauge needles and maintain firm pressure over injection sites for several minutes. Avoid massaging IM injection sites.
2. Maintain pressure for several minutes over venipuncture sites. Inform laboratory personnel of patient's bleeding tendencies.
3. Avoid arterial punctures. If it is necessary to obtain ABG values, consult physician or midlevel practitioner regarding use of an indwelling arterial line. If this is not possible, be certain to maintain pressure over the arterial puncture site and elevation for at least 10 minutes.
4. Monitor PT/INR levels and platelet counts daily. Consult physician for significant prolongation of the PT or for significant reduction in the platelet count.
5. Report bleeding to physician or midlevel practitioner. Note oral and nasal mucosal bleeding and ecchymotic areas, and test stools, emesis, urine, and gastric drainage for occult blood.
6. Use electric rather than safety razor for patient shaving. Provide soft-bristle toothbrush or sponge-tipped applicator and mouthwash for oral hygiene.
7. Avoid indwelling, large-bore gastric drainage tubes if possible, because they may irritate gastric mucosa or varices, causing bleeding to occur.
8. Administer fresh-frozen plasma and platelets as prescribed. Monitor carefully for fluid volume overload (see Excess *Fluid Volume*, p. 799).
9. Administer vitamin K as prescribed.
10. A postshunt coagulopathy may develop in some patients after peritoneal-venous shunt surgery. Monitor these patients closely (see fifth intervention of this diagnosis).
11. If fibrin split products (FSPs) are present in the blood and thrombocytopenia is significant, the patient may have DIC (see *Bleeding and Thrombotic Disorders: Disseminated Intravascular Coagulation*, p. 837).
12. When moving patient, avoid applying shearing forces to skin.
13. Keep sheets free of wrinkles. Keep clothing from bunching against patient's skin. Score patient's pressure ulcer risk and monitor skin integrity.
14. Dry skin well after morning care. Provide adequate lotion to skin, avoid massaging it in deeply, and rub gently.
15. Use paper tape if it is necessary to place tape directly on skin. If possible, use gauze to secure a dressing or IV line, and tape over the gauze to prevent it from unwrapping.

Ineffective tissue perfusion: renal *related to risk of diminished arterial flow secondary to increased preglomerular vascular resistance*

GOALS/OUTCOMES Patient has adequate renal perfusion as evidenced by urinary output greater than 0.5 ml/kg/hr.
NOC Circulatory Status

Fluid/Electrolyte Management
1. Consult physician or midlevel practitioner for serum sodium less than 120 mEq/L and urine sodium less than 10 mEq/L, associated with the development of HRS.
2. Consult physician or midlevel practitioner for significant increases in creatinine and potassium values. BUN level is not an accurate indicator of renal function, especially in the patient with hepatic failure, because alterations in hepatic function can cause decreased BUN values and GI bleeding results in increased BUN values.
3. Minimize infusion of sodium-containing fluids because they contribute to ascites and peripheral edema and may potentiate functional renal failure.
4. Report hypophosphatemia (mental confusion, metabolic acidosis, anorexia, cardiac dysrhythmias, hemolytic anemia, lethargy, and bone pain) to physician or midlevel practitioner.

5. Report hypomagnesemia (muscle weakness, nausea, vomiting, tremors, tetany, and lethargy) to physician or midlevel practitioner.
6. For additional information, see nursing diagnoses and interventions in *Acute Renal Failure*, p. 584, and *Fluid and Electrolyte Disturbances*, p. 37.

Impaired tissue integrity *related to chemical irritants (bile salts), impaired mobility, and fluid excess (tissue edema)*
- -

GOALS/OUTCOMES Patient's tissue remains intact; pruritus is relieved or reduced within 12 hours of this diagnosis.
NOC Comfort

Skin Surveillance
1. Bathe patient with a nonsoap cleanser. Apply an unscented, non–alcohol-containing lotion while skin is still moist.
2. Use a low-pressure mattress to minimize pressure on fragile tissues.
3. Initiate pressure ulcer prevention.
4. If patient is confused or obtunded, place the hands in soft gloves or mitts to minimize damage from scratching, and keep nails short.
5. Administer cholestyramine (e.g., Questran, LoCholest, Cholestid) as prescribed to reduce bile acids in the serum and skin and thereby relieve itching. Avoid administration of other oral medications within 2 hours of cholestyramine administration because they may bind with it in the intestine and reduce its absorption.

Deficient knowledge *related to lack of exposure to health care information; cognitive limitation secondary to hepatic encephalopathy*
- -

GOALS/OUTCOMES Within the 24-hour period before hospital discharge, patient states signs and symptoms of early hepatic encephalopathy, the importance of medical follow-up, the need to adhere to the prescribed diet, the importance of rest, infection control measures, availability of alcohol and drug treatment programs, medication instructions, and signs and symptoms of other complications.
NOC Knowledge: Disease Process, Knowledge: Diet, Knowledge: Medication, Knowledge: Substance Use Control, Risk Control Drug Use, Risk Control Alcohol Use.

Teaching: Disease Process
1. Stress importance of sufficient rest and adherence to prescribed diet.
2. *If hepatic failure is related to hepatitis B virus (HBV) infection:*
    a. HBV prophylaxis should be considered for sexual partners and household members with possible exposure to HBV (e.g., those who unknowingly shared a toothbrush or razor).
    b. Teach patient and exposure contacts practices that reduce the risk of exposure (e.g., condom use, having own personal grooming items). Prescreening for the presence of hepatitis B (HB) antibodies is encouraged if it does not delay treatment for greater than 14 days after last exposure.
    c. A dose of hepatitis B immune globulin (HBIG) is recommended immediately for sexual contacts and household contacts with possible blood and body fluid exposure. A second administration of HBIG vaccine should follow 1 month later.
    d. The HB vaccine series should be initiated for sexual and household contacts at risk. The first and second vaccines can be given at the same time the two HBIG vaccines are given. Make sure both vaccines are given in separate areas. The HB vaccines are to be given deltoid IM only. Stress importance of not sharing intimate items (e.g., razors, toothbrush, nail clippers).
3. *If hepatic failure is related to hepatitis C virus (HCV),* no prophylaxis is available to exposed persons. Therefore, baseline hepatitis C (HC) antibodies should be measured, and 1 month later a second sample should be drawn and tested. Based on results, an infectious disease consult may be indicated, along with possible treatment. It is important to note, however, that those with sexual exposure have less than a 5% chance of seroconversion. Those with exposure to blood, particularly through hollow-bore needles, have the greatest chance of seroconversion.
4. Inform patient about the availability of alcohol-treatment and drug-treatment programs if alcohol- and drug-related hepatic failure has occurred.
5. Explain the availability of support groups (i.e., Alcoholics Anonymous, Al-Anon) for patients and family members when hepatic failure is related to chronic alcohol ingestion.
6. Caution about the importance of avoiding over-the-counter medications without first consulting physician. Advise patient to confer with physician regarding use of NSAIDs, aspirin, and other medications that contain salicylates for minor aches and pains after hospital discharge.

7. Teach the signs and symptoms of infection: fever; unusual drainage from paracentesis or other invasive procedure sites; warmth and erythema surrounding the invasive sites; or abdominal pain. Have patient demonstrate technique for measuring oral temperature with type of thermometer used at home.

8. Teach the signs and symptoms of unusual bleeding, including prolonged mucosal bleeding, very large or painful bruises, and dark stools. Caution patient that, if possible, major dental procedures should be postponed until bleeding times normalize.

9. Inform patient about sodium restriction if ascites developed during the course of the illness.

10. Advise protein restriction if the patient has residual or chronic encephalopathy. Instruct patient to avoid constipation by increasing bulk in the diet or by using agents prescribed by physician.

11. Caution about the necessity of alcohol cessation for at least several months after complete recovery from the acute episode. After full recovery, one or two glasses of beer or wine a week are usually allowed if hepatic failure was not related to alcoholism or alcohol ingestion.

12. Instruct patient to weigh himself or herself daily and to report weight loss or gain of greater than 5 lb.

NIC Substance Use Treatment: Drug Withdrawal, Substance Use Treatment: Overdose, Substance Use Treatment: Alcohol Withdrawal, Medication Management, Nutrition Management

Risk for injury *related to invasive procedures*
- -

GOALS/OUTCOMES Patient does not sustain an injury related to liver biopsy, ICP monitoring, or other invasive procedures.
NOC Knowledge Health Promotion, Risk Control: Infection

Teaching Individual
1. Fully prepare patient emotionally and physically for the procedure.
2. Monitor patient closely after procedure; observe changes in vital signs that correlate with observations of patient.
3. Monitor dressing over puncture wounds for bleeding. Document amount, frequency of dressing changes, what types of dressings are applied, what the drainage looks like/smells like (if applicable), and what the wound looks like.
4. Monitor for fever.
5. If subject is encephalopathic, ensure airway is clear, and ensure that someone will accompany patient to and from procedure. Also ensure that a nurse will be with the patient when he or she is undergoing the procedure.

ADDITIONAL NURSING DIAGNOSES
As appropriate, see the following for additional nursing diagnoses and interventions: *Nutritional Support* (p. 117), *Mechanical Ventilation* (p. 99), *Prolonged Immobility* (p. 149), and *Emotional and Spiritual Support for the Patient and Significant Others* (p. 200).

PERITONITIS
PATHOPHYSIOLOGY
Peritonitis can be classified as *primary, secondary,* or *tertiary.* Primary peritonitis is a bacterial infection of the serosal membrane lining the abdominal cavity that occurs spontaneously without any apparent source of contamination, such as bowel perforation. The most common etiology of primary peritonitis is spontaneous bacterial peritonitis. Spontaneous bacterial peritonitis occurs most commonly in patients with cirrhosis of the liver with ascites and is associated with a 30% to 50% mortality rate. Bacterial seeding of ascitic fluid is believed to result from the translocation of enteric bacteria across the gut wall or mesenteric lymphatic vessels. Secondary peritonitis, the most common form of peritonitis, is an inflammation of all or part of the peritoneal cavity caused by diffuse microbial proliferation or chemical irritation from leakage of corrosive gastric or intestinal contents into the peritoneum. Ruptured appendix, leaky anastomoses from weight loss surgery (e.g., Roux-en-Y, gastric bypass), perforated peptic ulcer, bowel rupture related to ulcerative colitis or Crohn disease, pancreatitis, abdominal trauma, and ruptured abdominal abscesses are among the many etiologic factors associated with secondary peritonitis. Indwelling tubes and catheters, such as those used for postoperative drainage and peritoneal dialysis, are foreign bodies that compromise peritoneal integrity and permit the entry of infective organisms that can trigger peritonitis. Peritonitis is a leading

cause of morbidity in renal failure patients treated with peritoneal dialysis. Tertiary peritonitis represents persistent or recurrent infection following an apparently successfully treated episode of spontaneous bacterial peritonitis or secondary peritonitis. Tuberculosis peritonitis is rare in the United States but is worth mentioning as it is currently seen more frequently in patients with HIV disease and carries a high mortality rate (50% to 70%).

Regardless of the initiating factor, the inflammatory process is similar in every case. The initial reactions, which usually are triggered by histamine release, include hyperemia, edema, and vascular congestion. Fluid shifts from intravascular to interstitial spaces as a result of increased vascular permeability initiated by inflammatory mediators. The circulating blood volume is depleted, and hypovolemic shock may ensue. The transudated fluid contains high levels of fibrinogen and thromboplastin. The fibrinogen is converted to fibrin by the thromboplastin. Under normal conditions, the peritoneum has fibrinolytic abilities to stop the fibrin formation. When the peritoneum is weakened or injured, however, this ability is hampered and fibrin adhesions form around the damaged area. The fibrin deposits form a barrier that harbors and protects bacteria from the body's defenses, resulting in multiple pockets of infection and abscess formation. In most cases, the fibrin deposits dissolve. The continued presence of fibrin can lead to adhesions and potentially bowel obstruction. With severe inflammation, intra-abdominal sepsis may develop.

GASTROINTESTINAL ASSESSMENT: PERITONITIS
Goal of System Assessment
Identify early findings of peritoneal irritation.

History and Risk Factors
Inflammatory processes such as diverticulitis, appendicitis, or Crohn disease; obstructive events in the small bowel and colon; vascular events such as ischemic colitis, mesenteric thrombosis, or embolic phenomena; blunt or penetrating trauma, especially to hollow viscera; severe hepatobiliary disease; and continuous ambulatory peritoneal dialysis (CAPD). General risk factors include those related to poor tissue healing and infection (e.g., advanced age, diabetes, and vascular disease, advanced liver disease, malignancy, malnutrition, and debilitation). Some patients with severe peritonitis may present in overt septic shock.

Vital Sign Assessment
- Fever of greater than 38°C (100° to 101°F) is present in most cases.
- Tachypnea and tachycardia result from increased metabolic demands.
- Hypotension may be present due to dehydration from vomiting, fever, and third-space losses.
- Hypothermia may be present if the peritonitis advances to severe sepsis.

Abdominal Pain
- Abdominal pain may be quite severe, causing the patient to maintain a fetal position and resist any movement that aggravates the pain. Its onset can be sudden or insidious, with the location varying according to the underlying pathology.
- Nausea, vomiting, anorexia, diarrhea, and other changes in bowel habits also may be present and are reflective of GI dysfunction.
- Anorexia and nausea may precede the development of abdominal pain.

Observation
- Occasionally, mild-to-moderate ascites is observed, depending on the cause of the peritonitis.
- Respiratory rate is rapid, and the patient usually has a shallow ventilatory pattern to minimize abdominal movement and pain
- Restlessness and confusion occur because of impaired cerebral perfusion.

Auscultation
- Auscultation of all four quadrants usually reveals diminished or absent bowel sounds. The complete absence of bowel sounds suggests an ileus—a frequent complication of peritonitis.
- Breath sounds are diminished due to shallow respiratory pattern.

Palpation
- Palpation of the abdomen elicits tympany and tenderness that can be generalized or localized, depending on the nature and extent of infection.
- Rebound tenderness, guarding, and involuntary rigidity also may be present.
- The abdomen may feel firm and boardlike. Occasionally, the abdominal examination reveals an inflammatory mass.
- The abdomen is often distended, a finding that reflects a generalized ileus and may not be present if the infection is well localized.

Nutritional Assessment
- Evidence of malnutrition will be noted in the presence of chronic liver or renal disease.

Screening Labwork
- Abdominal paracentesis: ascitic fluid for cell count, Gram stain, and culture
- CBC: leukocytosis
- LFTs: elevated
- Serum chemistry
- Radiologic tests: abdominal radiograph, abdominal CT of the abdomen

Hemodynamic Measurements
- Hypovolemia with marked tachycardia, hypotension, low CO, decreased PAPs, and decreased urine output may occur due to massive fluid shifts from the intravascular space into the abdominal interstitium and peritoneum and from vasodilation caused by inflammatory mediators.
- Endotoxemic vasodilation is manifested by a low SVR, with an initial increase in HR and CO representing signs of septic shock.
- Persistent hypovolemia may result in a dangerously low MAP, thus impairing renal, cardiac, and cerebral perfusion.

Diagnostic Tests for Peritonitis

Test	Purpose	Abnormal Findings
Blood Studies		
Complete blood count (CBC) with differential Hemoglobin (Hgb) Hematocrit (Hct) RBC count (RBC) WBC count (WBC)	Assess for bacterial infection and anemia.	Leukocytosis ($>11,000$ cells/μl) with a shift to the left or elevation of immature neutrophils (bands).
Serum chemistry BUN Creatinine CO_2 Glucose Serum chloride Serum potassium Serum sodium Total bilirubin Serum amylase C-reactive protein Lactic acid/lactate	Assess for electrolyte imbalances and organ involvement	Elevated amylase and lipase with pancreas involvement (acute pancreatitis). Elevated BUN and creatinine with renal dysfunction. Elevated bilirubin with gallbladder disease. Elevated CO_2 with low Cl^- reflects metabolic alkalosis. Electrolyte losses, especially potassium with vomiting and diarrhea. C-reactive protein elevation indicates inflammation. Elevated lactate level may indicate sepsis/SIRS.

Continued

Diagnostic Tests for Peritonitis—cont'd		
Test	**Purpose**	**Abnormal Findings**
Diagnostic Paracentesis *Peritoneal Fluid Analysis*		
Peritoneal neutrophil count	This analysis is useful in confirming the diagnosis of bacterial peritonitis and assists in driving therapy.	WBC count >250 cells/μl with >50% polymorphonuclear leukocytes (PMNs) is an indication to begin antibiotic therapy.
Peritoneal total protein and LDH levels	Useful in confirming the diagnosis of bacterial peritonitis	Total protein >1 g/dl; ascitic LDL greater than serum LDL
Peritoneal glucose level	Useful in confirming the diagnosis of bacterial peritonitis	Decreased peritoneal fluid glucose level (<50 mg/dl)
Gram stain and culture	Identifies causative organism(s) to begin proper empiric or specific antibiotic therapy	*Spontaneous bacterial peritonitis:* monomicrobial infection; *E. coli, Klebsiella pneumoniae,* and *Streptococcus pneumoniae* are most common. *Secondary peritonitis:* multiple organisms will be present in peritoneal fluid Gram stain and culture.
Radiologic Procedures		
Abdominal radiograph Plain films	Identify the presence of dilated bowel and free air	Free air is present in most cases of perforation.
Abdominal computed tomography (CT) scan	Assess for an intra-abdominal source of infection	Abscess or mass may be identified.
Ultrasonography	Useful in locating small amounts of fluid, as well as in differentiating fluid collections in the abdomen	Loculated fluid, abscess, bile duct dilation, and pancreatitis may be identified.

Hematologic Studies

Leukocytosis will be present. A low total WBC count may indicate an exhausted bone marrow, with a poor prognosis. Initially, the Hgb and Hct values may be increased because of hemoconcentration, but they will decrease to baseline levels as normal intravascular volume is restored.

Blood Chemistry Studies

Depending on the severity of the patient's condition, blood electrolyte levels may be abnormal. If vomiting is present, metabolic alkalosis is expected. Serum albumin levels are often decreased due to increased capillary permeability and leakage. The underlying disease process affects chemistry studies (e.g., patients with pancreatitis, gallbladder disorders, and renal failure). Renal failure is a common complication of peritonitis and a major cause of death.

Radiologic Procedures

The abdominal radiograph study usually reveals dilation of the large and small bowel, with edema of the small bowel wall. Free air in the abdomen suggests visceral perforation. With abdominal CT, abscesses can be visualized and sometimes drained during the procedure, thus avoiding surgery. Free fluid in the abdomen on ultrasound suggests hemorrhage or ascites. **Nuclear Medicine Scans:** (Gallium, Indium, Technetium) are useful for persistent fever despite adequate antibiotic coverage and negative CT findings.

Diagnostic Paracentesis

Abdominal paracentesis involves the insertion of a catheter or trocar into the abdomen to obtain a specimen. Sterile saline is infused through the catheter, and the return fluid is analyzed for RBC, WBC, and bacteria content. If ascites is present, it may not be necessary to infuse saline because fluid can be removed directly for analysis. Paracentesis may be repeated

48 hours after the initiation of treatment to assess patient response. Multiple organisms on peritoneal or ascitic fluid Gram stain or culture are diagnostic of secondary peritonitis, whereas spontaneous bacterial peritonitis is caused by monomicrobial infection.

COLLABORATIVE MANAGEMENT

Management should be geared toward controlling the infectious source, eliminating bacteria and toxins, modulating the inflammatory process, and preventing organ system failure. Patients should be cared for in an intensive care setting, even if they do not appear critically ill initially.

Care Priorities

Care priorities begin with volume resuscitation, electrolyte replacement, and empiric antibiotic coverage. Medical, nursing, interventional, and surgical therapies should be complementary involving hemodynamic management, pulmonary support, and renal replacement therapy, and nutrition and metabolic support.

1. **Correct fluid and electrolyte imbalances:** Significant intravascular volume depletion may occur with peritonitis. In severely ill patients, fluid replacement should be guided by invasive hemodynamic monitoring. In most cases, crystalloids are used initially. If there is evidence of decreased intravascular proteins, colloids such as albumin are indicated. The use of IV albumin has also been shown to reduce the incidence of renal failure. If peritonitis is complicated by hemorrhage, PRBCs may be given. Electrolyte replacement, typically potassium, is implemented according to laboratory findings. (See *SIRS, Sepsis and MODS*, p. 924, for additional information.)

2. **Control peritoneal infection with antimicrobial therapy:** Initiate empiric broad-spectrum parenteral antibiotic therapy early for all suspected cases of peritonitis. Antibiotic therapy should be started as soon as the diagnosis is suspected. Suspicion is identified by clinical findings more than culture results because a large percentage of patients will exhibit negative cultures. Culture-negative patients must also receive antibiotic therapy because without it, severe sepsis and death may follow.

   - Third-generation cephalosporins are recommended in cases of spontaneous bacterial peritonitis initially, then tailor therapy in conformity with cultures. For secondary and tertiary bacterial peritonitis, broad-spectrum gram-negative and anaerobic coverage should be initiated, followed by definitive therapy based on culture sensitivities.
   - In severe hospital-acquired cases, imipenem, piperacillin-tazobactam, and a combination of aminoglycoside and metronidazole may be effective. Quinolones are also considered effective therapy.
   - The duration of antibiotic therapy must be individualized according to the infectious source, infection severity, underlying disease, and patient's response to therapy. Therapy for 5 to 10 days is sufficient for most patients.
   - The administration of intraperitoneal (IP) antibiotics should be considered over parenteral administration for patients with peritoneal dialysis–associated peritonitis. Aminoglycoside therapy should be avoided in patients with chronic liver disease due to an increased risk of nephrotoxicity.

3. **Control peritoneal infection with surgical procedure(s):** Surgical laparotomy is an important therapy in all cases of peritonitis. Surgical therapy allows for the removal of all intra-abdominal foreign material, and nonviable tissue can be débrided. Leaky anastomoses are identified and repaired. If present, bowel perforations and obstructions are corrected and abscesses are drained. This should remove the source of infection and prevent reinfection.

   - *Drains are placed laparoscopically.* Laparoscopy is currently used for diagnosis and determination of etiology.
   - *Open wound management of the abdomen* with scheduled reoperations is often advocated for severe disease. Open-abdomen technique may reduce the risk of abdominal compartment syndrome, and allow for better management of bowel edema and subsequent inflammatory changes in the postoperative period. Disadvantages of open-technique include alteration in respiratory mechanics and risk of abdominal contamination with nosocomial pathogens.
   - *Interventional therapies* include percutaneous drainage of abscesses and percutaneous and endoscopic stent placements. Ultrasound- and CT-guided percutaneous drainage

has been shown to be efficacious and safe and preferred in some cases, allowing for a delay in surgery until the acute process and sepsis can be resolved.

4. **Control pain resulting from peritoneal inflammation:** The degree of discomfort caused by peritonitis varies greatly. Opiate analgesics are used parenterally to ensure patient comfort but are given cautiously to avoid compromise of abdominal and respiratory function. These analgesics usually require frequent administration, with the dose titrated for each individual.

5. **Provide nutritional support:** Nutritional support is crucial for healing and survival. GI function is compromised and motility minimal or absent due to inflammatory processes.

- A large-bore nasogastric tube is inserted to reduce or prevent distention caused by obstruction or ileus. Placement of a small-bore enteric tube (nasoduodenal or NJ tube) is done to provide enteral (tube) feedings. Radiographic confirmation of correct placement should be done for all enteric tubes. Initially, the patient is placed on NPO status until some GI function is regained.
- If tolerated, jejunal feeding should be initiated early in the treatment course. Elemental feedings can be administered with or without bowel sounds present. More recent enteral feeding guidelines have challenged the validity of older guidelines for feeding intolerance. Gastric residual volumes exceeding 450 ml and absence of bowel sounds are no longer absolute contraindications for feeding. Newer feeding methods, such as "trickle feedings," may be better tolerated. If enteral feeding is not possible, total parenteral nutrition should be initiated. (See *Nutritional Support*, p. 117.)
- When resumption of bowel sounds or passage of flatus signals the return of GI motility, enteral nutrition with nonelemental (conventional) tube feedings can begin.

CARE PLANS FOR PERITONITIS

Deficient fluid volume *related to active loss secondary to fluid sequestration within the peritoneum*

GOALS/OUTCOMES Within 8 hours of this diagnosis, patient becomes normovolemic as evidenced by the following parameters: MAP 70 to 105 mm Hg, HR 60 to 100 bpm, normal sinus rhythm on ECG, CVP 2 to 6 mm Hg, urinary output ≥0.5 ml/kg/hr, warm extremities, peripheral pulses greater than 2+ on a 0 to 4+ scale, brisk capillary refill (less than 2 seconds), orientation to time, place, and person, and stable weight.
NOC Fluid Balance

Fluid/Electrolyte Management
1. Monitor BP every 1 to 4 hours, depending on patient stability. Be alert to MAP decreases of greater than 10 mm Hg from previous BP reading, indicative of possible sepsis.
2. Monitor HR and ECG every 1 to 4 hours, or more often if vital signs are unstable. Be alert to increases in HR, which suggest hypovolemia. Usually the ECG will show sinus tachycardia. In the presence of hypokalemia caused by prolonged vomiting or gastric suction, ECG may show ventricular ectopy, prominent U wave, and depression of the ST segment.

> **Safety Alert** *HR increases may be caused by fever, hypovolemia, and vasodilation related to sepsis.*

3. Maintain crystalloid therapy guided by invasive hemodynamic monitoring.
4. Measure CVP and CO at least every 4 hours, depending on stability of patient's condition. Be alert to low or decreasing CVP and CO. Inotropic therapy may be added to assist CO in conjunction with fluid replacement modalities.
5. Monitor BUN, creatinine, total protein, and albumin levels.
6. Albumin administration at 1 to 1.5 g/kg may be needed to replace losses due to capillary leak.
7. Measure urinary output hourly. Be alert to output less than 0.5 ml/kg/hr for 2 consecutive hours, which may signal intravascular volume depletion. Consult physician and increase fluid intake promptly if decreased urinary output is caused by hypovolemia and hypoperfusion.
8. Monitor patient for physical indicators of hypovolemia, including cool extremities, capillary refill greater than 2 seconds, decreased amplitude of peripheral pulses, and neurologic changes such as restlessness and confusion.

9. Estimate ongoing fluid losses. Measure all drainage from tubes, catheters, and drains. Note the frequency of dressing changes as a result of saturation with fluid or blood. Weigh the patient daily, using the same scales and method. Compare 24-hour body fluid output with 24-hour fluid intake, and record the difference.
10. Assess for signs of pulmonary edema due to overaggressive fluid replacement and increased capillary permeability caused by inflammatory mediators.

NIC Fluid Monitoring; Hemodynamic Regulation; Hypovolemia Management; Invasive Hemodynamic Monitoring; Shock Prevention; Dysrhythmia Management

Risk for infection *related to inadequate primary defenses (traumatized tissue, altered perfusion); tissue destruction; environmental exposure to pathogens*

GOALS/OUTCOMES Sepsis does not develop as evidenced by HR 60 to 100 bpm, RR 12 to 20 breaths/min, SVR 900 to 1200 dynes/sec/cm^{-5}, CI 2.5 to 4 L/min/m^2, normothermia, negative culture results, and orientation to time, place, and person.
NOC Infection Severity

Medication Management
1. Administer empiric broad-spectrum parenteral (IV) antibiotics early and in a timely fashion. Reschedule antibiotics if a dosage is delayed for longer than 1 hour. Recognize that failure to administer antibiotics on schedule may result in inadequate drug blood levels and treatment failure.
    a. Third-generation cephalosporins can be used in all cases for 5 to 10 days of therapy, such as cefotaxime.
    b. IP antibiotics should be considered for patients with peritoneal dialysis (PD) associated peritonitis since the PD catheter provides immediate access to the peritoneum.
    c. Avoid aminoglycoside therapy, which carries an increased risk of nephrotoxicity in patients with chronic liver disease.
2. A trail of antibiotic cessation should be considered for the patient with no defined infectious focus. Continued broad-spectrum antibiotics in these patients may allow resistant organisms to emerge.

Vital Signs Monitoring
1. Monitor vital signs and hemodynamic measurements for evidence of sepsis: increases in HR, RR, and CO (CI greater than 4 L/min/m^2) and a decrease in SVR (less than 900 dynes/sec/cm^{-5}). Check rectal or core temperature every 4 hours for increases. Be aware that hypothermia may precede hyperthermia in some patients.
2. Also note that older adults and those who are immunocompromised may not demonstrate a fever, even with severe sepsis.
3. If the patient has a sudden temperature elevation, obtain culture specimens of blood, sputum, urine, and other sites as prescribed. Monitor culture reports, and report positive findings promptly.

Wound Care
1. To minimize microbial growth, facilitate drainage of pus, GI secretions, old blood, necrotic tissue, foreign material such as feces, and other body fluids from wounds.
2. Evaluate wounds for evidence of infection (e.g., erythema, warmth, swelling, unusual drainage). Culture any unusual drainage.
3. Evaluate patient's orientation to time, place, and person and LOC every 2 to 4 hours. Document and report significant deviations from baseline.

NIC Hemodynamic Regulation; Temperature Regulation; Intravenous (IV) Therapy
See *SIRS, Sepsis and MODS*, p. 924, for additional information.

Hyperthermia *related to infectious process, increased metabolic rate, and dehydration secondary to peritonitis*

GOALS/OUTCOMES Patient's temperature remains within acceptable limits (36° to 38.9°C [97° to 102°F]) or returns to acceptable limits within 4 to 6 hours of this diagnosis. An open airway is secured in the event of hyperthermic seizures.
NOC Thermoregulation

Peritonitis

Temperature Regulation
1. Monitor rectal or core temperature every 2 to 4 hours.
2. If a hypothermia blanket is required, perform the following interventions:
   a. Protect the skin that is in contact with the blanket by placing a sheet between the blanket and patient.
   b. Inspect patient's skin every 2 hours for evidence of tissue damage caused by local vasoconstriction. Massage patient's skin every 2 hours to promote circulation and minimize tissue damage.
   c. Check patient's temperature at frequent intervals to ensure that sudden decreases (along with shivering) do not occur, which could increase metabolic demand.
3. If patient has a high fever (i.e., greater than 38.9°C [102°F]), consider tepid baths, which may be helpful in reducing the fever.
4. Administer antipyretics as prescribed.
5. Keep an appropriate-size oral airway and suction equipment in the patient's room for use in the event of seizure activity.

NIC Fever Treatment; Vital Signs Monitoring

Impaired tissue integrity *related to tissue destruction; surgical intervention with exposure to environmental pathogens*

GOALS/OUTCOMES By the time of hospital discharge, patient exhibits no further GI tissue destruction as evidenced by reduction in pain; return of bowel sounds and bowel function; and wound healing.
NOC Tissue Integrity: Skin and Mucous Membranes

Infection Control
1. See *Medication Management for Risk of Infection,* p. 811.
2. Adjust antibiotic therapy specific to culture sensitivity reports.
3. Monitor renal function for signs of nephrotoxicity secondary to antibiotic therapy.
4. Discuss repeat of paracentesis 48 to 72 hours following the initiation of antibiotic therapy to evaluate effectiveness of therapy.

Wound Care
1. Monitor for surgical site infection (warmth, tenderness, and purulent drainage).
2. If surgical wound is open:
   a. Consider VAC device, which applies localized negative pressure directly to the wound. This removes fluid that causes swelling, increases blood flow, and accelerates granulation tissue formation.
   b. Maintain dressing membrane, ensure adequacy of drainage, and monitor for granulation tissue formation.
   c. *Avoid wet-to-dry dressings* as they create a lack of physical barrier to bacterial entry; prompt tissue cooling in wounds, which heal best when kept normothermic; disrupt angiogenesis; and prolong inflammation.
3. Record volume and characteristics of drainage and obtain specimens as needed.
4. Assess for overall improvement within 24 to 72 hours. Failure to progress indicates recurrent, persistent, or new infectious focus.

Acute pain *related to biologic or chemical agents causing injury to the peritoneum and intraperitoneal organs*

GOALS/OUTCOMES Within 2 hours of this diagnosis, patient's subjective evaluation of discomfort improves, as documented by a pain scale. Nonverbal indicators of discomfort, such as grimacing, are absent.
NOC Pain Control

Analgesic Administration
1. Monitor patient for the presence of discomfort. Use a pain scale to rate discomfort.
2. Administer parenteral analgesics promptly, before pain becomes severe. Consistency and promptness in delivering analgesics also may help to decrease patient's anxiety, which can contribute to the severity of the pain. Rate the degree of pain relief obtained by using the pain scale. Be aware that opiate analgesics decrease GI motility and may delay the return of normal bowel function.
3. Modify patient's body position to optimize comfort. Many patients with severe abdominal pain find a dorsal recumbent or lateral decubitus bent-knee position more comfortable than other positions.
4. Monitor respiratory pattern and LOC hourly, because both may be depressed if large amounts of opiates are required to control the pain.

5.   Monitor HR and BP every 1 to 4 hours. Monitor CVP and PAOP every 4 hours, or more frequently in patients whose condition is unstable. Consult physician for significant deviations. Be aware that many opiates cause vasodilation and can result in serious hypotension, especially in patients with volume depletion.
6.   Evaluate effectiveness of the medication on an ongoing basis. On the basis of the patient's clinical response, discuss dose and drug manipulation with physician.
7.   Avoid administering analgesics to newly admitted patients before they have been fully evaluated by a surgeon, because analgesics can mask important diagnostic clues.

NIC Pain Management; Environmental Management: Comfort; Coping Enhancement; Simple Guided Imagery; Respiratory Monitoring

Imbalanced nutrition, less than body requirements *related to decreased intake secondary to impaired GI function*

GOALS/OUTCOMES Patient maintains baseline body weight, and nitrogen studies show a state of nitrogen balance within 5 to 7 days of this diagnosis.
NOC Nutritional Status: Food and Fluid Intake

Nutrition Management
1.   Monitor bowel sounds every 1 to 8h; report significant changes (i.e., sudden absence or return).
2.   Maintain NPO status during the acute phase of peritonitis with stomach decompression via NG tube.
3.   Initiate postpyloric (jejunal) elemental feedings within the first 24 to 48 hours. Gradually increase enteral intake when gastric motility returns.
4.   Initiate TPN if jejunal feedings are contraindicated or not tolerated.
5.   If patient has abdominal distention, measure and document abdominal girth every 8 hours. Distention can signal complications such as ileus or ascites.
6.   Administer histamine H_2-receptor antagonists as prescribed to reduce corrosiveness of gastric acid and prevent complications such as stress ulcers.
7.   Administer prescribed antiemetic medications as indicated.
8.   Ensure that gastric, intestinal, and other GI drainage tubes are functioning properly. Evaluate character of the drainage. Irrigate or reposition tubes as necessary. Patency and proper position of decompression tubes, such as the Miller-Abbott type, are essential for effective function.

NIC Nutritional Monitoring; Gastrointestinal Intubation; Total Parenteral Nutrition (TPN) Administration; Enteral Tube Feeding; Aspiration Precautions; Tube Care: Gastrointestinal

For additional information, see *Nutritional Support,* p. 117.

ADDITIONAL NURSING DIAGNOSES
For other nursing diagnoses and interventions, see the following as appropriate: *Hemodynamic Monitoring* (p. 75), *Prolonged Immobility* (p. 149), *Emotional and Spiritual Support of the Patient and Significant Others* (p. 200), and *SIRS, Sepsis and MODS,* p. 924.

SELECTED REFERENCES
AGA Institute: Medical position statement on acute pancreatitis. *Gastroenterology* 132:2019, 2007.
American Gastroenterology Association Institute: Technical review on acute pancreatitis. *Gastroenterology* 132(5):2022, 2007.
Barada K, et al: Upper gastrointestinal bleeding in patients with acute coronary syndromes. *J Clin Gastroenterol* 42(4):368, 2008.
Boyer TD, Haskal ZJ: AASLD practice guidelines: the role of transjugular intrahepatic portosystemic shunt in the management of portal hypertension. *Hepatology* 51(1):1–16, 2010.
Campsen J, Blei AT, et al: Outcomes of living donor liver transplant for acute liver failure. The A2ALL cohort study. *Liver Transplant* 14(9):1273, 2008.
Cappell MS: Acute pancreatitis: etiology, clinical presentation, diagnosis, and therapy. *Med Clin North Am* 92(4):889, 2008.

Peritonitis

Chavez-Tapia NC, Soares-Weiser K, Brezis M, et al: Antibiotics for spontaneous bacterial peritonitis in cirrhotic patients. *Cochrane Database Syst Rev.* http://www.mrw.interscience.wiley.com/cochrane/clsysrev/articles/CD002232/frame.html

de la Mora-Levy JG, Baron TH: Endoscopic management of the liver transplant patient. *Liver Transplantation* 11:1007–1021, 2005.

Evenson A, Fischer J: Current management of enterocutaneous fistula. *J Gastrointest Surg* 10:445, 2006.

Exenatide: U.S. Food and Drug Administration. http://www.fda.gov/cder/drug/infopage/exenatide/default.htm

Friedman S: Liver, biliary tract and pancreas disorders. In McPhee J, Papadakis M, editors: *Current medical diagnosis and treatment*, ed 48. New York, 2009, McGraw-Hill.

Ghany MG, Strader DB, Thomas DL, et al: AASLD practice guidelines: diagnosis, management and treatment of hepatitis C: an update. *Hepatology* 49(4):1335–1374, 2009.

Huber W, Umgelter A, Reindl W, et al: Volume assessment in patients with necrotizing pancreatitis: a comparison of intrathoracic blood volume index, central venous pressure and hematocrit, and their correlation to cardiac index and extravascular lung water index. *Crit Care Med* 36(8):2348, 2008.

Kamth PS, Kim WR: The model for end-stage liver disease (MELD). *Hepatology* 45(3):797, 2007.

Lee WM: November 2, 2008. State of the Art Lecture at the Moscone West Convention Center, American Association for the Study of Liver Diseases, San Francisco, California.

Lee WM, Squires RH Jr, et al: Acute liver failure: summary of a workshop. *Hepatology* 47:1401–1415, 2008.

Lindor KD, Gershwin MD, Poupon R, et al: AASLD practice guidelines: primary biliary cirrhosis. *Hepatology* 50(1):291–308, 2009.

Lloyd D, Gabe S, Windsor A: Nutrition and management of enterocutaneous fistula. *Br J Surg* 93(9):1045, 2006.

Lok ASF, McMahon B: AASLD practice guidelines: chronic hepatitis B update. *Hepatology* 50(3):1–36, 2009.

Marinis A, Gkiokas G, Anastasopoulos G, et al: Surgical techniques for the management of enterocutaneous fistulae. *Surg Infect* 10(1):1, 2009.

McPhee SJ: Disorders of the exocrine pancreas. In McPhee SJ, Ganong WF, editors: *Pathophysiology of disease: an introduction to clinical medicine*, ed 5. New York, 2006, McGraw-Hill.

McQuaid KR: Gastrointestinal disorders. In McPhee J, Papadakis M, editors: *Current medical diagnosis and treatment*, ed 48. New York, 2009, McGraw-Hill.

Minei J, Champine J: Abdominal abscesses and gastrointestinal fistula. In Feldman M, Friedman L, Brandt J, editors: *Sleisenger and Fordtran's Gastrointestinal and liver disease: pathophysiology, diagnosis, management*, ed 8, Philadelphia, 2006, Saunders Elsevier.

Ojiako K, Shingala H, Schorr C, et al: Famotidine versus pantoprazole for preventing bleeding in the upper intestinal tract of critically ill patients receiving mechanical ventilation. *Am J Crit Care* 17(2):142, 2008.

Peralta R, Genuit T, Napolitano LM, et al: Peritonitis and abdominal sepsis. *eMedicine.* http://emedicine.medscape.com/article/192329-overview

Polson J, Lee WM: AASLD position paper: The management of acute liver failure. *Hepatology* 41(5):1179–1197, 2005.

Rockey DC: Gastrointestinal bleeding. In Sleisenger MH, Feldman M, Fordtran JS, et al, editors: *Sleisenger and Fordtran's Gastrointestinal and liver disease: pathophysiology, diagnosis, management*, ed 8. Philadelphia, 2006, Saunders.

Rockey DC, Caldwell SH, Goodman ZD, et al: AASLD position paper: Liver biopsy. *Hepatology* 49(3):1017–1043, 2009.

Runyon BA: AASLD practice guidelines: Management of adult patients with ascites due to cirrhosis. *Hepatology* 49(6): 2087–2107, 2009.

Sass DA, Shakil AO: Fulminant hepatic failure. *Liver Transplantation* 11:594–605, 2005.

Schmidt LE, Larsen FS: MELD score as a predictor of liver failure and death in patients with acetaminophen-induced liver injury. *Hepatology* 45(3):789, 2007.

Sharma P, Rakela J: Management of pre-liver transplantation patients: part 1. *Liver Transplantation* 11(2):124–133, 2005.

Sharma P, Rakela J: Management of pre-liver transplantation patients: part 2. *Liver Transplantation* 11(3):249–260, 2005.

Singh R: Evaluation of nutritional status by different parameters and to predict spontaneous closure, morbidity and mortality in patients with enterocutaneous fistulas: a study of 92 cases. *Internet J Nutr Wellness* 6(1):7, 2008. www.cinahl.com/cgi-bin/refsvc?jid=3425&accno=2010062282

Siow E: Enteral versus parenteral nutrition for acute pancreatitis. *Crit Care Nurse* 28(4):19, 2008.

Spear M: Wet-to-dry dressings: evaluating the evidence. *Plast Surg Nursing* 28(2):92, 2008.

Stravitz RT: Critical management decisions in patients with acute liver failure. *Chest* 134:1092, 2008.

Thomson A: Nutritional support in acute pancreatitis. *Curr Opin Clin Nutr Metab Care* 11:261–266, 2008.

Twedell D: Acute pancreatitis. *J Cont Educ Nursing* 39(8):341, 2008.

Wiggins KJ, Craig JC, Johnson DW, et al: Treatment for peritoneal dialysis-associated peritonitis. *Cochrane Database Syst Rev.* http://www.mrw.interscience.wiley.com/cochrane/clsysrev/articles/CD005284/frame.html

Zaragoza AM, Tenias JM, et al: Prognostic factors in gastrointestinal bleeding due to peptic ulcer. *J Clin Gastroenterol* 42(7):786, 2008.

Zhao Y, Encinosa W: Hospitalizations for gastrointestinal bleeding in 1998 and 2006, Healthcare Cost and Utilization Project, Agency for Healthcare Research and Quality, Statistical Brief #65: 2008. http://www.hcup-us.ahrq.gov/reports/statbriefs/sb65.jsp

GENERAL HEMATOLOGY ASSESSMENT

Goal of Assessment

The goal of a basic hematology assessment is to identify assessment and historical factors that correlate with findings on the complete blood count (CBC) to assist in diagnosing a hematologic disorder. Correlation of findings helps with diagnosis and treatment of anemias, allergies, bleeding and clotting disorders, infections, and cancer (especially in patients requiring chemotherapy). The use of many medications and chemotherapy may have a negative effect on the bone marrow, resulting in reduced production of cells reflected on the CBC.

Observation

Changes in various blood components place patients at higher risk for infection, fatigue, weakness, lethargy, bleeding, and clotting. Patients may report:

- *General*: Chills, night sweats, altered mental status, confusion, restlessness, vertigo, visual changes
- *Pain*: Painful lymph nodes, painful joints, sore throat, sinusitis, headaches, abdominal pain
- *Respiratory*: Shortness of breath, exertional or chronic dyspnea, cough, hemoptysis, orthopnea
- *Cardiovascular*: Activity intolerance, dizziness, palpitations, chest discomfort, painful legs, swollen legs
- *Skin*: Unusual bruising, itching, paleness, jaundice, grayness, ulcers, difficulty stopping bleeding from small cuts
- *Musculoskeletal*: Swollen and/or tender joints, sore muscles, weakness
- *Gastrointestinal*: Decreased appetite, feeling of fullness, hematemesis, melena, black stools, "coffee grounds" stomach secretions, weight loss, diarrhea, constipation
- *Genitourinary*: Cystitis, hematuria, heavy menstrual periods, enlarged groin lymph nodes

History

Patients at risk of hematologic or immunologic problems may report having the following disorders:

- *Infections*: Recent or recurrent; prior blood transfusion
- *Allergies*: Foods, beverages, medications, plants, animals, birds, fish, detergents, household cleaners, fragrances, seasonal patterns of respiratory symptoms
- *Immunologic compromise*: Cancer, human immunodeficiency virus (HIV), liver or renal disorders; prior splenectomy, diabetes mellitus, rheumatoid arthritis, systemic lupus erythematosus, Sjögren syndrome, Hashimoto thyroiditis
- *Healing*: Prolonged bleeding or delayed healing with prior surgeries, including dental procedures
- *Presence of foreign bodies*: Prosthetic heart valves, inferior vena caval (IVC) filter, implantable defibrillators or other cardiac devices, vascular access devices
- *Social history*: Multiple sexual partners, excessive alcohol consumption, exposure to chemicals or radiation

- *Medications, including over-the-counter medications:* Aspirin, aspirin-containing drugs, nonsteroidal anti-inflammatory drugs (NSAIDs); glucocorticoids/steroids, anticoagulants, platelet inhibitors (e.g., clopidogrel), chemotherapy, hormone therapy, oral contraceptives

Commonly Reviewed Components of the Complete Blood Count (CBC)

Parameters	Significance	Normal Values
Hemoglobin (Hgb)	Protein in red blood cells containing iron which carries oxygen to tissues	14–18 g/dL (males) 12–16 g/dL (female)
Hematocrit (Hct)	The percentage of red blood cells in the bloodstream. When the Hct is too low, those with anemia may experience fatigue.	42%–52% (male) 37%–47% (female)
White blood cells (WBCs)	Cells of the immune system that protect the body from bacterial, fungal, and viral infections. Incidence of infection increases when WBCs are decreased.	5000–10,000/mm^3
Absolute neutrophil count (ANC)	The number of neutrophils (mature white cells) in the blood. Neutrophils are a type of WBC that help fight infection. When ANC decreases, the patient is neutropenic and more prone to infection. Risk of infection increases when the ANC falls below 2000 and the greatest risk is below 500 — a "right shift" on the WBC differential.	2000/mm^3 and above
WBC differential	Measures the percentage of each type of WBC in the total WBC count — a "left shift." Indicates a large percentage of WBCs are neutrophils; indicates the bone marrow has been stimulated by a severe infection to produce neutrophils to fight the infection. *Bands* are immature neutrophils. *"Right shift"*: Indicates a small percentage of WBCs are neutrophils, putting the patient at higher risk for an infection; neutropenia. *Eosinophilia:* Increased eosinophils indicate an allergic reaction is present. *Monocytes and lymphocytes:* Act as "backup" to the neutrophils. Percentages increase during infection when oncology patients begin bone marrow recovery. If levels do not rise and then fall in a normal pattern, this can be a indication the patient has a poor prognosis for recovery.	Neutrophils: 50%–62% Bands: 3%–6% Monocytes: 3%–7% Basophils: 0%–1% Eosinophils: 0%–3% Lymphocytes: 25%–40%
Platelets (thrombocytes)	Cells that form the matrix on which blood clots are formed	150,000–400,000/mm^3

Information specific to hematologic and/or immunologic findings for each section is presented in disease-specific sections. The basic assessment can be a part of every patient's assessment to determine the risk of development or presence of a hematologic or immunologic disorder.

ANAPHYLACTIC SHOCK

PATHOPHYSIOLOGY

Anaphylaxis (anaphylactic shock) is a potentially life-threatening condition resulting from an exaggerated or hypersensitive response to an antigen or allergen. The classic presentation occurs in a sensitized person (i.e., someone who has been exposed previously to the same antigen), within 1 to 20 minutes of exposure to the antigenic substance, most often drugs, foods, insect stings or bites, antisera, and blood products. The hypersensitive response results in airway inflammation that causes obstruction and respiratory distress, which can lead to respiratory arrest, with a relative hypovolemia caused by massive vasodilation. Fluids shift from the vasculature into interstitial spaces, creating a false hypovolemia or vasogenic (vasodilated) shock, which progresses to end-organ dysfunction secondary to tissue hypoxia from poor perfusion.

The hypersensitivity response occurs primarily on the surface of the mast cells of the lungs, small blood vessels, and connective tissue. The antigen combines with sensitized antibodies from previous exposure (usually immunoglobulin E [IgE] type) and attaches to basophils circulating in the blood. Inflammatory mediators are then released from the granules within the cells, including histamine, serotonin, kinins, and eosinophil and neutrophil chemotactic factors. *Histamine* is the primary mediator of an anaphylactic response. Activation of histamine receptors causes increased capillary permeability, increased pulmonary secretions, bronchoconstriction, and systemic vasodilation.

The antigen-antibody complexes activate production of prostaglandins and leukotrienes, which are termed *slow-reacting substances of anaphylaxis (SRSA)*—chemical mediators that produce systemic effects with potentially deleterious results, including profound shock. The *leukotrienes* produce severe bronchoconstriction and cause venule dilation and increased vascular permeability. The *prostaglandins* exaggerate bronchoconstriction and potentiate the effects of histamine on vascular permeability and pulmonary secretions. *Kinins* contribute to bronchoconstriction, vasodilation, and increased vascular permeability. Eosinophilic chemotactic factor of anaphylaxis (ECFA) is then released to attract eosinophils, which work to neutralize mediators such as histamine, but the amount of neutralization is ineffective in reversing the anaphylaxis. (See Figure 10-1 for a depiction of the pathophysiologic process of anaphylaxis.)

Researchers have made a distinction between "true anaphylaxis" and "pseudo-anaphylaxis" or an "anaphylactoid reaction." The symptoms, treatment, and mortality risk are identical, but "true" anaphylaxis results directly from degranulation of mast cells or basophils mediated by immunoglobulin E (IgE). Pseudo-anaphylaxis results from the other causes. Differential diagnosis is based on studying the allergic reaction.

ASSESSMENT: ANAPHYLACTIC SHOCK
Goal of System Assessment
- *Assess the symptoms*: Assess for ineffective breathing patterns, impaired gas exchange and airway obstruction, along with altered tissue perfusion related to vasodilation and third spaced intravascular fluids. Symptoms vary with means of antigen entry.
- *Classify severity of reaction*: Should be determined following initial assessment. Treatment must begin immediately; prior to when diagnostic test results are available. Shock may progress rapidly to circulatory collapse and cardiopulmonary arrest if improperly managed.
  - *Severity of reaction*: Varies with the means of antigen entry, the amount absorbed, rate of absorption, and the degree of hypersensitivity. Dramatic symptoms usually develop within minutes and progress rapidly. More rapid onset correlates with more severe symptoms.
- *Evaluate effectiveness of prior treatments*: Determine patient's prior treatment regime if asthmatic; classify which "step" of treatment has been needed to control symptoms; patient may need to move to the next step of treatment to maintain control (see *Acute Asthma Exacerbation*, p 354).

History and Risk Factors
Recent exposure to:
- *Pharmacologic agents*: Penicillin, anesthetics, vaccines, contrast media
- *Allergenic foods*: Seafood, shellfish, nuts, grains, dairy products
- *Insect bites or stings*: Wasps, hornets, bees, fire ants
- *Latex*
- *Recent blood transfusion*

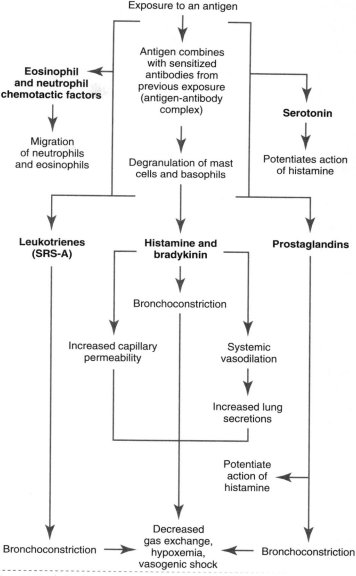

Figure 10-1 Pathophysiologic process of anaphylaxis. (Major chemical mediators are in boldface print.) *SRS-A*, Slow-reacting substance of anaphylaxis.

Vital Signs

- *Pulse oximetry:* Oxygen saturation is decreased from patient's baseline value.
- *Tachycardia* (heart rate [HR] greater than 140 beats/min [bpm]) and tachypnea (respiratory rate [RR] greater than 40 breaths/min)
- *Hypotension* may be present; hypotension is exacerbated by underlying vasodilation coupled with increased capillary permeability prompting third spacing of intravascular fluids.

Observation (see Table 10-1)

- Red to purple discoloration of face and body; "extreme flushing" with swelling of lips, eyelids, and face due to angioedema
- Tears coming from eyes with strained facial expression
- Severe reactions render patients unable to speak due to breathlessness
- Use of accessory muscles; fatigued, with or without diaphoresis
- Chest expansion may be decreased or restricted.
- Altered level of consciousness (LOC) (confusion, disorientation, agitation)
- Agitation is more commonly associated with hypoxemia while somnolence is associated with hypercarbia (elevated carbon dioxide level).
- *General early indicators* (occurring within seconds to minutes) include uneasiness, lightheadedness, tingling feeling, flushing, and pruritus.
- *General late indicators* (occurring within minutes) include rapid progression of urticaria involving large areas of skin; angioedema (tissue swelling; more commonly the eyes, lips, tongue, hands, feet, and genitalia); cough, hoarseness, dyspnea, and respiratory distress; lightheadedness or syncope; and abdominal cramps, diarrhea, and vomiting
- *Ingestion of antigen:* Cramping, diarrhea, nausea, and vomiting may precede systemic shock symptoms.
- *Inhalation of antigen:* Cough, hoarseness, wheezing, dyspnea
- *Allergic reaction:* Edema, urticaria, itching at the site of a bee sting or drug injection

Auscultation

- Wheezing bronchial breath sounds
- Chest may be nearly silent if airflow is severely obstructed.

Palpation

- Palpate to assess for chest expansion; chest may be hyperinflated if patient is asthmatic.
- Decreased tactile fremitus may be present if patient is asthmatic.

Table 10-1	SYSTEMIC EFFECTS OF ANAPHYLAXIS	
System	**Effects**	**Cause**
Neurologic	Apprehension; headache; confusion; decreased LOC progressing to coma	Vasodilation; hypoperfusion; cerebral hypoxia or cerebral edema occurring with interstitial fluid shifts
Respiratory	Dyspnea progressing to air hunger and complete respiratory obstruction; hoarseness; noisy breathing; high-pitched, "barking" cough; wheezes; crackles; rhonchi; decreasing breath sounds; pulmonary edema (some patients)	Laryngeal edema; bronchoconstriction; increased pulmonary secretions
Cardiovascular	Decreased BP leading to profound hypotension; increased HR; decreased amplitude of peripheral pulses; palpitations and dysrhythmias (atrial tachycardias, premature atrial beats, atrial fibrillation, premature ventricular beats progressing to ventricular tachycardia, or ventricular fibrillation); lymphadenopathy	Increased vascular permeability; systemic vasodilation; decreased cardiac output with decreased circulating volume; reflex increase in HR; vasogenic shock
Renal	Increased or decreased urine output; incontinence	Decreased renal perfusion; smooth muscle contraction of urinary tract
Gastrointestinal	Nausea, vomiting, diarrhea, abdominal cramping	Smooth muscle contraction of GI tract; increased mucus secretion
Cutaneous	Urticaria; angioedema (hands, lips, face, feet, genitalia); itching; erythema; flushing; cyanosis	Histamine-induced disruption of cutaneous vasculature; vasodilation, increased capillary permeability; decreased oxygen saturation

BP, Blood pressure; *HR,* heart rate; *GI,* gastrointestinal; *LOC,* level of consciousness.

Percussion

- May reveal hyperresonance (pneumothorax), a complication of asthma (if present)

Diagnostic Tests for Anaphylaxis

The diagnosis of anaphylaxis is based on presenting signs and symptoms. Treatment should be initiated before laboratory results are available.

Test	Purpose	Abnormal Findings
Arterial blood gas analysis (ABG)	Assess for abnormal gas exchange or compensation for metabolic derangements. Initially, Pao_2 is normal and then decreases as the ventilation-perfusion mismatch becomes more severe.	*pH changes:* Acidosis may reflect respiratory failure; alkalosis may reflect tachypnea; *Carbon dioxide:* Elevated CO_2 reflects respiratory failure; decreased CO_2 reflects tachypnea; rising Pco_2 is an ominous sign, since it signals severe hypoventilation which can lead to respiratory arrest. *Hypoxemia:* Pao_2 <80 mm Hg *Oxygen saturation:* Sao_2 <92%
Complete blood count (CBC) with WBC differential	WBC differential evaluates the strength of the immune system's response to the trigger of response	*Eosinophils:* Increased in patients not receiving corticosteroids; indicative of magnitude of inflammatory response *Hematocrit (Hct):* May be increased from hypovolemia and hemoconcentration
Tryptase level	Assesses for this chemical mediator released by mast cells following anaphylaxis	Increases within 1 hour following anaphylaxis and remains elevated for 4–6 hours
IgE levels	Used to confirm origin of the reaction is an allergic response	Levels are elevated if allergic response is present.
12-Lead electrocardiogram (ECG)	To detect dysrhythmias reflective of myocardial ischemia	Ischemic changes (ST depression) may be present as shock progresses.

COLLABORATIVE MANAGEMENT (see Figure 10-2)
Care Priorities

Prevention: The goal of management of patients with severe allergies is to control the allergic response using a stepped approach to therapies and/or to prevent exposure to the antigen. Ideally, patients should be educated regarding avoidance of the allergen, but for those with severe allergies, avoidance may not be possible for all substances, such as various substances in the air. For asthmatics, ideal control is attained when patients are free of daytime symptoms, do not awaken breathless or coughing at night, and have few or no limitations on activities. For those with allergies to insects, immunotherapy with hymenoptera venoms is used worldwide as an effective treatment for most patients hypersensitive to stings from bees, wasps, hornets, yellow jackets, or white faced hornets or bites from fire ants. A vaccine to prevent anaphylaxis from peanuts and tree nuts shows promise as a way to prevent allergic individuals from developing anaphylaxis. The Food and Drug Administration has not yet approved the vaccine.

When prevention fails, the potential for life-threatening respiratory failure is high during exacerbations unresponsive to treatment within the first hour. Management is directed toward decreasing bronchospasm and increasing ventilation. Other interventions are directed toward treatment of complications.

1. **Maintain a patent airway:** Early, rapid endotracheal intubation should be done to manage rapidly progressing laryngeal edema. Severe laryngeal edema may cause complete airway obstruction in minutes. A tracheostomy or an emergency cricothyroidotomy is necessary if endotracheal intubation is not possible.
2. **Provide supplemental oxygen:** Administered to support ventilation and aerobic metabolism. Amount and method of oxygen administration are guided by arterial blood gas (ABG) results. Often initiated at 6 L/min via nasal cannula or oxygen mask.

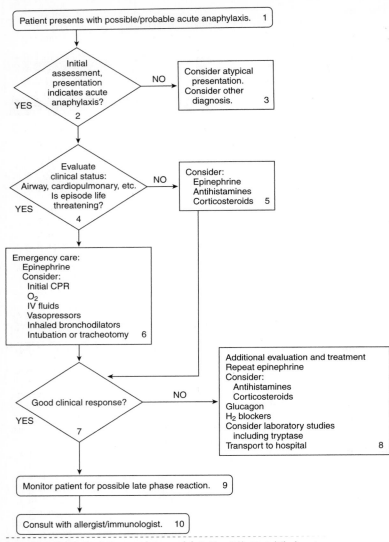

Figure 10-2 Algorithm for the treatment of acute anaphylaxis. (From Nicklas RA, et al: The diagnosis and management of anaphylaxis. *J Allergy Clin Immunol* 101(6 Pt 2):S465–S528, 1998.)

3. Manage vasodilation and increased capillary permeability
   a. *Epinephrine:* Epinephrine reverses anaphylaxis by increasing myocardial contractility, dilating bronchioles, constricting blood vessels, inhibiting histamine release, and counteracting histamine. Dosage and route vary.

 Safety Alert *Individuals taking beta adrenergic blocking agents such as propranolol may not respond as rapidly as expected to epinephrine and may require higher or additional dosing. Glucagon may help to counteract the effects of beta-blocking drugs.*

- *Standard adult dose:* 0.2 to 0.5 mg (0.2 to 0.5 ml of a 1:1000 solution) given intra-muscularly (IM) or subcutaneously (SC)
- *Alternate initial dose:* 0.1 mg (0.1 ml of a 1:1000 solution) may be administered.
- *Repeat dosage:* may be repeated every 10 to 15 minutes as needed
- *IV dosage:* preferred if patient is in shock and/or has severe airway obstruction: Initial dose of 0.1 to 0.25 mg (1.0 to 2.5 ml of 1:10,000 solution) over 5 to 10 minutes. The dose may be increased to 0.3 to 0.5 mg. Repeat every 5 to 15 minutes as needed.
- *IV infusion:* after initial dose, an IV drip of epinephrine 1.0 mg in 250 ml D_5W may be infused at 1 mcg/min and increased to 4 mcg/min (or more) as needed to achieve desired response.
- *Endotracheal (ET) tube:* 1.0 to 2.5 ml of 1:10,000 solution (1 mg epinephrine in 10-ml solution) into ET tube, followed by use of manual resuscitation (Ambu) bag. May repeat if needed.

   b. *Fluid resuscitation:* IV crystalloids (e.g., lactated Ringer, 0.9% normal saline) and/or colloids (e.g., albumin and plasma protein fraction) to increase intravascular volume. Colloids increase colloid osmotic pressure to help retain fluid in the blood vessels. May require rapid infusion of 2 to 3 L of fluids.

   c. *Vasopressors:* Used if fluid replacement does not increase blood pressure (BP). Drugs are titrated for the desired response (see Appendix 6). Usual dosages are as follows:
   - *Dopamine hydrochloride:* Effects are dose dependent. Increases cardiac contractility at 5 to 10 mcg/kg/min and systemic vascular resistance at 10 to 20 mcg/kg/min. Consider switching to norepinephrine if dose exceeds 20 mcg/kg/min.
   - *Norepinephrine:* Initial dosage is 2 to 8 mcg/min and can be increased to achieve the necessary BP.
   - *Phenylephrine:* Usual dosage is 40 to 60 mcg/min. Doses exceeding 200 mcg/min have been used.

   d. *Antihistamines: Diphenhydramine:* Usual dose is 20 to 50 mg, but 50 to 100 mg may be given IV or IM to relieve urticaria and abdominal cramping. IV H_2-antagonists (e.g., cimetidine, ranitidine) are also used.

   e. *Corticosteroids:* Used to help decrease release of chemical mediators that increase capillary permeability. *Hydrocortisone sodium succinate:* loading dose is 100 to 1000 mg IV; or *methylprednisolone sodium succinate:* loading dose is 125 to 250 mg IV. Followed by IV or oral (PO) corticosteroids for several days.

   f. *Inhaled bronchodilators (e.g., albuterol):* May be given for continued bronchospasm (see *Acute Asthma Exacerbation,* p. 354).

   g. *Glucagon IV bolus:* Use is controversial for counteracting effects of beta-blocking drugs or for other patients who have limited response to treatment. Relaxes smooth muscle and increases HR and force of contraction.

4. **ECG monitoring:** To detect dysrhythmias

CARE PLANS FOR ANAPHYLAXIS AND ANAPHYLACTIC SHOCK

Ineffective airway clearance *related to airway obstruction secondary to bronchoconstriction, increased secretions from the histamine response, and presence of leukotrienes and prostaglandins*

GOALS/OUTCOMES Within 20 minutes of treatment/intervention, patient has adequate spontaneous tidal and expiratory volumes as evidenced by easier breathing; audible breath sounds in expected range, and no adventitious breath sounds.

NOC Respiratory Status: Ventilation, Vital Signs Status, Respiratory Status: Airway Patency, Symptom Control Behavior, Comfort Level, Endurance

Airway Management

1. *Assess continuously for obstructed airway and increased respiratory effort:* Note increased pulmonary secretions, cough, expiratory wheezing, SOB, and dyspnea. Suction as needed. *Caution:* An oral airway provides airway support only as far as the posterior pharynx. If laryngeal edema is present, the oral airway cannot relieve symptoms because the obstruction is below the oral airway. If ET intubation is attempted and is not possible due to laryngeal edema, prepare for tracheostomy or cricothyroidotomy.

2. *Monitor for decreased breath sounds or changes in wheezing at frequent intervals:* Absent breath sounds in a distressed patient may indicate impending respiratory arrest. Identify patient requiring actual/potential airway

insertion. Consult physician and prepare for ET intubation if lingual edema is present and/or respiratory distress continues.

3. *Position patient for comfort and to promote optimal gas exchange:* High Fowler's position, with the patient leaning forward and elbows propped on the over-the-bed table to promote maximal chest excursion, may reduce use of accessory muscles and diaphoresis due to work of breathing. May not be possible with severe hypotension, as further decrease in BP may result.

Ventilation Assistance
1. *Monitor for signs of increasing hypoxia at frequent intervals:* Restlessness, agitation, and personality changes are indicative of severe reaction. Cyanosis of the lips (central) and nail beds (peripheral) are late indicators of hypoxia, but may be difficult to see with severe angioedema.
2. *Monitor for signs of hypercapnia at frequent intervals:* Confusion, listlessness, and somnolence are indicative of respiratory failure.
3. *Provide medications to abate allergic response:* Administer epinephrine and IV and inhaled bronchodilators as appropriate to attain control of deterioration.

NIC Airway Insertion and Stabilization; Airway Management; Anaphylaxis Management; Medication Administration, Medication Management, Respiratory Monitoring

---

Impaired gas exchange *related to alveolar-capillary membrane changes secondary to increased capillary permeability associated with histamine response*

GOALS/OUTCOMES Within 20 minutes of initiation of treatment/intervention, patient has adequate alveolar exchange of CO_2 or O_2 as evidenced by easier breathing, PaO_2 80 mm Hg or greater, and SpO_2 90% or greater.
NOC Respiratory Status: Ventilation

Anaphylaxis Management
1. *Monitor* FIO_2 *to ensure that oxygen is within prescribed concentrations.* If patient does not retain carbon dioxide, 100% nonrebreather mask may be used to provide maximal oxygen support. If the patient retains CO_2 and is unrelieved by positioning, lower-dose oxygen, bronchodilators and steroids, intubation, and mechanical ventilation may be necessary sooner than in patients who are able to receive higher doses of oxygen by mask.
2. *Monitor ABGs when continuous pulse oximetry values or patient assessment reflects progressive hypoxemia or development of hypercapnia.* Monitor and report ABG values with increasing $PaCO_2$ (greater than 50 mm Hg) or decreasing PaO_2 (less than 60 mm Hg) indicative of impending respiratory failure.
3. Administer antihistamines as prescribed.
4. Administer glucocorticoids as prescribed.
5. Position patient to alleviate dyspnea (assist patient to sitting position if BP is stable).
6. Stay with patient to promote safety and reduce fear. Use calm, reassuring approach.

NIC Respiratory Monitoring; Emotional Support; Medication Administration, Medication Management

---

Decreased cardiac output *related to decreased preload and afterload secondary to vasodilation and increased capillary permeability*

GOALS/OUTCOMES Within 4 hours of initiation of treatment, patient has adequate cardiac output (CO) as evidenced by BP 90/60 mm Hg or greater, strong peripheral pulses, CO 4 L/min or greater, CI 2.5 L/min/m^2 or greater, SVR 900 dynes/sec/cm^{-5} or greater, urinary output 0.5 ml/kg/hr or greater, and normal sinus rhythm on ECG.
NOC Circulation Status; Tissue Perfusion: Cardiac; Vital Signs

Hemodynamic Regulation
1. Assess for physical and hemodynamic indicators of decreased cardiac output:
   - Palpate peripheral pulses for decreasing amplitude.
   - Assess arterial BP or MAP for any decrease, an indicator of failed compensatory mechanisms.
   - Monitor SVR. A decrease (less than 800 dynes/sec/cm^{-5}) is associated with decreased afterload (vasodilation) and may precipitate decreased CO.
   - Monitor CO, ScVO2 and cardiac index if available. A CI of less than 2.0 L/min/m^2 and ScVO2 less than 80% are usually associated with hypoperfusion.

- *Hemodynamic measurements:* As vasogenic shock evolves, decreased arterial BP, mean arterial pressure (MAP), CO (less than 4 L/min), CI (less than 2.5 L/min), systemic vascular resistance (SVR) (less than 800 dynes/sec/cm^{-5}), and pulmonary artery wedge pressure (PAWP) (less than 5 mm Hg) are present from worsening vasodilation, progressive shifting of intravascular fluid to interstitial spaces, and decreasing venous return.

2. Monitor for dysrhythmias, such as atrial tachycardias, PVCs, ventricular tachycardia, and ventricular fibrillation, which may signal hypoxemia or occur as side effects of drugs such as aminophylline or epinephrine.
3. Monitor for increases and decreases in edema.

> **Safety Alert** *Continued swelling, despite treatment, may indicate ineffective treatment, overaggressive fluid therapy, or heart or kidney failure.*

4. Administer epinephrine as prescribed. Observe for therapeutic effects as evidenced by increased SVR, increased CO/CI, increased ScVO2, increased arterial BP and MAP, stronger peripheral pulses, warming of extremities, and increased urine output.
5. Administer fluid replacement therapy as prescribed, using a large-bore IV catheter. Colloids and crystalloids may be given together.

> **Safety Alert** *During fluid resuscitation, assess patient for indicators of fluid volume excess, including crackles with chest auscultation, presence of S_3 heart sounds, and jugular venous distention. If hemodynamic monitoring lines are present, be alert to increasing PAP, PAWP, and right atrial pressure (RAP).*

6. Prepare for possible vasopressor infusion if hypotension persists after fluid resuscitation and epinephrine administration.

NIC Anaphylaxis Management; Hypovolemia Management; Medication Administration, Medication Management, Cardiac Care: Acute

Altered tissue perfusion: peripheral, renal, and cerebral *related to hypovolemia secondary to fluid shift from the vascular space to the interstitial space*

GOALS/OUTCOMES Within 4 hours of initiation of treatment, patient has adequate perfusion as evidenced by strong proximal peripheral pulses, brisk capillary refill, warm extremities temperature, urinary output 0.5 ml/kg/hr or greater, uncompromised neurologic status, and no restlessness, listlessness, and unexplained anxiety.
NOC Tissue Perfusion: Abdominal Organs, Tissue Perfusion: Peripheral; Tissue Perfusion: Cerebral

Hypovolemia Management

1. Assess peripheral pulses. Report decreased amplitude of pulses.
2. Assess capillary refill. Delayed capillary refill (greater than 2 seconds) is likely with edema and decreased vascular volume.
3. Assess degree of peripheral edema.
4. Assess color and warmth of extremities. Report presence of coolness and pallor.
5. Monitor BP at frequent intervals. Be alert for indicators of hypotension such as BP readings greater than 20 mm Hg below patient's normal pressure, dizziness, restlessness, altered mentation, and decreased urinary output.
6. Monitor urine output hourly. Continuous CO monitoring using a noninvasive system or a pulmonary artery catheter may be needed to guide fluid resuscitation.
7. Observe for indicators of decreased cerebral perfusion such as anxiety, restlessness, confusion, and decreased LOC.

> **HIGH ALERT!** Changes in LOC may signal either decreased cerebral perfusion (tissue hypoxia) or increasing intracranial pressure (IICP) caused by interstitial swelling from capillary permeability.

8. Administer fluid and pharmacologic agents as prescribed (see previous nursing diagnosis).

NIC Hemodynamic Regulation; Anaphylaxis Management; Medication Administration, Medication Management

Impaired skin integrity *related to urticaria and angioedema secondary to allergic response*

GOALS/OUTCOMES Within 4 hours of initiation of treatment, patient states urticaria is controlled. Skin remains intact.
NOC Tissue Integrity: Skin and Mucous Membranes

Pruritus Management
1. Assess patient for urticaria (hives) and itching of hands, feet, neck, and genitalia.
2. Administer antihistamines as prescribed to relieve itching.
3. Discourage patient from scratching the skin. If unavoidable, teach patient to use pads of fingertips rather than nails.
4. Apply cool washcloths or covered ice as a soothing measure to irritated and edematous areas.

NIC Environmental Management: Comfort; Medication Administration

Deficient knowledge illness care: severe hypersensitivity reaction, its causes, and its symptoms *related to no prior exposure or incomplete understanding*

GOALS/OUTCOMES By the time of discharge from the critical care unit, patient demonstrates increased knowledge of severe hypersensitivity reactions as evidenced by verbalization of potential causative factors, symptoms of allergic reaction, need to inform health care providers of allergies, importance of wearing medical-alert identification, prescribed treatment modalities when in contact with allergen, and the necessity of informing primary health care provider immediately of any allergic symptoms.
NOC Knowledge: Treatment Regimen; Knowledge: Illness Care; Knowledge: Health Behavior; Knowledge: Disease Process

Teaching: Disease Process
1. Provide information about the antigenic agent that caused the anaphylaxis, including ways to avoid it in the future.
2. Explain need for wearing a medical-alert identification tag or bracelet to identify the allergy.
3. Give information about anaphylaxis emergency treatment kits. Teach patient self-administration technique and the importance of prompt treatment.
4. Stress the importance of seeking treatment immediately if symptoms of allergy occur, including flushing, warmth, itching, anxiety, and hives.
5. Explain the importance of identifying and checking all over-the-counter (OTC) medications for the presence of potential allergens.

NIC Health Education; Risk Identification; Teaching: Prescribed Medication

ADDITIONAL NURSING DIAGNOSES
Also see nursing diagnoses and interventions in *Hemodynamic Monitoring* (p. 75), *Emotional and Spiritual Support of the Patient and Significant Others* (p. 200), and *Mechanical Ventilation* (p. 99).

PROFOUND ANEMIA AND HEMOLYTIC CRISIS

PATHOPHYSIOLOGY
Anemia
Anemia reflects a reduction in total body hemoglobin (Hgb) concentration and is common in critically ill patients. By the third day in an intensive care unit (ICU), 95% of patients have reduced Hgb concentrations. As the Hgb decreases, the oxygen-carrying capacity of the blood

is reduced, resulting in tissue hypoxia unless compensatory mechanisms are adequate to assist the body with oxygen delivery. Anemia may be classified under one of three functional classes after initial evaluation of the CBC and reticulocyte index. (See Table 10-2 for functional classification.)

Hemolytic Crisis

Hemolytic crisis is an acute disorder that frequently accompanies hemolytic anemias. It is characterized by premature pathologic destruction (hemolysis) of red blood cells (RBCs). As RBC destruction accelerates, the oxygen-carrying capacity of the blood decreases, which results in a reduction in the amount of oxygen delivered to the tissues. This hypoxic state produces tissue ischemia and can progress to tissue infarction. Hemolytic episodes can be triggered by both emotional and physiologic states, including stress, trauma, surgery, acute infectious processes, and abnormal immune responses.

ASSESSMENT
Goal of System Assessment
Evaluate for decreased oxygen-carrying capacity with subsequent organ dysfunction due to decreased production or increased destruction or loss of RBCs.

Anemia
Risk factors: Advanced age; environmental exposure to certain chemicals, liver dysfunction, autoimmune or other immunologic disorders, malignancy (and its treatment), drug use (such as aspirin, NSAIDs, warfarin); diets low in protein and iron, iron or folic acid deficiency, B12 deficiency, chronic alcoholism, autoimmune disorders
Clinical presentation (chronic indicators)
- Pallor, melena, hematochezia, fatigue, weight loss, dyspnea on exertion, uremia, sensitivity to cold, intermittent dizziness, excessive menstruation, paresthesias
- *Chronic hemolytic anemia:* Jaundice, renal failure, hematuria, arthritis, increased incidence of gallstones, skin ulcers
Clinical presentation (acute indicators)
- Fever, chest pain, acute heart failure, confusion, irritability, tachycardia, orthostatic hypotension, dyspnea, tachypnea, frank bleeding, critical illness for longer than 3 days
Vital signs
- Tachypnea, orthopnea, tachycardia, fever

Table 10-2	FUNCTIONAL CLASSES OF ANEMIA WITH EXAMPLES	
Blood Loss/Hemolysis	**Decreased RBC Production**	**Maturation Disorders**
Autoimmune diseases Thrombotic Thrombocytopenia Purpura (TTP), Goodpasture's Syndrome, Systemic Lupus Erythematosus (SLE), Wegener's Granulomatosis	Damaged bone marrow: malignancy, lead poisoning, aplastic/hypoplastic anemia, chemotherapy, viruses	Abnormal RBC cytoplasm Phenylketonuria (PKU), G6PD
Abnormal hemoglobin Sickle cell disease, Hgb S, C D, E	Iron deficiency: malignancy, autoimmune disorders	Abnormal RBC nucleus
Abnormal RBC membranes Spherocytosis, hemolytic uremic syndrome, paroxysmal nocturnal hematuria	Erythropoietin deficiency: renal failure, malaria, thalassemias	Iron deficiency: dietary, chronic alcoholism
Bleeding/hemorrhage Physical trauma to blood (bypass, balloon, valves), antibodies (drug-induced antibodies), endotoxins (malaria, clostridia), GI bleed, trauma, rupture, excess menstruation	Inflammation/infection: chronic inflammatory disease; critical illness	
Excessive phlebotomies: lab sampling	Metabolic disturbance: pernicious anemia, hypothyroidism, megaloblastic anemia	

Observation
- Altered mental status, unusual fatigue or weakness
- Spider angiomas, unusual bleeding (i.e., stool, urine, emesis)
- Electrocardiogram (ECG) changes
- Monoarticular or polyarticular arthritis
- Smooth tongue, skin ulcers

Palpation
- Bone tenderness (especially rib and sternal areas), joint tenderness
- Enlargement of the liver and/or spleen

Auscultation
- Crackles associated with heart failure

Hemolytic crisis
Risk factors: Individuals with mild or chronic hemolytic anemia may be asymptomatic until they are exposed to a severe stressor, such as an acute infectious process, profound emotional upset, critical illness, surgery, or trauma. With added stress, hemolysis can accelerate to a crisis state in which patients experience organ congestion from massive amounts of hemolyzed blood cells, precipitating multiple organ dysfunction syndrome (MODS) and shock.

Clinical presentation (acute): Fever; abdominal, chest, joint, and back pain; jaundice; headache; dizziness; palpitations; shortness of breath (SOB); hemoglobinuria; lymphadenopathy; splenomegaly; and signs of peripheral nerve damage including paresthesias, paralysis, chills, and vomiting

Clinical presentation (chronic): Anemia; pallor; fatigue; dyspnea on exertion; mentation changes; icterus; bone infarctions; monoarticular and polyarticular arthritis; hematuria; renal failure; increased gallstone formation; skin ulcers and itching

Vital signs
- Tachypnea, tachycardia, hypertension

Observation
- Impaired growth and development, depending on severity and duration of anemia
- Jaundice; retinal detachment and associated vitreous hemorrhage
- SOB, with dyspnea on exertion
- Monoarticular or polyarticular arthritis
- Hemiplegia, paresthesias

Palpation
- Splenomegaly, hepatomegaly, lymphadenopathy or abdominal guarding
- Chronic skin ulcers, particularly in the ankle area

Auscultation
- Crackles associated with heart failure
- Murmurs related to valvular damage

Diagnostic Tests for Anemias and Hemolytic Crisis		
Test	**Purpose**	**Abnormal Findings**
Red blood cell count (RBCs)	Enumeration of the red cells found in each cubic millimeter of blood	Reduced; in hemolytic crisis, an increased number of premature RBCs (nucleated RBCs) will be present.
Hemoglobin (Hgb)	Hemoglobin content of RBCs	Decreased
Hematocrit (Hct)	Percentage of RBCs in relation to total blood volume	Decreased
Reticulocyte count, reticulocyte index, corrected reticulocyte	RBC precursors; measures how fast RBCs are produced in the bone marrow	Elevated: because of increased bone marrow production of RBCs due to blood loss or RBC destruction; also a sign of marrow recovery after chemotherapy.

Diagnostic Tests for Anemias and Hemolytic Crisis — cont'd

Test	Purpose	Abnormal Findings
Mean corpuscular volume (MCV) (subcategory of red cell indices) Macrocytic: MCV >100 mcg³ Microcytic: MCV <80 mcg³ Normocytic: MCV 80–100 mcg³	Morphologic classification of RBCs: average size of individual RBCs. Obtained by dividing HCT by total RBC count	Low in microcytic anemia; high in macrocytic anemia
Sickle cell test	Indicative of sickle cell anemia (trait, disease)	Presence of Hemoglobin S (Hgb S)
Hemoglobin (Hgb) electrophoresis	Screens for abnormal hemoglobins often present in hemolytic anemias Many hemoglobinopathies are interrelated. Disease expression is based on the degree of genetic abnormalities. Various combinations of abnormal hemoglobins are possible	Hemoglobins A_1, A_2, and F: Normal Hgb Hemoglobin C: Generally benign; May cause joint pain, splenomegaly and gallstones; may protect against malaria Hemoglobins D and E: Rarely occur "singly"; sometimes present with sickle cell disease or thalassemias Hemoglobin H: Causes premature destruction of RBCs and abnormal binding of O_2 to RBCs; causes alpha thallasemia Hemoglobin S: Most common abnormal hemoglobin, occurring in 10% of the African American population; causes sickle cell disease or sickle cell trait
Erythrocyte sedimentation rate (ESR), sedimentation rate or Biernacki reaction	Rate at which RBCs precipitate in a period of 1 hour: nonspecific measure of inflammation	Elevated in hemolytic anemia; decreased in sickle cell anemia, polycythemia and congestive heart failure
C_3 proactivator	Proactivator of complement 3 in the alternate pathway of complement activation	Increased in hemolytic anemia
Total iron-binding capacity (TIBC)	Measures the blood's capacity to bind iron with transferrin; also indirect test of liver function (rarely used for that) TIBC is typically measured along with serum iron to evaluate people suspected of having either iron deficiency or iron overload.	Normal or reduced, depending on the type of anemia
Ferritin	Iron stores: with damage to organs that contain ferritin (especially the liver, spleen, and bone marrow), ferritin levels can become elevated even though the total amount of iron in the body is normal.	Reduced with iron deficiency anemia; normal or elevated with anemia of critical illness; elevated with hemachromatosis
Transferrin	Used to determine the cause of anemia, to examine iron metabolism (for example, in iron deficiency anemia) and to determine the iron-carrying capacity of the blood.	Reduced with anemia of chronic inflammation, anemia of critical illness.

Continued

Diagnostic Tests for Anemias and Hemolytic Crisis—cont'd

Test	Purpose	Abnormal Findings
Transferrin saturation	The iron concentration divided by TIBC—a more useful indicator of iron status than iron or TIBC alone.	Reduced with anemia of chronic inflammation, anemia of critical illness.
Folate; folic acid	Measures folic acid in the blood	Reduced with nutritional deficiency leading to megaloblastic anemia.
Erythropoietin (EPO, EP)	Measures the amount of a hormone called erythropoietin (EPO) in blood; acts on stem cells in the bone marrow to increase the production of red blood cells; made by cells in the kidney, which release the hormone when oxygen levels are low.	Reduced with renal disease and normal in those who are critically ill who should have an elevated level if anemia of any cause is present. Reticulocyte response to EP has been shown to be reduced in many critically ill patients with elevated EP levels.
Vitamin B_{12}	Measures the amount of vitamin B_{12} in the blood; used with folic acid test, because a lack of either can cause megaloblastic anemia.	Reduced with pernicious or megaloblastic anemia.
Unconjugated bilirubin: free bilirubin, indirect bilirubin	Measures bilirubin that has not been conjugated in the liver. It gives an indirect reaction to the Van Den Bergh test.	Elevated in hemolytic anemia due to liver's inability to process increasing bilirubin released during hemolysis.
Serum lactic dehydrogenase isoenzymes (LDH_1 and LDH_2)	General indicator of the existence and severity of acute or chronic tissue damage and, sometimes, as a monitor of progressive conditions; monitor damage caused by muscle trauma or injury and to help identify hemolytic anemia	Elevated in hemolytic anemia because of their release when an RBC is destroyed.
Haptoglobin level	Used to detect and evaluate hemolytic anemia; not to diagnose cause of the hemolysis. Haptoglobin levels should be drawn prior to transfusion.	Decreased in hemolytic anemia due to increased binding of haptoglobin, which facilitates removal of increased Hgb from blood.
Peripheral blood smear	Microscopic examination of cells from drop of blood; investigates hematologic problems or parasites such as malaria and filaria	May reveal abnormally shaped RBCs, such as spherocytes. RBC hyperplasia (abnormal number) is present in nearly all cases of chronic hemolysis with intact bone marrow.
Bone marrow aspiration	Evaluates bone marrow status; diagnose blood disorders and determine if cancer or infection has spread to the bone marrow.	May reveal abnormal size, shape, or amounts of RBCs, WBCs or platelets
Coombs test: Direct antiglobulin test; Indirect antiglobulin test	Detects antibodies that may bind to RBCs and cause premature RBC destruction	Positive in antibody-mediated immunologic hemolysis.
Immunoglobulin levels	Measures the level of immunoglobulins, also known as antibodies, in the blood.	Elevated: autoimmune disorders, sickle cell; lower in immunocompromised states.

Diagnostic Tests for Anemias and Hemolytic Crisis—cont'd

Test	Purpose	Abnormal Findings
Glucose-6-phosphate dehydrogenase (G6PD) levels	Measures G6PD—enzyme levels are normal in newly produced cells but fall as RBCs age and only deficient cells are destroyed.	Decreased in G6PD deficiency, hemolysis Elevated: MI, liver failure, chronic blood loss, hyperthyroidism
Radiologic examinations	X-rays and bone scans Liver/spleen scans	Decreased density, aseptic necrosis of bones Hepatomegaly, splenomegaly, lesions

COLLABORATIVE MANAGEMENT: ANEMIAS
Care Priorities

1. **Oxygen therapy: Administered to relieve SOB or dyspnea:** Methods of oxygen delivery range from nasal cannulas, to various face masks, to mechanical ventilation in severe cases.
2. **Transfusions/blood component replacement:** Packed RBCs may be necessary in the management of profound anemia to help increase the blood's oxygen-carrying capacity. For patients who refuse blood transfusions, aggressive strategies to augment RBC production such as intravenous (IV) iron therapy and subcutaneous administration of erythropoietin may be implemented. These therapies may take up to 7 days or longer to promote significant improvement in the reticulocyte count and Hgb and hematocrit (Hct) levels. The oxygen-carrying capacity of banked blood is best when used within 14 days of collection. Blood transfused more than 21 days after collection has been linked to increased mortality rates in the critically ill, especially HIV-positive patients. Benefits must be weighed against risks, particularly in immunosuppressed patients.

RESEARCH BRIEF 10-1

In a multicenter, prospective study of 284 intensive care units (ICUs) in 213 U.S. hospitals, 4892 enrolled patients were used to quantify the incidence of anemia and red blood cell (RBC) transfusions in critically ill patients and to evaluate clinical outcomes in anemic patients related to RBC transfusions. Anemia was found to be common in the critically ill. While in the ICU, 44% of patients received at least one transfusion. Transfusion practice has remained almost unchanged in the past 10 years. Patients who received transfusions had more total complications, and those with multiple transfusions had longer hospital and ICU length-of-stay, with increased mortality. The number of RBC transfusions was an independent predictor of worse clinical outcome.

From Gould S, Cimino M, Gerber D: Packed red blood cell transfusion in the intensive care unit: limitations and consequences. *Am J Crit Care* 16:39–48, 2007.

---

3. **Volume replacement:** If patient is hypovolemic, aggressive fluid and/or blood replacement is mandatory to prevent profound hypotension and shock. Fluid challenges/boluses also assist in prevention of deposition of hemolyzed RBCs in the microvasculature.
4. **Elimination of causative factor:** Certain drugs and chemicals, cold temperatures, and stress can worsen many anemias, but most profoundly affected are hemolytic and aplastic anemias. Identifying and removing the causative agent can prevent life-threatening crisis. If the patient is bleeding, the cause of the bleeding must be addressed and the bleeding controlled.

5. **Folic acid supplement:** Necessary for RBC production. Supplements of 1 mg/day are used to treat megaloblastic anemia and, theoretically, to prevent hemolytic crisis in patients with hemolytic anemia. It is not effective in all patients with hemolytic anemia.
6. **Iron supplements:** Administered for iron-deficiency states to help increase production of normal-size RBCs. May be given intravenously or enterally. Iron levels must be normal to facilitate the action of erythropoietin injections.
7. **Epoetin alfa/erythropoietin, recombinant (Epogen/Procrit):** Stimulates production of rbcs in patients with bone marrow hypofunction/lack of production of RBCs, particularly when related to renal failure. Has been used as an alternative strategy in patients who refuse blood transfusions (in conjunction with IV iron, if needed) and in anemia associated with critical illness. Critically ill patients may or may not respond to erythropoietin.
8. **Vitamin B$_{12}$:** Administered by injections or IV infusion for management of pernicious anemia, a type of megaloblastic anemia caused by failure of the gastric mucosa to absorb vitamin B$_{12}$.
9. **Bone marrow transplantation:** Recommended for some patients with bone marrow malignancies, sickle cell disease, or aplastic anemia to provide a mechanism for regenerating normal RBC production.

CARE PLANS FOR ANEMIAS

Impaired gas exchange *related to lack of RBCs; hemoglobin abnormalities*

GOALS/OUTCOMES Within 3 to 24 hours of onset of treatment, patient has adequate gas exchange as evidenced by HR and RR within 10% of patient's baseline (or HR 60 to 100 bpm and RR 12 to 20 breaths/min), Hgb and Hct returned to patient's baseline (or Hgb greater than 12 mg/dl and Hct greater than 37%), oxygen saturation greater than 90%, and BP returned to patient's baseline (or greater than 90 mm Hg systolic within 24 hours of initiation of treatment).

NOC Respiratory Status: Gas Exchange; Tissue Perfusion: Pulmonary

Respiratory Monitoring
1. Administer supplemental oxygen, using appropriate device (i.e., nasal cannula, face mask/shield, or mechanical ventilation as necessary). Monitor oxygen liter flow. Provide for oxygen when patient is transported.
2. Monitor rate, rhythm, and depth of respirations.
3. Monitor for increased restlessness, anxiety, and air hunger.
4. Monitor oxygen saturation using pulse oximeter continuously. Consult with physician for persistent values less than 90% or, if oxygen saturation is chronically decreased, a sustained drop of greater than 10% of baseline.
5. Note changes in Sao$_2$, Svo$_2$, ScVO2, StO2 (if available) and changes in arterial blood gas (ABG) values, as appropriate.
6. Maintain large-bore (18-gauge) IV catheter(s) in case transfusion or rapid volume expansion is necessary. Administer intravenous fluids to maintain hydration.
7. Transfuse with packed cells (RBCs) (Table 10-3) as prescribed to facilitate oxygen delivery and assist in volume expansion, and/or implement aggressive strategy to augment RBC production.
8. Describe the purpose of blood product transfusion therapy to the patient and significant others.
9. Carefully evaluate dyspnea and chest pain in patients with sickle cell disease because of the possibility of pulmonary infarction.

NIC Airway Management; Oxygen Therapy; Circulatory Precautions; Cardiac Precautions

Activity intolerance *related to anemia/lack of oxygen-carrying capacity of the blood*

GOALS/OUTCOMES Within 24 hours of onset of treatment, patient's activity tolerance improves as evidenced by HR and RR returning to within 10% of baseline (or HR 60 to 100 bpm and RR 12 to 20 breaths/min) and BP returning to within 10% of patient's baseline (or systolic BP greater than 90% mm Hg). Within 24 hours of initiation of treatment, patient is able to assist minimally with self-care activities.

NOC Endurance; Activity Tolerance

Table 10-3 BLOOD AND BLOOD PRODUCTS*

Product	Volume	Infusion Time	Contents	Possible Complications
Whole blood (rarely used)	500 ml/unit	2–4 hours or <1 hour in emergency	All blood components. If fresh, processed with citrate-phosphate-dextrose (CPD)	Hepatitis, transmission of HIV (human immunodeficiency virus), CMV (cytomegalovirus), EBV (Epstein-Barr virus), and other organisms; transfusion reactions: all types
Packed red blood cells (RBCs)	200–250 ml/unit	1–4 hours or <1 hour in emergency	RBCs	See Whole blood
Fresh-frozen plasma	200–250 ml/unit	20 min to thaw; ½ to 1 hour or <½ hour in emergency	All clotting factors except platelets	See Whole blood
Platelets	35–50 ml/unit	Direct IV push at 30–50 ml/min; may combine or "pool" several bags into one; given in multiple units as quickly as possible	Platelets	Transfusion reaction: febrile or mild allergic; may need to premedicate with acetaminophen (Tylenol) or diphenhydramine HCl (Benadryl); rare instance of septic reaction
Cryoprecipitate	10–20 ml/unit	May need 10–30 units infused at 1 unit/min or 10–20 ml/min	Factor VIII, factor XIII, and fibrinogen	Small possibility of febrile or mild allergic reaction; rare instance of septic reaction
Granulocytes	300 ml/unit	1–2 hours; administer slowly for 5 minutes as test dose	White blood cells (WBC) extracted from 1 unit of whole blood	Transfusion reactions: all types; often ineffective in elevating WBC count
Leukocyte-poor and washed, frozen RBCs	250–300 ml/unit	2 hours or 1–2 hours in emergency	Red cells washed with saline (and possibly irradiated) to remove WBCs and protein from RBCs	Markedly reduced possibility of transfusion reactions: all types
Factor VIII concentrate	10–20 ml/unit	May need >10 units infused at 1 unit/min	Factor VIII (pooled from possibly thousands of donors)	Small possibility of febrile or mild allergic reaction; rare instance of septic reaction
Factor IX concentrate	20–30 ml/unit	May need >10 units infused at 1 unit/min	Factor IX (pooled from possibly thousands of donors)	Small possibility of febrile or mild allergic reaction; rare instance of septic reaction
Volume expanders Albumin (5% or 25%) Plasma protein fraction (PPF) Salt-poor albumin	Varies with each product	1 ml/min or as rapidly as tolerated in shock states	Reconstituted from human blood, plasma, or serum	Possible hypervolemia with rapid infusions, particularly with 25% albumin

*Use correct filter with each blood product; most filters can be used to administer 2–4 units; either piggyback or flush products with normal saline solution only.

Energy Management
1. Alternate periods of rest and activity to avoid stress that increases oxygen demand.
2. Collaborate with occupational therapy (OT), physical therapy (PT), and/or recreational therapy personnel in planning and monitoring an activity program as appropriate.
3. Determine patient's physical limitations. Focus on what patient can do, rather than on deficits.
4. Reposition patient slowly while monitoring effects on myocardial and cerebral perfusion.
5. Reduce fear, pain, and anxiety to decrease oxygen demand.
6. Determine causes of fatigue (e.g., treatments, pain, medications).
7. Monitor nutritional intake to ensure adequate energy resources.
8. Teach patient to avoid stressful situations, which can exacerbate symptoms of anemia and precipitate hemolytic crisis in patients with hemolytic anemia.
9. Teach signs of hypoxemia: altered mental status, activity intolerance, SOB, chest pain, and weakness.
10. Teach patient and significant others about the specific anemia affecting the patient.
11. See this diagnosis in *Prolonged Immobility*, p. 149.

NIC Activity Therapy; Teaching: Prescribed Activity/Exercise

Risk for impaired skin integrity *related to impaired oxygen transport secondary to chronic anemia*

GOALS/OUTCOMES Patient's skin remains intact during hospitalization.
NOC Tissue Integrity: Skin and Mucous Membranes

Pressure Management
1. Keep extremities warm to promote circulation and help prevent tissue hypoxia.
2. Perform a comprehensive appraisal of peripheral circulation (e.g., check peripheral pulses, edema, capillary refill, color, and temperature of extremity).
3. Monitor for sources of pressure and friction.
4. Monitor for infection, especially of edematous areas.
5. Use a bed cradle to reduce pressure of covers on extremities.
6. Monitor skin and mucous membranes for areas of discoloration and bruising.
7. Monitor skin for rashes, abrasions, excessive dryness, and moisture.
8. Provide adequate nutrition and nutritional supplements as appropriate. Negative nitrogen state or low serum protein or albumin increases the risk for skin breakdown.
9. Teach patient the signs of skin breakdown, since it can occur at any time with chronic anemia.
10. Instruct the patient on the importance of preventing venous stasis.
11. Teach patient about appropriate nutrition as discussed in *Nutritional Support*, p. 117.
12. Apply appropriate skin-saving dressing (e.g., Duoderm) or initiate aggressive skin care regimen to areas of breakdown.
13. For additional interventions, see *Wound and Skin Care*, p. 167.

NIC Pressure Ulcer Prevention; Skin Surveillance; Nutrition Management; Circulatory Precautions

COLLABORATIVE MANAGEMENT: HEMOLYTIC CRISIS
Care Priorities
1. **Oxygen therapy:** Administered to relieve SOB or dyspnea. Methods of oxygen delivery range from nasal cannulas, to various face masks, to mechanical ventilation in severe cases.
2. **Pain management:** Aspirin, acetaminophen, NSAIDs, narcotics, and sedatives may be necessary for relief of pain and anxiety associated with hemolytic anemia, particularly during hemolytic crisis.
3. **Volume replacement:** If patient is hypovolemic, aggressive fluid and/or blood replacement is mandatory to prevent profound hypotension and shock. Fluid challenges/boluses also assist in prevention of deposition of hemolyzed RBCs in the microvasculature
4. **Transfusions/blood component replacement:** Packed RBCs may be necessary in the management of profound anemia to help increase the blood's oxygen-carrying capacity. For patients who refuse blood transfusions, aggressive strategies to augment RBC production such as IV iron therapy and subcutaneous administration of erythropoietin

may be implemented. These therapies may take up to 7 days or longer to promote significant improvement in the reticulocyte count and Hgb and Hct levels. The oxygen-carrying capacity of banked blood is best when used within 14 days of collection. Blood transfused more than 21 days after collection has been linked to increased mortality rates in the critically ill, especially HIV-positive patients. Benefits must be weighed against risks, particularly in immunosuppressed patients.

5. **Red cell exchange therapy for sickle cell crisis:** Cytapheresis procedure used to replace sickled RBCs with normal RBCs for patients who are unresponsive to other treatments for sickle cell disease

6. **Thrombocytapheresis:** Cytapheresis procedure for patients experiencing symptoms of excessive thrombosis, to attempt rapid platelet reduction to decrease clotting before onset of MODS (see *Multiple Organ Dysfunction Syndrome* in *SIRS, Sepsis and MODS*, p. 924)

7. **Therapeutic phlebotomy:** Removal of 200 to 500 ml of whole blood from the patient when iron overload exists

8. **Corticosteroids:** Therapy used with limited success in management of hemolytic anemia.

9. **Splenectomy:** Removal of the spleen is sometimes recommended for patients suspected of having splenic sequestration crisis related to hemolytic anemia.

CARE PLANS FOR HEMOLYTIC CRISIS

Ineffective tissue perfusion: peripheral, cardiopulmonary, gastrointestinal, renal, and cerebral *related to interruption of arterial or venous blood flow secondary to formation of microthrombi*

GOALS/OUTCOMES Within 24 hours of institution of treatment, patient has adequate perfusion as evidenced by warm extremities, pink nail beds; peripheral pulses at least 2+ on a scale of 0 to 4+ or patient's baseline, capillary refill less than 2 seconds, BP within 10% of patient's normal range (or systolic BP greater than 90 mm Hg), HR and RR within 10% of patient's baseline (or HR 60 to 100 bpm, RR 12 to 20 breaths/min with a normal depth and pattern), oxygen saturation greater than 90%, urinary output 0.5 ml/kg/hr or greater, and orientation to time, place, and person.
NOC Circulation Status

Circulatory Care: Arterial Insufficiency

1. Initiate aggressive IV fluid volume replacement as prescribed to prevent deposition of hemolyzed RBCs in the microvasculature.

2. Assess extremities for inadequate peripheral perfusion: amplitude of peripheral pulses, coolness, pallor, and prolonged capillary refill. Use Doppler if unable to palpate pulses.

3. Evaluate chest pain. Note cardiac dysrhythmias and symptoms of decreased cardiac output. Monitor respiratory status for symptoms of heart failure.

4. Monitor vital signs frequently for signs of impending shock: increased HR and RR, increased restlessness and anxiety, and cool and clammy skin, followed by a decrease in BP.

5. Monitor abdomen for signs of decreased perfusion.

6. Keep lower extremities elevated slightly to promote venous blood flow.

7. Monitor ventilation and perfusion: assess ABG values for acidosis (i.e., pH less than 7.35, hypercarbia/CO_2 retention [$Paco_2$ greater than 45 mm Hg]), indicating hypoperfusion, and respiratory insufficiency. Assess for hypoxemia using continuous pulse oximetry and $ScVO2$ or $SVO2$ monitoring to detect decreased oxygen saturation. Consult physician or midlevel practitioner for sustained deterioration in status.

8. Monitor urinary output for decrease, which can signal decreased renal perfusion. Consult physician or midlevel practitioner for urine output less than 0.5 ml/kg/hr for 2 consecutive hours.

9. Monitor neurologic status every 2 to 4 hours, using the Glasgow Coma Scale (see Appendix 2).

10. Teach patient and significant others about hemolytic anemia, including the signs of impending hemolytic crisis, rendering information on the following:
    - *Indicators of impending hemolytic crisis:* Fever, abnormal pain, headache, blurred vision, dizziness, change in mentation, unsteady gait, palpitations, paresthesias, and paralysis
    - *Support groups:* Names, telephone numbers, and addresses of other persons/groups that can assist with support of people with hemolytic anemias
    - *Smoking cessation:* Support groups and programs that assist in stopping cigarette smoking to decrease vasoconstriction associated with nicotine intake
    - *Medications:* Drug name, dosage, frequency, and possible side effects, especially related to steroids: increased appetite, weight gain, "moon face," "buffalo hump," increased possibility of infection, headaches, and increased BP. Explain possible steroid-induced diabetes mellitus.

- *Prevention of infection:* Important if patient is on long-term steroid therapy or had a splenectomy. The patient should obtain an annual flu vaccine; practice good personal hygiene; obtain regular dental check-ups; and get adequate rest, sleep, and relaxation. For splenectomy, patients should have a pneumococcal vaccine and wear a medical-alert identification bracelet.

NIC Cardiac Care: Acute; Circulatory Care: Venous Insufficiency; Respiratory Monitoring; Shock Management: Cardiac; Cerebral Perfusion Promotion; Neurologic Monitoring; Peripheral Sensation Management; Fluid/Electrolyte Management; Fluid Management; Vital Signs Monitoring

Acute pain *related to tissue ischemia secondary to vessel occlusion; inflammation/injury secondary to blood within the joints*

GOALS/OUTCOMES Within 1 to 2 hours of initiating treatment, patient's subjective evaluation of discomfort improves as documented by a pain scale; nonverbal indicators of discomfort are reduced or absent.
NOC Pain Control; Pain Level

Pain Management
1. Monitor patient for signs of discomfort, including increases in HR, BP, and RR. Devise a pain scale with patient, rating discomfort from 0 (no pain) to 10.
2. Perform a comprehensive assessment of pain to include location, characteristics, onset/duration, frequency, quality, intensity or severity of pain, and precipitating factors.
3. Medicate for pain as prescribed. Assess effectiveness of medication using the pain scale. Confer with physician if pain relief is ineffective; devise an alternate plan for analgesia.
4. Recognize that components of chronic and acute pain are present and tolerance may be higher than expected for age and size. During a crisis, exacerbation of pain may be unpredictable due to intermittent vessel occlusion, so both baseline and breakthrough medications will be required to achieve pain relief.
5. If pain medication injections are frequent, consider an IV rather than an intramuscular (IM) route, when possible. While quick-acting, meperidine may not be drug of choice due to impact on renal function over time.
6. Administer adjuvant analgesics and/or medications when needed to potentiate analgesia.
7. Consider continuous infusion (alone or with bolus opioids) to maintain serum levels.
8. Collaborate with the physician if drug, dose, route of administration, or interval changes are indicated, making specific recommendations based on equianalgesic principles.
9. Consider complementary method of pain control such as relaxation techniques: guided imagery, controlled breathing, meditation, and listening to soft, soothing music. Use therapeutic/healing touch to relieve pain if practitioner is trained and patient agrees to participate. Alternatively, consult trained practitioner.
10. Control environmental factors that may add to discomfort (e.g., room temperature, light, noise).
11. Apply warm compresses to joints to increase circulation and thereby improve tissue oxygenation.
12. Apply elastic stockings to promote venous return and enhance circulation.
13. Teach patient to perform isometric or range-of-motion (ROM) exercises to promote circulation.
14. Help allay fears by reassuring patient that pain will decrease as the crisis subsides.
15. Provide emotional support to patient during the crisis episode. Reassure patient that the crisis is time-limited, and enable significant others to be with patient, if possible, during the crisis.
16. Teach patient to assess extremities daily for evidence of tissue breakdown or blood sequestration (i.e., swelling, erythema, tenderness) so that early interventions can be implemented in an attempt to prevent severe pain.

NIC Analgesic Administration; Medication Administration; Medication Administration: Intravenous (IV); Heat/Cold Application; Anxiety Reduction; Therapeutic Touch; Music Therapy; Meditation Facilitation

Risk for deficient fluid volume *related to failure of renal regulatory mechanisms of fluid and electrolyte balance secondary to microthrombi occluding the nephrons*

GOALS/OUTCOMES Patient's volume status returns to normal/baseline as evidenced by urinary output more than 0.5 ml/kg/hr, stable weight, BP within patient's normal range, HR 60 to 100 beats/min, RR 12 to 20 breaths/min, good skin turgor, moist mucous membranes, urine specific gravity 1.005 to 1.025, and central venous pressure (CVP) 4 to 6 mm Hg.
NOC Fluid Balance; Electrolyte and Acid-Base Balance

Fluid/Electrolyte Management

1. Monitor intake and output (I&O) hourly. Consult physician or midlevel practitioner for a urinary output less than 0.5 ml/kg/hr for 4 consecutive hours. Insert urinary catheter if patient is unable to void.
2. Monitor and document heart rate, rhythm, pulses, and blood pressure.
3. Evaluate efficacy of volume expansion by closely monitoring CVP. Overzealous volume expansion can lead to heart failure and pulmonary edema, with CVP greater than 20% to 25% of normal values.
4. Administer diuretics as prescribed in the well-hydrated patient with urine output less than 0.5 ml/kg/hr.
5. Assess patient for volume depletion, including poor skin turgor, dry mucous membranes, hypotension, tachycardia, and decreasing urine output and CVP.
6. Monitor electrolytes and serum osmolality. A universal increase in electrolytes and osmolality is indicative of dehydration. A universal decrease signals fluid overload.
7. Assess pH (normal range is 7.35 to 7.45) before replacing electrolytes. Acidosis and alkalosis alter electrolyte values. Replace potassium if the pH is outside the normal range.

NIC Electrolyte Monitoring; Fluid Management; Fluid Monitoring; Intravenous (IV) Therapy; Hypervolemia Management; Shock Management: Volume

ADDITIONAL NURSING DIAGNOSES

Uncontrolled pain, bleeding, and complications of hemolysis can be terrifying to the patient and significant others, who may fear that the patient will die. Chronic illness with episodic acute exacerbations may require more individualized intervention when handling long-term illness and its sequelae. See *Emotional Support of Patient and Significant Others*, p. 200.

BLEEDING AND THROMBOTIC DISORDERS

PATHOPHYSIOLOGY

Bleeding can result from qualitative (dysfunctional) or quantitative (lack of) abnormalities of platelets and/or coagulation factors, including proteins, in the plasma. Thrombocytopenia is common in the critically ill and, like anemia, necessitates differential diagnosis. The cause of thrombocytopenia, rather than simply the decreased numbers of platelets, poses the greatest threat to the critically ill patient. The four main causes of thrombocytopenia are as follows:

1. *Hemodilution:* related to administration of large amounts of retained fluids, IV fluids, multiple medications given in 50- to 100-ml "piggybacks," or blood/blood products
2. *Increased platelet destruction or consumption:* includes heparin-induced thrombocytopenia (HIT); antiphospholipid antibody syndrome (APAS) or lupus anticoagulant syndrome; idiopathic thrombocytopenic purpura (ITP); thrombotic thrombocytopenic purpura (TTP); hemolytic-uremic syndrome (HUS); febrile reactions; severe sepsis; hemolysis, elevated liver enzymes, and low platelet count (HELLP) syndrome. Disseminated intravascular coagulation (DIC) presents with a combined coagulopathy and platelet consumption.
3. *Platelet sequestration:* related to hypersplenism and hyperthermia
4. *Decreased production of platelets:* caused by alcohol (EtOH) abuse, bone marrow irradiation, bone marrow/stem cell disease, graft-versus-host disease, aplastic anemia, vitamin B_{12} or folate deficiencies, metastatic carcinoma, some renal diseases, leukemia, and myeloproliferative disorders

   Platelet destruction may be mediated by congenital autoimmune or alloimmune disorders, or by acquired immunologic or nonimmunologic mechanisms. Causative or related factors include septicemia, systemic inflammatory response syndrome (SIRS), pulmonary hypertension, extracorporeal circulation, thrombotic disorders, acute transplant rejection, severe allergic reactions, rheumatic disorders, intravascular catheters and prosthetics, fat emboli, acute respiratory distress syndrome (ARDS), and HIV infection. The most significant diagnostic finding associated with severe thrombocytopenia is presence of petechiae in dependent areas (i.e., back, ankles, posterior thighs of bedridden patients). Larger purpura such as ecchymoses and hematomas may also be present but are nonspecific for diagnosis of platelet disorders. Patients must be assessed for risk of bleeding with thrombocytopenia, considering the severity and cause as well as comorbid factors.

Coagulopathies leading to bleeding (with/without associated thrombi) may be caused by liver disease, vitamin K deficiency, pregnancy-induced hypertension associated with HELLP syndrome, or other defects of blood coagulation factors, such as hemophilia, von Willebrand disease, and DIC.

Patients prone to thromboembolic conditions include those with *platelet abnormalities,* including thrombocytosis, diabetes mellitus, hyperlipidemia, heparin-induced thrombocytopenia, systemic lupus erythematosus; *blood vessel defects* including venous disease/stasis, roughened surface of vascular endothelium (seen with arteriosclerosis, trauma, severe sepsis, SIRS, or infection), atrial fibrillation, grafts or other devices in place, hyperviscosity, TTP, hemolytic uremic syndrome, vasculitis; and those with *systemic illness and conditions,* including long bone fractures, orthopedic surgery, abdominal surgery, malignancy, pregnancy or postpartum (risk of venous thromboembolism is five times higher than for nonpregnant women), oral contraceptives, nephrotic syndrome, inflammatory bowel disease, slow/stagnant blood flow through the vessels (e.g., shock states, severe peripheral vascular disease), infusion of prothrombin complex, and sickle cell disease.

When patients are evaluated for a bleeding disorder, the process should include evaluation of platelets, deficiency of a single coagulation factor (factors VII, VIII, IX, X, or XI) or multiple coagulation factors, for endogenous or exogenous antibiotics in the circulation, and consumptive coagulopathy (e.g., ITP, TTP, vasculitis, hemolytic uremic syndrome, paroxysmal nocturnal hematuria, obstetric complication, trauma, liver disease). Adequate levels of calcium and vitamin K are also needed for adequate function of the clotting cascade.

Those suspected of having thromboembolic disease may require evaluation of coagulation factors, circulating antibodies, abnormal proteins (deficient protein C or S), and other endogenous chemicals.

Normal blood coagulation is activated most often as a result of injury to blood vessels, causing the following series of events:

1. *Reflex vasoconstriction:* Vascular spasm that decreases blood flow to the site of injury
2. *Platelet aggregation:* Accumulation of platelets that leads to formation of a platelet plug to help support the repair of the injury. If the damage to the vessel is small, the plug is sufficient to seal the injury. If the hole is large, a blood clot is necessary to stop the bleeding.
3. *Activation of plasma clotting factors:* Stimulation of factors that leads to the formation of a fibrin clot. The pathways that initiate clotting factors (Figure 10-3) include the following:
   a. *Intrinsic system:* Initiated by "contact activation" subsequent to an endothelial injury. The problem is "intrinsic" to the circulation, or begins with an injury to the blood or circulatory system.

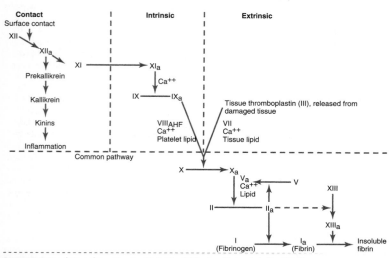

Figure 10-3 Coagulation pathway. (From Janz TG, Hamilton GC: Disorders of hemostasis. In Marx J, Hockberger R, Walls R, editors: *Rosen's Emergency medicine: concepts and clinical practice,* ed. 7. St. Louis, 2009, Mosby.)

 b. *Extrinsic system:* Initiated by tissue thromboplastin released from injured tissue. The problem is "extrinsic" to the circulation, or begins with an injury to tissue rather than within the blood system.

 c. *Common pathway:* The final part of the coagulation system, which completes the clot formation process begun by either the intrinsic or extrinsic pathway.

 d. *Clot retraction:* Several minutes after its formation, the clot contracts for 30 to 60 minutes to express most of the fluid from within the clot. The expressed fluid is called *serum*, because most of the clotting factors have been used or removed via the clot formation process. Serum is unable to clot. The absence of clotting factors differentiates *serum* from *plasma*.

4. *Growth of fibrous tissue:* Rubbery tissue that completes the clot within approximately 7 to 10 days after injury. This process results in permanent closure of the vessel injury. Both the intrinsic and extrinsic pathways are activated after rupture of a blood vessel. Tissue thromboplastin from the vessel initiates the extrinsic pathway, while contact of factor XII and platelets with the injured vessel wall traumatizes the blood and initiates the intrinsic pathway. The extrinsic pathway is able to form clots in as little as 15 seconds with severe trauma, whereas the intrinsic pathway requires 2 to 6 minutes for clot formation. Both are necessary to maintain clot.

HEPARIN-INDUCED THROMBOCYTOPENIA

PATHOPHYSIOLOGY

Heparin is the most widely used IV anticoagulant and one of the most frequently prescribed drugs in the United States. Heparin prevents the conversion of fibrinogen to fibrin. Heparin-induced thrombocytopenia (HIT), also called *heparin-induced thrombocytopenic thrombosis (HITT)*, white clot syndrome, or *heparin-associated thrombocytopenia (HAT)*, types I and II, occurs when heparin therapy causes either a mild to moderate (i.e., HAT type I) or severe (i.e., HAT type II) decrease in the number of freely circulating platelets. Platelets in affected patients exhibit unusual aggregation and can result in heparin resistance, arterial and venous thrombosis, and subsequent emboli in extreme cases (Figure 10-4). Depending on the source of the heparin received, HIT is reported in about 5% of all patients receiving heparin. Bovine (beef-based) heparin has been associated with HIT more frequently than other heparins. It is estimated that as many as 50% of patients on heparin may be asymptomatic but generate antibodies to heparin-platelet factor 4 (H-PF4), which increases the risk of HIT on their next exposure to heparin. HIT is not related to the heparin dosage and has been seen in patients receiving low-dose subcutaneous heparin, as well as in patients receiving simple heparin "flushes" to maintain patency of IV lines.

Two types of HIT have been described:

- *Mild to moderate, low morbidity:* Generally occurs 1 to 2 days after initiation of heparin. It may resolve within 5 days after symptoms begin. Platelets may decrease to levels as low as 100,000/mm^3 or may remain in the low-normal range. No treatment is required, and heparin therapy may be continued if the patient is asymptomatic.
- *High morbidity (immune-mediated):* Generally begins 5 to 7 days after initiation of heparin. Symptoms persist until heparin is discontinued. Platelets decrease to less than 100,000/mm^3. Thrombosis with subsequent embolization and bleeding is apparent. Complications may include pulmonary emboli, myocardial infarction, cerebral infarction, and circulatory impairment resulting in limb amputations. Mortality rate is 29%. Overall, 0.6% of all patients receiving heparin therapy develop thromboembolization.

ASSESSMENT
Goal of System Assessment
Evaluate for increased risk of inappropriate bleeding or clotting due to qualitative or quantitative dysfunction of platelets and clotting factors.

Risk Factors
Prior drug-induced or immunologic thrombocytopenia

Vital Signs
Tachypnea, tachycardia, hypertension

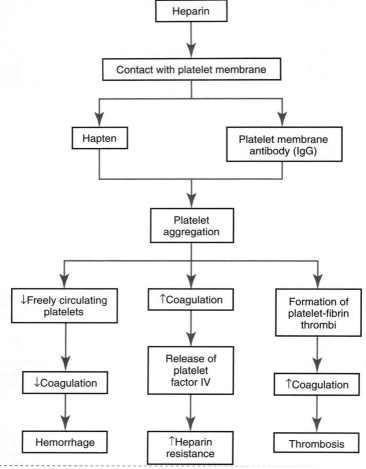

Figure 10-4 Heparin-induced thrombocytopenia. *IgG,* Immunoglobulin G.

Observation
Patients may present with high or low acuity states. Those without clinical symptoms with a slight decrease in platelets are much easier to manage than patients with severe, high morbidity. Extreme cases manifest arterial thrombosis of the distal aorta and proximal lower limb arteries. High morbidity patients present with:
- Petechiae, purpura, ecchymosis, gingival bleeding, hemoptysis, epixtaxis, bruising from mucosal surfaces or wounds
- Signs of arterial occlusion: cold, pulseless extremities
- Paresthesias; paralysis
- Severe chest pain and SOB, indicative of myocardial ischemia
- Diminished LOC, indicative of cerebral ischemia

Palpation
- Bone tenderness (especially rib and sternal areas)
- Enlargement of the liver and/or spleen

- Joint tenderness
- Enlargement of the liver and/or spleen
- Abdominal tenderness

Diagnostic Tests for Heparin-induced Thrombocytopenia

Test	Purpose	Abnormal Findings
Platelet count	Used to diagnose bleeding disorders or bone marrow disease	Mild to moderate: 100,000–150,000/mm³; severe: <100,000/mm³ caused by severe clumping or aggregation of platelets
Bleeding time	Measures how quickly blood clots, using platelets, coagulation factors, and small vessel vasospasm	Prolonged if platelets are <100,000/mm³
Platelet antibody screen	Identifies antibodies against platelets	Positive findings because of the presence of immunoglobulin G (IgG) platelet antibodies
Coagulation screening (prothrombin time [PT]; partial thromboplastin time [PTT], thromboplastin time)	PT — extrinsic pathway (Coumadin) PTT — intrinsic pathway (Heparin)	Normal, because the clotting factors that govern these test results are normal
Fibrinogen	Measures clot formation ability: may be ordered as a follow-up to an abnormal PT or PTT and/or an episode of prolonged or unexplained bleeding	May be low-normal or low due to increased consumption. Normal is 200–400 mg/dl
Fibrin degradation products: FDP, FSP, fibrin split products; fibrin breakdown products	Measures fibrin degradation products (which result from clots dissolving) in blood	Elevated to ≥40 mcg/ml because of fibrinolysis of platelet-fibrin thrombi. Normal is <10 mcg/ml
Platelet aggregation	Measures the rate and degree to which platelets form a clump	Results will be >100% (or high value of specific laboratory) because of release of platelet membrane antibody leading to "clumping."
Heparin-induced platelet aggregation	Adds patient platelet-poor plasma (as a source of immunoglobulin) to normal platelet-rich plasma in the presence of heparin to induce platelet aggregation	Reflects abnormal aggregation curve with decrease in the optical density in the aggregometer
Serotonin release testing and ELISA heparin PF4	Detects the presence of antibodies to PF4/heparin/TSP-1 complexes	Help in the differential diagnosis of HIT
Bone marrow aspiration	Evaluates bone marrow status; diagnose blood disorders and determine if cancer or infection has spread to the bone marrow.	Normal or increased number of megakaryocytes (platelet precursors), indicative of normal production of platelets or increased response to need for platelets

RESEARCH BRIEF 10-2

The investigators compared the outcomes of patients receiving activated protein C with or without bleeding precautions using the criteria defined by the PROWESS trial to those defined on the current drotrecogin alfa product labeling. Seventy-three patients received recombinant human activated protein C. The initial clinical trials for drotrecogin alfa (activated protein C) excluded only patients with specified bleeding disorders. Additional patients with bleeding disorders not specified received the drug. Results revealed fewer patients had a bleeding complication when the more extensive exclusion criteria from the PROWESS trial were used. Underlying bleeding disorders, higher APACHE score and presence of a bloodstream infection were the independent variables associated with mortality. Results suggest strict adherence to the PROWESS trial exclusion criteria would further limit serious bleeding events associated with the use of recombinant human activated protein C.

Gentry CA, Gross KB, Sud B, Drevets DA: Adverse outcomes associated with the use of drotrecogin alfa (activated) in patients with severe sepsis and baseline bleeding precautions. *Crit Care Med* 37(1):19–25, 2009.

COLLABORATIVE MANAGEMENT
Care Priorities

1. **Screen preheparin platelet count, and monitor platelets and amount of heparin needed:** A preheparin platelet count is made to establish baseline values. Daily platelet counts should be done for at least the first 4 days of heparin therapy. Subsequent counts are made every 2 days. If increasing amounts of heparin are needed to maintain therapeutic levels (i.e., PTT 40 to 60 seconds), heparin resistance should be suspected, which sometimes precedes HIT (see Figure 10-4).
   - *Consider stopping heparin therapy:* If the platelet count is greater than 100,000/mm³ and the patient is symptom-free, heparin is sometimes continued, but an alternate thrombin inhibitor may be recommended. Oral anticoagulation should begin immediately, if possible. If the platelet count is less than 100,000/mm³ and the patient develops bleeding or thrombosis: heparin must be discontinued immediately (including heparin flushes), alternate anticoagulant initiated, and subsequent complications managed as they occur. Use of low-molecular-weight heparins is contraindicated.
2. **Administer defibrinogenating agents if high morbidity symptoms are present:** Ancrod (Arvin) may be given to reduce the possibility of thrombosis.
3. **Prevent pulmonary emboli with a vena caval filter:** If patient experiences thrombosis with decrease or loss of perfusion to an extremity, the physician or midlevel practitioner may consider surgical insertion of a vena caval filter to reduce the risk of pulmonary emboli caused by clot migration from an extremity. See *Pulmonary Embolus*, p. 396.
   - *Warfarin, thrombolytics, and platelet inhibitors:* Streptokinase, urokinase, and alteplase (rtPA) have been used successfully to manage pulmonary emboli in HIT.
4. **Maintain anticoagulation, if needed, with a direct thrombin inhibitor:** Argatroban and hirudin, direct thrombin inhibitors, block thrombin generation needed for fibrin formation. They may be used alone or in combination with warfarin, as an alternate anticoagulation strategy for patients with HIT. Ximelagatran is the first orally available thrombin inhibitor. Bivalirudin is not licensed for use with HIT but can be used in patients undergoing percutaneous coronary interventions. If the patient needs further anticoagulation, warfarin sodium (Coumadin) should be considered. Platelet inhibitors are contraindicated, due to current platelet dysfunction.
5. **Consider use of newer anticoagulation agents in those who are difficult to manage:** New medications using recombinant DNA technology focus on each step of the coagulation process; many are under development. These agents are grouped into three stages of coagulation: initiation, propagation, and fibrin formation. Tissue factor pathway inhibitor (TFPI), nematode anticoagulant peptide, and factor VIIa target

initiation of coagulation. Soluble thrombomodulin, drotrecogin alfa (activated protein C), protein C concentrate, fondaparinux, and idraparinux inhibit clot propagation. Direct thrombin inhibitors (antithrombins) block fibrin formation for clot completion.

6. **Provide platelet transfusions for high morbidity patients who continue to bleed:** May be initiated after heparin therapy is discontinued if bleeding fails to subside.

7. **Provide plasma exchange for high morbidity patients who fail to respond to other therapies:** In severe cases, 2 to 3 L of plasma is removed and replaced with albumin, crystalloids, or fresh-frozen plasma to assist in decreasing bleeding by removing bound heparin from the body.

CARE PLANS: HEPARIN-INDUCED THROMBOCYTOPENIA

Ineffective protection *related to decreased platelet count with risk of bleeding and thromboembolization*

GOALS/OUTCOMES Within 24 hours of discontinuing heparin therapy, patient exhibits no signs of new bleeding, bruising, or thrombosis as evidenced by HR 60 to 100 bpm or within 10% of patient's baseline, RR 12 to 20 breaths/min with normal depth and pattern, systolic BP at least 90 mm Hg, and all peripheral pulses at patient's baseline or more than 2+ on a 0 to 4+ scale.

NOC Blood Coagulation

Bleeding Precautions

1. Assess patient at least every 2 hours for signs of bleeding, including hemoptysis, ecchymosis, petechiae on dependent areas, GI bleeding, hematuria, and bleeding from invasive procedure sites or mucous membranes. Monitor the patient closely for hemorrhage. Note Hgb and Hct levels before and after blood loss, and at least daily as indicated.

2. Assess for signs of internal bleeding including tachycardia and dysrhythmias, tachypnea and hypotension. Sustained increase in HR and RR or ECG changes, such as ST-segment depression or elevation, may precede hypotension.

3. Protect the patient from trauma that may cause bleeding. Do not use rectal temperatures to monitor for fever. Avoid IM injections and venous and arterial punctures as possible until bleeding time normalizes.

4. Perform a comprehensive assessment of peripheral circulation (e.g., check peripheral pulses, edema, capillary refill, and color and temperature of extremities) at least every 2 hours and assess patient for signs of thrombosis, including decreased peripheral pulses, altered sensation in extremities (i.e., paresthesias, numbness), pallor, coolness, cyanosis, or capillary refill time more than 2 seconds. Monitor extremities for areas of heat, pain, redness, or swelling.

5. Maintain adequate hydration to prevent increased blood viscosity and to help prevent constipation.

6. Administer stool softeners to help reduce straining with bowel movements, which may prompt rectal bleeding.

7. Monitor platelet count daily for significant changes. Consult physician or midlevel practitioner for values that remain less than 150,000/mm³ or below patient's baseline.

8. Monitor heparin dosage carefully. If increasing doses are required to maintain a therapeutic level (PTT 40 to 60 seconds or 2 to 2.5 times patient's baseline), consult physician or midlevel practitioner regarding possible heparin resistance, an early indicator of HIT. If heparin has been discontinued and new anticoagulants initiated, monitor appropriate values. If a direct thrombin inhibitor (e.g., Argatroban) is used alone, or in combination with warfarin, monitor PT and international normalized ratio (INR).

9. Assess patient's neurologic status hourly if platelet count decreases to less than 30,000.

10. Monitor for signs of MODS secondary to thrombosis or prolonged hypotension, if patient has hemorrhaged. (See *SIRS, Sepsis and MODS,* p. 924).

11. Teach patient and significant others about the basic pathophysiology of HIT, and instruct them to report this problem to all subsequent health care providers. Teach patient to wear a medical-alert bracelet to alert health care providers if patient becomes unable to speak.

NIC Surveillance: Safety; Vital Signs Monitoring

Deficient fluid volume (or risk for same) *related to active blood loss*

GOALS/OUTCOMES Patient becomes normovolemic within 24 hours of onset of treatment as evidenced by HR within patient's normal range or 60 to 100 bpm, RR 12 to 20 breaths/min with normal depth and pattern and urinary output at least 0.5 ml/kg/hr, and absence of abdominal discomfort, back pain, or pain from invasive procedure sites.

NOC Fluid Balance

Hypovolemia Management
1. Monitor patient for signs of hypovolemia, including increased HR and RR, decreased BP, increased restlessness or fatigue, and decreased urine output.
2. Administer supplemental oxygen if patient is actively bleeding.
3. Maintain accurate I&O record. Weigh daily and monitor trends.
4. Assess for intra-abdominal bleeding: note any abdominal pain, tenderness, guarding, or back pain.
5. Check excretions for occult blood, and observe for blood in emesis, sputum, feces, urine, nasogastric (NG) drainage, and wound drainage as appropriate.
6. Instruct the patient and/or family on the need for blood replacement as appropriate.
7. Replace lost volume with plasma expanders (e.g., albumin, hetastarch) or blood products as indicated. See Table 10-3 for more information.

NIC Electrolyte Management; Fluid Management; Fluid Monitoring; Intravenous (IV) Therapy; Bleeding Reduction: Gastrointestinal; Shock Management: Volume; Blood Products Administration

ADDITIONAL NURSING DIAGNOSES

Uncontrolled bleeding or thrombotic complications can be terrifying for the patient and significant others, who may fear that the patient will die. See nursing diagnoses and interventions in *Emotional and Spiritual Support of the Patient and Significant Others*, p. 200.

IMMUNE THROMBOCYTOPENIA PURPURA (ITP)

PATHOPHYSIOLOGY

Immune (often idiopathic) ITP is a disorder characterized by premature platelet destruction as well as impaired platelet production, resulting in a decrease in the platelet count to below 100,000/mm³. Normal platelet life span averages 1 to 3 weeks, whereas in ITP the platelet life span averages 1 to 3 days because of the presence of antiplatelet IgG and IgM antibodies, which destroy platelets in the reticuloendothelial system of the spleen. The coagulopathy is believed to be an autoimmune response and manifests as both an acute and a chronic problem.

Acute ITP is primarily a childhood disease, characterized by an abrupt onset of severe thrombocytopenia with evident purpura. Usually it occurs within 21 days following a viral infection. At the onset, platelets decrease to less than 20,000/mm³. The chronic form is typically a disease of adults ages 20 to 50 years, but it has occurred in a small percentage of children and elders. The chronic disease rarely resolves spontaneously, sometimes responds to treatment of the underlying disorder, and usually is not associated with infection but can be related to autoimmune disorders (e.g., systemic lupus erythematosus, rheumatoid arthritis) and neoplastic disorders (e.g., chronic lymphocytic leukemia, lymphoma). Women are affected three times more often than men. Petechiae and purpura are commonly seen on the distal upper and lower extremities. Patients may feel symptom-free until actual bleeding begins. Intracranial hemorrhage is a potential complication. Platelet counts decrease to as low as 5,000/mm³ in some patients but may be as high as 75,000/mm³ in others.

ASSESSMENT
Goal of System Assessment

Evaluate for increased risk of inappropriate bleeding or clotting due to qualitative or quantitative dysfunction of platelets and clotting factors

Risk Factors

- *Acute ITP*: History of antecedent viral infection occurring about 3 weeks before the hemorrhagic episode
- *Chronic ITP*: Insidious and sometimes associated with autoimmune hemolytic anemia, HIV disease, hemophilia, lymphoma, chronic lymphocytic leukemia, systemic lupus erythematosus, sarcoidosis, high-titer anticardiolipin antibodies, pregnancy, malabsorption and thyrotoxicosis. The cause is often unknown.

Vital Signs

- Tachypnea, tachycardia, hypotension, fever

Observation

- Petechiae, purpura, bruising on skin and mucous membranes, prolonged bleeding; intra-cranial hemorrhage occurs in less than 1% of patients if the thrombocytopenia is severe.
- Diminished LOC, indicative of intracranial hemorrhage
- Epistaxis, gingival bleeding, gastrointestinal (GI), genitourinary (GU), gynecologic (GYN) bleeding such as increased menstrual flow
- Retinal disturbances

Palpation

- Enlargement of the liver and/or spleen
- Lymphadenopathy, hepatomegaly, splenomegaly
- Joint tenderness

Diagnostic Tests for Immune Thrombocytopenia Purpura		
Test	**Purpose**	**Abnormal Findings**
Platelet count	Used to diagnose bleeding disorders or bone marrow disease	Decreased to 5000–75,000/mm³ (or lower) because of premature destruction. Normal range is 150,000–400,000/mm³.
Bleeding time	Measures how quickly blood clots, using platelets, coagulation factors, and small vessel vasospasm	Prolonged if platelets are less than 100,000/mm³
Platelet antibody screen	Identifies antibodies against platelets	Positive findings because of the presence of IgG and IgM antiplatelet antibodies
Coagulation screening (prothrombin time [PT]; partial thromboplastin time [PTT]; thromboplastin time)	PT – extrinsic pathway (Coumadin) PTT – intrinsic pathway (Heparin)	Normal, because these tests measure nonplatelet components of the coagulation pathway.
Complete Blood Count (CBC) with Differential	Measures RBCs, WBCs and platelets and the WBC differential	Decreased Hgb and Hct due to insidious blood loss or simultaneous hemolytic anemia (Evans syndrome) Normal WBC count: unless ITP is associated with another disease impacting differential leukocyte count.
Capillary fragility test: Rumpel-Leede Capillary-Fragility Test	Method to determine a patient's hemorrhagic tendency: assesses fragility of capillary walls: used to identify thrombocytopenia. Seldom used in current practice	Will show >1+, which signals that more than 11 petechiae were present in a 2.5-cm radial area on the skin after prolonged application of a BP cuff. Normal is 1+ or <10 petechiae
Bone marrow aspiration	Evaluates bone marrow status; diagnose blood disorders and determine if cancer or infection has spread to the bone marrow.	Biopsy will reveal megakaryocytes (platelet precursors) in normal or increased numbers with a "nonbudding" appearance, possibly indicating defective maturation or failure of platelet production

COLLABORATIVE MANAGEMENT: IMMUNE THROMBOCYTOPENIC PURPURA
Care Priorities
1. **Suppress immune response to reduce platelet destruction**
   - *Corticosteroid therapy:* Adrenocorticosteroids (e.g., prednisone 1 to 2 mg/kg/day) are effective in increasing the platelet count in 1 to 3 weeks after initiation of treatment. Effectiveness is attributed to suppression of phagocytic activity of the macrophage system (particularly the spleen), which increases the life span of the antibody-coated platelets. If improvement does not occur within 2 to 3 weeks, excessive doses of steroids are required, or if patient cannot tolerate tapering of steroids, splenectomy should be considered. "Normal" responders are able to have steroid dosage tapered over several weeks until platelets reach a sustained value of 50,000/mm^3. Relapse during or after tapering prednisone is a common occurrence.
   - *IV immunoglobulin (IVIG):* Given at 400 mg/kg/day for 2 to 5 consecutive days, resulting in increased platelet count in 60% to 70% of patients. Serum sickness (fever, chills, rash) is not uncommon between 9 to 14 days. It is less effective in patients with longstanding chronic ITP. The platelet level at initiation of treatment and incidence of serum sickness is not necessarily correlated to individual response. Duration of response may be longest in individuals who achieve the highest initial platelet increases.
   - *Danazol:* 400 to 800 mg/day has resulted in complete remission or partial improvement in 60% to 70% of patients in several studies. Use is controversial because other researchers have reported poor results and many untoward side effects.
   - *Splenectomy:* Treatment of choice in cases refractory to corticosteroid therapy. The condition stabilizes in 60% to 70% of patients who undergo splenectomy. The positive results are attributed to the removal of the site of destruction of the antibody-sensitized platelets. Prospective splenectomy candidates should have pneumococcal, meningococcal, and *Haemophilus influenzae* type B vaccinations before a planned splenectomy, to reduce the risk of postoperative infection with these organisms.
   - *Immunosuppression:* Various immunosuppressive drugs, including azathioprine, cyclophosphamide, methotrexate, vincristine, and cyclosporine, given alone or in combination with prednisone, have been used successfully in limited situations. A trial of immunosuppression therapy may be indicated in patients who fail to respond to splenectomy or in those who are too unstable to be surgical candidates.
   - *Anti-Rh immunoglobulin:* Low dose (200 to 1000 mcg) given IV for 1 to 5 days has been effective in limited studies. Success of treatment is attributed to sensitization of recipient RBCs, which results in low-grade hemolysis and blockade of the platelet destruction by the reticuloendothelial system.
   - *Colchicine:* A small percentage of patients refractory to other treatments may improve with 1.2 mg colchicine daily for 2 weeks or longer. The drug has been used successfully in limited studies.
   - *Plasmapheresis:* Several days of machine-assisted plasma exchange to remove approximately 1 to 1.5 times the total plasma volume per procedure and replace it with a suitable solution (e.g., colloids, crystalloids, plasma). Therapy is reserved for patients with life-threatening hemorrhage unresponsive to other measures. It is costly and of marginal benefit.
2. **Increase platelet count**
   - *Romiplostim:* A promising treatment approved for use in patients with chronic ITP who are refractory to corticosteroids, immunoglobulins, or splenectomy. A thrombopoeitin receptor agonist that stimulates bone marrow megakaryocytes to increase platelet production; 1 mcg/kg is given as a subcutaneous injection once weekly, titrated to a maximum dose of 10 mcg/kg to achieve a platelet count of greater than 50,000. Rare side effects include bone marrow fibrosis and reticulin formation.
   - *Platelet transfusions:* Platelets are given only in cases of life-threatening hemorrhage. The shortened platelet life span renders prophylactic transfusions ineffective.
   - *Vinca "alkaloid-loaded" platelets:* Transfusions of platelets "loaded" with vinblastine may reduce the phagocytic destruction of platelets in patients who fail to respond to other treatments.

CARE PLANS FOR IMMUNE THROMBOCYTOPENIC PURPURA
Ineffective protection *related to decreased platelet count, resulting in increased risk of bleeding*

GOALS/OUTCOMES Within 72 hours of onset of treatment, patient exhibits no clinical signs of new bleeding or bruising episodes. Secretions and excretions are negative for blood, and vital signs are within 10% of patient's normal range. Within the 24-hour period before discharge from intensive care, patient and significant others verbalize understanding of the indicators of potential or actual bleeding.
NOC Blood Coagulation

Bleeding Precautions
1. Monitor patient for bleeding and hemorrhage, including elevated HR and RR, decreasing BP, oozing from invasive procedure sites, bleeding mucous membranes, hematuria, and GU, GYN, and GI bleeding. Note Hgb and Hct levels before and after blood loss, as indicated.
2. Protect the patient from trauma that may cause bleeding. Avoid taking rectal temperatures.
3. Maintain fluid intake to prevent constipation and administer stool softeners to minimize straining.
4. Monitor skin or mucous membranes for pallor, discoloration, bruising, breakdown, erythema.
5. Monitor coagulation studies, including PT, PTT, fibrinogen, fibrin degradation products (FDP), fibrin split products (FSP), and platelet counts as appropriate.
6. Consult physician or midlevel practitioner for sustained low platelet values (less than 100,000/mm^3 or as appropriate for the individual).
7. Avoid administering NSAIDs (e.g., aspirin, ibuprofen). Teach patient to avoid all medications that potentially decrease platelet aggregation, especially aspirin or aspirin-containing products.
8. For severe menorrhagia, confer with physician regarding need for progestational hormones for suppression of menses. Assess blood loss by weighing perineal pads or tampons.
9. During the acute (bleeding) phase of ITP, teach patient to perform oral hygiene using sponge-tipped applicators soaked in water or dilute mouthwash to help prevent gum bleeding. Avoid hydrogen peroxide or lemon-coated swabs.
10. Teach patient that it is always safer to use an electric razor for shaving.
11. Instruct family member/caregiver about signs of skin breakdown, as appropriate.
12. Teach patient and significant others to recognize the signs of impending hemorrhage: more rapid pulse and breathing, easy bruising, painful joints, and blood in sputum, urine, or stool.

NIC Skin Surveillance

Decreased intracranial adaptive capacity: (or risk for same) *related to potential for intracranial hemorrhage (less than 1% of patients) secondary to decreased platelet level*

GOALS/OUTCOMES Throughout the hospitalization, patient remains free of symptoms of intracranial hemorrhage as evidenced by orientation to time, place, and person; normoreactive pupils and reflexes; patient's normal visual acuity, motor strength, and coordination; and absence of headache and other clinical indicators of IICP.
NOC Neurological Status

Neurologic Monitoring
1. Assess patient for initial signs of IICP, including diminished LOC, headaches, pupillary responses (e.g., unequal, sluggish/absent response to light), visual disturbances, weakness and paralysis, slow HR, and change in respiratory rate and pattern.
2. Monitor trend of Glasgow Coma Scale, ICP, and cerebral perfusion pressure (CPP).
3. Increase frequency of neurologic monitoring as appropriate.
4. Avoid activities that increase intracranial pressure (i.e., Valsalva, hyperthermia, pain, etc.). Administer stool softeners and cough suppressants as prescribed.
5. If initial signs of IICP are noted, consult physician immediately. Severe intracranial bleeding can lead to herniation. ICP can increase rapidly with severe bleeding, sometimes causing death within 1 hour of onset. Signs of impending herniation include unconsciousness, failure to respond to deeply painful stimuli, decorticate or decerebrate posturing, Cushing triad (i.e., bradycardia, increased systolic BP, widening pulse pressure), nonreactive/fixed pupils, unequal pupils, or fixed and dilated pupils. See *Traumatic Brain Injury*, p. 331 for more information about herniation.
6. Consult with physician or midlevel practitioner regarding management of IICP (see *Traumatic Brain Injury* p. XX for collaborative interventions for IICP). For additional interventions for IICP, see Box 3-7.

7. Teach patient to avoid Valsalva maneuver (e.g., straining at stool or when lifting; forceful and sustained coughing or nose blowing), which could cause intracranial bleeding.

8. Teach the importance of avoiding tobacco products (particularly cigarettes) and excessive caffeine, which may cause vasoconstriction. Constricted vessels may prevent platelets from circulating through portions of the capillary network.

NIC Cerebral Edema Management; Cerebral Perfusion Promotion; Intracranial Pressure (ICP) Monitoring; Neurologic Monitoring

Risk for deficient fluid volume *related to active loss secondary to intraabdominal bleeding or postsplenectomy intra-abdominal bleeding*

GOALS/OUTCOMES Patient remains normovolemic as evidenced by HR, RR, and BP within 10% of patient's normal range (or HR 60 to 100 bpm, RR 12 to 20 breaths/min with normal depth and pattern, systolic BP ≥90 mm Hg); urinary output at least 0.5 ml/kg/hr; and absence of abdominal pain or tenderness, back pain, and frank bleeding from the splenectomy incision.
NOC Fluid Balance

Fluid Management
1. Monitor fluid status, including I&O, and signs of hypovolemia, including increases in HR and RR and decreases in BP, and urinary output, restlessness, fatigue, and orthostatic vital signs.
2. Inspect for bleeding from mucous membranes, bruising after minimal trauma, oozing from puncture sites, and presence of petechiae. Maintain patent IV access.
3. Administer supplemental oxygen as necessary for postoperative status or active bleeding.
4. Replace lost volume with plasma expanders (e.g., albumin, hetastarch) and/or blood products as indicated. See Table 10-3 for information about blood products.
5. Inform patient of the importance of wearing a medical-alert bracelet and obtaining a pneumococcal vaccination if a splenectomy has been performed.

NIC Bleeding Precautions; Electrolyte Management; Fluid Monitoring; Hypovolemia Management; Intravenous (IV) Therapy; Shock Management: Volume; Blood Products Administration

Acute pain *related to joint inflammation and injury secondary to bleeding into the synovial cavity of the joint(s); postsplenectomy pain*

GOALS/OUTCOMES Within 4 hours of initiating treatment, patient's subjective evaluation of discomfort improves as documented by a pain scale, nonverbal indicators of discomfort are absent or decreased, and HR, RR, and BP are within 10% of patient's baseline.
NOC Pain Control

Pain Management
1. Devise a pain scale with patient, rating discomfort from 0 (no pain) to 10. Perform a comprehensive assessment of pain to include location, characteristics, onset/duration, frequency, quality, intensity or severity, and precipitating factors.
2. Ensure that patient receives appropriate analgesic care. Consult with physician or midlevel practitioner regularly until patient's pain is controlled. Avoid use of meperidine for pain relief in older adults or individuals with renal compromise; adverse effects are common.
3. Teach patient causes of the pain, how long it may last, and about discomforts from procedures.
4. Elevate patient's legs to decrease joint pain in the lower extremities. Avoid knee flexion. Support extremities with pillows, making sure bed is not "gatched" at the knee.
5. Teach patient to splint abdomen when coughing after splenectomy.
6. Evaluate patient's anxiety level, and provide emotional support to control fear and anxiety. If patient becomes agitated, evaluate potential causes including hypoxemia, poor pain or anxiety control, fluid and electrolyte imbalance, and alcohol or drug withdrawal, and intervene appropriately.
7. See *Pain*, p. 135, for additional pain interventions. Also see *Prolonged Immobility*, p. 149, for patients who are unable to move or who have limited movement.

NIC Analgesic Administration; Pain Management; Coping Enhancement; Anxiety Reduction

ADDITIONAL NURSING DIAGNOSES

Uncontrolled bleeding can be terrifying for the patient and significant others, who may fear that the patient will die. Refer to nursing diagnoses in *Emotional and Spiritual Support of the Patient and Significant Others*, p. 200, for appropriate interventions.

DISSEMINATED INTRAVASCULAR COAGULATION

PATHOPHYSIOLOGY

DIC is a syndrome characterized by overstimulation of the normal coagulation cascade, often related to severe sepsis or shock. DIC is a coagulopathy with potential to cause both profuse bleeding and widespread thrombosis leading to MODS. Inherent bodily control of bleeding requires a balance between procoagulants and thrombus formation, along with anticoagulants, inhibitors, and thrombolysis (see Figure 10-3, Table 10-4). The delicate balance may be upset by disease processes (Table 10-5), resulting in a cascade of uncontrolled coagulation and fibrinolysis. The abnormal clotting cascade that develops during DIC is as follows:

- Platelets and coagulation factors are activated by a disease stimulus and are rapidly consumed, particularly factors V and XIII and fibrinogen.
- Thrombin is formed very rapidly, and inherent inhibitors cannot stop the formation of the vast amounts of thrombin generated. Thrombin directly activates fibrinogen.
- Fibrin is deposited throughout the capillary beds of organs and tissues.
- The fibrinolytic system lyses fibrin and impairs thrombin formation.

Table 10-4	CLOTTING FACTORS: PRIMARY ACTIONS		
Coagulation Factor	**Thrombin-Sensitive/ Promotes Vasoconstriction**	**Vitamin K-Sensitive**	**Sites of Heparin Activity**
I Fibrinogen	✓		
II Prothrombin		✓	✓ IIa
III Tissue thromboplastin (tissue factor)			
IV Calcium			
V Proaccelerin (AC globulin [AC-g])	✓		
VI Not assigned			
VII Proconvertin stable factor (prothrombin accelerator)		✓	
VIII Antihemophilic factor A (antihemophilic factor [AHF], antihemophilic globulin [AHG])	✓		
IX Antihemophilic factor B (plasma thromboplastin component [PTC], Christmas factor)		✓	✓IXa
X Stuart-Prower factor (Stuart factor)		✓	✓Xa
XI Plasma thromboplastin antecedent (antihemophilic factor C)			✓ XIa
XII Hageman factor (contact factor)			
XIII Fibrin stabilizing factor	✓		
Other Factors			
Prekallikrein (Fletcher factor)			
High-molecular-weight kininogen (HMWK-Fitzgerald factor)			
Platelets			

Table 10-5 DISSEMINATED INTRAVASCULAR COAGULATION (DIC): PREDISPOSING CONDITIONS

Obstetric	GI Disorders	Tissue Damage	Infections	Hemolytic Processes	Vascular Disorders	Miscellaneous
Abruptio placentae	Cirrhosis	Surgery	Viral	Transfusion reaction	Shock	Fat or pulmonary embolism
Toxemia	Hepatic necrosis	Trauma	Bacterial	Acute hemolysis secondary to infection or immunologic disorder	Aneurysm	Snake bite
Amniotic fluid embolism	Acute fulminant hepatitis	Burns	Rickettsial		Giant hemangioma	Neoplastic disorders (esp. prostate, acute promyelocytic leukemia, lymphoma) Acute anoxia
Septic abortion	Pancreatitis	Prolonged extracorporeal circulation	Protozoal			
Retained dead fetus	Peritoneovenous shunts	Transplant rejection	Fungal			
Hydatidiform mole	Necrotizing enterocolitis	Heat stroke				

- FDPs (or FSPs) result from fibrinolysis, which changes platelet aggregation and inhibits fibrin polymerization. See Figure 10-3 for the normal coagulation pathway.

A predisposing event that damages the vascular endothelium initiates the clotting cascade. Studies reflect that both the intrinsic and extrinsic pathways are activated initially, resulting in an abnormal acceleration of the clotting process. Thrombocytopenia occurs because of thrombin production and microvascular thrombus formation.

ASSESSMENT
Goal of System Assessment
Evaluate for increased risk of inappropriate bleeding or clotting due to qualitative or quantitative dysfunction of platelets and clotting factors.

Risk Factors
Any clinical state or pharmacologic therapy (e.g., chemotherapy) that inhibits the removal of activated clotting factors, FDPs, and thromboplastin by the reticuloendothelial system. Any patient is at high risk following severe trauma or with systemic inflammatory response syndrome (SIRS), a severe infection, sepsis, severe sepsis, septic shock, or invasive procedures. Obstetrics patients with abruptio placenta, amniotic fluid embolism, or eclampsia release procoagulation factors, placing them at risk. DIC can occur as a paraneoplastic syndrome or oncologic emergency related to certain malignancies such as acute promyelocytic leukemia (APL), multiple myeloma, and some solid tumors. DIC may manifest as a profound bleeding/clotting disorder in the *acute* phase or as a less symptomatic *chronic* disorder.

In chronic (compensated) DIC, activation of coagulation and fibrinolysis does not occur rapidly enough to exceed the rate of production of clotting factors or inhibitors. The course of DIC depends on the intensity of the stimulus, coupled with the status of the liver, bone marrow, and vascular endothelium. Whether DIC leads to bleeding or to thrombosis is profoundly affected by the underlying disease process.

Vital Signs
- Tachypnea, tachycardia, hypotension

Observation
- *Bleeding with abrupt onset:* From invasive procedure sites and mucosal surfaces (e.g., oral, nasal, tracheal, gastric, urethral, vaginal, rectal); may include hematuria, petechiae, stools or gastric aspirate positive for occult blood, pallor, tachycardia, tachypnea, vertigo, hypotension, ecchymoses (e.g., on palate, gums, skin, conjunctivae), lethargy, irritability, or feeling of impending doom, and possible back pain and abdominal tenderness.
- Anxiety, restlessness
- Petechiae, purpura, ecchymoses, oozing blood, mottling
- Conjunctival hemorrhage and periorbital petechiae
- Acrocyanosis
- Joint pain, weakness
- SOB, ST-segment elevation/depression, T-wave inversion
- Grey Turner sign (flank ecchymoses)
- Hemoptysis, tarry stools, melena
- Decreased responsiveness, confusion, altered mentation, headaches
- *Abnormal thrombosis* may manifest with extremity pain, diminished pulses, oliguria or anuria, diminished or absent bowel sounds, severe chest pain with SOB (indicative of either myocardial infarction or pulmonary embolism), or paresis or paralysis (indicative of cerebral thrombus)

Palpation
- Hepatosplenomegaly
- Abdominal tenderness

Auscultation
- Diminished or absent bowel sounds
- Weakened or absent peripheral pulses

Diagnostic Tests for Disseminated Intravascular Coagulation

Test	Purpose	Abnormal Findings
Fibrin degradation products: FDP, FSP, fibrin split products; fibrin breakdown products	Measures fibrin degradation products (which result from clots dissolving) in blood	Increased (>10 mcg/ml) due to widespread fibrinolysis, which produces FDPs as the end product of clot lysis. Critical value: >40 ng/ml
D-dimer assay	Measures cleavage products of fibrin	Increased to >500 due to increased thrombin and plasmin generation. This is a rapid measurement technique, less sensitive than FDPs, and not recommended as a substitute for FDPs and fibrinogen determinations.
Fibrinogen	Measures clot formation ability: may be ordered as a follow-up to an abnormal PT or PTT and/or an episode of prolonged or unexplained bleeding	May remain normal or decrease in the early acute phase. As the process continues, fibrinogen levels will decrease. Normal range is 150–400 mg/dl.
PTT or activated partial thromboplastin time (aPTT)	Measure of the integrity of the intrinsic and common pathways of the coagulation cascade. The aPTT is the time, in seconds, for patient plasma to clot after the addition of an intrinsic pathway activator, phospholipid and calcium.	Prolonged (>40 seconds) because of activation of the intrinsic pathway, causing consumption of coagulation factors. Critical value: >70 seconds. In chronic DIC the value may be normal (25–35 seconds) or less than normal.
Prothrombin time (PT), International Normalized Ratio (INR)	Measure of the integrity of the extrinsic pathway of the coagulation cascade.	Prolonged (>15 seconds) because of activation of the extrinsic pathway, causing consumption of the extrinsic clotting factors. Critical value: >40 seconds.
Thrombin time, thrombin clotting time (TCT)	Test of the time it takes for a clot to form, measuring the conversion of fibrinogen to fibrin	Prolonged (>1.5 times the control value or >2 seconds in excess of a 9- to 13-second control value) because of rapid conversion of fibrinogen into fibrin.
Antithrombin III (AT-III), functional antithrombin III, antithrombin, activity and antigen	Evaluates whether the total amount of functional antithrombin is normal. Activity will be decreased with both type 1 and type 2 antithrombin deficiencies, so this test can be used as an initial screen for both. If the antithrombin activity is low, then the antithrombin antigen test is performed to determine the quantity of antithrombin present.	Decreased (<50% of control value using a plasma sample, or <80% using functional values) because of rapid consumption of this thrombin inhibitor. The action of AT-III is catalyzed by heparin.
Euglobulin clot lysis time (ECLT)	Measures overall fibrinolysis; measures fibrinogen activity via measurement of plasminogen and plasminogen activator, which assist in prevention of fibrin clot formations.	Decreased time is seen with DIC. Normal: lysis in 2–4 hours Critical value: 100% lysis in 1 hour
Platelet count	Used to diagnose bleeding disorders or bone marrow disease	Decreased (<140,000/mm³) because of rapid rate of platelet aggregation to form clots during DIC. Aggregation decreases the freely circulating platelets.

Test	Purpose	Abnormal Findings
Alpha$_2$-antiplasmin	Measures alpha$_2$-antiplasmin, which is an inhibitor that regulates the fibrinolytic system primarily by blocking the enzymatic activity of plasmin	Decreased because of rapid consumption due to large amounts of plasmin generated. When all alpha$_2$-antiplasmin is depleted, excessive hyperfibrinolysis (massive, rapid clot lysis) occurs.
Protamine sulfate test	Associated with the formation of excessive amounts of thrombin and secondary fibrinolysis.	Results are positive (normal: negative), indicative of presence of fibrin strands.
Peripheral blood smear	Microscopic examination of cells from drop of blood; investigates hematologic problems or parasites such as malaria and filaria	For visualization during microscopic examination of schistocytes and burr cells, which indicate the deposition of fibrin in the small blood vessels.

Diagnostic Tests for Disseminated Intravascular Coagulation—cont'd

COLLABORATIVE MANAGEMENT: DISSEMINATED INTRAVASCULAR COAGULATION
Care Priorities

1. **Treat the primary cause of the disease:** Aggressively treat the underlying cause. A primary disease promotes the development of DIC. If treatment of the disease fails, the mortality rate of DIC is high. When DIC occurs without apparent cause, the possibility of undiagnosed malignancy (e.g., prostate cancer or APL), a large abdominal aortic aneurysm, a progressive gram-negative bacterial infection, or hepatic cirrhosis should be explored. If the diagnosis is by laboratory tests alone, conservative management is appropriate. Other conditions and medication side effects should be considered (see Table 10-5).

2. **Manage abnormal clotting with continuous IV heparin therapy:** There are three conditions associated with DIC in which heparin may be effective:
   - Underlying malignancy/carcinoma
   - Acute Promyelocytic Leukemia (APL): a leukemia most often seen in young adults with acute myelocytic anemia, which may also be linked to patients who received radiotherapy for prostate cancer.
   - Purpura fulminans/extreme purpura, often seen with severe sepsis

   If used, the patient should have clinically obvious thrombosis. Low-dose therapy (5 to 10 units/kg/hr) is considered. Heparin binds to antithrombin, resulting in a strong anticoagulant effect. Use of higher-dose heparin in DIC is associated with a high risk of bleeding, and greater efficacy has not been documented. Heparin may be considered for serious bleeding or clotting when the condition underlying the DIC is not rapidly reversible and the patient's vascular system is surgically intact.

> **Safety Alert** *APL patients with DIC often experience accelerated symptoms of fibrinolysis (declotting) when receiving chemotherapy. If these individuals receive heparin, an antifibrinolytic agent such as epsilon- (ϵ-) aminocaproic acid (Amicar) may be added to decrease bleeding.*

3. **Manage abnormal bleeding due to fibrinolysis with antifibrinolytics:** ϵ-Aminocaproic acid (Amicar) and tranexamic acid (Cyklokapron) are used to inhibit fibrinolysis in patients who are bleeding as a result of a variety of causes. In patients with DIC, these agents should be used with extreme caution because they may convert a bleeding disorder into a thrombotic problem. When used in DIC, these agents are used in combination with heparin to minimize the potential for thrombosis. Failure rates with use are high.

4. **Consider use of thrombolytic agents for abnormal clotting:** Use of streptokinase, urokinase, and tissue plasminogen activator (rtPA) is not indicated for patients with thrombosis because these agents may facilitate excessive bleeding.

5. **Provide replacement of necessary blood components:** Clotting factors and inhibitors are replaced in the form of fresh-frozen plasma. The PT/INR may be the most accurate parameter(s) for guiding plasma replacement. Patients with markedly decreased fibrinogen levels may be given cryoprecipitate, which contains 5 to 10 times more fibrinogen than plasma contains. Thrombocytopenia in DIC may not be severe. The platelet count is usually more than 50,000/mm³. General replacement therapy guidelines indicate approximately 10 units of cryoprecipitate should be given for every 2 to 3 units of plasma. Platelet transfusions are used if the patient has impaired platelet production and profuse bleeding. AT-III concentrate has been used on a limited basis (see Table 10-3). More recently, DIC is being managed with antithrombin concentrate, activated protein C (APC) (drotrecogin alfa), tissue factor pathway inhibitor (TFPI), and synthetic serine protease inhibitors (e.g., aprotinin).
   - *RBC replacement:* Packed RBCs may be administered to increase oxygen-carrying capacity to maintain a Hgb value 7 to 9 mg/dl or greater than 20% below the patient's baseline if the patient is chronically anemic and symptomatic.
6. **Supplement vitamin K₁ (phytonadione) and folate:** Patients with DIC are at high risk for deficiency of these substances, and administration of both vitamins is recommended for most patients.
7. **Prevent viral infections resulting from immunosuppression with protease inhibitors:** Gabexate, nafamostat, and trasylol have been used.
8. **Manage hypotension related to heart failure, as appropriate:** If patient becomes severely hypotensive due to heart failure, the following drugs may be considered: milrinone, dobutamine, dopamine, epinephrine, and nitroprusside (see Appendix 6).

CARE PLANS: DISSEMINATED INTRAVASCULAR COAGULATION

Ineffective protection *related to bleeding resulting from overstimulation of the clotting cascade and rapid consumption of clotting factors*

GOALS/OUTCOMES Within 48 to 72 hours of initiation of treatment, patient is free of symptoms of bleeding as evidenced by absence of frank bleeding from invasive procedure sites and mucosal surfaces; secretions and excretions that are negative for blood; absence of large or increasing ecchymoses; decreasing purpura; and HR, RR, and BP within 10% of patient's baseline (or HR 60 to 100 bpm, RR 12 to 20 breaths/min, systolic BP greater than 90 mm Hg). **NOC** Blood Coagulation

Bleeding Precautions
1. Discuss bleeding history with patient or significant others. Assess prior incidences of bleeding from gums, skin, or urine; tarry/bloody stools; bleeding from muscles or into joints; hemoptysis, vomiting of blood, epistaxis, or prolonged bleeding from small wounds or after tooth extraction; or unusual bruising or tendency to bruise easily. Provide soft tooth brush.
2. Question patients about current medications, including over-the-counter (OTC) preparations, since many medications promote bleeding (Table 10-6).
3. Monitor coagulation tests daily. Consult physician or midlevel practitioner for abnormal values (Table 10-7).
4. Monitor closely for increased bleeding, bruising, petechiae, and purpura. Assess for internal bleeding by testing suspicious secretions (i.e., sputum, urine, stool, emesis, gastric drainage) for the presence of blood. Monitor for hemorrhage.
5. Monitor neurologic status (see Glasgow Coma Scale, Appendix 2) every 2 hours by assessing LOC, orientation, pupillary reaction, and movement and strength of extremities. Changes in status can indicate intracranial bleeding.
6. Use alcohol-free mouthwash and swabs for oral care to minimize gingival/gum injury. Use normal saline solution (NSS) or solution of NSS and sodium bicarbonate (500 ml NSS with 15 ml bicarbonate) to irrigate the oral cavity if irritated. Massage gums gently with a sponge-tipped applicator to help remove debris. Do not attempt to remove large clots from the mouth, to avoid profuse bleeding.
7. Use electric rather than safety razor for shaving patient.
8. Refrain from inserting objects into a bleeding orifice. Avoid taking rectal temperatures.
9. Protect the patient from trauma. Avoid unnecessary venipunctures and IM injections.
10. If patient undergoes an invasive procedure, manually hold pressure over the insertion site for 3 to 5 minutes for IV catheters and 10 to 15 minutes for arterial catheters or until bleeding subsides.

Table 10-6   MEDICATIONS THAT MAY PROMOTE BLEEDING

Medications that Inhibit Platelets or Cause Thrombocytopenia

Analgesics	Diuretic Agents	Other
Nonsteroidal anti-inflammatory agents (NSAIDs)	Sulfonamide derivatives	Antihistamines
Aspirin (acetylsalicylic acid)	Acetazolamide	Ethanol
Acetaminophen	Chlorpropamide	Heparin
Antipyrine	Chlorothiazide	Beta adrenergic blocking agents
Ibuprofen	Chlorthalidone	General anesthetics
Indomethacin	Clopamide	Local anesthetics
Fenoprofen	Diazoxide	Chemotherapeutic agents
Sodium salicylate	Furosemide	Vitamin E
Antirheumatic agents	Bumetanide	Estrogens
Oxyphenbutazone	Hydrochlorothiazide	Digitoxin
Phenylbutazone	Tolbutamide	Cimetidine
Hydroxychloroquine	Spironolactone	Levodopa
Gold salts	Mercurial diuretics	Propylthiouracil
Antimicrobials	Glycoprotein IIb/IIIa inhibitors	
Ampicillin	Abciximab	
Cephalothin	Eptifibatide	
Methicillin	Tirofiban	
Penicillin	Phenothiazines	
Pentamidine	Chlorpromazine	
Streptomycin	Promethazine	
Sulfonamides (antibiotics)	Trifluoperazine	
Chloramphenicol	Phosphodiesterase inhibitors	
Isoniazid	Caffeine	
Nitrofurantoin	Dipyridamole	
Rifampin	Theophyllines	
Trimethoprim	Antiplatelet drugs	
Anticoagulants	Aspirin (acetylsalicylic acid)	
Heparin	Ticlopidine	
Enoxaparin	Clopidogrel	
Dalteparin	Prostaglandins	
Thrombolytics	I_2	
Alteplase	D_2	
Reteplase	E	
Streptokinase	Sedative-hypnotics	
Urokinase	Benzodiazepines	
Anisoylated plasminogen streptokinase	Clonazepam	
Tenecteplase	Diazepam	
	Vasodilators	
	Nitroglycerin	
	Nitroprusside	

Continued

Table 10-6 MEDICATIONS THAT MAY PROMOTE BLEEDING—cont'd

Medications that Inhibit Vitamin K

Salicylates	Broad-Spectrum Antibiotics	Vitamins
Aspirin and aspirin-combination drugs	Sulfonamides	A
Other salicylates	Triple sulfa	E
Coumarins	Sulfamethoxazole	
Anisindione	Sulfasalazine	
Dicumarol	Sulfisoxazole	
Warfarin	Sulfamethoxazole-trimethoprim	
	Clindamycin	
	Gentamicin	
	Neomycin	
	Tobramycin	
	Vancomycin	
	Imipenem	
	Cefamandole	
	Cefoxitin	

Table 10-7 DISSEMINATED INTRAVASCULAR COAGULATION (DIC): LAB VALUES

Parameter	Normal	Acute DIC	Chronic DIC
Fibrinogen	150–400 mg/dL (adult)	Decreased	Normal or increased
Fibrin degradation	<10 mcg/ml	Positive (increased)	Positive (increased)
Platelet count	150,000–400,000/mm³ (adult)	Decreased	Normal or increased
Partial thromboplastin time (PTT); also known as activated partial thromboplastin time (aPTT)	25–35 seconds	Increased	Normal
Prothrombin time (PT)	11–15 seconds	Increased	Normal
Thrombin time	1.5 × Control value	Increased	Increased

11. Instruct the patient and/or family on signs of bleeding and appropriate actions.
12. Teach patient the importance of avoiding vitamin K–inhibiting and platelet aggregation–inhibiting medications or vitamin and dietary supplements (see Table 10-6), which promote bleeding.

NIC Infection Control; Infection Protection; Surveillance: Safety

Risk for deficient fluid volume *related to bleeding/hemorrhage*

GOALS/OUTCOMES Patient remains normovolemic as evidenced by HR and RR within 10% of patient's baseline (or HR 60 to 100 bpm and RR 12 to 20 breaths/min with normal depth and pattern; BP within patient's baseline (or systolic BP more than 90 mm Hg), warm extremities, distal pulses at least 2+ on a 0 to 4+ scale, urinary output more than 0.5 ml/kg/hr, and capillary refill less than 2 seconds. Within 24 hours of initiating treatment, patient verbalizes orientation to time, place, person, and self.
NOC Fluid Balance

Fluid Monitoring

1. Monitor every 2 hours for increases in HR and RR, decreased BP, and decreasing pulse pressure.
2. Measure urinary output every 2 to 4 hours. Consult physician or midlevel practitioner for output less than 0.5 ml/kg/hr.
3. Maintain accurate I&O record. Weigh daily, and monitor trends.
4. Increase measurement of vital signs and urine output to at least every 30 minutes for active bleeding. For profuse bleeding, check vital signs at least every 15 minutes. Inspect invasive procedure sites and dressings for bleeding.
5. Monitor CBC daily for significant alterations in Hct, Hgb, and platelets (Table 10-8).
6. Ensure that patient has typed and cross-matched blood available for transfusion.
7. Monitor coagulation studies (PT, PTT, fibrinogen, FDP/FSP, platelet counts), as appropriate.
8. Assess for signs of impending shock if the following signs are noted: increased HR and RR; decreased BP; or pallor, diaphoresis, cool extremities, delayed capillary refill, decreased pulse amplitude, restlessness, or disorientation.
9. Maintain at least one 18-gauge or larger IV catheter for use during shock management, at which time rapid infusion of blood products or IV fluids may be necessary.
10. Evaluate the effects of fluid therapy.

NIC Electrolyte Management; Fluid Management; Hypovolemia Management; Intravenous (IV) Therapy; Shock Management: Volume

Ineffective tissue perfusion (or risk for same): peripheral, cardiopulmonary, cerebral, gastrointestinal, and renal *related to blood loss or presence of microthrombi*

GOALS/OUTCOMES Patient has adequate perfusion as evidenced by peripheral pulses more than 2+ on a scale of 0 to 4+, brisk capillary refill (less than 2 seconds), BP within patient's normal range, CVP 2 to 6 mm Hg, and HR regular and less than 100 bpm. Patient is oriented to time, place, person, and self and has urinary output at least 30 ml/hr (0.5 ml/kg/hr) and oxygen saturation greater than 96%.
NOC Circulation Status

Shock Prevention

1. Assess and document peripheral perfusion every 2 hours, including temperature, sensation, pulses, and movement in extremities. Perform a comprehensive assessment of peripheral circulation (i.e., check peripheral pulses, edema, capillary refill, and color and temperature of extremities).

Table 10-8	COMPLETE BLOOD COUNT (CBC) VALUES	
Parameters	**Common Measurement Value**	**Population**
Red blood cells (RBCs)	4–5.5 million/mm^3 4.5–6.2 million/mm^3	Adult females Adult males
Hemoglobin (Hgb)	12–16 g/dl 14–18 g/dl	Adult females Adult males
Hematocrit (Hct)	37%–47%	Adult females
Mean corpuscular volume (MCV)	83–93 mcg^3	Adults
Mean cell hemoglobin (MCH)	26–34 pg	Adults
Mean cell hemoglobin concentration (MCHC)	31%–38%	Adults
White blood cells (WBCs)	4,500–11,000/mm^3	Adults
Differential White Blood Cells (Granulocytes)		
Segmented neutrophils (Segs)	54%–62%	Adults
Band neutrophils (Bands)	3%–5%	Adults
Eosinophils (Eos)	1%–3%	Adults
Basophils (Basos)	0–0.75%	Adults
Monocytes (Monos)	3%–7%	Adults
Lymphocytes (Lymphs)	25%–33%	Adults
Platelets	150,000–400,000/mm^3	Adults

2. Monitor vital signs frequently. Evaluate chest pain. Document cardiac dysrhythmias.
3. Monitor BP and assess for early signs of perfusion deficit at least every 2 hours, including dizziness, confusion, and decreased urinary output.
4. Monitor for decreased myocardial or pulmonary perfusion as evidenced by chest pain, ST-segment depression or elevation, T-wave inversion, SOB, dyspnea, and decreased oxygen saturation using continuous pulse oximetry.
5. Monitor CVP, observing for both high and low readings. Decreased pressures are indicative of hypovolemia/hemorrhage. Anticipate vasoconstriction with hypovolemia: CO may increase or decrease from normal range of 4 to 7 L/min, depending on cardiac contractility.
6. Monitor GI status by observing tolerance to diet or tube feedings, bowel habits (e.g., constipation, diarrhea), character of stool (e.g., tarry, bloody), and presence or absence of bowel sounds.

NIC Cardiac Care: Acute; Circulatory Care: Arterial Insufficiency; Circulatory Care: Venous Insufficiency; Respiratory Monitoring; Shock Management: Cardiac; Cerebral Perfusion Promotion; Neurologic Monitoring; Peripheral Sensation Management; Fluid/Electrolyte Management; Fluid Management; Vital Signs Monitoring

Impaired gas exchange (or risk for same) *related to loss of oxygen-carrying capacity through hemorrhage or pulmonary microembolus formation*

GOALS/OUTCOMES Patient's gas exchange is adequate as evidenced by PaO_2 at least 80 mm Hg, $PaCO_2$ 35 to 45 mm Hg, pH 7.35 to 7.45, RR 12 to 20 breaths/min with normal depth and pattern, oxygen saturation at least 90%, HR 60 to 100 bpm, SvO_2 at least 60%, and orientation to time, place, and person.
NOC Respiratory Status: Gas Exchange

Respiratory Monitoring
1. Assess respiratory status every 2 hours, noting rate, rhythm, depth, and regularity of respirations. Provide supplemental oxygen as appropriate.
2. Monitor for signs of respiratory failure: restlessness, anxiety, and air hunger indicative of hypoxemia; ABG values for increased $PaCO_2$ and decreased pH indicative of hypoventilation; or oxygen saturation less than 95% via pulse oximetry indicative of decreased ventilation. Consult physician or midlevel practitioner if signs of respiratory insufficiency are present.
3. Monitor $ScvO_2$ or SvO_2: steady increase or decrease from patient's normal level may indicate deterioration.
4. Assess lungs for bibasilar crackles (rales), indicative of pulmonary edema.
5. Monitor patient's respiratory secretions. Institute respiratory therapy treatments as needed.
6. Monitor for pulmonary embolus, including sharp, stabbing chest pain, dyspnea, pallor, cyanosis, pupillary dilation, rapid or irregular pulse, profuse diaphoresis, and anxiety. Assess need for supplemental oxygen, and consult physician immediately. Patients with severe pulmonary emboli may require mechanical ventilation. See *Pulmonary Embolus*, p. 396.
7. Assess patient for changes in sensorium (i.e., confusion, lethargy, somnolence), indicative of inadequate cerebral oxygenation or CO_2 retention (respiratory insufficiency).

NIC Airway Management; Oxygen Therapy; Respiratory Monitoring

Risk for injury *related to blood product administration*

GOALS/OUTCOMES Throughout transfusion and up to 8 hours after transfusion, patient does not exhibit signs of a blood transfusion reaction as evidenced by stable mentation, absence of fever and chills, normal appearance of skin (i.e., no flushing, rash, lesions), and baseline RR, BP, and HR.
NOC Risk Control

Surveillance: Safety
1. Check blood to be transfused with another professional to ensure the patient receives the correct blood. Verify the following: patient's name, patient's birthday and hospital number, blood unit number, blood expiration date, blood group, and blood type.
2. Discuss signs and symptoms of potential reaction with patient and family. Premedicate if there is a history of reaction or antibodies are present.
3. When blood products are being infused, check vital signs every 15 minutes for the first hour. Check patient frequently throughout the first 15 minutes of the transfusion to observe for signs of an acute hemolytic

transfusion reaction, including fever, chills, dyspnea, hypotension, flushing, tachycardia, back pain, hematuria, mentation changes, and shock.

4. Observe for transfusion reactions throughout the transfusion and during the 8-hour period afterward. If a transfusion reaction (Table 10-9) occurs, implement the following:
   - If the transfusion is in progress, stop the infusion immediately.
   - Maintain IV access with normal saline solution.
   - Maintain BP with a combination of volume infusion and vasoactive drugs, if indicated.
   - Monitor HR and ECG for changes. Treat symptomatic dysrhythmias as prescribed by a physician or midlevel practitioner.
   - Administer ordered diuretics and fluids to promote diuresis (urine output approximately 100 ml/hr).
   - Obtain blood and urine for a transfusion workup per institution blood bank protocol.
   - Perform blood cultures if patient exhibits signs of sepsis.
5. If an intravascular hemolytic reaction is confirmed, implement the following:
   - Monitor coagulation studies, including PT, PTT, and fibrinogen levels (see Table 10-7).
   - Monitor renal status by measuring the following: blood urea nitrogen (BUN), creatinine, potassium, and phosphate levels.
   - Monitor lab values for hemolysis: increased lactate dehydrogenase (LDH), bilirubin, and haptoglobin.
6. With massive transfusion for severe bleeding, manage hypocalcemia caused by citrated blood, hyperkalemia of uncertain etiology, hypothermia from refrigerated blood, ARDS, coagulopathy, and hemochromatosis (iron overload).

NIC Bleeding Precautions; Bleeding Reduction; Blood Products Administration

ADDITIONAL NURSING DIAGNOSES

The uncontrolled bleeding related to DIC can be terrifying to the patient and significant others, who may fear that the patient will die. Refer to nursing diagnoses in *Emotional and Spiritual Support of the Patient and Significant Others*, p. 200. For patients who manifest activity intolerance, see that nursing diagnosis in *Prolonged Immobility*, p. 149. For patients with sepsis or septic shock, see *SIRS, Sepsis and MODS*, p. 924.

Table 10-9	ACUTE TRANSFUSION REACTIONS	
Type	**Symptoms**	**Time Frame**
Acute intravascular hemolytic	Fever, chills, dyspnea, tachycardia, hypotension, back pain, flushing, hematuria, shock	After start of transfusion within 5–30 minutes
Acute extravascular hemolytic	Fever, elevated bilirubin, unusually low posttransfusion hematocrit and hemoglobin	Usually within 8 hours Delayed: 7–10 days
Allergic (mild)	Rash, hives pruritus	Within 1 hour
Anaphylactic	Dyspnea, shortness of breath, bronchospasms, tachycardia, flushing, hypotension, shock	Within 30 min–1 hour
Febrile	Fever, chills	Within 4 hours
Hypervolemic	Dyspnea, tachycardia, bibasilar crackles, jugular venous distention, possible hypertension, headache	Within 1–2 hours
Septic	Fever, chills, tachycardia, hypotension, vomiting, shock, muscle pain, cardiac arrest	Within 5 minutes–4 hours

SELECTED REFERENCES

Abraham J: Romiplostim for treating thrombocytopenia in chronic idiopathic thrombocytopenia purpura, *Commun Oncol* 5(12):651, 2008.

American Society of Anesthesiologists: Practice guidelines for perioperative blood transfusion and adjuvant therapies. *Anesthesiology* 105:198-208, 2006.

Circular of information: For the use of human blood and blood components. www.aabb.org/Content/About_Blood/Circulars_of_Information/aabb_coi.htm

Gentry CA, Gross KB, Sud B, Drevets DA: Adverse outcomes associated with the use of drotrecogin alfa (activated) in patients with severe sepsis and baseline bleeding precautions. *Crit Care Med*, 37(1):19-25, 2009.

Goldman L, Ausiello D, editors: *Cecil Medicine*, 23rd ed. Philadelphia, PA, 2007, Saunders Elsevier, chap 164.

Gould S, Cimino M, Gerber D: Packed red cell transfusion in the intensive care unit: limitations and consequences. *Am J Crit Care* 16(1):39, 2007.

Hebert P, Tinmouth A, Corwin H: Controversies in RBC transfusion in the critically ill. *Chest* 131:1583-1590, 2007.

Kelton J, Warkentin T: Heparin induced thrombocytopenia: a historical perspective. *Blood* 112(12):2607, 2008.

Klein H, Spahn D, Carson J: Red blood cell transfusion in clinical practice. *Lancet* 370:415-426, 2007.

Lim B, Henry D: Stroke syndrome secondary to hypercoagulability of lung cancer. *Commun Oncol* 5(11):595, 2008.

Marik P, Corwin H: Efficacy of red blood cell transfusion in the critically ill: a systematic review of the literature. *Crit Care Med* 36:2667-2674, 2008.

McMahon B: Malignancy-associated thrombosis. *Oncol Iss* 24(1):20, 2009.

Murphy G, Reeves B, Rogers C, et al: Increased mortality, postoperative morbidity, and cost after red blood cell transfusion in patients having cardiac surgery. *Circulation* 116:2544-2552, 2007.

Practice guidelines for blood transfusion: a compilation from recent peer-reviewed literature. http://www.redcross.org/www-files/Documents/WorkingWiththeRedCross/practice guidelinesforbloodtrans.pdf

Reeves B, Murphy G: Increased morality, morbidity, and cost associated with red blood cell transfusion after cardiac surgery. *Curr Opin Anaesthesiol* 21:669-673, 2008.

Rome S, Doss D, Miller K, et al: Thromboembolic events associated with novel therapies in patients with multiple myeloma: consensus statement of the IMF nurse leadership board. *Clin J Oncol Nursing* 12(3, suppl):21, 2008.

Sampson HA, Muñoz-Furlong A, Campbell RL, et al: Second symposium on the definition and management of anaphylaxis: summary report, Second National Institute of Allergy and Infectious Disease/Food Allergy and Anaphylaxis Network symposium. *J Allergy Clin Immunol* 117(2):391-397, 2006.

Simons FE: Anaphylaxis. *J Allergy Clin Immunol* 121(2 suppl):S402-S407, 2008.

Simons FE: Anaphylaxis: Recent advances in assessment and treatment. *J Allergy Clin Immunol* 124(4):625-636, 2009.

Yap C, Lau L, Krishnaswamy M, et al: Age of transfused red cells and early outcomes after cardiac surgery. *Ann Thorac Surg* 86:554-559, 2008.

Complex Special Situations

ABDOMINAL HYPERTENSION AND ABDOMINAL COMPARTMENT SYNDROME

". . . the end result of a progressive, unchecked increase in intra-abdominal pressure from a myriad of disorders that eventually leads to multiple organ dysfunction."

John Hunt, MD

PATHOPHYSIOLOGY

Intra-abdominal hypertension (IAH) occurs when the amount of intra-abdominal contents (through edematous bowel or fluid accumulating in the cavity) exceeds the distendable capability of the fascia. The result is an intra-abdominal hypertensive state. which can lead to abdominal compartment syndrome (ACS). As the fluid accumulates (due to bleeding, ascites, volume overload, and other causes), the resulting increase in pressure (change in compliance/change in volume) initially affects regional blood flow and results in impaired tissue perfusion, which is then associated with a systemic inflammatory response. The resulting ischemia and inflammatory response further causes capillary leakage and compression of the intra-abdominal viscera. If untreated, the continually elevated free fluid and measured pressure begin to compress blood vessels, causing organ dysfunction both inside and outside the abdomen, and lead to abdominal compartment syndrome. The inflammatory response promotes the release of cytokines, causing vasodilation and cell membrane dysfunction. The cell membrane loses integrity, which causes further inflammation, profound edema and ultimately cell death. The elevated pressure in the abdominal cavity generated by the severe increase in extra vascular fluid load increases the intra-abdominal contents (free water) and further impairs intestinal tissue perfusion as compression of the arteries and veins continues. This process underlies the multi-organ effects of rising intra-abdominal pressure (IAP). When the IAP rises above critical level, blood flow to the abdominal viscera and organs decreases and ACS is imminent.

Definitions

IAP refers to the pressure present within the abdominal cavity. The pressure within the cavity reflects the presence of extravascular fluids, which compress the blood vessels and organs in the abdominal cavity as well as displacing the diaphragm into the thoracic cage, which limits lung expansion. Elevated intrabladder pressure indirectly reflects high pressure within the abdominal cavity.

IAH is defined by the World Society of Abdominal Compartment Syndrome (WSACS) as a measured IAP of 12 mm Hg or greater, recorded three times using standardized measurement methods 4 to 6 hours apart and/or an abdominal perfusion pressure (APP) of less than 60 mm Hg (mean arterial pressure [MAP] minus intra-abdominal bladder pressure [IABP]), recorded using two standardized measurements 1-6 hours apart). These measurements should be evaluated in the context of clinical symptomatology.

An IAP of greater than 20 mm Hg reflects significant IAH almost universally.

An IAP of 18 mm Hg indicates a high probability of organ compromise.

An IAP of 15 mm Hg reflects moderate probability of organ compromise.

An IAP of 12 mm Hg reflects a lower probability of organ compromise.

Increased IAP may reflect a critical finding in patients with multiorgan dysfunction syndrome (MODS) or multisystem failure, which contributes to global hypoperfusion, aggravating the effects of increased IAP (Table 11-1).

ACS is defined as "intra-abdominal hypertension with a gradual and consistent increase in the IAP value of [equal to or greater than] 20 mm Hg," recorded by at least three standardized measurements taken 1 to 6 hours apart and in conjunction with at least one new onset organ dysfunction. ACS can be fatal and often complicates or results in a clinical condition refractory to treatment. The astute clinician suspects IAH and ACS when MODS is evolving and/or the patient presents with persistent lactic acidosis.

Historically, the belief of most critical care providers was that IAH and the more serious evolution of the state, ACS, was solely related to traumatic injury of the abdomen, including surgery. Within the last decade, the understanding of the pathophysiology involved in developing IAH and ACS has been enhanced by studies and revealed the prevalence in all critical patients; medical as well as surgical and trauma. The progressive conditions have been divided into two categories: primary or secondary abdominal hypertension disorders. The causes may differ, but outcomes are similar if either condition remains untreated.

Primary ACS is a condition associated with injury or disease in the abdominopelvic region that frequently requires early surgical or angioradiologic intervention. Any abnormal event that raises abdominal pressure can induce acute IAH, including blunt or penetrating abdominal

Table 11-1	PRESSURE AND SYMPTOM GRADE FOR INTRA-ABDOMINAL HYPERTENSION	
Graded Measurement	**Pressure Measurement and relevance**	**Physiologic Events and clinical signs**
Pressure Grade I	12–15 mm Hg Significant in the presence of organ dysfunction	Cytokine release and capillary leak Third spacing of resuscitative fluid Decreasing venous return and preload Early effects on ICP and CPP Abdominal wall perfusion decreases 42% Marked reduction in intestinal and intra-abdominal organ blood flow leading to regional acidosis and free radical formation.
Pressure Grade II	16–20 mm Hg Significant in most patients	Markedly decreased venous return, CO and splanchnic perfusion Increased SVR, CVP, PAWP Decreased blood pressure, pulse pressure and particularly systolic blood pressure Decreased TLC, FRC, RV. Increased vent pressures, hypercapnia, hypoxia Reduction to 61% of baseline mucosal blood flow and increasing gut acidosis Oliguria, anuria Increasing ICP and decreasing CPP
Pressure Grade III	21–25 mm Hg Significant in all patients	Hemodynamic collapse, worsening acidosis, hypoxia, hypercapnia, anuria. Inability to oxygenate, ventilate or resuscitate
Pressure Grade IV	>25 mm Hg Significant in all patients	Hemodynamic collapse, worsening acidosis, hypoxia, hypercapnia, anuria. Inability to oxygenate, ventilate or resuscitate

If both pressure and clinical symptoms are met for grade III and/or grade IV, patient has abdominal compartment syndrome.

trauma, abdominal aortic aneurysm (AAA), hemorrhagic pancreatitis, gastrointestinal (GI) obstruction, abdominal surgery resulting in retroperitoneal bleeding or secondary peritonitis, and with tight closure of abdominal incisions. Primary ACS also includes patients with abdominal solid organ injuries who were initially managed medically and then developed ACS. The condition has been relatively well understood by surgeons and their colleagues but is frequently misdiagnosed and/or untreated until surgical intervention is required.

Secondary ACS includes conditions that do not originate from abdominal injury that create IAH, including sepsis or any condition prompting capillary leak (e.g., major burns, and conditions requiring massive fluid resuscitation). A large multicenter study (Malbrain et al. 2005) found the prevalence of IAH was 54% among medical ICU patients and 65% in surgical ICU patients. This was remarkable, as most medical patients are not evaluated for or even considered recipients of IAH and ACS.

ACS treatments are the same regardless of the cause; however, the caregiver must be very careful in managing secondary ACS. The opportunity for early intervention may be lost with the subtle development of signs and symptoms of IAH and ACS. The lack of definitive signs often leads to delayed diagnosis and delayed recognition, and an urgent medical condition becomes an emergency surgical situation. Increased organ failure, increased mortality, increased resource utilization, and longer ICU lengths of stay may result. Similar to sepsis and severe sepsis, the greatest challenge is early recognition and diagnosis. Monitoring all high-risk patients would enable clinicians to trend the IAP, facilitating early, appropriate interventions when the syndrome is more likely to be responsive to medical therapy. The best management strategy is to prevent abdominal compartment syndrome via early monitoring, early medical interventions, and early surgical decompression if needed.

ASSESSMENT
Goal of System Assessment
To rapidly evaluate for significant primary and secondary IAH and correlating reduction of blood flow to other organs

History and Risk Factors
Patients with a history of abdominal trauma, abdominal surgery, intra-abdominal infection, damage control laparotomy with intra-abdominal packing, severe infection, sepsis, peritonitis, bleeding pelvic fractures, postoperative bleeding, massive retroperitoneal hematoma, liver transplantation, ruptured AAA, visceral tissue edema, pneumoperitoneum, hypovolemic or vasogenic shock or any patient with aggressive fluid resuscitation, acute ascites, and/or pancreatitis.

Vital Signs and Other Values
The following values may be increased:
- Heart and respiratory rates
- Intracranial Pressure (ICP)
- *Hemodynamic values:* Central venous pressure (CVP), pulmonary artery occlusive pressure (PAOP), systemic vascular resistance (SVR), inferior vena cava (IVC) pressure
- *Respiratory:* Pleural pressure, peak inspiratory pressure
- *Screening lab values:* $Paco_2$, serum creatinine, serum blood urea nitrogen (BUN)

The following values may be decreased:
- Systolic blood pressure (BP)
- *Respiratory:* tidal volume, Pao_2
- Cardiac output (CO)
- Urine output
- Cerebral perfusion pressure (CPP)
- Glomerular filtration rate (GFR)
- Abdominal Perfusion Pressure (APP)

Observation
Observe for upward trends in respiratory and heart rates (RR and HR, respectively) and decrease in urine output. Signs and symptoms are nonspecific and subtle and may be attributed to other clinical conditions (Table 11-1). Elevated IAP affects the cardiovascular, pulmonary, renal, and neurologic systems.

Cardiovascular: Hypotension may result from decreased CO, which results from IAH-induced vasoconstriction. Signs of shock, including pallor, tachycardia, and cool and clammy skin, may be present. Venous return is diminished due to compression of the IVC, resulting in loss of compliance (increased IVC pressure) and decreased preload (volume), which further reduces CO. Increased IAP compresses the aorta, resulting in elevated SVR (increased afterload), which reduces CO. The compensatory vasoconstriction affects blood flow to the hepatic and renal veins, leading to renal compromise, oliguria, and hepatic hypoperfusion; if untreated, kidney and liver failure can result.

Pulmonary: Respiratory distress results from the elevated abdominal pressure impeding diaphragmatic movement by forcing the diaphragm upward, which decreases functional residual capacity, promotes atelectasis, and decreases lung surface area. Tachypnea and increased work of breathing may be present. The worsening hypoxemia promotes elevated peak inspiratory pressures, with refractory hypoxemia and a poor P/F ratio, similar to acute respiratory distress syndrome (ARDS). Alternative ventilatory support is often required to maintain oxygenation and ventilation.

Neurologic: Altered mental status results from obstruction of cerebral venous outflow, leading to vascular congestion and increased ICP. Increased IAP increases intrathoracic pressure, which compresses the veins within the thoracic cavity, making it difficult for cerebral veins to drain properly. The combination of decreased CO and increased ICP can lead to decreased CPP, which prompts further deterioration in level of consciousness (LOC).

Renal: Renal dysfunction results as the increasing abdominal pressure compresses the bladder and urethra as well as the renal arteries and veins. Urine output decreases and serum Cr and BUN increase although they may not do so in proportion to each other (BUN/Cr ratio).

DIAGNOSTIC TESTS
Methods of Intra-Abdominal Pressure Measurement
The best method for measurement of IAP is controversial. The most common method is measuring the response of intra-bladder compliance to an instillation of 25 ml of sterile fluid by measuring the resulting pressure.

Direct intraperitoneal measurement: The most accurate method requires an intraperitoneal catheter inserted into the abdomen with a fluid manometer or pressure transducer attached to measure the pressure. This method requires expert catheter placement and is highly linked to infection.

Indirect methods: Bladder pressure is commonly used, while other methods are infrequently used. Indirect methods include gastric pressure measurement through gastrostomy or a nasogastric tube, intrarectal pressure measurement using an esophageal stethoscope catheter, or bladder pressure measurement through a urinary catheter.

Bladder pressure measurement: An indwelling urinary catheter is connected to either a pressure transducer or a fluid manometer to measure the pressure. Readings are reliable and easier to perform than direct intraperitoneal measurement.

The urinary bladder normally has a compliant wall. Many studies reveal compliance decreases when there is a high presence of intra-abdominal fluids, which increase the pressure in the abdominal cavity and compress the bladder, increasing resistance. When fluid is injected into the bladder pressure system, any decrease in bladder compliance is reflected by increased intra-bladder pressure. The procedure is generally easier and safer if a prepackaged closed bladder pressure system is used. If assembling the system without a prepackaged tool, use the urinary/Foley catheter with an aspiration or infusion port:

1. The nurse will connect a fluid filled pressure system to a transducer, then connect a needle to the distal end of the tubing (farthest from the transducer and after a stopcock).
2. The cable connecting the system to the monitor should allow for visualization of a small pressure (scale either auto or at 30 mm Hg).
3. The connected system will be inserted into the catheter infusion port.
4. After zeroing the system (transducer at the symphysis pubis and the stopcock will be turned off to the patient), the nurse will clamp the catheter drainage system just below the infusion port.
5. Using the stopcock, the system will be turned off to the monitor and 25 mls of sterile fluid (IV fluid is fine) will be injected rapidly into the infusion port on the urinary catheter. The stopcock will be then turned off to the injecting port, leaving a connected pressure system from patient to monitor.

6. Bladder pressure must be read during end expiration and the patient must be as flat as tolerated to facilitate accuracy. There is no dynamic waveform associated with bladder pressure. One should just observe the level of pressure in the first 10–20 seconds after fluid is instilled.

7. A normal value is generally considered between 0 and 5 mm Hg, although levels as high as 15 mm Hg are not unusual in the first 24 hours after abdominal surgery (see Table 11-1). If the pressures are elevated, document and repeat in the next hour using the same techniques. Inform the physician or midlevel practitioner if both measures are elevated.

8. Occlusion is then released and fluid is drained into the urine collection bag. Subtract the amount of fluid from the hourly output.

COLLABORATIVE MANAGEMENT
Care Priorities

1. **Prevent abdominal compartment syndrome:** Patients who have a high index of suspicion should have bladder pressure monitoring initiated in order to identify IAH earlier and possibly avoid decompressive laparotomy, which is the only documented evidence-based therapy for ACS (Box 11-1). There are many approaches that may be used to reduce IAH. These strategies are directed at reducing increased abdominal cavity volume or decreasing compliance. Therapies include:

Draining free intraperitoneal fluid: Paracentesis is performed by the advanced practitioner. Some centers may place a peritoneal drainage catheter and leave it in place if abdominal fluid accumulation is persistent and severe.

Volume replacement with small volumes of higher osmotic gradient IV fluids: More highly concentrated IV solutions (e.g., hypertonic [3%] saline, plasma, hextend, blood products) can sometimes facilitate fluid stabilization within the vasculature for longer periods of time than isotonic solutions.

Continuous renal replacement therapy (CRRT): Enables minute-to-minute control of intravascular fluid removal and replacement. Fluid management is more exact and CRRT was

---

Box 11-1	**MANAGEMENT OF ABDOMINAL COMPARTMENT SYNDROME**

1. Improvement of abdominal wall compliance
   - Sedation
   - Pain relief (Do not use fentanyl!)
   - Neuromuscular blockade
   - Body positioning
   - Negative fluid balance
   - Percutaneous abdominal wall component separation
2. Evacuation of intraluminal contents
   - Nasogastric suction
   - Rectal tube/enemas
   - Gastro/colonic prokinetic agents
   - Paracentesis
   - Percutaneous drainage of abscess/hematomas
3. Evacuation of peri-intestinal and abdominal fluids
   - Ascites evacuation in cirrhosis
   - CT- or US-guided aspiration of abscess
   - CT- or US-guided aspiration of hematoma
   - Percutaneous drainage of (blood) collections
4. Correction of capillary leak and positive fluid balance
   - Diuretics/colloids/hypertonic fluids
   - Hemodialysis/ultrafiltration
   - Dobutamine (Do not use dopamine!)
   - Ascorbic acid in burn patients

CT, computerized tomography; US, ultrasound.

Modified from Ivatury et al: In Vincent JL, editor: *Yearbook of intensive care and emergency medicine.* Berlin, 2008, Springer, p. 554.

thought to benefit the patient by removal of cytokines, but more recent evidence indicates that may not be of benefit (see *Continuous Renal Replacement Therapies*, p. 603).

Other options: Include the sedation and analgesic management of patients and ultimately the consideration of neuromuscular blockade or chemical paralysis

2. **Perform a decompressive laparotomy to relieve ACS:** Sudden release of the abdominal pressure may lead to further complications including ischemia-reperfusion injury, acute vasodilation, cardiac dysfunction, and arrest. Arteries and veins within the abdomen are suddenly able to expand to normal size and "refill" with normal blood volume. If the patient has insufficient volume to accommodate the renewed space within the vasculature, hypotension ensues. Patients should be hydrated with at least 2 L of intravenous (IV) fluid, which may include a "cellular protection cocktail," such as 25 grams of mannitol 12.5% given along with 2 ampules of bicarbonate per liter. IV fluids and vasopressors should be immediately available in case severe hypotension occurs as the abdomen is decompressed.

After opening the abdomen, temporary closure will be applied. The goal is to permanently close the abdomen as soon as possible. For most patients who require emergent opening of the abdomen for ACS, a vacuum-assisted closure device (abdominal wound VAC) attached to a negative pressure device is commonly applied. An open abdomen may precipitate loss of liters of volume. The modified negative pressure wound VAC facilitates open wound fluid and management and supports granulation of tissue, as well as local perfusion, which facilitates eventual closure of the open wound.

RESEARCH BRIEF 11-1

Tremblay and colleagues reported on 181 patients with an open abdomen over a 4-year period managed with silos, skin only or towel clip closure, open packing, and modified visceral packing—in fact, anything other than vacuum-assisted closure (VAC). Mortality and other complications were extremely high in this group compared to those with VAC: 14% developed enterocutaneous fistulas, 5% suffered wound dehiscence, and almost half of the patients in the series were left with large incisional hernias at discharge. The study concluded some method of vacuum-assisted technique should be applied in the majority of patients.

Tremblay LN, Feliciano DV, Schmidt J, et al: Skin only or silo closure in the critically ill patient with an open abdomen. *Am J Surg* 182:670, 2001.

CARE PLANS FOR ABDOMINAL COMPARTMENT SYNDROME AND INTRA-ABDOMINAL HYPERTENSION

Deficient fluid volume *related to either active intravascular fluid loss secondary to physical injury or a condition resulting in capillary leak syndrome with third spacing of fluids*

GOALS/OUTCOMES Within 12 hours of this diagnosis, patient is becoming normovolemic evidenced by MAP at least 70 mm Hg, HR 60 to 100 beats/min (bpm), normal sinus rhythm on ECG, CVP 6 to 12 mm Hg, CI at least 2.5 L/min/m², bladder pressure measurements of less than 15 mm Hg, APP at least 60 mm Hg, stroke volume variation (SVV) less than 15%, urinary output at least 0.5 ml/kg/hr, warm extremities, brisk capillary refill (less than 2 seconds), and distal pulses at least 2+ on a 0 to 4+ scale. Although hemodynamic parameters are helpful to determine adequacy of resuscitation, serum lactate and base deficit are required to evaluate cellular perfusion.
NOC Fluid Balance; Electrolyte and Acid-Base Balance

Fluid/Electrolyte Management
1. Monitor BP at least hourly, or more frequently in the presence of unstable vital signs. Be alert to changes in MAP of more than 10 mm Hg. Even a small but sudden decrease in BP signals the need to consult the physician or midlevel practitioner, especially with the trauma patient in whom the extent of injury is unknown.
2. Once stable, monitor BP at least hourly, or more frequently in the presence of any unstable vital signs. Be alert to changes in MAP of more than 10 mm Hg.

3. If massive fluid resuscitation was necessary for either the trauma patient or a patient with third-spaced fluid, the patient is at higher risk for IAH and should be observed closely for signs of decreased perfusion, respiratory distress, and deterioration in mental status.

4. In the patient with evidence of volume depletion or active blood loss, administer pressurized fluids rapidly through several large-caliber (16-gauge or larger) catheters. Use short, large-bore IV tubing (trauma tubing) to maximize flow rate. Avoid use of stopcocks, because they slow the infusion rate. Fluids should be warmed to prevent hypothermia.

5. Measure central pressures and CO continuously if possible, or at least every 2 hours if blood loss is ongoing. Calculate SVR and PVR if data is available at least every 8 hours — more often in unstable patients. Be alert to low or decreasing CVP and PAWP. Be aware that profound tachycardia (>120 bpm) will decrease the cardiac compliance and therefore normal pressure readings in this instance can be misleading. Also anticipate mild to moderate pulmonary hypertension, especially in patients with concurrent thoracic injury, such as pulmonary contusion, smoke inhalation, or early ARDS. ARDS is a concern in patients who have sustained major abdominal injury, inasmuch as there are many potential sources of infection and sepsis that make the development of ARDS more likely (see *Acute Lung Injury and Acute Respiratory Distress Syndrome*, p. 365).

6. Measure urinary output at least every 2 hours. Urine output less than 0.5 ml/kg/hr usually reflects inadequate intravascular volume in the patient with abdominal trauma. Decreasing urine output may also signify compression of the renal arteries in ACS.

7. Monitor for physical indicators of arterial hypovolemia, which may include cool extremities, capillary refill greater than 2 seconds, absent or decreased amplitude of distal pulses, elevated serum lactate, and base deficit.

8. Estimate ongoing blood loss. Measure all bloody drainage from tubes or catheters, noting drainage color (e.g., coffee grounds, burgundy, bright red). Note the frequency of dressing changes as a result of saturation with blood to estimate amount of blood loss by way of the wound site.

NIC Electrolyte Management; Fluid Management; Fluid Monitoring; Hypovolemia Management

Ineffective tissue perfusion: gastrointestinal *related to interruption of arterial or venous blood flow or hypovolemia secondary to physical injury or any condition resulting in third spaced fluid or development of ascites*

GOALS/OUTCOMES Within 12 hours of this diagnosis, patient is becoming normovolemic evidenced by MAP at least 70 mm Hg, HR 60 to 100 beats/min (bpm), normal sinus rhythm on ECG, CVP 6 to 12 mm Hg, Bladder pressure measurements of less than 15 mm Hg, APP at least 60 mm Hg, CI at least 2.5 L/min/m^2, SVV less than 15%, urinary output at least 0.5 ml/kg/hr, warm extremities, brisk capillary refill (less than 2 seconds), and distal pulses at least 2+ on a 0 to 4+ scale. There should be a normal bicarbonate or total serum CO$_2$. By the time of hospital discharge, patient has adequate abdominal tissue perfusion as evidenced by normoactive bowel sounds; soft, nondistended abdomen; and return of bowel elimination.

NOC Tissue Perfusion: Abdominal Organs

Circulatory Care: Arterial Insufficiency

1. Identify patients who are at high risk for IAH.

2. Monitor BP at least hourly, or more frequently in the presence of unstable vital signs.

3. Monitor HR, ECG, and cardiovascular status every 15 minutes until vital signs are stable.

4. Auscultate for bowel sounds hourly during the acute phase of abdominal trauma and every 4 to 8 hours during the recovery phase. Report prolonged or sudden absence of bowel sounds during the postoperative period, because these signs may signal bowel ischemia or mesenteric infarction, which requires immediate surgical intervention.

5. Evaluate patient for peritoneal signs (see Box 3-3, p. 249), which may occur initially as a result of injury or may not develop until days or weeks later, if complications caused by slow bleeding or other mechanisms occur.

6. Ensure adequate intravascular volume.

7. Evaluate laboratory data for evidence of bleeding (e.g., serial Hct) or organ ischemia (e.g., AST, ALT, lactic dehydrogenase [LDH]). Desired values are as follows: Hct greater than 28% to 30%, AST 5 to 40 IU/L, ALT 5 to 35 IU/L, and LDH 90 to 200 U/L.

8. Measure bladder pressure manually: See *Diagnostic Tests*, Bladder Pressure Measurement, p 864.

9. *Prepackaged closed system bladder pressure monitoring:* Complete bladder pressure monitoring systems became available in approximately 2004. The system remains completely closed throughout the injection of fluid into the bladder, making it more desirable as part of prevention of catheter-associated urinary tract infections.

10. Assess for changes in level of consciousness, possibly resulting from increased IAP, which may inadvertently affect the draining of the cerebral veins.

◢◣**Risk for infection** *related to inadequate primary defenses secondary to physical trauma, surgery, underlying infection, temporary closure of abdomen or insertion of urinary catheter for measurement of IAP; inadequate secondary defenses caused by debilitated condition, decreased hemoglobin or inadequate immune response; tissue destruction and environmental exposure (especially to intestinal contents); multiple invasive procedures*

GOALS/OUTCOMES Patient is free of infection as evidenced by core or rectal temperature less than 37.7°C (100°F); normal white blood cell count and no bandemia; HR less than 100 bpm; orientation to time, place, and person; and absence of unusual redness, warmth, or drainage at surgical incisions and drain sites.
NOC Immune Status; Infection Severity

Infection Protection
1. Note color, character, and odor of all drainage. Report the presence of foul-smelling or abnormal drainage. See Table 3-2 for a description of the usual character of GI drainage.
2. As prescribed, administer pneumococcal vaccine to patients with total splenectomy to minimize the risk of postsplenectomy sepsis.
3. If evisceration occurs initially or develops later, do not reinsert tissue or organs. Place a saline-soaked gauze over the evisceration, and cover with a sterile towel until the evisceration can be evaluated by the surgeon.
4. For more interventions, see this diagnosis in *Abdominal Trauma* (p. 245).

NIC Infection Control

ADDITIONAL NURSING DIAGNOSES
Also see *Major Trauma*, p. 235. For additional information, see nursing diagnoses and interventions in the following sections: *Hemodynamic Monitoring* (p. 75), *Prolonged Immobility* (p. 149), *Emotional and Spiritual Support of the Patient and Significant Others* (p. 200), *Peritonitis* (p. 805), *Enterocutaneous Fistula* (p. 778), *SIRS, Sepsis and MODS* (p. 927), and *Acid-Base Imbalances* (p. 1).

DRUG OVERDOSE
OVERVIEW/EPIDEMIOLOGY
Drug overdose and accidental poisonings are common events, varying widely with respect to drug class, victim profile, and clinical scenario. Over 2 million human toxic exposure cases are reported to poison control centers annually. The 5 million total reported cases at all sites is probably an underestimation due to underreporting and misdiagnosing. Most cases are unintentional, involve a single agent, and can be handled on site with help from a poison control center; however, 5% to 10% of emergency department visits and 5% of ICU admissions involve exposure to toxic substances.

Type, amount, and route of use of the drug determine the effects, management, outcome, prognosis, and physical presentation. Every drug has a threshold for occurrence of serious toxic effects. Drugs of abuse are more dangerous than prescription drugs, as they are uncontrolled and unregulated, with a haphazard nature of administration. The patient's history is often unavailable or of poor quality. Time is critical to successful treatment. A thoughtful and stepwise approach to laboratory testing, medical and nursing interventions, pharmacologic support, and general supportive measures is essential. No organ or body system is protected from the detrimental effects of drug overdose.

INGESTION OF UNKNOWN SUBSTANCES
Many patients with drug overdose first arrive to be seen with altered mental status and without a useful or reliable history. Identification of the ingested substance is difficult. Lab screening is done for common drugs of abuse, including amphetamines, barbiturates, benzodiazepines, cocaine, opioids, phencyclidine, and cannabinoids. Specific drug levels are available for salicylates, acetaminophen, digoxin, theophylline, iron, and lithium. When one of these drugs is not the offending agent, a number of signs and symptoms should be noted and tests done to determine the list of potential offending agents.

ASSESSMENT

It is beyond the scope of this chapter to include all the drugs and toxins leading to common presenting symptoms, but important clues to the poison may be gleaned from answering the following questions:

- *HR and rhythm:* Is the patient bradycardic or tachycardic? Is a dysrhythmia present?
- *Mental status:* Is the patient overall depressed or agitated? Is delirium present?
- *Temperature:* Is hypothermia or hyperthermia present?
- *Seizures:* Is the patient having seizures?
- *Eyes:* Are pupils showing miosis or mydriasis? Is nystagmus present?
- *Muscle tone:* Is the patient flaccid or rigid? Are dyskinesias present?
- *Lungs:* If respiratory failure is occurring, is it related to depression, aspiration, edema, hemorrhage, bronchospasm, or cardiac failure?
- *Arterial blood gas (ABG):* Is the pH acidotic or alkalotic?
- *Anion gap:* If abnormal, is it increased or decreased?
- *Blood glucose:* Is the patient hyperglycemic or hypoglycemic?
- *Psychosocial:* Does the patient have a history of psychiatric disorders, of drug abuse, or of depression? Is the patient on any drugs with narrow therapeutic windows, and is a list of current medications (including over-the-counter [OTC]) available?

Diagnostic Tests for Drug Overdose		
Drug	**Diagnostic Lab Tests**	**Specific Considerations**
Acetaminophen	Serum drug level	*Therapeutic level:* 10–20mcg/mL Draw level 4 hrs after ingestion. Subsequent levels are drawn according to the Rumack-Mathews nomogram until levels are below the predicted hepatotoxic range.
	Serum Na^+, K^+, CO_2, BUN, blood glucose, creatinine, liver enzymes, bilirubin; PT, coagulation studies; CBC; protein; amylase; ABGs	
Alcohol Amphetamines Benzodiazepines Phencyclidine	Blood level; urine drug screen	
Amphetamines Cyclic antidepressants	Serum K^+, Na^+, CO_2, BUN, glucose, creatinine, CBC, liver studies, cardiac enzyme levels with isoenzyme fractionations are monitored.	
Barbiturates	Serum drug level	
Barbiturates Benzodiazepines Cocaine Hallucinogens Opioids Phencyclidine Salicylates	Serum K^+, Na^+, CO_2, BUN, glucose, creatinine, CBC, ABGs, liver function studies	
Cocaine	Urinalysis provides a quantitative method for identifying the presence of a cocaine metabolite.	Assessing blood levels of cocaine is usually of little diagnostic value.
Hallucinogens	Serum plasma drug level.	
Opioids	Urine screening	

Drug Overdose

Continued

Diagnostic Tests for Drug Overdose—cont'd		
Drug	**Diagnostic Lab Tests**	**Specific Considerations**
Salicylates	Blood plasma level analyzed for presence of and amount	Repeat every 4 – 6 hours since the patient could have ingested sustained release drug
Cyclic Antidepressants	Blood plasma level; urine screen; gastric content analysis	

TREATMENT OPTIONS

Gastric decontamination is a general term referring to interventions used to prevent absorption of a toxin. Timely administration is essential for success. Best results are obtained if done within an hour of ingestion.

Activated Charcoal

Activated charcoal is a fine, insoluble, nonabsorbable powder that binds with many toxic drugs to enhance their elimination. Activated charcoal does not bind with lithium, potassium, potassium chloride, ethanol, iron, acidic or alkaline corrosives, or hydrocarbons. Use is common and well researched and has proved efficacy in the preabsorption and postabsorption phases. The dose is 1 g/kg initially, followed by repeat doses of 0.5 to 1 g/kg every 2 to 4 hours. Combining the first dose with sorbitol increases the tolerability of charcoal, may help relieve constipation associated with charcoal, but has not been shown to enhance drug elimination. Contraindicated in cases of bowel obstruction or perforation and in patients with depressed mental status unless intubated.

Gastric Lavage

Commonly known as "pumping the stomach," insertion of nasogastric tube with vigorous enteral irrigation is a decreasingly important adjunct for treatment of ingested overdose; no longer recommended as routine management by the American and European toxicology associations. If used, it must be done as soon as possible and has little benefit if more than 60 minutes has passed since ingestion. When using lavage, the airway must be protected and lavage should continue until the fluid is clear of fragments (usually requires about 5 L of fluid). Gastric lavage should not be attempted if it delays or interferes with activated charcoal administration in appropriate patients.

Large, life-threatening amounts of ingested toxin (which may be poorly bound to activated charcoal used prior to lavage) may justify use. Additionally, patients at risk for esophageal hemorrhage or perforation should not be lavaged.

Whole Bowel Irrigation

The administration of a polyethylene glycol balanced electrolyte solution to rapidly cleanse the bowel may be useful in cases where activated charcoal is ineffective, such as with ingestions of iron, lithium, and sustained released tablets. It may diminish the effectiveness of activated charcoal, should not be done concurrently, and is contraindicated when ileus, GI bleeding, bowel obstruction, or bowel perforation is present.

Extracorporeal Removal of Toxins

Techniques include all types of dialysis, hemoperfusion, exchange blood transfusion and plasmapheresis. These methods are most often used to remove methanol, ethylene glycol, lithium, theophylline, salicylates, and phenobarbital. May be used in extreme cases when other management strategies are ineffective for drugs which are not highly protein bound, which have a reasonable molecular size, are water soluble (rather than lipid soluble), have a limited volume of distribution, and are not highly charged or ionized. Hemofilters used for continuous renal replacement therapy are often able to accommodate larger sized molecules than conventional hemodialysis therapy.

COMMONLY ABUSED DRUGS

Acetaminophen (APAP)

Acetaminophen is one of the most commonly ingested drugs in overdose. Most patients admit taking this drug. Unintentional overdose may happen due to polypharmacy, wherein APAP is contained in one or more other medications being used. Unintentional overdose is more common in children. Signs and symptoms of toxicity vary significantly depending on the dose, time elapsed since ingestion, and whether overdose resulted from acute or chronic ingestion. Toxicity from acute ingestion may be asymptomatic for up to 12 hours.

Routes of administration: Oral (most common); rectal per suppository

Effects on Body Systems

Cardiovascular: Hepatic damage may prompt cardiac complications including dysrhythmias, ischemia, and injury (chest pain/pressure, nausea, shortness of breath [SOB], T-wave inversion, and ST-segment elevation on ECG).

Respiratory: Bronchospasm (wheezes and difficulty breathing) and tachypnea have been reported as a hypersensitivity reaction or as a side effect of N-acetylcysteine. See *Collaborative Management* section that follows.

Neurologic: Coma and seizures

Hepatic: Acute ingestion will cause hepatic necrosis, which can lead to liver failure. Hypoglycemia, right-sided abdominal pain, and nausea with vomiting may be noted, usually 1 to 2 days after ingestion.

Renal: Acute tubular necrosis with renal failure is seen in some cases but often resolves.

Associated findings: Hypophosphatemia, metabolic acidosis, hypothermia, thrombocytopenia, and hemorrhagic pancreatitis

Collaborative Management

Support of cardiovascular and respiratory systems: Supplemental oxygen should be given if ABG values indicate a trend toward respiratory failure. If the patient has an ineffective or absent breathing effort, mechanical ventilation is provided. Serial ECGs monitor for dysrhythmias. Symptomatic ventricular dysrhythmias and bradyarrhythmias are treated per Advanced Cardiac Life Support (ACLS) guidelines.

Removing acetaminophen from the patient: Intravenous N-acetylcysteine (Acetadote, Mucomyst-10, Mucosil-10, Mucosil-20) is the most current treatment, or a combination of activated charcoal and N-acetylcysteine (Mucomyst, NAC) can be administered orally or via a gastric tube. Activated charcoal effectively adsorbs APAP if given within 4 hours. Mucomyst prevents systemic toxicity; especially if given 8 to 10 hours after ingestion. Lavage is used only if less than 1 hour has elapsed since ingestion. Administration of the activated charcoal and NAC should not be delayed to perform lavage.

Treatment of nausea and vomiting: Fluid replacement therapy with lactated Ringer solution or D_5NS; antiemetics, such as promethazine hydrochloride (Phenergan).

Rewarming: A heating blanket is applied if patient has hypothermia.

Treatment of hypoglycemia: Usually done with a bolus of D_{50} and continuous infusion of D_5W, based on serum glucose results. Hypoglycemia occurs because of the potent hepatotoxic effects of acetaminophen.

Alcohol

Route of administration: Oral

Effects on Body Systems

Cardiovascular: Tachycardia, atrial fibrillation, cardiac arrest

Respiratory: Hypoventilation with acute intoxication, respiratory failure, aspiration

Neurologic: Confusion, aggressive behavior, irritability, tremors, hallucinations (especially auditory), memory loss, stupor, coma, seizures, loss of deep tendon reflexes (DTRs)

Renal: May have significant output initially; will demonstrate dehydration with acute intoxication

Associated findings: Dry oral mucosa, odor of alcohol on breath, hypoglycemia, hypothermia, lactic acidosis, hypokalemia

Collaborative Management

Support of cardiovascular and respiratory systems to prevent collapse: Oxygen supplementation; treatment of ventricular dysrhythmias and bradyarrhythmias according to ACLS guidelines.

Fluid/potassium replacement: Manage hypovolemia with IV fluid infusion. Include IV multivitamins (MVI) in fluid replacement, and provide thiamine IM to prevent Wernicke encephalopathy.

Removing alcohol from the patient: As alcohol is metabolized, the blood alcohol level decreases 15 mg/dl/hr according to recent literature (legal limit for driving is less than 100 mg/dl). Coma may occur if the level is greater than 300 mg/dl, but this is influenced by each individual's metabolic process and tolerance. When extreme amounts of alcohol have been absorbed into the system, the liver and kidneys may not be able to break down and excrete the alcohol. Hemodialysis may be used for a life-threatening intoxication.

Prevention of emesis: Antiemetics are given, and a gastric tube is inserted and maintained at low continuous suction.

Anticipation and treatment of withdrawal: Benzodiazepines are the drugs of choice for treating alcohol withdrawal. Lorazepam, which can be given IV, intramuscularly (IM), orally (PO), or sublingually (SL), is the preferred agent on most alcohol withdrawal protocols. Longer-acting agents (chlodiazepoxide and diazepam) are also used, because of the decreased risk of recurrent withdrawal and/or seizures. Oxazepam and lorazepam have a mechanism of metabolism that is less liver dependent and are useful in cases involving cirrhosis. Medications are given as needed for withdrawal symptoms. In patients at high risk for severe withdrawal symptoms, or if withdrawal would be dangerous, benzodiazepines may be given on a schedule. If withdrawal is severe and benzodiazepine doses become excessive, barbiturates may be added. Agents that have glutamate blocking properties, such as lamotrigine, memantine, and topiramate, are showing promise in alcohol detoxification.

Treatment of hypoglycemia: A bolus of D_{50} and continuous infusion of D_5W, based on serum glucose. Thiamine should be given before glucose to avoid sudden onset of heart failure and worsening neurologic impairment.

Treatment of delirium tremens (DTs): The most severe manifestation of withdrawal, which can result in death. Symptoms develop 48 to 96 hours after cessation of alcohol ingestion and include confusion, disorientation, delirium, agitation, severe diaphoresis, tachycardia, fever, and hypotension. DTs generally resolve within 3 to 5 days. Patients are sedated with benzodiazepines, allowed to rest and sleep, and oriented frequently to reality.

Treatment/prevention of seizures: Alcohol withdrawal seizures may occur in a range from the first 6 to 48 hours to late onset at 10 days after abstinence. Benzodiazepines are given to raise the seizure threshold during the withdrawal period. Additional seizure management should reflect institution protocol. If the patient has a history of a primary seizure disorder, an anticonvulsant agent may also be indicated.

Prevention of Wernicke-Korsakoff syndrome: Caused by thiamine deficiency and manifested by diplopia (the first real diagnostic clue), confusion, excitation, peripheral neuropathy, severe recent memory loss, impaired thought processes, and confabulation. Prophylactic administration of thiamine is recommended: IM thiamine on admission; supplemental oral thiamine; and multivitamins and multiminerals high in C, B complex, zinc, and magnesium. Multivitamins and minerals are given to prevent malnutrition related to inadequate food intake and malabsorption caused by alcohol's irritating effect on the GI tract.

Safety Alert *Ingestion of carbohydrates, either orally or parenterally, increases the body's demand for thiamine. For patients with a history of chronic alcohol ingestion, administration of thiamine should precede administration of glucose to prevent sudden profound thiamine deficiency and irreversible neurologic impairment.*

Amphetamines

Street names: Methamphetamine, speed, crystal meth, white crosses, ice, crank, ecstasy

Routes of administration: Oral, IV, IM, intranasal, smoked

Effects on Body Systems

Cardiovascular: Tachycardia, atrial and ventricular dysrhythmias, hypertension, myocardial ischemia and infarction, cardiovascular collapse

Respiratory: Hyperventilation and respiratory failure related to cardiovascular collapse

Neurologic: Confusion, aggressive behavior, hyperactivity, convulsions, delusions, irritability, tremors, hallucinations, memory loss, stupor, stroke, coma

Renal: Renal failure related to dehydration and rhabdomyolysis

Associated findings: Mydriasis, fasciculations, hyperthermia, thrombocytopenic purpura

Collaborative Management

Support of cardiovascular and respiratory systems to prevent collapse: Antidysrhythmic agents are given per ACLS guidelines to manage tachycardias. Ischemia is treated with nitrates; myocardial infarction is treated per ACLS guidelines for acute coronary syndromes.

Removing amphetamines from the patient: For oral ingestion, activated charcoal is administered orally or via gastric tube. Acidification of the urine with ammonium chloride helps clear amphetamine.

Treatment of hypertension: Antihypertensives such as nitroprusside (Nipride) or labetalol may be needed to decrease BP.

Prevention/treatment of seizures: IV diazepam 0.1 to 0.2 mg/kg is administered slowly and repeated every 5 minutes until sedation is achieved. Lorazepam is an alternative benzodiazepine.

Psychosis: Haldol 5 mg is given IM or IV. Repeat dose may be required to control behavior.

Treatment of hyperthermia: A cooling blanket, antipyretics, and iced IV fluids are used.

Treatment of dehydration: Done by fluid replacement, such as lactated Ringer solution and NS continuous IV infusions

Anticipation and treatment of rhabdomyolysis: Usually treated with sodium bicarbonate infusion, mannitol, or furosemide (Lasix)

Barbiturates

See Table 11-2.

Street names: Yellow jackets, reds, barbs

Routes of administration: Oral, IV, IM

Effects on Body Systems

Cardiovascular: Hypotension, bradycardia, cardiac arrest

Respiratory: Hypoventilation leading to respiratory failure and respiratory arrest

Neurologic: Symptoms may include headache, vertigo, dizziness, lethargy, ataxia, stupor, flaccidity, seizures, absent dolls-eye reflex, coma, loss of DTRs, and nystagmus (see Coma scale, which follows under *Classification of Barbiturate Intoxication* below.

Renal: Acute renal failure is possible.

Associated findings: Hypothermia, nausea, vomiting. Patient may experience opposite reactions of euphoria and excitability before the normal sedative effects occur. Withdrawal symptoms (tremors and convulsions) may occur.

Classification of Barbiturate Intoxication

Alert: No signs of CNS depression

Drowsy: CNS depression from alert to stuporous

Stuporous: Markedly sedated; responsive to verbal and tactile stimuli

Coma 1: Responsive to painful but not to verbal and tactile stimuli; no change in respirations or BP

Table 11-2	COMMON BARBITURATES	
Generic Name	**Common Brand Name**	**Half-life (hr)**
Amobarbital	Amytal	8–42
Secobarbital	Seconal	19–34
Pentobarbital	Nembutal	15–48
Phenobarbital	Luminal and others	24–140
Butabarbital	Butisol	34–42
Secobarbital/amobarbital	Tuinal	8–42

Note: Withdrawal symptoms can be correlated with the half-life of the drug that was used. Withdrawal from drugs with shorter half-lives produces more intense symptoms that last for shorter periods, whereas withdrawal from drugs with longer half-lives produces less intense symptoms that can be prolonged. Moreover, the severity of the withdrawal is directly related to the drug's dosage.

Coma 2: Unconscious; unresponsive to pain; no change in respirations or BP
Coma 3: Unresponsive to pain; slow, shallow, or rapid spontaneous respirations; low but adequate BP
Coma 4: Unresponsive to pain; apnea or inadequate BP, or both
Collaborative Management
Support of cardiovascular and respiratory systems to prevent collapse: Electrical rhythm is monitored; bradyarrhythmias are treated according to ACLS guidelines. After fluids are replaced, vasopressor therapy (see Appendix 6), including dopamine and norepinephrine bitartrate (Levophed), may be initiated for hypotension. Mechanical ventilation may be required, depending on the degree of hypoxia and CO_2 retention.
Removing barbiturates from the patient: If less than 1 hour since ingestion, gastric lavage may be initiated (provided there is no delay in the administration of activated charcoal). Activated charcoal is administered orally or via gastric tube to bind with the substance in the stomach; hemodialysis may be used if patient is in stage 4 coma. Sufficient sodium bicarbonate should be given to alkalinize the urine to a pH of 7.5.
Prevention/treatment of seizures: Phenytoin or diazepam may be given.
Sedation for withdrawal symptoms: Typically the barbiturate that was ingested is tapered gradually to zero.
Prevention of aspiration: A gastric tube is inserted, which is then connected to low suction.
Treatment of nausea and vomiting: Antiemetics are administered, usually IV promethazine hydrochloride.
Treatment of hypothermia: A warming blanket is used.

Benzodiazepines
See Table 11-3.
Routes of administration: Oral, IM, IV
Effects on Body Systems
Cardiovascular: Hypotension, tachycardia
Respiratory: Respiratory arrest
Neurologic: Drowsiness, ataxia, slurred speech, coma. Withdrawal may be manifested by seizures.
Renal: Renal failure because of rhabdomyolysis
Associated findings: Hypothermia

Table 11-3	COMMON BENZODIAZEPINES	
Generic Name	**Common Brand Name**	**Half-life (hr)**
Chlordiazepoxide	Librium and others	7–28
Diazepam	Valium and others	20–90
Lorazepam	Ativan	10–20
Oxazepam	Serax	3–21
Prazepam	Centrax	24–200*
Flurazepam	Dalmane	24–100*
Chlorazepate	Tranxene	30–100
Temazepam	Restoril	9.5–12.4
Clonazepam	Klonopin	18.5–50
Alprazolam	Xanax	12–15
Halazepam	Paxipam	14

*Includes half-life of major metabolites.
Note: Withdrawal symptoms can be correlated with the half-life of the drug that was used. Withdrawal from drugs with shorter half-lives produces more intense symptoms that last for shorter periods, whereas withdrawal from drugs with longer half-lives produces less intense symptoms that can be prolonged. Moreover, the severity of the withdrawal is directly related to the drug's dosage.

Collaborative Management

Support of cardiovascular system to prevent collapse: Electrical rhythm is monitored. Atrial fibrillation or flutter may be treated with digoxin or amiodarone, with initial rate control using diltiazem or beta-blockers. Severe supraventricular tachyarrhythmias may be treated with adenosine. Hypotension is treated with fluid replacement, followed by dopamine or norepinephrine (Levophed).

Support of respiratory system: Apnea monitoring and mechanical ventilation may be indicated. Flumazenil administration may be considered if hypoventilation ensues. Naloxone may be added if mixed ingestion, including opiates, is suspected.

Removing benzodiazepines from the patient: Gastric lavage is initiated if less than 60 minutes after ingestion; Activated charcoal is used to bind with the substance in the stomach.

Prevention of seizures: Phenytoin is administered.

Prevention of aspiration: Gastric tube is inserted, which is then connected to low intermittent suction.

Identification of rhabdomyolysis: Seizure activity and breakdown of muscle cause protein to precipitate in the kidneys, leading to renal failure. Increased BUN, creatinine, and urine protein values are noted. Prevention of seizures is the best treatment for prevention of rhabdomyolysis.

Treatment of hypothermia: A warming blanket is used if indicated.

Flumazenil administration: Sedative and respiratory depressant effects may be reversed by flumazenil (Romazicon). Repeat doses may be necessary, since the duration of action of many benzodiazepines exceeds that of flumazenil. Use with caution, especially in patients with possible multiple drug overdose. Flumazenil may precipitate seizures in benzodiazepine-dependent patients and causes arrhythmias in patients who also have high levels of cyclic antidepressants.

Cocaine

Street names: Crack, rock, freebase, snow
Routes of administration: Nasal or IV (cocaine, snow); smoked (crack, rock, freebase)
Effects on Body Systems

Cardiovascular: Hypertension; sinus tachycardia and sinus bradycardia; ventricular dysrhythmias such as premature ventricular contractions (PVCs), ventricular tachycardia, and ventricular fibrillation; myocardial infarction; heart failure; cardiomyopathy; acute endocarditis; and aortic dissection. Acute intoxication may result in profound hypotension and shock.

Respiratory: Sharp pleuritic pain, hemoptysis, pneumothorax, bronchospasm, pulmonary edema, and respiratory failure. Both lactic acidosis and metabolic acidosis have been seen.

Neurologic: The degree of CNS stimulation depends on the route and amount of drug taken. Headache, hyperexcitation, paranoia, delirium, hallucinations, tremors, and aggression may be seen. Mentation may vary from stimulated, euphoric, and excited states to delirium, stupor, and coma. Seizures are common, usually tonic-clonic, and may last for hours. Initially patients may seem well-coordinated, but later may show tremors and fasciculations as their condition deteriorates.

Renal: Renal failure can occur and has been related to profound hypotension and rhabdomyolysis.

Associated findings: Hyperthermia is common, and rectal temperatures may be elevated to as high as 43°C (109.4°F). Perforated nasal septum, track marks related to IV use, and mydriasis (dilated pupils) occur.

Indicators of withdrawal: Poor concentration, anergia, anhedonia, bradykinesis, sleep disturbance, decreased libido, intense cocaine craving, depression, and suicidal tendencies

Indicators of cocaine psychosis: Tactile and visual hallucination and paranoia

Peak Action

- Intranasal—20 to 60 minutes
- Oral—60 to 90 minutes
- IV—5 minutes
- Smoked —less than 5 minutes

Cutting agents: Cutting agents are substances mixed with pure cocaine to increase bulk. Cutting agents are often unknown but may include procaine, phencyclidine ("angel dust"),

Drug Overdose

amphetamine, quinine, talc, and strychnine. Agents used in the preparation of crack include powdered cocaine, water, baking soda, and lidocaine. Cutting agents can become emboli that shower into cerebral and pulmonary circulation, with subsequent effects.

Collaborative Management: Support of cardiovascular system to prevent collapse: Electrical rhythm is monitored. Supraventricular tachycardia and ventricular dysrhythmias are managed according to ACLS guidelines. Monitor ECG for ischemic changes or infarction pattern (T-wave inversion or ST-segment elevation or depression).

Support of respiratory system: Comatose patients are placed on mechanical ventilation.

Identification of route of administration and removing cocaine following oral ingestion: A radiograph of the GI tract may reveal a cocaine-filled condom. Surgery may be performed to remove it. Activated charcoal may be administered to bind with cocaine in the stomach, or a laxative or suppository may be given to facilitate rectal excretion. An approach under investigation is to flush cocaine from the circulation using IV ammonium chloride.

Treatment of hypotension or hypertension: Antihypertensives or vasopressors are administered as indicated.

Treatment of volume deficiency: IV fluid replacement is done, such as with lactated Ringer solution or D_5NS.

Prevention/treatment of seizures: Diazepam, phenytoin, or phenobarbital is administered.

Treatment of hyperthermia: A cooling blanket, ice, and/or acetaminophen is used. Core temperature is the most accurate measurement.

Prevention of aspiration: A gastric tube is inserted, then connected to low continuous suction.

Cyclic Antidepressants

Examples include amitriptyline hydrochloride (Elavil), doxepin hydrochloride (Sinequan), imipramine hydrochloride (Presamine, Tofranil), trimipramine maleate (Surmontil), nortriptyline (Pamelor, Aventyl), and desipramine (Norpramin).

Route of administration: Oral

Effects on Body Systems

Cardiovascular: Hypotension, sinus tachycardia, supraventricular tachycardia, ventricular dysrhythmias, conduction defects, myocardial infarction, cardiopulmonary arrest. Hypertension has been noted. Monitor ECG for widening QRS complex. Progressive QRS widening signals worsening toxicity.

Respiratory: Respiratory arrest, pulmonary edema, ARDS. Hyperventilation also has been noted.

Neurologic: Central nervous system depression, coma, seizures, delirium, hallucinations

Renal: Acute tubular necrosis; renal failure secondary to rhabdomyolysis

Pancreatic: Pancreatitis

Associated findings: Hyperthermia or hypothermia

Collaborative Management: If the patient is symptom free, monitor for a minimum of 6 to 8 hours, noting vital signs and width of QRS complex.

Support of cardiovascular system to prevent collapse: Electrical rhythm is monitored for at least 6 hours to enable assessment for a widening QRS complex, which is a signal of worsening toxicity. Supraventricular tachycardias are treated with adenosine or diltiazem; ventricular dysrhythmias are treated with antidysrhythmics such as amiodarone. Atropine and pacing may be indicated in the presence of symptomatic conduction defects.

Removing cyclic antidepressants from the patient: Activated charcoal is administered via gastric tube to bind with the ingested substance in the stomach.

Reversal of the effects of the drugs: IV sodium bicarbonate is used. An alternative approach is to promote a state of respiratory alkalosis by increasing respiratory rate via mechanical ventilation.

Prevention/treatment of seizures: Phenytoin and diazepam are administered.

Respiratory support: Mechanical ventilation is used. Pulmonary edema is treated with nitrates, morphine, diuretics, potassium replacement, and IPPB treatments.

Treatment of hypotension: Fluid replacement is carried out, followed by administration of dopamine and norepinephrine (Levophed) as indicated.

Treatment of hyperthermia or hypothermia: A cooling or a warming blanket is used as indicated.

Prevention of aspiration: A gastric tube is inserted, then connected to low intermittent suction.

Hallucinogens

Common agents: Lysergic acid diethylamide (LSD), mescaline, morning glory seeds, nutmeg
Routes of administration: Oral, IV, nasal, smoked
Effects on Body Systems: Effects will depend on the amount and type of drug ingested.
Respiratory: Apnea, respiratory arrest
Neurologic: Hallucinations and paranoid behavior patterns, tremors, seizures, coma
LSD: Patient may describe tasting or hearing colors or exhibit mental dissociation.
Mescaline: Sense of being followed by moving geometric shapes
Associated findings: Hyperthermia and diaphoresis. In addition, visual hallucinations may occur.
Collaborative Management: Support of cardiovascular system to prevent collapse: Manage BP and HR/rhythm according to ACLS guidelines.
Removing hallucinogens from patient: If oral ingestion was within 1 hour gastric lavage may be attempted, as long as activated charcoal therapy is not delayed. Activated charcoal is administered orally or via gastric tube to bind with the substance in the stomach.
Prevention of seizures: Anticonvulsants such as phenytoin or diazepam are administered.

Opioids

Examples of opioids include codeine, fentanyl, heroin, hydrocodone, hydromorphone hydrochloride (Dilaudid), levorphanol tartrate (Levo-Dromoran), meperidine hydrochloride (Demerol), methadone (Dolophine), morphine, opium, oxycodone hydrochloride (Percocet-5, Tylox, Oxycontin), and oxymorphone (Numorphan).
Routes of administration: Oral, IV, IM, smoked
Effects on Body Systems:
Cardiovascular: Profound hypotension, bradycardia, cardiovascular collapse, sudden death
Respiratory: Atelectasis, acute pulmonary edema, infiltrates related to aspiration complications, respiratory depression, apnea, hypoventilation, and bronchospasm
Neurologic: Range from decreased mental alertness to stupor and coma; pinpoint pupils, seizures
Renal: Renal failure has been associated with profound hypotension and rhabdomyolysis.
Associated findings: Track marks and scarring on arms and in hidden locations of the body, including between the toes and in the vessels underneath the tongue.
Collaborative Management
Support of cardiovascular system to prevent collapse: Electrical rhythm is monitored; bradyarrhythmias are treated per ACLS guidelines. Vasopressor therapy is initiated for hypotension after fluids have been replaced.
Removal of orally ingested opioids from patient: Activated charcoal is administered orally or via gastric tube to bind with the substance in the stomach.
Reversal of opioid effects: Administration of naloxone hydrochloride (Narcan) to manage respiratory depression. After the initial dose of naloxone, the patient's respiratory status must be monitored closely, since additional doses may be required. Respiratory depression and coma may occur when the effects of naloxone wear off and the opiate effects predominate. The half-life of naloxone is 60 to 90 minutes, and effects last 2 to 3 hours. If the narcotic effects last longer than the effects of the naloxone, the patient may slip into coma once the naloxone wears off. If persistent respiratory depression is present, a continuous naloxone infusion may be considered.
Treatment of drug withdrawal symptoms: Hallucinations are treated with haloperidol (Haldol).
Support of respiratory system: Pulmonary edema is treated with diuretics and restriction of IV fluid intake. An individual whose respiratory system is deteriorating is placed on apnea monitoring or mechanical ventilation.
Prevention of aspiration: A gastric tube is inserted, then connected to low continuous suction.
Prevention/treatment of seizure activity: Anticonvulsant therapy is done, such as phenytoin administration.
Prevention of rhabdomyolysis: See discussion in Benzodiazepines, p. 874.

Phencyclidine

Street names: PCP, angel dust, mist, peep, hog, crystal
Routes of administration: Oral, nasal, smoked

Effects on Body Systems

Cardiovascular: Hypertension, hypertensive crisis, tachycardia

Respiratory: Respiratory depression, respiratory arrest, laryngeal stridor, bronchospasm

Neurologic: Rage and "super-human strength" are hallmark signs. Ranges from hyperexcitability, hyperreflexia, muscle rigidity, and paranoid and psychotic behavior to stupor, seizures, and coma. Coma: eyes may be open in a blank stare, nystagmus, and pinpoint pupils.

Renal: Renal failure precipitated by rhabdomyolysis and myoglobinuria

Associated findings: Hypothermia or hyperthermia, hypoglycemia

Collaborative Management

Support of cardiovascular system to prevent collapse: Electrical rhythm is monitored and tachy-dysrhythmias are treated as previously discussed. Nitroprusside is used for antihypertensive therapy. Nitroglycerin may be given to treat ischemia.

Removal of phencyclidine from the patient: No specific antidote is available, although multiple administrations of charcoal to bind with the ingested substance in the stomach are standard practice. Charcoal is ineffective if phencyclidine was smoked, rather than swallowed. The first dose of charcoal may be accompanied with sorbitol. After ruling out the possibility of rhabdomyolysis, acidification of the urine with ammonium chloride or ascorbic acid to a pH around 5.5 is done.

Prevention/treatment of seizure activity: Phenytoin and diazepam are given. Diazepam is administered IV at an initial dose of 2 to 5 mg. May be repeated every 30 minutes until sedation is achieved. Haldol may be given 5 to 10 mg IV to control psychosis. The effects of Haldol usually occur within 5 to 10 minutes of administration.

Respiratory support: Pulmonary edema is treated with diuretics and restriction of IV fluid intake. Persons with hypoxia and respiratory distress require monitoring of pulse oximetry and may require mechanical ventilation.

Prevention of aspiration: A gastric tube is inserted, then connected to intermittent low suction.

Prevention of rhabdomyolysis: See discussion in Benzodiazepines, p. 874.

Treatment of hypothermia or hyperthermia: A warming or cooling blanket is used as appropriate.

Salicylates

Examples include aspirin, bismuth subsalicylate (Pepto-Bismol), and fendosal.

Routes of administration: Oral, rectal (suppository)

Effects on Body Systems

Respiratory: Hyperventilation, hyperpnea, pulmonary edema

Neurologic: Coma, cerebral edema (manifested by indicators of increased intracranial pressure [IICP]) (see Box 7-1)

Renal: Renal failure secondary to rhabdomyolysis

Hepatic: Liver dysfunction, hepatitis

Associated findings: Hyperthermia, bleeding, anemia, thrombocytopenia, hypokalemia, and tinnitus

Collaborative Management

Support of cardiovascular system to prevent collapse: Electrical rhythm is monitored. Ventricular dysrhythmias and bradyarrhythmias are treated per ACLS guidelines.

Removal of salicylates from the patient: Activated charcoal is administered orally or via gastric tube to bind with the substance in the stomach; several doses of activated charcoal may be necessary to achieve a 10:1 ratio of charcoal to salicylate. Hemodialysis may be necessary if the substance has been more extensively absorbed. Charcoal hemoperfusion may clear salicylates somewhat but cannot correct acid-base, electrolyte, and fluid problems associated with severe poisoning.

Fluid replacement: Replace fluids with lactated Ringer solution or NS 20 ml/kg over 1 to 2 hours. Sodium bicarbonate may be added at a rate of 1 mEq/kg/hr to promote forced alkaline diuresis.

Potassium replacement: See *Fluid and Electrolyte Imbalances: Hypokalemia*, p. 52.

Treatment of hyperthermia: A cooling blanket or applications of ice is used.

Treatment of cerebral edema: Hyperventilation (via mechanical ventilation) or mannitol is used.

Respiratory support: Mechanical ventilation is used as indicated.

Treatment of pulmonary edema: Nitrates, morphine, diuretics, potassium replacement, and intermittent positive pressure breathing (IPPB) are possible.

Prevention of aspiration: A gastric tube is inserted, then connected to low suction.
Replacement of blood loss: Through delivery of blood and blood products

Specific Antidotes for Common Drug Overdoses/Toxicities
Table 11-4 gives specific drug treatments for a few of the more common and critical drug overdoses not discussed in the preceding section.

CARE PLANS FOR ALL DRUG OVERDOSES
Ineffective airway clearance *related to presence of tracheobronchial secretions or obstruction; decreased sensorium*

GOALS/OUTCOMES Chest radiograph normalizes. Within 2 to 24 hours of intervention/treatment, patient has a patent airway and is free of congestion as evidenced by clear breath sounds over the upper airways and lung fields, RR 12 to 20 breaths/min with normal depth and pattern, Pao_2 at least 90 mm Hg, $Paco_2$ 35 to 45 mm Hg, pH 7.35 to 7.45, and Spo_2 at least 95%.

NOC Respiratory Status: Airway Patency; Aspiration Prevention; Respiratory Status: Ventilation

Respiratory Monitoring
1. Assess for respiratory distress hourly and as needed. Note secretions; stridor; gurgling; shallow, irregular, or labored respirations; use of accessory muscles of respiration; restlessness and confusion; and cyanosis (a late sign of respiratory distress).
2. Suction oropharynx, or use suction via endotracheal tube as needed.
3. Administer bronchodilators as appropriate.

Table 11-4	MANAGEMENT OF DRUG OVERDOSE/TOXICITIES
Target (toxic) Drug or Class	**Treatment or Antidote**
Acetaminophen	N-Acetylcysteine
Anticholinergics	Physostigmine
Arsenic, lead, mercury, or other heavy metals	Dimercaprol injection
Benzodiazepines	Flumezanil
Beta-blockers	Glucagon; beta agonists
Calcium channel blockers	Calcium IV, glucagon
Copper	Trientene
Cyanide	Sodium thiosulfate, sodium nitrite, amyl nitrite, hydroxocobalamin
Cyclic antidepressants	Sodium bicarbonate
Digitalis glycosides	Digoxin immune Fab
Heparin	Protamine
Insulin	Glucagon, dextrose, octreotide
Iron	Deferoxamine
Lead	Succimer, edetate calcium disodium (EDTA)
Methanol	Fomepizole, ethanol, folinic acid
Nitrites	Methylene blue
Opiates	Nalmefene, naltrexone, naloxone
Organophosphate insecticides	Atropine, pralidoxime
Warfarin	Vitamin K (IV or PO)

Drug Overdose

4. Monitor ABG values for evidence of hypoxia (Pao$_2$ less than 90 mm Hg) and respiratory acidosis (Paco$_2$ greater than 45 mm Hg, pH less than 7.35).
5. Monitor respiratory patterns; provide continuous apnea monitoring if available.
6. If patient has been placed on mechanical ventilation, monitor for indicators of airway obstruction (see *Mechanical Ventilation*, p. 99).
7. Monitor oxygen saturation continuously. Be alert to values less than 95% with response depending on patient's baseline and clinical presentation.
8. Monitor for nausea and vomiting. Evaluate effects of antiemetics.

NIC Airway Management, Aspiration Precautions

Hyperthermia *related to overdose of cocaine, hallucinogens, phencyclidine, salicylates, or cyclic antidepressants*

GOALS/OUTCOMES Optimally, within 24 to 72 hours of intervention, patient becomes normothermic.
NOC Thermoregulation

Safety Alert *With massive overdose, temperature regulation may never be achieved.*

Temperature Regulation
1. Monitor for hyperthermia: temperature greater than 38.3°C (greater than 101°F), pallor, absence of perspiration, and torso that is warm to the touch. If means are available, provide continuous monitoring of temperature. Otherwise, measure rectal, core, or tympanic temperature hourly and as needed.
2. Monitor effects of cooling blanket, cooling baths, and ice packs to the axillae and groin.
3. Maintain fluid replacement as prescribed. Monitor hydration status and trend of input and output (I&O).
4. Monitor neurologic status hourly and as needed until stabilized.
5. Monitor vital signs continuously or hourly and as needed until stabilized.
6. Administer and evaluate effects of antipyretic medications.

NIC Fever Treatment; Vital Signs Monitoring; Medication Prescribing

Deficient fluid volume *related to low intake or losses secondary to vomiting or diaphoresis and shock conditions*

GOALS/OUTCOMES Patient remains normovolemic as evidenced by urine output greater than 0.5 ml/kg/hr, moist mucous membranes; balanced I&O, BP within patient's normal range, HR less than 100 bpm, stable weight, CVP 8 to 12 mm Hg, and PAWP 6 to 12 mm Hg.
NOC Hydration; Fluid Balance

Fluid Management
1. Monitor hydration status. Note signs of continuing dehydration: poor skin turgor, dry mucous membranes, thirst, weight loss greater than 0.5 kg/day, urine specific gravity greater than 1.020, weak pulse with tachycardia, and postural hypotension.
2. If the patient has a pulmonary artery catheter:
   - Monitor SVR and pulmonary vascular resistance (PVR) as appropriate.
   - Monitor CO as appropriate.
   - Monitor PCWP/PAWP and central venous/right atrial pressures.
   - Administer positive inotropic/contractility medications.
3. Evaluate the effects of fluid therapy.
4. Assess for indicators of electrolyte imbalance, especially the presence of hypokalemia. Be alert to irregular pulse, cardiac dysrhythmias, and serum potassium level less than 3.5 mEq/L.
5. Monitor I&O hourly; assess for output elevated disproportionately to intake, bearing in mind the insensible losses.

6. Monitor laboratory values, including serum electrolyte levels and serum and urine osmolality. Note BUN values elevated disproportionately to the serum creatinine (indicator of dehydration rather than renal disease), high urine specific gravity, low urine sodium, and rising Hct and serum protein concentration. Optimal values are the following: serum osmolality 275 to 300 mOsm/kg, urine osmolality 300 to 1090 mOsm/kg, BUN 10 to 20 mg/dl, serum creatinine 0.7 to 1.5 mg/dl, urine sodium 40 to 180 mEq/24 hr (diet dependent), Hct 37% to 47% (female) or 40% to 54% (male), and serum protein 6 to 8.3 g/dl.
7. Maintain fluid intake as prescribed; administer prescribed electrolyte supplements.

NIC Fluid/Electrolyte Management; Surveillance; Hypovolemia Management

---

Disturbed sensory/perceptual perception: visual, tactile, auditory, kinesthetic, *related to chemical alterations secondary to ingestion of mind-altering drugs*

GOALS/OUTCOMES Within 48 hours of intervention, patient verbalizes orientation to time, place, and ¬person and is free of abnormal sensory and perceptual experiences.
NOC Cognitive Orientation; Distorted Thought Self-Control

Reality Orientation
1. Establish and maintain a calm, quiet environment to minimize patient's sensory overload.
2. Assess patient's orientation to time, place, and person. Reorient as necessary.
3. Explain procedures before performing them. Include significant others in orientation process.
4. Do not leave patient alone if agitated or confused.
5. Administer antianxiety agents as prescribed.
6. If patient is hallucinating, intervene in the following ways:
   - Be reassuring. Explain that hallucinations may be very real to patient but that they are not real, that they are caused by the substance that patient consumed, and that they will go away eventually.
   - Try to involve family and significant others, because patient may have more trust in them.
   - Explain that restraints are necessary to prevent harm to patient and others. Reassure patient that restraints will be used only as long as they are needed.
   - Tell patient that you will check on him or her at frequent intervals (e.g., every 5 to 10 minutes) or that you will stay at patient's side.

NIC Delusion Management; Environmental Management; Fall Prevention; Surveillance: Safety

---

Risk for violence: self-directed and/or other-directed *related to mind-altering drugs or depressed state*

GOALS/OUTCOMES Patient, staff, and patient's significant others are free of injury.
NOC Impulse Self-Control

Behavior Management
1. If patient's condition is stable, provide a sitter, or auxiliary staff member, such as an orderly or nursing assistant, to observe patient when awake.
2. Speak with patient in a quiet and calm voice, using short sentences.
3. Establish a therapeutic relationship with patient.
4. Encourage patient to take control over his or her own behavior.
5. Facilitate support by significant others.
6. Limit interventions.
7. Administer and evaluate effectiveness of sedation to calm patient.
8. Keep all sharp instruments out of patient's room. Follow agency protocol accordingly.
9. Develop appropriate behavior expectations and consequences, given the patient's level of cognitive functioning and capacity for self-control.

NIC Behavior Management: Self-Harm; Substance Use Treatment: Alcohol Withdrawal; Substance Use Treatment: Overdose, Suicide Prevention

ADDITIONAL NURSING DIAGNOSES

See nursing diagnoses and interventions in the following as appropriate: *Nutritional Support* (p. 117), *Mechanical Ventilation* (p. 99), *Hemodynamic Monitoring* (p. 75), *Prolonged Immobility* (p. 149), *Emotional and Spiritual Support of the Patient and Significant Others* (p. 200), *Acute Lung Injury and Acute Respiratory Distress Syndrome* (p. 365), *Acute Respiratory Failure* (p. 383), *Acute Coronary Syndromes* (p. 434), *Heart Failure* (p. 421), *Cardiomyopathy* (p. 482), *Dysrhythmias and Conduction Disturbances* (p. 492), *Aortic Aneurysm/Dissection* (p. 467), *Acute Renal Failure* (p. 584), *Status Epilepticus* (p. 668), *Hepatic Failure* (p. 785), *Acute Pancreatitis* (p. 762), *Fluid and Electrolyte Disturbances*, p. 37), and *Acid-Base Imbalances* (p. 1). In addition, see *Traumatic Brain Injury* for *Impaired Corneal Tissue Integrity* (p. 347).

HIGH-RISK OBSTETRICS

Most pregnant women are healthy and rarely in need of critical care. Obstetric complications account for less than 1% of intensive care unit (ICU) admissions and less than 0.5% of all deliveries. Despite this relatively low incidence, the acuity of obstetric critical care patients is high due to the unique pathophysiology and clinical disorders associated with the pregnant patient. Maternal mortality rates range from 5% to 20% when pregnant women require critical care. Obstetric patients may be admitted into critical care due to complications of obstetric conditions, such as eclampsia, or complications of an underlying medical condition such as heart disease. Those with obstetric conditions are admitted more frequently and generally have better outcomes than those admitted with underlying medical conditions. Approximately 75% of obstetric critical care patients are admitted to the unit postpartum (after delivery). Obstetric hemorrhage and pregnancy-induced hypertension are responsible for approximately 50% of obstetric ICU admissions. This chapter will focus on the hypertensive complications of pregnancy that may result in admission to a critical care unit.

Caring for a pregnant patient presents the unique challenge of caring for the mother and the fetus simultaneously. Although survival of the mother will take precedence over fetal survival in most cases, the optimal outcome is survival of both the mother and fetus. Two basic principles should underlie the care of the pregnant patient. First, maternal anatomic and physiologic changes occur during pregnancy to facilitate adequate blood flow to the fetus and protect the mother after delivery (Box 11-2). The pregnant patient may require hemodynamic monitoring, and the critical care nurse should be familiar with the different hemodynamic changes and pressure values in pregnancy and labor as outlined in Table 11-5. Second, the fetus is totally dependent on the mother for all of his or her oxygenation and growth needs, so any intervention performed on the mother will most likely affect the fetus. Despite the unique challenges presented by the critically ill obstetric patient, transfer of the patient to a critical care unit should not be delayed.

HYPERTENSIVE DISORDERS OF PREGNANCY

PATHOPHYSIOLOGY

Hypertensive disease occurs in up to 22% of pregnancies. Preeclampsia, eclampsia, and HELLP (Hemolysis, Elevated Liver enzymes, Low Platelets) are all part of a continuum of hypertensive disorders unique to pregnancy. The etiology of these diseases is probably related to early placental development. Risks to the baby include poor growth and prematurity. Risks to the mother include stroke, pulmonary edema, renal failure, liver rupture, and disseminated intravascular coagulation (DIC). The only definitive cure is delivery of the fetus and placenta. Signs and symptoms usually resolve within 24 to 48 hours after delivery. The overall goal of nursing care of the hypertensive pregnant patient is to avoid complications to the mother and deliver a healthy, mature neonate. (Refer to Box 11-3.)

Preeclampsia

Preeclampsia is defined as hypertension or BP at least 140/90 mm Hg accompanied by proteinuria during the second half of pregnancy. Preeclampsia occurs in 5% to 8% of all pregnancies. Preeclampsia is more common in first pregnancies and in nonwhite women from low socioeconomic backgrounds. *Eclampsia* is defined as seizures or coma during pregnancy following preeclampsia. Overall, preeclampsia and eclampsia are responsible for 15% of maternal deaths, with most deaths due to complications resulting from eclampsia.

Box 11-2   PHYSIOLOGIC ANATOMICAL CHANGES IN PREGNANCY

Body Position

Supine hypotension: After 20 weeks, supine positioning significantly reduces CO and uterine blood flow by compressing the inferior vena cava.

Lateral positioning or hip wedge under right or left hip is recommended to displace the gravid uterus to avoid supine hypotension.

Cardiovascular

Heart rate: 10 to 15 bpm increase from prepregnancy rate by 32 weeks

Blood pressure: 10 to 15 mm Hg decrease from prepregnancy value between 14 and 24 weeks returning to prepregnancy value by 37 to 40 weeks' gestation

Blood volume: 40% to 50% increase by 24 weeks

Stroke volume: 30% increase by 32 weeks

CO: 30% to 50% increase by 24 weeks

Fetal Circulation

More than 10% of maternal CO is diverted into the uterine circulation. Maternal CO increases by at least 25% during pregnancy. Fetal oxygenation is dependent on maintenance of sufficient maternal CO.

Gastrointestinal

Gastric motility: Decreased

Gastric emptying time: Decreased

IAP: Increased

These changes can cause increased risk of aspiration with general anesthesia.

Neck/Throat

Larynx: Displaced anteriorly; change prompts increased incidence of airway edema and bleeding, leading to failed intubation.

Pulmonary and Acid-Base Balance

Oxygen consumption: Increases

Functional residual capacity and volume: Decreased by elevated maternal diaphragm, resulting in increased risk of rapid development of hypoxemia and apnea compared to the nonpregnant patient

Acid-base imbalance: Respiratory alkalosis

Renal

Glomerular filtration rate: Increased by 50% at term

Preeclampsia is a systemic syndrome unique to pregnancy characterized by widespread arteriolar vasospasm resulting in increased peripheral vascular resistance. Areas of vasospasm cause breaks or roughened areas in the endothelial layer. These roughened areas trigger fibrin deposition and leakage of intravascular fluid into the extravascular space. Decreased colloid oncotic pressure contributes to fluid leakage and proteinuria. As preeclampsia worsens, blood flow through the rough vasospastic areas results in hemolysis and thrombocytopenia. The resulting end effect is decreased circulation and oxygenation to the maternal organ systems, the placenta, and the fetus. The physiologic process of vasospasm manifests in the development of the classic symptoms associated with preeclampsia: hypertension, proteinuria, headache, blurred vision, scotoma, epigastric pain, decreased urinary output, and increased liver enzymes.

Risk Factors for Preeclampsia Preeclampsia is more common in African American and Hispanic women and in women experiencing their first pregnancy at ages less than 18 years or older than 34 years. Additional risk factors for preeclampsia are pre-existing hypertension, diabetes, obesity, family history of preeclampsia, multifetal pregnancies, renal disease, connective tissue disease, and anti-phpholipid antibody syndrome.

Table 11-5	EXPECTED HEMODYNAMIC CHANGES DURING PREGNANCY, LABOR, DELIVERY, AND POSTPARTUM			
Hemodynamic Profile	**Third Trimester Changes Before Labor**	**% Additional Changes During Active Labor**	**Postpartal Measurements**	**Normal Values (Before Pregnancy)**
Cardiac output	↑ 25%–50% (L/min) (~7.5 L/min)	↑~10%	To prelabor value in 1 hr; normal in 10–14 days	5.0 L/min
Stroke volume (ml/beat)	↑ 20%–30% (~75–85 ml/beat)	↑~10%	To prelabor value in 24 hr; normal in 3–12 mo	65 ml/beat
Central venous pressure (mm Hg) Pulmonary artery pressures (mm Hg)	Unchanged	Data unavailable	Data unavailable	2–6 mm Hg
PA systolic	Unchanged	Data unavailable	Unchanged	15–25 mm Hg
PA diastolic	Unchanged	Data unavailable	Unchanged	6–12 mm Hg
PA wedge	Unchanged	Data unavailable	Unchanged	4–12 mm Hg
Systemic vascular resistance (dynes)	May ↓ up to 20%	Unchanged	To normal in 3–412 mo	800–1200 dynes/sec/cm^{-5}
Pulmonary vascular resistance (dynes)	May ↓ up to 25%	Data unavailable	Data unavailable	150–240 dynes/sec/cm^{-5}

Box 11-3	CLASSIFICATION OF HYPERTENSIVE STATES OF PREGNANCY

- *Gestational:* Mild hypertension that develops during pregnancy without additional PIH symptoms
- *Preeclampsia:* Hypertension that develops during pregnancy after 20 weeks' gestation (except in molar pregnancies) with proteinuria
- *HELLP syndrome:* Severe form of preeclampsia with hemolysis, elevated liver enzymes, and low platelets, which may lead to DIC. Rarely patients may be normotensive with HELLP.
- *Eclampsia:* Preeclampsia complicated by seizures
- *Chronic hypertension:* Hypertension that is present prior to pregnancy or develops before 20 weeks' gestation without a molar pregnancy
- *Chronic hypertension with PIH:* Preeclampsia and/or eclampsia superimposed on chronic hypertension

Mild Preeclampsia Mild preeclampsia is characterized by BP at least 140/90, proteinuria (2 g in a 24-hour urine specimen), and creatinine greater than 1.2 mg/dl without accompanying maternal symptoms such as headache, vision changes, or epigastric pain. The treatment for mild preeclampsia is generally hospitalization with bedrest in a lateral position and close observation of maternal and fetal status. Mild preeclampsia can rapidly move from a mild disease state to the severe preeclampsia, eclampsia, or HELLP syndrome. The critical care nurse should observe the mild preeclamptic pregnant patient closely for signs that the disease process is worsening, such as headache, vision changes, altered lab values, epigastric pain, or deterioration in fetal status.

Signs of mild preeclampsia include:
- *Hypertension:* BP at least 140/90 mm Hg, on two separate occasions, at least six hours apart, during the last half of pregnancy
- *Proteinuria:* Increased to greater than 2 g in a 24-hour urine specimen

Severe Preeclampsia Severe preeclampsia suggests a worsening degree of vasospasm within the maternal and fetal circulation as evidenced by the presence of headache, blurred vision, scotoma, epigastric pain in the right upper quadrant, altered lab values and indications of fetal status deterioration. Goals of nursing management for severe preeclampsia include controlling maternal BP, avoiding eclampsia and facilitating fetal oxygenation and delivery.

Magnesium sulfate is the drug of choice for eclamptic seizures, although 10% of patients receiving magnesium therapy will develop subsequent seizures. Numerous studies have demonstrated that magnesium sulfate is superior to diazepam, lorazepam, phenytoin, and "lytic cocktail" in the management of eclampsia.

Signs of severe preeclampsia include:

- *Hypertension:* BP at least 160/110 mm Hg
- *Proteinuria:* Increased to greater than 5 g in a 24-hour urine specimen
- *Interstitial Edema:* Third-spaced fluids manifest as edema
- *Serum creatinine:* Increased to greater than 2 mg/dl
- *Platelet count:* Rapidly decreasing platelet count
- *Oliguria:* Decreased to less than 500 ml/24 hr
- *Visual or cerebral disturbances:* Blurred vision, altered thought processes
- *Respiratory distress:* Cyanosis or noncardiogenic pulmonary edema
- *Intrauterine abnormalities:* Fetal growth restriction and/or oligohydramnios (decreased amniotic fluid)

Refer to Table 11-6 for more specific changes in physiology.

Eclampsia

The diagnosis of eclampsia is made when generalized seizures or coma develop in a preeclamptic woman. Less than 1% of preeclamptic women will become eclamptic. Eclampsia is responsible for most of the perinatal mortality attributed to the hypertensive disorders of pregnancy. The majority of eclampsia cases occur within the last 12 weeks of pregnancy. One fourth of eclampsia cases develop intrapartum, or during labor and delivery. Another one fourth of the cases develop postpartum, or following delivery, and may occur up to 6 weeks after delivery. Management of the eclamptic patient encompasses the same care goals as the severe preeclamptic with the addition of seizure management and any complications.

Safety Alert *Although critical care nurses frequently manage grand mal seizures of nonobstetric etiology, management of eclamptic seizure requires an obstetric nurse and physician at the bedside to monitor fetal and labor status.*

HELLP SYNDROME

PATHOPHYSIOLOGY

HELLP syndrome is an acronym for a unique pregnancy condition representing the most severe diagnosis of the preeclampsia continuum. HELLP is an abbreviation for hemolysis, elevated liver enzymes, and low platelets. HELLP syndrome occurs in up to 10% of patients with severe preeclampsia. The etiology of HELLP is uncertain. Worsening of systemic arteriolar vasospasm produces liver damage, subcapsular hematoma, and DIC. DIC in pregnancy may

Table 11-6	HEMODYNAMIC PROFILES IN OLIGURIC PATIENTS WITH PREECLAMPSIA			
Probable Etiology	**Pulmonary Artery Wedge Pressure**	**Systemic Vascular Resistance**	**Cardiac Output**	**Treatment**
Hypovolemia	Normal to decreased	Increased	Increased	Volume infusion
Spasm of renal arteries	Increased	Normal	Increased	Volume infusion Generalized vasodilation
Spasm of systemic arterial vessels	Increased	Increased	Decreased	Diuresis Arterial vasodilation

also be caused by placental abruption (abruptio placentae), dead fetus syndrome, septic shock, transfusion reaction, and amniotic fluid embolism. Maternal complications from DIC include ARDS and acute renal failure. The HELLP patient should be closely monitored for right upper quadrant pain or shoulder pain because these complaints may be indicative of liver hematoma or liver rupture. Hemodynamic monitoring may be required to manage patients with HELLP syndrome.

Diagnostic Tests for Hellp Syndrome	
Test	**Findings**
Complete blood count (CBC)	Hgb and Hct may be elevated (>35 Hct) and steadily rising with severe preeclampsia-eclampsia
Peripheral blood smear	Schistocytes or burr cells are present with HELLP syndrome
Urinalysis	Positive for protein spillage.
24 Hour urine collection	Mild/moderate: 0.3–5 g protein with normal urine output. Severe preeclampsia-eclampsia: >5 g protein with low urine output.
Serum albumin	Decreases as urine protein spillage increases. Severe: <2.5 mg/dl.
Liver enzymes	Aspartate transaminase (AST), alanine amino transferase (ALT), and lactate dehydrogenase (LDH) are elevated with severe preeclampsia-eclampsia and HELLP syndrome. Bilirubin may be elevated with HELLP.
Renal serum chemistry	Mild-moderate: BUN, creatinine, and uric acid levels may be elevated. Severe preeclampsia-eclampsia: BUN, creatinine, and uric acid will be elevated.
Platelet count	Mild-moderate: >100,000/mL. Severe preeclampsia-eclampsia and HELLP syndrome: <100,000/mL
Bleeding time	Prolonged when platelet count is <100,000/mm^3.
Fibrinogen	Decreased (<300 mg/dl).
Screening coagulation tests (PT, PTT, thrombin time)	Normal unless the patient develops HELLP syndrome that progresses to DIC, wherein all values are elevated.

COLLABORATIVE CARE

Collaboration between the critical care and obstetrics nurses is necessary in providing safe and comprehensive obstetric critical care. Nurses from each specialty bring unique and complementary knowledge and skills for patient management. Obstetric nurses have experience with fetal heart monitoring and interpretation, and critical care nurses have experience with managing patients requiring invasive monitoring, ventilatory support, and specific critical care procedures. A written protocol should be established to facilitate maternal transfer from the obstetric unit to the ICU or to an institution that can provide the appropriate level of care for both the mother and the fetus before and after delivery, based on the situation at hand. The protocol should also include planning and support for both obstetric and critical care nurses to work collaboratively to care for the patient. If the baby has been delivered, families may desire unrestricted visitation, or the mother may desire to have the baby remain in her ICU room. The collaborative team should develop a plan of care to address the physiologic, psychosocial, and family needs of the patient.

Preterm Complications: Timing of Delivery

Preeclampsia arising at 34 weeks' (or more) gestation is generally managed by delivery. Fetal viability, or the gestational age at which the fetus can survive outside the womb, is generally thought to be 24–25 weeks' gestation. After 34 weeks gestation, the majority of infants will avoid major complications from prematurity. Before 34 weeks, patients with severe preeclampsia-eclampsia require delivery unless the gestational age is less than 26 weeks, wherein attempts to prolong the pregnancy may be initiated. If the mother exhibits signs of HELLP syndrome, such as thrombocytopenia or epigastric or right upper quadrant pain, or has visual disturbances, delivery should be strongly considered regardless of fetal age, since the mother is at risk of life-threatening illness if delivery is delayed. Management of the severely preeclamptic patient will depend on three conditions: maternal status, fetal status, and gestational age. If the pregnancy is at least 34 weeks, delivery is planned as there is little benefit in prolonging gestation. If the pregnancy is 33 to 34 weeks, glucocorticoids are given to the mother to accelerate the development of fetal lung maturity. The glucocorticoids are given intramuscularly in two doses 12 hours apart with maximum effect achieved 24 hours after the second dose. Glucocorticoids are given to facilitate lung maturity. Both the maternal and fetal status must be closely monitored. If either deteriorates, definitive steps must be taken regarding plans for delivery. The medical team carefully and constantly weighs the benefits of delivery for the mother versus the risks of preterm delivery for the fetus. The decision to proceed to delivery in a preterm pregnancy should be made in consultation with the obstetrician, pediatrician, critical care physician, and neonatologist (if available).

The following are the factors to consider in choosing the best clinical placement for the patient based on availability of equipment, skills, and trained personnel:

- Is continuous electronic fetal monitoring available?
- Are there resources for the administration of and monitoring of medications for labor induction or augmentation, anesthesia, and analgesia?
- Are care providers appropriately trained to provide fetal resuscitation measures?
- Is timely access to operating rooms for emergency cesarean feasible?
- Are care providers able to provide maternal hemodynamic/cardiac/respiratory monitoring and treatment?
- Are there resources available for neonatal support should complications arise?

Preterm Labor

Most obstetric complications increase the risk of *preterm labor*, which is defined as labor that occurs prior to 37 weeks' estimated gestational age (EGA). Most infants between 35 and 37 weeks' gestation will transition to extrauterine circulation without difficulty. Signs and symptoms of preterm labor may be subtle and are likely to go unnoticed by nurses unfamiliar with labor assessment.

1. Routinely screen or observe for the following signs and symptoms of preterm labor:
    - Increase or change in vaginal discharge
    - Bloody vaginal discharge
    - Leakage of amniotic fluid
    - Signs and symptoms of urinary tract infection
    - Dull backache
    - Uterine cramping (menstrual-like cramps, intermittent or constant)
    - Pelvic pressure or pain (feeling that the baby is "pushing down")
    - Abdominal cramping with or without diarrhea
    - If the patient is unconscious, observe for restlessness or nonverbal indications of intermittent pain.
2. If patient has any signs or symptoms of labor, notify the physician or midlevel practitioner and:
    - Position mother in the lateral position (turn to the left or right side).
    - Encourage bladder emptying every 2 hours.
    - Report all new onset of contractions or any change in contraction pattern immediately to the obstetrician or midlevel practitioner, because cervical examination is the most accurate method for diagnosing preterm labor.
3. Monitor uterine contractions (preterm labor) and fetal status:
    - Preterm labor contractions may be infrequent, irregular, and painless or frequent, regular, and painful. Preterm labor, left undetected and untreated, can progress into an emergency delivery of a neonate within the critical care unit.
    - Tocolytics or medications are used to stop preterm labor, but they must be started early in the labor process to be effective.

Safety Alert *If frequent strong, painful uterine contractions continue, notify the obstetrician immediately as placental abruption may be occurring. Placental abruption refers to the detachment of the placenta from the wall of the uterus, which will result in life-threatening maternal hemorrhage. The only definitive treatment of a complete placental abruption is delivery of the fetus by cesarean section within minutes.*

4. **Provide fetal surveillance:** Fetal viability, or the gestational age at which the fetus can survive outside the womb, is generally thought to be 24 weeks' gestation. An electronic fetal monitor has two external devices, which are strapped to the maternal abdomen, and includes a transducer that records fetal HR and a tocodynamometer, or "toco," that records uterine activity. A continuous paper tracing can be produced for documentation. Volume control can be used to produce sound with each heartbeat or decreased to minimize noise, although most mothers enjoy hearing their baby's heartbeat and may become worried if the sound is muted.
   - *On admission:* Ultrasound, Doppler flow studies, biophysical profile, and amniotic fluid volume studies are ordered to evaluate fetal well-being. Between 14 to 24 weeks' gestation, the fetal heart rate (FHR) is generally evaluated with a Doppler or fetoscope. Note the absence of FHR by Doppler does not confirm fetal death.
   - *Initiating electronic fetal monitoring:* Monitoring of the FHR with an electronic fetal monitor typically is not begun until viability has been established. The timing of the initiation of electronic fetal monitoring will vary according to institutional protocol, medical provider, and/or patient situation.

Safety Alert *The use of an electronic fetal monitor requires an obstetric registered nurse with appropriate training and competency in fetal heart rate interpretation. This can be achieved by the requirement of having both a critical care and an obstetrics nurse at the patient's bedside. Having a labor nurse "on-call" if the critical care nurse notices an abnormal fetal heart rate or the onset of labor is not sufficient and compromises patient safety.*

- *Fetal nonstress testing:* A Non-Stress Test (NST) is a frequently ordered non-invasive test to monitor fetal status. NSTs are performed by the obstetric nurse who is trained in the procedure and interpretation of NST results. This test is used to determine fetal well-being and is reflective of fetal oxygenation and placental function. It is often ordered daily on patients who are stable and not in labor. The NST is an assessment of continuous FHR and uterine activity over a 20- to 30-minute period using an electronic fetal monitor. Test results are interpreted as reactive, nonreactive, equivocal, or unsatisfactory, based on the presence or absence of FHR accelerations or decelerations over a 20-minute period. A reactive NST indicates adequate fetal well-being. A nonreactive NST may indicate a problem with placental functioning or fetal oxygenation and should be followed up with additional testing.
- *Biophysical Profile:* The Biophysical Profile (BPP) uses a combination of NST and fetal parameters observed via ultrasound to measure fetal well-being. The fetus is scored either 0, 1, or 2 for each of five parameters: fetal breathing movement, gross fetal movement, fetal tone amniotic fluid volume, and NST test results. BPP results of 8–10 indicate a normal fetus (when amniotic fluid volume is adequate). BPP results of 4–5 are considered equivocal and BPP results of < 4 indicate are considered abnormal.
- *Amniocentesis:* Withdrawal of amniotic fluid under direct ultrasonography is called amniocentesis. Examination of amniotic fluid can be used to determine fetal maturity in pregnancies < 34 weeks. An LS (lecithin: sphingomyelin) ratio of > 2:1 represents fetal maturity.

Positioning of the Pregnant Patient

The supine position should be not be used with pregnant women after 20 weeks' EGA. At that time, the maternal vena cava is compressed by the growing maternal abdomen when the mother lies in a supine position. This effect is called "supine hypotension" and, if left unchecked, will lead to decreased blood return to the heart, decreased maternal BP, decreased CO, and subsequently to decreased blood flow to the uterus, placenta, and fetus. The appropriate position for the pregnancy patient is lateral positioning, which avoids the risk of supine hypotension and maximizes blood flow to the uterus, placenta, and fetus. Turning some pregnant women on the left side may improve CO more than the right side. Semi-Fowler's positioning with a hip roll tilting the maternal abdomen off of the vena cava is another acceptable position for the pregnant woman in the latter half of pregnancy.

Blood Pressure Control and Management

Control of maternal BP is essential to the care of the preeclamptic patient. The goal of therapy is to maintain BP less than 160 mm Hg systolic and less than 110 mm Hg diastolic. Sudden or extreme drops in maternal BP should be avoided as they may precipitate maternal stroke and/or decreased blood flow to the fetus. Venodilators are often used to lower BP. In pregnancy, the effect of the drug on the fetus must be considered. Antihypertensive agents used in pregnancy are chosen because of their ability to avoid vasodilation of placental vessels. The most commonly used antihypertensives are:

- Hydralazine 5 to 10 mg may be given every 10 to 15 minutes. Maximum dosage: 30 mg
- Labetalol 20 to 40 mg may be given every 10 to 15 minutes. Maximum dosage: 220 mg
- Labetalol should be used cautiously in patients with asthma and cardiac failure.
- Nifedipine 10 to 20 mg may be given every 30 minutes. Maximum dosage: 50 mg

Fluid Management

Severely preeclamptic patients are easily overloaded with IV fluid predisposing them to pulmonary edema. Strict observation of intake and output is warranted. Total fluid intake is typically maintained at 125 to 150 ml/hr. Hemodynamic monitoring may be indicated if pulmonary edema develops. Urine output of less than 100 ml/4 hr should be reported to the physician or midlevel practitioner.

A nonglucose solution should always be available as part of a fetal resuscitation protocol, and a bolus of 500 to 1000 ml of lactated Ringer or normal saline is usually given to improve maternal circulating volume and subsequently improve uterine perfusion and fetal oxygenation.

Pain Management

Generally speaking, medications used in pregnancy should be limited to Classes A and B whenever possible, to decrease potential negative effects on the fetus. The benefits of medications in Classes C, D, and E should be carefully weighed against the risk to the fetus. Butorphanol (Stadol), Nalbuphine (Nubain), and Fentanyl (Sublimaze) may all be given IM or as an IV bolus/IV push and are commonly given for pain relief during labor.

 Safety Alert *Meperidine (Demerol) and morphine are not often used due to their long half-life and potential to cause neonatal neurobehavioral depression, which may last several days.*

Neuraxial analgesia techniques (spinal, epidural, or combined spinal-epidural) are commonly used because they are more effective at relieving pain and do not cause respiratory depression in the mother or fetus. Medications used are generally a combination of local anesthetics and opioids, which produce greater pain relief with less motor block than local anesthetics alone. Lumbar epidurals may be given continuously or as a patient-controlled analgesia (PCA). Contraindications to neuraxial analgesia include allergy to local anesthetics, when the last dose of low-molecular-weight heparin has been within 12 hours, coagulation disorders, maternal shock, or infection at the insertion site. Common side effects of neuraxial analgesia include maternal hypotension and itching. Hypotension is generally treated with IV fluid boluses and/or IV Ephedrine. Ephedrine is the preferred vasopressor because it causes peripheral vasoconstriction without affecting the umbilical vessels. Loratadine (Claritin) or Cetirizine (Zyrtec) may be given to alleviate itching.

Prevention of Eclampsia/Seizure Management

Magnesium sulfate is the most effective anticonvulsant for preeclampsia, eclampsia, and HELLP syndrome, reflected by the Magpie Trial International Study Collaborative.

 Safety Alert *Magnesium sulfate is listed as a high-risk medication by The Joint Commission (formerly the Joint Commission on Accreditation of Healthcare Organizations [JCAHO], 2003). Obstetric nurses should be familiar with safety recommendations related to the administration of magnesium sulfate to pregnant or delivered patients.*

Magnesium is given IV as a loading (bolus) dose followed by a continuous drip. Magnesium works by decreasing the maternal seizure threshold and relaxes the uterine smooth musculature by decreasing or stopping uterine contractions. The patient receiving magnesium is at higher risk for postpartum hemorrhage due to uterine atony (failure of the uterus to contract after delivery). Magnesium is metabolized by the kidneys so a decrease in urine output will cause a subsequent rise in magnesium levels.

Administration of magnesium sulfate:

- Administer using an infusion pump. Two nurses should verify the infusion pump settings when magnesium is initiated or dosage changed.
- Magnesium solutions should be premixed and labeled in standard solutions.
- An initial loading dose of 4 to 6 g is given over 15 to 30 minutes followed by a maintenance dose of 2 to 3 g/hr.
- Magnesium therapy is continued after delivery for 12 to 24 hours. Side effects of magnesium include flushing, nausea, muscle weakness, headache, and toxicity.
- Magnesium levels greater than 8 mg/dl are associated with signs of toxicity; refer to Table 11-7.
- *If toxicity is suspected:* Discontinue infusion, administer oxygen, obtain stat magnesium level, and notify physician.
- The antidote for magnesium toxicity is calcium gluconate 10 mg of 10% calcium gluconate solution IVP over 10 minutes and should be readily available.
- Serum magnesium levels are drawn 2 hours following the loading dose, then every 6 hours.
- Continuously use electronic fetal monitoring.

 Safety Alert *The patient must be closely monitored during magnesium administration. It is recommended that the obstetric nurse be present at the bedside with the critical care nurse to monitor fetal and uterine response during magnesium therapy. The desired therapeutic level of magnesium is 5 to 8 mg/dl. If magnesium toxicity is suspected, discontinue the magnesium infusion, support oxygenation and notify the physician immediately (Simpson, 2004).*

Table 11-7	CLINICAL EFFECTS OF MAGNESIUM
Serum Magnesium Level	**Signs/Symptoms to Watch for**
1.7–2.4 mg/dL	Normal
5–8 mg/dL	Therapeutic
8–12 mg/dL	Loss of pateller reflexes
10–12 mg/dL	Somnolence
12–16 mg/dL	Respiratory difficulty and depression
15–17 mg/dL	Muscle paralysis
>18 mg/dL	Altered cardiac conduction
30–35 mg/dL	Cardiac arrest

Preparation for Delivery

Labor and delivery of the critically ill obstetric patient may occur either in the labor and delivery unit or the critical care unit, depending on several factors. A multidisciplinary discussion by medical specialists and nursing regarding the pros and cons of critical care versus the use of the delivery room or operating room setting will determine the best placement of the patient for optimal maternal and fetal care during labor and delivery.

Vaginal delivery is the safest method of delivery for the HELLP patient with a cervix that is favorable for induction of labor. Cesarean should be reserved for obstetric indications. The goal of delivery method is to minimize the incidence of complications. If operative delivery is the selected method of delivery, 5 to 10 units of platelets may be ordered preoperatively for a platelet count of less than 50,000 mm^3. The patient should be typed and cross-matched for blood and blood products to be used if hemorrhage and/or DIC develops intraoperatively or postoperatively. General anesthesia is typically selected, since regional anesthesia (entering the spine) is generally contraindicated with thrombocytopenia. Due to the potential for difficult intubation due to airway edema and hyperemia, fiberoptic intubation may be used. The patient will require close observation postoperatively for the first 24 to 48 hours.

Emergency Delivery in the Critical Care Unit

To improve communication and facilitate timely emergency response, the names, specialty, and pager/cell phone numbers of the medical and nursing care team members should be compiled on one sheet of paper or written on one specific white board in all of the units possibly involved in the care of the pregnant critical care patient. The teams would minimally include the medical and nursing personnel from critical care, labor and delivery, anesthesiology, neonatology, and possibly the nursery and respiratory therapists. Other medical specialists should be added as appropriate for the patient's condition. It is helpful to have core team members communicate every shift to discuss emergency plans and update the plan of care and discuss any possibility of emergent interventions.

CARE PLANS FOR THE HIGH-RISK OBSTETRIC PATIENT IN CRITICAL CARE

Ineffective protection *related to hemodynamic, hematologic, and neurologic changes associated with pregnancy-induced hypertension (PIH)*

GOALS/OUTCOMES Within 1 hour of development of severe preeclampsia, eclampsia, or severe HELLP syndrome, the pregnant patient (mother and child) is monitored intensively and prepared for delivery, to avoid life-threatening complications of pregnancy-induced hypertension.
NOC Blood Coagulation; Fetal Status: Intrapartum

Electronic Fetal Monitoring: Intrapartum
1. Verify HRs of mother and fetus prior to initiating electronic monitoring.
2. Monitor BP of mother at least every 5 minutes if severe hypertension or seizures have occurred. Monitor FHR for slowing, indicative of fetal distress.
3. Initiate fetal resuscitation measures to treat abnormal fetal heart rhythms, as appropriate. Note response to all supportive interventions.
4. Instruct woman and support person(s) about the need for monitoring and data to be obtained.
5. Keep physician informed of significant changes in FHR, interventions for abnormal patterns, fetal response, labor progress, and maternal response to interventions.
6. Administer anticonvulsive medications as ordered to control seizures.
7. Monitor magnesium levels, and be alert to hypermagnesemia: decreased respiratory rate and depth, loss of deep tendon reflexes.
8. Assist with application of forceps or vacuum extractor, as needed, during delivery.
9. Monitor the patient closely for hemorrhage if HELLP syndrome is present.
10. Note Hgb and Hct levels before and after blood loss, as indicated.
11. Monitor coagulation studies, including prothrombin time (PT), activated partial thromboplastin time (aPTT), fibrinogen, fibrin degradation products (FDPs), fibrin split products (FSPs), and platelet counts as appropriate.

NIC High-Risk Pregnancy Care; Surveillance: Late Pregnancy

Ineffective protection *related to potential for seizures and neurologic complications secondary to eclampsia or HELLP syndrome*

GOALS/OUTCOMES Throughout the hospitalization, patient remains free of seizures and neurologic complications as evidenced by orientation to time, place, and person; normoreactive pupils and reflexes; patient's normal visual acuity, motor strength, and coordination; and absence of headache and other clinical indicators of increased intracranial pressure (IICP).
NOC Fetal Status: Antepartum; Blood Coagulation; Fluid/Electrolyte Management

Seizure Precautions
1. Monitor for and document seizures. Protect patient from injury by initiating seizure precautions. When patient is seizing, turn her to the side to promote placental perfusion and prevent aspiration.
2. Assess patient for initial signs of increased ICP, including diminished LOC, headaches, abnormal pupillary responses (i.e., unequal; sluggish/absent response to light), visual disturbances, weakness and paralysis, slow HR, and change in respiratory rate (RR) and pattern. Patient may be experiencing problems related to seizure management, or may experience intracranial bleeding if platelets are extremely low.
3. Monitor trend of Glasgow Coma Scale if patient has difficulty awakening after seizures. If patient exhibits signs of magnesium toxicity, consult physician and consider calcium gluconate administration.
4. Increase frequency of neurologic monitoring as appropriate.
5. Assess the epidural site (as appropriate), if patient received epidural analgesia during labor and delivery. Patients with coagulopathy may develop an epidural hematoma, manifested by sensory or motor deficits, bowel or bladder dysfunction, or back pain. Report problems to the physician immediately. The epidural catheter should remain in place until coagulation studies normalize.
6. Avoid activities that increase ICP.
7. If initial signs of IICP are noted, consult physician immediately. Signs of impending herniation include unconsciousness, failure to respond to deeply painful stimuli, decorticate or decerebrate posturing, Cushing triad (i.e., bradycardia, increased systolic BP, widening pulse pressure), nonreactive/fixed pupils, unequal pupils, or fixed and dilated pupils. See *Traumatic Brain Injury, p. 333,* for more information about herniation. For additional interventions for IICP, see Box 3-7.

NIC Cerebral Perfusion Promotion; Neurologic Monitoring; Seizure Management

Risk for deficient fluid volume *related to active loss secondary to antepartum, postpartum, intraabdominal, or other bleeding*

GOALS/OUTCOMES Patient remains normovolemic as evidenced by HR, RR, and BP within 10% of expected normal range; urinary output 0.5 ml/kg/hr or greater and absence of epigastric or abdominal pain or tenderness, and frank bleeding resulting from HELLP syndrome.
NOC Fluid Balance

Fluid Monitoring
1. Monitor fluid status, including I&O, signs of hypovolemia, including increases in HR and RR, decreases in BP and urinary output, restlessness, and vital signs.
2. Initiate hemodynamic monitoring if necessary to assess shock state and/or manage hemodynamics.
3. Monitor Hgb and Hct as ordered. Postpartum, the uterus contracts and blood is released into the central circulation as it decreases in size. With a normal 500-ml vaginal delivery blood loss, often the Hgb and Hct increase despite the blood loss.
4. Inspect for bleeding from mucous membranes, bruising after minimal trauma, oozing from puncture sites, and presence of petechiae. Maintain patent IV access.
5. Administer supplemental oxygen as necessary for active bleeding.
6. Perform fundus checks and initiate gentle fundal massage to help the uterus remain firm and promote hemostasis.
7. Initiate bleeding control therapy as ordered. Methylergonovine, ergonovine, and carboprost may be used to manage prolonged bleeding or hemorrhage.
8. Replace lost volume with plasma expanders (e.g., albumin, hetastarch) and/or blood products as indicated. See Table 10-3 for information about blood products.

NIC Fluid Management; Fluid/Electrolyte Management; Surveillance: Late Pregnancy; Bleeding Reduction; Hypovolemia Management

Risk for infection *related to inadequate secondary defenses (HELLP syndrome causes liver dysfunction, which may impair the reticuloendothelial system phagocytic activity and portal-systemic shunting); multiple invasive procedures; stress and risks associated with pregnancy, labor, and delivery*

GOALS/OUTCOMES Patient is free of infection as evidenced by normothermia, HR less than 100 bpm, RR less than 20 breaths/min, negative culture results, WBC count less than 11,000/mm³, clear urine, and clear, thin sputum. **NOC** Immune Status; Infection Severity

Infection Protection

1. Monitor vital signs for evidence of infection (e.g., increases in heart and respiratory rates). Check rectal or core temperature every 4 hours for increases.
2. If temperature elevation is sudden, obtain specimens for blood, sputum, and urine cultures or from other sites as prescribed. Consult physician or midlevel practitioner for positive culture results.
3. Monitor CBC, and consult physician for significant increases in WBCs. Be aware that a normal or mildly elevated leukocyte count may signify infection in patients with liver dysfunction.
4. Evaluate secretions and drainage for evidence of infection (e.g., sputum changes, cloudy urine).
5. Evaluate IV, central line, and other site(s) for evidence of infection (i.e., erythema, warmth, unusual drainage).
6. Provide routine episiotomy care by spraying the area with warm water at least every 4 hours. Sitz baths are usually not possible with critically ill patients. Ice packs and topical anesthetics may be used to enhance comfort.
7. Provide daily breast care by cleansing the breasts with mild soap and water. Breast engorgement should be managed per physician's orders to help prevent infection and control pain. If left unrelieved, breast engorgement can result in stoppage of lactation. If breast-feeding is planned, breasts can be massaged and milk manually expressed or pumped.
8. Prevent transmission of infectious agents by washing hands well before and after caring for patient and by wearing gloves when contact with blood or other body substances is possible. Dispose of all needles and other sharp instruments in puncture-resistant, rigid containers. Keep containers in each patient room and in other convenient locations. Avoid recapping and manipulating needles before disposal. Teach significant others and visitors proper hand-washing technique. Restrict visitors with evidence of communicable disease.
9. Administer antibiotics as prescribed. Use caution and reduced dosage when administering antibiotics (especially aminoglycosides) to patients with low urinary output or renal insufficiency.

Compromised family coping *related to abnormal circumstances surrounding labor, delivery, and postpartum; creating need for mother to be separated from infant and other family members*

GOALS/OUTCOMES Patient and family demonstrate adequate coping behaviors and are facilitated in being together as soon as possible in the postpartal hospitalization. **NOC** Family Coping; Family Normalization

Coping Enhancement

1. Provide regular updates to family members about the condition of both mother and infant.
2. Invite family members to participate in care of the mother as possible.
3. Promote infant-mother bonding by allowing baby visitations in the ICU as soon as the conditions of mother and infant stabilize. Allow mother to feed baby if possible. Maintain infant safety if mother's condition is marginally stable.
4. Discuss feelings about labor, delivery, and complications with patient and family members. Relay information about the condition of the infant as often as possible, if mother is unable to visit with the baby.
5. If the infant or mother expires, provide all possible support measures for the patient and significant others, including pastoral care and referrals to community support groups or professional counseling.

NIC Family Involvement Promotion; Family Process Maintenance; Normalization Promotion

ONCOLOGIC EMERGENCIES

An *oncologic emergency* is defined as a life-threatening situation occurring as a manifestation of a malignancy or the result of antineoplastic treatment or tumor progression. Such emergencies most commonly arise from the ability of cancer to (1) spread by direct infringement on adjacent structures or metastasize to distant sites leading to thrombosis or hemorrhage, (2) produce abnormal amounts of hormones or cellular products leading to fluid and electrolyte imbalances and organ failure, (3) infiltrate serous membranes with effusion, (4) obstruct vessels, ducts, or hollow viscera, or (5) replace normal organ parenchyma. As more aggressive therapies are used in the treatment of these cancers, side effects are more intense and the use of critical care to manage such side effects will only increase.

Early recognition and intervention are essential to enhance positive outcomes. Once an oncologic emergency is recognized, the aggressiveness of management is influenced by the reversibility of the immediate situation, the probability of long-term survival, and the ability to provide effective supportive care.

Oncologic emergencies can be classified as hematologic, structural, metabolic, or side effects from treatment such as chemotherapy, radiation therapy, biologic therapy, surgery, or bone marrow transplantation. Neutropenic sepsis, tumor lysis syndrome (TLS), and superior vena cava syndrome (SVCS) will be discussed in this chapter as examples of oncologic emergencies seen in the critical care arena. When recognized early and managed appropriately, these acutely ill individuals have a high likelihood of recovery. An overview of additional oncologic emergencies, associated causes, and signs and symptoms is given in Table 11-8.

Cancer patients may require intensive care for several reasons: (1) overwhelming infection and sepsis, (2) structural complications of cancer or cancer treatment, or (3) metabolic complications of cancer or cancer treatment. Intensivists sometimes refuse admission to cancer patients needing critical care, which may result in denial of effective care for some deserving patients. A cancer patient may need admission to intensive care units for a variety of reasons. The outcomes of patients with hematologic malignancies, previously dismal, have improved over the last 10 years. The previously known indicators of poor outcome are no longer valid in view of recent advances in intensive care. A select group of patients with hematologic malignancies may be offered aggressive therapy for a limited duration and then prognosis can be reassessed. Cancer chemotherapy can produce toxicities affecting all major organ systems. Such patients may be admitted with acute organ dysfunction or years afterward for incidental illnesses. Knowledge of these toxicities is essential for early diagnosis, management, and prognostication in such patients. The postsurgical cancer patient has unique problems; the problems of these groups are discussed. The postsurgical cancer patient may need care ranging from monitoring alone after major surgery in some patients, to fully aggressive intensive care for postsurgical anastomotic dehiscence, mediastinitis, septic shock, and multiorgan dysfunction in others. The metabolic and mechanical complications commonly seen in nonsurgical cancer patients are also reasons for admission. Intensive care should be offered to all patients who have a reasonable chance of cure or supportive care of their disease. The intensivist must be able to recognize the potentially reversible critical illness among the various groups of cancer patients and discourage admission to terminally ill cancer patients. The intensivist must also be aware that the alleviation of the suffering in the last hours of the life of a terminal cancer patient is one of the functions of an ICU, once a decision to discontinue aggressive therapy has been taken, if there isn't time for transfer to a hospice.

NEUTROPENIC SEPSIS

PATHOPHYSIOLOGY

Neutropenia is defined as an abnormally low level of neutrophils in the blood. The normal level of neutrophils in human blood varies slightly by age and race. Infants have lower counts than older children and adults, and African Americans have lower counts than do whites or Asians. The average adult level is 1500 cells/mm^3 of blood. Neutrophil counts (in cells/mm^3) are interpreted as follows:

- Greater than 1000—Normal protection against infection
- 500 to 1000—Some increased risk of infection
- 200 to 500—Great risk of severe infection
- Lower than 200—Risk of overwhelming infection; requires hospital treatment with antibiotics

Untreated bacteremia in patients with neutropenia is fatal: septic shock is associated with a 50% to 70% mortality rate. Mortality is associated with causative organism, site of

Table 11-8 ONCOLOGIC EMERGENCIES DEFINED

Oncologic Emergency	Oncologic Causes	Definition	Signs and Symptoms
Disseminated intravascular coagulation (DIC) (See *Bleeding and Thrombotic Disorders,* p. 837)	Hematologic: Acute Promyelocytic Leukemia, prostate, pancreatic, liver, lung, metastatic cancers	Coagulopathy that develops when the normal balance between bleeding and clotting is disturbed. Excessive bleeding and clotting injures body organs, and causes anemia or death.	Petechiae, ecchymoses, hemorrhagic bullae, acral cyanosis, and focal gangrene in the skin and mucous membranes may be evident. Hemorrhages from incisions or catheter or injection sites, GI bleeding, hematuria, pulmonary edema, pulmonary embolism, progressive hypotension, tachycardia, absence of peripheral pulses, restlessness, convulsions, or coma may occur. Laboratory studies reveal a marked deficiency of platelets, low levels of fibrinogen and other clotting factors, prolonged prothrombin and partial thromboplastin times, and abnormal erythrocyte morphologic characteristics.
Neutropenic sepsis	Hematologic: Any cancer, bone marrow suppression due to chemotherapy, radiation, or targeted therapies	An abnormally low number of circulating neutrophils (absolute neutrophil count [ANC]) leading to predisposition to infections from endogenous flora from gut or skin. Signs of inflammation are often absent.	*Absent;* Febrile, infection Mild neutropenia (ANC 1000–1500): minimal risk of infection Moderate neutropenia (ANC 500–1000): moderate risk of infection Severe neutropenia (ANC <500): severe risk of infection. Symptoms of neutropenia include frequent infections and fevers. Infections can result in diarrhea, oral cavity ulcers, sore throats, burning during urination, and unusual redness around healing wounds.
Malignant pleural effusion	Structural: Breast, lung, GI, lymphoma, radiation to the chest wall, cardiotoxic chemotherapy, metastasis	Transudative or exudative in nature, excess fluid accumulates in the pleural cavity which limits lung expansion and impairs breathing. Chemical (sclerosing agents include tetracycline, bleomycin, talc, etc.) or surgical pleurodesis may be needed in the presence of hemodynamic compromise and recurrence of effusion. Very common, may require thoracoscopic intervention or radiation therapy.	Dyspnea, cough, chest (pleuritic) pain, cyanosis, hypotension, pulsus paradoxus progressing to hoarseness, hiccups, nausea, vomiting, engorged neck veins, distant heart sounds, edema, ascites, hepatosplenomegaly and hepatojugular reflex.

Continued

Table 11-8	ONCOLOGIC EMERGENCIES DEFINED—cont'd		
Oncologic Emergency	Oncologic Causes	Definition	Signs and Symptoms
Spinal cord compression (SCC) (See *Acute Spinal Cord Injury*, p. 264)	Structural: Breast, lung, renal, prostate, myeloma, epidural or bony metastasis, sarcoma, multiple myeloma, leukemia, thyroid cancer, lymphoma, melanoma, and GI malignancies	Compressive irregularity, displacement, or encasement of the spinal cord by metastatic or locally advanced cancer. Spinal cord compression constitutes a true emergency because the initial injury to the spinal cord will lead to permanent loss of neurologic function if the pressure of the tumor on the cord is not relieved quickly.	Earliest symptoms are sensory changes such as numbness, paresthesias, and coldness. When neurologic deterioration is rapid and the patient becomes paraplegic, function is rarely regained. Spinal cord compression is fatal only if it occurs in the cervical region of the spinal cord (C4 and above) and if it results in respiratory paralysis that is uncompensated by mechanical ventilation.
Superior vena cava syndrome (SVCS)	Structural *Malignant:* Lung, lymphomas, breast, mediastinal tumors, metastases from other solid tumors *Nonmalignant:* Indwelling catheter, thrombosis	Occurs due to obstruction to the blood flow caused by tumors, fibrosis, thrombosis and direct tumor invasion of great vessels. The treatment depends on the cause, so definitive tissue diagnosis is essential. Lymphoma or small cell carcinoma may respond to chemotherapy and will reduce obstruction. In chemotherapy-resistant tumors, radiotherapy and corticosteroids may provide relief in a significant number of patients.	Facial and upper extremity edema, facial plethora and tachypnea are most common clinical presentations. May develop slowly and progress to facial edema, venous engorgement and impaired consciousness due to brain edema, decreased cardiac output and upper airway edema. Death can occur from respiratory or circulatory compromise due to obstruction.
Hypercalcemia (See *Fluid and Electrolyte Disturbances*, p. 37)	Metabolic: Lung, breast, prostate, multiple myeloma, renal, head and neck cancers, T-cell lymphomas often due to metastases. In lymphomas and leukemias there is overproduction of activated vitamin D leading to hypercalcemia.	Most common metabolic complication of malignancies, occurring in 10% to 20% of all cancers. Develops when the rate of calcium mobilization from bone exceeds renal threshold for calcium excretion. Vigorous hydration with intravenous normal saline combined with the use of furosemide, is the standard therapy. Corticosteroids, diphosphonates, mithramycin and calcitonin can all reduce serum calcium levels by reducing bone resorption of calcium.	Nonspecific: may include polyuria, polydipsia, constipation, lethargy, confusion, nausea and anorexia progressing to somnolence and coma.

Oncologic Emergencies

| Syndrome of inappropriate antidiuretic hormone (SIADH) (See *SIADH*, p. 734) | Metabolic: Oat cell carcinoma of the lung: 80% of cancer cases. Other causes are CNS, or pulmonary disorders as well as pathologic reactions to various drugs. | Abnormal condition characterized by the excessive release of antidiuretic hormone (ADH) that alters the body's fluid and electrolytic balances. Prognosis depends on the underlying disease, promptness of diagnosis and treatment, and the response to treatment. Thus, if a tumor produces abnormal ADH, then surgery, radiation therapy, or chemotherapy may help by reducing tumor size. | Weight gain despite anorexia, vomiting, nausea, muscle weakness, and irritability. In some patients, SIADH may produce coma and convulsions. Most of the free water associated with this syndrome is intracellular. Other significant results include less than normal concentrations of blood urea nitrogen, serum creatinine, and albumin and a concentration of sodium in the urine higher than normal. |
| Tumor lysis syndrome (TLS) | Metabolic: Most common with hematologic, rapidly growing tumors such as lymphomas, multiple myeloma, leukemias. Also occur in small cell lung, breast, gastic, choriocarcinoma, testicular, melanoma, and hepatocellular cancer cells, particularly after chemoembolization. | Metabolic imbalance which occurs as a result of high tumor cell kill causing rapid release of normal intracellular products. Hemodialysis is initial treatment of choice to rapidly remove potassium, uric acid, and phosphate from serum, while correcting hypocalcemia. | Rapid change in electrolyte balance; dysrhythmics, altered ECG waveform, mentation changes, twitching, cramping, weakness, tetany, oliguria, flank pain, hematuria, weight gain, edema, nausea, vomiting, anorexia, and diarrhea. |

Sources: Recommendations for end-of-life care in the intensive care unit: A consensus statement by the American College of Critical Care Medicine. Crit Care Med 2008 36(3); Guidelines for evaluation of new fever in critically ill adult patients: 2008 update from the American College of Critical Care Medicine and the Infectious Diseases Society of America. Crit Care Med 2008 36(4). Clinical practice guideline: Red blood cell transfusion in adult trauma and critical care. Crit Care Med 2009 37(12); Dellinger RP, Levy MM, Carlet JM, et. al: Surviving Sepsis Campaign: International guidelines for management of severe sepsis and septic shock: 2008 [published correction appears in Crit Care Med 2008; 36:1394-1396]. Crit Care Med 2008; 36:296-327; National Comprehensive Cancer Network Clinical Practice Guidelines in Oncology, http://www.nccn.org; American Society of Clinical Oncology Practice Guidelines, http://www.asco.org; Oncology Nursing Society Practice Guidelines and Resources, http://www.ons.org/ClinicalResources/

infection, and the level and duration of neutropenia. The risk of infection is greater the faster the rate of decline of the neutrophil count and the longer the duration of neutropenia, especially if neutropenia lasts longer than 10 days. Infections in neutropenic patients typically take 2 to 7 days to respond to antimicrobial therapy. Fever (or any inflammatory response related to white cells or cytokines) may not be present in some infected neutropenic patients who are dehydrated or taking steroids or NSAIDs, and the possibility of infection must be considered in any neutropenic patient who is unwell.

ASSSESSMENT: NEUTROPENIC SEPSIS
History and Risk Factors
Granulocytopenia, immunosuppression, recent cancer treatment, diabetes, organ-related disease, age greater than 65 years, indwelling catheters, long hospital or ICU stays, loss of skin or mucosal integrity, malnutrition, hypothermia, intubation/mechanical ventilation, aspiration, alcoholism, renal failure, hepatic failure, chronic illness. The risk of death is twice as great for sepsis patients with cancer as for those without and is comparable to the risk observed in sepsis patients who are HIV positive.

THE FOUR STAGES OF SEPSIS
The progression of sepsis is subtle, rapid, and often deadly and usually broken down into four stages.

Stage 1. *Systemic inflammatory response syndrome (SIRS)* describes a systemic inflammation without a defined source of infection resulting from any major insult to the body, such as trauma, burns, or myocardial infarction, in which two or more of the following are present:
- HR at least 90 bpm
- Body temperature less than 36°C (96.8°F) or greater than 38°C (100.4°F)
- Tachypnea greater than 20 breaths/min or, on blood gas, a $Paco_2$ less than 32 mm Hg
- WBC less than 4000 cell/mm^3 or greater than 12,000 cells/mm^3 or the presence of greater than 10% immature neutrophils

Patients with SIRS can be routinely cared for on the medical-surgical floor but should be closely monitored for signs and symptoms of sepsis.

Stage 2. *Sepsis* is identified by the presence of two of the SIRS criteria in response to pathogenic microorganisms and associated endotoxins in the blood. However, in many cases of sepsis, the actual cause of infection is never identified. The delay in waiting for confirmation of infection can slow the treatment of sepsis; the most effective course of action once SIRS is identified and infection is suspected is to treat the infection and monitor the patient for signs and symptoms of organ failure, which will indicate that the condition has progressed to severe sepsis.

Stage 3. *Severe sepsis* occurs when a patient who meets the sepsis criteria shows one of the signs and symptoms of organ failure. Once severe sepsis is suspected, the patient requires aggressive treatment in a critical care area.

Stage 4. *Septic shock* is defined as severe sepsis plus hypotension (a systolic BP less than 90 mm Hg) that does not respond to fluid resuscitation. Septic shock is associated with a high mortality rate. The patient's chances of recovery are significantly reduced if, by this stage of sepsis, she or he has not already been transferred to the ICU.

Observation: Rapid Progression if Untreated
Signs and symptoms of infection may be absent due to decreased WBCs.
- *General:* fever, hypothermia, chills, pain
- *Neurological:* confusion, anxiety, restlessness, decreased level of consciousness, coma
- *Pulmonary:* tachypnea, rales, rhonchi, wheezes, dry cough, cyanosis, hypoxia, ARDS
- *Cardiovascular:* tachycardia, hypotension, fluctuating pulse pressure, thready pulse
- *Digestive:* nausea, vomiting, anorexia, decreased GI motility, GI bleed
- *Renal:* decreased urine output, anuria, renal failure
- *Integument:* warm, flushed changing to damp, cool, clammy

Diagnostic Tests for Neutropenic Sepsis

Test	Purpose	Abnormal Findings
Blood cultures (done baseline and every 24 hours if signs and symptoms of sepsis persist)	Check for bacteria or other microorganisms in a blood sample.	Gram-positive cocci: coagulase-negative staphylococci, Viridans streptococci and *Staphylococcus aureus* Gram-negative pathogens: *Escherichia coli*, *Klebsiella* spp., and *Pseudomonas aeruginosa*. Fungal: *Candida* spp., *Aspergillus* spp. Viral: Herpes simplex; respiratory syncytial virus
Cultures (throat, stool, urine, CV catheter, other sites of exudates) prior to antibiotics to determine pathogen	Determines source of infection	As above
Chest radiographic examination	Evaluates lung status	Pulmonary infiltrates, pulmonary edema
Complete blood count (CBC)	Evaluates the composition and concentration of the cellular components of blood	Increased WBC with infection, decreased WBC with sepsis; chemotherapy, radiation, leukemias
Chemistries — electrolytes, liver function tests	Evaluates blood chemistries and liver function	Increased BUN, creatinine reveal dehydration; Increase to decrease in glucose due to shock; increased transaminase, bilirubin, serum lactate in sepsis due to shock
Coagulation profile	Examines the factors most often associated with a bleeding problem	Prolonged PT, PTT
Pulse oximetry, ABGs	Measures oxygenation, acid-base balance	Respiratory alkalosis followed by metabolic acidosis
Electrocardiogram	Records the electrical activity of the heart.	Tachycardia, arrhythmias

Oncologic Emergencies

COLLABORATIVE MANAGEMENT

Fever (even low grade) is often the only reliable sign of infection in the neutropenic patient. No specific patterns of fever or clinical features can positively distinguish between fever due to infection and one of noninfectious cause. Therefore, all febrile neutropenic patients should be considered for the administration of empirical broad-spectrum antibiotics within 1 hour of presentation. Many patients are outpatients during their cancer treatments, and it is vital to their survival that they and their significant others be educated about early recognition (and timing during treatment) of neutropenia to minimize the risk of sepsis. All health care providers should be educated about this potential life-threatening situation and be aware of strategies to minimize risk to patients by systematically and regularly evaluating response to treatment and progress toward desired outcomes.

Because sepsis-related mortality is unacceptably high, the Society of Critical Care Medicine (SCCM) set a quality improvement goal to reduce mortality caused by severe sepsis and septic shock by 25%. Clearer definitions of sepsis, severe sepsis, and septic shock will help in achieving this goal, as will recently updated evidence-based management guidelines for severe sepsis and septic shock. To be effective, these definitions and guidelines need to be applied to the early identification and aggressive treatment of patients who have severe sepsis or septic shock. Early goal-directed therapy to achieve hemodynamic stabilization has been demonstrated to decrease mortality in patients who have septic shock. See **SIRS, Sepsis and MODS,** p. 927.

Care Priorities

1. **Manage hypovolemia:** Once severe sepsis or septic shock has been identified, the highest management priorities are to establish vascular access and initiate fluid resuscitation to improve tissue perfusion. Failure to manage global hypoxia can lead to MODS. Fluid resuscitation guidelines are defined by the Society of Critical Care Medicine and are a part of early goal-directed therapy (see *Sepsis, SIRS, and MODS,* p. 927).

2. **Restore tissue oxygenation:** Measurements commonly used are Svo_2, $Scvo_2$, and lactate levels. Low values indicate several possible causes of poor oxygenation, including inadequate oxygen delivery, high oxygen demand, or inability of tissues to extract oxygen from hemoglobin (see *Sepsis, SIRS, and MODS,* p. 927).

3. **Identify and manage the underlying infection:** Selection of an appropriate antimicrobial agent, often in the absence of microbiologic confirmation, requires consideration of patient-related characteristics such as drug intolerances, recently used antibiotics, previous infections, underlying disease, and clinical syndrome. Awareness of the prevalence of infections caused by specific organisms can provide clinicians with insight into appropriate empiric antimicrobial therapy. Pathogen resistance patterns in the hospital and community, along with hospital protocols to limit antibiotic resistance, also should be considered.

CARE PLANS FOR NEUTROPENIA

Ineffective protection: potential for life-threatening infections *related to reduced numbers and activity of WBCs.*

GOALS/OUTCOMES No fever, no clinical signs or symptoms of sepsis, no growth in blood, excrement or skin surface cultures
NOC Immune Status

Infection Control
1. Assess for signs and symptoms of infection, sepsis, septic shock.
   - Monitor temperature every 2 to 4 hours.
   - Monitor vital signs frequently for signs of impending shock: increased HR and RR, increased restlessness and anxiety, and cool and clammy skin, followed by a decrease in BP.
   - Monitor WBC and differential for evidence of infection and response to interventions.
   - Auscultate breath sounds for adventitious sounds or diminished breath sounds.
   - Observe all dressing sites daily for signs and symptoms of infection.
   - Observe all orifices daily for evidence of localized infection.
   - Assess areas of localized pain for erythema, swelling, exudate, or rebound tenderness.
2. Control environmental risks of infection
   - Strict handwashing.
   - Universal precautions.
   - Do not assign neutropenic patients with those known to be infected.
   - Monitor visitors for recent history of communicable disease and institute precautions as needed.
   - Clean all multipurpose equipment between patient use.
   - No live flowers kept in standing water.
3. Implement patient care routines to minimize infection,
   - Assist with daily bathing, oral and perineal hygiene; change linens daily.
   - Ensure sleep and nutritional needs are met to promote immune system recovery.
   - Sterile technique for insertion and care of IV catheters.
   - Encourage incentive spirometry or deep breathing and coughing.
   - Encourage ambulation if patient is able or turn every 2 to 4 hours to minimize skin breakdown or atelectasis.

NIC Cardiac Care: Acute; Circulatory Care: Arterial Insufficiency; Respiratory Monitoring; Shock Management: Cardiac; Cerebral Perfusion Promotion; Neurologic Monitoring; Fluid/Electrolyte Management; Vital Signs Monitoring

Decreased cardiac output *related to infection or sepsis-induced myocardial infarction*

GOALS/OUTCOMES Patient will have normal BP; patient will exhibit signs of adequate tissue perfusion as evidenced by adequate urinary output and normal mental status.
NOC Circulation Status

Hypovolemia Management
1. Monitor I&O hourly. Consult physician for a urinary output less than 0.5 ml/kg/hr for 4 consecutive hours. Insert urinary catheter if appropriate.
2. Monitor and document HR, rhythm, pulses, and BP.
3. Evaluate efficacy of volume expansion by closely comparing CVP, PAWP, and CO. Overzealous volume expansion can lead to heart failure and pulmonary edema.
4. Administer diuretics as prescribed in the well-hydrated patient with urine output less than 0.5 ml/kg/hr.
5. Assess patient for volume depletion, including poor skin turgor; dry mucous membranes; hypotension; tachycardia; and decreasing urine output, CVP, and CO.
6. Monitor electrolytes and serum osmolality. A universal increase in electrolytes and osmolality is indicative of dehydration. A universal decrease signals fluid overload.
7. Assess pH (normal range is 7.35 to 7.45) before replacing electrolytes. Acidosis and alkalosis alter electrolyte values. Replace potassium if the pH is outside the normal range.

NIC Electrolyte Monitoring; Fluid Management; Fluid Monitoring; Intravenous (IV) Therapy; Hypervolemia Management; Shock Management: Volume

Acute pain *related to fever, chills, headaches, myalgias, and arthralgias associated with neutropenia and infection*

GOALS/OUTCOMES Patient will not experience chills, temperature will stay below 38°C (100.4°F); patient will be able to perform activities of daily living without discomfort.
NOC Comfort Level

Pain Management
1. Administer acetaminophen as ordered for fever or mild discomfort.
2. Encourage restful environment.
3. Apply warmth to muscles or joints or cool compress to head as needed.
4. Administer meperidine 12.5 to 25 mg IV or other opiate or benzodiazepine as ordered for chills.
5. Monitor temperature 30 minutes after chill subsides.
6. Bathe patient and change linens after fever subsides.
7. Monitor platelet count as it may decrease with hypermetabolism of hyperthermia.
8. Monitor and document HR, rhythm, pulses, and BP.

NIC Analgesic Administration; Medication Administration; Medication Administration: Intravenous (IV); Heat/Cold Application; Anxiety Reduction; Therapeutic Touch; Music Therapy; Meditation Facilitation

ADDITIONAL NURSING DIAGNOSES
Refer to nursing diagnoses in *Emotional and Spiritual Support of the Patient and Significant Others* (p. 200). For patients who manifest activity intolerance, see that nursing diagnosis in *Prolonged Immobility* (p. 149). For patients with sepsis or septic shock, see *SIRS, Sepsis, MODS* p. 927.

SUPERIOR VENA CAVA SYNDROME

PATHOPHYSIOLOGY
The SVC is a low-pressure vessel between two immovable bone structures: clavicle and scapula. When mediastinal structures become edematous or mass-occupying lesions are introduced, there is insufficient room and the soft-walled SVC becomes occluded and surrounding lymph nodes become enlarged. SVCS is a disorder defined by internal or external obstruction of the SVC leading to reduced blood return to the right side of the heart. Venous congestion and low CO result.

Complications include laryngeal edema, cerebral edema, decreased CO with hypotension, and pulmonary embolism (when an associated thrombus is present). Potential issues include:
● Failure to establish the correct diagnosis and the underlying etiology
● Failure to initiate immediate treatment

Oncologic Emergencies

- Failure to recognize a thrombus in the SVC
- Failure to consult a medical oncologist and radiation therapist
- Failure to expeditiously diagnose and appropriately manage heparin-related complications

ASSESSMENT
Goal of Assessment
Minimize life-threatening complications of cancer and its treatment through early recognition and effective management.

History and Risk Factors
Malignancy: Primary intrathoracic malignancies are the cause of SVCS in approximately 87% to 97% of cases. The most frequent malignancy associated with the syndrome is lung cancer, followed by lymphomas and solid tumors that metastasize to the mediastinum. SVCS develops in approximately 3% to 15% of patients with bronchogenic carcinoma, and it is four times more likely to occur in patients with right- rather than left-sided lesions. Breast and testicular cancers are the most common metastatic malignancies causing SVCS, accounting for greater than 7% of cases. Metastatic disease to the thorax is responsible for SVCS in about 3% to 20% of patients.

Nonmalignant causes: The most common nonmalignant cause of SVCS in cancer patients is thrombosis secondary to venous access devices. Other nonmalignant causes include cystic hygroma, substernal thyroid goiter, benign teratoma, dermoid cyst, thymoma, tuberculosis, histoplasmosis, actinomycosis, syphilis, pyogenic infections, radiation therapy, silicosis, and sarcoidosis. Some cases are idiopathic.

Observation
Classic symptoms: Patients with SVCS most often present with complaints of facial edema or erythema, dyspnea, cough, orthopnea, or arm and neck edema. These classic symptoms are seen most commonly in patients with complete obstruction, as opposed to those with mildly obstructive disease.

Other associated symptoms: Other associated symptoms may include hoarseness, dysphagia, headaches, dizziness, syncope, lethargy, and chest pain. The symptoms may be worsened by positional changes, particularly bending forward, stooping, or lying down.

Common physical findings: The most common physical findings include edema of the face, neck, or arms; dilatation of the veins of the upper body; and plethora or cyanosis of the face. Periorbital edema may be prominent.

Other physical findings: Other physical findings include laryngeal or glossal edema, mental status changes, and pleural effusion (more commonly on the right side).

Diagnostic Tests for Superior Vena Cava Syndrome		
Test	**Purpose**	**Abnormal Findings**
Chest radiograph (CXR)	Evaluates lung status at baseline and every 24 hours if signs and symptoms of sepsis persist	Identify hilar, mediastinal masses, right middle lobe congestion, masses or nodes between clavicle and scapula
Spiral chest CT scan with contrast	Further evaluates lung status to help clarify findings from CXR.	Precisely identify location and size of masses around SVC; clarify growth versus compression
Magnetic resonance imaging (MRI) of the chest	Provides further data regarding the area of the superior vena cava	Precisely identifies location and size of masses around SVC
Doppler ultrasound of the vasculature	Noninvasively assesses the entire vascular tree to identify thrombosis or the effects of thrombolysis	Presence of thrombus or ineffective thrombolysis when therapies are rendered.

Diagnostic Tests for Superior Vena Cava Syndrome — cont'd		
Test	Purpose	Abnormal Findings
Contrast and radionuclide venography	Invasively assesses the entire vascular tree to identify thrombolysis; may be used to validate Doppler ultrasound findings	Presence of thrombus or ineffective thrombolysis when therapies are rendered.
Complete blood count (CBC): platelet count	Evaluates the composition and concentration of the cellular components of blood, particularly platelets	Declining platelet count may signal the presence of heparin-induced thrombocytopenia (HIT) or "white clot syndrome." If unmanaged, may lead to extremity gangrene and life-threatening venous thromboembolism.

COLLABORATIVE MANAGEMENT
Care Priorities

1. **Provide anticoagulation and thrombolysis:** Anticoagulation for SVCS has become increasingly important due to thrombosis related to intravascular devices. In certain situations, the device remains in place. Both streptokinase and urokinase have been used for thrombolysis, although urokinase has been more effective in lysing clots in this setting. Urokinase is given as a 4400 U/kg bolus followed by 4400 U/kg/hr, whereas streptokinase is administered as a 250,000 U bolus followed by 100,000 U/hr. The use of thrombolytic therapy is controversial for catheter-related thrombosis, however.

2. **Monitor for heparin-induced thrombocytopenia:** In particular, one must monitor platelet count and be vigilant should a rapid decline in platelets occur. This suggests the possibility of platelet-induced thrombocytopenia syndrome (white clot syndrome). This rare syndrome may lead to extremity gangrene and life threatening venous thromboembolism. Management requires urgent discontinuation of heparin and urgent evaluation by a hematologist for appropriate pharmacotherapy. Vascular surgical evaluation may also be indicated.

3. **Provide surgical intervention: stenting:** Placement of an expandable wire stent across the stenotic portion of the vena cava is an appropriate therapy for supportive care of SVCS symptoms when other therapeutic modalities cannot be used or are ineffective. Use of stents is limited when intraluminal thrombosis is present.

4. **Provide radiotherapy and/or chemotherapy:** Both radiotherapy and chemotherapy are treatment options for SVCS, depending on the tumor type. The specific drugs and doses used are those active against the underlying malignancy. Radiation therapy is the standard treatment of non–small cell lung cancer (NSCLC) with SVCS. Recent studies suggest that chemotherapy may be as effective as radiotherapy in rapidly shrinking small cell lung cancer (SCLC). Combination chemoradiation therapy may result in improved ultimate local control over chemotherapy alone in SCLC and non-Hodgkin lymphoma. Retrospective reviews of patients with SCLC have reported equivalent survival in patients with or without SVCS treated definitively with chemoradiation therapy.

> **Safety Alert** *Life-threatening symptoms, such as respiratory distress, are indications for urgent radiotherapy. A preliminary determination of the treatment goal (potentially curative or supportive only) is necessary prior to the initiation of treatment, even in the emergent setting.*

5. **Provide additional interventions to assist with maintaining patency of the SVC:** Balloon angioplasty is rare but may be considered in patients with SVCS, significant clinical symptoms, and critical SVC obstruction demonstrated by angiography.

Oncologic Emergencies

CARE PLANS FOR SUPERIOR VENA CAVA SYNDROME
Decreased cardiac output *related to reduced venous blood return to the heart*

GOALS/OUTCOMES Patient will show evidence of normal tissue perfusion and will not experience upper extremity edema.
NOC Circulatory Status; Tissue Perfusion: Cardiac; Tissue Perfusion: Peripheral; Tissue Perfusion: Pulmonary

Circulatory Care: Venous Insufficiency
1. Monitor I&O hourly. Consult physician for a urinary output less than 0.5 ml/kg/hr for 4 consecutive hours. Insert urinary catheter if appropriate.
2. Monitor and document HR, rhythm, pulses, and BP.
3. Evaluate efficacy of volume expansion by monitoring CVP and CO. Overzealous volume expansion can lead to heart failure and pulmonary edema, with CVP greater than 20% of normal values and CO less than 5 L/min.
4. Administer diuretics as prescribed in the well-hydrated patient with urine output less than 0.5 ml/kg/hr.
5. Assess patient for volume depletion, including poor skin turgor, dry mucous membranes, hypotension, tachycardia, CVP less than 2 mm Hg, and decreasing urine output.
6. Monitor electrolytes and serum osmolality. A universal increase in electrolytes and osmolality is indicative of dehydration. A universal decrease signals fluid overload.
7. Assess skin and mucous membranes for cyanosis and pallor, skin temperature for signs of change in perfusion.
8. Assist in care of patient receiving therapy to treat SVCS.

NIC Electrolyte Monitoring; Fluid Management; Fluid Monitoring; Intravenous (IV) Therapy; Hypervolemia Management; Shock Management: Volume

Impaired gas exchange (or risk for same) *related to decreased blood flow to the lungs*

GOALS/OUTCOMES Patient's gas exchange is adequate as evidenced by PaO_2 at least 90 mm Hg, $PaCO_2$ 35 to 45 mm Hg, pH 7.35 to 7.45, RR 12 to 20 breaths/min with normal depth and pattern, oxygen saturation at least 95%, HR 60 to 100 bpm, and orientation to time, place, and person.
NOC Respiratory Status: Gas Exchange; Vital Signs Monitoring

Respiratory Monitoring
1. Assess respiratory status every 2 hours, noting rate, rhythm, depth, and regularity of respirations.
2. Monitor for signs of respiratory failure: restlessness, anxiety, and air hunger indicative of hypoxemia; ABG values for increased $PaCO_2$ and decreased pH indicative of hypoventilation; or oxygen saturation less than 90% via pulse oximetry indicative of decreased ventilation. Consult physician if signs of respiratory insufficiency are present.
3. Monitor SvO_2: steady increase or decrease from patient's normal level may indicate deterioration.
4. Assess lungs for bibasilar crackles (rales), indicative of pulmonary edema.
5. Monitor patient's respiratory secretions. Institute respiratory therapy treatments as needed.
6. Monitor for pulmonary embolus, including sharp, stabbing chest pain, dyspnea, pallor, cyanosis, pupillary dilation, rapid or irregular pulse, profuse diaphoresis, and anxiety. Assess need for supplemental oxygen, and consult physician immediately. Patients with severe pulmonary emboli may require mechanical ventilation. See *Pulmonary Embolus*, p. 396.
7. Assess patient for changes in sensorium (i.e., confusion, lethargy, somnolence), indicative of inadequate cerebral oxygenation or CO_2 retention (respiratory insufficiency).

NIC Airway Management; Oxygen Therapy; Acid-Base Monitoring

TUMOR LYSIS SYNDROME

PATHOPHYSIOLOGY
Tumor lysis syndrome (TLS) is most commonly seen in individuals with rapidly growing tumors which are acutely responsive to chemotherapy due to the rapid release of intracellular contents into the bloodstream, leading to life-threatening concentrations of intracellular

electrolytes. If the resulting metabolic abnormalities remain uncorrected, patients may develop acute renal failure and sudden death resulting from a lethal dysrhythmia secondary to hyperkalemia.

The syndrome is caused by rapid lysis of malignant cells resulting in hyperuricemia, hyperkalemia, hyperphosphatemia, hypocalcemia, and an increase in BUN. These abnormalities can occur as early as 6 hours following chemotherapy and in the last 5 to 7 days after treatment. The hyperuricemia is caused by the massive release of intracellular nucleic acids and their metabolism by xanthine oxidase into uric acid. Urate crystals can form in the renal collecting ducts and result in acute renal failure. Similarly, potassium and phosphate are released from the tumor cells, and their excretion is hampered by the hyperuricemia. The best approach to management is to prevent its occurrence by proper hydration. Patients with the diagnosis of rapidly growing lymphoma, uric acid levels of greater than 10 mg/dl and a high blast count in leukemia, and a high lactate dehydrogenase level before treatment are at greatest risk of developing TLS.

TLS is also seen in small cell cancer of the lung and metastatic breast cancer. Because of clinicians' increased awareness of the tumor lysis syndrome during the past decade and the use of adequate prophylaxis prior to the initiation of chemotherapy, the number of cases has decreased. Occasionally, the syndrome occurs following treatment with radiation, glucocorticoids, tamoxifen, or interferon.

ASSESSMENT
History and Risk Factors
The typical patient at risk for TLS tends to be young (under 25 years of age), male, has an advanced, highly proliferative, high-grade disease (lymphoma, leukemia, etc.), often abdominal disease, and a markedly elevated lactic dehydrogenase level. Comorbid conditions include renal insufficiency and diabetes. Volume depletion, concentrated acidic urine pH, and excessive urinary uric acid excretion rates may also increase the risk.

TLS most commonly develops during the rapid growth phase of high-grade lymphomas and leukemia in patients with high leukocyte counts; it is less common in patients with solid tumors. The syndrome is often iatrogenic, caused by cytotoxic chemotherapy.

Observation
Signs and symptoms reflect electrolyte imbalance, coupled with those of acute renal failure. The syndrome is characterized by hyperuricemia, hyperkalemia, hyperphosphatemia, hypocalcemia, and oliguric renal failure (see *Fluid and Electrolyte Disturbances*, p. 37, and *Acute Renal Failure*, p. 584). The diagnosis of TLS is based on the development of increased levels of serum uric acid, phosphorus, and potassium; decreased levels of serum calcium; and renal dysfunction following chemotherapy

COLLABORATIVE CARE
Care Priorities
1. **Identify patients at risk and initiate prophylactic measures:** Patients at risk for TLS should be identified before the initiation of chemotherapy and should be adequately hydrated and given agents to alkalinize the urine. Treatment with allopurinol (IV or PO) may be instituted to minimize hyperuricemia. The recommended dosage of IV allopurinol ranges from 200 to 400 mg/m²/day. This regimen should be started 24 to 48 hours before the initiation of cytotoxic treatment. The dose may be equally divided into 6-, 8-, or 12-hour increments, but the final concentration should not exceed 6 mg/ml.
2. **Monitor electrolytes:** Serum electrolytes, uric acid, phosphorus, calcium, and creatinine levels should be checked repeatedly for 3 to 4 days after chemotherapy is initiated, with the frequency of monitoring dependent upon the clinical condition and the risk profile of the patient.
3. **Provide aggressive, immediate treatment of electrolyte imbalances and acute renal failure:** Once tumor lysis is established, treatment is directed at vigorous correction of electrolyte abnormalities, hydration, and hemodialysis (see *Fluid and Electrolyte Disturbances*, p. 37, and *Acute Renal Failure*, p. 584).

CARE PLANS FOR TUMOR LYSIS SYNDROME

Fluid volume excess *related to acute renal failure resulting from hyperuricemia with formation of uric acid crystals lodging in the kidneys*

GOALS/OUTCOMES Patient's volume status returns to normal/baseline as evidenced by urinary output at least 0.5 ml/kg/hr, stable weight, BP within patient's normal range, HR 60 to 100 bpm, RR 12 to 20 breaths/min, good skin turgor, moist mucous membranes, urine specific gravity 1.005 to 1.025, and CVP 2 to 6 mm Hg. Serum potassium, phosphorus, calcium, uric acid, BUN, and creatinine levels will be within normal limits.

NOC Electrolyte and Acid-Base Balance

Fluid/Electrolyte Management
1. Monitor intake and output hourly. Consult physician or midlevel practitioner for a urinary output less than 0.5 ml/kg/hr for 4 consecutive hours. Insert urinary catheter if appropriate.
2. Monitor electrolytes every 6 to 12 hours during high-risk period.
3. Monitor and document HR, rhythm, pulses, and BP.
4. Administer IV fluids before and after cancer treatment.
5. Administer allopurinol as prescribed to manage hyperuricemia.
6. Administer aluminum hydroxide as prescribed to manage hyperphosphatemia.
7. Administer cation-exchange resins as prescribed to manage hyperkalemia.
8. Assist with renal replacement therapies.
9. Administer diuretics as prescribed in the well-hydrated patient with urine output less than 0.5 ml/kg/hr.
10. Monitor electrolytes and serum osmolality. A universal increase in electrolytes and osmolality is indicative of dehydration. A universal decrease signals fluid overload.
11. Assess pH (normal range is 7.35 to 7.45) before replacing electrolytes. Acidosis and alkalosis alter electrolyte values. Replace potassium if the pH is outside the normal range.
12. Teach patients to restrict foods high in potassium and phosphorus and to increase fluid intake.

NIC Electrolyte Monitoring; Fluid Management; Fluid Monitoring; Intravenous (IV) Therapy; Hypervolemia Management; Shock Management: Volume

ADDITIONAL NURSING DIAGNOSES

Refer to nursing diagnoses in *Emotional and Spiritual Support of the Patient and Significant Others* (p. 200). For patients who manifest activity intolerance, see that nursing diagnosis in *Prolonged Immobility* (p. 149),

ORGAN TRANSPLANTATION

Solid organ transplantation remains a viable option for end-stage organ failure. As of February, 2010, there were nearly 106,000 people on the United Network for Organ Sharing (UNOS) organ transplant waiting list. The major constraint to meeting the demand for transplants is the availability of donated (cadaver) organs. Dialysis remains the main lifeline for kidney disease and mechanical devices for heart failure are becoming increasingly available throughout the United States. A small number of patients are living at home on mechanical ventilation. In general, those with liver, pancreatic, and lung disease remain dependent on organ transplantation to sustain life.

Several steps have been taken to alleviate the organ shortage. National laws mandate that families of every appropriate potential donor be offered the option to donate organs and tissues. In addition, the ongoing efforts of the National Organ Donation Collaborative and laws requiring all deaths to be reported to organ procurement agencies have prompted an increase in organ donations. Ongoing efforts of organ recovery coordinators and others to improve public awareness regarding organ donation will help reduce the shortage, along with use of extended donors.

Nationally, major improvements are being made to optimize organ distribution, improve procurement, and ensure good matches. Inclusion criteria for the waiting list are being standardized using listing criteria for all degrees of sickness (see Box 11-4). UNOS maintains a computerized registry of all patients awaiting organs for transplantations. Organs procured

Box 11-4   ALLOCATION OF THORACIC ORGANS

Status 1A
A patient is admitted to the transplant center and has at least one of the following:

A Mechanical circulatory support for acute hemodynamic decompensation that includes at least one of the following:
- Left or right ventricular assist device implanted within past 30 days
- Total artificial heart
- Intra-aortic balloon pump
- Extracorporeal membrane oxygenator

B Mechanical circulatory support for >30 days with significant device-related complications such as thromboembolism, device infection, mechanical failure, or life-threatening ventricular arrhythmias

C Mechanical ventilation

D Continuous infusion of a single high-dose inotrope or multiple inotropes with hemodynamic monitoring

E Patient does not meet the above criteria but has a life expectancy without a heart transplant of less than 7 days

Status 1B
A patient listed as status 1B has at least one of the following devices or therapies in place:

A Left and/or right ventricular assist device implanted for >30 days

B Continuous infusion of inotropes

Status 2
A patient who does not meet the criteria for status 1A or 1B is listed as a status 2.

Status 7
A patient listed as status 7 is considered temporarily unsuitable to receive a thoracic organ transplant.

From United Network for Organ Sharing (UNOS) for allocation of thoracic organs.
*For complete detailed criteria, see actual policy at www.UNOS.org.

within a region are shared first within that region. If a recipient cannot be found within the region, UNOS directs the organ to the recipient in another region with the greatest need. Organ recovery coordinators are always on call (24/7). They are responsible for arranging serologic testing, organ removal from donors, preservation of organs pretransplant, and distribution to recipients.

ASSESSMENT AND DIAGNOSTIC TESTING
General Evaluation for Transplantation
All solid organ recipients require multiple tests to evaluate readiness and appropriateness for transplantation as it relates to the patient's health status, comorbidities, pretransplantation disease processes, and donor matching. The general recipient evaluation includes:

Labwork
- *General laboratory assessment profiles* including biochemical, hematologic, lipid, hepatic, renal, thyroid studies, and urinalysis. If findings indicate several organs are impaired, the patient may be inappropriate for transplant, since immunosuppressive drugs can cause renal failure, those with heart disease may have a myocardial infarction in the postoperative period, those with lung disease may be unable to wean from mechanical ventilation, and those with liver disease may be immunocompromised and at higher risk for sepsis and metabolic complications, which cause capillary leak syndrome.
- *ABO blood typing:* Requires duplicate testing for accuracy and safety. Testing includes panel reactive antibody (PRA) and human leukocyte antigen (HLA) testing.

- *Virology screening:* HIV, hepatitis, herpes, cytomegalovirus (CMV), Epstein-Barr virus (EBV)
- *Other infectious diseases:* Toxoplasmosis, tuberculosis, resistant bacterial infections including *B. cepacia*
- *Cancer screening:* May include pap smears, prostate specific antigen (PSA), mammogram, colonoscopy, and chest radiography

Diagnostic Testing

- *Pulmonary evaluation:* Oxygenation assessment and chest radiograph
- *Cardiac and vascular evaluation:* Exercise stress test and Doppler imaging for patients with a history of diabetes, coronary artery disease, claudication, cerebrovascular accident
- *Nutritional evaluation:* Body mass index (BMI) less than 16 (cachexia) and BMI greater than 30 are associated with poorer outcomes.
- *Osteoporosis screening:* Osteoporosis may place a patient at higher risk for complications following transplantation, as maintenance medication may increase the severity, which increases the probability of bone fractures.
- *Dental examination:* Poor oral hygiene may be a source of infection.
- *Ultrasound of gallbladder:* Presence of gallstones increases the probability of need for cholecystectomy following transplantation.
- *Psychosocial evaluation:* The patient must have an adequate support system to participate in post-transplant medical care and life maintenance activities. Patient must also be ready to comply with all aspects of medical care, including medications, diet, exercise, and refraining from substance use and abuse.
- *Financial evaluation:* The financial burden associated with organ transplantation is significant. The patient must have appropriate resources in place to cover the costs.

Organ-Specific Evaluation

- *Cardiac:* Cardiac catheterization (right and left heart), cardiopulmonary exercise testing, cardiac magnetic resonance imaging (MRI) or positron emission tomography (PET) scan and MVo_2 testing
- *Lung:* Computed tomography (CT) scan to define the anatomy, ventilation-perfusion scan, 6-minute walk test, ABG, continuous pH testing, smoking cessation readiness, and ability to remain "smoke free"
- *Liver:* Alpha-fetoprotein, CA 19-9 tumor markers for hepatocellular carcinoma and cholangiocarcinoma. Liver biopsy may be performed to determine staging or presence of disease. Abdominal imaging and GI testing assess portal vein system and hepatic vasculature. A GI evaluation is done to assess for bowel diseases. *Alcohol consumption screening:* to assess for usage patterns and readiness to stop drinking alcohol. If use persists in those whose need for liver transplant is directly related to alcohol, the person is unable to qualify for organ transplantation. A complete battery of tests is performed to determine the cause and acuity of liver failure.
- *Kidney:* Specific urine testing for preoperative baseline, screen for hypercoagulopathy, abdominal imaging for anatomic and renal vessel assessment
- *Pancreas:* Complete testing referred to in the cardiac section, as well as full assessment of diabetes status. Initial screening includes performing a hemoglobin A1C test to assess for average blood glucose level over the past 8 weeks.

ORGAN-SPECIFIC CRITERIA FOR TRANSPLANTATION
Cardiac

Table 11-9 summarizes the selection criteria that patients must meet before they can be considered for cardiac transplantation.

Lung

Lung transplant candidates generally have a life expectancy of less than 18 months, are supplemental oxygen dependent, have severe exercise intolerance, are under 65 years of age, and report poor quality of life.

Indications: In adults, irreversible, progressively disabling, end-stage pulmonary disease (ESPD) encompassing a wide variety of etiologies. The majority of lung transplants are performed for chronic obstructive pulmonary disease (COPD), which is the most common

Table 11-9	SELECTION CRITERIA FOR TRANSPLANTATION CONSIDERATION
Inclusion Criteria	**Exclusion Criteria**
• End-stage heart failure • Refractory and intolerable symptoms; New York Heart Association classes III–IV • Failure of maximal medical treatment (e.g., digoxin, diuretics, vasodilators, ACE inhibitors, beta-blockers) • 1-year survival expectancy <50% and poor short-term prognosis or poor functional capacity • Age <60–70 • Left ventricular ejection fraction 20%–35% • Chronic, unstable angina • Peak O_2 consumption 14 ml/kg/min • Onset of atrial fibrillation • Decreasing cardiac output • Cachexia, BMI < 16 • Refractory ventricular dysrhythmias • Otherwise good health	*Relative* • Active substance abuse • Active infection associated with ventricular assist • Psychological/social issues related to support or finances • Age greater than 65–70 yr • History of cancer in remission *Absolute* • Complicated IDDM with end-organ damage • Poor compliance • Severe obesity • Pulmonary hypertension: PVR >6 Wood Units • Comorbid diseases • Active infection (until resolved) and infection with highly resistant organisms which are nearly impossible to eradicate • Irreversible liver and kidney dysfunction • Active peptic ulcer disease • Coexisting cancer • Symptomatic peripheral and cerebral vascular disease • Severe osteoporosis • Amyloidosis

IDDM, Insulin-dependent diabetes mellitus; *PVR,* pulmonary vascular resistance.

cause, followed by idiopathic pulmonary fibrosis (IPF), pulmonary hypertension, and cystic fibrosis (CF). Four groupings of lung diseases which may result in transplantation are:

1. *Nonbronchiectatic:* Obstructive lung conditions or changes in the upper and lower airways NOT resulting from an infectious process, including emphysema, chronic bronchitis, alpha₁-antitrypsin disease and bronchiolitis obliterans syndrome (BOS), a disease associated with chronic transplant rejection. BOS and chronic bronchitis can evolve into bronchiectasis. Most recently, the BODE index was introduced (BMI, Obstruction of airflow severity, Dyspnea severity as measured by the modified Medical Research Council dyspnea scale, Exercise capacity). Patients scoring greater than 5 on the BODE index should be referred for transplant.

2. *Bronchiectatic:* Obstructive lung conditions resulting from abnormal dilation and thickening of the walls in the bronchi and bronchioles, which result from recurrent inflammation, leading to mucus retention. Diseases include CF and severe chronic bronchitis, which result in chronic bacterial pneumonia.

3. *Interstitial:* Restrictive lung disease resulting from chronic inflammation of the lower airways, including IPF, diseases related to occupational exposure to toxins (asbestos, coal, or organic dust, crystalline silica), histiocytosis X, and sarcoidosis. Patients who have been irradiated and/or undergone chemotherapy for a nonpulmonary condition and who then develop lung disease are considered on an individual basis. Not all centers accept patients with pulmonary fibrosis associated with connective tissue disease.

4. *Pulmonary vascular:* Pulmonary hypertension resulting from vascular disease that severely increases pulmonary vascular resistance, which leads to right-sided heart failure and chronic hypoxia. Pulmonary hypertension may be primary (idiopathic pulmonary vascular disease) or secondary to a shunt associated with heart disease, thromboembolism, connective tissue disease, or parenchymal disease.

Contraindications

Relative

1. *Advanced age:* Historically, patients older than 65 years of age have a higher mortality rate, but centers vary with candidate acceptance. Generally, the age limit for heart-lung transplantation is 50 years, for bilateral sequential lung transplantation is 60 years, and for single lung transplantation is 65 years.

2. *Ventilator dependence:* Not a contraindication as an entity, but as the time on the ventilator extends, patients are at higher risk of other contraindications, such as infection, or development of MODS, muscle atrophy, and other concerns surrounding deconditioning, which impacts success of attaining a functional lifestyle following transplantation.
3. *Corticosteroid therapy:* Low dose is now acceptable, while high dose may be viewed as an absolute contraindication.
4. *Infection:* CF patients may be excluded if infected with the highly resistant organism *B. cepacia* because of inability to eradicate the organism with antibiotics; those with active tuberculosis are generally not candidates, as well as CF patients with *Aspergillus fumigatus*. Infection with nontuberculous *Mycobacteria* is not a contraindication.
5. *Body weight:* Patients with BMI less than 16 likely have a poor nutritional status, which impairs healing. Those with BMI greater than 30 are at higher risk of developing postoperative atelectasis and pneumonia.
6. *Associated organ dysfunction:* Patients with left ventricular systolic or diastolic dysfunction may not be a candidate if disease is severe, with bilirubin of greater than 2 mg/dl and with connective tissue diseases.

Absolute
1. Malignancy within the past 2 years (except cutaneous squamous and basal cell tumors)
2. Noncurable, chronic, extrapulmonary infection (e.g., chronic hepatitis B or C, HIV)
3. Untreatable advanced organ dysfunction of another body system
4. Current cigarette smoking (must be smoke free for at least 6 months)
5. Poor rehabilitation potential (based on evaluation of issues mentioned in relative contraindications)
6. Significant psychosocial problems, substance abuse, or history of nonadherence to past medical therapies or disease management programs

Liver

Indications Currently, any patient who has chronic or acute liver disease that leads to the inability to sustain a normal quality of life or that results in life-threatening complications should be considered a candidate for liver transplant. Complications that warrant liver transplantation generally include recurrent variceal hemorrhage, intractable ascites, spontaneous bacterial peritonitis, refractory encephalopathy, severe jaundice, and sudden deterioration in status. Reduced-size, split, and living-related liver transplantation continue to expand the number of donors, yet these efforts still fail to meet the demand for organs.

- *Chronic end-stage liver disease:* Hepatitis C, hepatitis B, alcoholic cirrhosis, primary biliary cirrhosis, primary sclerosing cholangitis, hepatocellular carcinoma, autoimmune hepatitis, metabolic disease (e.g., Wilson disease, inborn errors of metabolism), and other liver diseases (generally, types of hepatitis).
- *Fulminant hepatic failure (FHF):* Severe impairment of hepatic failure in the absence of preexisting liver disease. Those exposed to, or who ingest toxins, or toxic doses of illicit drugs or medications (e.g., acetaminophen toxicity) are included in this group. Hepatotoxic drugs include acetaminophen (paracetamol), salicylates (aspirin, Pepto-Bismol), methanol (wood alcohol), isoniazid, intravenous tetracycline, chlorinated hydrocarbons, and sodium valproate. The most common drug involved is acetaminophen, and, in some locations, it is the most common cause of FHF. Other diseases that may cause FHF include heart failure, cardiomyopathy, sepsis, shock,cyanotic heart disease, obstructive lesions of the aorta, vascular occlusions, myocarditis, Hodgkin disease, and severe asphyxia.

Contraindications
Absolute
- Spontaneous bacterial peritonitis (or other active infection)
- Active alcohol or other substance abuse
- Extra hepatic malignancy that does not meet "cure" criteria
- Severely advanced cardiac or pulmonary disease
- Extreme psych/social situations that prohibit adherence to immunosuppressive therapies
- Severe portopulmonary hypertension (moderate and mild pulmonary hypertension are acceptable, and are sometimes included in the indication criteria)
- Hepatocellular carcinoma lesion(s) greater than 5 cm or more than three lesions present

Relative
- Chronic renal failure (may require a combined liver/kidney transplant)
- Advanced cachexia
- Large hepatocellular cancers/tumors: More advanced than stage II, as described by the UNOS-modified American Joint Committee on Cancer [AJCC] classification
- Medication-resistant hepatitis B viral cirrhosis (HBV)
- Portal and mesenteric vein thrombosis
- History of prior cancer not meeting full AJCC cure criteria
- Active infections
- MODS
- Age: Physiologic age, rather than chronologic age, is used.

Kidney
Indications
- Chronic end-stage kidney disease
- Dependency on dialysis

Contraindications
Absolute
- Active or current malignancy
- Goodpasture disease or systemic lupus erythematosus (can damage the transplanted kidney)
- Active infection
- Obesity
- Significant peripheral vascular disease
- End-stage diseases of other organs
- Active systemic vascular disease
- Noncompliance
- Active substance abuse
- Untreated psychiatric illness or mental incapacity
- Active peptic ulcer disease
- Limited life expectancy

Pancreas
Preexisting advanced renal disease is observed in significant numbers of pancreas transplantation candidates. Many pancreas transplantation candidates may benefit from a combined pancreas/kidney transplant.
- *Islet cell:* A novel, less invasive harvesting of pancreatic cells for transplantation is in limited use. The islet cells are the islets of Langerhans (alpha, beta, and delta). Islet cells are isolated from a donor pancreas or from patient's own pancreas after the pancreatectomy. It is specially processed then infused into the patient via the portal vein. A neovascularization process takes place. The islet cells begin to produce insulin shortly after transplantation. No further discussion will take place in this chapter.

Indications
- Type 1 diabetes with chronic poor metabolic control
- Patients requiring a total pancreatectomy
- Mean duration of diabetes 23 to 27 years
- C-reactive peptide less than 0.8 ng/ml
- Frequent or severe metabolic complications, e.g., hypoglycemia/hyperglycemia and ketoacidosis
- End-organ failure with numbness of extremities, lethargy, nausea, dizziness, blurred or poor vision

Contraindications
Relative
- Evidence of significant secondary complications of type 1 diabetes, including peripheral neuropathy, retinopathy, gastroparesis, nephropathy, and coronary artery disease, which may impede the success of the transplant
- Type 2 diabetics are seldom evaluated.

Absolute
- Active cancer or history of cancer
- Severe cardiac, vascular, or pulmonary insufficiency
- Active/chronic hepatitis B
- Severe psychiatric or substance abuse issues

ORGAN DONORS

The mainstay of organ supply is the deceased donor or (cadaveric) donation. Nationwide, approximately 30% of all deceased organ donors are trauma patients. Evaluation of the trauma patient as a potential organ donor is critical to maximizing the availability of deceased donor organs for transplantation. Regional transplant centers vary in absolute and relative criteria for excluding potential organ donors. Early criteria limited evaluation to ideal donors aged 10 to 50 years without comorbid conditions. In response to the increasing demand for organs, donation from an expanded donor pool reflects restrictions that have loosened considerably. Organs are now often harvested from patients younger than 10 years old and older than 50 years. Factors such as hepatitis C or active bacterial infection are no longer absolute contraindications. "Nonideal" donors are often used for specific recipients.

There are relatively few absolute contraindications, and most potential donors are reviewed on an individual or a case-by-case basis. Additional absolute and relative contraindications are assessed for donation of specific organs. Some organs must be transplanted within a very short time following brain death, while other organs can be preserved for much longer periods of time. The following are types of organ donors:

Donation after Brain Death

The patient has sustained an irreversible brain injury causing cessation of brain function, including the brain stem. The patient is brain dead but is kept "alive" with a ventilator for organ recovery. Diagnosing brain death consists of an absence of neurologic function, apnea, irreversibility, and physiologic confirmatory tests.

Donation after Cardiac Death

The death is declared on a basis of cardiopulmonary criteria (irreversible cessation of circulatory and respiratory function). The patient may have sustained catastrophic brain injury that is not anticipated to progress to brain death (stroke or trauma). If the family decides to remove the patient from the ventilator to allow for natural death, they may be offered the opportunity for organ donation. Natural death would need to occur within 1 hour of removal from the ventilator. The organs are harvested once the patient is pronounced. The donation should not hasten the death, and the transplant procurement team would enter the operating room after the patient is pronounced dead and will not be a part of the end-of-life care. Donation can also be considered if there is an unplanned cardiac arrest.

Living Donors

Living donors are considered for kidney and liver transplants. The evaluation process is very critical for living donors. Postoperative care for the donor and donor family must also be clearly prioritized. Those considerations are:
1. Ensure there is a maximum benefit to the recipient and minimum risk to the donor.
2. Physical and psychosocial health of the donor is evaluated.
3. Potential donors should not be pressured or coerced by the recipient or others.
4. The donor should be seen separately in the absence of the prospective recipient.
5. Risk to the donor should be carefully considered.
6. Informed consent is complete, neutral, and not coerced.
7. Do not overestimate the benefits of donating.
8. Do not underestimate the risk.
9. Understand donor motivation.
10. Donors should be informed of the potential financial costs they will incur and the amount of time they will be away from work.
11. Emotional well-being of the donor and family is of high priority.
    a. Postoperative pain may prompt feelings of anxiety and remorse.
    b. Donors are concerned about the recipient.
    c. Postdonation depression is common.

Paired and Chain Donations

Paired donation is an opportunity for a live donation when a direct related donation is not possible. Transplant centers strategically manage a group of potential recipients and potential live donors so that a donor can give to an unrelated person, while the unrelated person's donor can give to their related person. What could be a complex chain of exchanges ("swaps") if worked out, could benefit a larger number of individuals.

LABORATORY AND DIAGNOSTIC TESTS

- Varies from center to center

General Screening for Organ Donors

- Basic laboratory values (e.g., CBC, electrolytes, glucose, ABG)
- ABO blood typing
- HLA typing
- Blood cultures
- Sputum Gram stain, culture, and sensitivities
- Urinalysis, culture, and sensitivities
- HIV, EBV, CMV, human T-cell leukemia virus type 1 (HTLV-1), and hepatitis B and C virus serologies
- Venereal disease research laboratory (VDRL) test or rapid plasma reagent (RPR) test
- Inguinal lymph nodes tested for evaluation of recipient sensitivity

Heart Donor

- ECG
- Chest radiograph
- Echocardiogram
- Cardiac catheterization (male older than 40 years or female older than 45 years, or younger if other cardiovascular risk factors present)
- Creatine kinase (CK), isoenzyme of CK with muscle and brain subunits (CK-MB), and troponin levels

Lung Donor

- ABG on 100% F_{IO_2}; then, serial ABGs
- Chest radiograph
- Bronchoscopy

Pancreas Donor

- Serial blood glucose determinations
- Amylase and lipase levels

Liver Donor

- LFTs
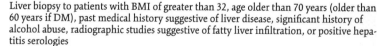
- Liver biopsy to patients with BMI of greater than 32, age older than 70 years (older than 60 years if DM), past medical history suggestive of liver disease, significant history of alcohol abuse, radiographic studies suggestive of fatty liver infiltration, or positive hepatitis serologies
- PT
- aPTT

Kidney Donor

- Electrolytes
- BUN
- Creatinine (Cr)

PRIORITY/WAITING LISTS/MEDICAL URGENCY DETERMINATION

Heart

Demographics including age, ethnicity, gender, and location, with ABO type, height, weight, diagnosis, and medical urgency, are matched with the donor information (weight, age, distance to transplant center, and need for prospective cross-match).

Lungs

The Lung Allocation Score (LAS) is a numerical scale (0 to 100) computed from a list of criteria and is updated every 6 months. People who are most likely to die before transplantation and have a chance of greater survival after transplantation are the candidates given the highest scores on the list. Along with the LAS, blood type, age, and distance from the donor are used to determine priority for the organ. Also under consideration is the bilirubin level and changes in this level while on the waiting list. A current bilirubin of at least 1.0 mg/dl or an increase by at least 50% during a 6-month time period increases the candidate's risk of dying while on the list. Pediatric and adolescent patients have priority over adults. LAS testing is updated every 6 months.

Kidneys

Living donor allocation/timing is dependent on availability and matching. The waiting time may be quicker than for a deceased donor. Waiting times can vary from 2 to 5 years for a deceased donor. Recipients must have a GFR of no more than 20 to earn time. Recipient is either active or inactive. There is no urgent status. Extended criteria donors (ECDs) are on the rise. Considerations include ABO type, HLA antibodies, cross-match, and PRAs. PRAs can be tested as frequently as monthly. A new algorithm is on the horizon: Life Years from Transplantation (LYFT). It will attempt to pair the donor and recipient combination that will achieve the greatest survival benefit relative to dialysis.

Liver

Status 1 is a patient in the ICU with life expectancy of less than 7 days with acute liver failure, hepatic artery thrombosis, primary graft nonfunction or acute decompensated Wilson disease.

MELD Score: Model for End-stage Liver Disease (MELD) is a score ranging from 6 (less ill) to 40 (gravely ill) used to prioritize liver transplant candidates at least 12 years of age. It is predictive of risk of 3-month mortality from liver disease. The number is calculated using a formula that considers three blood studies: bilirubin (measures liver excretion of bile); INR (international normalized ratio), which measures the ability of the liver to manufacture clotting factors; and creatinine, which measures kidney function. Bile excretion and the ability to synthesize clotting factors are impaired by chronic liver disease. Renal impairment is often associated with liver disease. A numerical scale is used for liver allocation for chronic liver disease only. Only Status 1 patients (have sudden, severe onset of liver failure with a life expectancy of a few hours to days without a transplant) are excluded from MELD scoring. Status 7 patients are inactive.

Pancreas

Waiting lists and allocation of organs vary by institution and are generally based on time waiting and PRA level. Frequent evaluation is necessary, every 6 months or per program standard.

PHARMACOTHERAPY
Post-Transplant Immunosuppression

Goals of therapy include:
1. Prevent rejection
2. Improve graft survival
3. Improve patient survival
4. Maintain quality of life

Immunosuppression therapy prevents rejection and is required indefinitely post transplant. Immunosuppression agents have their own risks: infection, malignancy, toxicity, and patient compliance. Finding the balance between saving the graft and preventing complications is a lifelong challenge.

Levels of Immunosuppression Therapy

Induction: Immunosuppression, usually in high doses, in the initial period of organ transplantation wipes out T cells completely. Commonly used drugs typically consist of corticosteroids and monoclonal and polyclonal antibodies: orthoclone OKT3, antithymocyte globulin (ATG), basiliximab, daclizumab, alemtuzumab.

Maintenance: Maintenance dose of immunosuppression for transplant patients in a stable condition serves to maintain a gradual process of healing and to prevent a rejection. The potential for weaning patients off some of their medication therapies is a high priority. Commonly used drugs are corticosteroids, calcineurin inhibitors (CNIs), antiproliferative agents, and mammalian target of rapamycin (mTOR) inhibitors.

Rejection: Immunosuppression, usually in high doses for a patient whose organs are acutely rejecting. Commonly used drugs are corticosteroids and polyclonal and monoclonal antibodies: OKT3, ATG, basiliximab, daclizumab, and alemtuzumab.

Desensitization: Therapies to reduce newly formed or preexisting alloantibodies. Commonly used drugs are IV IG, rituximab, and cyclophosphamide. Plasmapheresis mechanically removes antibodies but does not deal with the original problem.

Categories of Drugs

Interleukin 1 Inhibitors

Corticosteroids. Used to treat and prevent rejection and to suppress production of cytotoxic T-lymphocytes from noncytotoxic precursor cells. Evidence indicates that steroids may prevent release of interleukin (IL)-1 and IL-2. IL-1 is released by the macrophages and promotes differentiation of helper T cells. The release of IL-2 promotes differentiation of cytotoxic cells and helps to reduce or prevent edema, to promote normal capillary permeability, and to prevent vasodilation. They can be used for maintenance to prevent rejection or as part of an acute rejection protocol. Side effects are numerous, including mood changes, sodium retention, blurred vision, fragile skin, bleeding, glucose intolerance, increase in appetite and subsequent weight gain, osteoporosis, and "moon face" appearance from an accumulation of fatty tissue on cheeks and upper back.

Methylprednisolone: Used as an induction agent with dose range from 250 to 1000 mg at the time of transplantation and for the next three doses. The dose is reduced to 35 mg by mouth (PO) every 12 hours . until biopsy or per program protocol. It is commonly weaned by 5mg at each dosage until a maintenance dose of 0–10 mg daily is achieved. It is also used prior to poly/monoclonal antibody therapy for cytokine release syndrome. *Dosage:* Solu-Medrol: 125 mg IV every 12 hours for three doses. Taper to as low a dose as tolerated.

Calcineurin Inhibitors (CNIs)

Cyclosporine (Sandimmune, Neoral, Gengraf): Inhibits production and release of lymphokines and generation of cytotoxic and plasma cells by blocking the response of cytotoxic T-lymphocytes to IL-2. Cyclosporine is metabolized by the cytochrome P-450 enzyme system in the liver. Careful monitoring of cyclosporine drug levels, with concomitant dose adjustments, is necessary when cyclosporine is used with other drugs. It is eliminated by the liver and is not dialyzed out.

Dosage is dependent on the type of transplant and on whether the modified or nonmodified formulation is used and is dependent on the practitioner, patient status, and biopsy results. Side effects include kidney and renal dysfunction, excessive hair growth, hypertension, diarrhea, swelling and tenderness in gums, hand tremors, and increased risk of infections and tumors.

Tacrolimus (Prograf): Blocks T-cell activation genes via a similar mechanism to cyclosporine but is more potent than CSA. It is also metabolized by the cytochrome P-450 enzyme system in the liver. It is used as a **first-line drug** (used first) or replaces cyclosporine if there are multiple rejections while on cyclosporine. It inhibits T-lymphocyte activation.

Dosage depends on trough blood levels, organ function, and rejection status. It is cleared through the liver and depends on liver function. *Dosage:* dependent on type of transplant given in continuous drip, converted to an oral dose every 12 hours after GI function has returned. Trough levels are initially 8 to 15 ng/ml then maintenance of 5 to 15 ng/ml. It is not dialyzed out and should be given on an empty stomach without other medications. Side effects are dose related and diminish when dose is decreased. They include hyperkalemia, nephrotoxicity, glucose intolerance, hypertension, nausea, diarrhea, infections, and lymphoproliferative disorders.

Antiproliferative Agents

Mycophenolic acid: Mycophenolate mofetile (MMF; Cellcept): Currently a first-line immunosuppressant that inhibits immunologically mediated inflammatory responses. It inhibits the proliferation of T and B-lymphocytes, the production of antibodies, and the generation of cytotoxic T cells. Dosed at 1.0 to 1.5 g every 12 hours IV/PO, no blood level monitoring is required. Preferred administration is on an empty stomach, if given PO. Side effects include diarrhea, vomiting, headache, tremor, insomnia, dizziness, leukopenia, and anemia. Use chemo precautions during administration. Do not open, crush, or chew tablets.

Mycophenolic acid (Myfortic): Delayed release. Indication, efficacy, and adverse effects profile are the same as for MMF. Dosing is 720 mg taken orally every 12 hours. Do not open, crush, or chew tablets.

Azathioprine (Imuran): Interferes with gene transcription. It is used in combination to prevent rejection. WBC counts are monitored, and dosage is adjusted accordingly. It is taken daily at bedtime. Maintenance dosage is 1 to 3 mg/kg/day, to a maximum of 150 to 175 mg/day. Side effects include decreased WBC count and platelets, bone marrow suppression, toxic hepatitis, hair loss, mouth sores, and muscle wasting. Decrease or hold if WBC count is less than 5.

Mammalian Target of Rapamycin (mTOR) Inhibitors mTOR is a key regulatory kinase in the process of cell division and thus inhibited with this group of drugs. Inhibitors improve renal profile when replacing CNIs that are more damaging to the kidneys.

Sirolimus (Rapamune): Prevents rejection. This inhibits T- and B-lymphocyte activation and proliferation and also has antineoplastic effects. Oral loading dose is 6 mg/day followed by a maintenance dose of 2 mg/day regulated by blood level assessment, divided into two doses given every 12 hrs. Some centers do administer the drug once daily. Therapeutic trough blood levels are seen between 8 and 15 ng/ml. It is associated with impaired wound healing, so it is not used during induction in the post-transplantation period. Other side effects include peripheral edema, hypertension, fever, headache, mouth ulcers, acne, rash, interstitial pneumonitis, hyperlipidemia, leukopenia, and thrombocytopenia.

Everolimus (Certican): Very similar to Sirolimus in mechanism of action and side effect profile. Dosage is 0.5 mg to 1.5 mg orally twice daily. The therapeutic drug level range is 3 to 8 ng/ml.

Monoclonal Antibodies

OKT3 (Orthoclone): Treats rejection. OKT3 is a murine (mouse) monoclonal antibody that recognizes and binds the CD3 receptor present on all mature T cells. Anti-CD3 is a homologous antibody that reacts with and blocks the function of the chemical (T3) complex on the surface of the T-lymphocytes. The T3 complex is responsible for the T-lymphocyte's identification of a transplanted organ as foreign and the attempts to reject it. OKT3 binds to the T3 antigen on the surface of the T cells, enhancing phagocytosis and entrapment of the cells in the spleen and liver. The T-lymphocytes are removed from the circulation by this process in approximately 10 to 15 minutes. Dose at 5 mg given IV push over 1 minute every day for 10 to 14 days. It is associated with cytokine release syndrome that occurs during the first 2 days of therapy, manifested as high fever, chills, tremor, and pulmonary edema. When receiving OKT3, patients are premedicated with acetaminophen, H_2-receptor antagonist, and hydrocortisone (before) and diphenhydramine (1 hour before).

Other side effects are diarrhea, vomiting, headache, tremor, insomnia, dizziness, leukopenia, tachycardia, pyrexia, and anemia. Associated with higher infection and malignancy rates, especially CMV, CD3 levels are measured to maintain adequate levels of OKT3.

Basiliximab (Simulect): Immunosuppressive monoclonal antibody, used at induction, that specifically binds to and blocks the IL-2 receptor alpha chain on the surface of the activated T-lymphocytes. It inhibits IL-2 activation of T-lymphocytes. Anti-CD25, it does not treat rejection. *Dosage:* 20 mg within 2 hours of transplantation surgery and repeated 4 days after transplant. Most common side effects are GI disorders.

Daclizumab (Zenapax): Action similar to Basiliximab. *Dosage:* 1 mg/kg/dose for 5 doses, the first dose within 24 hours of transplant, then at intervals of 14 days 4 doses.

Rituximab (Rituxan): Targeted against CD20 antigen on B-lymphocytes. It prevents and treats humoral rejection. *Dosage:* 375 mg/m^2 × 1 dose for humoral rejection or 375 mg/m^2 dose every week for 4 doses for post-transplant lymphoproliferative disorder (PTLD). Patient is premedicated with acetaminophen and diphenhydramine. Start at 50 mg/hr and ramp up, as tolerated.

Alemtuzumab (Campath, MabCampath, or Campath-1H): Used in the treatment of chronic lymphocytic leukemia (CLL) and T-cell lymphoma. Alemtuzumab targets CD52, a protein present on the surface of mature T-lymphocytes, but not on the stem cells from which these lymphocytes were derived. Used in organ transplant patients as induction therapy and for rejection in a very small population.

Alemtuzumab has been associated with infusion-related events including hypotension, rigors, fever, shortness of breath, bronchospasm, chills, and/or rash. Other serious infusion-related events were syncope, pulmonary infiltrates, ARDS, respiratory arrest, cardiac arrhythmias, myocardial infarction, and cardiac arrest.

Polyclonal Antibodies

Antilymphocyte sera (anti–lymphocytic globulin [ALG] or anti–thymocyte gamma-globulin [ATGAM or thymoglobulin]): Used for induction and rejection. The antilymphocyte antibodies in the sera are useful in the treatment of steroid-resistant rejection and are potent suppressors of cell-mediated immunity. They are directed against many different antigens on the surface of human lymphocytes and affect immunity via reduction of T-lymphocytes. Associated with cytokine release syndrome that occurs during the first 2 days of therapy, manifested as high fever, chills, tremor, and pulmonary edema. When receiving ATGAM or thymoglobulin, patients are premedicated with acetaminophen, H_2-receptor antagonist, and hydrocortisone (before) and diphenhydramine.

Others

Intravenous immune globulin (IVIG): Use for desensitization and treatment of humoral rejection. *Dosage:* 1 to 2 g/kg, start at low rate (0.05 to 0.06 mg/kg/hr) and titrate up as tolerated. Premedicate with acetaminophen and diphenhydramine. Side effects include back pain, headache, chills, fevers, bronchospasms, and hypotension.

Antibiotics: Cefazolin or a similar antibiotic is given until the chest tubes are removed.

Antivirals: Valganciclovir (Valcyte): Prophylaxis and treatment for CMV. CMV remains the major cause of morbidity and mortality with cardiac transplantation patients. *Dosage:* Induction 900 mg every 12 hrs x 21 days, maintenance and prevention 450 to 900 mg orally daily for 3 to 6 months post event.

Acyclovir: Prophylaxis and treatment for herpes virus. *Dosage:* 5 to 10 mg/kg IV every 8 hours for 7 to 10 days or 200-800 mg orally, 2-5 x a day depending on active infection or suppressive therapy.

Antifungal: Mycostatin, Nystan, Fluconazole: For potential secondary *Candida* infections related to immunosuppression. *Dosage:* 5 ml swish-and-swallow or Mycelex troche three times daily beginning after extubation.

Prevention of pneumocystic pneumonia (PCP): Bactrim, TMP/SMX, pentamidine, dapsone

Other side effect or preventive medications: Antiulcer medications, aspirin, BP management, stool softener, insulin, cholesterol lowering, calcium phosphorus, magnesium, and osteoporosis medications

In-hospital Medications Used Postoperatively

Inotropic medications: Nitroglycerin to decrease preload; nitroprusside (Nipride) to decrease afterload; dobutamine to increase contractility/CO; epinephrine to increase HR and contractility; norepinephrine (Levophed) to increase BP; milrinone (Primacor) to increase contractility/CO and decrease afterload; dopamine for renal perfusion in smaller doses (controversial), and increase HR and BP at higher doses; and isoproterenol (Isuprel) to increase HR and decrease pulmonary vascular resistance. Theophylline may also be used for increasing HR and decreasing PVR.

Pain: Fentanyl is commonly used because it is short acting and, unlike morphine, does not cause histamine-mediated hypotension.

Pretransplant and Post-transplant Sensitization Poor outcomes, such as CAD, PTLD, and an increased incidence of rejection, have been associated with pretransplant sensitization. Positive PRA levels detect circulating HLA and reflect level of sensitization. Pregnancy, blood transfusion, ventricular assist devices, or previous transplants can trigger sensitization. Elevated PRA levels increase the difficulty of finding an HLA-compatible donor organ. HLA compatibility will enhance graft survival and reduce infection and malignancies related to aggressive immunosuppression. Plasmapheresis may decrease sensitization and reduce PRA levels.

COLLABORATIVE MANAGEMENT
Care Priorities

1. **Prevent Infection.** Infection control is paramount because of immunosuppression therapy. Immunosuppressed patients are vulnerable to bacterial (*Staphylococcus, Streptococcus, Klebsiella, Pseudomonas*) viral (CMV, EBV, herpes simplex, varicella zoster) and fungal infections (*Aspergillus, Candida, Cryptococcus*, histoplasmosis, Coccidioides, pneumocystis, and *Toxoplasma gondii*). Prophylactic antibiotics and antivirals are used.

Steps to reduce infection postoperatively and beyond:

1. Isolation. Keep door closed, and limit visitors; no employees or visitors with active infection are allowed; avoid taking care of other patients with infections.
2. Survey wound sites for infection.
3. Vital signs and temperature on a regular basis. Temperature greater than 99.2°F may be sign of infection.
4. Perform a thorough clinical physical assessment.
5. Review blood work and radiographs.
6. Provide antifungal mouth rinses.
7. Perform sterile wound dressing changes.
8. Discontinue invasive and tubes as soon as possible.
9. Facilitate early extubation.
10. Provide early optimal nutrition.
11. Use a leukocyte filter for blood administration or use leukocyte-reduced blood.
12. Provide education to the patient and significant others regarding infection prevention.

2. **Prevent organ rejection.** Graft or organ rejection is the leading concern with transplantation. A transplanted organ originates from a donor who is genetically different from the recipient (the exception is a kidney/liver from an identical twin). The organ contains foreign antigens that trigger an immune response in the recipient, which leads the organ to reject that foreign object. Historically, rejection has been classified as hyperacute, accelerated acute, acute, or chronic (Table 11-10). An untreated rejection response results in complete destruction of the organ. Table 11-11 describes the clinical presentation for various types of acute organ rejection.

When the body detects the presence of a foreign substance, the immune system mounts a defense with nonspecific inflammation and phagocytosis. Antibody-mediated (humoral) and cell-mediated immune responses work together to defend after exposure to an antigen. Antibody-mediated immune response stimulates B-lymphocyte activity. When an antigen is encountered, the B-lymphocyte enlarges, divides, and differentiates into a plasma cell that produces and secretes antigen-specific immunoglobulins, or antibodies. The formation of this antigen-antibody complex triggers events that augment the nonspecific responses of inflammation and phagocytosis. Cell-mediated immune response involves T-lymphocytes. T-lymphocytes recognize a foreign antigen on the surface of the macrophage, bind to the antigen, enlarge, and produce a sensitized clone, which migrates through the body to the site of the antigen. When the sensitized T cell combines with the antigen, chemicals are released that kill foreign cells directly and facilitate phagocytosis and the inflammatory response.

Graft-versus-host disease: A rejection process whereby there is a transplant of functioning allogeneic T cells into an immunocompromised host, such as a bone marrow transplant.

Table 11-10	CHARACTERISTICS OF ORGAN REJECTION BY CATEGORY	
Type of Rejection	**Characteristics**	**Outcome**
Hyperacute	Occurs immediately Antibody-mediated Result of preformed circulatory antibodies	Usually irreversible and untreatable Preventable with crossmatching
Accelerated acute	Occurs 3–5 days after transplant Antibody-mediated Rapid loss of function Fever and oliguria	Irreversible and untreatable Preventable with crossmatching
Acute	Primarily T cell–mediated Possible presence of humoral component Occurs weeks, months, or years after transplant	Treatable and reversible multiple episodes affect long-term graft survival
Chronic	Develops slowly over months to years Probably a combination of cellular and humoral-mediated processes	Untreatable; eventually leads to graft loss

Table 11-11	**CLINICAL PRESENTATION WITH ACUTE ORGAN REJECTION**
Organ	**Clinical Presentation**
Heart	10–14 days after transplantation. Indicators include fever, anxiety, lethargy, low back pain, atrial or ventricular dysrhythmias, gallop, pericardial friction rub, jugular venous distention, hypotension, and decreased CO late in rejection.
Lung	Expected during the first 21 days after surgery, with increased frequency and severity 6–8 wks after transplantation. Classic rejection: decreased lung ventilation and perfusion alveolar exudate containing desquamated pneumocytes and inflammatory cells Atypical rejection: decreased ventilation without blood flow reduction; ventilation-perfusion imbalances, and respiratory insufficiency with shunting Vascular rejection: increased vascular resistance; decreased blood flow to graft
Liver	4–10 days after transplantation. Indicators include malaise; fever; abdominal discomfort; swollen, hard, tender graft; tachycardia; RUQ or flank pain; cessation of bile flow; change in bile fluid from golden to colorless; jaundice; elevated PT, bilirubin, transaminase, and alkaline phosphatase.
Kidney	Occurs in the immediate postop period and seen as fever, pain over graft, decreased urine output, edema with increase in creatinine. Renal scan or Doppler is used for a quick look at blood flow to the kidneys. Patients may even need dialysis for a short time until the kidney functions.
Pancreas	Time of rejection occurrence varies. Patient may have hyperglycemia, pancreatitis, pain over graft. Open biopsy may be necessary to diagnose rejection.

Vasculopathy: Chronic rejection phenomena. Changes are seen in the allograft vessels. This is a diffuse disease that affects the full wall thickness of the arteries and not just the intralumen, as occurs in atherosclerosis in the heart.

DIAGNOSIS AND ASSESSMENT OF REJECTION

Rejection is assessed in many ways, with biopsy being the most invasive direct assessment. Biopsy of the transplanted organ provides the means of diagnosing rejection, its severity, and the possibility of response to antirejection therapy. Tiny pieces of muscle tissue are removed for pathologic examination to assess for tissue rejection.

Heart

Biopsy is performed in a cardiac catheterization lab/biopsy lab or surgery. The cannulation site is generally the right internal jugular or sometimes the femoral vein. Biopsy samples are graded according to one of several grading systems. Biopsies are generally performed at 7 and 14 days after surgery and at specified intervals thereafter.

The following assist in assessment for rejection of the transplanted heart:

- *Vital signs and heart sounds:* May reveal decreased stroke volume, CO, cardiac tones, and BP and presence of S_3 and S_4 sounds, pericardial friction rub, extrasystole, and crackles
- *Echocardiogram:* Used to assess chamber size, wall thickness, ejection fraction, thrombus formation, valve function, and systolic and diastolic function
- *Chest radiograph:* Will reveal increased dimensions of the heart late in rejection
- *ECG:* Will show presence of atrial and ventricular dysrhythmias and decreased QRS voltage
- *CBC:* Will show increased total lymphocyte count
- *Intravascular ultrasound (IVUS):* Used to evaluate vasculopathy of the coronary arteries
- *Blood analysis of rejection:* Currently only used to assess cardiac rejection, AlloMap detects the absence of acute cellular rejection in clinically stable heart transplant patients. The test uses a peripheral blood sample and has replaced biopsies in many institutions. Studies are currently ongoing for lung patients, with other organs targeted in the future.

Lung

- *Transbronchial biopsy:* Not particularly helpful in detecting rejection; the morbidity risk increases with open biopsy.
- *Biopsy grading*
    - Grade 0: No acute cellular rejection

- Grade 1: Minimal acute cellular rejection
- Grade 2: Mild acute cellular rejection
- Grade 3: Moderate acute cellular rejection
- Grade 4: Severe acute cellular rejection

The following assist with assessment of the transplanted lung:

- *Symptoms:* Cough (although it goes away in the initial stages), dyspnea, fatigue, fever, flulike symptoms
- *Chest radiograph:* Changes indicative of rejection are noted.
- *Leukocyte and absolute T-lymphocyte counts:* Rise during rejection
- *Vital signs and hemodynamics:* Can change suddenly with increases in PVR, HR, BP, SVR, and CO
- *ABG values:* Decrease in Pao_2 and increase in $Paco_2$ occur with rejection. Decrease in PFTs.
- *Infection:* The most significant cause of post-transplant morbidity and mortality because the lung is the most immunogenic of the solid organs and it is the only solid organ exposed to the outside air

Kidney

- *Renal biopsy:* Determines presence, type, and severity of rejection
- *Kidney biopsy grading* (Table 11-12)

The following signs assist in assessment for rejection of the transplanted kidney:

- *Symptoms:* Fever, pain over graft, edema
- *BUN and creatinine values:* Will increase from previous 24-hour levels and continue to rise until rejection is reversed
- *24-Hour urine collection:* Will exhibit a change in components (e.g., decreases in creatinine clearance, total amount of creatinine excreted, and urinary sodium excretion; increase in protein excretion)

Table 11-12	BANFF DIAGNOSTIC CATEGORIES FOR RENAL ALLOGRAFT BIOPSIES
Acute Active Rejection	
1. Normal	
2. Antibody mediated rejection: Immediate (hyperacute), Delayed (accelerated acute)	
3. Borderline changes: No intimal arteritis is present, but there are foci of mild tubulitis	
4. Acute/active rejection	

Type Grade	Histopathologic findings
IA	Significant interstitial infiltration (>25% parenchyma affected) and foci of moderate tubulitis (>4 mononuclear cells/tubular cross section or group of 10 tubular cells)
IB	Significant interstitial infiltration (>25% parenchyma affected) and foci of moderate tubulitis (>10 mononuclear cells/tubular cross section or group of 10 tubular cells)
IIA	Cases with mild to moderate intimal arteritis
IIB	Cases with severe intimal arteritis comprising >25% of the luminal area.
III	Cases with transmural arteritis and/or arterial fibrinoid change and necrosis of medical smooth muscle cells
5. Chronic/sclerosing allograft nephropathy	

Grade	Histopathologic findings
I: Mild	Mild interstitial fibrosis and tubular atrophy without (a) or with (b) specific changes suggesting chronic rejection
II: Moderate	Moderate interstitial fibrosis and tubular atrophy (a) or (b)
III: Severe	Severe interstitial fibrosis and tubular atrophy and tubular loss (a) or (b)
Other	Changes not considered to be due to rejection

- *Renal scan:* Will exhibit decreased blood flow
- *Kidney assessment:* May reveal a firm, large kidney that may be tender on palpation
- *Renal scan:* Evaluates blood flow to the kidney and rate of excretion of substances into the bladder

Liver

Several methods are used to obtain liver samples, including laparoscopic liver biopsy, percutaneous image-guided liver biopsy, and open surgical liver biopsy.

Laparoscopic liver biopsy: Using trocars (shafts with three-sided points), small incisions are made in the abdomen to enable insertion of the laparoscope. Using the monitor to facilitate viewing, the physician uses instruments within the laparoscope to remove tissue samples from one or more parts of the liver. This type of biopsy is used when samples from specific parts of the liver are required.

Percutaneous liver biopsy: A local anesthetic is first administered to numb the area on the body's right side. Through a small incision near the rib cage, a special biopsy needle is inserted to retrieve liver tissue. In some cases, ultrasound imaging or computed axial tomography (CAT) scans of the liver may be used to help guide the needle to a specific spot. This biopsy method is often used when the disease process is localized to discrete spots in the liver.

Open surgical liver biopsy: Open liver biopsies are done by a surgeon using a biopsy needle or through surgical excision of a small piece of liver tissue. This is generally used during another surgical procedure, because less invasive techniques are available.

The following signs assist in diagnosis of rejection of the transplanted liver (Table 11-13):

- *Symptoms:* Light-colored stools, dark-colored urine, jaundice of the sclera or skin, fever, right upper quadrant pain, fatigue, malaise, and pruritus
- *Serum bilirubin level:* Total bilirubin will rise in relation to baseline postoperative level.
- *Transaminase level:* Will increase from baseline; may be markedly elevated early in rejection
- *Alkaline phosphatase level:* Will increase from baseline
- *Prothrombin time:* Will be prolonged
- *CBC:* May reveal decreased platelet count and increased total lymphocyte count

Pancreas

Open biopsy is the only means by which a definitive diagnosis can be made.

The following signs also assist in the diagnosis of rejection of the transplanted pancreas:

- *Symptoms:* Pain over pancreas graft; malaise, fever, and hyperglycemia
- *Fasting and 2-hr postprandial plasma glucose:* Levels will be increased above normal ranges.
- *Serum amylase:* Levels may be elevated, indicating presence of pancreatitis, an inconsistent marker of rejection.
- *Serum creatinine:* Elevated
- *C-reactive peptide (serum and urine):* Levels may be decreased.
- *Pancreas radioisotope flow scan:* Determines organ viability; decreased flow may indicate rejection.

Table 11-13	**LIVER TRANSPLANT DATABASE (LTD GRADING SCHEME)**
Grade	**Criteria**
A0	No rejection
A	Rejection without bile duct loss
1	Rejection infiltrate in some, but not all of the triads, confined within the portal spaces
2	Rejection infiltrate involving all of the triads, with or without spillover into the lobule. No evidence of centrilobular hepatocyte necrosis, ballooning or dropout.
3	Infiltrate in some or all of the triads, with or without spillover into the lobule, with or without inflammatory cell linkage of the triads, associated with centrilobular hepatocyte ballooning or necrosis and dropout

Organ Transplantation

CARE PLANS FOR ORGAN TRANSPLANTATION

Risk for injury *related to organ rejection related to inadequate immunosuppressant drug levels*

GOALS/OUTCOMES Within 48 hours after the transplant, patient verbalizes accurate information about the signs and symptoms of rejection. Within 72 hours after initiation of medications, patient and significant others verbalize accurate information regarding the prescribed immunosuppressive agents, the side effects that can occur, and precautions that should be taken. Patient demonstrates ability to relax, discusses anxiety related to the rejection, and exhibits increased involvement in his or her own care.

NOC Immune Status

Environmental Risk Protection
1. Assess patient's knowledge of drug therapy.
2. Provide patient with verbal and written information for the type of immunosuppressive agent that has been prescribed. Discuss the generic name, trade name, purpose, usual dosage, route, side effects, and precautions.
3. Monitor blood levels as appropriate for drug.
4. Instruct patient to take medication at designated time(s) each day. Never withhold immunosuppressant without consulting with physician or midlevel practitioner.
5. Monitor for signs of rejection, as appropriate for each specific organ.
6. Reinforce necessity of regularly scheduled appointments with transplant coordinator. Encourage patient to bring a significant other to the visit.

NIC Teaching: Disease Process; Teaching: Individual; Teaching: Prescribed Medication. Additional, optional interventions include Discharge Planning; Medication Management; and Weight Management.

Risk for infection (lungs and heart most common) *related to immunosuppression*

GOALS/OUTCOMES Patient is free of infection as evidenced by normothermia; absence of erythema, swelling, and drainage of catheter and wound sites; absence of adventitious breath sounds or cloudy and foul-smelling urine; negative results of urine, wound drainage, and blood cultures; and WBC count 4,500 to 11,000/mm^3.

NOC Immune Status

Infection Protection
1. Patient is to wear mask when outside immediate living area, in public areas, or near construction or during "cleaning" of environment.
2. Notify physician/transplant coordinator immediately if temperature greater than 99.5°F, WBC count increasing, patient complaints of malaise, or there is any obvious infection.
3. Avoid placement of indwelling catheters; if necessary, remove as soon as possible.
4. Assess and document condition of indwelling IV sites and other catheter sites every 8 hours. Be alert to swelling, erythema, tenderness, and drainage. Consult physician for any of these findings.
5. As prescribed, obtain blood, urine, and wound cultures when infection is suspected.
6. Be alert to WBC count greater than 11,000/mm^3 or less than 4500/mm^3. A below-normal WBC count with increased band neutrophils on differential (shift to the left) may signal acute infection.
7. Inspect graft wound for erythema, swelling, and drainage. Consult physician or midlevel practitioner for significant findings.
8. Record volume, appearance, color, and odor of urine. Be alert to foul-smelling or cloudy urine, frequency and urgency of urination, and patient complaints of flank or labial pain, all of which are signs of renal-urinary infection.
9. Auscultate lung fields every 8 hours, noting presence of rhonchi, crackles, and decreased breath sounds.
10. Use meticulous aseptic technique when dressing and caring for wounds and catheter sites.
11. Obtain specimens for urine cultures once a week during patient's hospitalization and once a month after hospital discharge.

NIC Infection Control. Additional, optional interventions include Airway Management; Exercise Promotion and Therapy Medication Management; Respiratory Monitoring; Teaching: Disease Process; Tube Care: Urinary; and Vital Signs Monitoring.

Deficient knowledge *related to post-organ transplant care*

GOALS/OUTCOMES Within 24-hour period before discharge from the hospital, the patient and one family member will verbalize understanding of his or her disease, as well as the necessary lifestyle changes.
NOC Knowledge: Illness Care; Knowledge: Health Resources

Teaching: Disease Process
1. New condition, procedure, treatment
2. Complexity of treatment
3. Emotional state affecting learning (anxiety, denial, or depression)
4. Unfamiliarity with information resources
   - Provide physical comfort for the learner and a quiet atmosphere without interruption.
   - Establish objectives and goals for learning at the beginning of the session.
   - Assist the learner in integrating information into daily life. Allow learner to practice new skills. Allow patient to take their own medications and vital signs in the hospital.
   - Provide information using various mediums (e.g., explanations, discussions, demonstrations, pictures, written instructions, computer-assisted programs, and videotapes).
   - Encourage questions, and include significant others as often as possible. Document progress of teaching and learning.

Impaired oral mucous membranes *related to treatment with immunosuppressive medication*

GOALS/OUTCOMES Patient's oral mucosa, tongue, and lips are pink, intact, and free of exudate and lesions. Patient states that he or she can swallow without difficulty within 24 hours after treatment for altered oral mucous membrane.
NOC Oral Hygiene; Tissue Integrity: Skin and Mucous Membranes

Oral Health Restoration
1. Inspect the mouth daily for signs of exudate and lesions; consult physician if they are present. Teach patient to perform self-inspection of mouth.
2. Teach patient to brush with a soft-bristle toothbrush and nonabrasive toothpaste after meals and snacks.
3. To help prevent monilial infection, provide patient with mycostatin prophylactic mouthwash for "swish and swallow" after meals and at bedtime.

NOC Oral Health Maintenance; Oral Health Promotion

Impaired skin integrity (or risk for same): herpetic lesions, skin fungal rashes, pruritus, and capillary fragility *related to treatment with immunosuppressive medications*

GOALS/OUTCOMES Patient's skin is intact and free of open lesions or abrasions.
NOC Tissue Integrity: Skin and Mucous Membranes

Skin Surveillance
1. Assess for and document daily the presence of erythema, excoriation, rashes, or bruises on patient's skin.
2. Assess for and document the presence of rashes or lesions in the perineal area, inasmuch as herpetic lesions are common in the immunosuppressed patient.
3. Inspect the trunk area daily for the presence of flat, itchy rashes. Skin fungal rashes are common in the immunosuppressed patient.
4. Teach patient the importance of daily skin care with water, nondrying soap, and lubricating lotion.
5. Use nonallergenic tape when anchoring IV tubing, catheters, and dressings.
6. Assist patient with changing position at least every 2h; massage areas that are susceptible to breakdown, particularly areas over bony prominences.

NIC Pressure Ulcer Prevention. Additional, optional interventions include Bathing; Bleeding Precautions; Cutaneous Stimulation; Exercise Promotion and Therapy Electrolyte Monitoring; Exercise Promotion: Stretching; Fluid/Electrolyte Management; Infection Control; Infection Prevention; Medication Management; Nail Care; Nutrition Management; Perineal Care; Surveillance; and Vital Signs Monitoring.

Organ Transplantation

SYSTEMIC INFLAMMATORY RESPONSE SYNDROME (SIRS), SEPSIS, SEPTIC SHOCK, AND MULTIPLE ORGAN DYSFUNCTION SYNDROME (MODS)

PATHOPHYSIOLOGY

SIRS is a state of generalized, uncontrolled inflammation. Inflammation is a complex response initiated by mechanical, ischemic, chemical, or microbial sources. Signs of systemic inflammation such as fever and leukocytosis characterize SIRS. A patient with sepsis presents with at least two of the SIRS criteria: an abnormal body temperature, elevated HR and RR, and an altered WBC count as well as a suspected or proven source of infection. Sepsis with one or more organ dysfunctions is considered severe sepsis. Septic shock is severe sepsis with cardiovascular dysfunction (primary loss of vascular tone) that does not respond to fluid resuscitation.

Over the past 30 years, understanding the malignant, destructive, uncontrolled inflammatory and coagulation process has become the primary focus in the management of patients exhibiting signs and symptoms of severe sepsis that can ultimately result in MODS. The process leading from SIRS to MODS to organ failure is a continuum that often begins with the same event (Table 11-14). The SIRS initiates a process of relative hypovolemia. To the unsuspecting practitioner, the early signs of arterial hypoperfusion may be masked by the patient's near normal appearance resulting from compensatory vasoconstriction (maintaining BP). If SIRS and/or sepsis is managed aggressively in the early stages, studies reveal that the incidence of MODS is decreased. The American College of Chest Physicians (ACCP)/Society of Critical Care Medicine (SCCM) Consensus Conference first initiated one suggested approach to the identification of profound and uncontrolled inflammatory response in 1992. These guidelines have been modified and updated several times, with the most recent revisions reflected in the 2008 Surviving Sepsis Campaign International Guidelines (Table 11-15). Some of the more specific recognized signs and laboratory profiles are listed in Table 11-16.

The purpose of the inflammatory response is to protect the body from further injury and promote rapid healing. Vasodilation with increased microvascular permeability, neutrophil activation and adhesion, and enhanced coagulation initially occur in a balanced framework. The vascular response is initiated at the cellular level by histamine, prostaglandins, bradykinin, and numerous other mediators.

The term *sepsis* implies, to many practitioners, an infectious process that has facilitated a systemic inflammatory response (SIRS). Sepsis is typically not associated with a simple infection requiring antibiotic management to resolve without hospitalization. In addition to infection, sepsis is associated with multiple injuries in trauma patients and other patients with significant inflammation such as those with pancreatitis. Critically ill patients with sepsis resulting from infection are often not easily managed, with microorganisms that require considerable skill to control. Microorganisms commonly seen in the critically ill include gram-negative enteric pathogens (e.g., *Escherichia coli*, *Klebsiella* spp., *Enterobacter* spp., *Pseudomonas aeruginosa*), *Staphylococcus aureus*, coagulase-negative staphylococci, *Enterococcus* spp., and *Candida* spp. Antibiotic-resistant bacteria (e.g., methicillin-resistant *S. aureus* [MRSA]) are commonly seen.

Table 11-14	SYSTEMIC INFLAMMATORY RESPONSE SYNDROME (SIRS) If 2 or More of the Following are Present, the Patient Meets Criteria for SIRS:
1	Temperature >38°C or <36°C
2	Heart rate >90 beats/min
3	Respiratory rate >20 breaths/min or $Paco_2$ <32 mm Hg
4	White blood cell (WBC) >12,000 cells/mm³ or <4000 cells/mm³ or >10% immature (band) forms

Adapted from Levy MM, Fink MP, Marshall JC, et al: 2001 SCCM/ESICM/ACCP/ATS/SIS International Sepsis Definitions Conference. *Crit Care Med* 31:1250–1256, 2003.

Table 11-15   ASSESSMENT FINDINGS FOR THE PATIENT WITH SEPSIS IN THE EARLY HYPERDYNAMIC STAGE

Clinical indicator	Cause
Cardiovascular	
Increased HR (>100 beats/min)	Sympathetic/autonomic nervous system (SANS) stimulation
Decreased BP (<90 mm Hg systolic, MAP <65 mm Hg)	Vasodilation
CO >7 L/min; CI >4 L/min/ m², CVP <8 mm Hg	Hyperdynamic state secondary to SANS stimulation
SvO_2 >80%	Decreased utilization of oxygen by cells
PAWP usually <6 mm Hg	Venous dilation; decreased preload
SVR <900 dynes/sec/cm^{-5}	Vasodilation
Strong, bounding peripheral pulses	Hyperdynamic cardiovascular system (Keeping in mind that patients with preexisting cardiomyopathy will have minimal elevation in cardiac output and drop in SVR)
Respiratory	
Tachypnea (>20 breaths/min) and hyperventilation	Metabolic acidosis which leads to decreases in cerebrospinal fluid pH that stimulate the central respiratory center
Crackles	Interstitial edema occurring with increased vascular permeability
$PaCO_2$ <35 mm Hg	Tachypnea and hyperventilation
Dyspnea	Increased respiratory muscle work
Renal	
Decreased urine output (<0.5 ml/kg/hr)	Decreased renal perfusion
Increased specific gravity (1.025–1.035)	Decreased glomerular filtration rate
Cutaneous	
Flushed and warm skin	Vasodilation
Metabolic	
Increasing body temperature (usually >38.3°C [100.9°F])	Increased metabolic activity; release of pyrogens secondary to invading microorganisms; release of interleukin-l by macrophages
pH <7.35 Lactic acid >2.5	Metabolic acidosis occurring with accumulation of lactic acid
↑ Blood sugar or at times profound hypoglycemia	Release of glucagon; insulin resistance
Neurologic	
Changes in LOC	Decreased cerebral perfusion and brain hypoxia
Fluid	
↑ Fluid retention	↑ ADH, ↑ aldosterone

ADH, Antidiuretic hormone; *beats/min,* beats per minute; *BP,* blood pressure; *CO,* cardiac output; *CI,* cardiac index; *HR,* heart rate; *LOC,* level of consciousness; *PAWP,* pulmonary artery wedge pressure; *SVR,* systemic vascular resistance.

SIRS, Sepsis, and MODS

Table 11-16 ASSESSMENT FINDINGS FOR THE PATIENT WITH SEPSIS IN THE LATE STAGE

Clinical Indicator	Cause
Cardiovascular	
Extreme tachycardia with S_3 sound, sinus arrhythmia and atrial fibrillation with rapid ventricular response	Compensatory attempt by sympathetic nervous system to maintain CO
Profound hypotension	Decreased stroke volume. Diastolic BP may remain high because of vasoconstriction
CO <4 L/min; CI <2.5 L/min/m²	Failure of compensatory mechanisms
PAWP usually >12 mm Hg	Increased left ventricular end-diastolic pressure (LVEDP) because of increased residual volume from decreased stroke volume
SVR >1200 dynes/sec/cm^{-5}	Vasoconstriction
Weak or absent peripheral pulses	Decreased peripheral perfusion because of decreased CO
Svo_2 <60%	Decreased oxygen binding to hemoglobin because of acidosis
Respiratory	
Increased >30 breath/min (even at late stage) or decreased respiratory rate <12 breaths/min	Metabolic acidosis and acute lung injury lead to tachypnea, whereas central respiratory center depression can cause hypopnea
Decreased respiratory rate (<12 breaths/min) and depth	Central respiratory center depression
Crackles, rhonchi, wheezes	Accumulation of lung secretions
Increased Fio_2 required to maintain Pao_2 (possible ARDS)	Ventilation/perfusion mismatch and decreased lung compliance
Renal	
Decreased urine output progressing to anuria	Decreased renal perfusion and tubular ischemia
Low urinary excretion of sodium, with possibly decreased fractional excretion of sodium; if patient develops acute tubular necrosis, sodium excretion typically increases	Activation of the aldosterone mechanism and release of ADH, which stimulate sodium and water retention
Cutaneous	
Cool, pale skin or cyanosis	Sustained vasoconstriction
Neurologic	
Decreased LOC, coma	Severe hypoxia and metabolic derangements leading to reversible encephalopathy.
Hematologic	
Oozing from previous venipuncture sites	Development of DIC caused by stimulation of coagulation process, and fibrinolysis
Acid-Base Status	
pH <7.35; $PaCO_2$ >45 mm Hg; HCO_3^- <22 mEq/L (or less than expected)	Mixed acid-base disorder: respiratory acidosis and metabolic acidosis

ARDS, Acute respiratory distress syndrome; *ADH*, antidiuretic hormone; *CI*, cardiac index; *CO*, cardiac output; *DIC*, disseminated intravascular coagulation; *LOC*, level of consciousness; *PAWP*, pulmonary artery wedge pressure; *SVR*, systemic vascular resistance.

In some cases, regulatory mechanisms fail and uncontrolled systemic inflammation overwhelms the body's normal protective response. This leads to systemic vasodilation, arterial hypotension, a generalized increase in vascular permeability, extravascular fluid sequestration, increased hematologic cellular aggregation with microvascular obstruction, which greatly accelerates consumption of coagulation products. The process is now considered to be severe sepsis.

Severe sepsis is the compounding of sepsis by comorbid conditions, wherein the inflammatory response to a nidus of infection or inflammation is fulminating and out of control. A new view of severe sepsis is evolving. Severe sepsis has recently been viewed as endothelial dysfunction resulting from overwhelming inflammatory mediation, in conjunction with profound, unopposed coagulation. The capillary vasculature sustains a significant injury by a cascade of events that ends in capillary occlusion. The more massive the occlusion, the greater is the potential for organ failure, as cellular level circulation requires a functional capillary network for delivery of oxygen and nutrients and removal of cellular metabolic waste products. When infection or other injury prompts an initially widespread inflammatory response, or SIRS, the normally smooth surface of microvascular (capillary) endothelium is roughened or damaged by the response. Release of inflammatory mediators prompts vasodilation with increased capillary permeability. Microscopically, the endothelium resembles a road riddled with tiny "potholes." Systemic mediators are released to facilitate healing of the endothelium, which is aimed at "filling the tiny potholes." The four main factors associated with severe sepsis that may evolve to septic shock are hyperinflammation, hypercoagulation, microvascular obstruction, and increased endothelial permeability.

Because endothelial damage is generalized, the extensive or hyperinflammatory response leads to accelerated formation of microclots on the non–smooth capillary endothelium, consuming platelets and inhibiting clot lysis (fibrinolysis). This progresses to uncontrolled alterations in the vascular tone with vasodilation in the large vessels (where BP is measured). Both vasodilation and constriction occur in capillaries, where oxygen delivery takes place. Stimulated by products of antigen ingestion, activated neutrophils and other humoral mediators combine, activate, and potentiate an ongoing vascular endothelial injury with a concomitant proinflammatory, procoagulating, antifibrinolytic response. Among other mediators, an increased presence of tissue factor (TF) persistently stimulates thrombin, which ultimately increases fibrinogen conversion to fibrin and promotes platelet aggregation. Coupled with microvascular clotting, the process limits oxygen delivery and may lead to organ ischemia. Unopposed, this process may lead to a profound consumptive coagulopathy (DIC), diminished distal blood flow, and cell death by activated cellular suicide (apoptosis). The blood flow necessary to maintain tissue oxygenation and aerobic metabolism, nutrient transfer, and metabolic waste removal is profoundly threatened.

Excessive thrombin production and a secondary decrease in endothelial production of plasminogen activator, thrombomodulin, protein C, and, ultimately, activated protein C, illustrate the overwhelming response that separates simple infection from severe sepsis. The endothelial regulation of appropriate blood flow requires a balance of vasodilators (i.e., nitric oxide) and vasoconstrictors (e.g., endothelin). In severe sepsis, when the balance cannot be maintained, the corresponding maldistribution of blood flow and loss of vascular tone at the macrovascular and microvascular levels result in both ischemia and hyperemia in the cells supplied by the same capillary beds. In addition, myocardial depressant factor is released and may contribute to the loss of the compensatory CO, which is required to keep blood moving through the vascular beds.

Severe sepsis accompanied by hypotension that does not respond to volume infusion is called *septic shock*. Impaired perfusion may cause lactic acidosis, oliguria, or acute alterations in mental status. Genetic predisposition and other factors compound severe sepsis, leading to MODS as well as multiple organ failure (MOF) and may be fatal. MODS is diagnosed when two or more vital organ systems become dysfunctional.

ASSESSMENT: SIRS, SEPSIS, SEVERE SEPSIS, SEPTIC SHOCK AND MODS
Goal of System Assessment
Evaluate for hypermetabolism, progressive tissue hypoxia, and prevention of organ dysfunction.

History and Risk Factors

- Multiple presentations to emergency department or physician's office for the same complaint
- Infection, sequential infections, any indwelling catheters, malnutrition, immunosuppression, bone marrow suppression, advanced age (more than 65 years old), infants
- Recent traumatic injuries, or surgical or invasive procedures; presence of intravascular devices or artificial joints
- Chronic health problems (e.g., liver or renal disease, diabetes mellitus, rheumatic heart disease)
- Underlying diseases or conditions such as splenectomy, IV substance abuse

Vital Signs

- Patients may present with tachycardia, tachypnea, hyperthermia or hypothermia, and hyperglycemia or hypoglycemia. Hypoglycemia is being increasingly recognized and is thought to be related to depletion of glycogen stores, increased cellular glucose utilization, and/or impaired gluconeogenesis. Criteria for diagnosis of sepsis are evolving.
- *SIRS:* In 2003, Levy and colleagues revised the 1992 ACCP/SCCM guidelines to reflect that the diagnosis of SIRS was based on the presence of two or more of the following: tachypnea (RR greater than 20 breaths/min), hypocarbia (less than 32 mm Hg), tachycardia (HR greater than 90 bpm), temperature greater than 38°C (100.4°F) or less than 36°C (96.8°F), WBC count greater than 12,000/mm³ or less than 4000/mm³, or greater than 10% immature (band) forms. Older adults may manifest normal or slightly decreased temperature.
- *Sepsis:* In 2004, the SCCM developed the following definition of sepsis—A documented or suspected infection with some of the following: fever, hypothermia, HR greater than 90 or more than 2 standard deviations (SDs) above the normal for age, tachypnea, altered mental status, hyperglycemia greater than 120 mg/dl in absence of diabetes, leukocytosis, leukopenia, normal WBC count with greater than 10% immature forms (bands), plasma C-reactive protein level more than 2 SDs above normal, and decreased protein C level (see Tables 11-15 and 11-16).
  1. *Hemodynamic measurements:* The hemodynamic presentation varies with fluid balance and cardiac function of the patient. The Scvo₂ (reflecting tissue use of oxygen) in early stages may be low to normal. Serum lactate levels in conjunction should measure adequacy of tissue oxygenation with methods of monitoring central or local hemoglobin saturation to determine the degree of anaerobic metabolism present and the effects of resuscitation. Lactate is produced when poor circulation and oxygenation prompt cells to initiate anaerobic metabolism. Placement of a central catheter to measure both pressures on ventricular filling, as well as the saturation of hemoglobin after blood has passed the capillaries, may be an important component of monitoring for these patients.
  2. *Tissue metabolic dysfunction:* Use of Svo₂ and/or Scvo₂
     - Scvo₂ (obtained by measuring a blood sample in the right atrium). Levels are generally about 5% to 13% higher than Svo₂ levels.
     - Threats to tissue oxygenation occur, such as a decrease in blood flow from hypovolemia or low CO (relative to tissue demand). The compensatory mechanism is to release more oxygen from hemoglobin (shift to right), which reflects a lower than normal measured Scvo₂.
     - In early sepsis, the lower the Scvo₂, the more the tissue viability may be at risk. As sepsis progresses, elevated Scvo₂ may reflect inability of tissues to utilize oxygen. As sepsis evolves to severe sepsis and septic shock, Scvo₂ levels do not fall, but rather increase. Return of Scvo₂ to normal may indicate improvement of blood flow, but in late sepsis it may also indicate that shunting is worsening due to vasopressors, microvascular occlusion and obstruction, and other issues interfering with oxygen utilization. The pathologic increase in measured Scvo₂ occurs frequently in septic shock. Differentiation from improving status is vital.
       - Lactate level should be reviewed to assess progress, as increases in Scvo₂ are not always indicative of improvement.
     - *Severe sepsis, septic shock, and MODS:* Terminal heart failure, with decreasing HR and BP, pump failure exhibited by a significant drop in BP, a narrowing of the pulse pressure, and an increase in filling pressures. This often presents with a

normal to high (60% to 80%) Scvo$_2$ and a decrease in tissue oxygenation (Sto$_2$) related to failure of the tissues to uptake and utilize oxygen. Although not widely available, Sto$_2$ is the most accurate reflection of true localized tissue oxygenation. Occlusion of the capillaries (microcirculation) limits oxygen utilization at the cellular level, causing failure of the hemoglobin to release oxygen even though the oxygen is desperately needed (evidenced by the presence of worsening metabolic acidosis and increasing Scvo$_2$).

Observation and Other Assessment Findings

- *Early signs reflective of SIRS and sepsis:* Anxiety, continuous agitation, discomfort in excess of condition. Vasodilation may create a "healthy" flushed appearance of the skin, which may be warm or hot to touch.
- *Signs of severe sepsis, septic shock, and MODS:* Flushed skin that changes to pallor; edema of face, neck, torso, sacrum, and extremities; deteriorating LOC with possible obtundation or unresponsiveness as cerebral perfusion is failing; rales caused by heart failure; respiratory failure requiring endotracheal intubation and mechanical ventilation; oliguria; diminished bowel sounds; and diminished peripheral pulses. Vasodilation may maintain warm to hot skin ("warm shock") until patient totally decompensates with cool to cold, clammy skin ("cold shock").

Diagnostic Tests for SIRS, Sepsis, Severe Sepsis, Septic Shock and MODS

The diagnosis of the various stages of the continuum of sepsis is based on signs and symptoms, testing for causes of infection, degree of perfusion deficit associated with shock and presence of organ failure. Treatment should be initiated before laboratory results are available.

Test	Purpose	Abnormal Findings
Complete blood count (CBC) with WBC differential	WBC differential evaluates the strength of the immune system's response to the trigger of response and whether infection may be present.	*WBC Differential:* White blood cell count may be normal, elevated, or decreased. The presence of >10% of bands indicates an inflammatory response. *Hematocrit (Hct):* May be increased from hypovolemia and hemoconcentration.
Blood cultures and antibiotic sensitivity testing of isolates	To identify if a microorganism has moved into the bloodstream to cause a systemic infection, and if so, which antibiotics will be most effective to eradicate the organism.	Possible presence of an organism; Approximately one third of patients with sepsis do not have an identified organism present in the bloodstream.
Culture and antibiotic sensitivity testing of suspect infection sites (e.g., urine, sputum, blood, intravenous [IV] lines, incisions)	To identify the original source of the infection.	Results are correlated with blood cultures to validate where the systemic infection causing a massive inflammatory response originated.
Arterial blood gas analysis (ABG)	Assess for abnormal gas exchange or compensation for metabolic derangements. Initially Pao$_2$ is normal and then decreases as the ventilation-perfusion mismatch becomes more severe.	*pH changes:* Acidosis may reflect respiratory failure; alkalosis may reflect compensatory tachypnea seen in early stages. *Carbon dioxide:* Elevated CO$_2$ reflects respiratory failure; decreased CO$_2$ reflects tachypnea; rising Pco$_2$ is an ominous sign, since it signals severe hypoventilation which can lead to respiratory arrest. *Hypoxemia:* Pao$_2$ <80 mm Hg Oxygen saturation: Sao$_2$ < 92%

SIRS, Sepsis, and MODS

Continued

Diagnostic Tests for SIRS, Sepsis, Severe Sepsis, Septic Shock and MODS—cont'd

Serum lactate level	Assesses for degree of anaerobic metabolism present. Anaerobic metabolism ensues when capillary beds are unable to effectively perfuse tissues and organs.	Increases to >4 mmol/L indicate the presence of significant capillary occlusion. Normal is <2 mmol/L
Blood chemistry or biochemical profile	To screen for changes associated with the stress response. In stress states (e.g., infection, trauma, hypoxia), hormones are released to increase generation of additional glucose from nonglucose products (gluconeogenesis) and create insulin resistance.	Hyperglycemia is common but may improve as the liver fails, since the liver has a key role in gluconeogenesis. If catecholamines (e.g., norepinephrine, phenylephrine) are given to increase blood pressure, this may prolong hyperglycemia, since catecholamines create insulin resistance.
Clotting studies	Assesses for presence of activation of the clotting cascade and for consumptive coagulopathy such as DIC.	If clotting cascade is activated, reflects decreased platelets (>50% drop over 3 days is an indicator of severe sepsis), increased prothrombin time (PT), increased partial thromboplastin time (PTT), increased international normalized ratio (INR), and increased fibrin split products.
Radiographs	Chest radiograph to check for pneumonia or acute respiratory distress syndrome (ARDS) prior to computed tomography (CT) scanning of the lung. Other radiographs are done to assess underlying condition.	Positive findings helps to either detect the source of infection or inflammation, and the presence of MODS.
Computed tomography (CT)	Lung CT is more reflective of changes in the pulmonary microcirculation, and most accurately depicts extravascular lung water. Also used to assess for abnormalities such as intra-abdominal abscess or perforated viscus.	Positive findings helps to either detect the source of infection or inflammation, and the presence of MODS.
12-Lead ECG	To detect dysrhythmias reflective of myocardial ischemia	Ischemic changes (ST depression) may be present as shock progresses
Biomarkers of sepsis	Presence of various levels of >100 distinct molecules have been suggested to be helpful in the diagnosis of sepsis. Biomarkers are used as part of screening, diagnosis, risk stratification and evaluating the response to therapy.	The ability to use a biomarker varies with each patient, and with the stage of the sepsis syndrome during which the value was drawn. There are no universally accepted biomarkers, but the more commonly recognized mediators include tumor necrosis factor (TNF), interleukin 6 (IL-6), procalcitonin (PCT) and presence of various endotoxins from gram-negative bacteria.

RESEARCH BRIEF 11-2

A select group of expert researchers convened to develop a methodology for identification and validation of the significance of the overwhelming number of biomarkers suggested to be pertinent to the diagnosis of sepsis. The group identified the need for standardization of biomarker methodologies, more extensive integration of biomarkers into clinical studies, especially in helping to assess the presence of various markers in early sepsis, need for increased rigor in studies, and development of consistent collaboration among investigators, regulatory agencies, and both the pharmaceutical and biomarker industries. The study concluded biomarkers had the potential to transform sepsis from a physiologic syndrome to a group of separate disorders with goal-directed therapy for each; thus improving the prognosis for patients with all types of sepsis.

Marshall JC, Reinhart K, for the International Sepsis Forum: Biomarkers of sepsis. *Crit Care Med* 37(7):2290-2298, 2009.

COLLABORATIVE MANAGEMENT
Care Priorities

1. **Manage hypovolemia with IV isotonic fluids.** IV volume expansion is implemented to maintain adequate ventricular filling pressures and volume, which are compromised with increased capillary permeability and vasodilation. Crystalloid solution such as lactated Ringer or normal saline can be used. Although colloids (albumin and fresh-frozen plasma) have also been used, there is no benefit to such an approach. Current guidelines recommend use of packed RBC transfusion and dobutamine drip if Svo_2 remains less than 70% after initial fluid resuscitation.

2. **Manage the infection immediately.** *Antibiotics should be administered within 1 hour of patient presenting with severe sepsis or septic shock.* Every effort should be made to draw blood cultures prior to antibiotic administration

3. **Use early goal-directed therapy to prevent or slow patient progression to MODS and MOF.** Treatment should be done in accordance with the following sepsis bundles (www.ihi.org/sepsis). According to current ACCP/SCCM guidelines, the following are points of early goal-directed therapy:
   - Immediate fluid resuscitation should be performed if not already done. The goal is to infuse no less than 1 L, or 20 ml/kg, via fluid bolus if tolerated. The rate of fluid infusion should be reduced if filling pressures rise without improvement in overall circulation.
   - All blood for labwork for sepsis profile should be drawn (serum lactate, blood culture, biomedical profile, CBC with differential, coagulation profile, biomarkers such as presence of tumor necrosis factor [TNF], IL-6, or procalcitonin [PCT] if available) and then repeated every 2 to 4 hours initially to assess for progress.
   - Antibiotics should be administered within 1 hour of patient presenting with severe sepsis or septic shock.
   - Place oximetry capable central line or PICC line and obtain CVP and $Scvo_2$ or PA pressures and Svo_2 if BP is unresponsive to fluids and/or serum lactate is elevated > 4 mg/dl.
   - Vasopressors are administered for MAP less than 65 mm Hg during fluid resuscitation and after adequate fluid resuscitation.
   - Inotropes and/or packed RBCs (when appropriate) are used for central venous oxygen saturation less than 70% after fluid replacement.
   - Increase myocardial contractility using positive inotropic drugs (e.g., dopamine, dobutamine, epinephrine): May be given to augment cardiac contractility and CO. In the late stages of sepsis, positive inotropic drugs may be given with vasodilators such as nitroprusside and nitroglycerin, which decrease preload and afterload by dilating veins and arteries, to assist in the management of terminal heart failure. Given there is both vasodilation and vasoconstriction present throughout the circulation, it is

difficult to predict the most effective strategy for support of circulation. Some institutions may attempt noncatecholamine inodilator medications such as milrinone to provide inotropic support as well as decreasing resistance to ventricular ejection.

- Early resuscitation must be completed within 6 hours of the diagnosis of sepsis, severe sepsis, and septic shock.

4. **If early resuscitation fails, or the patient presents in septic shock or MODS, the second group of therapies is instituted in conjunction with or immediately following early goal-directed therapy.**

Support ventilation and oxygenation if patient develops acute lung injury (ALI) or ARDS. Mechanical ventilation: Intubate and place on low tidal volume, pressure-controlled ventilation if high-flow oxygen or noninvasive positive pressure ventilation fails to stabilize ventilation. If on volume control ventilation, plateau pressure (p_{Plat}) should be on average less than 30 cm H_2O for ventilated patients. Lung protective ventilation with low tidal volume (6 to 8 ml/kg of ideal body weight) is recommended. Assist control volume- or pressure-controlled ventilation may be initiated (see *Mechanical Ventilation*, p. 99).

Maintain the Blood Pressure. Vasopressors (e.g., dopamine, norepinephrine): May be administered in cases when optimal left ventricular preload fails to restore adequate tissue perfusion (i.e., the initial MAP is very low or MAP is persistently less than 60 mm Hg). If dopamine and epinephrine are ineffective, phenylephrine, vasopressin, and high-dose epinephrine may be used. The goal of therapy is to optimize CI through providing a balance of promoting venous return, augmenting cardiac contractility, and creating the ideal level of resistance to ventricular ejection.

Consider corticosteroids. In stress situations, the normal adrenal gland output of cortisol is approximately 250 to 300 mg over 24 hours. Use of corticosteroids remains controversial. IV hydrocortisone should be given only to adult septic shock patients after it has been confirmed that their BP is poorly responsive to fluid resuscitation and vasopressor therapy and cortisol levels are low. Most important, all patients on chronic steroid replacements such as those with rheumatoid arthritis on daily prednisone have to receive high doses of IV steroids while in shock. Corticosteroids also help to control inflammation (see *Acute Adrenal Insuffficiency (Adrenal Crisis)*, p. 696).

- Administer 100 mg of hydrocortisone in 100 ml of isotonic sodium chloride solution by continuous IV infusion at a rate of 10 to 12 ml/hr. Infusion may be initiated with 100 mg of hydrocortisone as an IV bolus.
- An alternative method of hydrocortisone administration is 50 mg as an IV bolus every 6 hours.
- The infusion method maintains plasma cortisol levels more adequately at steady stress levels, especially in the small percentage of patients who are rapid metabolizers and who may have low plasma cortisol levels between the IV boluses.

Treat the Problems. Provide antibiotics to control infection: Broad-spectrum antibiotic coverage for sepsis (often directed at gram-negative sepsis) should be initiated prior to identifying a specific microorganism if patients exhibit physiologic changes and positive signs and symptoms. Cultures should be obtained prior to initiating antibiotics unless doing so would considerably delay treatment. Obtain at least two blood cultures, one percutaneously and another through invasive IV lines that have been in place more than 48 hours prior to antibiotic administration. Timely administration of appropriate antibiotics is critical to patient outcome. Choice of antimicrobial depends on the organ and organisms involved. Physicians and midlevel practitioners will prescribe ceftriaxone and zithromycin or levofloxacin for severe community-acquired pneumonia, whereas health care–acquired pneumonia may need to be treated with broader-spectrum antibiotics that cover drug-resistant pathogens. Such antibiotics may include ceftazidime, meropenem, vancomycin, and aminoglycosides. The effectiveness of the antibiotics should be reevaluated daily and use should be anticipated for 7 to 10 days. Use of the fewest possible antibiotics reduces the possibility of development of a superinfection with an opportunistic organism including fungus (*Candida*), infection with a resistant organism (MRSA, VRE) or development of *Clostridium difficile* ("C. diff")–associated diarrhea (CDAD). Treatment of infection helps control the inflammatory response.

Control the source of the infection: Other methods for controlling the source of infection should be weighed carefully for risks and benefits. Identifying the source of infection is as critical. Localizing and draining an abscess or removing new pleural fluid collections and discontinuing infected indwelling catheters are keys to improved mortality.

Other pharmaceutical agents: For many years, researchers and clinicians have been looking for a miracle medication that will stop the vicious cycle of events that occurs in severe sepsis and leads to MODS. Unfortunately, many of the medications only affected one of many major cascades, such as the anti-TNF medications. Recombinant human activated protein C (Xigris™) has been shown to reduce mortality in patients with an APACHE II score greater than 25 or those who are at high risk of dying from sepsis. It is not recommended for patients with an APACHE score less than 20. Absolute contraindications are related to the high risk of bleeding.

Control blood glucose: Use IV insulin therapy to keep blood glucose below 180 mg/dl, with a target of 150 mg/dl. Use of intensive insulin therapy to lower blood glucose to 80 to 110 mg/dl is no longer recommended, as septic shock patients often become hypoglycemic. (See *Hyperglycemia,* p. 711.)

Provide nutritional support: Current SCCM recommendations for enteral feedings/nutritional support in the critically ill include short- and medium-chain fatty acids and branched-chain amino acids administered to stop protein catabolism. The short- and medium-chain fatty acids are absorbed more readily and metabolized more easily than long-chain fatty acids. They may be given orally (e.g., MCT Oil, which is a proprietary name for triglycerides of medium-chain fatty acids), as part of enteral feeding, or via the IV route (e.g., intralipid solutions). Branched-chain amino acid solutions are used in sepsis, as they are metabolized by muscle rather than the liver and can therefore be used in the presence of organ failure. (See *Nutritional Support,* p. 117.)

CARE PLANS FOR SIRS, SEPSIS, AND MODS

Deficient fluid volume   *related to active loss from vascular compartment secondary to increased capillary permeability and shift of intravascular volume into interstitial spaces and relative hypovolemia resulting from vasodilation*

GOALS/OUTCOMES Within 4 hours of initiation of therapy, patient is normovolemic as evidenced by peripheral pulses greater than 2+ on a 0 to 4+ scale, stable body weight, urine output 0.5 ml/kg/hr or greater, mean BP 60 mm Hg or greater (or within patient's normal range), sustained systolic BP 90 mm Hg or greater or within patient's normal range, and absence of edema and adventitious lung sounds. CVP is 2 to 6 mm Hg (add 3 mm Hg to normal if patient is on positive pressure ventilation), PAWP is 6 to 12 mm Hg, CO is 4 to 7 L/min, SVI is 30 to 40 ml/min /m3, SVV is less than 15% and calculated SVR is 900 to 1200 dynes/sec/cm^{-5}.

NOC Fluid Balance; Electrolyte and Acid-Base Balance

Hemodynamic Regulation

1. Monitor hemodynamic pressures, using noninvasive or invasive methods to assess CO, stroke volume index (SVI) and stroke volume variation (SVV) if available. If a pulmonary artery catheter is used, PAWP, CO, and SVR are measured. During the early stage of sepsis, filling pressures (PAWP and CVP) may be normal to low, but as biventricular dysfunction occurs, these pressures may increase. If the patient manifests a compensatory increase in CO, the calculated SVR may initially be low, but the calculated value may rise as the CO drops.

2. Initiate early goal-directed therapy to support the CO and BP as prescribed, including IV fluids, positive inotropic agents. Vasopressors are used if inotropic agents and fluid resuscitation fail to stabilize the BP (see *Collaborative Management,* p. 932). Fluid replacement therapy is given to maintain a CVP of 2 to 6 mm Hg or PAWP of 6 to 12 mm Hg. Assess CVP and/or PAWP and lung sounds at frequent intervals during fluid replacement to detect evidence of fluid overload: crackles, wheezing, and increasing CVP and/or PAWP.

3. Assess fluid volume by monitoring BP, peripheral pulses, and urine output hourly. Report failure of early goal-directed therapy to stabilize mean BP to greater than 60 mm Hg or sustained systolic BP to 90 mm Hg or greater or within patient's normal range. Weigh patient daily; monitor I&O every shift, noting 24-hour trends. Report urine output less than 0.5 ml/kg/hr. The patient's weight may actually increase with fluid volume deficit because of a shift of intravascular volume into interstitial spaces.

4. Assess for interstitial edema as evidenced by pretibial, sacral, ankle, and hand edema, as well as crackles on auscultation of lung fields.

5. Position patient supine with the legs elevated to increase venous return and preload.

NIC Fluid/Electrolyte Management; Hypovolemia Management; Fluid Management; Shock Management: Volume

Decreased cardiac output *related to negative inotropic changes in the heart (late stage) secondary to effects of tissue hypoxia, worsening during late septic shock*

GOALS/OUTCOMES Within 8 hours of initiation of therapy, patient has improved CO as evidenced by peripheral pulses greater than 2+ on a 0 to 4+ scale, stable body weight, urine output 0.5 ml/kg/hr or greater, mean BP 60 mm Hg or greater (or within patient's normal range) sustained systolic BP 90 mm Hg or greater or within patient's normal range, and absence of edema and adventitious lung sounds. CVP is 2 to 6 mm Hg (add 3 mm Hg to normal if patient is on positive pressure ventilation), PAWP is 6 to 12 mm Hg, CO is 4 to 7 L/min, CI greater than 2.5 L/min/m^2, calculated SVR is 900 to 1200 dynes/sec/cm^{-5}. SVI is 30 to 40 ml/min/m$_3$, SW is less than 15% and Scvo$_2$ or Svo$_2$ 60% to 80%.
NOC Cardiac Pump Effectiveness; Circulation Status

Cardiac Care: Acute
1. Assess patient for signs of decreased CO: decreasing BP, increasing HR, decreasing amplitude of peripheral pulses, restlessness, decreasing urinary output, and increasing PAWP.
2. Administer positive inotropic agents (e.g., dobutamine) as prescribed to augment cardiac contractility.
3. If continuous or intermittent CO monitoring is not in place, assess CVP at least every 4 hours. Observe for development of premature ventricular complexes (PVCs), which may occur with hypoxia, and extreme tachycardia. Dysrhythmias and hypoxia may further reduce CO.
4. Monitor Scvo$_2$ or Svo$_2$ continuously; report values outside of normal range.

NIC Hemodynamic Regulation; Invasive Hemodynamic Monitoring; Fluid/Electrolyte Management

Ineffective tissue perfusion: cerebral, renal, and gastrointestinal *related to hypovolemia secondary to mixed vasodilation and constriction interruption of arterial and venous blood flow secondary to vasoconstriction and thrombus obstruction*

GOALS/OUTCOMES Within 24 hours of initiating therapy, patient has improved perfusion as evidenced by orientation to time, place, and person; peripheral pulses greater than 2+ on a 0 to 4+ scale, stable body weight, urine output 0.5 ml/kg/hr or greater, mean BP 60 mm Hg or greater (or within patient's normal range) sustained systolic BP 90 mm Hg or greater or within patient's normal range, and absence of edema and adventitious lung sounds. CVP is 2 to 6 mm Hg (add 3 mm Hg to normal if patient is on positive pressure ventilation), PAWP is 6 to 12 mm Hg, CO is 4 to 7 L/min, CI greater than 2.5 L/min/m^2, calculated SVR is 900 to 1200 dynes/sec/cm^{-5}. SVI is 30 to 40 ml/min/m^3, SVV is less than 15% and Scvo$_2$ or Svo$_2$ 60% to 80%.
NOC Circulation Status

Circulatory Precautions
1. Assess for changes in LOC as an indicator of decreasing cerebral perfusion.
2. Assess for the following signs of decreasing renal perfusion: urine output less than 0.5 ml/kg/hr and increased BUN, serum creatinine, and serum potassium levels.
   - Monitor arterial BP continuously for signs of deteriorating circulatory status related to cardiac failure or hypovolemia. Systolic BP will be decreased because of decreased CO, and the diastolic BP may be low secondary to vasodilation or normal to high secondary to compensatory vasoconstriction.
   - Assess peripheral pulses, temperature, color of skin, and capillary refill. With hypoperfusion, pulse amplitude decreases, extremities are cool because of vasoconstriction, skin color is pale or mottled because of decreased perfusion, and capillary refill is delayed.
3. Monitor cellular oxygen consumption (Vo$_2$) as an indicator of tissue perfusion. With sepsis, cellular oxygen delivery is decreased (precapillary vasoconstriction), and thus cellular oxygen use is decreased. Mixed venous blood oxygen saturation (Svo$_2$) is elevated.
4. Administer vasoactive drugs as prescribed. CVP monitoring using a centrally placed central line or peripherally inserted line is a good alternative. The goal range is CVP of 2 to 6 mm Hg (add 3 mm Hg when positive pressure ventilation is utilized). Pulmonary artery catheters are associated with high risk and are not used as often for management of septic patients. When in place, SVR and CO can be assessed to determine the drug effects. Optimally, SVR will increase to at least 900 dynes/sec/cm^{-5}, CO will be 4 to 7 L/min, and CI will be 2.5 to 4 L/min/m^2. Fluid boluses are administered rapidly to obtain the goal.
5. Assess for evidence of decreasing splanchnic (visceral) circulation, including decreased or absent bowel sounds, elevated serum amylase level, and decreased platelet count.

NIC Cerebral Perfusion Promotion; Circulatory Care; Fluid/Electrolyte Management; Oxygen Therapy; Hemodynamic Regulation; Shock Management; Nutrition Management; Hemodialysis Therapy

Impaired gas exchange *related to alveolar-capillary membrane changes secondary to interstitial edema, alveolar destruction, and endotoxin release with activation of histamine and kinins*

GOALS/OUTCOMES Within 4 hours of initiation of therapy, patient's Pao_2 is greater than 80 mm Hg, $Paco_2$ is less than 45 mm Hg, pH is 7.35 to 7.45, and the lungs are clear.
NIC Respiratory Status: Gas Exchange; Electrolyte and Acid-Base Balance

Ventilation Assistance
1. Assess for and maintain a patent airway by assisting patient with coughing or by suctioning the trachea as necessary.
2. Assess all ABG values. Be alert to decreasing Pao_2, increasing $Paco_2$, and acidosis (decreasing pH). Monitor patient for the presence of dyspnea, hypopnea, and restlessness.
3. Listen to breath sounds hourly and with each change in patient condition. The presence of crackles may indicate fluid accumulation.
4. If patient exhibits evidence of inadequate gas exchange (e.g., Pao_2 less than 60 mm Hg while patient is on 100% oxygen via nonrebreather mask) but mental status remains stable, attempt noninvasive positive pressure ventilation (NPPV). If NPPV fails, prepare for the probability of endotracheal intubation.
5. If patient has been placed on mechanical ventilation, monitor inspiratory peak and plateau pressures for increasing trends, which may signal decreasing compliance and development of ARDS. As ARDS develops, an increasing Fio_2 (at least 0.50) and increasing levels of PEEP are required to maintain adequate Pao_2 (at least 60 mm Hg) (see *Acute Lung Injury and Acute Respiratory Distress Syndrome*, p. 365, and *Mechanical Ventilation*, p. 99).
6. Monitor end-tidal CO_2 trends for changes indicative of development of ARDS, hypoperfusion, and misplacement of the endotracheal tube.
7. Turn patient every 2 hours to maintain optimal ventilation-perfusion ratios and to prevent atelectasis.

NIC Acid-Base Management: Metabolic Acidosis; Oxygen Therapy; Respiratory Monitoring; Artificial Airway Management; Invasive Hemodynamic Regulation

Ineffective breathing pattern *related to decreased lung expansion secondary to central respiratory depression occurring in late shock*

GOALS/OUTCOMES Within 2 hours of initiating respiratory support, patient has an effective breathing pattern as evidenced by normal limits of inspiratory-expiratory ratio (1:1 to 1:2); tidal volume (at least 6 ml/kg); and maximal inspiratory pressures (less than 20 cm H_2O).
NOC Respiratory Status: Ventilation

Respiratory Monitoring
1. Monitor for decreasing respiratory rate, depth, and air movement. Ensure that patient demonstrates adequate air movement by noting presence of breath sounds over all lung fields.
2. Assist patient into a comfortable position to facilitate respirations. Depending on patient's hemodynamic stability, the optimal position may be a 15- to 30-degree head of the bed elevation.
3. Assess/measure tidal volume and inspiratory force. Be alert to tidal volume less than 4 ml/kg and inspiratory force less than 20 cm H_2O as indicators of an ineffective breathing pattern.
4. If patient exhibits respiratory depression/ineffective breathing pattern, prepare for the probability of endotracheal intubation. (See *Acute Respiratory Failure*, p. 383.)

NIC Oxygen Therapy; Mechanical Ventilation

Ineffective thermoregulation *related to illness with concomitant endotoxin effect on hypothalamic temperature-regulating center*

GOALS/OUTCOMES Within 24 hours of initiation of treatment, patient becomes normothermic.
NOC Thermoregulation

Temperature Regulation
1. Monitor patient's temperature continuously or at frequent intervals. Use temperature probe (rectal, bladder, or esophageal) for continuous monitoring of core temperature. Body temperature can range from 38.3° to 40.6°C (101° to 105°F) in the early stage of sepsis and can be less than 35.6°C (96°F) in the late stage. Patients

with immunodeficient states on chronic steroid therapy, or high-dose steroids, may have a normal or low temperature. Be alert to shaking chills early in sepsis as temperature increases, and to profuse chills as temperature decreases late in sepsis. Temperatures up to 103°F may be allowed in the septic patient, as increased temperature may help control bacteremia. The following are weighed for each patient to determine the extent of treatment that should be used to decrease fever (e.g., acetaminophen administration):
- Useful effects of a fever — decreased viral and bacterial replication
- Harmful effects of a fever — increased cardiac workload and increased oxygen consumption
2. Administer antimicrobials as prescribed. Discuss appropriate antibiotic therapy. Observe for untoward effects, including renal toxicity, ototoxicity, allergic reactions, anaphylaxis, pseudomembranous colitis (Clostridium difficile associated diarrhea), overgrowth of normal flora, and superimposed infectious processes of the skin, urinary tract, or respiratory tract. Large doses of antibiotics may cause the release of endotoxins from dying bacteria, which may potentiate the progression of septic shock.
3. Administer antipyretic agents as prescribed.
4. For patients with hyperthermia, use tepid baths, which decrease body temperature by releasing internal heat. Cooled IV fluids also may decrease core temperature. In addition, a cooling blanket may be prescribed to reduce the metabolic rate, thereby decreasing myocardial oxygen demand. Avoid "chilling," which will cause shivering and thus increase myocardial oxygen demand and cardiac workload.
5. In the presence of hypothermia, use warm blankets to increase body temperature. Heating devices can damage ischemic cells in peripheral tissues and usually are avoided.

NIC Fever Treatment; Temperature Regulation; Environmental Management

Imbalanced nutrition: less than body requirements *related to increased need secondary to increased metabolic rate*

GOALS/OUTCOMES Within 48 hours of initiation of treatment, patient has adequate nutrition as evidenced by stable weight, serum albumin 3.5 g/dl, prealbumin 20 to 30 mg/dl, retinol-binding protein 4 to 5 mg/dl, urine urea nitrogen 10 to 20 mg/dl, and a state of nitrogen balance as determined by nitrogen studies.
NOC Nutritional Status

Nutrition Management
1. Monitor laboratory findings for serum albumin, prealbumin, retinol-binding protein, and nitrogen studies.
2. Administer nutritional supplements as prescribed.
3. Assess and record weight and nutritional intake daily. Consult with nutritional services for calorie count.
4. Observe for and document areas of tissue breakdown, which may indicate a negative nitrogen state.
5. If patient is receiving oral feedings, assess for the presence of bowel sounds at least every 8 hours. Paralytic ileus can occur secondary to an ischemic bowel.
6. If the patient is receiving continuous gastric tube feedings, assess for residual feeding at least every 4 hours. (See *Nutritional Support*, p. 117.)
   - Enteral feedings are recommended whenever possible, and the choice of feeding formula is determined based on the individual patient. However, formulas with supplemental omega-3 fatty acids such as gamma-linoleic acid (GLA) and eicosapentaenoic acid (EPA) are recommended. TPN is administered to patients unable to tolerate enteral feedings. Standard TPN solutions are not metabolized well in the septic state. Branched-chain amino acid solutions and short- to medium-chain fatty acid solutions may be used (e.g., MCT Oil or FreAmine HBC).

NIC TPN Administration; Enteral Tube Feeding

ADDITIONAL NURSING DIAGNOSES
Also see nursing diagnoses and interventions in *Hemodynamic Monitoring* (p. 75), *Acute Lung Injury and Acute Respiratory Distress Syndrome* (p. 365), *Emotional and Spiritual Support of the Patient and Significant Others* (p. 200), and *Bleeding and Thrombotic Disorders: Disseminated Intravascular Coagulation* (p. 849).

SELECTED REFERENCES

American Academy of Pediatrics and the American College of Obstetricians and Gynecologists: *Guidelines for perinatal care*, ed 6. Washington, DC, 2007, ACOG and AAP.

American College of Obstetricians and Gynecologists: ACOG Practice Bulletin No. 33: Diagnosis and management of preeclampsia and eclampsia. *Obstet Gynecol* 99:159-167, 2002.

American College of Obstetricians and Gynecologists: ACOG Practice Bulletin Number 70: *Intrapartum fetal monitoring*. Washington, DC, 2005, ACOG.

Arbour R: Clinical management of the organ donor. *AACN Clin Issues* 16(4):551, 2005.

Association of Women's Health, Obstetric and Neonatal Nurses: *Fetal heart monitoring principles and practices*. Washington, DC, 2003, AWHONN.

Cairo M: Preventing and managing tumor lysis syndrome: a case review, Special Report. April 2006.

Campbell PT, Rudisill PT: Psychosocial needs of the critically ill obstetric patient: the nurse's role. *Crit Care Nursing Q* 29(1):77-80, 2006.

Celli BR, Cote CG, Marin JM, et al: The body-mass index, airflow obstruction, dyspnea and exercise capacity index in chronic obstructive pulmonary disease. *N Engl J Med* 350:1005-1012, 2004.

Cheatham ML, White MW, Sagraves SG, et al: Abdominal perfusion pressure: a superior parameter in the assessment of intra-abdominal hypertension. *J Trauma* 49:621-627, 2000.

Christie JD, Edwards LB, Aurora P, et al: Registry of the International Society for Heart and Lung Transplantation: Twenty-fifth Official Adult Lung and Heart/Lung Transplantation Report, 2008. *J Heart Lung Transplant* 27:957-969, 2008.

Coiffier B, Altman A, Pui CH, et al: Guidelines for the management of pediatric and adult tumor lysis syndrome: An evidence based review. *Journal of Clinical Oncology* 26 (16): 2767-2778, 2008.

Coppage KH, Sibai BM: Treatment of hypertensive complications in pregnancy. *Curr Pharmaceut Design* 11(6):749-757, 2005.

Crespo-Leiro MG, Alonso-Pulpon L, et al: Malignancy after heart transplantation: incidence, prognosis, and risk factors. *Am J Transplant* 8(5):1031, 2008.

Cupples S, Ohler L: *Transplant nursing secrets*. Philadelphia, PA, 2003, Mosby.

Decker E, Coimbra C, Weekers L, et al: A retrospective monocenter review of simultaneous pancreas-kidney transplantation. *Transplant Proc* 41(8):3389-3392, 2009.

Dellinger RP, Carlet JM, Masur H, et al: Surviving Sepsis Campaign: guidelines for management of severe sepsis and septic shock. *Crit Care Med* 32:858-873, 2004.

Dellinger RP, Levy MM, Carlet JM, et al: Surviving Sepsis Campaign: international guidelines for management of severe sepsis and septic shock: 2008 [published correction appears in *Crit Care Med* 36:1394-1396, 2008]. *Crit Care Med* 36:296-327, 2008.

Demartines N, Schiesser M, Clavien PA: An evidence-based analysis of simultaneous pancreas-kidney and pancreas transplantation alone. *Am J Transplant* 5(11):2688-2697, 2005.

Doenges, ME, Moorhouse MG, Murr AC: *Nurse's pocket guide: diagnosis, prioritized interventions, and rationales*. Philadelphia, 2008, FA Davis.

Duley L: The global impact of pre-eclampsia and eclampsia. *Semin Perinatol* 33(3):130-137, 2009.

Ely EW, Kleinpell RM, Goyette RE: Advances in the understanding of clinical manifestations and therapy of severe sepsis: an update for critical care nurses. *Am J Crit Care* 12(2):120-135, 2003.

Flounders J: Superior vena cava syndrome. *Oncol Nursing Forum* 30(4):E84, 2003.

Gonwa TA, McBride MA, Anderson K, et al: Continued influence of preoperative renal function on outcome of orthotopic liver transplant (OLTX) in the US: where will MELD lead us? *Am J Transplant* 6(11):2651-2659, 2006.

Haddad B, Sibai BM: Expectant management in pregnancies with severe preeclampsia. *Semin Perinatol* 33(3):143-151, 2009.

Hambli M, Sibai BM: Hypertensive disorders of pregnancy. In Gibbs RS, Karlan BY, Haney AF, Nygaard IE, editors: *Danforth's obstetrics and gynecology*, ed 10. Philadelphia, 2008, Lippincott Williams & Wilkins.

Higdon M, Higdon J: Treatment of oncologic emergencies. *Am Fam Physician* 74:1873, 2006.

Hunt S, Haddad F: The changing face of heart transplantation. *J Am Coll Cardiol* 52(8):587, 2008.

Itano J, Taoka K, editors: *Core curriculum for oncology nursing*, ed 4. St. Louis, 2005, Elsevier Saunders.

Joint Commission on Accreditation of Healthcare Organizations: *National patient safety goals*. Oakbrook, IL, 2003, Author.

Kucukardali Y, Cancir Z, et al: Oncologic emergencies that need supportive care in ICU. *Internet J Oncol* 1(2), 2002.

Kuklina E, Ayala C, Callaghan W: Hypertensive disorders and severe obstetric morbidity in the United States. *Obstet Gynecol* 113(6):1299-1306, 2009.

Kulkarni AP: An overview of critical care in cancer patients. *Indian J Crit Care Med* 11:4–11, 2007.

Lam S, Partovi N, et al: Corticosteroid interactions with cyclosporine, tacrolimus, mycophenolate, and sirolimus: fact or fiction? *Ann Pharmacother* 42, 2008.

Leeman L, Fontaine P: Hypertensive disorders of pregnancy. *Am Fam Physician* 78(1):93–100, 2008.

Levy MM, Fink MP, Marshall JC, et al: 2001 SCCM/ESICM/ACCP/ATS/SIS International Sepsis Definitions Conference. *Crit Care Med* 31:1250–1256, 2003.

Long T, Sque M, et al: What does a diagnosis of brain death mean to family members approached about organ donation? A review of the literature. *Progr Transplant* 18(2):118, 2008.

Lowdermilk DM, Perry SE: *Maternity and women's health care*, ed 9. St Louis, 2007, Mosby Elsevier.

Magee LA, von Dadelszen P: The management of severe hypertension. *Semin Perinatol* 33(3): 138–142, 2009.

Malbrain ML: Abdominal perfusion pressure as a prognostic marker in intra-abdominal hypertension. In Vincent JL, editor: *Yearbook of intensive care and emergency medicine*. Berlin, 2002, Springer-Verlag, pp. 792–814.

Malbrain ML, et al: Intra-abdominal hypertension in the critically ill: it is time to pay attention. *Curr Opin Crit Care* 11(2):156–171, 2005.

Marik PE, Wood K, Starzl TE: The course of type 1 hepato-renal syndrome post liver transplantation. *Nephrol Dial Transplant* 21(2):478–482, 2006.

Marshall J, Reinhart K: Biomarkers of sepsis. *Crit Care Med* 37(7):2290–2298, 2009.

Miller H, Lyman G, editors: Neutropenia: overview and current therapies. *Clin Cornerstone* 8(suppl 5), 2006.

Mulligan MS, Shearon TH, et al: Heart and lung transplantation in the United States 1997–2006, *Am J Transplant* 8(4):977, 2008.

National Guideline Clearinghouse: Tuffnell DJ, Shennan AH, Waugh JJ, Walker JJ. The management of severe pre-eclampsia/eclampsia. London (UK): Royal College of Obstetricians and Gynaecologists; 2006 Mar. 11 2006. http://www.guideline.gov/summary/summary.aspx?ss=15&doc_id=9397&nbr=5033

Nelson D, Privette D, et al: Recognizing sepsis in the adult patient. *Am J Nursing* 109(3), 2009.

Norwitz E, Hsu C, Repke J: Acute complications of preeclampsia. *Clin Obstet Gynecol* 45(2):308–329, 2002.

Ohler L, Cupples S: *Core curriculum for transplant nurses*. Philadelphia, 2008, Mosby.

Orens JB, Estenne M, Arcasoy S, et al: International Guidelines for the Selection of Lung Transplant Candidates: 2006 Update: a consensus report from the Pulmonary Scientific Council of the International Society for Heart and Lung Transplantation. *J Heart Lung Transplant* 25:745–755, 2006.

Ponfret EA, Fryer JP, et al: Liver and intestine transplantation in the United States, 1996–2005. *Am J Transplant* 7(5):1376, 2007.

Repke JT, Sibai BM: Preeclampsia and eclampsia. *OBG Manage* 21(4):45–55, 2009.

Rivers E, Ahrens T, editors: Improving outcomes for severe sepsis shock tool for early identification of at-risk patients and treatment protocol. *Crit Care Clin* 24(3, suppl):2008.

Rivers E, Nguyen B, Havstad S, et al: Early goal-directed therapy in the treatment of severe sepsis and septic shock. *N Engl J Med* 345:1368–1377, 2001.

Said A, Einstein M, et al: Liver transplantation: an update. *Curr Opin Gastroenterol* 23(3): 292, 2007.

Shapiro JM: Critical care of the obstetric patient. *J Intens Care Med* 21(5):278–286, 2006.

Shelton B, Ziegfeld C, Olsen M, editors: *Manual of cancer nursing*, ed 2. Philadelphia, 2004, Lippincott, Williams & Wilkins.

Sibai BM: Diagnosis, prevention and management of eclampsia. *Obstet Gynecol* 105(2):402–409, 2005.

Sibai BM, Barton JR: Expectant management of severe preeclampsia remote from term: patient selection, treatment and delivery. *Am J Obstet Gynecol* 196(6):514.e1–9, 2007.

Simpson KR: Critical illness during pregnancy: considerations for evaluation and treatment of the fetus as the second patient. *Crit Care Nursing Q* 20(1):20–31, 2006.

Simpson KR: Obstetrical accidents involving intravenous magnesium sulfate: recommendations to promote patient safety. *Maternal Child Nursing J* 20(3):160–171, 2004.

Simpson KR, Creehan PA: *Perinatal nursing*. Philadelphia, 2007, Wolters-Kluwer/Lippincott Williams & Wilkins.

Steinbrook R: Organ donation after cardiac death. *N Engl J Med* 357(3):209, 2007.

The Magpie Trial Collaborative Group: Do women with pre-eclampsia, and their babies benefit from magnesium sulphate? The Magpie Trial: a randomized placebo-controlled trial. *Lancet* 359:1877–1890, 2002.

Tremblay LN, Feliciano DV, Schmidt J, et al: Skin only or silo closure in the critically ill patient with an open abdomen. *Am J Surg* 182:670, 2001.

Trzeciak S, Dellinger RP, Parrillo JE, et al: Early microcirculatory perfusion derangements in patients with severe sepsis and septic shock: relationship to hemodynamics, oxygen transport, and survival. *Ann Emerg Med* 49:88-98, 2007.

United Network for Organ Sharing (UNOS): UNOS Web site. http://www.unos.org/.

United Network for Organ Sharing: MELD/PELD calculator documentation. http://www.unos.org/waitlist/includes_local/pdfs/meld_peld_calculator.pdf.

Vincenti F, Schena FP, et al: A randomized, multi-center study of steroid avoidance, early steroid withdrawal or standard steroid therapy in kidney transplant recipients. *Am J Transplant* 8(2):307, 2008.

Witcher PM: Promoting fetal stabilization during maternal hemodynamic instability or respiratory insufficiency. *Crit Care Nurs Q* 29(1):70-76, 2006.

World Society on Abdominal Compartment Syndrome: Consensus definitions and recommendations. http://www.wsacs.org.

Zeeman GG, et al: A blueprint for obstetric critical care. *Am J Obstet Gynecol* 188(2):532-536, 2003.

1 Heart and Breath Sounds

Assessing Heart Sounds

Sound	Auscultation Site	Timing	Pitch	Clinical Occurrence	End-Piece/ Patient Position
S_1 (M_1 T_1)	Apex	Beginning of systole	High	Closing of mitral and tricuspid valves; normal sound	Diaphragm/patient supine
S_1 split	Apex	Beginning of systole	High	Ventricles contracting at different times because of electrical or mechanical problems (e.g., longer time span between M_1 T_1 caused by right bundle branch heart block, or reversal [T_1 M_1] caused by mitral stenosis)	Same as S_1
S_2 (A_2 P_2)	A_2 at second ICS, RSB; P_2 at second ICS, LSB	End of systole	High	Closing of aortic and pulmonic valves; normal sound	Diaphragm/patient supine
S_2 physiologic split	Second ICS, LSB	End of systole	High	Accentuated by inspiration; disappears on expiration. Sound that corresponds with the respiratory cycle because of normal delay in closure of pulmonic valve during inspiration. It is accentuated during exercise or in individuals with thin chest walls; heard most often in children and young adults	Same as S_2
S_2 persistent (wide) split	Second ICS, LSB	End of systole	High	Heard throughout the respiratory cycle; caused by late closure of pulmonic valve or early closure of aortic valve. Occurs in atrial septal defect, right ventricular failure, pulmonic stenosis, hypertension, or right bundle branch heart block	Same as S_2

Assessing Heart Sounds—cont'd

Sound	Auscultation Site	Timing	Pitch	Clinical Occurrence	End-Piece/ Patient Position
S$_2$ paradoxical (reversed) split (P$_2$ A$_2$)	Second ICS, LSB	End of systole	High	Because of delayed left ventricular systole, the aortic valve closes after the pulmonic valve rather than before it. (Normally, during expiration, the two sounds merge.) Causes may include left bundle branch heart block, aortic stenosis, severe left ventricular failure, MI, and severe hypertension.	Same as S$_2$
S$_2$ fixed split	Second ICS, LSB	End of systole	High	Heart with equal intensity during inspiration and expiration because of split of pulmonic and aortic components, which are unaffected by blood volume or respiratory changes. May be heard in pulmonary stenosis or atrial septal defect.	Same as S$_2$
S$_3$ (ventricular gallop)	Apex	Early in diastole just after S$_2$	Dull, low	Early and rapid filling of ventricle, as in early ventricular failure, heart failure. Common in children, during last trimester of pregnancy, and possibly in healthy adults >50 yr of age	Bell/patient in left lateral or supine position
S$_4$ (atrial gallop)	Apex	Late in diastole just before S$_1$	Low	Atrium filling against increased resistance of stiff ventricle, as in heart failure, coronary artery disease, cardiomyopathy, pulmonary artery hypertension, ventricular failure. May be normal in infants, children, and athletes	Same as S$_3$

A, *aortic; ICS,* Intercostal space; *LSB,* left sternal border; **M,** *mitral; MI,* myocardial infarction; **P,** pulmonic; *RSB,* right sternal border; **T,** tricuspid.

Commonly Occurring Heart Murmurs

Type	Timing	Pitch	Quality	Auscultation Site	Radiation
Pulmonic stenosis	Systolic ejection	Medium-high	Harsh	Second, ICS, LSB	Toward left shoulder, back
Aortic stenosis	Midsystolic	Medium-high	Harsh	Second, ICS, RSB	Toward carotid arteries
Ventricular septal defect	Late systolic	High	Blowing	Fourth ICS, LSB	Toward RSB
Mitral insufficiency	Holosystolic	High	Blowing	Fifth-sixth ICS, left MCL	Toward left axilla
Tricuspid insufficiency	Holosystolic	High	Blowing	Fourth ICS, LSB	Toward apex
Aortic insufficiency	Early diastolic	High	Blowing	Second, ICS, RSB	Toward sternum
Pulmonary insufficiency	Early diastolic	High	Blowing	Second, ICS, LSB	Toward sternum
Mitral stenosis	Mid-late diastolic	Low	Rumbling	Fifth ICS, left MCL	Usually none
Tricuspid stenosis	Mid-late diastolic	Low	Rumbling	Fourth ICS, LSB	Usually none

ICS, Intercostal space; *LSB,* left sternal border; *MCL,* midclavicular line; *RSB,* right sternal border.

Assessing Normal Breath Sounds

Type	Normal site	Duration	Characteristics
Vesicular	Peripheral lung	I > E	Soft and swishing sounds. Abnormal when heard over the large airways
Bronchial	Trachea and bronchi	E > I	Louder, coarser, and of longer duration than vesicular. Abnormal if heard over peripheral lung
Bronchovesicular	Sternal border of major bronchi	E = I	Moderate in pitch and intensity. Abnormal if heard over peripheral lung

I, Inspiration; *E,* expiration.

Assessing Adventitious Breath Sounds

Type	Waveform	Characteristics	Possible Clinical Condition
Coarse crackle		Discontinuous, explosive, interrupted. Loud; low in pitch	Pulmonary edema, pneumonia in resolution stage
Fine crackle		Discontinuous, explosive, interrupted. Less loud than coarse crackles, lower in pitch, and of shorter duration	Interstitial lung disease; heart failure; atelectasis
Wheeze		Continuous, of long duration, high-pitched, musical, hissing	Narrowing of airway; bronchial asthma; COPD
Rhonchus		Continuous, of long duration, low-pitched, snoring	Production of sputum (usually cleared or lessened by coughing or suctioning)
Pleural friction rub		Grating, rasping noise	Rubbing together of inflamed parietal linings; loss of normal pleural lubrication

COPD, chronic obstructive pulmonary disease.

Assessing Respiratory Patterns

Type	Waveform	Characteristics	Possible Clinical Condition
Eupnea		Normal rate and rhythm for adults and teenagers (12–20 breaths/min)	Normal pattern while awake
Bradypnea		Decreased rate (<12 breaths/min); regular rhythm	Normal sleep pattern; opiate or alcohol use; tumor; metabolic disorder
Tachypnea		Rapid rate (>20 breaths/min); hypoventilation or hyperventilation	Fever; restrictive respiratory disorders; pulmonary emboli
Hyperpnea		Depth of respirations greater than normal	Meeting increased metabolic demand (e.g., sepsis, MODS, SIRS, and exercise)
Apnea		Cessation of breathing; may be intermittent	Intermittent with CNS disturbances or drug intoxication; obstructed airway; respiratory arrest if it persists
Kussmaul		Deep, rapid (>20 breaths/min), sighing, labored	Renal failure, DKA, sepsis, shock
Cheyne-Stokes		Alternating patterns of apnea (10–20 sec) with periods of deep and rapid breathing. Lesions located bilaterally and deep within cerebral hemispheres	Heart failure, opiate or hypnotic overdose, thyrotoxicosis, dissecting aneurysm, subarachnoid hemorrhage, IICP, aortic valve disorders; may be normal in older adults during sleep
Central neurogenic hyperventilation		Rapid (>20 breaths/min), deep, regular. Lesions of midbrain or upper pons thought to be source of pattern	Primary injury (ischemia, infarction, space-occupying lesion); secondary injury (IICP, metabolic disorders, drug overdose)
Apneustic		Deep, prolonged inspiration, followed by 20–30 sec pause and short expiration. Lesion located in lower pons	Anoxia, meningitis, basilar artery occlusion
Cluster		Irregular breaths occurring in clusters with periods of apnea. Overall pattern irregular. Lesion located in lower pons or upper medulla	Primary and secondary neurologic injury may produce this respiratory pattern
Atoxic (Biot)		Irregular deep or shallow breaths. No discernible pattern. Lesion located in medulla	Primary and secondary neurologic injury may produce this respiratory pattern

CNS, central nervous system; DKA, diabetic ketoacidosis; IICP, increased intracranial pressure; MODS, multiple organ dysfunction syndrome; SIRS, systemic inflammatory response syndrome.

2 Glasgow Coma Scale

Parameter	Patient Response	Score
Best eye opening response (record "C" if eyes closed due to swelling)	Spontaneously	4
	To speech	3
	To pain	2
	No response	1
Best motor response (record best upper limb response to painful stimuli)	Obeys verbal command	6
	Localizes pain	5
	Flexion — withdrawal	4
	Flexion — abnormal	3
	Extension — abnormal	2
	No response	1
Best verbal response (record "E" if endotracheal tube is in place or "T" if tracheostomy tube is in place)	Conversation — oriented × 3	5
	Conversation — confused	4
	Speech — inappropriate	3
	Sounds — incomprehensible	2
	No response	1
Total Score	**Interpretation**	
15	Normal	
13–15	Minor head injury	
9–12	Moderate head injury	
3–8	Severe head injury	
4–7	Coma	
3	Deep coma or brain death	

Cranial Nerves: Assessment and Dysfunctions

Cranial Nerve	Type	Functions	Assessment/Dysfunctions
I Olfactory	Sensory	Smell	Anosmia; cannot distinguish familiar odors; will affect ability to taste; test each nostril separately;
II Optic	Sensory	Sight Visual acuity Visual fields Fundus	Blindness; blurred vision; partial vision; loss of full visual field; distorted vision; test each eye separately; a blind eye does not have a pupillary direct light reflex, but has a consensual light reflex;
III Oculomotor	Motor	Pupillary constriction Elevation of upper eyelid Extraocular movements	Ptosis, diplopia, unequal pupils; abnormal pupillary constriction to light; strabismus; loss of pupillary consensual light reflex.
IV Trochlear	Motor	Downward and inward movement of eye	Diplopia, visual disturbances with downward gaze
V Trigeminal	Sensory and motor	*Sensory:* Facial, scalp, anterior two thirds of tongue, lips, teeth, proprioception for mastication, corneal reflex *Motor:* Temporal and masseter muscles (jaw clenching and lateral movement for mastication)	Loss of corneal reflex; abnormal blinking of eyes; Paresis or paralysis of muscles of mastication, decreased facial sensation; unable to clench teeth or weakly clenches teeth;
VI Abducens	Motor	Lateral eye movement	Eye will not move laterally; Cranial nerves III, IV and VI are tested together for full "6 pointed star configuration" eye movements.
VII Facial	Sensory and motor	*Sensory:* Taste in anterior two thirds of tongue, proprioception for face and scalp *Motor:* Facial expression, lacrimal and salivary glands	Loss of taste in anterior two thirds of tongue Paresis or paralysis of facial muscles, facial droop, cannot open eyes against resistance; reduced or absent saliva and tears
VIII Acoustic	Sensory	*Cochlear division:* Hearing *Vestibular division:* Balance	Tinnitus, deafness; test one ear at a time Vertigo, nystagmus; nausea, sweating, hypotension and vomiting can indicate vestibular dysfunction

Cranial Nerve	Type	Functions	Assessment/Dysfunctions
IX Glossopharyngeal	Sensory and motor	*Sensory:* Taste in posterior one third of tongue; pain, touch, heat, cold in tongue, tonsils, soft palate, and pharynx *Motor:* Elevation of the soft palate, movement of pharynx, secretion and vasodilation of parotid glands for saliva; gag reflex	Loss of taste, pain, touch, heat, and cold in posterior one third of tongue, tonsils, and soft palate Paresis or paralysis of soft palate and pharynx, dysphagia, dysarthria, loss of gag reflex; coughing with oral intake;
X Vagus	Sensory and motor	*Sensory:* Muscles of pharynx, larynx, esophagus, thoracic and abdominal viscera; external ear, mucous membranes of larynx, trachea, esophagus, thoracic and abdominal viscera; lungs (stretch receptors), aortic bodies (chemoreceptors), respiratory/GI tract (pain receptors) *Motor:* Muscles of pharynx, larynx, esophagus, thoracic and abdominal viscera; respiratory/GI tract (smooth muscle), pacemaker and cardiac atrial muscle	Similar to dysfunction of glossopharyngeal; parasympathetic nerve fibers may fail to normally inhibit heart rate; may have slow peristalsis and lack gastric and pancreatic secretions, prompting digestive disorders. Loss of gag reflex and difficulty swallowing; coughing with oral intake; palate may have abnormal arch when patient says "Ah"; Speech defects (inability to articulate syllables clearly); hoarseness of voice;
XI Spinal accessory	Motor	Sternocleidomastoid and trapezius muscles	Paresis or paralysis of sternocleidomastoid and trapezius muscles; Inability to turn head or shrug shoulders
XII Hypoglossal	Motor	Tongue movement	Paresis or paralysis of the tongue; cannot protrude/ "stick out" tongue from the mouth

4 Major Deep Tendon (Muscle-Stretch) Reflexes

Reflex	Innervations	Examination Technique	Normal Response
Biceps	C5, C6	Arm partially flexed at elbow, palm down. Place thumb or finger on biceps tendon. Strike finger with reflex hammer	Contraction of biceps muscle Flexion at elbow
Triceps	C6, C7	Arm flexed at elbow, palm toward body, arm pulled slightly across body. Strike triceps tendon with reflex hammer above elbow	Contraction of triceps muscle Extension of arm at elbow
Brachioradialis	C5, C6	Hand resting on abdomen, palm slightly pronated. Strike radius with reflex hammer 3–5 cm above wrist	Contraction of brachioradialis muscle Flexion and supination of forearm
Achilles (ankle jerk)	S1, S2	Leg flexed at knee, dorsiflex the foot. Strike Achilles tendon with reflex hammer	Plantar flexion of foot
Quadriceps (knee jerk)	L3, L4	Leg flexed at knee. Strike patellar tendon with reflex hammer	Contraction of quadriceps muscle Extension of knee

Grading of Deep Tendon Reflexes	
Scale (0 to 4+)	**Interpretation**
4+	Very brisk, hyperactive, repetitive, rhythmic flexion and extension (clonus); indicative of disease
3+	Brisker than average; may be normal for certain individuals or may indicate disease
2+	Average/normal
1+	Diminished response or low normal
0	No response

5 Major Superficial (Cutaneous) Reflexes

Reflex	Innervations	Examination Technique	Normal Response
Abdominals			
Above/upper Below/lower	T8, T9, T10 T10, T11, T12	Using tongue blade or wooden end of cotton-tipped applicator, lightly stroke abdomen in each quadrant, outer-to-inner direction, toward umbilicus	Contraction of abdominal muscles Umbilicus deviates (pulls) toward the stimulus
Bulbocavern-ous (male)	S3, S4	Pinch glans penis or apply pressure over bulbocavernous muscle behind scrotum	Scrotum will elevate toward the body
Corneal	Cranial nerves V and VII	Using wisp of cotton, lightly touch cornea	Eyelids will quickly close
Cremasteric (male)	L1, L2	Lightly stroke inner aspect of thigh	Testicle on side stroked will elevate
Gag	Cranial nerves IX and X	Using tongue blade, lightly touch posterior pharynx	Gagging or retching
Perianal	S3, S4, S5	Stroke tissue surrounding anus with blunt instrument, or examine rectum by gently inserting gloved finger	Anal puckering with external stimuli. Tightening of anal sphincter with internal examination

Inotropic and Vasoactive Medication Infusions

	MEASUREMENTS					
Medications	**HR**	**PAWP**	**SVR**	**Cardiac Output**	**Dosage**	**Effects**
Inotropes/ Vasoactives						***Main Effect: Increase cardiac contractility and change vascular resistance***
Dopamine hydrochloride (Intropin)	—↑	—	—	—↑	Low dose 1–2 mcg/ kg/min	Major effect may be to *increase* urine output; may potentiate effect of diuretics
	—↑	—	—	↑↑	Moderate dose 2–10 mcg/ kg/min	Major effect is to increase contractility
	—	—	↑↑	—	High dose >10 mcg/ kg/min	Can cause tissue necrosis and sloughing if infiltration occurs
Dobutamine (Dobutrex)	—↑	—↓	—↓	↑↑	2.5–10 mcg/ kg/min	Overall effect is improved CO; may cause tachycardia and dysrhythmias as side effects
Isoproterenol (Isuprel)	↑↑	—↓	↓↓	↑↑	2–10 mcg/ min	Significant increase in myocardial oxygen consumption; can produce ventricular tachycardia and fibrillation
Epinephrine	↑↑	↑↑	↓↑	↑↑	0.5–1 mg IV push for cardiac arrest	May induce ventricular ectopy
					1–4 mcg/min for inotropic support	Can exacerbate myocardial ischemia Can prompt supraventricular and ventricular dysrhythmias
					2–20 mcg/ kg/min	Main effect is vasoconstriction of peripheral blood vessels
Inamrinone lactate (Inocor)	—↑	↓	↓	↑	Loading dose: 0.75 mg/kg; then 5–10 mcg/kg/min	
Milrinone lactate (Primacor)	—↑	↓	↓	↑	50 mcg/kg given over 10 min; start infu-sion of 0.375–0.75 mcg/kg/ min	"Inodilator" medication used most often as the first step in managing acute decompen-sated heart failure.

MEASUREMENTS						
Medications	**HR**	**PAWP**	**SVR**	**Cardiac Output**	**Dosage**	**Effects**
Levosimendan (Simdax)	—↑	↓	↓	↑↑↑	Loading dose: 24 mcg/kg followed by 0.1–0.2 mcg/kg/min for 24 hours	A calcium sensitizer used to treat patients with acute decompensated heart failure (CHF).
Vasopressors						**Main effect: Constriction of arteries and veins (vasoconstriction)**
Methoxamine hydrochloride (Vasoxyl)	—	↑	↑↑↑	—	3–5 mg	*Potent vasoconstrictor, used rarely; increases myocardial oxygen demand*
Norepinephrine (Levophed)	↑↓	↑	↑↑↑	↑	2–12 mcg/min	*Potent vasoconstrictor. Contra-indicated when hypotension occurs secondary to hypovolemia. Can cause tissue necrosis and sloughing if infiltration occurs. Increased myocardial oxygen demand without increased coronary artery flow can cause myocardial ischemia and infarction*
Phenylephrine (Neo-Synephrine)	—	↑	↑↑↑	—	100–180 mcg/min	*Potent vasoconstrictor, may cause dysrhythmias or trigger reflex bradycardia*
Vasopressin	↑	—	↑↑	—	0.02–0.1 unit/min	Used to augment other vasopressors; Higher doses cause marked splanchnic vasoconstriction
Vasodilators						**Main effect: Dilation of arteries and/or veins (vasodilation)**
Sodium nitroprusside (Nipride)	—↑	↓	↓↓	—	Starting dose of 0.5–0.8 mcg/kg/min; titrate up to 10 mcg/kg/min	Drug is photosensitive; keep infusion container protected from light. Thiocyanate (a metabolite of nitroprusside) toxicity can occur after 72 hr. Monitor thiocyanate levels daily, being alert to levels >10 mg/dl and or signs of metabolic acidosis
Nitroglycerin (Tridil, Nitrostat)	—↑	↓↓	↓	—	Starting dose of 0.5 mcg/min; titrate up to 200 mcg/min	Absorbed by standard plastic IV tubing. Use special polyvinyl chloride tubing. Ensure that the drug is diluted for IV use

—, No effect; ↑, minimal effect; ↑↑, moderate effect; ↑↑↑, major effect; *CO*, cardiac output; *HR*, heart rate; *IV*, intravenous; *PAOP*, pulmonary artery occlusive pressure; *SVR*, systemic vascular resistance.

Sample Relaxation Technique

Give the patient the following instructions:

1. Sit quietly in a comfortable position. Close your eyes.
2. Relax all your muscles, starting at your feet and progressing to your facial muscles. Focus your attention on one body area at a time while you relax the muscles in that area.
3. Breathe through your nose. As you breathe out, say the word "one" silently to yourself. Become aware of your breathing. Continue this process for about 20 minutes.
4. Do not worry whether you are achieving deep relaxation. Maintain a passive attitude and permit relaxation to occur at its own pace. If distractions interfere, see your thoughts floating away like clouds. Continue breathing and repeating the word "one."

8

Abbreviations Used in This Manual

A—aortic valve
AACN—American Association of Critical Care Nurses
AAL—anterior axillary line
ABA—American Burn Association
ABG—arterial blood gas
ACC—American College of Cardiology
ACCP—American College of Chest Physicians
ACE—angiotensin-converting enzyme
ACh—acetylcholine
AChR—acetylcholine receptors
ACLS—advanced cardiac life support
ACS—abdominal compartment syndrome
ACT—activated clotting time
AD—autonomic dysreflexia
ADA—American Diabetes Association
ADH—antidiuretic hormone
ADL—activity of daily living
AED—automatic external defibrillator
AEG—atrial electrogram
AF—atrial fibrillation
AHA—American Heart Association
AIDS—acquired immunodeficiency syndrome
AIS—acute ischemic stroke
ALI—acute lung injury
ALP—alkaline phosphatase
ALT—alanine aminotransferase
AM—akinetic mutism
AMA—American Medical Association
AMI—acute myocardial infarction
ANA—American Nurses Association
ANP—atrial natriuretic peptide
APAS—antiphospholipid antibody syndrome
APSAC—anisoylated plasminogen streptokinase activator complex
aPTT—activated partial thromboplastin time
ARDS—acute respiratory distress syndrome
ARF—acute respiratory failure; acute renal failure
ARS—adjective rating scale
ASA—acetylsalicylic acid (aspirin)
ASO—antistreptolysin O
AST—aspartate aminotransferase
AT—antithrombin

AT_1—receptor antagonist
ATGAM—antithymocyte gamma globulin
atm—atmosphere (standard)
ATN—acute tubular necrosis
ATP—adenosine triphosphate
AV—atrioventricular; arteriovenous
AVM—arteriovenous malformation
AVNRT—atrial-ventricular nonreciprocating tachycardia
AVRT—atrial-ventricular reciprocating tachycardia
BAL—bronchoalveolar lavage
BEE—basal energy expenditure
BIS—bispectral index
BMI—body mass index
BP—blood pressure
bpm—beats per minute
BS—bowel sounds
BSA—body surface area
BUN—blood urea nitrogen
C—centigrade
Ca^{2+}—calcium
CABG—coronary artery bypass grafting
CAD—coronary artery disease
CAPD—continuous ambulatory peritoneal dialysis
CASHD—coronary atherosclerotic heart disease
CAVH—continuous arteriovenous hemofiltration
CBC—complete blood cell count
CBF—cerebral blood flow
CD—Cotrel-Dubousset
CDC—Centers for Disease Control and Prevention
CDI—central diabetes insipidus
CHF—congestive heart failure
CI—cardiac index
CIE—counterimmunoelectrophoresis
CJD—Creutzfeldt-Jakob disease
CK—creatine kinase
Cl^-—chloride
CK-MB—creatine kinase–myocardial band
CM—cardiomyopathy
CMV—cytomegalovirus; controlled mechanical ventilation
CNS—central nervous system
CO—cardiac output; carbon monoxide

CO₂—carbon dioxide

COPD—chronic obstructive pulmonary disease

CPAP—continuous positive airway pressure

CPK—creatine phosphokinase

CPP—cerebral perfusion pressure; coronary perfusion pressure

CRRT—continuous renal replacement therapy

CRT—cardiac resynchronization therapy

C&S—culture and sensitivities

CSF—cerebrospinal fluid

CT—computed tomography

cTnI—cardiac troponin I

CVA—cerebrovascular accident; costovertebral angle

CVC—central venous catheter

CVP—central venous pressure

CVVH—continuous venovenous hemofiltration

CVVHD—continuous venovenous hemofiltration with dialysis

CVVHDF—continuous venovenous hemodiafiltration

CXR—chest radiograph

CyA—cyclosporine

DAI—diffuse axonal injury

DCM—dilated cardiomyopathy

DFI—diffusion-weighted imaging (or DWI)

DI—diabetes insipidus

DIC—disseminated intravascular coagulation

DKA—diabetic ketoacidosis

DM—diabetes mellitus

DNR—do not resuscitate

Do₂—oxygen delivery

DOE—dyspnea on exertion

DPAHC—durable power of attorney for health care

DPL—diagnostic peritoneal lavage

DTR—deep tendon reflex

DVT—deep vein thrombosis

EACA—epsilon-(ε)aminocaproic acid

EBV—Epstein-Barr virus

ECG—electrocardiogram

ECHO—electrocardiography

EEG—electroencephalogram

EFA—Epilepsy Foundation of America

ELISA—enzyme-linked immunosorbent assay

EMI—electromagnetic interference

EPS—electrophysiologic studies

ESR—erythrocyte sedimentation rate

ET—endotracheal

ETCO₂—end-tidal carbon dioxide

ETOH—alcohol

ETT—endotracheal tube

F—Fahrenheit

FAST—focused assessment with sonography for trauma

FDP—fibrin degradation product

FEF—forced expiratory flow

FEV—forced expiratory volume

FHF—fulminant hepatic failure

FIO₂—fraction of inspired oxygen

Fr—French

FRC—functional residual capacity

FSP—fibrin split product

FVC—forced vital capacity

GABA—gamma-(γ) aminobutyric acid

GBS—Guillain-Barré syndrome

GCS—Glasgow Coma Scale

GERD—gastroesophageal reflux disease

GI—gastrointestinal

GKI—glucose-potassium-insulin

G6PD—glucose-6-phosphate dehydrogenase

GU—genitourinary

H₂O—water

HAT—heparin-associated thrombocytopenia

HCM—hypertrophic cardiomyopathy

HCO₃⁻—bicarbonate

Hct—hematocrit

HDL—high-density lipoprotein

HELLP—hemolysis, elevated liver enzymes, low platelet count

Hgb—hemoglobin

HHS—hyperglycemic hyperosmolar syndrome

HITT—heparin-induced thrombocytopenia thrombosis

HIV—human immunodeficiency virus

HOB—head of bed

HPO₄—phosphate

HR—heart rate

HRS—hepatorenal syndrome

HSV—herpes simplex virus

HUS—hemolytic-uremic syndrome

HVPG—hepatic venous pressure gradient

HVWP—hepatic vein wedge pressure

IABP—intra-aortic balloon pump

IAP—intra-abdominal pressure

ICA—internal cerebral artery

ICD—implantable cardioverter-defibrillator

ICH—intracerebral hematoma

ICP—intracranial pressure

ICS—intercostal space

ICU—intensive care unit

IE—infective endocarditis

I/E—inspiration/expiration

IER—in expected range

IgG—immunoglobulin G

IHSS—idiopathic hypertrophic subaortic stenosis

IICP—increased intracranial pressure

IM—intramuscular

INR—international normalized ratio

I&O—intake and output

IPD—intermittent peritoneal dialysis; intracranial pressure dynamics

IPPB—intermittent positive-pressure breathing
IRV—inverse ratio ventilation
ITP—idiopathic thrombocytopenic purpura
IV—intravenous
IVP—intravenous pyelogram
JNC VII—Joint National Committee VII
JT—junctional tachycardia
JVD—jugular vein distention
K⁺—potassium

K^+—potassium
kcal—kilocalorie
KCl—potassium (K) chloride (Cl⁻)
kg—kilogram
KUB—kidney, ureter, bladder
L—liter; lumbar
LAD—left anterior descending (coronary artery)
LAP—left atrial pressure
LDH—lactate dehydrogenase; also abbreviated LD
LDL—low-density lipoprotein
LIS—locked-in-syndrome
LMW—low molecular weight
LOC—level of consciousness
LOS—length of stay
LP—lumbar puncture
LR—lactated Ringer's
LUQ—left upper quadrant
LUT—lower urinary tract
LV—left ventricular
LVEDP—left ventricular end-diastolic pressure
LVH—left ventricular hypertrophy
m—meter
M—mitral valve
MAP—mean arterial pressure
MCA—middle cerebral artery
MCL—modified chest lead; midclavicular line
MCS—minimally conscious state
MCT—medium-chain triglycerides
MCV—mean corpuscular volume
Mg²⁺—magnesium
MG—myasthenia gravis
mg—milligram
MI—myocardial infarction
MODS—multiple organ dysfunction syndrome
mOsm—milliosmole
MPAP—mean pulmonary artery pressure; also abbreviated PAM
MRA—magnetic resonance arteriogram
MRI—magnetic resonance imaging
MS—multiple sclerosis
MSO₄—morphine sulfate
MUGA scan—multiple-gated acquisition scan
Na/Na⁺—sodium
NaCl—sodium chloride/saline

NCV—nerve conduction velocity
NDI—nephrogenic diabetes insipidus
NG—nasogastric
NHO—National Hospice Organization
nl—normal
NMBA—neuromuscular blocking agent(s)
NPO—nothing by mouth
NRS—numeric rating scale
NSAID—nonsteroidal anti-inflammatory drug
NSTEMI—non-ST-segment elevation myocardial infarction
NTG—nitroglycerin
nvCJD—new variant Creutzfeldt-Jakob disease
OT—occupational therapist
OTC—over-the-counter
P—pulmonic valve
PA—pulmonary artery
PAC—premature atrial complexes
Paco₂—carbon dioxide (arterial pressure)
PAD—pulmonary artery diastolic
Pao₂—oxygen (arterial pressure)
PAP—pulmonary artery pressure/positive airway pressure
PASG—pneumatic antishock garment
PAT—paroxysmal atrial tachycardia
PAW—pulmonary artery wedge
PAWP—pulmonary artery wedge pressure
PBV—percutaneous balloon valvuloplasty
PCA—patient-controlled analgesia
PE—pulmonary embolus
PEEP—positive end-expiratory pressure
PEG—percutaneous endoscopic gastrostomy
PEJ—percutaneous endoscopic jejunostomy
PET—positron emission tomography
PIH—pregnancy-induced hypertension
PJC—premature junctional complexes
PK—pyruvate kinase
PMI—point of maximal impulse
PN—parenteral nutrition
PND—paroxysmal nocturnal dyspnea
PO—by mouth
PO₄—phosphates
PPF—plasma protein fraction
Pplat—plateau pressure
PRA—panel-reactive antibody
PRBCs—packed red blood cells
PSB—protected specimen brush
PSV—pressure support ventilation
PSVT—paroxysmal supraventricular tachycardia
PT—physical therapy; physical therapist; prothrombin time
PTCA—percutaneous transluminal coronary angioplasty
PTH—parathyroid hormone
PTT—partial thromboplastin time
PVC—premature ventricular complex; peripheral venous catheter

PVR—pulmonary vascular resistance
PWI—perfusion-weighted imaging
RAP—right atrial pressure
RBC—red blood cell
RCM—restrictive cardiomyopathy
RDA—Recommended Daily Allowance; Recommended Dietary Allowance
rHuEPO—recombinant human erythropoietin
RLA—Rancho Los Amigos
ROM—range of motion
RPE—rate perceived exertion
RR—respiratory rate
RRT—renal replacement therapy; registered respiratory therapist
rtPA—recombinant tissue plasminogen activator
RV—right ventricle
RVP—right ventricular pressure
SA—status asthmaticus
SAH—subarachnoid hemorrhage
SAS—subarachnoid space
SBP—systolic blood pressure
SCCM—Society of Critical Care Medicine
SCI—spinal cord injury
Scvo$_2$—central venous oxygen saturation
SGOT—serum glutamic oxaloacetic acid transaminase
SGPT—serum glutamic pyruvic transaminase
SIADH—syndrome of inappropriate antidiuretic hormone
SIMV—synchronized intermittent mandatory ventilation
SIRS—systemic inflammatory response syndrome
Sjo$_2$—jugular venous oxygen saturation
SOB—shortness of breath
Spo$_2$—pulse oximetry oxygen saturation
SQ—subcutaneous; also abbreviated SC
SS—sensory stimulation
STEMI—ST-segment elevation myocardial infarction
Sto$_2$—tissue oxygen saturation
STSG—split-thickness skin graft
SV—stroke volume
Svo$_2$—mixed venous oxygen saturation

SVR—systemic vascular resistance
T—tricuspid valve
TBSA—total body surface area
TCD—transcranial Doppler
TdP—torsades des pointe
TE—thrombotic emboli
TEA—tranexamic acid
TEC—transluminal extraction catheterization
TEE—total energy expenditure; transesophageal echocardiography
TENS—transcutaneous electrical nerve stimulation
TIA—transient ischemic attack
TIBC—total iron-binding capacity
TIPS/TIPSS—transjugular intrahepatic portal-systemic shunt
TMP—transmembrane pressure
TNA—total nutrient admixtures
TNF—tumor necrosis factor
TOF—train-of-four
TPA—tissue plasminogen activator
TPN—total parenteral nutrition
TSF—triceps skinfold thickness
UF—ultrafiltration
URI—upper respiratory infection
UTI—urinary tract infection
VAD—venous access device; ventricular assist device
VAS—visual analog scale
VC—vital capacity
VCJD—variant (new) Creutzfeld-Jakob disease
VEDP—ventricular end-diastolic pressure
VF—ventricular fibrillation
VLDL—very low-density lipoprotein
VMA—vanillylmandelic acid
Vo$_2$—oxygen consumption
VS—vital signs/vegetative state
VSD—ventricular septal defect
VT—ventricular tachycardia
Vt—tidal volume
WBC—white blood cell
WNL—within normal limits
WPW—Wolff-Parkinson-White syndrome

Index

Page numbers followed by "t" indicate tables; page numbers followed by "f" indicate figures.

W

Z